GRS

Geriatrics Review Syllabus

Sixth Edition

Syllabus/Book 1

A Core Curriculum in Geriatric Medicine

The Chief Editors were Peter Pompei, MD, and John B. Murphy, MD; Syllabus Editors were Colleen Christmas, MD, Steven R. Counsell, MD, G. Paul Eleazer, MD, Anne R. Fabiny, MD, and Susan Schultz, MD; Question Editors were William J. Burke, MD, Alison A. Moore, MD, MPH, and Gail M. Sullivan, MD, MPH; Consulting Editor on Ethnogeriatrics was Carmel Dyer, MD; Consulting Editor on Pharmacotherapy was Todd P. Semla, PharmD, MS; Special Advisors were James T. Pacala, MD, MS, and Stephanie Studenski, MD, MPH; Consulting Question Reviewers were Itamar B. Abrass, MD, and Jane F. Potter, MD; Medical Writers were Barbara B. Reitt, PhD, ELS(D), and Dalia Ritter; Indexer was L. Pilar Wyman; and Managing Editor was Andrea N. Sherman, MS.

Many thanks to Fry Communications for assistance in organizing the *Geriatrics Review Syllabus* material onto an editorial content management Web site and all production work including typesetting, graphic design, CD-ROM development, and printing. With more than 60 years in the information industry, Fry offers printing and ancillary services to publishers and other content providers.

Citation: Pompei P, Murphy JB, eds. *Geriatrics Review Syllabus: A Core Curriculum in Geriatric Medicine.* 6th ed. New York: American Geriatrics Society; 2006.

Geriatrics Review Syllabus: A Core Curriculum in Geriatric Medicine, 6th Edition. Cataloging in publication data is available from the Library of Congress.

Library of Congress Control Number: 2005938012

ISBN Number Book 1: 978-1-886775-13-8

TABLE OF CONTENTS

LIST OF FIGURES

LIST OF TABLES

ACKNOWLEDGMENTS

As the editors, it is our pleasure and privilege to acknowledge the many people who have made the *Geriatrics Review Syllabus: A Core Curriculum in Geriatric Medicine*, 6th Edition (*GRS6*) possible.

We express our gratitude to the Syllabus Editors: Colleen Christmas, MD; Steven R. Counsell, MD; G. Paul Eleazer, MD; Anne R. Fabiny, MD; Susan K. Schultz, MD; and to the Question Editors: William J. Burke, MD; Alison A. Moore, MD, MPH; and Gail M. Sullivan, MD, MPH; all of them devoted countless hours to the development of this program. We are thankful for the assistance from our Special Advisors: James T. Pacala, MD, MS; and Stephanie Studenski, MD, MPH; as well as our Consulting Editors: Carmel Bitondo Dyer, MD; and Todd P. Semla, PharmD, MS. Special thanks also to our Consulting Question Reviewers: Itamar B. Abrass, MD; and Jane F. Potter, MD. We also appreciate the outside chapter review by David H. Stern, MD. On behalf of all these editors, we thank the contributing authors for lending us their expertise in the various fields of medicine covered in this publication.

We thank Andrea Sherman, MS, *GRS* Managing Editor, for her guidance, organization, and coordination overseeing the administrative, editorial, and distribution aspects of the program. Her tireless dedication to ensuring that the *GRS* is of the highest quality and to making sure the train runs on time is instrumental to our success. So too, Barbara B. Reitt, PhD, ELS(D), is an extraordinary medical editor whose fine hand is evident throughout the *GRS* and whose wise guidance on production is always on target. Thanks also go to Dalia Ritter for editing the first round of questions and critiques, helping us to ensure that these are consistent with the questions that you will face on secure Board exams, and to L. Pilar Wyman for her comprehensive index of the *GRS*, which contributes greatly to its ease of use.

We wish to express our appreciation for their ongoing support to the AGS Board of Directors and to Linda Hiddemen Barondess, AGS Executive Vice President; Nancy Lundebjerg, MPA, Associate Vice President, Education, Communications and Special Projects; Elvy Ickowicz, MPH, Senior Director, Education, Communications, and Special Projects; Linda Saunders, MSW, Senior Director, Professional Education and Special Projects; and Dennise McAlpin, Manager, Professional Education and Special Projects.

We also give special thanks to the administrative assistants and secretaries of the editors and contributing authors for their contributions and assistance in preparing the initial drafts of the chapters, questions and critiques. We want to express thanks to our patients, who keep us honest and teach us so much. Finally, and most importantly, we thank our families.

Peter Pompei, MD
John B. Murphy, MD
Chief Editors

EDITORIAL BOARD

Consulting Question Reviewers

Itamar B. Abrass, MD
Professor and Division Head,
Gerontology and Geriatric Medicine
University of Washington
Harborview Medical Center
Seattle, WA

Jane F. Potter, MD
Harris Professor of Geriatric Medicine
Chief, Section on Geriatrics and Gerontology
Department of Internal Medicine
University of Nebraska Medical Center
Omaha, NE

CONTRIBUTING CHAPTER AUTHORS

Sumaira Z. Aasi, MD
Assistant Professor
Department of Dermatology
Yale University School of Medicine
New Haven, CT

Harold P. Adams, Jr., MD
Professor and Director
Division of Cerebrovascular Diseases, Department of
    Neurology
University of Iowa Hospitals and Clinics
Iowa City, IA

Reva N. Adler, MD, MPH
Medical Director, STAT Centre and At-home
    Supports
Vancouver Hospital & Vancouver Community Health
    Services
Clinical Associate Professor, Division of Geriatric
    Medicine
University of British Columbia
Vancouver, BC

Marc E. Agronin, MD
Director of Mental Health Services
Miami Jewish Home and Hospital for the Aged
Assistant Professor of Psychiatry
Miller School of Medicine at the University of Miami
Miami, FL

Cathy A. Alessi, MD
Associate Director
Clinical Programs: Geriatric Research, Education and
    Clinical Center, Sepulveda Division
Veterans Administration Greater Los Angeles
    Healthcare System
Professor, University of California, Los Angeles
Multicampus Program in Geriatric Medicine and
    Gerontology
Sepulveda, CA

Neil B. Alexander, MD
Professor, Division of Geriatric Medicine
Department of Internal Medicine
Research Professor, Institute of Gerontology
University of Michigan
Director, VA Ann Arbor Health Care System Geriatric
    Research, Education and Clinical Center
Ann Arbor, MI

Wilbert S. Aronow, MD
Clinical Professor of Medicine
Divisions of Cardiology, Geriatrics, and
    Pulmonary/Critical Care
Westchester Medical Center and New York Medical
    College
Valhalla, NY
Adjunct Professor of Geriatrics and Adult
    Development
Mount Sinai School of Medicine
New York, NY

Priscilla Faith Bade, MD, MS
Associate Professor of Internal Medicine
University of South Dakota School of Medicine
Rapid City, SD

Cynthia Barton, RN, MSN
Gerontological Nurse Practitioner
Memory and Aging Center
Assistant Clinical Professor, School of Nursing
University of California, San Francisco
San Francisco, CA

Marc R. Blackman, MD
Chief, Endocrine Section
Laboratory of Clinical Investigation
National Center for Complementary and Alternative
    Medicine
National Institutes of Health
Bethesda, MD

Caroline S. Blaum, MD, MS
Associate Professor of Internal Medicine
Division of Geriatric Medicine
University of Michigan
Research Scientist, Ann Arbor DVAMC Geriatric
    Research, Education and Clinical Center
Ann Arbor, MI

Harrison G. Bloom, MD
Senior Associate
International Longevity Center, USA
Associate Clinical Professor
Brookdale Department of Geriatrics and Adult
    Development
Mount Sinai School of Medicine
New York, NY

Chad Boult, MD, MPH, MBA
Professor of Public Health
Director, Lipitz Center for Integrated Health Care
Johns Hopkins Bloomberg School of Public Health
The Johns Hopkins University
Baltimore, MD

Cynthia J. Brown, MD
GRECC Investigator
Medical Director
Falls Prevention and Mobility Clinic
Birmingham/Atlanta VA Geriatric Research, Education
    and Clinical Center
Assistant Professor
University of Alabama at Birmingham
Birmingham, AL

David M. Buchner, MD, MPH
Chief, Physical Activity and Health Branch, Division of
    Nutrition and Physical Activity
Centers for Disease Control and Prevention
Atlanta, GA

Lynda C. Burton, ScD
Associate Professor
Department of Health Policy and Management
The Johns Hopkins Bloomberg School of Public
    Health
Baltimore, MD

David Bush, MD
Director, Cardiac Catheterization Laboratory
Johns Hopkins Bayview Medical Center
Associate Professor of Medicine
Division of Cardiology
The Johns Hopkins University School of Medicine
Baltimore, MD

Erin L. Cassidy, PhD
Research Associate
Department of Psychiatry and Behavioral Sciences
Stanford University School of Medicine
Palo Alto, CA

Gurkamal S. Chatta, MD
Associate Professor of Medicine
Division of Hematology-Oncology
University of Pittsburgh
Pittsburgh, PA

Colleen Christmas, MD
Assistant Professor of Medicine
Division of Geriatric Medicine and Gerontology
The Johns Hopkins University School of Medicine
Baltimore, MD

Anne L. Coleman, MD, PhD
Professor of Ophthalmology and Epidemiology
Frances and Ray Stark Chair of Ophthalmology
Jules Stein Eye Institute
University of California, Los Angeles
Los Angeles, CA

Leo M. Cooney, Jr., MD
Humana Foundation Professor of Geriatric Medicine
Chief, Section of Geriatric Medicine
Yale University School of Medicine
New Haven, CT

G. Willy Davila, MD
Chairman, Department of Gynecology
Head, Section of Urogynecology and Reconstructive
    Pelvic Surgery
Cleveland Clinic Florida
Ft. Lauderdale, FL

Margaret A. Drickamer, MD
Associate Professor of Medicine (Geriatrics)
Yale University School of Medicine
New Haven, CT

Catherine E. DuBeau, MD
Associate Professor of Medicine
Section of Geriatrics
University of Chicago
Chicago, IL

Pamela W. Duncan, PhD
Professor, College of Medicine
Career Health Scientist—Department of Veteran
    Affairs
Director of Department of Veterans Affairs Center of
    Excellence in Rehabilitation Outcomes
Department of Aging and Geriatrics Research
Co-Director, Institute of Aging
Department of Aging and Geriatric Research
University of Florida
Gainesville, FL

G. Paul Eleazer, MD
Director, Division of Geriatrics
University of South Carolina School of Medicine
Columbia, SC

E. Wesley Ely, MD, MPH
Associate Professor of Medicine
Associate Director of Aging Research
Tennessee Valley Geriatric Research, Education and
    Clinical Center
Allergy, Pulmonary and Critical Care
Vanderbilt University School of Medicine
Nashville, TN

William B. Ershler, MD
Director Institute for Advanced Studies in Aging and
  Geriatric Medicine
Washington, DC

Terry T. Fulmer, PhD, RN
The Erline Perkins McGriff Professor and Dean
College of Nursing
New York University
New York, NY

Angela Gentili, MD
Associate Professor of Internal Medicine
Director, Geriatrics Fellowship Training Program
VA Medical Center/Virginia Commonwealth
  University
Richmond, VA

Thomas M. Gill, MD
Associate Professor of Medicine
Yale University School of Medicine
New Haven, CT

Lisa J. Granville, MD
Professor and Associate Chair
Department of Geriatrics
Florida State University College of Medicine
Tallahassee, FL

David A. Gruenewald, MD
Associate Professor of Medicine
Division of Gerontology and Geriatric Medicine
Department of Medicine
University of Washington School of Medicine
Staff Physician, Geriatrics Research, Education and
  Clinical Center
VA Puget Sound Health Care System
Seattle, WA

Arthur E. Helfand, DPM
Professor Emeritus
Temple University School of Podiatric Medicine
Retired Chair, Department of Community Health,
  Aging & Health Policy
Adjunct Professor, Department of Medicine
Temple University School of Medicine
Philadelphia, PA

Kenneth W. Hepburn, PhD
Professor and Associate Dean for Research
School of Nursing
University of Minnesota
Minneapolis, MN

Kevin Paul High, MD, MSc
Associate Professor of Medicine
Sections of Infectious Diseases and
  Hematology/Oncology
Wake Forest University School of Medicine
Winston Salem, NC

Gordon L. Jensen, MD, PhD
Director, Vanderbilt Center for Human Nutrition
Professor of Medicine
Vanderbilt University Medical Center
Nashville, TN

Donald A. Jurivich, DO
Chief, Section of Geriatric Medicine
Vitoux Associate Professor of Medicine
University of Illinois at Chicago Medical School
Chicago, IL

Jennifer M. Kapo, MD
Assistant Professor of Clinical Medicine
Division of Geriatrics
University of Pennsylvania
Philadelphia, PA

Judith D. Kasper, PhD
Professor, Department of Health Policy and
  Management
The Johns Hopkins University Bloomberg School of
  Public Health
Baltimore, MD

Jurgis Karuza, PhD
Visiting Professor of Rochester Medical Center
Rochester, NY
Professor and Chair, Psychology Department
State University College at Buffalo
Buffalo, NY

Paul R. Katz, MD
Professor of Medicine
Chief, Division of Geriatrics
University of Rochester School of Medicine and
  Dentistry
Rochester, NY

Catherine Lee Kelleher, MD
Nephrology Division
Denver Health Medical Center
University of Colorado Medical Center
Denver, CO

Gary J. Kennedy, MD
Professor of Psychiatry and Behavioral Science
Albert Einstein College of Medicine
Director, Division of Geriatric Psychiatry
Montefiore Medical Center
Bronx, NY

Anne M. Kenny, MD
Associate Professor of Medicine
UConn Center on Aging
University of Connecticut Health Center
Farmington, CT

Douglas P. Kiel, MD, MPH
Associate Professor of Medicine
Harvard Medical School Division on Aging
Director, Medical Research
HRCA Research and Training Institute
Boston, MA

Kurt Kroenke, MD
Professor of Medicine
Indiana University School of Medicine
Senior Scientist
Regenstrief Institute for Health Care
Indianapolis, IN

C. Seth Landefeld, MD
Professor of Medicine
Chief, Division of Geriatrics
Director, UCSF/Mount Zion Center on Aging
University of California, San Francisco
Associate Chief of Staff, Geriatrics and Extended Care
San Francisco VA Medical Center
San Francisco, CA

Melinda S. Lantz, MD
Director of Psychiatry
Jewish Home and Hospital
Assistant Professor, Department of Geriatrics and
    Adult Development
Mount Sinai School of Medicine
New York, NY

Robert Dean Lindeman, MD
Professor Emeritus of Medicine
University of New Mexico School of Medicine
Albuquerque, NM

David A. Lipschitz, MD, PhD
Professor of Geriatrics
Chair, Donald W. Reynolds Department of Geriatrics
University of Arkansas for Medical Sciences
Little Rock, AR

Dan L. Longo, MD
Scientific Director
National Institute on Aging
Baltimore, MD

Courtney H. Lyder, ND, GNP
University of Virginia Medical Center Professor
Chairman, Department of Acute and Specialty Care
University of Virginia School of Nursing
Charlottesville, VA

Constantine G. Lyketsos, MD, MHS
Professor of Psychiatry and Behavioral Sciences
Co-Director, Division of Geriatric Psychiatry and
    Neuropsychiatry
The Johns Hopkins University and Hospital
Baltimore, MD

William L. Lyons, MD
Assistant Professor
Section of Geriatrics and Gerontology
Department of Internal Medicine
University of Nebraska Medical Center
Omaha, NE

Edward R. Marcantonio, MD, SM
Associate Professor of Medicine
Harvard Medical School
Director of Research
Division of General Medicine and Primary Care
Beth Israel Deaconess Medical Center
Boston, MA

Coleman O. Martin, MD
Clinical Associate
Department of Neurology
University of Iowa Hospitals and Clinics
Iowa City, IA

Alvin M. Matsumoto, MD
Professor, Department of Medicine
University of Washington School of Medicine
Division of Gerontology and Geriatric Medicine
Director, Clinical Research Unit
Associate Director, Geriatric Research, Education, and
    Clinical Center
VA Puget Sound Health Care System
Seattle, Washington

Robert McCann, MD
Professor of Medicine
University of Rochester School of Medicine and
    Dentistry
Highland Hospital Department of Medicine
Rochester, NY

Barbara E. Moquin, PhD(c), MSN, APRN
Senior Nurse Specialist (Research)
National Center for Complementary and Alternative
  Medicine
National Institutes of Health
Division of Intramural Research
Bethesda, MD

R. Sean Morrison, MD
Hermann Merkin Professor of Palliative Care
Professor of Geriatrics and Medicine
Vice-Chair for Research
Brookdale Department of Geriatrics and Adult
  Development
Mount Sinai School of Medicine
New York, NY

Thomas Mulligan, MD
Ruth S. Jewett Professor of Medicine
Chief, University of Florida Division of Geriatrics
Director, Geriatrics Research, Education and Clinical
  Center
North Florida/South Georgia Veterans Health System
Gainesville, FL

David W. Oslin, MD
Associate Professor
Geriatric and Addiction Psychiatry
University of Pennsylvania
Philadelphia, PA

Stacie T. Pinderhughes, MD
Assistant Professor
Albert Einstein College of Medicine
Medical Director
Harlem Community Hospice of Continuum
  Healthcare
New York, NY

Peter Pompei, MD
Associate Professor of Medicine
Stanford University School of Medicine
Stanford, CA

James S. Powers, MD
Associate Professor of Medicine
Vanderbilt University Medical Center
Nashville, TN

Karen M. Prestwood, MD
Associate Professor of Medicine
UConn Center on Aging
University of Connecticut Health Center
Farmington, CT

Peter V. Rabins, MD
Professor of Psychiatry, Medicine, Mental Health and
  Health Policy and Management
Johns Hopkins Medical Institution
Baltimore, MD

John W. Rachow, PhD, MD
Assistant Clinical Professor
Department of Medicine
University of Iowa College of Medicine
Iowa City, IA

Paula A. Rochon, MD, MPH
Associate Professor
Department of Medicine and Health Policy
  Management and Evaluation
University of Toronto
Senior Scientist and Assistant Director
Kunin-Lunenfeld Applied Research Unit
Baycrest Centre for Geriatric Care
Scientist, Institute for Clinical Evaluative Sciences
Toronto, ON

David Sarraf, MD
Assistant Clinical Professor of Ophthalmology
Jules Stein Eye Institute, UCLA School of Medicine
  and the Greater Los Angeles
VA Healthcare Center
Assistant Professor of Ophthalmology
Martin L. King Medical Center/Charles R. Drew
  University of Medicine
Los Angeles, CA

Todd P. Semla, PharmD, MS
Clinical Pharmacy Specialist
Department of Veterans Affairs
Pharmacy Benefits Management & Strategic Health
  Group
Hines, IL
Associate Professor
Department of Psychiatry and Behavioral Sciences
The Feinberg School of Medicine
Northwestern University
Chicago, IL

Kenneth Shay, DDS, MS
Director of Geriatric Programs
Office of Geriatrics and Extended Care
VA Central Office, Washington, DC
Adjunct Professor of Dentistry
University of Michigan School of Dentistry
Ann Arbor, MI

Javaid I. Sheikh, MD
Professor
Department of Psychiatry and Behavioral Sciences
Stanford University School of Medicine
Stanford, CA
Chief of Staff
VA Palo Alto Health Care System
Palo Alto, CA

Gary W. Small, MD
Parlow-Solomon Professor of Psychiatry and
 Biobehavioral Sciences
Director, UCLA Center on Aging
University of California, Los Angeles
Los Angeles, CA

Stephanie A. Studenski, MD, MPH
Professor, Department of Medicine (Geriatrics)
Staff Physician
Veterans Affairs Pittsburgh Geriatric Research,
 Education and Clinical Center
Pittsburgh, PA

Mark A. Supiano, MD
Professor and Chief, Division of Geriatric Medicine
University of Utah Health Science Center
Director, Veterans Affairs Salt Lake City
Geriatric Research, Education and Clinical Center
Executive Director, University of Utah Center on
 Aging
Salt Lake City, UT

George Triadafilopoulos, MD
Clinical Professor of Medicine
Division of Gastroenterology and Hepatology
Stanford University School of Medicine
Stanford, CA

Bruce R. Troen, MD
Associate Professor of Medicine
Miller School of Medicine
University of Miami
Geriatric Research, Education and Clinical Center
Miami Veterans Affairs Medical Center
Miami, FL

Andrew C. Warren, MB, BS, DPhil
Attending Physician, Sheppard Pratt Hospital
Associate Professor of Psychiatry
The Johns Hopkins University School of Medicine
Baltimore, MD

Debra K. Weiner, MD
Associate Professor of Medicine, Psychiatry and
 Anesthesiology
University of Pittsburgh School of Medicine
Pittsburgh, PA

Kristine Yaffe, MD
Associate Professor
Departments of Psychiatry, Neurology, Biostatistics
 and Epidemiology
University of California, San Francisco
Chief, Geriatric Psychiatry
San Francisco Veterans Administration Medical Center
San Francisco, CA

CONTRIBUTING QUESTION AND CRITIQUE AUTHORS

Reva N. Adler, MD, MPH
Medical Director, STAT Centre and At-home
  Supports
Vancouver Hospital and Vancouver Community
  Health Services
Clinical Associate Professor
Division of Geriatric Medicine
University of British Columbia
Vancouver, BC

Kathryn A. Atchison, DDS, MPH
Professor and Associate Dean for Research
School of Dentistry
University of California, Los Angeles
Los Angeles, CA

Sidney T. Bogardus, Jr., MD
Associate Professor of Medicine
Yale University School of Medicine
New Haven, CT

Kenneth Brummel-Smith, MD
Charlotte Edwards Maguire Professor of Geriatrics
Chair, Department of Geriatrics
Florida State University College of Medicine
Tallahassee, FL

Susan Charette, MD
Assistant Clinical Professor
Division of Geriatrics
Department of Medicine
University of California, Los Angeles
Los Angeles, CA

Pejman Cohan, MD
Assistant Professor of Medicine
Co-Director, Pituitary Program
School of Medicine
University of California, Los Angeles
Los Angeles, CA

Leo M. Cooney, Jr., MD
Humana Foundation Professor of Geriatric Medicine
Chief, Section of Geriatric Medicine
Yale University School of Medicine
New Haven, CT

Robert S. Crausman, MD, MMS
Chief Administrative Officer
Rhode Island Board of Medical Licensure and
  Discipline
Providence, RI

James Cummins, MD
Staff Psychiatrist
OhioHealth Behavioral Health
Columbus, OH

Margaret A. Drickamer, MD
Associate Professor
Yale University School of Medicine
New Haven, CT

Edmund H. Duthie, Jr, MD
Professor of Medicine (Geriatrics/Gerontology)
Chief, Division of Geriatrics and Gerontology
Medical College of Wisconsin
Lead Physician, Geriatrics Section, Consultant Care
  Division
VA Medical Center, Milwaukee
Milwaukee, WI

Carmel Bitondo Dyer, MD
Associate Professor of Medicine
Baylor College of Medicine
Director, Geriatrics Program
Harris County Hospital District
Houston, TX

Michelle S. Eslami, MD
Associate Professor of Medicine
Division of Geriatrics
David Geffen School of Medicine
University of California, Los Angeles
Los Angeles, CA

Mark H. Fleisher, MD
Associate Professor of Psychiatry
Medical Director, Adult Community Psychiatry Clinics
Director, Neurodevelopmental Psychiatry
University of Nebraska College of Medicine
Omaha, NE

Alastair J. Flint, MB
Professor of Psychiatry
University of Toronto
Head, Geriatric Psychiatry Program
University Health Network
Toronto, ON

David G. Folks, MD
Professor of Psychiatry
University of Nebraska College of Medicine
Omaha, NE

Christine Himes Fordyce, MD
Medicare Medical Director
Group Health Cooperative
Seattle, WA

Andrea R. Fox, MD, MPH
Associate Director
Clinical Care GRECC
VA Pittsburgh Healthcare System
Associate Professor of Medicine
University of Pittsburgh
Pittsburgh, PA

Angela Gentili, MD
Associate Professor of Internal Medicine
Director, Geriatrics Fellowship Program
VA Medical Center/Virginia Commonwealth
    University
Richmond, VA

Mary Kane Goldstein, MD, MS
Associate Director for Clinical Services
Geriatrics Research Education and Clinical Center
VA Palo Alto Health Care Systems
Professor of Medicine
Center for Primary Care and Outcomes Research
Stanford University
Palo Alto, CA

Shelly L. Gray, PharmD, MS, BCPS
Director, Geriatric Pharmacy Program
Associate Professor, School of Pharmacy
Seattle, WA

Nathan Herrmann, MD
Professor, Department of Psychiatry
University of Toronto
Head, Division of Geriatric Psychiatry
Sunnybrook & Women's College Health Science
    Centre
Toronto, ON

Kevin Paul High, MD, MSc
Associate Professor of Medicine
Sections on Infectious Diseases and
    Hematology/Oncology
Wake Forest University School of Medicine
Winston Salem, NC

Michele Iannuzzi-Sucich, MD
Family Practice and Geriatrics
Modena Family Practice
Modena, NY

Gail Ishiyama, MD
Assistant Professor
Department of Neurology
Division of Neurotology
University of California, Los Angeles
Los Angeles, CA

Thomas Vincent Jones, MD, MPH
Associate Editor
The Merck Manuals
Merck & Co, Inc.
Blue Bell, PA

Fran E. Kaiser, MD
Chief Executive Officer
Kaiser and Associates Consulting
Clinical Professor of Medicine
University of Texas Southwestern Medical School
Dallas, TX
Adjunct Professor of Medicine
St. Louis University School of Medicine
St. Louis, MO

Anne Kenny, MD
Associate Professor of Medicine
UConn Center on Aging
University of Connecticut Health Center
Farmington, CT

Mary B. King, MD
Assistant Professor of Medicine
University of Connecticut School of Medicine
Geriatrician, Hartford Hospital
Division of Geriatric Medicine and Gerontology
Hartford, CT

George A. Kuchel, MD
Director, University Connecticut Center on Aging
Chief, Division of Geriatric Medicine
University of Connecticut Health Center
Farmington, CT

Robert K. Lee, DPM
Assistant Clinical Professor
David Geffen School of Medicine
University of California, Los Angeles
Los Angeles, CA

Michael C. Lindberg, MD
Director of Clinical Inpatient Services
Department of Medicine
Hartford Hospital
Clinical Associate Professor
University of Connecticut School of Medicine
Hartford, CT

Shari M. Ling, MD
Clinical Research Branch
National Institute on Aging
Intramural Research Program
Baltimore, MD

Constantine G. Lyketsos, MD, MHS
Professor of Psychiatry and Behavioral Sciences
Co-Director, Division of Geriatric Psychiatry and
    Neuropsychiatry
The Johns Hopkins University and Hospital
Baltimore, MD

Mathew S. Maurer, MD
The Advanced Cardiac Care Center
Columbia University
Irving Assistant Professor of Medicine
Director, Clinical Cardiovascular Research Laboratory
    for the Elderly
Columbia University College of Physicians and
    Surgeons
New York, NY

Ellen McMahon, MD
Assistant Professor
University of Massachusetts Medical School
Oak Bluffs, MA

Lynn McNicoll, MD
Assistant Professor of Medicine
Geriatrician
Division of Geriatrics
Rhode Island Hospital
Providence, RI

Daniel Ari Mendelson, MS, MD
Assistant Professor of Medicine
Division of Geriatrics
University of Rochester School of Medicine and
    Dentistry
Medical Director
Acute Care for Elders Unit, Highland Hospital
Medical Director
Visiting Nurse Service of Rochester and Monroe
    County
Rochester, NY

Laura Mosqueda, MD
Director of Geriatrics
Professor of Family Medicine
Ronald W. Reagan Endowed Chair in Geriatric
    Medicine
University of California, Irvine School of Medicine
Orange, CA

Benoit H. Mulsant, MD
Professor of Psychiatry
Center for Addiction and Mental Health
University of Toronto
Toronto, ON

Arash Naeim, MD, PhD
Assistant Professor of Medicine
University of California, Los Angeles
Los Angeles, CA

Joseph G. Ouslander, MD
Professor of Medicine and Nursing
Director, Division of Geriatric Medicine and
    Gerontology
Chief Medical Officer
Wesley Woods Center of Emory University
Director, Emory Center for Health in Aging
Research Scientist
Birmingham/Atlanta VA Geriatric Research, Education
    and Clinical Center
Atlanta, GA

Ronald Frederick Pfeiffer, MD
Professor and Vice Chair
Department of Neurology
University of Tennessee Health Science Center
Memphis, TN

James T. Pacala, MD, MS
Associate Professor
Distinguished University Teaching Professor
Department of Family Medicine and Community
    Health
University of Minnesota Medical School
Minneapolis, MN

Joe W. Ramsdell, MD
Professor and Head
Division of General Internal Medicine/Geriatrics
University of California, San Diego
UCSD Medical Center
San Diego, CA

Anthony E. Ranno, PharmD
Clinical Education Consultant
Pfizer Inc.
Sherwood, OR

Michael W. Rich, MD
Associate Professor of Medicine
Washington University School of Medicine
Director, Cardiac Rapid Evaluation Unit
Barnes-Jewish Hospital
St. Louis, MO

Debra Saliba, MD, MPH
Research Associate
VA Health Services Research and Development
Center for the Study of Healthcare Provider Behavior
Sepulveda, CA

Gary Schiller, MD
Department of Medicine
Division of Hematology/Oncology
School of Medicine
University of California, Los Angeles
Los Angeles, CA

Nancy Shafer Clark, MD
Assistant Professor, Medicine and Geriatrics
University of Rochester
Rochester, NY

Alan M. Singer, DPM
Department of Medicine
Division of Podiatry
University of California, Los Angeles
Los Angeles, CA

Upinder Singh, MD
Clinical Associate Professor
School of Medicine, UNR
Chief of Geriatrics
Southwest Medical Associates
Sierra Health Services
Las Vegas, NV

Monica Stallworth Kolimas, MD
Faculty, Harvard Division on Aging
Shattuck House, Harvard University
Boston, MA

David H. Stern, MD
Specialized Ambulatory Geriatric Evaluation Clinic
(S+AGE)
Sherman Oaks, CA

Gwen K. Sterns, MD
Chief, Department of Ophthalmology
Rochester General Hospital
Clinical Professor of Ophthalmology
University of Rochester Eye Institute
Rochester, NY

Dennis H. Sullivan, MD
Director, Geriatric Research Education and Clinical
  Center
Central Arkansas Veteran's Healthcare System
Vice Chairman and Professor
Donald W. Reynolds Department of Geriatrics
University of Arkansas for Medical Sciences
Little Rock, AR

Mark Supiano, MD
Professor and Chief, Division of Geriatric Medicine
University of Utah Health Science Center
Director, VA Salt Lake City Geriatric Research,
  Education and Clinical Center
Executive Director, University of Utah Center on
  Aging
Salt Lake City, UT

Robert A. Sweet, MD
Associate Professor of Psychiatry
Vice-Chair, Institutional Review Board
University of Pittsburgh
Pittsburgh, PA

David C. Thomas, MD, MS
Associate Professor of Medicine and Rehabilitation
Department of Medicine, Division of General Internal
  Medicine
Medical Director, Ambulatory Care/Outpatient
  Services
Mount Sinai School of Medicine
New York, NY

Corina M. Velehorschi, MD
Adjunct Professor of Psychiatry
University of Western Ontario
Windsor Regional Hospital
Windsor, ON

Katherine Ward, MD
Assistant Clinical Professor
Division of Geriatric Medicine
University of California, Los Angeles
Los Angeles, CA

Michael R. Wasserman, MD
Senior Care of Colorado
Assistant Clinical Professor
University of Colorado Health Science Center
Denver, CO

Barbara E. Weinstein, PhD
Executive Officer, Clinical Doctoral Programs
The Graduate Center, CUNY
Professor, Lehman College, CUNY
Bronx, NY

Steven P. Wengel, MD
Chair, Department of Psychiatry
University of Nebraska Medical Center
Omaha, NE

PROGRAM GUIDELINES

CONTINUING EDUCATION CREDITS

Accreditation

The American Geriatrics Society (AGS) is accredited by the Accreditation Council for Continuing Medical Education (ACCME) to provide continuing medical education (CME) for physicians.

CME Credit Hours

The AGS designates this educational activity for a maximum of **75 Category I credits toward the American Medical Association (AMA) Physician's Recognition Award (PRA)**, provided that the answers are submitted for computer scoring and at least 70% of the questions are answered correctly. Each physician should claim only those credits that he/she actually spent in the activity. Diplomates of the American Board of Internal Medicine who are recertifying may also obtain Maintenance of Certification credits from the *GRS6*. This is in addition to Category 1 credit and is more fully described below.

The *GRS6* is accredited for physicians wishing to earn AMA PRA CME credits through December 2008. The AGS will review the program in November 2008, and a determination regarding extension of CME credits through December 31, 2009, will be announced in January 2009.

The *GRS6* has been reviewed and is acceptable for up to **75 Prescribed credits from the American Academy of Family Physicians**, provided that the answers are submitted for computer scoring and at least 70% of the questions are answered correctly. The initial approval of the *GRS6* for 75 Prescribed credits is for the period January 1, 2006, to December 31, 2007. The AGS will apply for renewal of Prescribed credits for the period January 1, 2008, to December 31, 2009, following the review of the *GRS6* for currency of content in mid-2007.

The **American Osteopathic Association** (AOA) has determined that the *GRS6* is eligible for up to **75 hours in Category 2-B of AOA CME**, through December 31, 2009, provided that the answers are submitted for computer scoring and at least 70% of the questions are answered correctly.

Instructions for Submitting Answer Sheets for CME Credit

CME credit hours are awarded to participants on a one-time basis after participants submit the answer sheet enclosed with the *GRS6* and if the program is successfully completed by answering 70% of the questions correctly. The type of CME credit requested must be indicated on the answer sheet. Upon program completion, the answer sheet must be submitted in the envelope addressed to Program Management Services, Inc. (PMSI).

Notification of CME Examination Performance

PMSI will evaluate answers and mail an individualized performance report to each participant. For those who successfully complete the program, a CME certificate will be enclosed with the report. For those who do not successfully complete the program, another answer sheet will be enclosed with an offer of the opportunity to take the examination again. Both types of notices will be sent within 3–4 weeks of submission. All score results are considered confidential.

Questions about CME certificates should be directed to PMSI at 1-800-232-4422.

User Eligibility for CME Credits

Each copy of the *GRS6* program is valid for CME credits only for one participant.

Maintenance of Certification Credits

For those applying for ABIM Maintenance of Certification (MOC) credits, please see the *GRS6* CD-ROM program guidelines. MOC credits are *only* available through the *GRS6* CD-ROM program and by using its electronic submission form. MOC credits are not offered by completing the enclosed paper exam answer sheet.

QUESTION ANALYSIS

AGS will post an analysis of participant performance on the Syllabus Questions to the AGS Web site (http://www.americangeriatrics.org) once 250 answer sheets have been scored.

USER EVALUATION

The AGS would appreciate participants' comments about the *GRS6* program through the user evaluation enclosed with the program. Comments and suggestions will be taken into consideration by those planning the next edition.

CONGRUITY OF CONTENT BETWEEN SYLLABUS AND QUESTIONS

Since the *Syllabus* chapters and the questions with critiques are written by different authors, questions may not always correlate directly with the *Syllabus*. In the event that a question's content is not addressed in the correlating chapter, its answer is fully supported in the question critique.

UPDATES AND ERRATA

Important updates, such as medication alerts, will be posted as necessary on the AGS Web site: http://www.americangeriatrics.org.

Please report any errata to: info.amger@american geriatrics.org, Attention: *GRS* Managing Editor. Identified errata will be posted on the AGS Web site: http://www.americangeriatrics.org.

AGS GERIATRICS RECOGNITION AWARD

The Geriatrics Recognition Award (GRA) was developed by the AGS to encourage health care profession-als to acquire special knowledge and keep abreast of the latest developments in geriatrics through continuing education programs. The GRA demonstrates a health care professional's commitment to providing quality care to patients by participating in continuing education programs in geriatrics. It provides professional recognition of a health care professional's special knowledge in geriatrics sought by many employers.

CME credits earned from successfully completing the *GRS6* may be applied toward the GRA. To receive more information and an application, please provide your mailing address to the American Geriatrics Society CME Department, Empire State Building, Suite 801, 350 Fifth Avenue, New York, NY 10118, telephone (212) 308-1414, fax (212) 832-8646.

GRS6 ONLINE (Web version)

The *GRS6* will soon be available online via the Web through institutional subscriptions. Subscribers can purchase yearly access to the full *GRS6* Syllabus along with the questions and critiques for all of their students and faculty to use through their institution intranets. For more information on this great teaching resource, please call Elvy Ickowicz at 212–308–1414 or e-mail her at eickowicz@americangeriatrics.org.

INTRODUCTION

The core mission of the American Geriatrics Society (AGS) is to promote the optimal health, function, and well-being of older persons. Through the *Syllabus*, we advance this goal by providing health care providers with a current fund of knowledge that is evidence based and incorporates the most recent advances in health care. In 1989 the AGS published its first *Geriatrics Review Syllabus (GRS)*. This publication was enormously successful and has become the standard resource in the field of medicine to assist clinicians in staying current and providing the best possible care to their older patients. We update the *GRS* to keep pace with advances in medical knowledge. It is with a great sense of accomplishment that the AGS publishes this sixth edition (*GRS6*) authored largely by AGS members who are leaders in the field of geriatric medicine.

The *GRS6* is available as a 3-volume set of books or in CD-ROM format. Book 1 contains the *Syllabus* of 59 chapters, annotated references that allow the interested reader to pursue topics in greater depth, and an appendix with assessment instruments and practical resources. Book 2 contains 263 case-oriented, multiple-choice questions and is accompanied by an answer sheet for those participating in the continuing education program. Book 3 repeats the questions and contains answers, supporting critiques, and references, providing an effective self-assessment tool. The CD-ROM format comprises the entire program.

The *Syllabus* is divided into five sections—Current Issues in Aging, Approach to the Patient, Syndromes, Psychiatry, and Diseases and Disorders—that encompass 59 chapters. Each chapter provides a synopsis of the current thinking about a particular topic or field. The goal of the *GRS* editorial board is to provide a comprehensive resource that covers the scope of geriatric medicine. Accordingly, discussions of certain subjects that are well-covered in other resources are kept brief, and participants are referred to more in-depth discussions in an annotated bibliography. In compiling the bibliography, the Editorial Board has made every attempt to restrict the references to journals listed in Index Medicus. By intention, *GRS6* focuses on recent developments since the publication of the fifth edition rather than on basic principles of caring for older persons. Finally, little attention is devoted to topics that are core components of medicine and are not unique to the care of older persons; this information can be found in standard medical texts.

The Question Editors, using questions drafted by a team of question writers, have developed an entirely new set of 263 case-oriented, multiple-choice self-study questions. These questions are designed to complement material in the *Syllabus* chapters, and they draw on the entire knowledge base of geriatric medicine, rather than limiting themselves to the text of the *GRS Syllabus*. We recommend that participants prepare for answering these questions by first carefully reading through the *Syllabus* chapters. Any material addressed in the questions that is not discussed in the chapters is amply discussed in the critiques. The questions have been developed independently of any specialty board and will not be a part of any secure board certification examination.

GRS6 is the result of a major collaborative effort by AGS members and staff. The Editorial Board selected over 100 authors to develop the 59 chapters and 263 questions with answers, explanations, and references.

All *GRS* authors were encouraged to include information on health disparities among racial and ethnic minorities in those areas where accurate data exist. Although there has been an increase in the understanding of the health outcomes and diseases among older minorities, these populations remain insufficiently studied. Clinicians must recognize the differences between various ethnic groups and are encouraged to be sensitive to cultural issues in the care of older persons. *Doorway Thoughts: Cross-Cultural Health Care for Older Adults* (a series of volumes also published by the AGS) is a useful companion to the *GRS* for readers who are interested in exploring cultural issues in more depth.

Topics for inclusion were carefully selected by the editorial team. Authors were chosen on the basis of their in-depth knowledge of a particular area and their ability to condense large amounts of information into clinically applicable, succinct essays. Editors and authors are experienced in caring for geriatric patients and emphasize the geriatrics perspective in the preparation of manuscripts, bibliographies, and questions.

With each new edition, the *Syllabus* has included increasing amounts of information about drugs commonly used in treating older adults, though no effort is made to provide comprehensive coverage of available drugs for each disease or disorder. (See the AGS *Geriatrics At Your Fingertips*, published annually, for details about individual agents.) When *Syllabus* authors have chosen to discuss specific drugs, we have made certain that the information provided was up to date at the time of publication and that any mentions of uses not specifically approved by the U.S. Food and Drug Administration (so called "off-label" uses) are so tagged.

Another product supplementing the *GRS* is the AGS *GRS Teaching Slides*, available as a subscription through the AGS Web site. The slide presentations in

Microsoft® Power Point® are based on *GRS* chapters and suitable for faculty, fellows, residents, and students. Each presentation is designed for approximately a 1-hour seminar and may be used as a stand-alone lecture or to complement the lecturer's personal teaching materials.

Chapters new to *GRS6* include those on perioperative care, cultural aspects of care, persistent pain, and diabetes mellitus. Also new to the *GRS* are key points provided at the beginning of each chapter. The Appendix offers material that clinicians find useful in clinical practice.

The *GRS* self-assessment program provides participants with the option of applying for 75 Continuing Medical Education (CME) credits through the American Medical Association, American Academy of Family Physicians, and American Osteopathic Association. For information on self-scoring or submitting answer sheets for CME credit, please see the Program Guidelines (p 000). In addition to the CME credit offered by successfully completing the *GRS6*, the American Board of Internal Medicine (ABIM) has approved the CD-ROM version of the *GRS6* self-assessment program for 100 lifelong learning points for ABIM diplomates who are enrolled in the Maintenance of Certification program.

We hope the *GRS* will meet our goal of improving participants' knowledge base in geriatrics and thus enhancing the practice patterns of clinicians who care for older persons by providing a self-study tool that is current, concise, scholarly, and clinically relevant. We encourage your comments and suggestions, as the AGS continually strives to better serve its members, other health professionals, and the older persons they treat.

Learning Objectives

At the conclusion of this program, participants will be better able to:

• Describe the general principles of aging and the biomedical and psychosocial issues of aging;

• Discuss legal and ethical issues related to geriatric medicine;

• Evaluate the financing of health care for older persons;

• Identify the basic principles of geriatric medicine, including assessment, pharmacology, prevention, exercise, palliative care, rehabilitation, and sensory deficits;

• Diagnosis and manage geriatric syndromes, including dementia, delirium, urinary incontinence, malnutrition, osteoporosis, falls, pressure ulcers, sleep disorders, pain, dysphagia, and dizziness;

• Use state-of-the-art approaches to geriatric care while providing care in hospital, office-practice, nursing-home, and home-care settings;

• Apply relevant information from the fields of internal medicine, neurology, psychiatry, dermatology, and gynecology to the care of older patients;

• Adjust patient care in the light of evidence-based data regarding the particular risks and needs of ethnic, racial, and sexual patient groups; and

• Employ evidence-based data to increase the effectiveness of teaching geriatrics to all health professionals.

DISCLOSURE OF FINANCIAL INTERESTS

As an accredited provider of Continuing Medical Education, the American Geriatrics Society continuously strives to ensure that the education activities planned and conducted by our faculty meet generally accepted ethical standards as codified by the ACCME, the Food and Drug Administration, and the American Medical Association's Guide for Gifts to Physicians. To this end, we have implemented a process wherein everyone who is in a position to control the content of an education activity has disclosed to us all relevant financial relationships with any commercial interests as related to the content of their presentations and under which we work to resolve any real or apparent conflicts of interest. Faculty conflicts of interest in this particular CME activity have been resolved by having the content independently peer reviewed before publication by the Editorial Board and Question Review Committee.

The following faculty (and/or their spouses/ partners) have reported real or apparent conflicts of interest that have been resolved through a peer review content validation process.

Harold Adams, MD
Dr. Adams has received speaking honorarium from Bayer (aspirin) and has received research grants from Bristol-Meyers-Squibb (clopidogrel).

Marc E. Agronin, MD
Dr. Agronin is a member of the Speaker's Bureau for Janssen (risperidone) and for Forest Laboratories (escitalopram oxalate).

William J. Burke, MD
Dr. Burke serves as a paid consultant and is a member of the Speakers Bureau for Forest Pharmaceuticals (psychopharmacology) and for Cyberonics (depression). He receives grants from Cyberonics (depression) and Merck (Alzheimer disease).

Anne L. Coleman, MD, PhD
Dr. Coleman receives grant support from Pfizer.

Catherine E. DuBeau, MD
Dr. DuBeau serves as a paid consultant and is a symposium speaker for Astellas (solifenacin), Indevus (trospium chloride), Novartis (darifenacin), and is a symposium speaker for Watson (oxybutynin).

William B. Ershler, MD
Dr. Ershler receives grant support and is a member of the Speaker's Bureau for Amgen.

Anne R. Fabiny, MD
Dr. Fabiny discloses that her spouse/partner serves as a paid consultant to Abgenix (bone and mineral metabolism).

Lisa J. Granville, MD
Dr. Granville serves as a paid consultant for Novartis and Pfizer in the area of incontinence.

Nathan Herrmann, MD
Dr. Herrmann serves as a paid consultant and is a member of the Speaker's Bureau for Janssen (risperidone).

Fran E. Kaiser, MD
Dr. Kaiser was CEO of Kaiser and Associates Consulting when she began work on the GRS-6 and is currently an employee of Merck & Co., Inc.

Gary J. Kennedy, MD
Dr. Kennedy discloses that he receives grant support and is a member of the Speaker's Bureau for Forest Laboratories (escitalopram), and is a member of the Speaker's Bureau for Pfizer (sertraline).

Melinda S. Lantz, MD
Dr. Lantz receives grant support from Bristol-Myers Squibb (aripiprazole) and from Forest Laboratories (memantine).

Courtney H. Lyder, ND, GNP
Mr. Lyder is a member of the Speaker's Bureau for ConvaTec (wound dressings), and for Hil-Rom (mattress replacements).

Constantine G. Lyketsos, MD, MHS
Dr. Lyketsos receives grant support and speaking honorarium from Forest, serves as a paid consultant and is a member of the Speaker's Bureau for Novartis, receives grant support and speaking honorarium from Pfizer, and receives speaking honorarium from GlaxoSmithKline.

Alison A. Moore, MD, MPH
Dr. Moore owns shares of Merck stock.

Thomas Mulligan, MD
Dr. Mulligan owns significant shares of Pfizer stock, and receives grant support from Ascend (dihydrotestosterone) and Solvay (testosterone).

Benoit H. Mulsant, MD
Dr. Mulsant is a member of the Speaker's Bureau for Pfizer (sertraline), and is a paid consultant and a member of the Speaker's Bureau for Forest Labortatories (citalopram, escitalopram).

Joseph G. Ouslander, MD
Dr. Ouslander serves as a paid consultant, receives grant support and is a member of the Speaker's Bureau for Pfizer (tolterodine).

Peter V. Rabins, MD
Dr. Rabins is a member of the Speaker's Bureau for Pfizer, AstraZeneca, Janssen, Eli Lilly, and Forest Laboratories.

Anthony E. Ranno, PharmD
Dr. Ranno is an employee of Pfizer (sertraline).

Michael W. Rich, MD
Dr. Rich is a member of the Speaker's Bureau for Merck & Co. (simvastatin, losartan) and receives grant support from Bristol-Myers Squibb (irbesartan).

Todd P. Semla, PharmD, MS
Dr. Semla serves as a paid consultant for Omnicare and Ovations (a part of United Healthcare) Pharmacy and Therapeutics Committees, and his spouse is employed by and holds shares of Abbott Laboratories.

Javaid I. Sheikh, MD
Dr. Sheikh is a member of the Speaker's Bureau for Pfizer, Forest, and Janssen Pharmaceutica.

Gary W. Small, MD
Dr. Small is a member of the Speaker's Bureau for Pfizer (donepezil) and Novartis (rivastigmine). He is a significant shareholder in MFI (educational information), and holds a license with Siemens for FDDNP-PET.

Stephanie Studenski, MD, MPH
Dr. Studenski serves as a paid consultant for Wyeth and receives grants from Eli Lilly and Co. and Ortho-Biotech for studies of measurement of physical function.

Dennis H. Sullivan, MD
Dr. Sullivan receives grant support from Bristol-Myers Squibb (megase).

George Triadafilopoulos, MD
Dr. Triadafilopoulos serves as a paid consultant, receives grant support, and is a member of the Speakers Bureau for Astra-Zeneca (omeprazole), Pfizer (celecoxib), TAP (lansoprazole). He is also a paid consultant and member of the Speaker's Bureau for Santarus (omeprazole).

Kristine Yaffe, MD
Dr. Yaffe serves as a paid consultant for Novartis.

The following faculty have returned disclosure forms indicating that they (and/or their spouses/partners) have no affiliation with, or financial interest in, any commercial interest that may have direct interest in the subject matter of their presentation(s):

Sumaira Aasi, MD

Itamar B. Abrass, MD

Reva N. Adler, MD, MPH

Cathy A. Alessi, MD

Neil B. Alexander, MD

Wilbert S. Aronow, MD

Kathryn A. Atchison, DDS, MPH

Priscilla F. Bade, MD, MS

Cynthia Barton, RN, MSN

Marc R. Blackman, MD

Caroline Blaum, MD

Harrison G. Bloom, MD

Sidney T. Bogardus, Jr., MD

Chad Boult, MD, MPH, MBA

Cynthia J. Brown, MD

Kenneth Brummel-Smith, MD

David M. Buchner, MD, MPH

Lynda C. Burton, ScD

David Bush, MD

Erin L. Cassidy, PhD

Susan Charette, MD

Gurkamal S. Chatta, MD

Colleen Christmas, MD

Pejman Cohan, MD

Leo M. Cooney, Jr., MD

Steven R. Counsell, MD

Robert S. Crausman, MD, MMS

James Cummins, MD

G. Willy Davila, MD

Margaret A. Drickamer, MD

Pamela W. Duncan, PhD

Edmund H. Duthie, Jr., MD

Carmel Bitondo Dyer, MD

G. Paul Eleazer, MD

E. Wesley Ely, MD, MPH

Michelle S. Eslami, MD

Mark H. Fleisher, MD

Alastair J. Flint, MB

David G. Folks, MD

Christine Himes Fordyce, MD

Andrea R. Fox, MD, MPH

Terry T. Fulmer, RN, PhD

Angela Gentili, MD

Thomas M. Gill, MD

Mary K. Goldstein, MD, MS

Shelly L. Gray, PharmD, MS

David A. Gruenewald, MD

Arthur E. Helfand, DPM

Kenneth W. Hepburn, PhD

Kevin P. High, MD, MSc

Chris Himes, MD

Michelle Iannuzzi-Sucich, MD

Gail Ishiyama, MD

Gordon L. Jensen, MD, PhD

Thomas V. Jones, MD, MPH

Donald A. Jurivich, DO

Jennifer M. Kapo, MD

Jurgis Karuza, PhD

Judith Kasper, PhD

Paul R. Katz, MD

Catherine Lee Kelleher, MD

Anne Kenny, MD

Douglas P. Kiel, MD, MPH

Mary B. King, MD

Kurt Kroenke, MD

George A. Kuchel, MD

C. Seth Landefeld, MD

Robert K. Lee, MD

Michael C. Lindberg, MD

Robert D. Lindeman, MD

Shari M. Ling, MD

David A. Lipschitz, MD, PhD

Dan L. Longo, MD

William L. Lyons, MD

Edward R. Marcantonio, MD, SM

Coleman O. Martin, MD

Alvin M. Matsumoto, MD

Matthew S. Maurer, MD

Robert M. McCann, MD

Ellen McMahon, MD

Lynn McNicholl, MD

Daniel A. Mendelson, MD

Barbara E. Moquin, PhD, MSN, APRN, BC-P

R. Sean Morrison, MD

Laura Mosqueda, MD

John B. Murphy, MD

Arash Naeim, MD, PhD

David W. Oslin, MD

James T. Pacala, MD, MS

Ronald F. Pfeiffer, MD

Stacie T. Pinderhughes, MD

Peter Pompei, MD

Jane F. Potter, MD

James S. Powers, MD

Karen M. Prestwood, MD

John W. Rachow, MD, PhD

Joe W. Ramsdell, MD

Paula A. Rochon, MD, MPH

Debra Saliba, MD, MPH

David Sarraf, MD

Gary Schiller, MD

Susan K. Schultz, MD

Nancy Shafer-Clark, MD

Kenneth Shay, DDS, MS

Alan M. Singer, DPM

Upinder Singh, MD

Monica Stallworth-Kolimas, MD

David H. Stern, MD

Gwen K. Sterns, MD

Gail M. Sullivan, MD, MPH

Mark A. Supiano, MD

Robert A. Sweet, MD

David C. Thomas, MD

Bruce R. Troen, MD

Corina M. Velehorschi, MD
Katherine Ward, MD
Andrew C. Warren, MB, BS, DPhil
Michael R. Wasserman, MD

Debra K. Weiner, MD
Barbara E. Weinstein, PhD
Steven P. Wengel, MD

CURRENT ISSUES IN AGING

CHAPTER 1—DEMOGRAPHY

KEY POINTS

- The aging of baby boomers, ethnic differentials in aging, and particularly increases in the old-old age group will significantly shift the composition of older adult population in the United States.

- The older segment of the U.S. population is changing: (a) becoming better educated; (b) becoming better off financially (though ethnic minorities lag behind white Americans); and (c) altering living arrangements, especially with the growth of assisted living.

- Population heterogeneity continues to increase, with wider variations in ethnicity, functional ability, and chronic conditions.

- Among older adults, heart disease, cancer, and stroke remain the leading causes of death, and age-specific conditions such as Alzheimer's disease are becoming more common; other diseases (influenza, pneumonia) become more lethal than among younger adults.

DEMOGRAPHIC TRENDS

In 2000 about one in eight Americans living in the United States was aged 65 or older, but by 2030 that rate is expected to be one out of every five. This major demographic shift has prompted numerous concerns regarding U.S. social and health policy in recent years. Not only will the sheer number of older adults increase dramatically, but the composition and characteristics of the older population will also change. Although clinicians are primarily concerned with the needs of individual patients, some of the attributes that an older patient brings to the patient-physician relationship are a function of the cohort to which he or she belongs. Aging baby boomers (the generation born between 1940 and 1960) are expected to have a major impact on the health and social service systems of the United States, although the exact nature of this impact remains unclear.

During the 20th century the U.S. population under age 65 tripled, while the age group 65 years and older increased by a factor of more than 11, growing from 3.1 million in 1900 to 35.6 million in 2002. This group will more than double by the middle of the next century, to 82 million people, with most of this growth occurring between 2010 and 2030. The United States is not unique in its growing share of older people. At present it is surpassed by many other developed countries, including Italy, Japan, Germany, Sweden, and the United Kingdom, where the proportion of people aged 60 and older is already at 20% or above.

The older population of the United States is not evenly distributed geographically. Half of persons aged 65 or older live in nine states, led by California, Florida, New York, and Texas. The midwestern states, however, have the highest percentages of older persons living alone (30% or greater). The older U.S. population is predominantly white, but the proportion of older persons of other races is expected to grow from about one in 10 currently, to two in 10 in the next 50 years. The number of older black Americans is expected to triple in this period, whereas the size of the older Hispanic American population, which is growing much faster, may exceed that of the older black population within 30 years.

LIFE EXPECTANCY

In the United States the average life expectancy is currently highest for white women, followed by that for black women and white men, who have nearly identical in life expectancies, and black men (Table 1.1). Women who survive to age 65 can, on average, expect to live to age 84, and those surviving to age 85 can expect to live to age 92. Up to age 85, the life expectancy of white American men and women exceeds that of their black counterparts. At age 85, these racial differences in life expectancy largely disappear. There is disagreement about whether these findings reflect errors in documenting age (for older black Americans) or a true cross-over in mortality rates.

The exact number of centenarians in the United States is difficult to gauge, but their numbers are growing and are expected to be over 800,000 by 2050. For persons born in 1899, the odds against living to 100 were 400 to 1; for persons born in 1980, the odds are estimated at 87 to 1.

SOCIOECONOMIC STATUS

Improvements in the Social Security system and the adoption of Medicare have had an important impact on the economic well-being of older persons in the United States. In the early 1960s, 35% of people aged 65 or older had incomes below the federal poverty

Table 1.1—Years of Life Expectancy at Birth and Ages 65, 75, 85, by Gender and Race, 2000

	All Races			White			Black		
	Both sexes	Male	Female	Both sexes	Male	Female	Both sexes	Male	Female
At birth	76.9	74.1	79.5	77.4	74.8	80.0	71.7	68.2	74.9
Age 65	17.9	16.3	19.2	17.9	16.3	19.2	16.2	14.5	17.4
Age 75	11.3	10.1	12.1	11.3	10.1	12.1	10.5	9.4	11.2
Age 85	6.3	5.6	6.7	6.2	5.5	6.6	6.3	5.7	6.5

SOURCE: Data from *National Vital Statistics Report.* 2002; 51(3):2. Available at http//www.cdc.gov/nchs/ (accessed July 2005).

level, and only 70% received Social Security pensions. By the early 1970s, over 90% of older people received Social Security retirement benefits (accounting for at least 50% of income for 63% of beneficiaries, and 90% or more of income for 26%), and 97% were covered by Medicare. The percentage of older people with incomes below the poverty line today is about 10%. Another 6.5% are classified as "near poor," that is, with an income between the poverty level and 125% of this level. For impoverished seniors (generally having an income well below the poverty line), Medicaid plays a key role in filling in the gaps in Medicare by covering prescription drugs, nursing-home and other long-term care services, and health care services not covered by Medicare, as well as paying for Medicare premiums and cost sharing. Currently there are approximately 4.5 million seniors enrolled in both Medicare and Medicaid (ie, "dual eligibles").

Although the overall economic position of older people in the United States has improved significantly over the past three decades, these gains have not been shared by all. Poverty rates among older people are higher among black Americans (22%), Hispanic Americans (22%), persons aged 85 and older (12%), those who never finished high school (21%), those living in rural areas (13%) and central cities (14%), and those living alone (21%). Rates in some groups of older persons are much higher—half of older black American women living alone are poor, for example.

Older workers have declined as a share of the U.S. work force, and this trend is expected to continue. In 1950, 60% of men aged 65 to 69 were still in the work force, whereas in 1990, 28% of the same age group were working. Overall, in the early 1990s, 16% of older men and 8% of older women were working. Today, more than half of those who continue to work do so part time and largely by choice, rather than because of restricted opportunities for full-time work.

Compared with their parents at the same age, baby boomers typically have higher income, are preparing for retirement at largely the same pace, and have accumulated more private wealth. On the whole, boomers are on track to have higher incomes in retirement than their parents and appear much less likely to live in poverty after they retire.

One of the most dramatic changes in the older U.S. population of the future will be in levels of educational attainment. Between 1970 and 2001, the percentage of those aged 65 or older who completed high school increased from 28% to 70%. By 2030, 83% of older people will have completed high school. The percentage with a bachelor's degree or more will have increased to 24% from the current level of 15%. Education is closely related to lifetime economic status, and, as many studies have shown, those with more education generally are in better health and at lower risk of disability than those with low levels of educational attainment. There is also speculation that the better-educated older baby boomers will be both more activist health care consumers and more demanding of the health care system. Today, approximately 50% of U.S. households have personal computers, but Internet use is much more common among persons under the age of 55. Despite concerns about the accuracy of much of the health and medical information available on various Internet Web sites, the use of these alternative information sources is likely to grow. In addition, pharmaceutical companies are increasingly marketing directly to consumers as a means of developing demand.

LIVING ARRANGEMENTS AND MARITAL STATUS

Among Americans living in the United States who are aged 65 to 74 years, two thirds are married and living with their spouse; in contrast, only about one fifth of those aged 85 and older are living with their spouse (Table 1.2). Not surprisingly, given older women's greater life expectancy, older men are far more likely to be married than are older women. Conversely, widowhood is much more common among older women; 56% of women aged 75 to 84 and 82% of women aged 85 and older are widows.

Older men and women who live alone, often having lost a spouse, usually prefer to remain independent and continue living alone as long as their health

Table 1.2—Marital Status and Living Arrangement of Medicare Beneficiaries, by Age, 2000 (beneficiaries as a percentage of total in each age group)

	All (%)			Male (%)			Female (%)		
	65–74	75–84	85+	65–74	75–84	85+	65–74	75–84	85+
Marital status									
Married	64.1	49.1	21.9	79.0	70.5	50.9	51.7	34.2	9.8
Widowed	21.0	41.4	70.4	7.2	19.9	41.8	32.5	56.2	82.3
Other	14.9	9.5	7.7	13.8	9.6	7.3	15.8	9.6	7.9
Living arrangement									
Lives alone	24.5	33.6	38.8	14.9	20.1	28.9	32.6	43.0	42.9
With spouse	62.6	46.8	18.4	76.8	67.5	43.5	50.7	32.4	8.0
With children	6.8	9.6	14.9	2.5	4.9	9.4	10.4	12.9	17.2
With others	4.7	4.7	5.1	4.3	3.7	4.2	5.1	5.4	5.5
In nursing home	1.4	5.3	22.8	1.5	3.8	14.0	1.2	6.3	26.4

SOURCE: Data from *Medicare Current Beneficiary Survey*, 2000; Table 1.2. Available at http://www.cms.hhs.gov/mcbs/PubCNP00.asp (accessed October 2005).

and economic means allow them to do so. Many of those who live alone have families or friends nearby, and about three in five have lived in the same place for 10 years or more. These persons may also be vulnerable, however. They are more likely than older people who live with others to use community services and to report greater levels of loneliness and social isolation.

THE OLDER FOREIGN-BORN POPULATION

In 2000, there were 3.1 million foreign-born persons aged 65 or older in the United States. More than one third (39%) of this older foreign-born group are from Europe, and another 31% are from Latin America; 22% are from Asia, and 8% are from other parts of the world. In the future, the older foreign-born resident is more likely to be from Latin America or Asia. Almost two thirds of the older foreign-born group have lived in the United States for more than 30 years. About one third of them live in the western states.

Older foreign-born persons are more likely than their native counterparts to live in family households. Eight of 10 older foreign-born men are married; nearly half of older foreign-born women are widowed. Older foreign-born women are much more likely than older foreign-born men to live alone. The poverty rate is higher for the older foreign-born population than for the older native population. Households with older foreign-born householders participate in means-tested programs at higher rates than households with older native householders.

ASSISTED-LIVING FACILITIES

Assisted living represents one of the fastest-growing trends in residential settings for older people in the United States. This type of facility seeks to fill the need for greater supervision and assistance than may be possible in a private home while avoiding the detrimental aspects of institutional care. Approximately 800,000 people were estimated to be living in 33,000 assisted-living facilities in the United States in 2002. A typical assisted-living resident is a woman between 75 and 85 years of age who is mobile but needs assistance with about two activities of daily living (ADLs). Residents move to assisted-living residences from a variety of settings. Just under half (46%) come from their home, 20% come from another assisted-living residence, 14% come from a hospital, and 10%, from a nursing home. The average length of residency is 2 years. (See also the section on assisted living in "Community-Based Care," p 131, and the AGS statement on assisted living in the Appendixes, p 494.)

TRENDS IN NURSING-HOME USE

The 1999 National Nursing Home Survey showed 1.6 million residents in 18,000 homes and an 87% occupancy rate. The rate per thousand population for those aged 65 and over was 429.2: 108 per 1000 for those aged 65 to 74, 429.7 for those 75 to 84, and 182.5 for those 85 years and over. Nationally, the percentage of older people residing in nursing homes has remained fairly constant, at about 5% overall, rising to 20% of persons aged 85 and older. The lifetime chance of ever being in a nursing home is much higher, however, at nearly 1 in 2. In part, this is due to increased use of nursing homes for short stays for recovery and rehabilitation following hospital discharge, stays that are paid for by Medicare if preceded by a 3-day hospital stay. The resident population is older and more disabled today. Over the past decade, the proportion of residents aged 85 and older has risen from 49% to 56% for women, and 29% to 33% for men; the proportion needing help with three or more ADLs rose from 72% to 83%.

The rate of all full-time equivalent employees for all facilities was 53.2 per 100 beds, with a slightly higher rate for voluntary nonprofit and government-owned facilities than for proprietary nursing homes. The rate per 100 beds for registered nurses was 7.6; for licensed practical nurses, 10.6; and nurse's aides and orderlies, 32.9.

In the past 10 years, nursing homes have put more resources into developing special care units, and almost one fifth of all nursing homes now have one. Two thirds of these units are for Alzheimer's disease and other dementias. Studies comparing the performance of these units with that of traditional units have not shown that residents of special units receive more direct care or experience better outcomes.

TRENDS IN HEALTH AND FUNCTIONING

The burden of disease and disability is greater for older people than for those under age 65. In the United States in 2000, 84% of persons aged 65 or older had one or more chronic conditions. Hypertension is the most common chronic condition reported, followed by

arthritic symptoms, heart disease, chronic obstructive pulmonary disease, and cancer (Figure 1.1). Although 80% of very old persons (aged 85 and older) report two or more chronic conditions, only 36% report being in fair or poor health (Figure 1.2). There is great heterogeneity in health status among older people (Table 1.3). Data on self-assessed health, which has been shown in several studies to correlate highly with mortality and risk of functional decline, illustrate this. Among white non-Hispanic Americans aged 65 to 74, 18% regarded their health as excellent and another 31% as very good; 13% indicated only fair health and 5%, poor health (Table 1.3). As might be expected, the percentages who viewed their health as only fair or poor increases with age. Also, self-reports of only fair or poor health were higher for older black and Hispanic Americans than for older white Americans.

Functional disability also increases with age and is closely associated with chronic disease. In the United States, the majority of people under the age of 85 report no difficulty in ADLs or instrumental activities of daily living (IADLs); much lower proportions of those aged 85 and older report little or no difficulty (Figure 1.3). Older women exhibit a higher percentage of limitations at all ages than older men do. Differ-

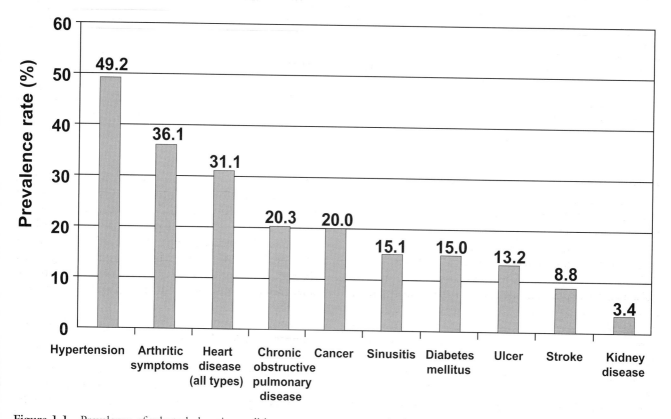

Figure 1.1—Prevalence of selected chronic conditions among persons aged 65 and over, all races.

SOURCE: Data from Data Warehouse on Trends in Health and Aging: Health Status and Chronic Conditions, 1997–2001, from the National Health Interview Survey. Estimates for 2000–2001. See http://www.cdc.gov/nchs/agingact.htm (accessed October 2005).

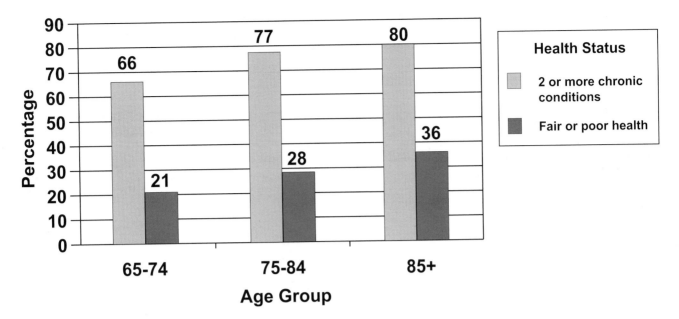

Figure 1.2—Percentage of all Medicare beneficiaries with two or more chronic conditions and self-reporting fair or poor health, by age group, 2000.

SOURCE: Data from Medicare Beneficiary Survey, 2000. See http://www.cms.hhs.gov/mcbs/ (accessed October 2005).

Table 1.3—Perceived Health of Medicare Beneficiaries, by Age and Race or Ethnicity, 2000

	White, non-Hispanic (%)			Black, non-Hispanic (%)			Hispanic (%)		
	65–74	75–84	85+	65–74	75–84	85+	65–74	75–84	85+
Excellent	18.23	13.79	11.19	10.93	7.42	8.31	13.17	12.86	8.19
Very good	31.06	26.97	22.98	22.58	18.73	17.13	21.61	17.48	20.56
Good	31.87	32.96	31.30	35.05	34.84	30.70	30.06	32.11	28.46
Fair	13.40	18.78	25.82	24.31	29.85	30.90	25.26	29.08	32.48
Poor	5.44	7.50	8.70	7.13	9.56	12.97	9.91	8.47	10.32

SOURCE: Data from *Medicare Current Beneficiary Survey*, 2000; Table 2.3. Available at http://www.cms.hhs.gov/mcbs/PubCNP00.asp (accessed October 2005).

ences between racial and ethnic groups exist as well. Among those aged 70 and older, black Americans are 1.5 times as likely as white Americans to be unable to perform one or more ADLs.

In the United States older persons who need assistance with functioning in routine ADLs rely first and foremost on family. In 1995, of those providing assistance to community-dwelling persons aged 70 or older, 73% were unpaid or informal helpers. Nine out of 10 informal or unpaid caregivers were family members, one fourth were spouses, and about half were children. Half of these informal caregivers resided with the person receiving help. Estimates of the use of paid helpers vary across studies, but use is consistently found to be higher among persons living alone and to rise with increasing age.

Deaths of older persons make up nearly 75% of all deaths in the United States. About one fifth of all deaths occur at age 85 or older, but this proportion is expected to grow. For many decades, heart disease, cancer, and stroke have been the leading causes of death among people 65 or older, accounting for six out of 10 deaths (Table 1.4). Causes of death vary by race, ethnicity, and gender, however. Diabetes mellitus was the fourth leading cause of death among older Hispanic and black Americans, while ranking sixth for older white Americans. Alzheimer's disease ranked seventh among all causes of death.

Some causes of death usually associated with younger people also are of concern in the older population. In the United States, older men have motor vehicle accident death rates two to three times those of older women, overall and within racial and ethnic groups. The highest suicide rates among older people are for white men (43.7 per 100,000, compared with 6.5 per 100,000 for older white women), who are more likely to commit suicide than die in a motor vehicle crash.

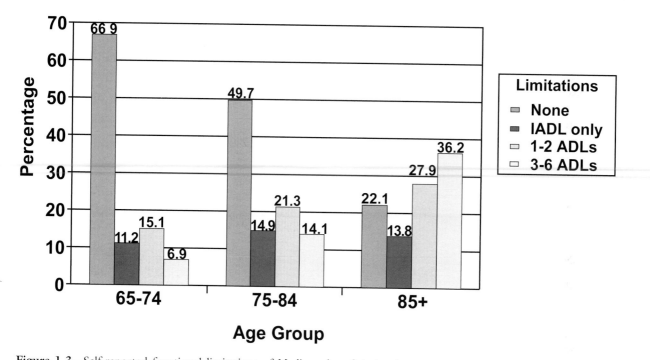

Figure 1.3—Self-reported functional limitations of Medicare beneficiaries, by age group, 2000. Key: ADLs = activities of daily living; IADL = instrumental activity of daily living.

SOURCE: Data from Medicare Beneficiary Survey, 2000; Table 2.1. See http://www.cms.hhs.gov/mcbs/ (accessed October 2005).

Table 1.4—Leading Causes of Death and Numbers of Deaths, for Persons Aged 65 and Over, 1999

Rank	Cause of Death	Number of Deaths	% of Deaths
	All Causes	1797,331	100.0
1	Diseases of heart	607,265	33.8
2	Malignant neoplasms	390,122	21.7
3	Cerebrovascular diseases	148,599	8.3
4	Chronic lower respiratory disease	108,112	6.0
5	Influenza and pneumonia	57,282	3.2
6	Diabetes mellitus	51,843	2.9
7	Alzheimer's disease	44,020	2.4
8	Unintentional injuries	32,219	1.8
9	Nephritis, nephrotic syndrome, and nephrosis	29,938	1.7
10	Septicemia	24,626	1.4

SOURCE: *Health, United States, 2002 With Chartbook on Trends in the Health of Americans.* Hyattsville, MD: National Center for Health Statistics; 2002:132 (Table 33).

TRENDS IN DISABILITY

There are conflicting opinions about whether rates of disability in the United States are declining among people aged 65 and over. Some studies suggest a decline in the past decade in the proportion unable to do some activities (one or more ADLs or IADLs), but there is also evidence for an increase in the proportion unable to perform one or more ADLs. Differences in study populations and measures contribute to conflicting findings. The measurement of disabilities varies across studies, and assessments of the presence and severity of disability can differ when histories are taken from an older person, the family caregiver, or the physician.

Trends in disability are of special interest because increases in life expectancy overall and for people aged 65 and older have led to debate over whether these additional years will be free of disability. Studies of active life expectancy, which use mortality and disability estimates to project disability-free years, suggest an advantage for persons with more education. Because of their greater total life expectancy, older women also experience both greater active life expectancy and more years of disability than do older men. It has also been suggested that if there is a limit to increases in life expectancy, increases in disability-free years could produce a *compression of morbidity*, with the period of disability prior to death gradually compressed as active life expectancy (or disability-free years) increases. Increases in active life expectancy must occur if compression of morbidity is to be achieved, but debate continues regarding whether there is a maximum human life span, and whether compression of morbidity is possible if total life expectancy continues to increase.

As more longitudinal studies are conducted and other evidence is brought to bear, the trend in active life expectancy among older people may become clearer. Regardless of its true direction, however, preventing and reducing disability among older people remains a major objective of much geriatrics research.

The assumption has been that disability is irreversible, but studies show that up to one third of persons who experience disability in a basic ADL recover. Age less than 85 years, good nutritional status, and greater mobility are all associated with increased likelihood of recovery from basic ADL disability.

TRENDS IN HEALTH CARE

On average, older people in the United States have more contacts with health care professionals than do younger adults, from a mean of 10 per year among those aged 65 to 74, to nearly 15 per year among those aged 85 and older. Those who assess their health as fair or poor have twice as many contacts per year as do persons in excellent or good health. Older adults accounted for 20% of the hospital discharges and used a third of the days of care in 1970; in the year 2000 they made up close to 40% of discharges and used almost one-half of the hospital days. Variations in length of stay can be considerable, however.

Diseases of the heart were the leading discharge diagnosis in the United States for older people, with heart disease and stroke together accounting for more than one fourth of all hospital discharges among older men and women aged 85 and older. Malignant neoplasms were the next most common discharge diagnosis, followed by pneumonia and bronchitis. Fracture-related hospitalizations were more common among women than men and accounted for nearly 10% of discharges for those aged 85 and older.

Home-health care, including medical treatment, physical therapy, and homemaker services, is an alternative to institutional care for older people. Nursing care is the most commonly used service (85% of older home-health patients received nursing care in 1996), and 29% of patients use homemaker services. Medicare has been a major payer for home-health care (nearly half of expenses in 1996), and changes in payment methods have resulted in a dramatic drop in use of these services (both in the numbers of persons served and visits per user).

Prescription drugs have become a major component of medical treatment. Eighty percent of older people in the United States are using one or more prescribed medicines; among those with three to five ADL limitations, 93% use at least one.

OTHER ISSUES

The older U.S. population is among the most heterogeneous subgroups, encompassing the entire spectrum of health and functioning, from the bedridden Alzheimer's patient to the marathon runner. One of the important unresolved questions is whether gains in longevity after age 65 are accompanied by gains or declines in years of disability-free life. It is unlikely that one answer will fit this large and diverse group. There are many questions in other areas as well. While levels of education continue to rise, so do rates of early retirement. Will the increasing numbers of better-educated, longer-lived persons contribute to the larger society, and in what ways? Will the sheer numbers of older people strain to the breaking point the medical care system and public programs that finance health care and retirement, as some analysts fear? Or will improvements in health behavior, medical breakthroughs, and financial prosperity diminish these threats?

Under any scenario, chronic illness will remain a constant in the lives of many older people. Physicians treating this population face the challenge not only of treating chronically ill persons but of assisting all older people in preventing or at least delaying the onset of chronic disease.

ANNOTATED REFERENCES

■ Administration on Aging, U.S. Department of Health and Human Services. *A Profile of Older Americans: 2002.* Available at http://www.aoa.gov/prof/statistics/profile/2002profile.pdf (accessed October 2005).

This report contains current statistics on the older population in the following categories: future growth, marital status, living arrangements, racial and ethnic composition, geographic distribution, income, poverty, housing, employment, education, health, health care, and disability.

■ American Association of Retired People (AARP). Public Policy Institute Releases—Topics in Health and Wellness: Disabilities; Spring 2005.

The topics cover disability reports as well as quality of health care, wellness, disease prevention, and health care policy.

■ Federal Interagency Forum on Aging-Related Statistics. *Older Americans 2000: Key Indicators of Well-Being.* Washington, DC: U.S. Government Printing Office; August 2000. Available at http://www.agingstats.gov/chartbook2000/default.htm (accessed October 2005).

This report covers 31 key indicators selected by the Forum to portray aspects of the lives of older Americans and their families. It is divided into five subject areas: population, economics, health status, health risks and behaviors, and health care.

- Gill TM, Robison JT, Tinetti ME. Predictors of recovery in activities of daily living among disabled older persons living in the community. *J Gen Intern Med.* 1997;12(12):757–762.

  The disability rate for the geriatric population is typically presented in a static, point-prevalence form. Clinicians can benefit from knowing factors that predict recovery of activities of daily living (ADL) function in their disabled elderly patients. This study is one report from Project Safety, a community-based study that followed 213 disabled elderly persons for 2 years. Fifty-nine (28%) were considered to have recovered their ADL functions. A large number (24) of possible predictors of recovery were subjected to analysis to determine whether any association existed between the demographic, psychosocial, sensory, functional, physical performance, clinical, or nutritional status of the study subjects and their recovery of function. Using bivariate and multivariate analysis, the researchers found that four factors are independently associated with recovery: age of 85 years or younger, Mini–Mental State Examination score of 28 or better, high mobility, and good nutritional status. Interestingly, some variables that did not predict recovery were whether a person lived alone, scored as depressed on a measure of depression, or had specific conditions, such as diabetes mellitus, heart disease, stroke, arthritis, or urinary incontinence.

- Hall MJ, Owings MF. 2000 National Hospital Discharge Survey. *Advance Data from Vital and Health Statistics,* No. 329, June 19, 2002. Available at http://www.cdc.gov/nchs/data/ad/ad329.pdf (accessed October 2005).

  This report presents information about hospital utilization during 2000 as well as trend data for selected variables.

- Manton KG, Stallard E, Corder LS. The dynamics of dimensions of age-related disability 1982 to 1994 in the U.S. elderly population. *J Gerontol A Biol Sci Med Sci.* 1998;53(1):B59–B70.

  Declines in chronic disability were observed in National Long Term Care Survey data from 1982 to 1994. Seven dimensions described changes in the age dependence of 27 activities of daily living, instrumental activities of daily living, and physical performance measures in community-dwelling and institutionalized persons. Disability declines were correlated with reductions in selected health conditions over the study period.

- Stone R. *Long-Term Care for the Disabled Elderly: Current Policy, Emerging Trends and Implications for the 21st Century.* New York: Milbank Memorial Fund; 2000.

  This report describes long-term care for disabled elderly people in terms of key trends and projections for service need, issues in service and work force availability, and problems in financing. It concludes with a discussion of current and emerging trends in long-term-care policy.

Lynda Burton, ScD
Judith D. Kasper, PhD

CHAPTER 2—BIOLOGY

KEY POINTS

- Aging changes are caused by multiple factors, including genetics, wear and tear, oxidative and glycative damage, and environmental factors.

- Animal models have shown that maximum life span can be extended by caloric restriction, genetic mutations, and genetic manipulation.

- Human studies indicate that hereditary factors account for approximately 10% to 58% of longevity.

- Genetic factors may regulate aging or life span through a variety of mechanisms, including insulin signaling, control of oxidative damage, predisposition to (or suppression of) age-associated diseases (including cancer), DNA maintenance, and altered gene expression at the level of transcription or translation, or both. There may be no "master control" or single pathway that controls senescence.

Knowledge about age-dependent changes in cellular and organ function is important in the care of older persons. The rate of physiologic aging varies from person to person, with large interindividual variations. At the cellular and molecular levels, provocative scientific findings have begun to unravel the question of why we age. Some determinants of longevity now can be understood in terms of gene expression. Importantly, temporal expression of aging resembles a rheostatic switch with small incremental changes. Attempts to answer questions about what controls the rheostatic switch and the rate of senescence have resulted in several theories on aging (Table 2.1).

CHARACTERISTICS OF AGING

Common traits of aging processes include the following:

- Mortality increases with age after maturation, and the increases become exponential with increasing age.

Table 2.1—Representative Theories of Aging

Theory	Synopsis	Support
Oxidative stress	The result of homothermia and metabolism is the accumulation of protein, lipid, and DNA damage mediated through highly reactive, oxygen-derived substances (free radicals).	Mutations in oxidative stress pathway can extend life span. Mutations of genes in other pathways (including in mammals) that increase longevity also exhibit enhanced resistance to stress and oxidative damage.
Chromosomal alterations	Deletions, mutations, translocations, and polyploidy have been suggested as age-acquired chromosomal instabilities that contribute to gene silencing or expression of disease-related genes, such as those seen in cancer.	Mitochondrial DNA mutations of genes in the oxidative stress pathway may contribute to reduced resistance to oxidative stress. However, the practical impact in normal nondiseased aging may be minimal.
Immunologic	Time-acquired deficits, primarily in T-cell function, predispose elderly persons to infections and cancer.	Impact upon diseases associated with aging, but not apparently directly related to a healthy organismic aging
Neuroendocrinologic	The cortisol surge leading to death in spawning salmon has served as a model for explaining the decline of humans after their maximal reproductive years.	No direct support in humans
Developmental-genetic	Because the maximum life span appears fixed, a genetically programmed induction of senescence is thought to occur, resulting in the activation or suppression of specific "aging" genes.	Longevity in humans appears heritable. However, evolution selects for reproductive fitness to maintain the species, not for postreproductive senescence.
Metabolic and insulin signaling, caloric restriction	Alterations in body size and composition, and in insulin-signaling pathways act independently and in concert to extend life span.	Caloric restriction and mutations in insulin-signaling pathways in a wide variety of species (yeast, worms, flies, rodents) enhance resistance to oxidative stress and extend life span.

- The biochemical composition of tissue changes with age; examples are lipofuscin and extracellular matrix cross-linking, protein oxidation, and altered rates of gene transcription.
- Physiologic capacity decreases.
- The ability to maintain homeostasis diminishes, especially with regard to adaptive processes under physiologic stress.
- The susceptibility and vulnerability to disease increase.

Loss of physiologic reserve and decreased homeostatic control may be a consequence of changes in allostasis and development of homeostenosis. *Allostasis*, "maintaining stability through change," refers to the normal response to stress, that is, the activation of the neuroendocrine, immune, and autonomic systems with a stressor, such as a surgical operation. The responses to the stress include changes in cortisol, epinephrine, and cytokines that are adaptive in the short run but that may be harmful if prolonged. *Allostatic load* refers to the effects of prolonged or overactive allostatic response. A possible example of allostatic load is the relationship between the subtle increase in cortisol levels seen in many older people, possibly leading to hippocampal damage and memory loss. Conversely, it has been hypothesized that brief or recurrent exposures to stress such that specific signaling pathways and expression of genes are stimulated or suppressed, or

both, may be beneficial and ultimately promote longevity of an organism. This phenomenon is known as *hormesis* and is likely to be found occurring alongside examples of allostatic load. Hormesis has been observed in a variety of organisms (yeast, flies, worms, rodents) and in human cells in vitro.

Homeostenosis is the altered response to physiologic stresses often seen in older people. Examples include decreased ability to manage fluid and electrolyte derangements, including diminished thirst perception, decreased glomerular filtration, and changes in the renin-aldosterone system, urinary concentrating, and dilutional capacity.

One axiom of aging had been the irreversibility of changes that occur over time, and although this is generally true, the rate of aging can be influenced by environmental and genetic factors. Thus, the prevention of deleterious changes with age and the reversal of certain aspects of senescence are promising possibilities.

THEORIES OF AGING

The oxidative stress theory is one widely accepted explanation of the aging process. This theory posits that oxygen converted during metabolism into superoxide anions, hydrogen peroxide, and hydroxyl radicals causes damage over time. Untoward events are indiscriminate and cumulative. Key observations include the following:

- Free-radical damage to lipids, protein, and DNA have been found in aging heart, liver, and kidney tissue.

- Short-lived species accumulate this damage quickly.

- Transgenic animal models that concurrently overexpress copper and zinc superoxide dismutase and catalase have extended life spans.

- Antioxidant compounds such as vitamin E can enhance the average life span in animal models. Interestingly, the expression of human SOD (super oxide dismutase) gene in *Drosophila* neurons has been found to increase life span by 40%, which suggests that the central nervous system plays a key role in longevity.

- Caloric restriction, which extends life span, and single gene mutations that increase longevity enhance resistance to oxidative stress in yeast, worms, flies, and rodents.

Skeptics of the oxidative stress theory point out that knockout of the SOD gene does not accelerate aging. This observation attests to redundant systems that counter damage. On a pragmatic level, no evidence exists that antioxidants delay human senescence or disease. In fact, sufficient levels of these compounds may not reach critical areas such as the brain to prevent age-associated oxidant injury.

Mitochondria play a key role in biologic aging. Damage induced by free radicals results in mitochondrial-DNA (mtDNA) mutations in muscle and brain. These lead to defective mitochondrial respiration and further oxidant injury, which creates a cycle of damage and continued loss of mitochondrial function. Mitochondrial mutations and defective respiration have been linked to neurodegeneration in conditions such as Alzheimer's disease and Parkinson's disease. Given maternal inheritance of mtDNA, human longevity potentially is linked to the maternal genome.

Longevity is greater in family members of extremely old humans. Epidemiologic studies of twins suggest that heritability of life span is between 22% and 33%. Similar studies in families yield a wider range of estimates, between 10% and 58%. If this is true, the question is "Which genes are responsible for longevity?" It has been proposed that genes regulate the rate of aging (longevity assurance) and disease acquisition (disease-resistance genes). Genes also exist for damage repair. Thus, the human life span may depend upon multiple components that counter deleterious changes. The question remains whether a "master switch" is turned on over time so as to down-regulate repair mechanisms or perhaps exude a systemic factor for aging.

Differences in life spans observed among various mammalian species suggest a developmental-genetic theory of aging. Some aspects of aging resemble developmentally regulated programs; however, it is difficult to understand why evolutionary pressures would preferentially select senescence, unless a genetically controlled program for aging might be a mechanism to assure gene-pool turnover. On the other hand, genetically regulated programs that delay the onset of aging might be selected in human evolution if this enhanced the reproductive years. There is a growing literature documenting the association of single nucleotide polymorphisms with longevity in humans. Some of these gene alleles are actually associated with increased prevalence of disease at younger ages, suggesting that they may be examples of antagonistic pleiotropy (exerting deleterious effects early in life, but beneficial effects at later ages). Irrespective of potential selective evolutionary pressures, comparable longevity between monozygotic and not dizygotic twins hints that normal aging is influenced by a genetic program. Genetic disorders leading to accelerated aging, such as that seen in Hutchinson-Gilford progeria syndrome (HGPS) and Werner's syndrome, provide insight into the genetic components of processes associated with aging, such as alopecia, arteriosclerosis, osteoporosis, and skin atrophy. One of the progeria conditions, Werner's syndrome, is due to a perturbation on chromosome 8 and is linked to a gene that codes for a helicase. This enzyme is responsible for unwinding DNA during replication and repair. Chromosomal instability appears to mediate cumulative cellular pathology that contributes to death in the middle-aged adult. It has been discovered that mutations in the lamin A gene on chromosome 1 result in HGPS. Lamins are a family of nuclear intermediate filament proteins that establish and maintain the shape and strength of the interphase nucleus. HGPS fibroblasts exhibit abnormalities of the nuclear membrane. Lamin A mutations also cause at least six other genetic disorders, including forms of muscular dystrophy and cardiomyopathy. Clearly, both HGPS and Werner's syndrome, as well as accelerated aging observed in trisomy 21 syndrome (Down syndrome), indicate that the phenotype of human senescence has several genetic loci that can mediate the pace of aging.

Although indirect evidence supports a genetic link to the rate of aging, little direct evidence exists for a genetic program that actively triggers the aging processes. Indeed, animal models show that environmental manipulations, such as caloric restriction, can significantly extend life span. Thus, the relationship between environmental factors and gene expression appears to drive the aging process.

CELLULAR CHANGES WITH AGE

Senescence induces functional changes in cells. Perturbations are observed in cells with full replicative potential, as well as in those in a postmitotic state. Cells with proliferative capacity, such as lymphocytes and fibroblasts, typically demonstrate diminished proliferative potential over time. For instance, cultured lymphocytes from human blood start to divide after being provided a growth stimulus (plant lectin, phytohemagglutinin, and interleukin-2). The onset of proliferation is slower in old than in young donor lymphocytes, and the peak number of dividing cells is lower in elderly donor lymphocytes. The main reason for loss of lymphocyte proliferation with age is decreased secretion of interleukin-2 and expression of T-cell populations that have an altered affinity for this cytokine. Mixed populations of T cells from old donors express a high percentage of memory cells that exhibit different proliferative characteristics than naive T cells, which are more plentiful in young donor samples.

To circumvent concerns about mixed subpopulation dynamics characteristic of polyclonal T-cell cultures, researchers have stimulated single T-cell clones from young and elderly donor cells. In these instances, the cloning efficiency of T cells from old donors is reduced, with many fewer of them reaching benchmarks of 20, 30, and 40 population doublings than young donor cells that have identical cell surface markers. Thus, it appears that age alters both the population dynamics of T-cell growth and individual cellular capacity to sustain clonal expansion. The net result is diminished T-cell responses with age, which could account for the increasing infection and cancer rates observed over the human life span.

The loss of proliferation in cultured cells is broadly known as *clonal senescence*. Other cell types, such as endothelial and fibroblast cells, also exhibit loss of proliferative potential over time during in vitro tissue culture. A well-established model for replicative senescence entails serial passage of fetal or primary fibroblasts in well-defined cell culture media. At a certain point, these cells enlarge and no longer divide. A number of studies have suggested that donor fibroblasts from old individuals undergo fewer population doublings than do donor cells from young individuals. However, an important consideration is that the loss of replicative potential varies among aged individuals. Thus, a wide range exists whereby some young donor cells divide only a few times and old donor cells replicate comparably to many young donor cells. Furthermore, other studies fail to reveal a reproducible age-related alteration in donor cell proliferative capacity and demonstrate no change in replicative capacity when cells from the same individuals are examined at older ages. Skin biopsy experiments suggest an age-dependent accumulation of senescent fibroblasts as indicated by staining for β-galactosidase; however, the percentage of these cells in old donor skin is surprisingly small. Furthermore, this putative marker of senescence may be indicative of quiescent or damaged cells rather than the age of the cell. The body of evidence implies that changes in function other than loss of proliferation contribute to cellular aging.

Evidence indicates that age results in perturbations in gene expression and signal transduction. The in vitro senescence models of cellular aging demonstrate alterations in certain membrane receptors as well as transmembrane signaling molecules. For example, levels of interleukin-2 and its receptor are reduced in clonally senescent T cells as well as freshly isolated T cells from old donors; telomere length, T-cell receptor signaling, and expression of the *bcl* 2 gene are also decreased.

It is possible that cellular senescence evolved as a mechanism of tumor suppression and that aging is an antagonistically pleiotropic manifestation of evolutionary pressures to prevent malignant transformation. Consequently, cellular senescence is good for the organism, and aging may be the price we pay to avoid, for the most part, cancer. However, even this concept has been qualified by the demonstration that senescent cells can foster the growth of premalignant and malignant epithelial cells in culture and the tumorigenesis of these cells in mice. Although these findings seem to be at odds with the beneficial effects of cellular senescence, they are themselves another example of antagonistic pleiotropy, wherein a process that has evolved to protect us against cancer in fact may predispose us to cancer later in life.

DNA AND GENE EXPRESSION DURING SENESCENCE

DNA Mutations or Deletions

The concept that age alters the integrity of DNA, primarily through mutations, originally led to the somatic mutation theory of aging. That aging results in DNA template errors, thus leading to errors in or loss of gene expression, has not held up experimentally. However, certain "hot spots" of DNA change have been observed in human and animal aging. These hypermutable DNA foci are thought to accumulate changes that produce functional cellular problems over time. Structural changes in DNA range from deletions to aberrant expansions. These changes occur in both somatic and germ cells. Importantly, several hypermutable areas are juxtaposed with key regulatory elements, such as the insulin gene and oncogene *ras1* locus. Changes over vast distances of DNA sequences can affect downstream gene activity, which suggests that age-related changes observed in nonfunctioning DNA areas can potentially exert untoward effects on critical regulatory genes.

A similar concern exists with age-dependent changes in mtDNA. The circular mtDNA is reported to undergo a mutation rate that is 10,000-fold greater in elderly than in younger adult tissue. A nearly exponential increase in mtDNA mutations occurs over time, with up to 10% of extremely old donor tissue exhibiting deletions. Because mitochondria and mtDNA are amply redundant, subtle, if any, age-dependent changes in respiratory chain activities are noticed, and it is most likely that aging results in a reduced functional reserve of energy production.

Telomeres

Perhaps the most provocative data concerning DNA changes with age relates to chromosomal end points. These chromosomal tips contain redundant DNA sequences or tandem repeats that cannot be replicated by DNA polymerase. To solve this problem, a ribonucleoprotein called *telomerase* deals with end chromosomal replication.

A fundamental problem observed in aged donor cells with replicative potential is that their telomeres shorten. Telomere shortening and loss of telomerase activity has been observed during clonal senescence of fibroblasts and T cells. Telomeric DNA loss is also a function of donor age. The consequence of this diminished activity is thought to be alterations in the immune system and deficient wound healing.

Conversely, telomerase hyperactivity is linked to cellular transformation and cancer. Given the relationship of telomeres to aging and cancer, some have proposed measurement of telomere length and telomerase activity as potential clinical markers of human aging and oncogenesis. Thus, targeted disruption of telomerase activity would be important as cancer therapy, whereas reactivation of this enzyme might reverse age-dependent changes in replicative potential. Such an approach may have to be tumor specific, since some cancerous cells do not have telomerase.

Gene Expression

Age affects gene expression at several levels. Age-related changes depend upon the cellular state, such as quiescence, proliferation, or physiologic stress. When side-by-side comparisons of gene expression from mature adult and aged donors are conducted, the rates of gene expression either decrease, stay the same, or increase in elderly donors. An important and, as yet,

unresolved consideration is whether differences in gene expression with age are functionally significant. The inability of cells to withstand physiologic stress with age is the strongest evidence that changes in stress-related gene expression contribute to poor functional outcomes.

A variety of mechanisms can influence gene expression with aging. For instance, mutations in DNA sequences in or around certain genes can influence their expression. Similar effects can be expected from latent viral infections (eg, herpes viruses), as well as from accumulation of environmentally induced cell damage. Targets for altered gene expression and aging would be reduced activity of transactivators, enhanced activity of DNA silencers or repressors, and intrinsic changes in RNA polymerase activity.

Because the overall total messenger ribonucleic acid (mRNA) content does not appear to change with age, aging has been characterized as a state with a decline in mRNA turnover and transcriptional rate. RNA polymerase per se does not appear to change with age, so most of the change in mRNA expression appears to be due to changes in the gene-promoter regions. Gene promoters are areas of DNA upstream of the target gene that have constitutively and inducibly bound DNA-binding proteins. Through proper assemblage of these DNA-binding proteins, DNA conformational changes that enhance RNA polymerase recruitment and efficiency are affected. Expected age-dependent changes would include alterations in DNA-protein interactions (transcription factors), accumulation of proteins interfering with DNA binding proteins, and unfavorable conformations of DNA during transcriptional activation. Importantly, there is no evidence that age leads to an increased error rate during transcription and translation.

In sum, the primary changes in gene expression with age are as follows:

- decreased transcription rates for key genes;
- decreased mRNA turnover;
- decreased inducibility of genes, such as immediate early genes, acute phase reactants, and stress genes.

Constitutive levels of gene expression remain intact.

The ability to detect different patterns of gene expression has been facilitated by the development of microchip DNA arrays. Printing hundreds to thousands of DNA templates corresponding to specific genes on a small glass slide or nitrocellulose paper makes possible rapid screening of mRNA samples from young and old donor cells for decreases or increases in gene expression. Messenger RNA levels from primary skin fibroblasts from young (prepubescent), middle-aged (37 years old), and elderly (90 to 96 years old) donors were analyzed by this technique. Table 2.2 lists significant changes in gene expression when middle-aged and elderly donor dermal fibroblasts are compared at similar stages of cell proliferation, albeit during asynchronous growth. Typically, aging alters the morphology of the nucleus, including multilobulation and irregular membranes. Micronucleation is commonly noted in old donor cells, and more cells from elderly donors than from young donors manifest abnormal chromosomal DNA content.

Of 6000 known human genes analyzed, only 61 or 1% showed changes in expression between young and middle-aged donors. Most of these changes were reduced gene expression involving cell cycle progression and maintenance or repair of the extracellular matrix. The functional consequence of declining gene expression related to cell cycle is possibly to predispose elderly individuals to increased DNA strand breaks and other chromosomal instabilities.

When gene expression in fibroblasts from progeria donors and elderly donors are compared, some interesting linkages between normal and premature aging are manifest. For example, down-regulation of bone- and joint-associated genes is found in normal aged and progeric individuals. Cathepsin C, a lysosomal protease, is similarly down-regulated sixfold in aged donors and likely contributes to dermal changes with senescence. A tumor-suppressor gene, BARD1, is down-regulated 4.5-fold with age and may account for age-related increases in breast cancer. Because the most extensive gene-expression data are derived from human fibroblasts, information about changes in gene expression with age that are specific to other tissues may reveal additional underlying mechanisms of senescence and increased susceptibility to disease.

Not all genes examined during senescence are found to be attenuated in their expression. Curiously, basal expression of genes related to the stress response is up-regulated in aged donor cells. One of these genes, alpha-B-crystallin, is associated with the maintenance of the cellular cytoskeleton. The consequence of up-regulation of gene expression in human aging remains to be determined. Possibly these changes are simply adaptations to accumulated ravages of environmental or metabolic (oxidative) stress.

Some of the most definitive age-dependent changes in gene expression are observed when aged donor cells are analyzed during different forms of physiologic stress. This observation is perhaps not surprising, given clinical observations that elderly persons often respond less well than young adults to physiologic stress, such as infections, environmental extremes, and hypoxic events.

CELLULAR DEFENSE MECHANISMS

Age results in altered responses to physiologic stress. Cells have specific reactions to thwart injury and death. Damage may result from ultraviolet light, heat, lack of oxygen, absent nutrients, and metabolic oxidants. Cells have multiple strategies to cope with various forms of stress by means of stress-inducible transcription factors. For instance, ultraviolet radiation affects the transcription factor NF-κB, whereas thermal stress causes the transcription factor heat-shock factor (HSF1) to be activated. The thermal stress response can also be

Table 2.2—Changes With Age in Fibroblast Gene Expression or Cell Senescence, or Both

Class of Gene	Decreased Expression	Increased Expression
Cell cycle control proteins	B-Myb Cyclins A, B, D, F Select protein kinases	
Extracellular matrix and cytoskeleton	A1 (III) procollagen	Alpha-B-crystallin, metalloproteinase 3 & 10, collagenase, fibronectin, TIMP2 (tissue inhibitor of metalloproteinase)
Fatty acid metabolism		Prostaglandin synthase
Disease-related genes	BARD1*	
Stress-inducible genes	Small-molecular-weight heat-shock proteins under physiologic stress levels	Small-molecular-weight heat-shock proteins at baseline or constitutive levels
Cytokines, growth factors, growth regulatory genes, transcription factors	c-fos, IGF-1, TGFβ, IL-6 Id 1, 2, & 4 EPC1 Microphthalmia-associated transcription factor (Mitf)	IGFBP2, 3, & 5 IL-1α & β IL-15

NOTE: B-Myb = transcription factor involved in the regulation of cell survival, proliferation, and differentiation; EPC1 = early population doubling level cDNA; Id = inhibitor of differentiation or DNA binding; IL = interleukin; IGF-1 = insulin-like growth factor 1; IGFBP= IGF binding protein; TGFβ = transforming growth factor β.

* Breast cancer 1 (*brca1*) is a tumor-suppressor gene; BARD1 is a BRCA1-associated RING domain 1 (BARD1).

evoked by hypoxia, heavy metals, and other types of injury. Damaged intracellular proteins trigger the cytoplasm-located transcription factor to translocate to the nucleus and bind to a gene promoter region containing consensus nucleotide sequences GAA. HSF1 binding to the heat-shock element increases RNA polymerase activity, leading to elevated expression of mRNAs for various heat-shock proteins.

Heat-shock proteins have multiple functions. They primarily function as chaperones to allow protein trafficking and organelle transmembrane transport. Other functions include refolding damaged proteins and newly synthesized polypeptides. Heat-shock proteins interact with transcription factors, such as the steroid receptor, and serve as a type of molecular brake or attenuator of the transcription factor when conditions do not require its activation. During stress, increased need of heat-shock proteins causes the protein synthetic machinery to exclusively translate mRNA for heat-shock proteins. These proteins protect enzymatic function under stress. In short, heat-shock proteins assure proper protein levels and function so that cells may survive. Once overexpressed, their efficacy is sustainable, as witnessed by the increased ability of cells to withstand subsequent lethal stress.

The study of the human heat-shock response is an excellent paradigm for understanding how aging affects basic responses to cellular injury. One reason is that all species studied thus far have consistently revealed age-related decrements in various components of the heat-shock response. This fact illustrates how inducible responses, rather than constitutive responses, go awry with age.

The primary age-dependent defect of the heat-shock response occurs in the transcriptional trigger. Age causes approximately a 50% reduction in observable DNA binding after stress of old donor cells. Loss of HSF1–DNA binding with age appears to be multifactorial. This age-dependent change in stress-inducible HSF1 binding results in marked reduction in the rate of mRNA production for all the heat-shock proteins. No one knows exactly what levels are necessary for full protection from cell death; however, levels are likely proportional to the degree and duration of cell stress. In other words, higher levels of heat-shock proteins are needed if the cellular stress is severe, whereas lower levels are capable of handling mild to moderate stress. Most importantly, increased susceptibility to cell death results from altered heat-shock gene expression. For example, heat-shocked human lymphocytes from elderly donors aged 75 years and older result in earlier cell death and involve more cells than young donor lymphocytes. Despite this observation, controversy exists whether age represents a defect in apoptosis or programmed cell death. When fibroblasts are serially passaged, the cells passaged very late minimally produce heat-shock genes when thermally stressed, yet these cells are resistant to another form of death, namely, serum deprivation. These seemingly paradoxical observations are reconcilable when one considers that apoptosis can occur through several pathways, not all of which are equally affected by age.

Observations regarding senescence and cell stress demonstrate an emerging principle, that inducible responses requiring enhanced gene expression are attenuated by aging. The attenuation of inducible stress responses may be due to the accumulation or overexpression of heat-shock proteins in the nonstress state, which raises a provocative question, whether senescent cells are in a state of low-grade stress.

One concern is whether age results from elevated expression of certain genes, perhaps triggered by some internal chronometer. So far, no clear evidence exists for genes that evoke the senescence phenotype. However, experiments with nematode aging show that manipulation of *daf-2*, a mutation that confers longevity, may result in secretion of a factor that regulates the pace of aging. Similarly, in *Drosophila* studies, manipulation of the methuselah gene, which is homologous with G-regulatory proteins, can extend life span. By comparison, the decline in estrogen levels in aging women has been cited as a waning systemic factor that prevents bone, brain, and vascular deterioration. However, there is no hormonal factor known to extend human life span, and it is not clear whether changes in the hormonal axis with aging influence the rate of aging or merely represent an adaptive response to intrinsic tissue changes.

CELL DEATH

Experimental investigations have assessed the impact of aging on cell death. Cell death may occur by necrosis or apoptosis. In the former case, massive cell injury results in chromatin clumping and disorderly breakdown of cellular components. On the other hand, apoptosis is an active suicidal mechanism in response to external or internal stimuli. Apoptosis is essential to tissue maintenance, and it is especially important in down-regulating immune responses, such as clonally expanded lymphocytes, when infections resolve. Age-dependent problems with apoptosis could result in leukemias, lymphomas, and abnormal tissue repair.

Apoptosis is recognized by compaction and segregation of chromatin adjacent to the nuclear membrane, condensation of the cytoplasm, and nuclear fragmentation. DNA "ladders," detected in acrylamide gels, represent the orderly enzymatic degradation of DNA. Membrane-bound apoptotic bodies are phagocytized. Gene products activate and block apoptosis. For instance, cysteine proteases (ICE, CPP32, and ICH-1) initiate apoptosis, whereas *bcl-2* and HIAP (human inhibitor of apoptosis protein) block or prevent apoptosis.

It has been suggested that apoptosis plays a role in neurodegenerative diseases associated with aging. The neuronal loss observed in Alzheimer's disease is possibly due to cytotoxicity of aggregated β-amyloid, which can induce apoptosis in cultured cells. Putative toxins such as free radicals created during neuronal transmission have also been implicated in neuronal cell death seen in Parkinson's disease; however, the exact role of apoptosis in aging and diseases of aging remains an area of ongoing research.

CALORIC RESTRICTION AND METABOLIC AND INSULIN SIGNALING

Dietary restriction without malnutrition can increase both the average and maximum life spans in a wide variety of species, including yeast, worms, flies, spiders, fish, hamsters, rats, and mice. Although calories are severely restricted (up to 40%), essential nutrients such as vitamins and minerals are maintained at levels equivalent to those found in ad libitum diets. The diet-restricted animals exhibit a delay in the onset of physiologic and pathologic changes with aging. These include hormone and lipid levels, female reproduction, immune function, nephropathy, cardiomyopathy, osteodystrophy, and malignancies. Size, weight, fat percentage, and some organ weights are markedly less in calorically restricted animals. Leanness per se is not necessarily an important feature in life span extension (see below). However, small body weight early in life is a predictor of longevity in genetically heterogeneous mice. Caloric restriction in rhesus monkeys leads to reductions in body temperature and energy expenditure, consistent with changes seen in rodent studies in which aging is retarded by dietary restriction. Calorie restriction also increased high-density lipoprotein and retards the postmaturational decline in serum dehydroepiandrosterone sulfate in the rhesus monkeys. However, it is too soon to assess whether life span is affected in these primates, given that they can live 50 years or more. Caloric restriction in mice retards the age-associated accumulation of mtDNA mutations. Perhaps very importantly, caloric restriction reduces oxidative damage in flies, rodents, and primates.

In yeast, the benefits of caloric restriction are mediated by the enzyme Sir2. Overexpression of Sir2 in both yeast and worms enhances longevity. Sir2 belongs to the sirtuin family of proteins, which are present in other animals and humans. Screening of sirtuin-activating compounds (STACs) has revealed that resveratrol, a plant polyphenol that is commonly found in red wine, potently activates Sir2 and thereby prolongs life span in yeast. Furthermore, resveratrol also enhances life span in fruit flies and worms, and does so without impairing reproduction. Resveratrol has also been found to exert anti-inflammatory, antioxidant, anticancer, and vasoactive effects upon human cells. These studies hold out the possibility that STACs may act to enhance life span in humans. They may also explain some of the potential benefits of red wine consumption and lay the foundation for the development of calorie restriction mimetics to be used in humans.

There are multiple single gene mutations that extend life span in yeast, worms, flies, and rodents. Many of the products of these genes appear to play roles in metabolic and insulin-signaling pathways and also enhance the organism's resistance to oxidative stress. Animals lacking expression of the growth hormone–releasing hormone are long lived, but are small and exhibit delayed puberty. Similarly, knockout of the growth-hormone receptor results in small subfertile animals that are long lived. Growth hormone acts via the insulin or insulin-like growth factor 1 (IGF-1) pathway. In worms, flies, and mice, mutations in insulin receptor substrate (IRS) genes, the insulin receptor, and the IGF-1 receptor enhance longevity. A study in transgenic rats suggests that caloric restriction may also act, in part, independently of the GH-IGF-1 axis. The first single gene mutation that was described in worms to extend life span is in the AGE-1 gene, which appears to code for the homologue of the human phosphoinositol-3-kinase gene, which in turn is a downstream effector of IGF-1. In worms, a neuron-specific mutation in the insulin-signaling system extends life span. In addition, reducing the activity of heat-shock factor 1 (HSF-1) shortens life span, whereas overexpression of heat-shock protein 70F increases life span in worms. Interestingly, HSF-1 is required for insulin–IGF-1 signaling. Mice with a knockout of the insulin receptor specifically in adipose tissue are longer lived. Furthermore, mice heterozygous for a knockout of the IGF-1 receptor (homozygous knockouts are lethal) are longer lived, while exhibiting normal fertility and essentially normal size. These mice display increased resistance to oxidative stress, as do many of the long-lived mutants noted above. Polymorphisms in the IGF-1 receptor gene and the phosphoinositol-3-kinase gene result in lower plasma IGF-1 levels in humans and are more represented in long-lived individuals. Therefore, there appears to be an evolutionarily conserved endocrine regulation of aging by insulin-like signals. Though more research is needed, these pathways represent potential targets for drug development that may delay or even prevent physiologic and pathologic concomitants of aging.

ANNOTATED REFERENCES

- Bordone L, Guarente L. Caloric restriction, SIRT1 and metabolism: understanding longevity. *Nat Rev Mol Cell Biol.* 2005;6(4):298–305.

  This review summarizes recent findings that provide insight into the mechanisms whereby caloric restriction has resulted in a consistent robust increase in the maximal length of life in mammalian species.

- Campisi J. Senescent cells, tumor suppression, and organismal aging: good citizens, bad neighbors. *Cell.* 2005;120(4):513–522.

  This article reviews the evidence that some mammalian tumor-suppressor mechanisms contribute to aging. It explores how senescence is a manifestation of antagonistic pleiotropy, whereby early survival is enhanced by curbing cancer, but at the price of limiting longevity.

- Damjanovich S, Gaspar R Jr, Bene L, et al. Signal transduction in T lymphocytes and aging. *Exp Gerontol.* 2003;38(3):231–236.

  This report reviews signal transduction pathways in immune cells during aging and the utility of these cells to serve as a model for examining aging in other systems.

- Finkel T. Ageing: a toast to long life. *Nature.* 2003;425(6954):132–133.

  This editorial discusses insights into the mechanism of aging, with regard to the sirtuin family of proteins. There is evidence of life prolongation in yeast through the expression of the Sir2 gene. The relationship between caloric restriction and aging and the effects of resveratrol are summarized.

- Longo VD, Finch CE. Evolutionary medicine: from dwarf model systems to healthy centenarians? *Science.* 2003;299(5611):1342–1346.

  This article examines the similarity in alterations in insulin-signaling pathways ranging from yeast to mice that extend life span.

- Troen BR. The biology of aging. *Mt Sinai J Med.* 2003;70(1):3–22.

  This article reviews the cellular biology of aging, including the role of evolution, multiple theories of aging, and the potential interplay between cellular senescence and organismic aging. The beneficial paradox may be that the maximum life span potential of humans may have been achieved, in part, because of our ability to grow old.

Bruce R. Troen, MD
Donald A. Jurivich, DO

CHAPTER 3—PSYCHOSOCIAL ISSUES

KEY POINTS

- The older adult faces many psychosocial issues. Stressors can be modified or mediated by factors both internal and external to the individual. Positive modification of the stressors can improve outcomes.

- Stressors such as caregiving, loss and grief, and changes in social status and social roles are more common in the lives of older adults; successful adaptation to stressors can improve health outcomes; unsuccessful adaptation can lead to health declines.

- Implementing healthy behaviors can be beneficial, regardless of age.

- Social networks and positive interpersonal relationships can significantly moderate age-related stressors and lead to improved health.

Appreciating the role and scope of psychosocial aspects of aging improves clinicians' ability to address and treat factors that have important bearing on the overall well-being of older persons. Health events have broad ramifications. When they are viewed within a frame-work that includes both the stressors and the means to ameliorate the impact of stress, other factors besides the treatment of the disease itself can be seen to need clinical attention.

Stressors are any demands that call forth a physiologic, behavioral, or emotional response; often, such demands are perceived as threats. Unchecked stressors can lead to negative outcomes directly related to the situation as well as to more indirect negative outcomes across the whole spectrum of physical and mental health, economic welfare, and family life. Given the range of demands posed by the stressors, it is evident that they can greatly affect a person's physical and mental health, including every aspect of his or her well-being. The person's ability to function in the world may be reduced; the enthusiasm the person brings to and the pleasure he or she takes from social interaction may also be reduced. The use the person makes of financial, health, and social service resources may also be strongly affected.

Figure 3.1 offers a framework for considering the complex interaction of physical and psychosocial factors shaping the outcomes of stressors confronting older persons; the figure also structures the material presented in this chapter. The chapter briefly discusses

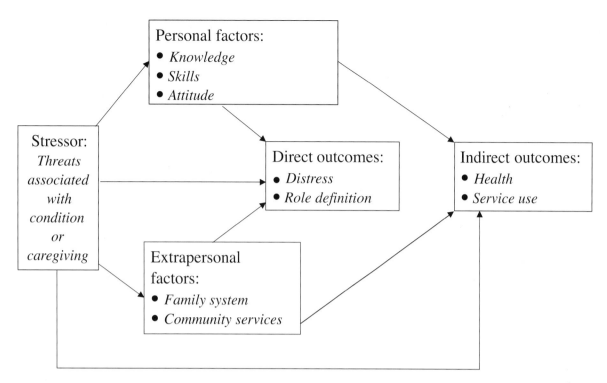

Figure 3.1—Stress theory model

common psychosocial threats faced by older persons, but it is principally focused on immutable and mutable factors that bear on the direct and indirect outcomes of stress situations, all with an eye to offering the clinician important tools for treatment as well as targets for therapeutic intervention. The chapter highlights findings from social science research that indicate ways in which unchangeable facts about a person's life (eg, gender) contribute to the outcome of stress situations—and to a person's ability to respond to them. In particular, the chapter discusses mediators and moderators, factors that can serve to filter, though not entirely protect against, the impact of stress through different mechanisms. Mediators involve the older person's perceptions of and responses to the stress situation. Moderators—which may be constituents of an older person's environment or behaviors in which the person engages—can be thought of as acting on the stressor itself to lessen its intensity or buffer its effect; they also affect a person's ability to respond to the stressor. Assisting older persons to see and work toward health outcomes that impact the quality of their life is an appropriate and effective clinical strategy for helping them to confront declines in physical health and the issues of mortality.

STRESSORS

The older person faces a great number and variety of stressors that are produced by a broad range of events and conditions. The stressors may be chronic, or they may have sudden, dramatic onset. They may be based in diseases or they may be of a more social nature. A chronic stressor may be health related (eg, the pain and mobility limitation of arthritis) or it may be psychologic (eg, the prolonged worry over a chronically ill spouse). An acute stressor might also be physical or psychologic (eg, learning of a newly diagnosed medical condition or experiencing the unexpected death of a close friend). Other stress demands include changes in social identity due to role loss in retirement or the function-driven need to move to a more supportive living arrangement. Losses in physical capacity and reserve may place demands on the person, not only because he or she perceives them as threats or increased physical demands, but also because of their accompanying psychologic component, the perception that he or she may have diminished capacity to respond to other demands. Always in the background for older persons are the various risk factors for incident or recurrent morbidity and mortality.

Some risk factors—particularly those involving behaviors over which the person (with some encouragement, teaching, and counseling) might exert control—may be modifiable. Other risk factors, such as gender and race, are not modifiable and produce accumulated assaults that may amplify other stressors. The increasing incidence of diseases with age means that the number and frequency of stressors are likely to increase as a person ages.

Caregiving

Caregiving is nearly endemic; more than 44 million Americans care for family members of all ages. Gender is an important factor; more than 70% of all caregivers are women. Many older persons are caregivers for a family member. Chronic diseases affect a large proportion of elderly persons, and much of the care they receive is provided by family members, especially spouses. The burden of caregiving for dementing disorders like Alzheimer's disease is typical. Dementia caregivers spend many hours each day in caregiving activities, and they do so for many years (20% are caregivers for more than 5 years). Such caregiving exacts a heavy toll. Caregivers are at twice the risk as their noncaregiving peers for adverse physical and mental health outcomes and more than twice as likely to be taking psychotropic medications. Social isolation, family disharmony, and economic hardships are common sequelae of caregiving.

Caregivers need training, information, and support, and they should be regularly observed for signs of the known effects of caregiving. Attention to family dynamics may also be useful in identifying issues contributing to stressors that are modifiable. A number of intervention programs (eg, those providing education, counseling, and cognitive-behavioral therapy) have proven effective in ameliorating the stress associated with caregiving. Disease-specific support activities offer only modest relief but may be the conduit for more focused help.

Loss and Grief

Being widowed, especially for women, is a common occurrence in old age; so, too, are deaths in one's extended family and larger social network. More than 1 million spouses will be widowed in the United States in 2003; by 2030, more than 1.5 million spouses will be widowed annually. In 2000, 8.3% of those between 65 and 74 years of age were widowed; 22.7% of those older than 75 were widowed. Other losses, such as sensory and functional losses imposed by the onset of chronic or acute illnesses, also produce grief. Such losses are generally understood to be among the major negative life events, and they place a substantial demand on a person. For most, the intense experience of grief lasts 6 to 12 months, generally a time of withdrawal and depression. After about a year, a more accepting period ensues, during which a re-emergence into a social milieu occurs or a less affecting form of more permanent memorialization of the lost person is established. Acknowledgment and monitoring of the grieving process and active treatment for the depression associated with loss can help in avoiding prolongation of this process. (See also "Depression and Other Mood Disorders," p 269.)

Role Loss and Acquisition

People typically encounter a large number of role shifts in aging. They leave work and social roles that may have provided economic rewards as well as status. For example, the Social Security administration made 1.8 million new awards in 2001, a year in which 2 million Americans turned 65. The average age of retirement has been in steady decline, dropping to slightly under 62 years of age in 1995–2000 (down more than 5 years since 1950–1955). Within relationships, roles may change, and wage-earning spouses, after retirement, may find themselves in significantly greater contact with each other. Grandparenthood and great-grandparenthood provide both new demands and opportunities. Functional losses may place older persons in help-seeking rather than help-providing roles, or, as noted above, another's losses may place one in a caregiving role. These role changes can be stressful and can negatively affect mental or physical health. Retirement planning can help make these positive experiences. The clinician's assessment of an older person's role loss and acquisition may suggest the need for interventions.

Social Status

Three factors are consistently associated in the United States with a broad range of negative psychosocial and physical outcomes: being nonwhite, being a woman, and being poor or poorly educated (usually a surrogate for being poor). They should serve as warnings for clinicians, as the presence of one or more of these factors may add to the person's stress load. They may also affect the kinds of coping mechanisms the person has available. Lack of disposable income, for example, may exclude the use of some formal services or involvement in community activities that come with a fee. Cultural status may present other challenges; women from some cultures, for example, may face special barriers to exercising in public.

Race has a direct bearing on health stresses and longevity in old age. A 65-year-old black American man can expect to live nearly 2 years less than a 65-year-old white American man (a pattern mirrored among black American and white American women). A person's ethnic or cultural background and community context may substantially affect the outlook she or he brings to bear on a situation, the kinds of moderating activities she or he deems acceptable, and the importance she or he places on various outcomes. Older persons may understand disease through frameworks specific to other cultures, and treatment may need to include or rely principally on culturally centered options. A concept like autonomy that has become so central in issues of patient choice and advance directives has a different weight and value in cultures where choice belongs more to the community as a whole (as with some American Indian groups) or to a community or family leader (eg, in Hmong societies). Choices like hospice care may be viewed in some cultures as tantamount to wishing for and bringing about the death of the person. A procedure like autopsy may strongly violate cultural or religious beliefs. The clinician is advised to proceed attentively in cross-cultural situations. (See also "Cultural Aspects of Care," p 51.)

MEDIATORS

Mediators shape a person's responses to stress. They are the internal and external resources the person can bring to bear to assess and interpret the stress, to assess his or her own capacities for addressing it, and to formulate a coping response to it. Many key mediators are modifiable through psychosocial intervention. Instruction and information can affect the person's understanding of a situation. Various forms of psycho-education have been shown to be effective in enhancing an older person's sense of mastery within a stress situation and in increasing his or her awareness and use of formal services. Family counseling and therapy can strengthen older person's involvement with his or her social network.

Self-efficacy Beliefs

A number of constructs have been studied that relate to a person's sense of his or her own ability to manage situations. The concept of self-efficacy is comparable to concepts such as mastery, internal locus of control, resilience, and competence, and although it is singled out here, it resembles these in representing a key personal quality to be considered when dealing with an older person facing any stress situation. Self-efficacy is an important consideration for the mental and physical health of older persons for two reasons.

First, there is a relationship between strong or positive self-efficacy and a number of important health and mental health outcomes (Table 3.1). A large number of longitudinal studies—most notably the MacArthur study of "successful" or healthy aging—have produced a coherent set of conclusions about self-efficacy. The way a person approaches a situation—whether it be a specific threat, like the onset of an acute condition, or a more pervasive one, like change of life roles or decline in physical performance—affects the eventual outcome. Of particular note in Table 3.1 is the broad range of effects of strong self-efficacy beliefs, which influence physical and mental health as well as overall function. In addition, self-efficacy seems to contribute to a person's ability to be actively engaged in life, an important moderating factor.

Table 3.1—Physical and Mental Health Impacts of Self-Efficacy Beliefs

Strong self-efficacy beliefs

- Buffer the effects of stress exposure on physical and mental health
- Contribute to overall physical performance, independently of ability
- Help maintain good function
- Slow functional decline among those with poor physical performance
- Contribute to good choice making, good performance, and persistence of effort (especially in women)
- Contribute to increased productivity

Weak self-efficacy beliefs

- Are associated with declines in functional status, especially in those with decreased physical performance

The second reason self-efficacy is important is that it is modifiable. It can be weakened by repeated assaults and poor outcome, but it can also be strengthened. Among the strategies effective for strengthening self-efficacy are the following:

- performance accomplishment (seeing oneself succeed in a series of increasingly difficult tasks);
- vicarious learning and social modeling (seeing others like oneself succeed in a targeted area);
- encouragement (being persuaded to undertake a targeted activity); and
- reinforcement (experiencing pleasure from success).

A number of training programs aimed at improving specific performance (eg, reducing the fear of falling or increasing adherence to an exercise regimen following a heart attack) have succeeded by working to strengthen participants' self-efficacy beliefs in the targeted area. Strong self-efficacy beliefs appear to be better predictors of performance than are measures of physical ability. In falls prevention studies, for example, those with strong self-efficacy beliefs related to falling were found to show reduced fear of falling, despite low objective measures for risk of falling. Self-efficacy appears to play an important role in coping and overall well-being in older persons. Clinicians should assess the older person's sense of his or her own competence and intervene, where possible, to strengthen it.

Coping Strategies

A number of theorists have studied the manner in which older persons meet and address the accumulated challenges of aging. Cultivating an emotional response to a stressor can mediate its effect and produce a better outcome. Thus, invoking confidence and optimism in the face of bad news helps a person to meet the challenge and strengthens the likelihood of a positive outcome. One strategy older people may use consists of selection, optimization, and compensation. In this strategy, as people age, they begin to hone down the number and kinds of things in which they engage on the basis of what they believe they do well, selecting activities in which they are more likely to succeed. They also reframe the way they judge their own performance, looking, for example, at people their own age or older for a source of comparison. They do the selected things more, and they derive optimal credit for doing them. As losses continue and performance diminishes, people employ compensatory strategies that allow them to put their remaining performance capacities in the best light possible. A person known for preparing elaborate dinners might, for example, choose a simpler main course (selection) that she does well and has prepared many times (optimization) and surround it with numerous but very simple courses and side dishes as a way of favorably setting it off (compensation). Other coping strategies (eg, assimilation, accommodation, immunization, or resilience) also build essentially on the notion of reframing the self or one's performance in order to provide positive reinforcement and to reinforce self-esteem. Clinicians should attempt to learn how their patients typically form successful responses to challenges and help them to address new challenges in these same terms.

Social Involvement

Like people at all ages, older persons are faced with developmental tasks and challenges. In Erikson's theory of staged development, the task of old age is integration—putting the pieces together in a way that both celebrates and continues to act on the learning and accomplishments of life. In this conception, and consistent with many other findings, involvement (sometimes termed *productivity*) plays an important role. Becoming more involved, actively seeking out ways to contribute to and participate in the broader world, even engaging in paid work are all mediators that can lead to better outcomes. Taking part, making a contribution—through volunteering, productive (sometimes paid) labor, active family roles (especially child care), and participation in group activities—are all associated with older persons' continued well-being.

In terms of the framework of factors affecting health outcomes, social involvement can be understood as a positive, problem-focused coping response, a way of filtering the effects of a stressor by strengthening the connection of the person to the community (affirming the person's value in the community). Older theories of normal aging saw disengagement—the systematic withdrawal of ties to the social world—as normative. In current thinking, however, such disengagement is not encouraged and might even be considered an abnormal behavior. At the very least, there is an association between lack of social involvement and affective disorders such as depression.

MODERATORS

Moderators are components of a person's life or behaviors in which the person engages that act to affect the demands of the various stressors he or she faces. Moderators may be in place before the onset of a stressor or they might be developed in response to it. A person who has a long history of exercise already has a good base of conditioning to deal with an emergent condition affecting mobility (eg, arthritis). Alternately, making a decision to begin to exercise, to control diet or alcohol consumption, or to cease smoking is a possible—and healthy—response to stressors ranging from the onset of illness to a realization that one has slowed down. These healthy behaviors directly moderate the effect of the threat or demand and contribute to better physical and mental health outcomes. Having a strong social network and calling on it in a time of crisis (rather than withdrawing) may help moderate age-related demands (for example the loss of a loved one).

The literature points to three major activities that moderate stress or demand and that appear to contribute to healthy aging: social involvement, spiritual or religious activity, and engaging in healthy behaviors. Older persons' activities in these areas should be assessed regularly and encouraged, as appropriate.

Social Networks

The older person's social network is a critical resource for overall well-being, and social isolation is a powerful risk factor for broad declines and mortality. The effect of their social networks on older persons' overall well-being has been extensively studied, and the results of these studies are conclusive (Table 3.2). The literature points to the importance of quality over quantity but does not discount the latter. The closeness of social relationships is most important; thus, a well-functioning marital or familial relationship—a relationship that provides a person with a confidante—will offer the kinds of support and protection suggested in Table 3.2. Dysfunctional close relationships—those characterized by negative and conflict-filled interactions—appear to work in the contrary direction. The size of an older person's social network appears to work in both directions. On the one hand, having a larger social network offers the opportunity for greater involvement

Table 3.2—Physical and Mental Health Impacts of Robust Social Networks

- Reduced mortality risks
- Better physical health outcomes
- Better mental health outcomes
- Reduced risk of ADL disability or decline
- Increased likelihood of ADL recovery
- Buffered impact of major negative life events
- Promotion of strong self-efficacy beliefs
- Assistance that does not preclude self-care but that may increase risk of new or recurrent ADL disability (especially in men)

NOTE: ADL = activities of daily living.

and contribution; on the other hand, it presents the likelihood of experiencing a greater number of losses within the network (because of death or increased disability).

A robust social network both mediates and moderates age-related stresses. Social networks provide emotional and instrumental help in times of crisis. Families help older persons, for example, weather the death of a spouse or close friend, but they also provide direct and indirect help when more functional losses occur. The social network can provide a person under stress with a context within which to envision and frame responses to various demands. Social networks seem to exert a positive effect on older persons by strengthening their self-efficacy beliefs (the person feels valued within the social network, and this contributes to a sense of self-value). It also provides opportunities for taking action to address demands (eg, calling on family for specific functional assistance, spending more time with children following the death of a spouse, increasing time spent with friends following retirement).

The literature is clear that the provision of such help is positive and contributes to recovery, unless it sends the wrong message. Too much instrumental assistance provided to older people (particularly men) by the social network may contribute to continued disability. Rather than being encouraged to work toward restored function, a person may receive too much help or not be encouraged to self-care and may, therefore, accept a modifiable condition as permanent. Thus, although assistance from the social network should be encouraged, it should be done with attention to promoting maximum function by the person receiving the help.

Spiritual or Religious Involvement

Studies have consistently demonstrated two important facts about religion and older people. First, religion plays a more important part in the lives of older persons; older persons are more actively involved than

younger persons in attending religious services and in carrying out regular private religious practices. More than 50% of older persons report frequent attendance at religious events (with little variation by gender or race). Second, there are consistent positive relationships between religious involvement and indicators of good health. Whether religious activity contributes to social integration, promotes involvement, or assists in the developmental tasks of aging, it seems clear that it is a positive force—at least for those already inclined to it.

Healthy Behaviors

Implementing positive behaviors (eg, exercise; controlling intake of food, tobacco, and alcohol; and active relaxation or stress-reduction techniques) have all been shown to have positive effects on overall well-being, no matter at what age they are begun. Although these are physical behaviors, they often rely on and benefit from strong psychosocial mediators, particularly self-efficacy and social networks. Clinicians should use these mediators when proposing older persons begin or strengthen healthy behaviors. It can help to invoke a person's understanding of benefits and appreciation of his or her own proven ability to make change while at the same time offering suggestions about how the targeted behavior might contribute to a strong social network (eg, "you could walk every day with your daughter," "you and your husband could take the healthy cooking class together").

ANNOTATED REFERENCES

- Aneshensel CS, Pearlin LI, Mullan JT, et al. *Profiles in Caregiving: The Unexpected Career*. San Diego, CA: Academic Press, Inc; 1995.

  This book provides an excellent explication of the Pearlin stress model. It does so in the context of applying the model to the situation of family dementia caregivers. Valuable in itself, this application can readily be extrapolated to other caregiving and self-care situations, offering a more general model of stress and possible methods to intervene effectively.

- Blazer DG. Self-efficacy and depression in late life: a primary prevention proposal. *Aging Ment Health*. 2002;6(4):315–324.

- Fry PS, Debats DL. Self-efficacy beliefs as predictors of loneliness and psychological distress in older adults. *Int J Aging Human Dev*. 2002;55(3):233–269.

  These two articles, in conjunction, illustrate the linkage among late-life stresses, a mediator and a moderator identified in the chapter (self-efficacy and spirituality), and an important late-life outcome, depression. The first article is one of many articles by this author detailing the issues that older people face with depressive disorders and the prevalence and incidence of these disorders among elderly persons. Of particular interest, this article offers a proposal for strengthening self-efficacy as a preventive technique against depression in older persons. The second article reports on a small study that documents the inverse association between spiritual self-efficacy and loneliness and psychologic distress.

- Crowther MR, Parker MW, Achenbaum WA, et al. Rowe and Kahn's model of successful aging revisited: positive spirituality—the forgotten factor. *Gerontologist.* 2002;42(5):613–620.

  This article integrates the findings from many studies establishing and delineating the importance of religion and spirituality in the lives of older persons and linking this important dimension of their lives to positive health outcomes.

- Levenstein S, Smith MW, Kaplan GA. Psychosocial predictors of hypertension in men and women. *Arch Intern Med.* 2001;161(10):1341–1346.

  This article reports on a cohort of 2357 adults followed since 1974 in the Alameda County longitudinal study. The article provides a good illustration of the association of psychosocial variables highlighted in the chapter—race, income, education, social status—with an adverse health outcome in later life.

- Pinquart M, Sorensen S. Associations of stressors and uplifts of caregiving with caregiver burden and depressive mood: a meta-analysis. *J Gerontol B Psychol Sci Soc Sci.* 2003;58(2):P112–P128.

  The literature on family caregiving for older persons is voluminous; this meta-analysis provides an overview of the

strategies used to study and intervene with caregiver burden and depression and of the outcomes of these studies. The meta-analysis reinforces the concept that the outcomes of a stress process are multifaceted and subject to moderators and mediators. A good companion piece to this article is that by Brodaty H, Green A, Koschera A. Meta-analysis of psychosocial interventions for caregivers of people with dementia. *J Am Geriatr Soc.* 2003;51(5):657–664.

- Rowe JW, Kahn RL. *Successful Aging.* New York: Pantheon Press; 1998.

  This book summarizes the results of the MacArthur Foundation study of aging in America. This study followed a large cohort of healthy young-old persons over the course of several years. It identified a number of key factors that promote healthy or successful aging, most notably, social involvement and the maintenance of self-efficacy. The study has led to a number of more scientific presentations of results, principally in the *Journal of Gerontology.*

- Smith J, Maas I, Mayer KU, et al. Two-wave longitudinal findings from the Berlin aging study: introduction to a collection of articles. *J Gerontol B Psychol Sci Soc Sci.* 2002;57(6):P471–P500.

  This essay introduces four related articles emanating from the work of Paul and Margaret Baltes in the two-wave Berlin Aging Study. The overview essay and the subsequent findings quantitatively explore the selection, optimization, and compensation theory advanced by the Baltes to explain how older persons cope with the decrements in function that are associated with aging.

  Kenneth W. Hepburn, PhD

CHAPTER 4—LEGAL AND ETHICAL ISSUES

KEY POINTS

- Four guiding ethical principles of American medical practice are beneficence, nonmaleficence, justice, and the respect for autonomy.

- A physician may evaluate a patient's *capacity* to make decisions; *competence* is a legal term implying that a court has taken action.

- Substituted judgment is the process of constructing what a person would have wanted.

- Living wills are advance directives that describe the decisions a person would make under specified circumstances.

Normative ethics is the inquiry into the standards of what we see as right or wrong action. It focuses on the question "What *ought* I do?" Medical ethics is based on a utilitarian ethical structure; that is to say, it is not based on deontological overarching moral imperatives

(as a religious ethic would be), but rather seeks the answer to the *ought* question through the principles that are applied in the context of the clinical situation with the goal of providing the greatest beneficence (ie, maximizing good consequences and minimizing bad consequences). These principles are tethered to values and perspectives that are unique to each culture and that may differ, depending on whether one is talking about a specific case (situational ethics) or about public policy.

The four guiding principles for American medical practice most often cited are the following: respect for autonomy, nonmaleficence, beneficence, and justice. How each of these principles guides the practice of medicine today is different from even 50 years ago. These principles and their application also differ widely within various subcultures within the American culture.

The primacy of individual autonomy is a foundation of American culture, from the early pioneers to modern medical practice. Respect for individuals' autonomy should include respect for their right to subjugate their individualism to family, culture, or religion. In many cultures, family structure dictates who will be the decision maker for individuals within that family, and that person is deferred to even when the individual involved retains the ability to make his or her own decisions. However, even when such dictates are absent, clinicians all too often consult with and defer decisions to the adult child of an elderly patient who is capable making decisions him or herself.

Nonmaleficence is, in essence, the Hippocratic "do no harm." What a culture or an individual may view as harm differs widely. The most frequently cited conflict between mainstream and subculture perspectives is that concerning blood transfusions for a Jehovah's Witness. For a Jehovah's Witness, blood transfusion causes more harm than the alternative, even if that alternative is death. But views of harm will also vary from individual to individual. Understanding the values of subcultures within our society may help to give us clues as to the spectrum of the values that underlie that individual's perspective on harm. Similarly, what constitutes beneficence, doing more good than harm, is very culture bound as well as specific to the individual. (See "Cultural Aspects of Care," p 51.)

Finally, the concept of justice and health care in our society is still very ambiguous. There is not a recognized right to health care in this country. The distribution of health care benefits and the use of health care technologies continue to be very uneven and reflect biases regarding gender, age, race, and ethnic origin. Researchers have neglected to include older adults in their study population, and the lack of knowledge on the relative effectiveness of interventions when they are used for older patients may lead to the under- or overutilization of interventions in this age group. Furthermore, assumptions that equate age with chronic illness and comorbidity may deny beneficial treatment to healthy elderly patients. Patients from groups that have long been denied many of the benefits of our society, especially our health care dollars, may be more reluctant than more historically privileged patients to step back from aggressive treatments because of a perception of continued prejudice.

It is important to keep these differences in mind when considering the following discussions of ethical decision making and its application to the individual patient. These are, in a true utilitarian sense, guiding principles, not moral imperatives. Just as the "laws" of medical science differ from case to case, these principles need to be used as they apply to each individual situation.

DECISIONAL CAPACITY

Because of the nature of the diseases affecting older persons, clinicians are often called on to assess a person's decision-making capacity and to use other, appropriate sources of decisional authority when that capacity is impaired. Although the focus of much of the literature has been on clinicians' assessments of patients' capacity to make medical decisions, clinicians are also asked to render opinions on patients' ability to make decisions about other matters, such as managing money, writing a will, continuing to drive, or possessing firearms. It is important to use the correct terminology in discussing the physician's responsibility. A physician may evaluate a patient's capacity to make decisions, but *competence* and *incompetence* are legal terms, and they imply that a court has taken a specific action.

Assessment of Patients' Decisional Capacity

Assessing the patient's ability to understand the consequences of a decision is the overarching principle used in making a judgment of decisional capacity. To make a medical decision, the patient must be able to understand the basic information about his or her condition and the probable outcomes of the disease and of various potential interventions. This requires the ability to understand the disease process; the proposed therapy and alternative therapies; the advantages, adverse effects, and complications of each therapy; and the possible course of the disease without intervention. The patient needs to be able to understand the broad consequences of accepting, deferring, or rejecting a proposed intervention. Admittedly, even physicians cannot predict the full implications of complex medical decisions, since they can rarely know all the consequences of an intervention or the precise natural history of an illness. Nonetheless, the patient should be able to make decisions that are based on his or her beliefs and values. Therefore, it is often most helpful for the clinician to explore a patient's hopes and fears and to help the patient clarify his or her goals so that the treatment options that are offered are based on these goals. Cultural differences of the members of ethnic minority groups can make assessing decision-making capacity a more difficult task than it already is. Capacity assessment involves abstract concepts not easily communicated in another language. It also involves interpreting value judgments on the basis of what is considered reasonable; this may differ according to culture. Clinicians must avoid assuming on the basis solely of ethnic background that a patient holds certain beliefs and evaluate each patient by considering his or her own biopsychosocial circumstances.

The capacity to make a living will is similar to that of being able to make treatment decisions, although it is somewhat more complicated, since the patient is being asked to think in the abstract, with a "what if?" frame of reference. The ability to choose a health care proxy (see below) is much less complex, and even fairly impaired patients are often able to choose someone to make decisions for them.

The requirements are even less stringent for *testamentary competence* (the ability to make a last will and testament). In general, a person's ability to decide how he or she wishes to dispose of belongings after death is felt to be preserved even when the person is very cognitively incapacitated in other ways. As long as the person can identify the individuals involved, is not delusional or in other ways psychiatrically ill such that judgment is impaired (eg, paranoia), and is capable of understanding the consequence of signing the will, he or she is considered to have testamentary competence.

Table 4.1 summarizes the elements of decisional capacity in each of these four areas.

Standardized Tests of Decisional Capacity

Traditional tests of cognitive function have some, but limited, utility in determining decisional capacity. An overall score on the Folstein Mini–Mental State Examination (MMSE) of 10 or less indicates such diminished cognitive ability that it is unlikely that the person retains decisional capacity. Some deficits uncovered by the use of the MMSE may be relevant (eg, immediate memory, attention, word finding, understanding simple verbal or written instructions, and ability to express simple ideas in writing). Others are not (eg, calculation and visuospatial relationships). As we come to appreciate the influence of frontal lobe dysfunction on a patient's capacity to function, especially to perform complex activities of independent living, we are also coming to appreciate the influence that the cognitive domains tested with executive function have on decisional capacity. Executive functions include problem solving, planning (including appreciating consequences of an action), initiation, capacity to monitor one's own behavior, and inhibition of inappropriate behaviors. The Executive Interview 25-item examination (EXIT 25) of executive function has been shown to correlate well with subjective measures of decisional capacity. Observation of the patient while completing tasks on the examination may reveal poor insight, impulsivity, intrusion of irrelevant material, poor self-monitoring, and impaired ability to form and follow through on a plan. Clinicians may make similar observations by observing a patient draw a clock.

Specific tests of decisional capacity have been developed. The Capacity to Consent to Treatment Instrument asks the person to read two vignettes and then decide between two treatment options. The Competency Assessment Test helps judge the person's ability to understand advance directives. Both instruments deal with hypotheticals, thereby adding more abstraction than is necessary for deciding real-time issues. The MacArthur Competency Assessment Tool—Treatment tests the person's ability to make a specific decision and has the advantage of dealing with real-time decisions. Assessment of decisional capacity is a functional assessment; therefore, there is no substitute for critical observation of the process itself.

Principles Governing Decision Making for Patients Who Lack Decisional Capacity

The hierarchy of decision-making strategies for those making the decisions for incapacitated patients is as follows: 1) respect their last competent indication of their wishes, 2) use substituted judgment, and 3) determine their best interests (ie, an analysis of benefits versus burden). Table 4.2 summarizes the hierarchy.

The last competent indication of wishes is most relevant in cases when patients are able to foresee that they will become incapacitated and can foresee what decisions will need to be made. Patients entering the terminal phase of an illness who know that at some point they will become confused or unconscious can

---

Table 4.1—Decisional Capacity

Medical decisions
- Ability to understand relevant information
- Ability to understand the consequences of the decision
- Ability to communicate a decision

Decisions of self-care
- Ability to care for oneself *or*
- Ability to accept the needed help to keep oneself safe

Finances
- Ability to manage bill payment
- Ability to appropriately calculate and monitor funds

Last will and testament
- Ability to remember estate plans
- Ability to express logic behind choices

Table 4.2—Hierarchy of Decision Making

Patient's current wishes
- If the patient has decisional capacity, this ALWAYS takes precedence

Substituted judgment
- Done by the surrogate decision maker only when the patient is not fully capable of making the decision
- Based on the patient's prior values and wishes
- Advance directive is used as guide
- Patient input is used when possible even if the patient is not fully capable of making the decision

Beneficence
- Done by the surrogate decision maker when the patient lacks decisional capacity and evidence does not exist for substituted judgment
- Weighing of benefits and burdens as based on the patient's present indications of pleasures and burdens
- Input from caregivers is very important

give very clear advance directives (also called *advance care plans* in some contexts) stating their preferences for care. As long as the circumstances remain substantially as predicted, other persons should not be allowed to reverse these decisions.

Substituted judgment is the process of constructing what the person would have wanted if he or she had been able to foresee the circumstances and give directions for care. In theory, those who know the person best and understand what his or her fears, pleasures, and goals were (ie, what the patient's rationale for a decision would have been) can provide substituted judgment. This is usually, but not always, the next of kin. A patient can appoint someone to hold durable power of attorney for health affairs (designating that person as what is also referred to as a *health care agent* or *proxy*). The patient chooses the person who can best represent him or her. Any such surrogate makes decisions only if the patient has become incapable of making decisions. The person granted durable power of attorney takes precedence over the next of kin.

The best-interest standard or the principle of beneficence guides physicians in making a medical decision for an incapacitated patient on the basis of the benefits and burdens an intervention poses for that person. When there is no expressed wish by the patient and no one to offer substituted judgment, then the surrogate decision maker must weigh the benefits and the burdens of treatment for that person in order to make a decision. Such analysis is best done by someone who is very aware of what gives that patient pleasure, what causes agitation, fear, pain, or discomfort, and how the patient reacts to a change in setting, use of restraints, and similar matters.

Conservatorships and Living Wills

In the absence of next of kin or durable power of attorney for a patient lacking decisional capacity, the court may appoint a conservator (called a *guardian* in some states). There are usually two types of conservatorship: conservator of finance and conservator of person. Incompetence in matters of finance is usually determined either by the demonstrated incapacity of the patient to manage financial matters (eg, unpaid bills, uncashed checks) or through specific testing by either an occupational therapist or a neuropsychologist. A conservator of person is required when the patient has demonstrated that he or she can no longer make personal decisions (such as medical decisions) or care for him- or herself to the point that the patient endangers him- or herself and cannot understand and accept the need for help (eg, neglecting oneself or risking injury).

Living wills are advance directives that attempt to demonstrate what decisions a person would make under certain circumstances. Most living wills address a couple of hypothetical clinical situations (eg, vegetative state, terminal illness) and four possible treatment options (cardiopulmonary resuscitation, respirator therapy, artificial feeding and hydration, and dialysis). A living will has limited utility because of its vagueness and lack of generalizability to the decisions that most commonly need to be made. Some living wills offer a detailed set of hypothetical case scenarios and treatment decisions, but these can be difficult for patients to understand and may not add information about the person's rationale for decisions. An individual's reaction to a hypothetical event may differ from how he or she will deal with reality. Nonetheless, a living will can be used as evidence of preferences as one is trying to construct how a patient who lacks decisional capacity might have felt about an intervention.

The Role of the Incapacitated Patient in Decision Making

Even when patients may not be fully capable of making decisions, often they can still participate in decision making at many levels. A task assessment of decision-making ability around a specific issue is always appropriate. A patient with even very little cognitive ability can give some indication when something causes discomfort or displeasure or when something brings pleasure. The surrogate decision maker must consider these indications when analyzing the benefits and burdens of an intervention. Case law supports the idea that the patient's indications of preference should be given consideration.

The perceived relative burden of an intervention may vary from one person to the next because of differences in mental status and ability to cope with change or disability. A demented patient who is accustomed to one environment will have a much harder time adjusting to hospitalization and may need restraints in order to undergo even something as simple as intravenous antibiotic therapy. The relative benefit of this therapy should be weighed against the burden of hospitalization for such a patient.

It is nearly impossible to perform some interventions without the cooperation of the patient. If the conservator recommended a cataract operation but the patient refuses to cooperate, for instance, it is doubtful that the procedure could be performed. In other situations it may be hard to justify doing a major invasive procedure against the will of an alert and mildly to moderately impaired person, even though it could be done. An example is a patient with frontal lobe dementia who adamantly refuses cardiac surgery. A surrogate decision maker must consider the present status of the patient and the patient's wishes, concerns, pleasures, and pains. Even though a person may not be intellectually capable of consenting to (or refusing) a treatment, on some level his or her assent may be needed in order to carry out that treatment.

Temporary Loss of Decisional Capacity

Patients may temporarily lose the ability to make decisions during acute confusional states, acute psychotic episodes, periods of unconsciousness from anesthesia or illness, or during an acute central nervous system event. Although in these cases the patients can be expected to regain this ability over time, the rules described above still apply. Decisions that the patient has made before becoming temporarily incapacitated should be respected. A patient may reverse his or her do-not-resuscitate status while undergoing anesthesia with the understanding that it can be reinstated postoperatively. However, a patient who has stated that he would never agree to resuscitation should not have this reversed by a family member during a temporary confusional state due to an intercurrent illness.

When using either substituted judgment or best-interest standards in surrogate decision making for a patient with a transient loss of decisional capacity, the decision maker should err on the side of more aggressive intervention if there are situations where the patient's wishes are not known or the circumstances are substantively different from what the patient had anticipated.

Informed Consent for Research

The new emphasis on the quality of consent obtained for participants in research must extend to the vulner-

able populations of elderly persons. Still, it is imperative that researchers study dementia and related problems so that the care of these patients may improve. The two most vulnerable populations are those with cognitive impairment, by virtue of their inability to understand the study or their role in it, and institutionalized patients, who may feel coerced to consent. Research involving vulnerable populations needs to be particularly well designed and focused on issues of importance to that population because of their lack of free will in having others agree to their participation.

Guidelines developed by the American Geriatrics Society for informed consent for research on cognitively impaired persons are shown in Table 4.3.

DECISIONS NEAR THE END OF LIFE

Although the issues discussed in this section focus on the period near the end of life, the decision-making process and ethical principles described are the same for all medical decisions. All patients make decisions, consciously or subconsciously, concerning treatment of minor conditions, adherence with medical regimens, and related issues by weighing competing values and needs. When a person is faced with a terminal illness or a chronic, disabling, or progressive disease, decision

Table 4.3—AGS Guidelines for Research Using Cognitively Impaired Persons as Subjects

- The research must be justified on scientific, clinical, and ethical grounds but can be focused on conditions other than dementia itself.

- The capacity to give consent should be assessed for each individual for each research protocol since decision-making capacity is task specific and some cognitively impaired individuals will be able to give consent.

- Advance consent to participate in research given prior to the loss of decisional capacity should, in general, be respected.

- The traditional surrogates for decision making can be used to obtain consent.

- Research protocols that involve more than minimal risk or do not have a likelihood of direct benefit for the subjects should be offered only to persons who are able to consent or who have an advance directive consenting to participate in research. Exceptions might be made for exceptionally promising treatments, but this should be reviewed at a national level.

- Surrogates can refuse participation or withdraw the person from participation if the surrogate determines that the research protocol is not what the person intended to consent to or is not in the person's best interest, even if there is advance consent.

- Only in very unusual circumstances would the refusal to participate of even an incapacitated patient be overridden.

NOTE: AGS = American Geriatrics Society.

SOURCE: Data from AGS Ethics Committee. Informed consent for research on human subjects with dementia. *J Am Geriatr Soc.* 1998;46(10):1308–1310.

making becomes more acute and focused. Patients, families, and physicians must attempt to balance benefits and burdens when making many health care decisions. This difficult task is further complicated by the fact that only probabilities of the benefits and burdens can be known, not certainties.

See also the section on end-of-life decision making in "Cultural Aspects of Care" (p 54).

Forgoing and Discontinuing Interventions

A patient's right to refuse unwanted treatment was confirmed by the Supreme Court of the United States in the 1991 case of *Cruzan* v. *Director, Department of Health of Missouri.* This refusal can occur before the intervention has been instituted or after it is in place. There is no ethical or legal distinction made between these two situations, often referred to in the more dramatic terms of *withholding* or *withdrawing* therapies. For example, in the case of uremia, a patient with kidney failure may decline to begin dialysis, thus increasing the risk of death from uremia. Alternatively, a patient may try dialysis for a period of time, even years, and then choose to stop this treatment and die from uremia. The same principle holds for discontinuing ventilatory support for a patient. The patient will die from his or her underlying respiratory disease whether ventilatory support is never started or if it is discontinued. The act of extubating a patient with the expectation that he or she will die is difficult for many clinicians because of the proximity of the act performed by the clinician and the death of the patient, but the decision is informed by the same ethical principles as is the decision to discontinue dialysis or to decline other medical interventions.

Clinicians and families often feel uncomfortable when a patient declines tube feeding and intravenous fluids. Case law, as well as the *Cruzan* case, characterizes these methods of delivering food and fluid as medical interventions; therefore, they are subject to the same ethical right of refusal that applies to any other medical interventions. Many people worry that the terminally ill patient will suffer without these interventions, but accumulated experience in hospice care has shown that it is usually easier to make someone comfortable without them: intravenous and gastric administration of food and fluid can cause discomfort through decreased gastric emptying and gastric distention, the need to replace intravenous lines or nasogastric tubes, and fluid overload as membranes become more permeable. These interventions may dampen or eliminate some of the natural comfort measures that occur, such as the release of endorphins.

Interventions That May Hasten Death

Palliative care, defined here as interventions that are given in order to relieve discomfort or suffering, may at times have the unintended effect of hastening death. We have come to accept that there may be two effects of a treatment, one (intended) effect of palliation, and the other possible (unintended) effect of hastening death. This is sometimes referred to as *the rule of double effect*. The intention of the application of the medical intervention is not to hasten death, but to palliate symptoms. Aggressive pain management, when respiratory depression is foreseeable but not intended, is generally seen as an ethical practice. Further, most evidence shows that gradually increasing narcotic dosage does not hasten death. The rule of double effect has been extended by some to cover the use of terminal sedation (without hydration) in cases where any level of consciousness will constitute continued suffering, as is frequently the case in death from head and neck cancer, for example.

Physician-assisted suicide and euthanasia occur when an intervention is made with the clear intention of ending the patient's life. The underlying motivation of patients who wish to hasten death varies. In population-based surveys, people commonly cite fear of pain and of other suffering (such as shortness of breath, anorexia, nausea, constipation, insomnia, and anxiety) as the reason for considering physician-assisted suicide. Fear of being dependent or a burden to others is mentioned at least as often. Other motivating factors that physicians mention are depression, problems with personal relationships, spiritual issues, grief, and sleep disorders.

In the United States, unlike in some other countries that have addressed this issue, only physician-assisted suicide (and not euthanasia) is being considered for legalization. Because suicide is an act committed by the person who will suffer the consequences, it is felt that such a death is more clearly voluntary than a death that results from another person's administration of a lethal intervention. Although the Supreme Court has ruled that there is not a constitutional right to physician-assisted suicide, it did not rule that it is unconstitutional, either. Each state has been left to make its own laws in this regard. Some states have yet to act; many have made physician-assisted suicide explicitly illegal. Oregon has had legalized physician-assisted suicide since 1997. Experience there has shown that relatively few terminally ill patients request physician assistance with suicide. In the first 3 years after legalization, 91 patients out of 90,000 who died in Oregon availed themselves of physician-assisted suicide, yielding a rate of 1 per 1000 deaths. Prominent motivating factors were loss of autonomy and determination to control the way in which one dies.

Ability to Predict Time of Death

Despite increasingly sophisticated prediction models, especially for patients who are critically ill, patients still rely on their clinician's judgment for most assessments of prognosis. Instruments such as the APACHE III (the third version of the acute physiology and chronic health evaluation scoring system), which uses a combination of age, diagnosis, cause of acute illness, and a scale of physiologic parameters to predict mortality risk in acute illness, are unable to address issues of the burden of treatment or the patient's quality of life. Long-range predictions for patients with slowly deteriorating conditions are even more difficult. Physicians must certify that a patient has 6 months or less to live in order for that patient to qualify for the Medicare hospice benefit. Similarly, the Oregon Death with Dignity Act asks physicians to predict, using reasonable judgment, whether a terminal illness will produce death within 6 months. Patients often seek a precise prognosis from their clinicians as they weigh the benefits and burdens of interventions and consider quality-of-life issues as well as survival. Unfortunately, neither clinician judgment nor prediction rules have proven accurate in predicting prognosis under these circumstances.

The Continuum of End-of-Life Decisions Based on Goals

Decisions near the end of life are not all-or-nothing choices. The absence or presence of do-not-resuscitate orders (more accurately referred to as do-not-attempt-resuscitation orders) is often misinterpreted as instruction to the clinician either to do everything or to do nothing. This dichotomy is false.

Other medical interventions for seriously ill patients with similar prognoses may have very different outcomes. For example, a patient with New York Heart Association Class 4 heart failure from a cardiomyopathy may ask not to receive cardiopulmonary resuscitation but might choose to accept placement of an automatic implantable cardiovascular defibrillator or be given a "dobutamine holiday." A patient who is dying from lung cancer might weigh the relative burdens and benefits of antibiotic treatment for pneumonia before deciding whether to treat the infection. The benefits and burdens of enteral feeding are highly influenced by the condition being treated. Most studies that have been done on the utility of enteral feeding for patients who aspirate have grouped all patients with feeding tubes together, which may not be appropriate. These scenarios illustrate some of the variables:

- Patient 1 has had surgery for a localized pharyngeal cancer followed by radiation. The procedure has left the patient freely aspirating, making it difficult for him to take sufficient calories by mouth. The patient's overall prognosis is still uncertain.
- Patient 2 has Parkinson's disease and still functions well. His pharyngeal muscle coordination is slow, and he recurrently chokes on his food, especially thin liquids.
- Patient 3 has end-stage Alzheimer's disease. Although she has evidence of aspiration on a swallowing examination and has had two documented pneumonias that are probably related to aspiration, she is seems comfortable when she eats. One of her few remaining discernible pleasures is eating.

The balance between benefits and burdens is very different for each of these patients. Enteral feeding may or may not prolong their lives, and restrictions on eating could have a different meaning for each. The recommendations by clinicians to each patient or patient's surrogate might include everything from feeding-tube placement and avoidance of taking food or drink by mouth to oral intake, as tolerated, for pleasure and the use of antipyretic medications for fevers. Before a choice is made, the patient or family must first clarify their priorities. The clinician can then decide how different approaches can best meet these goals.

SPECIAL ETHICAL ISSUES IN DEMENTIA

Although most of the topics discussed above intimately involve the ethics of caring for cognitively impaired persons, some areas of particular concern for this population merit further discussion.

Truth Telling

The ethics of truth telling has evolved considerably through the last half of the 20th century in mainstream American culture, breaking with the longstanding tradition of paternalism in medicine that advocated withholding bad news from patients in order to do no harm. In many other cultures, telling the truth is still not felt to be appropriate. In the United States, however, telling a patient that he or she has a dementing illness may be the last area of controversy about truth telling. Increasingly, both professional and lay people agree that patients with dementia should be given a chance to understand what is happening to them. The opportunity for the older person with early dementia to prepare legal documents (powers of attorney, a will, advance directives), to address personal issues, and to make plans is important. As therapies become available and research advances, it is imperative that persons with dementia be informed of their options and given the opportunity to voice their preferences, even though they may no longer be capable of giving fully informed consent.

Autonomy

Ensuring personal safety and avoiding harm to others are important concerns in caring for patients with dementia. Because of the very nature of the disease process and its effect on recent memory, patients may not perceive how they have changed; they may not be able to recognize when their problem interferes with their ability to make decisions. Some patients with dementia may not understand the consequences of their actions and may have difficulty planning because of frontal lobe dysfunction. This puts them at risk for behaviors that may endanger themselves or others, including unsafe driving, the continued possession of firearms, wandering, and socially inappropriate behaviors. Their care needs may exceed what their caregivers can provide, and they may be unable to understand the rationale for seeking help at home or for a sitter, day care, or nursing-home care. The clinician plays a crucial role in being able to objectively recognize when this has happened and to help the family or others to take the necessary steps to protect the patient and others.

Definition of Personhood and Advance Directives

Adults with intact decisional capacity not only have the right to make their own decisions but also always have the right to change their minds. Even when they become unconscious, their last competent statement was usually made close to the event, often with full knowledge of the decisions that will need to be made; the likelihood is low that their rationale for the decision or that their goals, fears, and pleasures had changed significantly. If life experiences do mold their thinking, or if new interventions or approaches to problems occur, they can alter their directive to fit with these changes. A person with a progressive cognitive disorder can change substantially over time. What brings pleasure and what causes fear or pain can change substantially from year to year; almost certainly a patient's perceptions change greatly as the disease progresses. The demented person is unable to comprehend the future and slowly becomes more and more disconnected from the past. In some ways, the person with advancing dementia becomes suspended in time:

the person loses his or her connection to previous and future selves, the essence of what many define as personhood. A demented person is tied to the decisions and perceptions of a previous self whom he or she may not even remember. The decisions made by this prior "self" may inform current decision making, even though that person did not know what he or she would need or want at this time. Therefore, conflict can arise between the previous directives made by that patient and what is best for the demented patient in the here-and-now (ie, what gives the patient pleasure and what may disturb him or her).

Genetic Testing and Alzheimer's Disease

Relatives of persons with Alzheimer's disease are increasingly interested in knowing their risk of having the disease. For relatives of those who have a clear autosomal dominant, known single-gene mutation, as is the case with Huntington's chorea, genetic testing has proven useful when accompanied by safeguards of counseling and follow-up. In familial, early-onset Alzheimer's disease, several gene mutations have been found that cause clusters of Alzheimer's disease in families. For those clusters where the mutation is known, mapping and phenotyping may be helpful in conjunction with counseling. For most familial clusters, however, the genes responsible have not been identified, and testing is not useful.

The value of testing is less certain in the case of apolipoprotein E alleles, which may influence a person's susceptibility or probability of having Alzheimer's disease sometime in the future. Many people with the high-risk alleles do not get the disease, and many without it do. As long as there is no intervention that has been shown to significantly alter the course of the dementing process, it does not seem advisable to create anxiety when the predictive value of the test is so low.

See also "Dementia" (p 221).

ETHICS IN THE NURSING HOME

Although the ethics that apply to the treatment of patients in other settings apply to patients in the nursing home, some issues are brought more acutely into focus because of the setting and the concentration of patients with chronic and end-stage disease.

Treatment Decisions

Until policymakers and clinicians paid attention to the resuscitation status of patients in nursing homes, residents were assumed not to be candidates for attempted resuscitation. It was rarely, if ever, attempted. Studies that have looked at the outcomes of attempted resuscitation of patients in long-term-care facilities show that it is used infrequently and is associated with low long-term survival. However, the number of patients in long-term-care settings for short-term recuperation and rehabilitation has grown, which may change the statistics concerning the utility of attempted resuscitation of nursing-home patients.

Staff perceptions of the utility of resuscitation efforts differ by profession. Nursing staff strongly prefer to limit interventions in this setting, especially for older patients and those with cognitive impairments. On the other hand, physicians tend to overestimate the benefit of interventions for these patients and sometimes hesitate to honor a do-not-resuscitate request for those who are not clearly terminally ill. Patient participation in the process is variable. Federal legislation requires the systematic inquiry into advance directives for all patients in institutions receiving federal funds. With the advent of this more systematic approach to discussions about treatment status, nursing homes have transferred fewer patients to acute-care settings, and yet patient and family satisfaction have not declined.

Regulatory agencies have encouraged enteral feeding of patients in nursing homes to prevent nutritional deficits in patients who may be failing to get enough nourishment by eating. Although the motives for enacting these regulations were compassionate, the usefulness of enteral feeding, especially for patients with advanced dementia, is questionable. Also, it is not ethical to use enteral feedings for a patient capable of taking oral sustenance but who may not be getting enough nutrition because a facility fails to provide patients with the help they need in eating. (See "Malnutrition," p 174.)

Restraints

The use of restraints in the long-term-care setting has become closely regulated and monitored. Studies have shown that using physical restraints has little, if any, value in preventing injuries from falls. Less restrictive alternatives are usually available. Clinicians and patients' surrogates must consider several factors in deciding whether to use restraints. If the patient is engaging in activities that might harm other residents or staff, and when intervention is ineffective or the patient's surrogate refuses it, then the institution's responsibility to protect others may require that it send the patient elsewhere.

Conflicts of Interest

The allocation of resources in nursing homes is closely linked to the ability of nursing-home care to prevent complications of chronic illness. When staffing falls

below a critical level, pressure ulcers, functional decline, depression, agitation, and the need for restraints may increase. Appropriate activities to meet the patient's physical, cognitive, and emotional needs, although sometimes referred to as the "hotel" functions or "recreation," are also part of the good medical care of these patients. The role of the nursing-home medical staff in monitoring and participating in this process needs further clarification.

MISCELLANEOUS ISSUES

Driving

Older persons with physical and cognitive impairments have as high a risk of motor vehicle collisions per mile driven as do teenage drivers. Physicians face complex ethical problems when caring for older patients who endanger themselves and others by driving. The conflicting values are powerful: respect for the patient's autonomy, duty to protect the patient from harm, duty to protect others from predictable danger, and respect for patient-doctor confidentiality. Educating the patient and family members is often the key to developing a practical solution. Legal requirements regarding physician reporting of unsafe older drivers vary from state to state. In some states, physicians are required to report patients who may be unsafe; in other states they are permitted to do so; and in a few states, reporting may be considered a violation of patient-physician confidentiality. (See also the section on the older driver in "Assessment," p 49.)

Ethics and Health Care Financing

The ethical issues regarding the financing of health care have become much more salient in an era of rapidly rising costs and managed care. Health care professionals need to be aware of the forces, both positive and negative, exerted by payment structures on the nature of the care delivered. Ideally, providers, aware of these forces, will take maximum advantage of the positive forces and work to guard against the negative forces when caring for patients. The two major care payment structures to health care providers, fee-for-service and capitation, influence care differently.

Fee-for-Service Structures

Fee-for-service (FFS) care means that the provider receives payment for each service rendered. The built-in advantage of an FFS method is that providers have an incentive to be thorough in diagnosing and treating of patients; the more services a physician provides (and documents), the more he or she is paid.

Patients receiving FFS care may be more reassured that the doctor is doing everything possible to care for them. The potential disadvantage of FFS care is overtreatment of patients, resulting in unnecessary iatrogenic morbidity and mortality as well as increased costs.

About 85% of older adults receive care from "traditional" Medicare, a system that compensates physicians under an FFS arrangement (see "Financing, Coverage, and Costs of Health Care," p 32). Medicare FFS providers have relative incentives to provide covered benefits and disincentives to perform noncovered services. The primary method of controlling overall costs in an FFS system is to carefully delineate which services are covered and to discount payments for those services. The catalogue of Medicare-covered services is published as the *Current Procedural Terminology* coding system. One of the most common areas where physicians may feel pressured to stretch the truth, or to lie outright, is in the coding of conditions and procedures in order to make sure that patients will not be left liable for bills.

Capitation Structures

Capitation means prepayment for the care of a patient population on the basis of the number of patients, regardless of the amount of care the physician provides. Under the Medicare Advantage option (formerly the Medicare Plus Choice option), which is selected by about 15% of Medicare beneficiaries, health plans (not individual providers) receive capitation from the Centers for Medicare and Medicaid Services (formerly the Health Care Financing Administration) on the basis of the number of enrollees (see "Financing, Coverage, and Costs of Health Care," p 32). Capitation arrangements provide incentives for the prevention of serious (and costly) conditions, commonly through the use of disease management programs, health promotion efforts, and care management. Analysts describe capitated care as proactive and FFS as reactive. The chief concern regarding capitation is an inherent underservice bias; the less that is spent on the patient, the more the provider or plan may profit. Physicians receiving capitation, or any other incentive to restrict costs, have an ethical obligation not to undertreat their patients.

ANNOTATED REFERENCES

■ AGS Ethics Committee. Informed consent for research on human subjects with dementia. *J Am Geriatr Soc.* 1998; 46(10):1308–1310.

The AGS Ethics Committee outlined nine positions, each with accompanying rationale, as guidelines for appropriateness of the informed-consent process in research using persons who have dementia. The positions encompass discussions of types of research, surrogate consent, advance consent on the part of the potential subject, and need for subject's assent to participate.

■ Marson DC. Loss of competency in Alzheimer's disease: conceptual and psychometric approaches. *Int J Law Psychiatry.* 2001; 24(2–3):267–283.

This is a review of the literature on competency and Alzheimer's disease. The author looks at the cognitive changes that happen with progression of the disease, the psychometric measures of these cognitive functions, and their impact on decisional capacity.

■ Post SG, Whitehouse PJ. Fairhill guidelines on ethics of the care of people with Alzheimer's disease: a clinical summary. Center of Biomedical Ethics, Case Western Reserve University, and the Alzheimer's Association. *J Am Geriatr Soc.* 1995; 43(12):1423–1429.

Drawn from the content of discussions with patients and families, these guidelines discuss ethical issues of common concern for patients with dementia. Topics covered include truth telling, driving privileges, respecting choices (autonomy, capacity, and competence), dilemmas of behavioral control (including wandering, use of physical restraints, polypharmacy), and death and dying (thresholds of quality of life).

■ Quill TE, Lee BC, Nunn S. Palliative treatments of the last resort: choosing the least harmful alternative. *Ann Intern Med.* 2000;132(6):488–493.

Using clinical examples, the authors discuss five alternatives that may effect the time of death of patients in the terminal stages of illness: forgoing any therapies that might be life sustaining, accelerating opioid therapy for pain, physician-assisted suicide, stopping eating and drinking, and terminal sedation without hydration.

■ Sullivan AD, Hedberg K, Fleming DW. Legalized physician-assisted suicide in Oregon—the second year. *N Engl J Med.* 2000;342(8):598–604.

This is an analysis of the patients who had been reported to have been given lethal doses of medicine in the second year of legalized physician-assisted suicide in Oregon. Percentage of deaths and patients' underlying diagnoses are discussed.

■ The Hastings Center. *Guidelines for the Termination of Life-Sustaining Treatment and the Care of the Dying.* Bloomington, IN: Indiana University Press; 1987.

This is an older reference, but one that has stood the test of time. It has excellent definitions of terminology and straightforward presentation of the issues involved in care of the dying patient, surrogate decision making, and end-of-life decisions.

Margaret A. Drickamer, MD

CHAPTER 5—FINANCING, COVERAGE, AND COSTS OF HEALTH CARE

KEY POINTS

- Medicare Part A covers hospital, skilled nursing home, and home-health and hospice services; Medicare Part B covers physicians, nurse practitioners, social workers, psychologists, therapists, laboratory tests, and durable medical equipment. Medicare Part D (optional) covers some of the cost of prescription medications.

- Medigap supplemental insurance plans are available that cover Medicare Part A and Part B deductibles and co-insurance costs, as well as preventive care and other health-related goods and services.

- The Medicare Personal Plan Finder (http://www.medicare.gov/MPPF/home.asp) can assist patients in selecting a Medigap plan or Medicare HMO and in comparing nursing facilities and home-health-care agencies.

- Medicaid is a joint federal and state program that provides supplemental health insurance (including long-term custodial care in nursing homes) to people of all ages who have low incomes and limited savings.

In 1965 the U.S. government passed legislation designed to improve access to acute health care for people who are old, disabled, or poor. During the decades that followed, the resulting Medicare and Medicaid programs expanded, evolved, and spawned thousands of supplemental commercial insurance plans. Today, a complex and often confusing array of personal payments, public programs, and private insurance plans (see Figure 5.1) pays for and thereby determines much of the health care that older Americans receive.

This chapter describes, through the eyes of patients and providers, how these programs influence the day-to-day care of older people. It illustrates their effects during a year in the life of Mrs. Rose Murat, an imaginary 79-year-old retired schoolteacher who lives with her 83-year-old husband in a small older home. Mrs. Murat has hypertension, coronary artery disease, and mild heart failure, for which she takes hydrochlorothiazide, metoprolol, lisinopril, and nitroglycerine. Her total out-of-pocket payments for these medications are $104.67 per month.

OUTPATIENT CARE

At the end of her quarterly office visit, Mrs. Murat asks for advice on joining a health maintenance organization (HMO) that has been marketing a Medicare health plan in her county. She is impressed by the HMO's offer of free eyeglasses, hearing aids, and preventive check-ups, all of which she has purchased out-of-pocket in the past. Her options, summarized in Table 5.1, are as follows: staying with traditional fee-for-service (FFS) Medicare as her only coverage; keeping FFS Medicare and applying for either Medicaid or supplemental ("medigap") coverage; or exchanging her FFS Medicare coverage for membership in the Medicare HMO. Depending on the Murats' income, savings, and state of residence, they may also qualify for a Medicare assistance program that pays for some combination of their Medicare premiums, deductibles, and co-insurance costs. Some older Americans may have additional health insurance options through the federal Department of Veterans Affairs or through their (or their spouses') present or previous employer or union.

Medicare is a federal insurance program run by the Centers for Medicare and Medicaid Services (CMS) that pays health professionals and organizations to provide acute health care for Americans who are 65 and older, disabled, or suffering from end-stage renal disease. As originally enacted, Medicare comprises two separate FFS plans (Part A and Part B), each of which pays predetermined amounts for specified health-related goods and services that are needed by its beneficiaries. More than 80% of older Americans are covered by both plans.

Medicare Part A uses regional insurance companies ("intermediaries") to pay hospitals, nursing homes, home-care agencies, and hospice programs for the Medicare-covered services they provide. Older Americans (and their spouses) who have had Medicare taxes deducted from their paychecks for at least 10 years are entitled to coverage through Part A without paying premiums. Others may be able to purchase Part A coverage (for $189 to $343 per month, depending on how long they had Medicare taxes deducted from their paychecks).

Medicare Part B uses other regional insurance companies ("carriers") to pay physicians, nurse practitioners, social workers, psychologists, rehabilitation therapists, home-care agencies, ambulances, outpatient facilities, laboratory and imaging facilities, and suppliers of durable medical equipment for the Medicare-covered goods and services they provide. At age 65, people become eligible for Part B coverage if they are entitled to Part A coverage or if they are citizens or permanent residents of the United States. To obtain this coverage, eligible persons must enroll in Part B and pay premiums ($78 per month), usually by agreeing to have them deducted from their monthly Social Security checks.

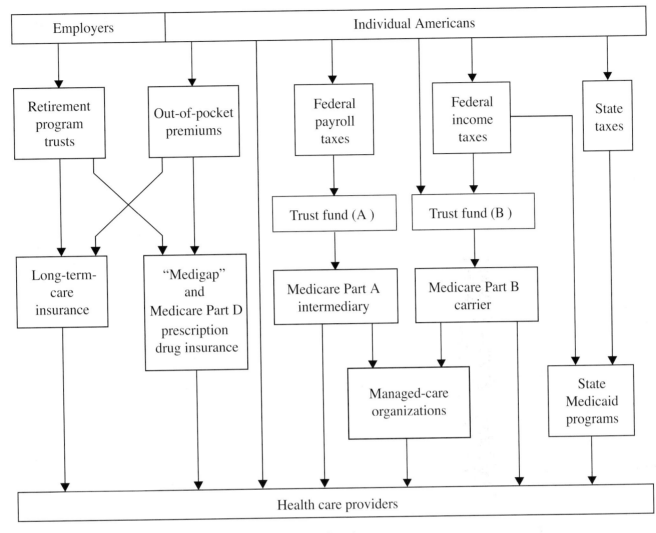

Figure 5.1—The flow of funds for the health care for older Americans.

Physicians must choose whether to participate in the FFS Medicare program. For each Medicare-covered service performed, a participating physician will submit a claim to the Part B carrier, accept Medicare's fee for the service (80% of its preestablished "allowed" amount), and bill the patient or her secondary insurer for no more than a 20% co-insurance payment. For services not covered by Medicare, the physician may bill the patient, if the patient agrees in advance in writing. Physicians who do not participate in Medicare can bill patients directly for up to 15% more than 95% of Medicare's allowed amounts. The patients pay the physicians and then submit their requests to Medicare for partial reimbursement (ie, for 80% of 95% of the allowed amounts). Some physicians choose to enter into "private contracts" with older patients. Under these contracts, Medicare (and medigap insurance plans) pay nothing, and patients pay physicians the full amount of the fees specified by the contracts.

Neither Part A nor Part B of the Medicare program covers periodic physical examinations, outpatient medications, dental care, hearing aids, eyeglasses, foot care, orthopedic shoes, cosmetic surgery, care in foreign countries, or custodial long-term care at home or in nursing homes. Part B covers some preventive services (see Table 5.1).

Beneficiaries pay out-of-pocket for:

- monthly premiums for Part B ($78),
- annual deductible for Part B ($110),
- the deductible for Part A ($912 per benefit period, ie, the first 60 days following an admission),
- co-insurance payments (usually 20%) for goods and services for which Medicare or other insurance pays only a portion, and
- the full cost of those goods and services that are not covered by Medicare or other insurance, including outpatient prescription medications.

Table 5.1—Health Insurance Coverage for Older Americans

Covers the cost of:	FFS Medicare		Supplemental Coverage		Medicare HMO Plan [b]
	Part A	Part B	Medicaid [a]	Medigap Policy	
Hospitals	100% [c]	—	$912	$912	100%
Postacute care in SNF	100% [d]	—	—	—	100%
Hospice	100% [e]	—	—	—	—
Home care ("medically necessary")	100%	100%	—	—	100%
Durable medical equipment	80% [f]	80% [f]	20%	20%	100%
Diagnostic laboratory tests	—	100%	—	—	100%
Diagnostic imaging tests	—	80%	20%	20%	100%
Physicians, nurse practitioners	—	80%	20%	20%	100%
Outpatient PT, OT, ST	—	80%	20%	20%	100%
Outpatient services, supplies	—	80%	20%	20%	100%
Emergency care	—	80%	20%	20%	100%
Ambulance services	—	80%	20%	20%	100%
Preventive services	—	g	20%	20%	g, h
Outpatient mental health care		50%	50%	50%	100%
Custodial care in nursing home	—	—	100%	—	—
Hearing, vision services	—	—	i	i	i
Outpatient medications	—	—	i	i	i
Additional costs to patient:					
Deductibles	$912 [j]	$110 [k]	—	i	i
Monthly premiums	—	$78	—	i	i

NOTE: FFS = fee for service; HMO = health maintenance organization; OT = occupational therapy; PT = physical therapy; SNF = skilled nursing facility; ST = speech therapy.

a Under the Balanced Budget Act of 1997, state Medicaid programs were given the option whether or not to pay deductibles and co-insurance costs.

b Some Medicare Advantage plans require members to pay deductibles and copayments.

c After the beneficiary or secondary insurer pays the deductible amount ($912).

d For the first 20 days of SNF care following a hospital stay of at least 3 days.

e Patient makes copayments of $5.00 per outpatient prescription and 5% of cost of respite care.

f When patient is receiving Medicare-covered home care.

g 100% of allowed cost of fecal occult blood test, Pap smear interpretation, prostate-specific antigen test, blood tests for diabetes and cardiovascular disease, and influenza and pneumococcal vaccinations; 80% of allowed cost of mammograms and clinical examination of breast and pelvis (no deductible applies); after the annual Part B deductible has been paid, 80% of allowed cost of a general physical examination at age 65, glaucoma screening, sigmoidoscopy or colonoscopy or barium enema, digital examination of rectum (men), measurement of bone mass, hepatitis B vaccination, and diabetic education and equipment.

h Some Medicare Advantage plans cover additional preventive services.

i Benefits and costs vary widely among medigap insurance plans and state Medicaid plans.

j Per benefit period (first 60 days following hospital admission).

k Annual.

In 2003, the U.S. Congress passed and President George W. Bush signed a sweeping Medicare reform bill that included an option (Medicare Part D) for beneficiaries to purchase insurance coverage for prescription medications beginning in 2006. If Ms. Murat were to choose this option, she would pay annual premiums ($420), deductibles ($250), and co-insurance (25% of her remaining medication expenses = $250). Her total out-of-pocket medication costs would be reduced 26% from $1250 to $920 per year (from $104.67 to $76.67 per month).

Medicaid is a joint federal and state program that provides supplemental health insurance to people of all ages who have low incomes and limited savings. The exact criteria for Medicaid eligibility and the benefit packages provided by Medicaid programs vary considerably from state to state. Most programs pay Medicare Part B premiums, and some pay Medicare deductibles and co-insurance costs. Most important, Medicaid pays for long-term custodial care in nursing homes for those who qualify. Several states have begun offering fixed capitation payments to managed-care organizations that are willing to provide Medicaid and Medicare benefits to residents who are "dually eligible" (for Medicaid and Medicare).

Medigap supplemental plans fill some of the holes in the insurance coverage provided by Medicare Part A and Part B. Private insurance companies offer FFS medigap plans of ten types (A through J), classified according to the benefits they cover. For new Medicare beneficiaries at age 65, the premiums for A-level (basic) plans across the United States range from $40 to $125 per month. These policies cover a person's Part A and Part B co-insurance costs, for example, 20% of Medicare's allowed fees for durable medical equipment and physicians' services. (In Minnesota, Wisconsin, and Massachusetts, A-level medigap policies are required by law to cover more than just the costs of Medicare co-insurance.) B-level plans cover Part A and Part B co-insurance, plus the Part A deductible ($912 per benefit period). Each successive level of medigap policy provides additional benefits and costs more. J-level plans cover co-insurance, deductibles, care in foreign countries, preventive services, and some of the cost of medications—at a cost of $175 to $400 per month. Consumers can obtain less expensive medigap coverage by purchasing plans that require the insured to pay high deductibles (F- and J-level plans only) or plans that cover the services of only selected physicians and hospitals ("Medicare SELECT" policies). Medigap policies do not cover long-term care, dental care, eyeglasses, hearing aids, or private-duty nursing.

Within 6 months of their initial enrollment in Medicare Part B, beneficiaries are entitled to purchase any medigap policy on the market at advertised prices. After this open enrollment period, medigap insurers can refuse to insure individual beneficiaries or charge them higher premiums because of their past or present health problems.

Medicare HMOs hold contracts with CMS specifying that, for each Medicare beneficiary they enroll, they will provide at least the standard Medicare benefits in return for fixed monthly capitation payments. In order to attract enrollees, most Medicare HMOs also cover additional benefits and charge low or no premiums, deductibles, and copayments. The HMOs achieve cost savings by managing their enrollees' use of services within their networks of providers, with whom they negotiate price discounts in return for patient volume. Each January the HMOs have the option of

changing their premiums, benefits, and provider networks—or of discontinuing their Medicare plans altogether.

Each November, beneficiaries covered by Medicare Part A and Part B have the option of joining any Medicare HMO operating in their area; they cannot be denied enrollment because of any health problems except end-stage renal disease. Enrollees must continue to pay their monthly Medicare Part B premiums, and they must obtain their health care from the HMO's provider network. They have the option of leaving the HMO at any time and going back to the FFS Medicare program. The primary advantages and disadvantages of each of Mrs. Murat's options are outlined in Table 5.2. Extensive information about all the options is available to consumers at each state's medical assistance office, at 1-800-MEDICARE (1-800-633-4227) or 1-877-486-2048 for hearing-impaired TTY users, and at the Medicare Personal Plan Finder (http://www.medicare.gov/MPPF/home.asp).

Managed Care

Mrs. Murat's provider of primary care, knowledgeable about her health and prognosis, can help her to choose the plan(s) that will cover the goods and services that she needs, both now and in the future. If she can obtain what she is likely to need from the HMO's network of providers, joining the HMO might be her best option, because it will allow her to obtain "free" eyeglasses, hearing aids, and preventive services and to avoid paying the usual Medicare premiums, deductibles, and co-insurance. Data about the quality

Table 5.2—Advantages and Disadvantages of Four Types of Health Insurance

Type of Insurance	Primary Advantages	Primary Disadvantages
FFS Medicare (Parts A, B, and D)	Traditional Medicare benefits, choice of any provider that participates in the Medicare program, partial coverage for prescription medications	Cost of co-insurance, deductibles, noncovered goods and services (eg, eyeglasses, hearing aids)
Medicaid	Coverage of co-insurance, deductibles, and some benefits* not covered by Medicare	Choice of providers restricted to a single network in some states
Medigap insurance	Coverage of co-insurance, deductibles, and some benefits** not covered by Medicare	Out-of-pocket monthly premiums range from $40 to $400, depending on the coverage provided by the policy purchased
Medicare Advantage plan (eg, HMO)	Traditional Medicare benefits plus coverage of additional goods and services**	Choice of providers restricted to a single network; potential for changes in premiums, copayments, deductibles, benefits, and providers at the discretion of the plan

NOTE: FFS = fee for service; HMO = health maintenance organization.

* Benefits vary from state to state.

** Benefits vary from plan to plan.

of care and the satisfaction of other enrollees in all the local Medicare HMOs are available at the Medicare Personal Plan Finder.

In the event that she needs health care that is not available from the HMO's network, or if she is reluctant to change providers, retaining the flexibility of her traditional Medicare coverage (which covers her use of any provider that participates in the Medicare program) might be a better choice, especially if she also qualifies for Medicaid or buys a medigap policy. Information from Medicare's information line or from the Medicare Personal Plan Finder would help her compare the prices and coverage of the medigap policies available in her area.

The primary care provider's recommendations to Mrs. Murat are likely to be influenced by the characteristics of the different plans she is considering. For instance, if the primary care provider is not in the HMO's service network, he or she would point out to Mrs. Murat that her enrollment in the HMO would require her to select a new primary care provider. If the primary care provider is in the HMO's network, Mrs. Murat's enrollment would change (ie, probably reduce) the payment for her care. As shown in Table 5.3, the payments would depend on the type of HMO involved. If it is a group or independent practice association (IPA) model, the HMO may pay providers "discounted FFS," that is, less than Medicare Part B would pay for each service. Or it may pay primary providers a fixed capitation amount each month to cover specified services. If these services are limited to primary ambulatory care, the capitation amount will be relatively small. The HMO may reward primary providers with end-of-the-year bonus payments if they have limited their referrals to specialists and their admissions to hospitals. If the covered services also include specialty and inpatient care, the capitation amounts will be considerably larger, and the provider will have incentives to use these services judiciously because he or she will have to pay for them, at least in part.

Fee for Service

Under the Medicare FFS system, providers obtain the fairest possible reimbursement by understanding and following CMS's payment system, which is based on evaluation and management (E&M) codes (see Table 5.4).

For each Medicare-covered service provided, the provider submits to the regional Medicare carrier the appropriate E&M code and the international classification of disease (ICD) code that indicates the diagnosis for which the service was provided. Entries in the medical record, which are subject to audit, must document that the data collection and medical decision-making aspects of the service conform to standards established for the E&M code submitted. By providing and documenting services efficiently, providers can maximize their FFS reimbursements within the (tight) limits imposed by the Medicare fee schedules.

Regardless of the payment mechanism, the crucial question is whether the amount of payment suffices to support high-quality care. For example, if capitation rates are below the aggregate cost of the services they are intended to cover, the provider will feel pressure to take on more patients and limit the amount of service that each patient receives. Similarly, if FFS amounts are too small, the provider will feel pressure to schedule more visits and procedures and to reduce the time devoted to each patient. Each provider should, therefore, monitor carefully and continuously the many changing elements in the practice environment (eg, payment schedules, covered services, expenses, patients' and families' expectations, population demographics) to help determine the numbers and types of services that are appropriate for each older patient.

INPATIENT CARE

Four months later, Mrs. Murat awakes dysarthric and unable to feel her left hand. Her face is asymmetric, and her left arm and left leg are weak. Her husband calls 911; the ambulance rushes her to the nearest emergency department, where the physician on duty diagnoses a right hemispheric stroke and admits her to the hospital.

Managed Care

If Mrs. Murat had joined the Medicare HMO, the HMO would pay for the ambulance, emergency, and

Table 5.3—How Medicare HMOs Pay Providers of Health Care

| | Type of HMO | | |
	Staff Model	Group Model	IPA Model
Providers	Employees	One large group practice	Many small independent practices
Method of payments	Salary	FFS or capitation*	FFS or capitation*

NOTE: FFS = fee for service; HMO = health maintenance organization; IPA = independent practice association.

* The services covered by the capitation payments range from "primary care only" in some plans to "medications and all acute care" in others.

Table 5.4—Fee-for-Service Reimbursement by Medicare, Year 2005

E&M Service	E&M code	"Allowed" Amount ($)*	%	CMS Payment ($)**
Comprehensive office visit, new patient	99205	179	× 0.80 =	143
Detailed office visit, established patient	99213	55	× 0.80 =	44
Detailed office visit (mental health problem), established patient	99213	55	× 0.50 =	28
Comprehensive office consult	99245	230	x 0.80 =	184
Comprehensive inpatient consultation***	99255	201	× 0.80 =	161
Complex hospital admission	99223	161	× 0.80 =	129
Complex hospital follow-up visit	99233	81	× 0.80 =	65
Comprehensive nursing facility initial assessment	99303	111	x 0.80 =	89
Detailed nursing facility follow-up visit	99313	82	× 0.80 =	66
Comprehensive initial home visit	99345	205	× 0.80 =	164
Detailed follow-up home visit	99349	114	× 0.80 =	91
Home-health certification	G0180	77	x 0.80 =	62
Care plan oversight	99375	131	× 0.80 =	105

NOTE: E&M = evaluation and management; CMS = Centers for Medicare and Medicaid Services.

* For physicians who participate in Medicare; amounts vary by location (see http://www.cms.hhs.gov/physicians/mpfsapp/ for local rates and annual updates).

** For eligible services provided by nurse practitioners, payment is 85% of the amount shown.

*** Hospital or nursing facility consultation.

physician services; in most cases, it would pay the hospital a prenegotiated lump sum or a per diem fee to cover all of her inpatient care. The amount of this lump sum would be determined by the diagnosis-related group (DRG) of her discharge diagnosis, in this case stroke. If the admitting hospital had no contract with her HMO, Mrs. Murat would probably be transferred to a hospital in the HMO's provider network as soon as she was medically stable. Depending on the HMO's benefit package, she might be responsible for copayments and deductibles for some of these services.

Fee for Service

If Mrs. Murat had retained traditional Medicare as her only health insurance, she would have to pay Medicare's required deductibles ($110 per year under Part B for the ambulance and the emergency medical care, plus $912 under Part A for the hospital admission) and co-insurance amounts (20% of Medicare's allowed charges by physicians and the ambulance service). She would also have to pay any ambulance charges in excess of Medicare's approved fee. If she had supplemented her Medicare coverage, her Medicaid or private medigap coverage would cover some of these deductibles and co-insurance payments. She would not be transferred to another hospital for insurance reasons.

The hospital would submit its claim for emergency and inpatient care, which would be based on the DRG of her discharge diagnosis, to Medicare's Part A regional intermediary insurance company. The involved physicians and the ambulance service would submit their E&M coded claims to Medicare's Part B regional insurance carrier. The intermediary and the carrier would pay their shares of these costs and, if Mrs. Murat had supplemental coverage, they would forward requests for payment of the balances to the state Medicaid program or her medigap insurance company. Ultimately, CMS would reimburse the intermediary from the Medicare Part A Trust Fund and the carrier from the Medicare Part B Trust Fund.

POSTACUTE REHABILITATION

After 4 days of stabilization, evaluation, and rehabilitation, Mrs. Murat is deemed stable enough for discharge from the acute-care hospital. She has improved somewhat, but she is still mildly hemiparetic and dysarthric, and she is apathetic and easily fatigued. Because her days in the hospital are fewer than the average number of hospital days associated with the DRG of her discharge diagnosis (ie, 5.9 days) and because her discharge diagnosis is one of those listed in Table 5.5, CMS regards her "early" discharge as a "transfer." This permits CMS to reduce the amount it pays the hospital for her care. The consulting neurologist advises her and her husband that her progress during the next few weeks will determine her potential for functional recovery. Mr. Murat asks the neurologist to recommend a rehabilitation facility for his wife.

Table 5.5—Primary Diagnoses for Which "Early" Discharges from Hospitals Are Regarded as "Transfers" to Postacute Care

Primary Diagnosis	DRG Number	Hospital Days, National Average
Degenerative nervous system disorders	12	8.1
Specific cerebrovascular disorders, except transient ischemic attack	14	5.9
Seizure and headache with complications and comorbidities	24	5.0
Seizure and headache without complications and comorbidities	25	3.2
Chronic obstructive pulmonary disease	88	5.1
Simple pneumonia and pleurisy with complications and comorbidities	89	6.0
Simple pneumonia and pleurisy without complications and comorbidities	90	4.1
Amputation for circulatory system disorders, except upper limb and toe	113	12.3
Circulatory disorders with acute myocardial infarction and major complications, discharged alive	121	6.4
Circulatory disorders with acute myocardial infarction without major complications, discharged alive	122	3.7
Heart failure and shock	127	5.3
Peripheral vascular disorders with complications and comorbidities	130	5.7
Peripheral vascular disorders without complications and comorbidities	131	4.2
Major joint and limb reattachment procedures for lower extremity	209	5.1
Hip and femur procedures except major joint with complications and comorbidities	210	6.8
Hip and femur procedures except major joint without complications and comorbidities	211	4.9
Fractures of hip and pelvis	236	5.2
Pathological fractures and musculoskeletal and connective tissue malignancy	239	6.3
Cellulitis with complications and comorbidities	277	5.7
Cellulitis without complications and comorbidities	278	4.3
Diabetes mellitus	294	4.6
Nutritional and miscellaneous metabolic disorders with complications and comorbidities	296	5.2
Nutritional and miscellaneous metabolic disorders without complications and comorbidities	297	3.4
Kidney and urinary tract infections with complications and comorbidities	320	5.3
Kidney and urinary tract infections without complications and comorbidities	321	3.8
Red blood cell disorders	395	4.4
Organic disturbances and mental retardation	429	10.0
Extensive operating room procedure unrelated to principal diagnosis	468	13.0
Tracheostomy for face, mouth, and neck diagnoses	483	39.6

NOTE: DRG = diagnosis-related group.

Managed Care

If she had joined the Medicare HMO, Mrs. Murat's insurance coverage would include postacute rehabilitative care, probably at a nursing home in the HMO's provider network rather than at a rehabilitation facility. Some nursing homes concentrate such high-acuity patients in transitional (or postacute) care units and provide them with coordinated rehabilitative (physical, occupational, and speech), social, and nursing services. Most homes, lacking such units, offer only custodial care supplemented by rehabilitative services as needed. The HMO would also cover the physician's postacute services, but the Murats may be responsible for a deductible and copayments.

Fee for Service

If Mrs. Murat could participate in rehabilitative therapy, Medicare Part A would pay for 20 days of postacute rehabilitation, in either a rehabilitation facility or a transitional (postacute) care unit of a nursing home. Upon her admission to either type of postacute care unit, rehabilitation professionals would evaluate Mrs. Murat's functional status, establish a plan for her care, and certify her as needing one of 26 levels of intensity of care according to the resource utilization group system (RUGS). Her RUGS category would determine the daily rate that Medicare Part A would pay the facility for the first 2 weeks of her care as long as she was demonstrating progress in rehabilitation.

After 2 weeks, a nurse would reevaluate her status, update her plan of care, and adjust her RUGS category and thereby adjust Medicare's payments to the facility for the next 2 weeks. Under this prospective payment system (PPS), the facility would be responsible not only for Mrs. Murat's nursing, rehabilitative, and social services, but also for the costs of her medications, laboratory tests, and visits to an emergency department not resulting in admission to the hospital.

Using nursing-home rates, Medicare Part B would pay 80% of the allowed charges for the postacute medical care provided by her physician. Any postacute care related to an inpatient surgical procedure would be the responsibility of the surgeon, who would receive a "global fee" to cover the surgery and all postoperative surgical care. The Murats would need to satisfy Medicare Part B's $110 annual deductible and then make 20% co-insurance payments for the physician's care. Their out-of-pocket expenses would be reduced or eliminated by any Medicare supplements in effect, such as Medicaid, medigap, or long-term-care coverage.

More than 3 million Americans have long-term-care insurance policies, but these policies pay for less than 2% of all nursing-home care. The high premiums for these policies, combined with consumers' uncertainty about needing long-term care in the future and their doubts about the policies' ability to cover the costs of long-term care in the future, have limited the growth of the long-term-care insurance sector. Many middle-aged Americans believe they will retain good health and independence into old age; they appear to be relying on a combination of good fortune, social insurance (ie, Medicaid), and their personal assets to see them through their later years. Those who are interested in long-term-care insurance can obtain information by reading "Choosing Long-Term Care: A Guide for People with Medicare" (CMS Publication No. 02223) or "A Shopper's Guide to Long-Term Care Insurance" (available from state insurance departments or the National Association of Insurance Commissioners, 2301 McGee St., Suite 800, Kansas City, MO 64108-3600).

HOME-HEALTH CARE

During the first 10 days of rehabilitative therapy, Mrs. Murat regains her ability to speak, and her left arm becomes stronger. During the following 8 days, however, she makes few additional gains. After 18 days, she is still unable to walk, cook, bathe, or dress herself without help. Her lack of continued progress toward functional independence will probably make her ineligible for coverage of additional rehabilitative services in either the HMO or the FFS Medicare program. The Murats will have to purchase any future physical therapy or occupational therapy on their own.

To obtain long-term care for her functional deficits, they will need to choose between a home-health agency and a custodial nursing home. If she returns home, neither the HMO nor the FFS Medicare program will be likely to pay for a home-health aide unless she is homebound and requires the services of a registered nurse or rehabilitation therapist. Local community agencies, however, may be able to offer assistance. The Murats' choice of a home-health agency could be informed by comparisons of their local agencies' recent clinical performance—available at Home Health Compare (http://www.medicare.gov/HHcompare/home.asp).

Managed Care

If Mrs. Murat's condition made her homebound and dependent on skilled professional services, her HMO probably would pay a home-health agency a fixed fee to provide her with the services and equipment necessary to treat her primary diagnosis. The HMO would also provide her with the services of a primary care physician.

Fee for Service

In the FFS environment, if Mrs. Murat were homebound and dependent on skilled professional services, the traditional Medicare Part A would pay any Medicare-certified home-health agency a fixed fee to provide her with the services and equipment necessary to treat her primary diagnosis. Medicare Part B would pay her primary care physician 80% of the allowed charges for house calls, office visits, and care plan oversight services. In addition, Medicare Part B will pay her physician for home-health certifications and recertifications. The Murats would be responsible for the annual Part B annual deductible ($110) and the 20% co-insurance payments, unless they had supplemental coverage through Medicaid, a medigap policy, or a long-term-care policy. (See also "Community-Based Care," p 125.)

PACE

If a health care organization in the area had contracted with CMS and the state Medicaid agency to create a Program for All-inclusive Care of the Elderly (PACE), it could provide community-based long-term care for "dually eligibles" (people eligible for both Medicare and Medicaid) whose disabilities qualified them for custodial care in a nursing home. (See also "Community-Based Care," p 125.) If she were eligible for Medicaid and she enrolled in PACE, Mrs. Murat would attend an adult day health care center several days each week and receive comprehensive outpatient, inpatient, acute, and long-term care from a salaried interdisciplinary team composed of a physician, a nurse, a social worker, rehabilitation therapists, and other members of the PACE staff.

Nursing-Home Care

Three months after Mrs. Murat returns home, Mr. Murat, now 84 years old, suffers a myocardial infarction and is no longer able to care for his wife at home. Their daughter logs on to Nursing Home Compare (http://www.medicare.gov/NHcompare/home.asp) to shop for a nursing home. After comparing the local facilities' nurse-to-resident ratios, results of recent quality-of-care inspections, and rates of pressure ulcers and behavior problems, she arranges for her mother to enter a high-quality nursing home in her neighborhood, at least until Mr. Murat recovers.

Managed Care

If Mrs. Murat had joined the Medicare HMO, one of the HMO's physicians would provide her primary care in the nursing home. Unless she was covered by Medicaid or a long-term-care policy, however, she and her husband would be responsible for the nursing home's per diem charges for room, board, and other basic services, usually about $100 per day. After "spending down" their savings at this rate, the Murats might become sufficiently impoverished to qualify, if they had not qualified previously, for Medicaid coverage. If the Murats owned their house, some states would put a lien on it in order to recover some of its payments to the nursing home when the house was eventually sold.

Fee for Service

The FFS Medicare program would pay 80% of the allowed charges submitted by her physician for visits to the nursing home. The Murats would be responsible for the annual Medicare Part B deductible ($110) and the 20% co-insurance payments. Medicare would not cover any of the nursing home's per diem charges.

Hospice Care

After residing in the nursing home for 6 months, Mrs. Murat suffers a massive stroke that leaves her physiologically stable, but in a persistent vegetative state.

Her husband reports that she had always said she would not want to go on living in such a condition if there were little hope of recovery. Although she is unable to swallow thin liquids, her husband says she would not want to be fed through any sort of tube. Her physician says that, with oral feeding, she is likely to live for several weeks. With the understanding that she will receive palliative care without life-prolonging interventions, her husband agrees to enroll her in a hospice program.

Enrollment in hospice would require the traditional FFS Medicare program (Part A) to pay a Medicare-certified hospice program a daily fee that would cover all care of her terminal diagnosis, including home care, medications, equipment, respite, counseling, and social services even if she had enrolled in (and remained in) the Medicare HMO.

If she had remained in the FFS Medicare program, Part B would pay her primary care physician, 80% of the allowed charges for home or office visits and care plan oversight services. Mr. Murat would be responsible for the 20% co-insurance and for small copayments for outpatient prescription medications, and respite care.

Changes in the Federal Financing of Health Care

The complex and evolving combinations of coverage and programs create difficult choices for older Americans and powerful incentives for the providers of their health care. The U.S. Congress and CMS continue to revise the Medicare program.

The Balanced Budget Act of 1997

In 1997 Congress passed, and President Bill Clinton signed, the Balanced Budget Act (BBA 97) through which they intended to limit future growth in the cost of the Medicare program, improve the quality of the health care it provides, and expand the number and variety of managed-care plans from which Medicare beneficiaries could choose. It authorized five types of "Medicare Plus Choice" (recently renamed "Medicare Advantage") plans:

- Medicare HMOs (IPA, group, or staff model)—insurance companies that accept capitation payments from CMS and provide or purchase Medicare-covered health services;

- Preferred provider organizations (PPOs)—alliances of providers that accept capitation payments and deliver Medicare-covered health services to their enrolled patients;

- Provider-sponsored organizations (PSOs)—partnerships of physician groups and hospitals that accept capitation payments and deliver Medicare-covered health services to their enrolled patients;

- Private FFS plans—plans that may charge beneficiaries a premium, pay providers more liberally than the original Medicare FFS program does, and allow physicians to charge their patients copayments of up to 15%;

- Medical savings accounts (MSAs)—accounts into which Medicare beneficiaries can make tax-deductible contributions and out of which they can withdraw funds to purchase routine health-related goods (including medications) and services (including long-term-care insurance) from any Medicare provider. Linked to the MSA is a catastrophic insurance policy that limits the individual beneficiary's expenses for health care to $6000 per year.

Perhaps because of the risks and uncertainties involved, very few PPOs, PSOs, private FFS insurance companies, or MSA providers have entered into Medicare Advantage contracts with CMS. Citing inadequate capitation payments and burdensome administrative requirements, many HMOs have withdrawn from the Medicare market, constricted their service areas (eliminating many rural counties), reduced the scope of the benefits they cover, and increased the premiums, deductibles, and copayments for which their enrollees are responsible. The total number of Medicare beneficiaries enrolled in Medicare Advantage plans declined from 6.4 million (17%) in 1999 to 4.6 million (11%) in 2003. As a result, nearly 2 million older Americans had to select new health plans and new health care providers. Between 2003 and 2005, the number of enrolled beneficiaries increased to 4.9 million.

Federal actuaries projected that BBA 97 would save the Medicare program $116 billion during 1998–2003 and extend the life of the Medicare Part A Trust Fund until 2023. The specific actions by which BBA 97 attempted to control costs include restricting Medicare benefits (eg, home care), reducing payments to providers (eg, hospitals and HMOs), and requiring CMS to begin risk-adjusting the capitation rates at which it paid managed-care plans.

CMS pays each managed-care plan a monthly county-specific capitation fee for each of its Medicare enrollees, an amount based on CMS's recent average adjusted per capita cost (AAPCC) for FFS Medicare beneficiaries in the county. The AAPCC amounts range from about $450 per month in many rural counties to more than $800 per month in some urban areas. Before BBA 97, the payment formulas adjusted these capitation amounts only for enrollees' age, sex, Medic-aid enrollment status (yes or no), and living situation (nursing home or independent residence). BBA 97 required that CMS also begin adjusting capitation amounts according to enrollees' risk of requiring expensive health care. This results in higher capitation payments for high-risk enrollees and lower payments for low-risk enrollees.

The current risk-adjustment method is based on the diagnoses associated with beneficiaries' health care during a recent 12-month period. If a hospital or outpatient provider designated as a reason for providing a health care service a diagnosis included in CMS's list of 61 "selected significant disease" groups, CMS would increase the amount of its capitation payment for that beneficiary during the following year. For example, if a beneficiary received care for heart failure during the 12 months from July 2004 to June 2005, CMS would adjust its capitation payments for the beneficiary during 2006 to provide the extra funds typically needed to care for people who have heart failure. In order to make this risk-adjustment system cost-neutral, CMS offsets the diagnosis-related increases in capitation payments by reducing its capitation payments for beneficiaries who have not received care for diagnoses in the 61 disease groups during this 12-month period. CMS is incorporating this risk-adjustment method into its formula for computing its capitation rates gradually over several years. In 2004, 30% of the capitation amounts were determined by diagnoses; during subsequent years, this percentage will increase to 100%.

BBA 97 provisions for improving the quality of health care for older Americans include:

- the Quality Improvement System for Managed Care (QISMC),

- the Healthcare Employers' Data Information System (HEDIS), which requires Medicare Advantage plans to monitor and report to CMS their rates of compliance with selected processes and outcomes of health care (eg, mammography and immunization against influenza),

- the Medicare Health Outcomes Survey, which requires Medicare Advantage plans to contract with third parties to survey a sample of their members and report information to CMS about their health status, functional ability, and satisfaction with their recent health care.

CMS summarizes the information generated by all three systems and makes it available at the Medicare Personal Plan Finder to help older Americans make informed choices about Medicare's FFS program and its various managed-care options.

Balanced Budget Revision Act of 1999

Within the first 18 months of the enactment of BBA 97, the quality of health care for older Americans began to erode, and the decreases in the payments to providers proved to be steeper than projected. For example, Medicare payments for home-health care decreased by 45% between 1997 and 1999. In response, Congress passed the Balanced Budget Revision Act at the end of 1999. This legislation restored some of the budget cuts made 2 years earlier, including $4.5 billion to Medicare Advantage plans.

Medicare Modernization Act of 2003

The contentious Medicare Prescription Drug Improvement and Modernization Act of 2003 required dramatic changes in the nature and scope of the Medicare program during the following years, including:

- The creation of an optional ("Medicare Part D") program covering prescription medications.
- Subsidies for employers who continue to provide their retirees with insurance that covers prescription medications.
- Elimination of coverage for prescription medications by Medicaid.
- Competition between traditional FFS Medicare and Medicare Advantage plans.
- Higher premiums for Medicare Part B to be paid by beneficiaries with higher incomes.
- Expanded coverage for preventive services.
- Increased reimbursement rates to physicians and hospitals in rural areas.

The results of this act will be determined by the specific programs that it spawns and by subsequent legislative and administrative reactions during the years after its enactment.

The Future of Medicare and Medicaid

CMS is now conducting dozens of demonstration projects designed to improve the quality and outcomes of care for beneficiaries with chronic conditions. In most of these demonstrations, CMS is paying provider and managed-care contractors capitated monthly fees for providing case management or disease management services to beneficiaries with specified chronic conditions, such as heart failure, diabetes mellitus, or other "special needs." Many of these demonstrations are based on the principle of "pay for performance," which stipulates that CMS will pay the capitation fees only to the extent that the contractor attains pre-agreed standards of performance, eg, performing certain diagnostic tests, reducing Medicare's overall FFS payments, and satisfying beneficiaries with the services they provide.

The aging of the baby-boom generation, technology-driven increases in health care spending, and a decline in the number of workers per Medicare beneficiary will contribute to serious financial challenges for the Medicare program in the years ahead. Similarly, imminent sharp increases in the number of older Americans with serious disabilities will soon surpass states' ability to pay for their long-term care. To meet these challenges, the nation needs visionary leaders, committed professionals, and rapid major changes in its systems for providing and paying for health care.

ANNOTATED REFERENCES

- American Geriatrics Society. Information on the Medicare Prescription Drug, Improvement, and Modernization Act 2003 (Public Law No: 108-173). Available at http://www.americangeriatrics.org/policy/medicare_info.shtml (accessed October 2005).

  This exhaustive resource describes the Medicare Modernization Act of 2003 and its implications for providers and beneficiaries.

- Centers for Medicare and Medicaid Services, Department of Health and Human Services. Medicare Modernization Act. Available at http://www.cms.hhs.gov/medicarereform (accessed October 2005).

  This is an informative, user-friendly Web site that provides a summary and the text of the Medicare Modernization Act of 2003, as well as periodic addenda that describe revisions to the act.

- Centers for Medicare and Medicaid Services, Department of Health and Human Services. *Medicare: Resident and New Physician Guide: Helping Health Professionals Navigate Medicare.* 7th ed. Rockville, MD: US Government Printing Office; 2003.

  This well-written handbook provides detailed information about most facets of the Medicare program.

- Emmer S, Allendorf L. The Medicare Prescription Drug, Improvement, and Modernization Act of 2003. *J Am Geriatr Soc.* 2004;52(6):1013–1015.

  This is a clear description of the major provisions and implications of the Medicare Modernization Act of 2003.

- Ettinger WH Jr. The Balanced Budget Act of 1997: implications for the practice of geriatric medicine. *J Am Geriatr Soc.* 1998;46(4):530–533.

  This article provides a succinct summary of the major provisions of the Balanced Budget Act of 1997, the most significant piece of federal health care legislation since the creation of Medicare and Medicaid in 1965. It defines the four new channels through which Congress authorized the Centers for Medicare and Medicaid Services to purchase health care for Medicare beneficiaries: provider-sponsored organizations, preferred provider organizations, private fee-for-service plans, and medical savings accounts. It also describes Medicare's new coverage of screening tests, telemedicine services, and care provided by geriatric nurse practitioners, physician assistants, and clinical nurse specialists.

■ Health Care Financing Administration. *2004 Guide to Health Insurance for People with Medicare.* Rockville, MD: US Government Printing Office; 2004. Pub. No. HCFA-02110. Available in regular and large print at http://www.Medicare.gov/publications/home.asp (accessed October 2005).

This well-written handbook provides detailed information about the coverage, the costs, and the purchase of Medicare supplemental (medigap) insurance policies. An introductory section describes the Medicare program and explains how different medigap policies fill its gaps in coverage. A "beyond the basics" section answers most questions about selecting and using medigap policies and lists telephone numbers, addresses, and a Web site for obtaining additional information.

■ Health Care Financing Administration. *Medicare and You 2005.* Rockville, MD: US Government Printing Office; 2004. Pub. No. HCFA-10050. Available in regular and large print at http://www.Medicare.gov/publications/home.asp (accessed October 2005).

This clear, easy-to-read booklet is intended to help older people use the Medicare program. It describes Medicare's structure, function, and covered services, and it gives sound advice about purchasing supplemental (medigap) insurance and joining Medicare Advantage plans. It also lists telephone numbers, addresses, and a Web site for obtaining more specific information about Medicare in any area of the country.

■ Medicare: The Official U.S. Government Site for People with Medicare. Available at http://www.medicare.gov (accessed October 2005).

This is an informative, user-friendly Web site that supplies consumers and professionals with extensive information about most aspects of the Medicare program. It provides detailed side-by-side comparisons of the available Medicare Advantage plans, medigap insurance policies, home-health care agencies, and nursing homes in each community in the United States.

Chad Boult, MD, MPH, MBA

APPROACH TO THE PATIENT

CHAPTER 6—ASSESSMENT

KEY POINTS

- Geriatric assessment is a multifaceted approach to the care of the older adult with the goal of promoting wellness and independent function.

- Assessment of function includes the physical, cognitive, psychologic, and social domains.

- Tools that are time efficient and valid are available to the clinician for use in a variety of settings to evaluate the older person's status in all these domains.

- Time tends to be a less important element than the skills of the clinician in facilitating successful communication with older patients.

Geriatric assessment is a multifaceted approach to the care of the older adult with the goal of promoting wellness and independent function. Function is defined broadly to encompass the physical, cognitive, psychologic, and social domains. The scope of the assessment of any individual domain depends on the site of care, the patient's level of frailty, time constraints, the goals of care, and the availability of a multidisciplinary team. The essential aspects of geriatric assessment should be performed routinely in all sites of care, whether the ambulatory setting, the emergency department, the hospital, the nursing home, or the home. Whenever possible, assessments should be performance based. An informant, ideally a caregiver or family member who lives with the patient, is often required to provide or to verify pertinent historical information about the older patient's day-to-day functioning.

THE ROUTINE OFFICE VISIT

Efficient strategies are required to incorporate geriatric assessment into routine office practice. One such strategy entails rapid screening of targeted areas (Table 6.1), followed by comprehensive assessment in areas of concern. Many of the initial screens can be completed by trained office staff; some can be completed by the patients themselves while seated in the waiting area or at home prior to the visit. The use of a "rolling" assessment, which targets at least one area for screening during each office visit, should be considered. Finally, in the absence of specific target symptoms, parts of the routine examination, such as auscultation of the chest and palpation of the abdomen, can be

Table 6.1—Rapid Screening Followed by Assessment and Management in Key Domains

Domain	Rapid Screen	Assessment and Management
Functional status	Answers "Yes" to one or more of the following: Because of a health or physical problem, do you need help to: (a) shop? (b) do light housework? (c) walk across a room? (d) take a bath or shower? (e) manage the household finances?	Assess all other activities of daily living listed in Table 6.3 Evaluate cognitive function and mobility using performance-based tests Assess social support Consider use of adaptive equipment
Mobility	"Timed Get Up and Go" test: unable to complete in less than 20 seconds	Treat underlying musculoskeletal or neurologic disorder Refer to physical therapy
Nutrition	Answers "Yes" to "Have you lost more than 10 lbs over the past 6 months without trying to do so?" OR body mass index $(kg/m^2) < 20$	See "Malnutrition," p 174
Vision	If unable to read a newspaper headline and sentence while wearing corrective lenses, test each eye with Snellen chart; unable to read greater than 20/40	See "Visual Impairment," p 149
Hearing	Unable to hear a 40-dB tone at 1000 or 2000 Hz in both ears or at either of these frequencies in one ear, as determined by use of a hand-held AudioScope	See "Hearing Impairment," p 155
Cognitive function	3-item recall: unable to remember all three items after 1 minute	Administer Folstein Mini–Mental State Examination
Depression	Answers "Yes" to "Do you often feel sad or depressed?"	Administer 15-item Geriatric Depression Scale (see the Appendix, p 496)

replaced by aspects of geriatric assessment, such as observation of gait, balance, and transfers.

PATIENT-CLINICIAN COMMUNICATION

Because of the demands of a busy clinical practice, the time available for office visits is often constrained. Time tends to be less important, however, than the skills of the clinician in facilitating communication with older patients. Table 6.2 lists several simple strategies that may be used to enhance communication. (See also the table on communication in "Hearing Impairment," p 159.) To accommodate the high prevalence of sensory deficits among older persons, particular attention should be given to the environment of the examination room. The use of simple, inexpensive amplification devices with lightweight earphones can be especially effective, even for the severely hearing-impaired person. During the course of the interview, the clinician should go beyond the customary clinical inquiries by asking open-ended questions such as, "What would you like me to do for you?" Finding out what the patient wants can be a prime mechanism for solving potential problems, generating trust, and improving mutual satisfaction in the patient-clinician relationship.

PHYSICAL ASSESSMENT

The importance of a full, appropriately detailed physical examination cannot be overstated. Many older adults cannot see well enough to report signs of disease or have cognitive impairment that prevents them from being able to accurately report symptoms. The clinician cannot assume that "no news is good news" in the care of older adults.

Functional Status

Functional status refers to the person's ability to perform tasks that are required for living. These tasks, usually referred to as activities of daily living (ADLs), are listed in Table 6.3. When assessing function, ask whether the patient is independent or requires the help of another person to complete the tasks. Bathing is typically the basic ADL with the highest prevalence of disability, and disability in bathing is often the reason why older persons receive home aide services. To identify patients with "preclinical" disability, that is, those who do not yet require personal assistance but who are at risk for becoming disabled, ask about perceived difficulty with the tasks and whether the

Table 6.2—Effective Strategies to Enhance Communication

- Use a well-lit room and avoid backlighting.
- Minimize extraneous noise and interruptions.
- Carefully introduce yourself to establish a friendly relationship.
- Face the patient directly, sitting at eye level.
- Address the patient by his or her last name.
- Speak slowly.
- Inquire about hearing deficits and raise the volume and lower the tone of your voice accordingly.
- If necessary, write questions in large print.
- Allow sufficient time for the patient to answer.
- Touch the patient gently on the hand, arm, or shoulder during the conversation.

Table 6.3—Activities of Daily Living

Self-care
Bathing	Toileting
Dressing	Grooming
Transferring from bed to chair	Feeding oneself

Instrumental
Using the telephone	Doing laundry
Preparing meals	Doing housework
Managing household finances	Shopping
Taking medications	Managing transportation

Mobility
Walking from room to room
Climbing a flight of stairs
Walking outside one's home

patient has changed the way he or she completes the task because of a health-related problem or condition. Assess the use of any assistive devices, such as a cane or walker, as well as duration and circumstances of use.

Outside of a rehabilitation setting, performance-based testing of most of the self-care and instrumental ADLs is not practical. Hence, performance-based testing of functional status focuses primarily on mobility, including transfers, gait, and balance. Ask the patient to stand from the seated position in a hard-backed chair while keeping his or her arms folded. Inability to complete this task suggests lower extremity, or quadriceps, weakness and is highly predictive of future disability. Once he or she is standing, observe the patient walk back and forth over a short distance, ideally with the usual walking aid. Abnormalities of gait include path deviation; diminished step height or length or both; trips, slips, or near falls; and difficulty with turning. The tasks of rising from the chair, walking 10 feet (3 meters), turning around and returning to the chair, turning, and then sitting back down in the chair make up the "Timed Get Up and Go" test. Persons who can complete this sequence of maneuvers in less than 10 seconds have intact mobility; those who take 20 seconds or longer require further evaluation.

An alternative assessment strategy is to measure gait speed as a predictor of future disability. A gait speed of 0.80 m per second allows for independent community ambulation; a speed of 0.60 m per second allows for community activity without the use of a wheelchair. These norms indicate that patients who can walk 50 feet in your office corridor in 20 seconds or less should be able to walk independently in normal activities.

Balance can be tested progressively by asking the patient to stand first with his or her feet side by side, then in semi-tandem position, and finally in tandem position. Difficulty with balance in these positions predicts an increased risk of falling. Although standardized instruments, such as the Tinetti Performance-Oriented Mobility Assessment, may be used to quantify impairments in gait and balance, a qualitative assessment is usually sufficient to make recommendations about the need for an assistive device, such as a cane or walker. When assessing gait and balance, particularly in older women, clinicians should observe for the use of proper footwear, that is, flat, hard-soled shoes. (Also see the Appendix, p 497, for falls-assessment guidelines.)

Finally, clinicians can often glean useful functional information by observing their older patients as they complete simple tasks, such as unbuttoning and buttoning a shirt or blouse, picking up a pen and writing a sentence, taking off and putting on shoes, touching the back of the head with both hands, and climbing up and down from an examination table.

Nutrition

Poor nutrition in the older person may reflect concurrent medical illness, depression, dementia, inability to shop or cook, inability to feed oneself, or financial hardship. Aside from visual inspection for signs of malnutrition, older persons should have their weight and height measured routinely. A low body mass index (ie, kg/m^2 < 20) or an unintentional weight loss of more than 10 pounds in 6 months suggests poor nutrition and requires further evaluation. (See "Malnutrition," p 174.)

Vision and Hearing

Although visual impairment from cataracts, glaucoma, macular degeneration, and abnormalities of accommodation usually worsens with age, older persons are often unaware of their visual deficits. Asking about difficulty with driving, watching television, or reading may uncover a problem with vision. As a brief performance-based screen, an older patient can be asked to read (using corrective lenses, if applicable) a short passage from a newspaper or magazine, with the caveat that low literacy is not an uncommon problem among older persons. Significant impairment in vision can be confirmed through the use of a Snellen chart or Jaeger card; the inability to read greater than 20/40 is the standard criterion. (See "Visual Impairment," p 149.)

The high prevalence of hearing loss among older persons and its association with depression, dissatisfaction with life, and withdrawal from social activities make it an important target for assessment. Hearing loss is usually bilateral and in the high-frequency range. Hearing should be assessed routinely during the history-taking session and can be assessed more formally using a hand-held AudioScope. Inability to hear a 40-dB tone at 1000 or 2000 Hz in both ears or at either of these frequencies in one ear is considered abnormal and, in the absence of cerumen impaction, warrants a discussion about referral for formal audiometric testing. (See "Hearing Impairment," p 155.)

COGNITIVE ASSESSMENT

The prevalence of cognitive decline doubles every 5 years after the age of 65 and approaches 40% to 50% at age 90. Most patients with dementia do not complain of memory loss or even volunteer symptoms of cognitive impairment unless specifically questioned. Older persons with cognitive impairment, even in the absence of dementia, are at increased risk for accidents, delirium, medical nonadherence, and disability. Therefore, an important feature of every assessment of an older adult, especially those aged 75 years and older, is a brief cognitive screen.

Because short-term memory loss is typically the first sign of dementia, the best single screening question is recall of three words after 1 minute. Anything other than perfect recall should lead to further testing. An alternative strategy adds orientation to day of the week, month, and year to the three memory items. A cut-off of three or more errors has a sensitivity and specificity of nearly 90% for a diagnosis of dementia. The most commonly used instrument for formal testing of cognition is the Folstein Mini–Mental State Examination (MMSE), which assesses orientation, registration and recall, attention and calculation, language, and visual-spatial skills. Although scores on the MMSE need to be interpreted in the context of educational attainment, race and age, scores lower than 24 generally warrant further evaluation for possible dementia.

An often overlooked area of cognition, which is essential for proper goal-directed behaviors, is executive function. The clock-drawing test is valuable because it assesses executive control and visual-spatial skills, two domains of cognition that are otherwise not tested or incompletely tested by the MMSE. In the clock-drawing test, the patient is asked to draw the face of a clock and to place the hands correctly to indicate 2:50 or 11:10. The clock-drawing test is combined with the three-item recall in the Mini-Cog Assessment Instrument for Dementia, a brief screening test that has been recently developed and validated. The Mini-Cog also has the advantage over the MMSE of being both very sensitive and specific when used with those patients whose native language is not English and those with less than a high school education.

Another useful question to assess executive function is asking the patient to name as many four-legged animals as possible in 1 minute. Fewer than 8 to 10 animals or repetition of the same animals is abnormal and suggests the need for further evaluation.

PSYCHOLOGIC ASSESSMENT

Although the prevalence of major depression among community-dwelling older persons is only about 1% to 2%, a large number of older persons suffer from significant symptoms of depression below the severity threshold of major depression as defined by the fourth edition of the *Diagnostic and Statistical Manual of Mental Disorders*. These subthreshold depressive symptoms, which often include somatic complaints such as poor sleep and fatigue, increase the risk of physical disability and slower recovery after an acute disabling event. They are also associated with a significant increase in the cost of medical services, even after accounting for the severity of chronic medical illness. Hence, clinicians should have a high index of suspicion for depressive symptoms and a low threshold for treatment. The best single question to ask is, "Do you often feel sad or depressed?" An affirmative response warrants further evaluation of other depressive symptoms, perhaps through the use of a standardized instrument such as the 15-item Geriatric Depression Scale (see the Appendix, p 496).

Anxiety and worries are also important symptoms in older patients and are often a manifestation of an underlying depressive disorder. Finally, because older persons are particularly likely to experience the loss of a loved one, special efforts should be made to recognize and manage the consequences of bereavement. (See "Depression and Other Mood Disorders," p 269.)

SOCIAL ASSESSMENT

The social assessment consists of several elements, including ethnic, spiritual, and cultural background, the availability of a personal support system, the need for a caregiver and his or her role, presence of caregiver burden, the safety of the home environment, the patient's economic well-being, the possibility of elder mistreatment, and the patient's advance directives. Although a comprehensive social assessment may not be feasible in a busy office practice, clinicians caring for older patients should be mindful of these aspects of an older patient's life. Some older persons, for example, may be illiterate, uneducated, or have a poor command of English, making it difficult for them to navigate through the complexities of the current health care system. Clinicians can uncover important clues to unmet needs by inquiring about the availability of help in case of an emergency. For frail older persons, particularly those who lack social support, referral to a visiting nurse may be helpful in assessing home safety and level of personal risk. (See "Psychosocial Issues," p 16, "Cultural Aspects of Care," p 51; "Elder Mistreatment," p 86.)

QUALITY OF LIFE

During the past decade, *quality of life* has been embraced as a convenient catchphrase to denote important patient outcomes other than death and traditional physiologic measures of morbidity. Although a gold standard does not exist, most instruments designed to measure quality of life include various aspects of physical, cognitive, psychologic, and social function. Perhaps the most commonly used instrument is the Short Form-36 Health Survey (SF-36), which includes 36 items organized into eight domains—physical function, role limitations due to physical health, role limitations due to emotional health, bodily pain, social functioning, mental health, vitality, and general health perceptions. The SF-36 has been tested extensively among community-living persons and hospitalized patients, but it may not be suitable for use among the oldest-old persons, especially those who are frail, because of floor effects and insensitivity to clinically important changes in health status.

When assessing quality of life, ask about patient preferences regarding medical care and goals of care. Goals can be multiple, diverse, and sometimes conflicting. There is striking heterogeneity among older patients with respect to physiologic function, health status, belief systems, cultural and ethnic backgrounds, values, and personal preferences. The successful management of chronic conditions, such as diabetes mellitus, arthritis, and heart failure, requires that patients, families, and clinicians work collaboratively to define the specific problems, to elicit personal preferences, and to establish the goals of care. A patient's cultural and ethnic heritage will have an important role in her understanding of her illness, its meaning in her life, and her response to it. It is crucial, therefore, for the physician to have an appreciation of that heritage and the role it plays in the patient's understanding of health and illness. (See "Cultural Aspects of Care," p 51.) Treatment plans that include patient preferences have been shown to enhance adherence and increase satisfaction, and they have the potential to improve patient outcomes.

ASSESSING THE OLDER DRIVER

Evaluating the older driver presents a difficult challenge to the physician. The automobile is the most important, and often the only, source of transportation for older persons. Yet a variety of age-related changes, chronic conditions, and medications place the older person at risk for automobile accidents. Although the absolute number of crashes involving older drivers is low, the number of crashes per mile driven and the likelihood of serious injury or death are higher than for any age group other than those aged 16 to 24 years.

To their credit, the vast majority of older persons make prudent adjustments in their driving behaviors by avoiding rush hour or congested thoroughfares or by not driving at night or during adverse weather conditions. Nonetheless, impaired older persons who continue to drive represent an important safety hazard not only to themselves but also to other drivers, passengers, and pedestrians. Pertinent risk factors for automobile accidents include poor visual acuity (less then 20/40) and contrast sensitivity; dementia, particularly deficits in visual-spatial skills and visual attention; impaired neck and trunk rotation; and poor motor coordination and speed of movement. Alcohol and medications that adversely affect alertness, such as narcotics, benzodiazepines, antihistamines, antidepressants, antipsychotics, sedatives, and muscle relaxants, may impair driving skills and increase crash risk. Hence, caution is warranted when initiating or adjusting the dose of these medications, and patients should be warned about potential adverse effects on driving safety.

Any report of an accident or moving violation should trigger an assessment of the patient's driving capacity. Discuss safety concerns honestly with the older driver, and ideally with a spouse or other family member as well, particularly when the patient lacks insight into his or her driving limitations. Alternative modes of transportation should be considered. Recommendations to stop driving, however, should not be proffered lightly, since driving cessation can lead to a decrease in activity level and an increase in depressive symptoms. Referral for a formal driving evaluation by a skilled occupational therapist may be helpful in confirming unsafe driving behaviors or, perhaps, in suggesting interventions such as adaptive equipment to correct for specific physical disabilities. In the interest of public safety, physicians should know their state's law on reporting impaired drivers. In most states, physicians are encouraged, and in some states mandated, to report their concerns to the licensing agency. (See also the section on driving in "Legal and Ethical Issues," p 30.) An excellent reference for physicians caring for older drivers is *The Physician's Guide to Assessing and Counseling Older Drivers*. Developed by the American Medical Association in cooperation with the National Highway Traffic Safety Administration, it was recently made available free of charge. Visit the Web site: http://www.ama-assn.org/ama/pub/category/10791.html to view the publication, download it, or order a printed copy.

COMPREHENSIVE GERIATRIC ASSESSMENT

Comprehensive geriatric assessment (CGA) is a process intended to determine a patient's medical, psychosocial, and functional capabilities and limitations, with the goal of developing an overall plan for treatment and long-term follow-up. Because CGA typically requires a highly trained team of geriatricians, geriatric nurse clinicians, physical and occupational therapists, geriatric psychiatrists, and social workers, it is expensive and time consuming. Success generally requires the geriatric team to take over the direct care of the patient. An extended period of intensive team involvement with ongoing care is essential to assure the efficacy of the intervention. When the geriatric team assumes a purely consultative role (ie, without a role in implementing the recommendations), CGA is unlikely to be successful in improving patient outcomes.

CGA has had its greatest success in terms of improving function and reducing nursing-home placement and hospital readmissions, in inpatient geriatric units that are staffed by highly trained professionals. Accumulating evidence, however, suggests that preventive home visitation programs may also be beneficial. A meta-analysis of randomized trials demonstrated that these programs decrease nursing-home admissions and reduce functional decline if the interventions are based on comprehensive geriatric assessment with extended follow-up, include multiple follow-up home visits, and target persons at lower risk for death.

ANNOTATED REFERENCES

■ Cohen HJ, Feussner JR, Weinberger M, et al. A controlled trial of inpatient and outpatient geriatric evaluation and management. *N Engl J Med.* 2002;346(12):905–912.

This landmark clinical trial evaluated the effectiveness of geriatric evaluation and management in outpatient clinics and inpatient units among nearly 1400 predominantly male patients, aged 65 years or older, who were seen at 11 Veterans

Affairs medical centers and had at least two potential markers of frailty. The results revealed modest but significant benefits of the geriatric evaluation and management inpatient units on basic activities of daily living, physical performance, and four domains of quality of life. In contrast, the outpatient geriatric clinics offered relatively little benefit. There was no improvement in survival related to either inpatient or outpatient geriatric evaluation and management. Over the course of a year, the two programs were cost-neutral relative to usual care. The investigators speculate that improvements in usual care over the past two decades could account for the absence of a survival benefit, which had been documented in two prior single-site trials.

■ Fried LP, Tangen CM, Walston J, et al. Frailty in older adults: evidence for a phenotype. *J Gerontol A Biol Sci Med Sci.* 2001;56(3):M146−M156.

Increasingly, frailty is recognized as a geriatric syndrome, distinct from disability and comorbidity, which results from a multisystem reduction in reserve capacity and confers high risk for adverse outcomes. The investigators of this report developed an operational definition (or "phenotype") of frailty that is based on the presence of three or more of the following criteria: unintentional weight loss, self-reported exhaustion, weakness, low physical activity, and slow gait speed. Using data from the Cardiovascular Health Study, the investigators provide preliminary evidence to support the predictive validity of the proposed phenotype. If further validated in subsequent studies, the standardized phenotype could be a valuable tool for clinicians to identify and manage affected individuals and for researchers to evaluate the consequences and causes of frailty.

■ Gill TM, Kurland B. The burden and patterns of disability in activities of daily living among community-living older persons. *J Gerontol A Biol Sci Med Sci.* 2003; 58:70−75.

In this longitudinal study, the investigators interviewed 754 nondisabled community-living persons aged 70 years or older monthly for 2 years to determine the presence and severity of disability in four key activities of daily living: bathing, dressing, walking, and transferring. The investigators found that disability is a dynamic process with considerable diversity, particularly among persons who are physically frail by virtue of slow gait speed. For example, 42% of nondecedents who were physically frail had multiple months or episodes of disability over 2 years, with no single pattern representing the disability experience of more than half the participants. These findings provide strong evidence to support an emerging paradigm of disability as a reversible, and often recurrent, event.

■ Mouton CP, Esparza YB. Ethnicity and geriatric assessment. In: Gallo JJ, Fulmer T, Paveza GJ, et al., eds. *Handbook of Geriatric Assessment.* 3rd ed. Gaithersburg, MD: Aspen Publishers, Inc., 2000:13−27.

As the U.S. population of older persons becomes increasingly diverse in terms of ethnicity and race, clinicians must become better attuned to cultural factors that may influence assessment, such as educational attainment, language, and attitudes about illness and treatment. This informative chapter discusses ways that geriatric assessment can be modified for patients from diverse ethnic groups. The authors discuss several general issues, including the heterogeneity of ethnic groups; the reliability, validity, and use of assessment instruments; strategies to enhance communication; and the elicitation of beliefs and attitudes about illness. They focus on culturally competent assessment in relation to physical function, cognitive impairment, depression, social and economic issues, and ethics in medical decision making.

■ Smeeth L, Fletcher AE, Stirling S, et al. Randomised comparison of three methods of administering a screening questionnaire to elderly people: findings from the MRC trial of the assessment and management of older people in the community. *BMJ.* 2001;323(7326):1403−1407.

In this remarkable study set in the United Kingdom, the investigators compared three different methods of administering a screening questionnaire to a sample of nearly 33,000 persons aged 75 years or older, using a randomized design. The response rate was significantly higher for the postal questionnaire (83.5%) than for face-to-face interviews by a lay interviewer (73.9%) or nurse (75.9%). The proportion of missing or invalid responses was low overall (2.1%), but was greater for the postal questionnaire than for the other two methods. Counterintuitively, the specificity of the screening questions was higher than the sensitivity for vision, hearing, depression, and cognition, although the values differed little by mode of administration. Although the ongoing randomized trial will ultimately determine whether health outcomes differ by screening method, the results of this report provide strong evidence to support the use of a postal questionnaire as a feasible, efficient strategy to identify potentially modifiable impairments, problems, and conditions in a defined population of older persons.

■ Studenski S, Perera S, Wallace D, et al. Physical performance measures in the clinical setting. *J Am Geriatr Soc.* 2003;51(3):314−322.

Several epidemiologic studies have demonstrated that simple tests of physical performance are effective at stratifying risk for functional decline, health care utilization, and death among large, population-based samples of community-living older persons. In this prospective cohort study, evidence is provided to support the utility of physical performance tests in the primary care setting. Gait speed alone and a composite measure of physical performance, which included gait speed, chair stands, and progressive balance, predicted hospitalization and decline in function and health status over 12 months among persons aged 65 year or older in two outpatient settings. These results, coupled with those of prior studies, provide strong support for the use of performance-based tests as geriatric "vital signs" in everyday clinical practice.

Thomas M. Gill, MD

CHAPTER 7—CULTURAL ASPECTS OF CARE

KEY POINTS

- Cultural competence is a nuanced understanding of the role of culture in our lives.
- The culturally astute clinician remains alert to the differences among individual patients from a given culture and guards against stereotyping on the basis of ethnic or cultural affiliation.
- Communication and clinical care are enhanced when the patient and provider make an effort to negotiate a common understanding of causation, diagnosis, and treatment while maintaining respect for the beliefs and constructs of both individuals.

As the cultural diversity of older Americans continues to grow, it will become increasingly important for clinicians caring for older adults to develop an approach to working with older adults from a broad range of cultural groups. The purpose of this chapter is to assist clinicians in developing and improving their skills during intercultural patient encounters. The chapter also appears in volume 1 of *Doorway Thoughts,* published by the American Geriatrics Society (see the annotated references at the end of the chapter). Other chapters in *Doorway Thoughts* demonstrate how the general approach outlined here in each topic relates to working with patients in seven specific minority cultural groups. It is very important to keep in mind when using *Doorway Thoughts* that although the cultural information offered in each chapter is accurate *in general,* the beliefs, traditions, customs and preferences of individuals in all cultural groups vary widely. The astute clinician *never* assumes that any person's cultural background dictates his or her health choices or behavior. The culturally literate clinician remains alert to the differences among individual patients and families from a given culture and on guard against stereotyping an older person on the basis of his or her ethnic or cultural affiliation.

DOORWAY THOUGHTS IN CROSS-CULTURAL HEALTH CARE

The key concepts discussed in this chapter are "doorway thoughts"—factors that the culturally competent practitioner reflects upon before walking through the doorway of any examining, consultation, or hospital room. These factors can shape intercultural health care encounters and relationships for good or for ill. Cultural and historical facts and issues relating to the members of an entire minority group can be in play in any cross-cultural encounter or relationship. The practitioner should be sensitive to the possibility that they may affect their relations with individual patients and families and may also affect patients' willingness or ability to understand, accept, and adhere to prescribed regimens.

The quality of any encounter between a clinician and a patient from different ethnic or cultural backgrounds depends on the clinician's skill and sensitivity. Questions about the individual patient's attitudes and beliefs should be worked naturally and carefully into the clinical interview. The clinician must remember that no culture is monolithic; attitudes and beliefs vary widely from one individual to another within a single cultural group. Prior familiarity with a patient's cultural background will not suffice, for it is inaccurate to assume that a person's outlook is inflexibly determined by his or her cultural heritage. The concepts presented here are intended to serve as guides in choosing appropriate questions, and not as a rigid list of cultural attributes or clinical scenarios.

PREFERRED TERMS FOR CULTURAL IDENTITY

The terms referring to specific cultural or ethnic groups can change over time, and individuals in any one group do not always agree on the terminology that is appropriate. It is important to learn what the individual patient's preferred term is for his or her cultural identity and to use that terminology in conversation with the patient, as well as in his or her health records.

FORMALITY

Attitudes regarding the appropriate degree of formality in a health care encounter differ widely among cultural groups. Learning what a new patient's preferences are with regard to formality and allowing that preference to shape the relationship is always advisable. Initially, a more formal approach is likely to be appropriate.

Addressing the Patient

The patient's correct title (eg, Dr., Reverend, Mr., Mrs., Ms, Miss) and his or her surname should be used unless and until he or she requests a more casual form of address. Another important issue is to determine the correct pronunciation of the person's name.

Addressing the Health Provider

It is also important to learn how the patient would prefer to address the clinician and to allow his or her preference to prevail. For example, in some cultures, trust in the physician depends on his or her assuming an authoritative role, and informality would undermine the patient's trust. This is an aspect of the clinical relationship where the clinician's personal preferences can be relinquished.

LANGUAGE AND LITERACY

- What language does this individual feel most comfortable speaking? Will a medical interpreter be needed?
- Does this patient read and write English? Another primary language? If so, which one(s)?
- If the patient is not literate, does he or she have access to someone who can assist at home with written instructions?

It is worthwhile to consider these questions early in the health care relationship to determine whether interpretation services are needed and to make certain that communication with the patient is effective. Even those who use English fluently may wish to discuss complicated issues in their native language. It is the clinician's responsibility to explain medical terms and to ask the patient for explanations of any cultural or foreign terms that are unfamiliar.

RESPECTFUL NONVERBAL COMMUNICATION

Body position and motion is interpreted differently from one cultural group to another. Specific hand gestures, facial expression, physical contact, and eye contact can hold different meanings for the patient and the clinician when their cultural backgrounds differ. The clinician should watch for particular body language cues that appear to be significant and that might be linked to cultural norms that are important to the patient, in order to cultivate sensitivity to the conditions that make the flow of communication feel easy and effective.

Conservative body language is an advisable choice early in a relationship with a patient or when in doubt about a patient's background or preferences; assume a calm demeanor, avoid expressive extremes such as very vigorous handshakes, a loud and hearty voice, many hand gestures or, on the other hand, an impassive facial expression, avoidance of eye contact, standing at a distance. Remain alert for signals that the person is comfortable or uncomfortable. Directly asking the

patient questions about body language may also help. It is very important to avoid making negative judgments about a patient that are rooted in unconscious cultural assumptions about the meaning of his or her gestures, facial expressions, or body language.

The distance from others that individuals find comfortable varies, depending in part on their cultural background. The clinician should determine what distance seems to be the most comfortable for each patient and, whenever practicable, allow the patient's preference to establish the optimal distance during the encounter.

ELEPHANTS IN THE ROOM

Are there any issues that are critical to the success of the health care encounter that are present but that go unspoken? Remain alert for the possibility that such issues are indeed present. Examples include

- a lack of trust in health care providers and the health care system,
- a fear of medical research and experimentation,
- fear of medications or their side effects, and
- unfamiliarity or discomfort with the Western biomedical belief system.

In general, sensitivity to the possibility that such issues are in play is advised in all intercultural patient encounters.

HISTORY OF TRAUMATIC EXPERIENCES

Is the patient a refugee or survivor of violence or genocide? Are family members missing or dead? Have patients or family members been tortured? Such experiences could negatively affect the health care encounter without the clinician's knowledge unless relevant questions are included among standard questions about the patient's history.

It is important for clinicians to remember that in some historical periods and jurisdictions, health care providers have participated in torture and genocide. For example, during World War II, Nazi medical personnel were responsible in concentration camps for selecting individuals for gassing, supervising the gassing process, and administering lethal injections to inmates in "hospitals." The methods and tools of torture employed have sometimes resembled legitimate clinical procedures and tools. Patients who have survived such experiences may not feel safe in medical or governmental settings, and contact with all clinicians may invoke feelings of vulnerability, fear, panic, or anger. Great sensitivity is necessary in providing health care for these individuals.

ISSUES OF IMMIGRATION

Immigration Status

Some individuals may be residing in North America without the protection of appropriate immigration documents. Clinicians may wish to assure each patient that information given within the medical encounter will be kept in the strictest confidence.

History of Immigration or Migration

The history of the movements of a whole ethnic or cultural group can affect the attitudes and behavior of an individual in that group even when he or she has not immigrated to North America from another country. In addition, understanding the specific migration history of a person often provides insight into the key life transitions informing his or her outlook. Knowing how a person came to reside in North America can be important. The time and effort the clinician invests in learning more about a minority group's history and current situation can be repaid not only in a better relationship with the individual patient but also in an enhanced appreciation of the factors affecting clinical relationships with all patients from that group.

ACCULTURATION

Acculturation is defined as a process in which members of one cultural group adopt the beliefs and behaviors of another group. Acculturation of a group may be evidenced by changes in language preference, adoption of common attitudes and values, and gradual loss of separate ethnic identification. Although acculturation typically occurs when a minority group adopts the habits and language patterns of a dominant group, acculturation may also be reciprocal between groups.

It is essential to keep principles of acculturation in mind during any intercultural health encounter. Begin by determining how long a person has lived in North America and whether he or she was born here. However, remember that the degree to which the person is acculturated to Western customs and attitudes is the consequence of many factors, and not just of the number of years since he or she immigrated. Older adults who follow the traditions of their cultural group may have been born outside of the United States or Canada, may be recent arrivals to the continent, or may even be lifelong North American residents.

A patient's level of acculturation may greatly impact not only his or her health behavior but also preferences in end-of-life planning and decision making. Acculturation can also be an issue dividing family members, and a person's resistance to or ease of acculturation may be a matter of pride or shame and guilt. Developing sensitivity about the issues of acculturation for one's older minority patients is a key element in effective intercultural health care. Asking patients directly about their adherence to cultural traditions can be useful.

TRADITION AND HEALTH BELIEFS

People from non-Western cultural groups may not conceive of illness in Western terms. Some may have highly developed concepts of the causes of health and disease that are incompatible with the concepts that form the foundations of Western medicine. Non-Western paradigms include beliefs that illnesses have spiritual causation or are the result of imbalance among bodily humors, or that they are caused by a person's actions in past lives, to name but a few.

Patients may be making unexamined assumptions that are based on traditional beliefs, and these can cause confusion or create misunderstanding. The more the clinician knows about specific traditions, the more he or she can avoid such problems.

In addition, patients holding traditional beliefs may be using alternative remedies (eg, rituals, herbal preparations) that they do not mention, and questions about such practices should be included among other questions about the patient's history. It is unrealistic to expect that a patient will simply "adapt" to Western approaches to health and health care, just as it is impractical to expect the clinician to accept a new paradigm of wellness and disease. Clinical communication and efficacy will be enhanced when patients and providers make an effort to negotiate a common understanding of causation, diagnosis, and treatment for a specific health problem while maintaining respect for the beliefs and constructs of both individuals.

ATTITUDES TOWARD NORTH AMERICAN HEALTH SERVICES

Some minority patients may not feel comfortable in customary North American health care settings. Explanations for the discomfort, distrust, or uneasiness of some include lack of familiarity with Western practices, dissatisfying previous encounters with the health care system, or the belief that insensitivity or discrimination is inevitable for anyone in the cultural or ethnic group. Such feelings may result from having been stereotyped or treated insensitively or even unfairly by clinicians in the past. Sensitive exploration of these issues with patients is often both worthwhile and necessary. Generally, the clinician meeting a new patient from an ethnic or cultural minority group should be alert for signs of guardedness that signal an underlying lack of comfort or trust.

CULTURE-SPECIFIC HEALTH RISKS

Epidemiologic and medical research has identified numerous differences among ethnic and cultural populations with regard to specific health risks. The clinician who treats many patients from a specific group is advised to make every effort to stay abreast of the latest findings in relevant areas.

APPROACHES TO DECISION MAKING

The influence of specific cultures on approaches to health decision making has been the subject of many studies. Western bioethics emphasize individual autonomy in all health decisions, but for many other cultures, decision making is family or community centered. Autonomy principles allow competent persons to involve others in their health decisions or to cede those rights to a proxy decision maker. The clinician should ask patients if they prefer to make their own health decisions or if they would prefer to involve or defer to others into the decision-making process. Some may wish to assign the decision-making authority wholly to another individual or a group. In some cultures, the definition of family may include fictive kin. In families where the degree of acculturation of the generations differs, the older person may defer to or depend on younger relatives, even though the tradition might suggest that the reverse would occur.

Establishing an understanding of each patient's decision-making preferences early in the clinical relationship will, in most instances, promote better communication and avoid the difficulties inherent in trying to address the issues at a time of crisis. When the patient's and clinician's cultural backgrounds differ, careful exploration of the issues is all the more important because the clinician cannot proceed as if he or she and the patient are starting from common assumptions.

ATTITUDES REGARDING DISCLOSURE AND CONSENT

Cultural attitudes toward truth telling and disclosure of terminal diagnoses vary widely. In some cultures, it is commonly believed that patients should not be informed of a terminal diagnosis, as this may be injurious to health or hasten death. Obtaining informed consent from patients with this belief may prove to be difficult.

There is no consensus in bioethics concerning the rigorous application of full clinical disclosure in every situation. However, it is generally agreed that incorporating a patient's beliefs concerning disclosure and truth telling into clinical planning whenever possible is desirable. Some patients may prefer not to know if they are terminally ill and ask that family members or other caregivers receive all diagnostic information and make all treatment decisions. It is advisable to explore each patient's preferences regarding disclosure of serious clinical findings early in the clinical relationship and to reconfirm these wishes at intervals.

GENDER ISSUES

Each culture has intricate traditions and structures with regard to gender roles. Societies seemingly based on the same patriarchal or matriarchal model may vary widely in their expressions of the model. A person's gender influences the sorts of experiences he or she has had, not only within the family but in the community and health care system as well. Another level of complexity may be added to health care encounters when an older adult's group struggles with conflicting traditional and contemporary views on gender roles. Cultural norms for men and women can profoundly influence their health behavior, and these norms for the genders vary widely from one culture to another. These norms also affect decision making, disclosure, and consent.

It is highly advisable for the clinician to explore each patient's attitudes regarding the interplay among gender, autonomy, and personal decision making early in the patient-provider relationship, to confirm his or her preferences at intervals, and to follow the individual patient's wishes whenever possible.

END-OF-LIFE DECISION MAKING AND CARE INTENSITY

Culture is an important influence in a person's formation of his or her attitudes toward supportable quality of life, approach to suffering, and beliefs about medical feeding, life-prolonging treatments, and palliative care. Some cultures value a direct struggle for life in the face of death, and both patients and families will expect an intensive approach to treatment. Other cultures ardently avoid direct confrontation of death and dying and will prefer to leave such decisions to the clinician. Still others will take a direct approach to death and dying but will reject too aggressive an approach.

Research has shown that physicians and patients from shared cultural backgrounds have similar values in these areas; the implications of such findings for clinicians and patients from differing backgrounds are obviously important. Both physicians and patients bring their own attitudes and beliefs to any clinical encounter. It is important for clinicians to be aware of their personal views and cultural set when discussing end-of-life plans with patients and to respect patients' beliefs and preferences even when they are different from their own.

In negotiating end-of-life decisions with a patient whose background is different from his or her own, the clinician must listen especially carefully to the patient's goals and concerns and exert every effort to avoid making culture-based assumptions that do not apply. For example, the assumption that "no one would want to live in that condition" or that "everyone would want treatment in this situation" is likely to be faulty. To ensure that end-of-life plans and decisions reflect an individual's rights and wishes, the clinician must strive to understand the older person's overall approach to life and death, and as far as possible provide care that is congruent with that approach.

ATTITUDES TOWARD ADVANCE DIRECTIVES

The use of advance directives and health care proxies has become more common on the past 20 years, but research indicates that the use of written directives may be more common among older persons in the dominant North American culture than among older persons in minority cultural groups. It is advisable in intercultural situations, when discussing attitudes and beliefs regarding written directives with a patient, to be sensitive to the possibility that some minority older persons will prefer to use alternatives—verbal directives or directives dictated to family members or others— and others will need to avoid any such discussion so as to observe proscriptions against talking about death. In view of the fact that preferences for care intensity may also differ according to cultural background, patients should also be given the opportunity to indicate the interventions they do want as well as those they do not want in any written or verbal directive used.

CULTURAL COMPETENCE: A FINAL WORD

There is no gold standard definition of cultural competence. Most definitions emphasize a careful coordination of individual behavior, organizational policy, and system design to facilitate mutually respectful and effective cross-cultural interactions.

Cultural competence combines attitudes, knowledge base, acquired skills, and behavior. It is an approach, not a technique. Cultural competence is not a form of "political correctness." Ideally, it is a nuanced understanding of the determining role that culture plays in all of our lives and of the impact culture has on every health care encounter, for both the clinician and the patient.

Cultural competence cannot be achieved exclusively by reading, but we hope that this chapter will provide clinicians who care for older persons from all minority groups with basic information and a foundation for further investigation. We would encourage clinicians to view each intercultural encounter as an opportunity to learn more, not only about the individual patient and his or her culture, but also about themselves. We also recommend that clinicians learn more about the impact of culture on health decisions by reading the publications listed in the annotated references, exploring available Web sites, and attending workshops. We also urge clinicians to work with the entire interdisciplinary health care team, including administrators, to promote cultural competence in the health care organizations where they practice. Finally, we encourage clinician educators to develop their own teaching materials and educational programs designed to meet the needs of specific communities.

ANNOTATED REFERENCES

■ American Geriatrics Society, Adler R, Kamel H. *Doorway Thoughts: Cross-Cultural Health Care for Older Adults*. Vol. 1. Boston, MA: Jones and Bartlett; 2004.

> This book addresses the health care issues raised by the increasingly multicultural state of North American society. It focuses on the ways clinicians who care for older adults can develop an understanding of various ethnic and cultural groups that will enhance their ability to care for older minority patients. Chapters address the cross-cultural health care issues that relate to all older patients as well as to those from the following groups: African Americans, American Indians and Alaska Natives, Asian Indian Americans, Chinese Americans, Hispanic Americans, Japanese Americans, and Vietnamese Americans. Volume 2 in the series, to appear in 2006, contains chapters on Arab Americans, Cambodian Americans, Filipino Americans, Haitian Americans, Korean Americans, Pakistani Americans, Portuguese Americans, and Russian Americans.

■ Blackhall LJ, Murphy ST, Frank G, et al. Ethnicity and attitudes toward patient autonomy. *JAMA*. 1995;274(10):820–825.

> This influential paper was the first of its kind in the medical literature to report the findings of a survey conducted with 200 older persons from specific ethnic groups in Los Angeles, California. Study data revealed that Korean Americans and Mexican Americans were far less likely than European Americans or black Americans to believe that a patient should be told of a terminal prognosis or make decisions regarding end-of-life treatment and that they were more likely than other groups to believe that family members should receive information and make health decisions for older relatives facing illness with a grave prognosis.

- Bowman KW, Singer PA. Chinese seniors' perspectives on end-of-life decisions. *Soc Sci Med*. 2001; 53(4):455–464.

   This study draws on data from semi-structured interviews with 40 Chinese adults over 64 years of age living in Toronto. Study participants had low acculturation as measured on the Marin Acculturation scale. Many expressed beliefs that the future is preordained and held indifferent or negative attitudes toward the use of advance directives. Respondents expressed the opinion that advance care planning should be avoided in order to prevent distress. Most believed that they would not want life-sustaining treatment if terminally ill, citing a wish neither to suffer personally nor to inflict suffering on family. They stressed the importance of family consensus in decisions regarding end-of-life treatments. These findings have broad implications for practice, pointing to the potential limitations of the use of advance directives or single proxy decision makers when working with this population of older adults.

- Cykert S, Joines JD, Kissling G, et al. Racial differences in patients' perceptions of debilitated health states. *J Gen Intern Med*. 1999;14(4):217–222.

   This study compares self-reported perceptions of debilitated health states of European and African Americans. Sixty-four consecutive patients (ages 50 to 75) who met criteria for breathing impairment were surveyed in a community hospital pulmonary medicine clinic while awaiting appointments. The measurements of interest were individuals' strengths of preference for a range of theoretical limitations in physical function. In multivariate analysis, self-identified African American cultural background was found to be the only predictor of high acceptance of bed-to-chair limitation and permanent facility placement. These results suggest that attitudes and values should be explored carefully when crafting health care plans for older adults facing severe limitations.

- Vydelingum V. South Asian patients' live experience of acute care in an English hospital: a phenomenological study. *J Adv Nurs*. 2000;32(1):100–107.

   This qualitative investigation explored the experience of individuals of South Asian descent from a variety of religious and cultural backgrounds while hospitalized for 6 days or more on acute-care units. All participants were born outside of the United Kingdom. Key findings include extreme patient loneliness and isolation (significantly exacerbated by language barriers), covert practice of religious and cultural rituals (so as not to alienate staff and fellow patients of European descent), mismatched dietary choices (eg, for vegetarians and Muslims requiring halal meats), and dissatisfaction with information exchange and arrangements at discharge.

Reva N. Adler, MD, MPH

CHAPTER 8—PHYSICAL ACTIVITY

KEY POINTS

- Promoting physical activity is one of the most important and effective preventive and therapeutic interventions in older adults.

- The health benefits of physical activity accrue independently of other risk factors and are generally proportional to the amount of physical activity.

- Clinical guidelines identify a role for physical activity in the management of numerous conditions, including cardiovascular and chronic lung disease, diabetes mellitus, hypertension, obesity, osteoporosis, knee osteoarthritis, and falls.

- Adults should engage in a brisk walk, or an equivalently intense aerobic activity, for at least 10 minutes at a time, for a total of at least 30 minutes a day, on at least 5 days a week.

- A useful clinical approach to promoting physical activity is to adopt the 5-A framework (assess, advise, agree, assist, and arrange).

Physical activity is defined as bodily movement produced by skeletal muscles that expend energy. Exercise is a subset of physical activity that involves a structured program designed to improve one or more components of physical fitness. The primary attributes of physical activity are type (mode), frequency, duration, and intensity. Promoting physical activity is one of the most important and effective preventive and therapeutic interventions in older adults. There is conclusive evidence that regular aerobic activity has large health benefits. Resistance training and balance training also have important health benefits in older adults. Flexibility training is important for maintaining the range of motion required to do physical activities.

PREVENTIVE HEALTH EFFECTS

Regular physical activity has beneficial effects on most, if not all, organ systems. Consequently, it prevents a large number of diseases. Physical activity reduces the risk of cardiovascular disease, high blood pressure, stroke, some lipid disorders, non-insulin-dependent diabetes mellitus, obesity, osteoporosis, colon cancer, and breast cancer. There is substantial evidence that physical activity also reduces the risk of fall injuries, sarcopenia, depression, and anxiety disorders. There is some evidence that physical activity reduces the risk of sleep problems, cognitive impairment, osteoarthritis, and back pain.

Consistent with its broad physiologic effects, regular physical activity decreases both cardiovascular and noncardiovascular mortality in older adults. The mortality benefit is large. Some studies report that inactive adults have mortality rates that are twice as high as those of active adults.

Observational studies consistently report that regular physical activity substantially delays the onset of functional limitations and loss of independence (disability). For example, an analysis of Established Population for Epidemiologic Studies of the Elderly (EPESE) data showed that inactive, nonsmoking women at age 65 have 12.7 years of active life expectancy, compared with 18.4 years of active life expectancy for highly active women. Higher levels of physical activity are associated with fewer years of disability preceding death.

The health benefits of physical activity accrue independently of other risk factors. For example, sedentary overweight smokers experience health benefits from increasing physical activity, even if they continue to smoke and do not lose weight.

The health benefits of physical activity are generally proportional to the amount of physical activity. When activity is performed above minimum thresholds for frequency, duration, and intensity, health benefit depends mainly upon the volume (energy expenditure) of aerobic activity. The dose-response relationship between physical activity and disease risk varies by disease in a manner that is incompletely understood. Cardiovascular disease risk decreases with volume of aerobic activity over a wide range of volume. Blood pressure shows little dose-response effect, as most of the effect of activity on blood pressure occurs at low levels of activity. The effect of activity on bone density is less related to volume of aerobic activity and more related to resistance training and high-impact activities.

ECONOMIC EFFECTS

Habitually active adults have lower medical expenditures. One study estimated direct medical expenditures in adults attributable to inactivity as being $330 per person in 1987 ($825 in 2002 dollars). Evidence is growing that medical expenditures decline in sedentary older adults who become more active. In one study comparing older adults who remained sedentary with sedentary older adults who became active 3 or more days each week, the active group was found to have a decline in medical expenditures averaging about $2200 a year. Data on the cost-effectiveness of promoting physical activity in older adults is promising but

limited, and it varies by intervention. One study of subsidized exercise classes reported cost savings of around $175 per participant per year.

THERAPEUTIC EFFECTS

Physical activity has therapeutic benefits in the management of a wide variety of chronic conditions. Selected clinical guidelines for the use of physical activity in managing common chronic conditions are shown in Table 8.1. In addition, clinical practice guidelines identify a role for physical activity in the management of the following conditions: dementia, persistent pain, heart failure, syncope, reflex sympathetic dystrophy, possible venous thromboembolism, back pain, some sleep disorders, and constipation.

It is possible that physical activity will assume a prominent role in the management of mental health conditions in older adults. There is substantial evidence that both aerobic activity and resistance training improve symptoms of depression. Physical activity should be considered as an adjunct to medication and psychotherapy for older adults with depressive illness, pending more studies clarifying which patients can be prescribed activity as a substitute for medication and psychotherapy. Cognitive ability is positively correlated with higher levels of physical activity and fitness. Ongoing research is testing if, and how much, physical activity can improve cognitive function.

The therapeutic use of exercise to reverse low fitness, physical functional limitations, and disability has been carefully studied over the past 20 years. Randomized trials of exercise in sedentary older adults show that aerobic capacity, muscle strength, flexibility, and balance can be improved by appropriate forms of exercise. Several evidence-based reviews conclude that exercise has a beneficial effect on functional limitations (restrictions in basic physical actions such as walking). Although some exercise studies report only small improvements in functional limitations, most randomized trials prescribe just 3 or 4 days of exercise each week, for only 3 to 12 months. Generally, the benefits of exercise are most demonstrable in older adults with low fitness and clinically significant functional limitations. However, a study of relatively healthy older adults, using a highly sensitive physical performance measure of functional limitations, found that 6 months of aerobic exercise and strength training caused a 14% improvement in functional limitations. These results suggest that relatively healthy adults experience some functional gains with exercise. Other studies suggest that, after an initial boost in function due to exercise, exercisers show a decline in function, but have a slower

Table 8.1—Selected Guidelines That Include Recommendations for Physical Activity

Topic	Guideline Source	Activity Recommendation
Cardiovascular disease	American Heart Association	Aerobic, strength, and flexibility training are recommended in the treatment of atherosclerotic cardiovascular disease. Both moderate and vigorous intensity aerobic activities are effective.
Hypertension	American College of Sports Medicine	"Dynamic aerobic training reduces resting BP in individuals with normal BP and HTN." "Resistance training performed according to ACSM guidelines reduces BP in normotensive and hypertensive adults."
Type 2 diabetes mellitus	American Diabetes Association	"To improve glycemic control, assist with weight maintenance, and reduce risk of CVD, we recommend at least 150 min/week of moderate-intensity aerobic physical activity . . . and/or at least 90 min/week of vigorous aerobic exercise. . . ." "In the absence of contraindications, people with type 2 diabetes should be encouraged to perform resistance exercise three times a week."
Falls	American Geriatrics Society, British Geriatrics Society, American Academy of Orthopaedic Surgeons	"Older people who have recurrent falls should be offered long-term exercise and balance training."
Osteoarthritis	American Geriatrics Society	Aerobic, strength, and flexibility training are recommended in the management of osteoarthritis.
Osteoporosis	American College of Sports Medicine	Weight-bearing aerobic activities, activities that involve jumping, and resistance exercise are recommended to preserve bone health in adults.
Major depression	Institute for Clinical Systems Improvement	"Among individuals with major depression, exercise therapy is feasible and is associated with significant therapeutic benefit, especially if exercise is continued over time."
Persistent pain	American Geriatrics Society	". . . there is strong evidence that participation in regular physical activity reduces the pain and enhances the functional capacity of older adults with persistent pain."
Dementia	American Academy of Neurology	"Walking and light exercise appear to reduce wandering, aggression and agitation. . . ."
Heart failure	European Society of Cardiology	". . . regular exercise can safely increase physical capacity by 15–25%, improve symptoms and perception of quality of life in patients with stable class II and II heart failure (level of evidence B)."
Cholesterol	National Cholesterol Education Program Expert Panel (3rd Report)	"For management of atherogenic dyslipidemia, emphasis in management should be given to life-habit modification—weight control and increased physical activity."
Obesity	U.S. Preventive Services Task Force	"There is fair to good evidence that high-intensity counseling—about diet, exercise, or both—together with behavioral interventions aimed at skill development, motivation, and support strategies produces modest, sustained weight loss . . . in adults who are obese. . . ."

NOTE: ACSM = American College of Sports Medicine; BP = blood pressure; CVD = cardiovascular disease; HTN = hypertension.

SOURCES: (1) Fletcher GF, Balady GJ, Amsterdam EA, et al. Exercise standards for testing and training: a statement for healthcare professionals from the American Heart Association. *Circulation.* 2001;104:1694–1740, and Pollock ML, Franklin BA, Balady GJ, et al. Resistance exercise in individuals with and without cardiovascular disease: benefits, rationale, safety, and prescription. An advisory from the Committee on Exercise, Rehabilitation, and Prevention, Council on Clinical Cardiology, American Heart Association. *Circulation.* 2000;101:828–833. (2) Pescatello LS, Franklin BA, Fagard R, et al. American College of Sports Medicine position stand: exercise and hypertension. *Med Sci Sports Exerc.* 2004;36:533–553. (3) Sigal RJ, Kenny GP, Wasserman DH, et al. Physical activity / exercise and type 2 diabetes. *Diabetes Care.* 2004;27(10):2518–2539. (4) American Geriatrics Society, British Geriatrics Society, and American Academy of Orthopaedic Surgeons Panel on Falls Prevention. Guideline for the prevention of falls in older persons. *J Am Geriatr Soc.* 2001;49(5):664–672. (5) Exercise prescription for older adults with osteoarthritis pain: consensus practice recommendations: a supplement to the AGS Clinical Practice Guidelines on the management of chronic pain in older adults. *J Am Geriatr Soc.* 2001;49(6):808–823. (6) Kohrt WM, Bloomfield SA, Little KD, et al. American College of Sports Medicine position stand: physical activity and bone health. *Med Sci Sports Exerc.* 2004;36:1985–1996. (7) Institute for Clinical Systems Improvement (ICSI). *Major Depression in Adults in Primary Care.* 8th ed. Bloomington, MN: Institute for Clinical Systems Improvement (ICSI);2004:17–18. (8) AGS Panel on Persistent Pain in Older Persons. The management of persistent pain in older persons. *J Am Geriatr Soc.* 2002;50(6):S205–S224. (9) Doody RS, Stevens JC, Beck C, et al. Practice parameter: management of dementia (an evidence-based review). Report of the Quality Standards Subcommittee of the American Academy of Neurology. *Neurology.* 2001;56:1154–1166. (10) Remme WJ, Swedberg K. Guidelines for the diagnosis and treatment of chronic heart failure. *Eur Heart J.* 2001;22:1527–1560. (11) *Third Report on the National Cholesterol Education Program (NCEP) Expert Panel on Detection, Evaluation and Treatment of High Blood Cholesterol in Adults (Adult Treatment Panel III).* National Institutes of Health, NIH Publication No. 01-3670, Washington, DC: May 2001. (12) U.S. Preventive Services Task Force. Screening for obesity in adults: recommendations and rationale. *Ann Intern Med.* 2003;139(11):930–932.

rate of loss than nonexercisers. There are too few studies to determine whether physical activity in sedentary older adults has a beneficial effect on disability (ability to do activities of daily life such as personal care and work).

RECOMMENDED AMOUNTS OF PHYSICAL ACTIVITY

Aerobic Activity

An adult can achieve recommended levels of aerobic activity by doing either vigorous or moderate activity. The vigorous-intensity recommendation, developed in the 1980s, is to engage in at least 20 minutes of vigorous physical activity on 3 or more days each week. The moderate-intensity recommendation, published in 1995 by the Centers for Disease Control and Prevention (CDC) and the American College of Sports Medicine (ACSM), is that "every US adult should accumulate thirty minutes or more of moderate intensity physical activity on most, preferably all, days of the week." An alternative statement of the recommendation, which better communicates the meanings of some of its terms, is this: Adults should engage in a brisk walk, or an equivalently intense aerobic activity, for at least 10 minutes at a time, for a total of at least 30 minutes a day, on at least 5 days a week.

Several comments help to clarify these two recommendations. First, moderate-intensity physical activity is defined as aerobic activities that expend 3.0 to 6.0 METS (metabolic equivalents; ie, 4 to 7 kcal/min). The standard example of a moderate-intensity activity is brisk walking at 3 to 4 miles per hour. Vigorous activities, such as running, expend more than 6.0 METS. Many activities allow a broad range of intensity of effort, so they can be performed as either moderate or vigorous activities, including cycling, swimming, backpacking, skiing, stair climbing, and volleyball. Second, only activity bouts of at least 10 minutes in duration count toward meeting either recommendation. Third, any physical activity, not just exercise, can count toward meeting the recommendations, including occupational activity, leisure-time activity, domestic activity such as gardening, and transportation activity. Fourth, daily physical activity is preferable, in part because there are beneficial acute effects of physical activity such as reduction in blood pressure. Daily activity is also recommended on the basis of the philosophy that the body is designed to be active every day. Finally, greater amounts of physical activity produce greater health benefits. It is inappropriate to cite the recommendations as meaning that "a person only needs 30 minutes a day."

Despite some evidence that vigorous activity has greater health benefit and some evidence that even low-intensity activities have benefit, the recommendations reflect consensus that moderate intensity is the minimum threshold for substantial health benefits. Despite the fact "more is better" and that a minimum of 60 minutes of moderate activity has been suggested, the recommendations reflect consensus that substantial health benefits accrue from 30 to 60 minutes of moderate activity.

Resistance Training

Adults should perform resistance training activities of the major muscle groups on 2 or 3 days each week, with at least 48 hours of rest in between. For all adults, ACSM recommends resistance training of moderate intensity that is sufficient to develop and maintain muscular fitness and fat-free mass. Selected adults may prefer high-intensity training instead. Dynamic resistance training (as opposed to static training) is recommended for most adults.

Flexibility Training

Activities that develop and maintain musculoskeletal flexibility and that are performed a minimum of twice a week are recommended. Unlike aerobic activities and resistance training, flexibility training by itself does not have substantial health benefits. It is recommended because regular physical activity requires an adequate range of motion, and flexibility training permits and facilitates the types of physical activity that have health benefit.

Balance Training

Unlike aerobic activity, resistance training, and flexibility training, balance training is not recommended for all adults. Balance training is currently recommended only for adults at increased risk of falls, as explained below.

PHYSICAL ACTIVITY LEVELS IN OLDER ADULTS

Older adults are the least active age group. In 2001, 11% of adults aged 65 and over reported strength training activities at least twice a week, and only 6% met both strength training and aerobic recommendations. However, trend data show increasing levels of physical activity in older adults over time. In 1990, 30% of adults aged 75 and over met either the strength training or aerobic recommendation, compared with 35% in 2000. In 1988, 41% of adults aged 70 and over were sedentary (reported no leisure-time physical activity), compared with 30% in 2002.

RECOMMENDING PHYSICAL ACTIVITY TO OLDER ADULTS

Preference for Moderate-Intensity Aerobic Activity

The vast majority of sedentary and insufficiently active older adults should gradually increase moderate aerobic activity, especially walking, so as to meet the recommendation for moderate intensity. Moderate exercise is associated with lower cardiovascular risk, lower risk of musculoskeletal injury, and, in comparison with vigorous exercise, a higher adherence to training. Most older adults prefer moderate-intensity activities. A target between 30 and 60 minutes of moderate activity on 5 to 7 days each week is appropriate for most older adults.

The traditional emphasis on walking for older adults is appropriate. The obvious advantages of walking are that it requires no special skills, equipment, or facilities. The risk of injury is relatively low. One study has reported that higher amounts of walking are not associated with a higher injury risk. Walking is the most common physical activity reported by older adults.

Importance of Resistance Training

Age-related decreases in skeletal muscle mass and quality, termed *sarcopenia*, contribute to functional limitations and dependence in older adults. Sarcopenia is more than just disuse atrophy, as even highly trained athletes lose muscle mass with age. The biologic mechanisms for sarcopenia are incompletely understood. Neurogenic mechanisms may involve the loss of neurons for a variety of reasons, such as exposure to heavy metals, loss of blood supply, and mechanical damage. Denervated muscle fibers can be reinnervated by axonal sprouting of remaining motor neurons, but the process appears to be incomplete, so that cycles of denervation and reinnervation result in net loss of fibers. Myogenic mechanisms include the possibility that repair processes for contraction-induced muscle damage are impaired with aging. General mechanisms of cell damage may involve skeletal muscle, including damage of skeletal muscle mitochondria by free radicals.

Epidemiologic studies report that regular physical activity reduces age-related loss of muscle mass. Randomized controlled trials have demonstrated that resistance training increases muscle mass and thereby counteracts sarcopenia. Early studies of resistance training prescribed vigorous training similar to that prescribed for young adults. Subsequently, it has been demonstrated that less training has both physiologic effects on muscle function and health benefits. Larger gains in strength are typically reported by studies using weight machines. For older adults with good fitness, weight machines are usually the most feasible and safest training method. Randomized trails have also tested resistance training programs that use body weight or free weights, such as weight cuffs or dumbbells. These programs are more appropriate for adults with lower fitness levels, where lower amounts of weight provide adequate exercise stimulus. In theory, resistance in a home-based program can be adjusted on the basis of the progressive overload principle, and, given sufficient repetitions, strength should increase steadily. In practice, these programs typically report smaller gains in strength.

Other Considerations

With older adults, there is more emphasis on doing the minimum amount of all recommended types of activity: aerobic activities, resistance training, flexibility training, and (if at increased risk of falling) balance training. It is appropriate to encourage older adults to join exercise classes that mix aerobic, resistance, and flexibility training.

The traditional guidance to increase level of physical activity gradually over time is highly appropriate for older adults. Injury risk is minimized, and the experience is more pleasant. Focus group studies report that older adults view increasing physical activity as an extremely difficult task. It is appropriate to break this task up into stages, with intermediate goals. Adults with lower fitness should be permitted more time to adapt to each stage.

Older adults should be strongly encouraged to reduce sedentary behavior and get some activity each week, even if less than the minimum recommended. Illustrative of the dose-response relationship of activity and health, many studies show that levels of activity below minimum recommendations have health benefits in older adults.

For many older adults, exercise has a therapeutic role in one or more chronic conditions, as well as its traditional preventive role. Most commonly, integrating preventive and therapeutic recommendations involves essentially following public health recommendations, with specific preferences for modes of activity. For example, aquatic exercise classes are chosen for adults with arthritis, weight-bearing exercise is chosen for adults with osteoporosis, and rotation of exercise modes is chosen for adults with obesity to minimize risk of orthopedic injury. As chronic conditions become more severe, therapeutic considerations typically are the main determinants of the activity recommendation, such as pulmonary rehabilitation for adults with moderate to severe lung disease.

CONSIDERATIONS IN OLDER ADULTS WITH LOW FITNESS

For aerobic activities, a different definition of intensity is necessary for adults with low fitness. Intensity is defined, not as absolute energy expenditure in METS, but relative to the person's level of fitness, as judged by the heart-rate response to exercise. Moderate-intensity activity has a heart-rate response in the range of 55% to 69% of maximal heart rate (220 – age for men; 220 – [0.6 × age] for women), and vigorous intensity is the range greater than 69% of maximal heart rate. With this definition of intensity, unfit older adults need not do a brisk walk or equivalently intense activity to meet the moderate recommendation. Rather, the person should walk at a speed that causes a heart rate response in the range of moderate intensity.

Physical activity should be increased very gradually in adults with low fitness. Initially, short bouts of activity are appropriate. Activity bouts less than 10 minutes are acceptable. It is not necessary to specify a minimum heart rate.

Older adults in community-based long-term-care programs and residents of long-term-care facilities benefit from physical activity. Supervised classes of a few months' duration cause improvements in fitness and functional limitations, even in older adults who are physically frail or who have incontinence or mild dementia. Physical activity may improve sleep and decrease agitation. Exercise programs for nursing-home residents may include strength training, even high-intensity training. Randomized trials show strength training to be safe, increase strength, improve functional limitations, and increase amount of spontaneous activity.

OBESITY

The obesity epidemic has placed a great deal of attention on the role of physical activity in maintaining a healthy body weight. Public health recommendations advise that weight loss should be achieved by both reducing caloric intake and increasing energy expenditure. Possibly, regular physical activity during weight loss may be more important for older adults. Obesity increases the risk of many chronic diseases and of functional limitations in older adults, but it also has the beneficial effects of increasing bone and muscle mass. Weight loss is accompanied by loss of bone and muscle mass. Exercise during weight loss, particularly resistance training, should theoretically reduce loss of bone and muscle mass. For older adults advised to lose weight, a reasonable approach is to meet the moderate recommendations for 30 minutes or more and to limit caloric intake. Physical activity level then can be gradually increased as necessary to achieve and maintain a healthy weight.

OSTEOPOROSIS, FALLS, FRACTURES, AND BALANCE TRAINING

Regular physical activity by older adults has a modest effect in slowing age-related loss of bone mass. Evidence indicates that resistance and high-impact exercises are most beneficial. Weight-bearing aerobic activities can also provide the mechanical loading that maintains bone mass.

In older adults at increased risk for falling, randomized trials demonstrate that falls can be prevented by multicomponent interventions targeting factors such as sedative use, environmental hazards, and poor balance. Increasing physical activity is regarded as an effective component of falls prevention programs. Solid evidence of the effectiveness of exercise in falls prevention comes from a meta-analysis of a series of exercise studies in New Zealand, which reported that exercise reduces both falls and fall injuries by 35% to 45%. One meta-analysis of randomized trials reported that aerobic activity, resistance training, and balance training are all associated with reduced risk of falling. Balance training is specifically recommended in clinical practice guidelines for falls prevention in adults at increased risk. There is no experimental evidence that exercise reduces either total fractures or hip fractures. However, a meta-analysis of epidemiologic studies reported that physical activity reduces the risk of hip fracture by up to 50%.

A variety of balance training interventions have been studied. Some exercises focus on maintaining balance over a narrow base of support, such as a tandem stand or one-leg stand. Other exercises train dynamic balance, such as ability to do a tandem walk. Some programs have separate balance exercises. Others propose that some stretching and strengthening exercises be done in a manner that also improves balance. An example of the latter is the program described in the books *Exercise: A Guide from the National Institute on Aging* (http://www.niapublications.org/exercisebook/index.asp) and *Exercise: Getting Fit for Life* (http:www.niapublications.org/engagepages/exercise.asp).

Balance training is typically designed so that exercises are graduated in difficulty, and adults progress to more difficult exercise as training improves balance. For example, a tandem walk is easiest when holding on to a table and becomes progressively harder with arms in any position, arms close to the body, and arms close to the body while holding a weight.

Tai Chi Chuan is often mentioned as a form of exercise that improves balance and prevents falls. Although the original study of Tai Chi reported almost a 50% reduction in falls, a follow-up study reported a (nonsignificant) 25% reduction. A reasonable summary of the evidence is that Tai Chi remains a promising intervention that is popular, fun, and social, and it is appropriate for the balance training component of a falls prevention program.

THE RISKS OF PHYSICAL ACTIVITY

Although the benefits of physical activity far outweigh the risks, promoting physical activity should include strategies for minimizing risk. The main risk of physical activity is musculoskeletal injury. Several factors affecting musculoskeletal injury risk are modifiable and offer opportunities for risk management. The risk of injury is higher with vigorous exercise, with higher volume of exercise, and with obesity. The risk of injury is less with higher fitness, supervision, protective equipment such as bike helmets, and in well-designed exercise environments. The principle that physical activity should be increased gradually over time is widely regarded as critical for reducing risk of injury. Vigorous activity, such as running and participation in vigorous sports, should be recommended only to older adults who are accustomed to these activities or who have sufficient fitness, experience, and knowledge to perform vigorous activities and prevent injuries associated with them. ACSM recommends that older adults begin resistance training with one set of 10 to 15 repetitions of each exercise, rather than the 8 to 12 repetitions for younger adults. To complete more repetitions, training must begin with less resistance (relative to maximal strength), which should reduce injury risk.

The risk of both exercise-related myocardial infarction and sudden death is greatest in individuals who are the least active. Sedentary adults should avoid isolated bouts of vigorous activity and should increase activity gradually over time.

PROMOTING PHYSICAL ACTIVITY

A general clinical approach to promoting physical activity is shown in Figure 8.1. *Healthy People 2010* recommends that clinicians counsel physically inactive adults to increase their physical activity level. However, the U.S. Preventive Services Task Force regards the efficacy data on counseling as difficult to interpret. A wide variety of interventions have been studied, and the results are mixed. The U.S. Preventive Services Task Force has recommended high-intensity counseling about diet and exercise, together with behavioral interventions, for obese adults with a body mass index of 30 or greater.

One clinical approach to promoting physical activity is to adopt the 5-A framework (assess, advise, agree, assist, and arrange), which has been used in behavioral interventions such as smoking cessation. Because of the importance of physical activity, the clinician assesses an older patient's level of physical activity at least once a year and provides a specific recommendation about physical activity. The clinician and patient collaboratively agree on goals for physical activity. The clinician provides assistance. Counseling is one option; other options include self-help materials, referral to community programs, and referral to medically supervised programs.

Older adults typically feel overwhelmed by recommendations calling for substantial and immediate life-style changes. A stepwise approach is often appropriate. It allows the person to take small steps toward a tangible goal and feel rewarded upon meeting it, before moving on to the next, more ambitious goal.

Pedometers have become popular in promoting walking. Pedometers can be useful in providing feedback and monitoring progress toward physical activity goals. However, it is not appropriate to prescribe a universal step goal, such as 10,000 steps a day. Recommendations specify a minimum bout of 10 minutes, so many of the steps recorded by a pedometer do not count toward physical activity recommendations. Further, pedometers can miscount steps in older adults with slower gaits. However, some adults find step counters to be helpful in tracking activity levels and use them appropriately to ensure that every day includes an adequate amount of brisk walking. Some weight-management approaches use bouts of activity less than 10 minutes or low-intensity activity, or both, to increase caloric expenditure. Pedometers can be useful in tracking progress to caloric expenditure goals.

Research highlights the importance of the physical and social environment in promoting physical activity. Studies report that people with access to recreational facilities are twice as likely to get recommended levels of physical activity. People are more likely to commute to work by bicycle or by walking if they live in a city center with a variety of destinations, such as grocery stores and restaurants, and have good access to public transportation. The medical care system should work in tandem with the community to promote environments that encourage physical activity. Clinicians should be aware that there are effective community-level interventions to promote physical activity. The Guide to Community Preventive Services identifies six recommended or strongly recommended community-level interventions proven effective in increasing physical activity. These are community-wide campaigns, prompts to increase usage of stairs, individually adapted behavior change programs implemented in groups of adults, school-based physical education, interventions

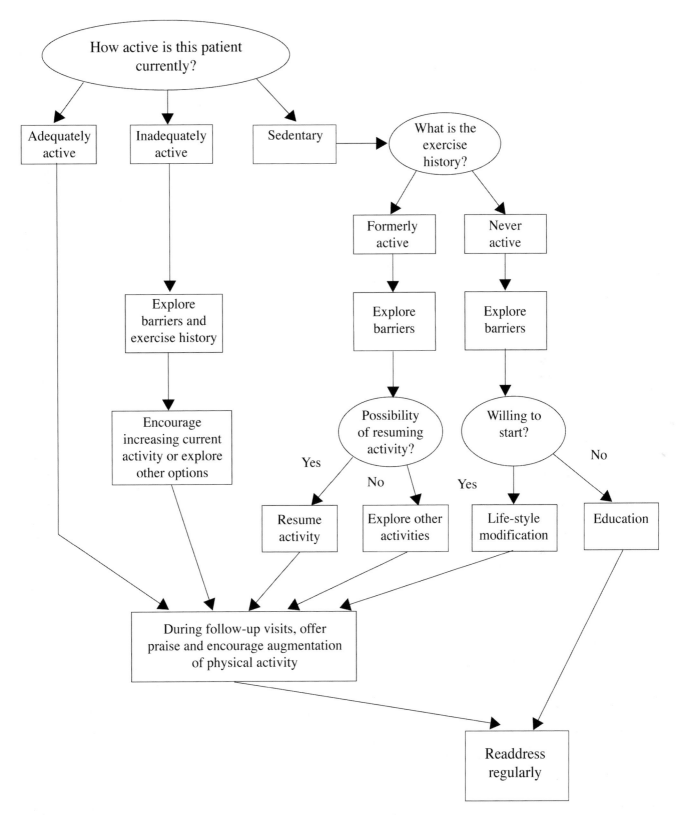

Figure 8.1—Framework for discussions about physical activity with the older patient.

SOURCE: Christmas C, Andersen RA. Exercise and older patients: guidelines for the clinician. *J Am Geriatr Soc.* 2000;48(3):321. Reprinted by permission of Blackwell Science, Inc.

that increase nonfamily social support such as programs that arrange walking groups, and enhanced access to recreational facilities (eg, parks and trails) combined with outreach to promote awareness of facilities.

ANNOTATED REFERENCES

■ Balfour JL, Kaplan GA. Neighborhood environment and loss of physical function in older adults: evidence from the Alameda County Study. *Am J Epidemiol.* 2002;155(6): 507–515.

The main focus of this report was to provide evidence that environmental factors influence functional limitations in older adults. The study found that six neighborhood problems (traffic, noise, crime, trash and litter, lighting, and public transportation) were associated with higher risk of loss of physical function over 1 year. More neighborhood problems were also associated with lower physical activity levels. Like other cohort studies, the study also found that higher levels of physical activity were associated with lower risk of disability. The study suggests the neighborhood environment affects the risk of loss of physical function in older adults, and one mechanism by which the environment affects function is by influencing physical activity levels.

■ Nelson ME, Layne JE, Bernstein MJ, et al. The effects of multidimensional home-based exercise on functional performance in elderly people. *J Gerontol A Biol Sci Med Sci.* 2004;59(2);154–160.

A genre of community exercise programs for older adults has become popular over the past decade. These programs include strength training using body weight, cuff weights or dumbbells or both, balance training, aerobic activities that do not involve expensive equipment, and stretching exercises. As these programs do not require a gym or fitness facility, they can be done at home or in settings like senior centers. This randomized trial of one such program, in 72 adults aged 70 years and over, illustrates that these programs can have beneficial effects. The study found that 6 months of home-based exercise improves dynamic balance and functional performance, as measured by the Physical Performance Test

and the Established Population for Epidemiologic Studies of the Elderly (EPESE) short physical performance battery.

■ Penninx BW, Messier SP, Rejeski WJ, et al. Physical exercise and the prevention of disability in activities of daily living in older persons with osteoarthritis. *Arch Intern Med.* 2001;161(19):2309–2316.

This report from the Fitness Arthritis and Seniors Trial (FAST) appears to provide the first data from a randomized trial that exercise by sedentary older adults reduces the incidence of disability. The study recruited adults aged 60 and over with knee osteoarthritis and free of activities of daily living (ADL) disability; it randomized participants to 18 months of aerobic exercise, resistance exercise, or attention control. Risk of incident disability during follow-up was reduced by both aerobic exercise (relative risk = .60) and by resistance training (relative risk = .53). Lowest risk of ADL disability was associated with the highest adherence to exercise. These data support the value and importance of both aerobic training and strength training in older adults.

■ Tanasescu M, Leitzmann MF, Rimm EB, et al. Exercise type and intensity in relation to coronary heart disease in men. *JAMA.* 2002;288(16);1994–2000.

This report from the Health Professionals' Follow-up Study analyzed the relationship between physical activity and risk of coronary heart disease (CHD) in 44452 U.S. men aged 40 through 75 at the start of the study. After 12 years of follow-up, the study reported that total physical activity, running, weight training, and walking are each associated with reduced risk of CHD. The results illustrate some themes of physical activity and health. First, moderate-intensity walking has health benefits. Second, both moderate and vigorous aerobic activities have health benefits, though vigorous aerobic activity has greater benefit. Third, there is increasing evidence for the benefit of resistance training on CHD risk. Fourth, the beneficial effects of physical activity on health are independent of other risk factors. In particular in this study, effects were found to be independent of body mass index. Finally, cardiovascular disease risk decreases with volume of aerobic activity over a wide range of volume.

David M. Buchner, MD, MPH

CHAPTER 9—PREVENTION

KEY POINTS

■ The clinician has available a growing number of preventive services that have been shown to be effective in the care of older persons.

■ It is important to consider all relevant issues in determining which conditions to screen for, the appropriate screening interval, and when (if ever) to discontinue screening in an older patient.

■ Many factors need to be taken into account when recommending for or against screening for various cancers in the older person.

■ Several system-based approaches can be employed for optimal implementation of preventive services (eg, trained office staff, computer reminders).

As the population ages and the average active life expectancy increases, issues of primary and secondary prevention become increasingly important. The prevalence of undetected, correctable conditions and comorbid diseases is high in older adults. Moreover, a growing number of older adults are highly motivated about disease prevention and health promotion. The clinician provides the information and opportunity for preventive care that helps older patients to maintain functional independence for as long as possible. Additionally, clinicians must understand the significant heterogeneity of the aging population. Recommendations for screening community-dwelling, cognitively and functionally intact individuals will necessarily be quite different from those dealing with functionally dependent and cognitively impaired nursing-home residents with multiple comorbidities.

Many findings from research on preventive care and the appropriate components of periodic health examinations are inconclusive. In addition, older persons are typically not included in clinical trials of preventive strategies, which has limited the clinician's ability to adjust guidelines for preventive practices for patients aged 65 and older on the basis of new scientific findings. Primary care physicians are consequently compelled to rely on clinical judgment in planning the preventive care of their older patients.

A number of factors, including age, functional status, comorbidity, patient preference, socioeconomic status, and the availability of care, affect health care decisions of the older adult. Unlike chronologic age, physiologic age may be determined by self-rated health and overall medical condition. Classifications that are based on life expectancy, physiologic age, and functional status may facilitate medical decision making with older patients. For example, the clinician might strongly recommend fecal occult blood testing (FOBT) to a healthy, functionally independent patient; discuss the potential pros and cons of FOBT and offer the test to a chronically ill, partially dependent patient; and actually recommend against FOBT for a severely frail, demented patient. It is important to consider all relevant issues in determining which conditions to screen for, the appropriate screening interval, and when (if ever) to discontinue screening in an older patient.

The risks of screening and its follow-up diagnostics and treatments (eg, perforation from colonoscopy; impotence or incontinence from prostate surgery) need more emphasis when discussions regarding screening recommendations occur. Also, attention to all-cause mortality, as opposed to disease-specific mortality, must be taken into account. For example, finding a preventable cancer that might result in death in 5 to 10 years if not detected early is of no benefit (and can result in actual harm and considerable cost) in an individual whose life expectancy is less than 5 years. It is important, too, that the values, beliefs, and preferences of older patients be factored into discussions, as should issues regarding quality of life.

Attention to the underlying principles of primary and secondary prevention is important for patients of any age. Screening measures should be systematically performed when the prevalence and morbidity or mortality of the condition outweighs both the economic cost and potential consequences of a falsely positive or negative test result. Some recommendations may be applicable only to high-risk individuals, not to the general population. (See also the discussion of cancer screening in "Oncology," p 482, and definitions of terms used to assess screening tests in the Appendix, p 502.)

Increasingly important is the clinician's responsibility to counsel against the often grossly exaggerated and unproven claims of the anti-aging industry. The dollar costs and potential psychologic and physical damage associated with this burgeoning area are staggering and very worrisome.

RECOMMENDED PREVENTIVE SERVICES

A number of preventive services have been shown to be effective in the care of older persons and are widely endorsed. Table 9.1 summarizes these preventive activities, which are discussed below.

Screening

Obesity or Malnutrition

Routine measurement of height and weight can be used to calculate body mass index (BMI = kg/m^2). Obesity has been defined in men as a BMI $\geq$ 27.8 and in women as a BMI $\geq$ 27.3. An unintentional weight loss of 10 pounds in 6 months can indicate malnutrition or a serious occult illness. (See also "Malnutrition," p 174.)

Hypertension

The prevalence of hypertension increases with advancing age. The treatment of hypertension in older adults has been associated with a reduction in morbidity and mortality from left ventricular hypertrophy, heart failure, myocardial infarction, and stroke. However, older adults are more susceptible to adverse effects of antihypertensive therapy, such as hyponatremia, hypokalemia, depression, confusion, or postural hypotension. (See also "Hypertension," p 361.) This susceptibility is especially true for the oldest-old patients and those with multiple comorbidities and taking multiple medications.

Vision and Hearing Deficits

Uncorrected refractive errors, glaucoma, cataracts, and macular degeneration account for most undetected

Table 9.1—Evidence-Based Preventive Services Recommended for Older Adults

Preventive Activity	Frequency	Condition to Detect or Prevent
Screening		
Height and weight	at least annually	Obesity, malnutrition
Blood pressure	at least annually	Hypertension
Vision testing	annually	Visual deficits
Hearing ability	annually	Hearing impairment
Depression questionnaire	*	Depression
Alcoholism questionnaire	*	Alcoholism
Serum lipids (with prior MI, angina)	annually	Recurrent CAD
Abdominal ultrasonography (men aged 65–75 years who have ever smoked)	once	Abdominal aortic aneurysm
Bone density measurement	*	Osteoporosis
Glucose (with hypertension or hyperlipidemia)	*	Type 2 diabetes mellitus
Mammography	every 2–3 years	Breast cancer
Pap smear	at least every 3 years**	Cervical cancer
Fecal occult blood testing *and/or*	annually	Colorectal cancer
flexible sigmoidoscopy *or*	every 3–5 years	
colonoscopy	once	
Counseling to encourage:		
Smoking cessation	every visit	COPD, many cancers, CAD
Regular dental visits	annually	Malnutrition, oral cancers, edentulism
Low-fat, well-balanced diet	annually	Obesity, CAD
Adequate calcium intake	annually	Osteoporosis
Physical activity	annually	Immobility, CAD, osteoporosis
Injury prevention	annually	Injurious falls, motor vehicle crashes, burns, other injuries
Immunization		
Influenza vaccination	annually	Influenza
Pneumococcal vaccination	†	Pneumococcal disease
Tetanus booster	every 10 years	Tetanus
Chemoprophylaxis		
Aspirin therapy	daily	Recurrent MI, TIA, or stroke

Note: CAD = coronary artery disease; COPD = chronic obstructive pulmonary disease; MI = myocardial infarction; TIA = transient ischemic attack. For updates from the U.S. Preventive Services Task Force, see http://www.ahrq.gov/clinic/prevenix.htm (accessed July 2005).

* The optimal interval for screening is unknown.

** May stop screening at age 65 if patient has had regularly normal smears up to that age; if never tested prior to age 65, may stop after two normal annual smears.

† Vaccinate immunocompetent patients once at age 65; revaccination after 7–10 years may be appropriate.

visual disorders. Routine screening with a Snellen chart is recommended by the U.S. Preventive Services Task Force (USPSTF). Undetected hearing loss can lead to social isolation and may indicate other underlying disorders. The USPSTF recommends periodically questioning older adults about their hearing and counseling them about the availability of hearing aid devices. The evidence for routine audiometry as a screening tool is unproven. (See also "Visual Impairment," p 149, and "Hearing Impairment," p 155.)

Depression

Depression is a disease with significant morbidity and mortality in the older age group. Treatment can be highly effective. The USPSTF recommends screening of the general adult population. Importantly, they add the recommendation that clinicians who do screen for depression have systems in place to assure accurate diagnosis, effective treatment, and follow-up. There are several reliable and valid depression screening instruments for older persons, including the Geriatric Depression Scale. (See the Appendix, p 496; see also "Depression and Other Mood Disorders," p 269).

Alcoholism

All older adults should be screened for alcohol abuse at least once and whenever a drinking problem is suspected. Screening questionnaires such as the CAGE (see Table 39.1, p 301) can be useful in detecting alcohol problems. (See also "Alcohol and Drug Abuse," p 298.)

Dyslipidemia

There is good evidence that in elderly persons with prior myocardial infarction or angina, correcting lipid abnormalities (ie, levels of low-density lipoprotein ≥ 130 mg/dL, of high-density lipoprotein ≤ 35 mg/dL, of triglycerides ≥ 200 mg/dL) lowers the risk of recurrent cardiac events. These persons should be screened for lipid abnormalities; treatment goals for those found to have dyslipidemia should be low-density lipoprotein levels of < 100 mg/dL, high-density lipoprotein levels of > 40 mg/dL, and triglyceride levels of < 200 mg/dL. There is no evidence that screening older adults who are clinically free of coronary artery disease (CAD) or who have few cardiac risk factors for primary prevention of CAD is effective. (See also "Cardiovascular Diseases and Disorders," p 344.)

Abdominal Aortic Aneurysm

The USPSTF recommends one-time screening for abdominal aortic aneurysm (AAA) by ultrasonography in men aged 65 to 75 years who have ever smoked. Evidence shows that screening for AAA and surgical repair of large AAAs (≥ 5.5 cm) in men aged 65 to 75 years who have ever smoked (current and former smokers) leads to decreased AAA-specific mortality. Because of the potential harms of screening and early treatment (including an increased number of surgeries with associated clinically significant morbidity and mortality), the USPSTF makes no recommendation for or against screening for AAA in men aged 65 to 75 years who have never smoked. Since women have a low prevalence of large AAAs, the USPSTF recommends against routine screening for AAA in women.

Osteoporosis

The USPSTF now recommends that women aged 65 and older be screened routinely for osteoporosis by the use of bone density measurements. For those at high risk for osteoporotic fractures, the task force recommends beginning screening at age 60. Clinician counseling regarding adequate calcium intake, smoking cessation, exercise, and avoidance of falls is also recommended. (See also "Osteoporosis and Osteomalacia," p 210.)

Breast Cancer

Despite considerable controversy regarding the efficacy of screening mammography, almost all government-sponsored groups, medical societies, and advocacy groups do recommend routine mammography for women aged 65 and older. How often to screen and at what age to stop remain unresolved. Mammography every 2 to 3 years for older women with an active life expectancy of 5 or more years is a reasonable guideline. For high-risk individuals, yearly screening is prudent. Medicare covers annual screening mammograms.

Clinician breast examination is not uniformly recommended for screening, and breast self-examination has not been shown to be efficacious.

(See also the section of breast cancer in "Oncology," p 485.)

Cervical Cancer

Approximately 40% of new cases of invasive cervical cancer and deaths from cervical cancer occur in women aged 65 years and over. The Papanicolaou smear is most cost-effective in older patients who have previously had incomplete screening. Between 4% and 8% of cervical cancers are found in the cervical stump in women who have undergone incomplete hysterectomy. Regular Pap smears every 1 to 3 years are recommended for all women who are or have been sexually active and who have a cervix. Medicare has covered triennial screening without age limit since 1990. The appropriate cut-off age for screening remains controversial, although most experts recommend cessation of screening after age 65 if the patient has had a history of regularly normal smears. In older women never previously screened, screening can cease after two normal Pap smears are obtained 1 year apart.

Colorectal Cancer

Although evidence is not yet definitive, screening for colorectal cancer by colonoscopy is the preferred method for older persons. The entire colon can be examined expeditiously by an experienced endoscopist and any appropriate biopsies can be obtained.

Medicare will pay for a screening colonoscopy every 10 years for all beneficiaries. In addition, Medicare provides coverage for annual FOBT and biennial flexible sigmoidoscopy. A double-contrast or air-contrast screening barium enema may be substituted for either a screening flexible sigmoidoscopy or a screening colonoscopy. When FOBT is recommended, instructions regarding proper diet, medication usage, and vitamin usage before and during stool collections and proper collection technique are crucial in order to avoid false positives and negatives. "Virtual" colonoscopy, a new method using thin-section, helical computed tomography, is currently under investigation as a screening tool for colorectal cancer.

Studies have refuted the concept that a low-fat, high-fiber diet plays a role in preventing colorectal cancer. Although epidemiologic data suggest that aspirin or nonsteroidal anti-inflammatory drugs may be protective against colorectal cancer, there is insufficient evidence to support the routine use of these medications for primary prevention. However, for individuals wanting to maximize prevention and having no contraindications, one aspirin daily is reasonable and justifiable. This does not replace screening, FOBT, sigmoidoscopy, or colonoscopy.

(See also the section on colon cancer in "Oncology," p 486.)

Counseling

Smoking Cessation

Smoking cessation at any age reduces rates of chronic obstructive pulmonary disease, many cancers, and CAD. All older adult smokers should be encouraged to and helped with smoking cessation at each office visit. (See also "Alcohol and Drug Abuse," p 298, and "Respiratory Diseases and Disorders," p 326.)

Dental Care

Many common problems can be detected and effectively treated by regular dental visits, including periodontitis, xerostomia, and oral cancers. (See also "Oral Diseases and Disorders," p 319.)

Dietary Counseling

The importance of a well-balanced diet should be addressed routinely with older adults. An appropriate diet is high in fruits and vegetables and low in fat and salt, and it has adequate calcium content. Also, it is important not to overly restrict the diet of those who are underweight or frail. Restrictions in these situations can be counterproductive and lead to increased morbidity. (See also "Malnutrition," p 174.)

Physical Activity

Increasing evidence supports the importance of physical activity for both physical health and sense of well-being. Physical activity has been associated with greater mobility and lower rates of CAD and osteoporosis. Older adults should be counseled about an exercise program that balances modalities of flexibility (eg, stretching), endurance (eg, walking or cycling), strength (weight training), and balance (eg, Tai Chi or dance therapy). (See also "Physical Activity," p 56.)

Injury Prevention

The USPSTF recommends counseling older persons on measures to reduce the risk of falling (see also "Falls," p 201, "Gait Impairment," p 195, and the appendix, p 497 for details about preventing falls), safety-related skills and behaviors, and environmental hazard reduction. Safety-related behaviors include the regular use of seat and lap belts in automobiles, regular driving tests, and avoidance of alcohol use while driving or operating machinery. Environmental hazard reduction might include lowering hot-water temperature to prevent serious burns, installing smoke detectors, and, in homes of demented persons, installing alarms and automatic shut-off features on appliances, and removing or safely storing firearms. A home safety checklist or formal environmental assessment by a physical or occupational therapist can facilitate injury prevention.

Immunizations

Medicare covers the costs of influenza, pneumococcal, and tetanus immunizations.

Influenza Vaccine

The current influenza vaccine is a killed virus that is moderately immunogenic, with estimated efficacy rates of 70% for illness and 90% for mortality. Multiple evaluations of the vaccine's efficacy reveal that, although it incompletely protects against disease, it clearly reduces rates of respiratory illness, hospitalization, and mortality in the elderly age group. Annual vaccine administration must be provided because of antigenic drift and the short-lived (4 to 5 months) protection provided by the vaccine. Current recommendations are that all patients aged 65 or over or those under age 65 with underlying medical illnesses be immunized annually between October and mid-November, but any time from September to the end of influenza season is appropriate. Medical personnel and caregivers for high-risk patients should also be immunized. Potential adverse effects include fever, chills, myalgias, and malaise, but these are rare. Contraindications include anaphylactic egg hypersensitivity or allergic reactions following occupational exposure to egg protein. Live, attenuated influenza vaccines have been developed, appear to be more effective, and are likely to be approved for widespread use in the near future.

In outbreak situations, chemoprophylaxis can protect against influenza during the 2 weeks immediately after immunization until the antibody response is mounted, or in persons who cannot receive the vaccine. Amantadine, rimantadine, zanamivir[OL], and oseltamivir are all effective for influenza A, but they differ greatly with regard to cost, adverse effects, mechanism of action, and mode of delivery. Only the neuraminidase inhibitors zanamivir and oseltamivir have activity against influenza B. Zanamivir is administered via a disk-inhaler system; the others are taken orally.

Treatment of influenza is also possible with any of the four drugs and reduces the duration of illness by about 1 to 1.5 days, if started within 24 hours of symptom onset. Again, only the neuraminidase inhibitors can be used for treatment of influenza B. Resistance to amantadine and rimantadine can develop rapidly in many persons during the course of treatment; resistance to the neuraminidase inhibitors is less well characterized at this time.

Pneumococcal Vaccination

Pneumococcal vaccination is indicated for all persons aged 65 years or older and many persons under age 65 with comorbid conditions. If ≥ 5 years has elapsed since the first dose and the patient was vaccinated before the age of 65, repeat vaccination is indicated. Studies show that adverse events following revaccination are rare and mild. Thus, an unknown vaccination history should prompt administration of the pneumococcal vaccine. (*When in doubt, vaccinate!*) The vaccine does not prevent mucosal disease such as sinusitis and has unclear efficacy for preventing pneumonia. However, there is strong evidence that suggests that the vaccine reduces the risk of invasive disease (ie, bacteremia) and that it is cost-effective for older immune-competent adults.

Although the protective efficacy of the pneumococcal vaccine is estimated to be only 60% to 70% and studies have revealed mixed results regarding benefits in high-risk older adults, all patients aged 65 years and older should receive one dose of 0.5 mg IM. Studies suggest that people may benefit from revaccination every 7 to 10 years. Other than local soreness, adverse effects are usually minimal.

Tetanus Vaccination

More than 60% of tetanus infections occur in persons aged 60 years of age and older. There is evidence that the absorbed tetanus and diphtheria toxoids provide long-term protection 35 years after the primary series or booster. Older adults who have never been vaccinated should receive two doses, 0.5 mg IM 1 to 2 months apart, followed by an additional dose 6 to 12 months later. The optimal interval for booster doses is not established; the USPSTF and Canadian Task Force recommend booster vaccinations every 10 years. Local pain and swelling or, rarely, hypersensitivity may accompany vaccination. A neurologic or hypersensitivity reaction to a previous dose is an absolute contraindication.

OTHER PREVENTIVE SERVICES TO CONSIDER

A number of other preventive activities are recommended by assorted specialty organizations even though the evidence for effectiveness is lacking. Some of these preventive measures are listed in Table 9.2. In the face of unproven effectiveness for each of these procedures, clinicians must weigh the potential benefits of the preventive procedure against the potential risks of unnecessary treatment. Procedures that are particularly pertinent and controversial in the older adult population are discussed below.

Screening

Skin Cancer

The USPSTF recommends neither for nor against annual skin examination to detect early skin cancers because of a lack of research-proven effectiveness. However, the relatively low cost associated with annual skin examinations and the low costs and morbidity

Table 9.2—Potentially Beneficial Services Lacking Evidence

Preventive Activity	Condition to Detect or Prevent
Screening	
Skin inspection	Skin cancer
Mental status examination	Dementia
Blood glucose	Diabetic complications
Thyrotropin	Hypo- and hyperthyroidism
PSA *or* digital rectal examination *or* both	Prostate cancer
Serum lipids (without apparent CAD)	MI, angina
Nutritional supplementation, vitamins, antioxidants	Cancer, atherosclerosis
Chemoprophylaxis	
Aspirin therapy	Initial MI or stroke, or colon cancer

NOTE: CAD = coronary artery disease; MI = myocardial infarction; PSA = prostate-specific antigen.

[OL] Not approved by the U.S. Food and Drug Administration for this use.

associated with treatment (eg, excision, cryotherapy) of false positives makes the decision to screen considerably less weighty for skin cancer than for prostate cancer. The USPSTF does recommend counseling high-risk patients (those who are light-skinned or with a past history of skin cancer) to avoid sun exposure and to use protective clothing when outdoors. (See also "Dermatologic Diseases and Disorders," p 309.)

Dementia

Although routinely screening for dementia in the general older population is not recommended by the USPSTF, clinicians should be alert to detect new cases as early as possible since a combination of medications, education, and counseling can benefit patients and their families.

For primary prevention, aggressively controlling cardiovascular and cerebrovascular risk factors (eg, hypertension, hyperlipidemia) may be helpful for both vascular and Alzheimer's dementias. There is some evidence that staying mentally active (eg, reading, pursuing new areas of learning, working crossword puzzles) may be beneficial in prevention as well. Estrogen and nonsteroidal anti-inflammatory agents are not efficacious in Alzheimer's prevention. Statins are currently under investigation and cannot at this time be routinely recommended for prevention of Alzheimer's disease. (See also "Dementia" p 221.)

Diabetes Mellitus

The increased prevalence of diabetes mellitus with age and the consequent morbidity burden warrants consideration for screening. Routine screening of asymptomatic adults for diabetes is not recommended by the USPSTF; however, the USPSTF does recommend screening for type 2 diabetes in those individuals with hyperlipidemia, as a method to improve an individual's risk estimates for coronary heart disease. (See also "Diabetes Mellitus," p 382.)

Thyroid Disease

The prevalence of subclinical and clinical hyperthyroidism and hypothyroidism increase with advancing age. The USPSTF does not recommend routine screening but acknowledges that screening may be performed on the basis of the high prevalence of the disease and the likelihood that its symptoms will be overlooked in older adults. The preferred test is the immunometric assay that is sensitive to thyrotropin. (See also "Endocrine and Metabolic Disorders," p 368.)

Prostate Cancer

Randomized controlled trials of screening by prostate-specific antigen or digital rectal examination, currently in progress, should provide valuable information on the efficacy of these modalities. Until the results of those trials are known, however, patients should be counseled about the implications of an elevated prostate-specific antigen level or a mass detected by digital rectal examination and the potential adverse effects (surgery, incontinence, impotence) of treating false or even true positives. The American College of Physicians supports selective testing in 50- to 69-year-old men, provided that optimistic assumptions are used and the risks, benefits, and uncertainties are understood. With evidence currently available, it is difficult to justify screening in men aged of 70 and over. Medicare covers the cost of prostate cancer screening. (See also "Prostate Disease," p 423.)

Nutritional Supplementation

For a discussion of vitamin and mineral supplements and antioxidants, see "Malnutrition," p 174.

Chemoprophylaxis: Aspirin Therapy

Aspirin therapy up to 500 mg per day has not been consistently shown to reduce myocardial infarction or cardiovascular mortality. The adverse bleeding effects of aspirin increase with age, although the absolute serious adverse-effect rate of dosages ≤ 325 mg per day is low. Older adults with risk factors for myocardial infarction or stroke may be more appropriate for prophylaxis with aspirin. (See also "Cardiovascular Diseases and Disorders," p 344.)

See also the section on infective endocarditis in "Infectious Diseases" (p 339) for the use of antibiotics to prevent infective endocarditis and prosthetic device infections in at-risk patients.

PREVENTIVE SERVICES NOT INDICATED IN OLDER ADULTS

Table 9.3 lists services that have been shown not to be effective in preventing certain conditions or their adverse outcomes. There is excellent evidence that the general screening modality of the annual complete history and physical examination is not any more effective for improving outcomes than a more targeted approach of individual screening, counseling, immunoprophylaxis, and chemoprophylaxis. Current evidence does not support specific screening for lung, pancreatic, ovarian, bladder, or hematologic malignancies for the general population. However, promising

Table 9.3—Preventive Services That Have Been Demonstrated Not to Be Beneficial

Annual complete history and physical examination
Screening for specific diseases
    Lung cancer
    Pancreatic cancer
    Ovarian cancer
    Bladder cancer
    Hematologic malignancies
Routine laboratory testing
    Annual complete blood cell count
    Annual blood chemistry panel
    Annual electrocardiogram
    Annual chest radiography
Chemoprophylaxis
    Hormone replacement therapy

new screening modalities, such as helical low-density computed tomography of the chest for lung cancer and homocystinemia for heart disease, are being actively developed and investigated.

Recent evidence has demonstrated that the risks of estrogen-progestin combinations significantly outweigh any potential benefits and therefore should not be recommended. (See the section on estrogen replacement therapy in "Endocrine and Metabolic Disorders," p 379.)

DELIVERY OF PREVENTIVE SERVICES

A well-organized systems-based approach using various personnel, sites, and communication methods may narrow the gap between the knowledge of age-appropriate practice recommendations and the implementation of preventive measures. Lack of time and inadequate reimbursement are only two of the barriers faced by clinicians. Overcoming these barriers commonly involves the assistance of paramedical personnel and the use of technology. A nurse or trained office assistant may be able to adequately explain a screening procedure such as FOBT and its implications in terms of follow-up diagnostic testing. Reminders can be used to prompt clinicians to offer selected screening tests and improve adherence to recommendations. Mailed or computer-generated reminders can be used to enhance screening rates for procedures such as mammography, colorectal cancer screening, and influenza vaccination. Automated telephone technology

may be useful to deliver behavioral interventions for improving medication adherence, dietary modification, and physical activity among sedentary persons. Primary and secondary preventive services may be provided at a variety of sites, including ambulatory clinics, assisted-living and long-term-care facilities, mobile vans, and supermarket-based pharmacies.

The implementation and evaluation of novel approaches for preventive practice are clearly warranted if progress is to be made in this increasingly important field. The more the primary care physician is able to rely upon others to help explain and perform preventive maneuvers, the greater the likelihood that the patient adherence will improve as well.

ANNOTATED REFERENCES

■ Agency for Healthcare Research and Quality. Preventive Services. Available at http://www.ahrq.gov/clinic/prevenix.htm (accessed October 2005).

    Routinely updated literature searches and critical reviews with revised recommendations continue to make this the best source for evidence-based guidelines. Recommendations of the USPSTF, however, are conservative and therefore can be justifiably modified depending upon the setting and population being addressed.

■ Bloom H. Prevention. In: Cassel CK, Leipzig RM, Cohen HJ, et al., eds. *Geriatric Medicine: An Evidence-Based Approach.* 4th ed. New York: Springer-Verlag; 2003: 169–184.

    This chapter presents a comprehensive overview of preventive approaches and practices in the care of the older population. Included are tables outlining the recommendations of key prevention-oriented organizations and specialist organizations regarding primary and secondary prevention for persons aged 65 and older.

■ Walter LC, Covinsky KE. Cancer screening in elderly patients: a framework for individualized decision making. *JAMA.* 2001;285(21):2750–2756.

    This article delineates the complexity of decision making regarding cancer screening in older persons. The authors argue credibly that many factors need to be taken into account when recommending for or against screening for various cancers. Such factors include estimated life expectancy, potential harmful as well as beneficial screening outcomes, and detecting cancers that would never have become clinically significant. Also emphasized is the importance of the patient's own values and preferences in decision making.

Harrison G. Bloom, MD

CHAPTER 10—PHARMACOTHERAPY

KEY POINTS

- Age-associated changes in body composition, metabolism, and pharmacodynamics make benzodiazepine use by older adults especially hazardous.

- Risk factors associated with inappropriate prescribing and overprescribing include having more than one prescriber, poor record keeping, and the use of more than one pharmacy.

- Recent evidence suggests that underprescribing of indicated medications for older patients is a bigger problem than the prescribing of inappropriate medications.

- Cardiovascular drugs, diuretics, nonsteroidal anti-inflammatory drugs (NSAIDs), hypoglycemics, atypical antipsychotics, and anticoagulants are the drug classes most often associated with preventable adverse drug events.

- Collaboration with pharmacists and access to up-to-date drug information can help the clinician to minimize the total number of medications and doses prescribed to individual patients and avoid important drug-drug and drug-disease interactions.

Persons aged 65 years or older are prescribed the highest proportion of medications in relation to their percentage of the U.S. population. Currently, approximately 13% of the U.S. population is aged 65 years or older; this age group purchases 33% of all prescription drugs. These figures are expected to increase to 25% and 50%, respectively, by the year 2040.

Drugs are the most common treatment for acute and chronic diseases. They are also used to prevent many of the diseases and disorders experienced by the older adult. Pharmacotherapy that is successful requires the correct drug at the correct dosage, for the correct disease or condition, for the correct patient. Unfortunately, achieving these goals is not simple or easy. Many other factors come into play, including the patient's other disease states, other medications, adherence, beliefs, functional status, physiologic changes due to aging and disease, and ability to afford the medication. The basic principle of prescribing for older patients—briefly, start low, go slow—is repeated often. However, even the best clinicians who carefully adhere to this principle will encounter patients who have negative outcomes from one or more of their medications.

The principles of pharmacotherapy have not changed significantly during the past 20 years, but drug treatment has become more complex. More drugs are available every year, some with a new pharmacologic profile or mechanism of action. In addition, physicians must contend with expanded indications for available agents, both those that are approved by the U.S. Food and Drug Administration (FDA) and those that are off-label. Physicians also must be responsive to frequent changes in the managed-care formulary, the scientific advances in the understanding of drug-drug interactions (ie, the cytochrome P-450 system), the change of many drugs from prescription to nonprescription, and the boom in an unregulated third class of medications called *nutriceuticals,* that is, nutritional supplements, alternative medicines, and herbal preparations. Finally, very little information is available about the use of these unregulated medications in older patients—particularly, sick older patients on other medications.

AGE-ASSOCIATED CHANGES IN PHARMACOKINETICS

Pharmacokinetic studies define the time course of a drug and its metabolites throughout the body with respect to four parameters: absorption, distribution, metabolism, and elimination. The effects of aging on each parameter have been studied, and the resulting generalizations have been incorporated into the principles of prescribing for the older patient.

Absorption

Aging does not affect drug absorption via the gastrointestinal tract to any clinically significant degree. The rate of absorption may be slowed with age, but the extent of absorption remains unchanged. Consequently, the peak serum concentration of a drug in the older patient may be lower and the time to reach it delayed, but the overall amount absorbed (*bioavailability*) does not differ in younger and older patients. Exceptions include drugs that undergo an extensive first-pass effect (eg, nitrates); they tend to have higher serum concentrations or increased bioavailability, since less drug is extracted by the liver as a consequence of decreased liver size and blood flow.

Factors that have a greater impact on drug absorption include the way a medication is taken, what it is taken with, and a patient's comorbid illnesses. For example, the absorption of many fluoroquinolones (eg, ciprofloxacin) is reduced when they are taken with divalent cations such as calcium, magnesium, and iron that are found in antacids, sucralfate, dairy products, or vitamins. Enteral feedings interfere with the absorption of some drugs (eg, phenytoin). An increase in gastric pH from proton-pump inhibitors, H_2 antagonists, or antacids may increase the absorption of some drugs, such as nifedipine and amoxicillin, and decrease the absorption of other drugs, such as the imidazole antifungals, ampicillin, cyanocobalamin, and indinavir. Agents that promote or delay gastrointestinal motility, such as stimulant laxatives and metoclopramide, can, in theory, affect a drug's absorption by increasing or decreasing the time spent in the segment of the intestinal tract necessary for dissolution or absorption. Another mechanism that can increase or decrease drug absorption is the inhibition or induction of enzymes in the gastrointestinal tract (this is discussed on p 76, in the section on drug interactions).

Distribution

Distribution refers to the locations in the body a drug penetrates and the time required for the drug to reach those locations. Distribution is expressed as the volume of distribution (Vd), with units of volume (eg, liters) or volume per weight (eg, L/kg).

Age-associated changes in body composition can alter drug distribution. In older patients, drugs that are water soluble (*hydrophilic*) have a lower volume of distribution, as older people have less body water and lean body mass. Drugs affected include ethanol and lithium. Digoxin, which distributes and binds to skeletal muscle, has been reported to have a reduced volume of distribution in older persons because of the reduced muscle mass of older adults. Drugs that are fat soluble (*lipophilic*) have an increased volume of distribution in older persons because they have greater fat stores than do younger persons. Thus, it takes longer for an older patient taking a lipophilic drug to reach a steady-state concentration and longer for the drug to be eliminated from the body. Examples of fat-soluble drugs include diazepam, flurazepam, thiopental, and trazodone.

The extent to which a drug is bound to plasma proteins also influences its volume of distribution. Albumin, the primary plasma protein to which drugs bind, is often decreased in older patients; thus, a higher proportion of drug is unbound (free) and pharmacologically active. Drugs that bind to albumin and whose unbound fraction has been shown to be increased in elderly persons include ceftriaxone, diazepam, lorazepam, phenytoin, valproic acid, and warfarin. Normally, additional unbound drug is eliminated; however, age-related decreases in the organ systems of elimination may result in the accumulation of unbound drug in the body. Phenytoin provides an example of the way an increase in unbound drug can lead to an unnecessary and potentially harmful dosage increase. A patient with a low serum albumin (≤ 3

g/dL) whose phenytoin dose is increased because his or her total phenytoin concentration is subtherapeutic may develop symptoms and signs of phenytoin toxicity after a dose increase because the concentration of free phenytoin is elevated.

Metabolism

The liver is the most common site of drug metabolism, but metabolic conversion also can take place in the intestinal wall, lungs, skin, kidneys, and other organs. Aging affects the liver by decreasing liver blood flow as well as decreasing liver size and mass. Consequently, in the older patient the metabolic clearance of drugs by the liver may be reduced. Drug clearance is also reduced with aging for drugs that are subject to the phase I pathways or reactions, which include hydroxylation, oxidation, dealkylation, and reduction. Most drugs metabolized through phase I pathways may be converted to metabolites of lesser, equal, or greater pharmacologic effect than the parent compound (eg, diazepam). Drugs metabolized through the phase II pathways are converted to inactive compounds through glucuronidation, conjugation, or acetylation (eg, lorazepam). Medications subject to phase II metabolism are generally preferred for older patients, as their metabolites are not active and will not accumulate.

Age and gender differences also have been reported. For example, oxazepam is metabolized faster in elderly men than in elderly women. The reason is unknown. Nefazodone concentrations have been reported to be 50% greater in older women, but no differences were found between older men and younger persons.

In drug metabolism, factors other than aging can exaggerate or override the effects of aging. For example, hepatic congestion due to heart failure decreases the metabolism of warfarin, resulting in an increased pharmacologic response. Smoking stimulates monooxygenase enzymes and increases the clearance of theophylline even in older patients.

Elimination

Elimination refers to a drug's final route(s) of exit from the body. For most drugs, this involves elimination by the kidney as either the parent compound or as a metabolite or metabolites. Terms used to express elimination are a drug's *half-life* and its *clearance*.

A drug's half-life is the time it takes for its plasma or serum concentration to decline by 50%, for example, from 20 µg/mL to 10 µg/mL. Half-life is usually expressed in hours. Steady state is reached when the amount of drug entering the systemic circulation is equal to the amount being eliminated. For a drug administered on a regular basis, 95% of steady state in the body is achieved after five half-lives of the drug.

Clearance is usually expressed as volume per unit of time (eg, L/hour or mL/minute) and represents the volume of plasma or serum from which the drug is removed (ie, cleared) per unit of time. Clearance may also be expressed as volume per weight per unit of time (L/kg/hour). Half-life and clearance can also refer to metabolic elimination.

The effects of aging on kidney function have been studied to a greater extent than have the effects of aging on liver function. Glomerular filtration declines as a consequence of a decrease in kidney size and renal blood flow and a decrease in functioning nephrons. On average, kidney function begins to decline when people reach their mid-30s, with an average decline of 6 to 12 mL per minute per 1.73 m^2 per decade. Follow-up studies (conducted in men only) over 10 to 15 years found three normally distributed groups: those whose creatinine clearance declined to the extent that it was clinically significant; a second group whose creatinine clearance declined to the extent that it was statistically but not clinically significant; and a third group whose creatinine clearance did not change. Renal tubular secretion also declines with age.

Serum creatinine is not an accurate reflection of creatinine clearance in elderly patients. Because of the age-related decline in lean muscle mass, the older person's production of creatinine is reduced. The decrease in glomerular filtration rate counters the decreased production of creatinine, and serum creatinine stays within the normal range, not revealing the change in creatinine clearance.

The conservative approach in treating the older patient is to calculate the appropriate dose for renally eliminated medications as if the patient's kidney function actually has declined with aging. Measuring a patient's 24-hour creatinine clearance would be the most accurate way to determine the appropriate dose, but this is time consuming and requires an accurate 24-hour urine collection. An 8-hour collection time has been shown to be accurate but has not been widely accepted.

To initially estimate a patient's creatinine clearance (CrCl), the clinician can use the Cockroft and Gault equation (see below).

$$CrCl = \frac{(140 - age) \times weight}{72 \times serum\ creatinine}$$

Weight in kg; serum creatinine in mg/100 mL; 85% less in women.

The equation is widely applied, but it has limitations. First, not all patients experience a significant age-related decline in renal function, and for them, the equation would underestimate creatinine clearance. Second, for patients whose muscle mass is reduced beyond that of normal aging, the creatinine clearance would be overestimated. This would apply to persons whose serum creatinine is less than normal, that is, < 0.7 mg/dL. It has been suggested that 1 mg/dL be substituted for a low serum creatinine. However, normalizing the serum creatinine has not been shown to be a precise estimate, and it generally underestimates the actual creatinine clearance.

In cases in which the patient's kidney function may be impaired but estimates of function are uncertain, the clinician should consider the following:

- Avoid drugs that are entirely dependent on renal elimination and with which accumulation would result in toxicity (eg, imipenem).
- If the use of such an agent cannot be avoided, obtain an accurate measure of kidney function (eg, an 8- or 24-hour creatinine clearance).
- Monitor serum or plasma concentrations of the drug (eg, aminoglycosides).

AGE-ASSOCIATED CHANGES IN PHARMACODYNAMICS

The pharmacodynamic action of a drug—that is, its time course and intensity of pharmacologic effect—may change with the increasing age of the patient. An excellent example of such pharmacodynamic changes in older persons has been demonstrated with the benzodiazepines. Older persons have been found to have more sedation and lower performance than younger persons on a psychomotor test following a single dose of triazolam. These differences are attributed to pharmacokinetic changes, that is, to significantly higher plasma triazolam concentrations that are due to reduced clearance in the elderly persons. However, a different pattern has been found for nitrazepam: The pharmacokinetics of nitrazepam (an intermediate-acting benzodiazepine similar to lorazepam) were found to be no different in young and older persons after a single 10-mg dose; yet, 12 hours and 36 hours after a 10-mg dose, older persons were found to make significantly more mistakes on a psychomotor test than when they had taken placebo. Younger persons did not demonstrate significant impairment at any time. In addition, even with short-term use, young and elderly patients may experience impaired balance and posture following a single dose of a benzodiazepine.

It is uncertain whether the age-associated pharmacokinetic changes of morphine account for the increased level and prolonged duration of pain relief experienced by older patients. In older adults, morphine has been shown to have a smaller volume of distribution, higher plasma concentrations, and longer clearance than in younger adults. Older patients achieve pain relief at least equivalent to younger patients at half the intramuscular dose, and they have an increased duration of pain relief. Thus, the dose or frequency, or both, of morphine given intramuscularly or by intravenous infusion should be lower, at least initially, in older patients.

Pharmacodynamic and pharmacokinetic changes, alone or together, generally result in an increased sensitivity to medications by the older adult. In some patients, particularly those who are frail, the use of lower doses, longer intervals between doses, and longer periods between changes in dose are ways to successfully manage drug therapy and decrease the chances of medication intolerance or toxicity. Disease- and drug-specific monitoring are also necessary to ensure a successful outcome.

OPTIMIZING PRESCRIBING

Optimizing drug therapy for older adults means achieving the balance between overprescribing and underprescribing of beneficial therapies. Overprescribing of drug therapies not only refers to the use of multiple medications but also implies a lack of appropriateness in medication selection, dose, or use. One survey found that 40% of nursing-home residents had an order for at least one potentially inappropriate medication. Analyses of national medication use surveys in the ambulatory setting have consistently shown that > 20% of older patients received at least one potentially inappropriate medication, with at least one potentially inappropriate medication prescribed at 8% of office visits. Furthermore, nearly 4% of office visits and 10% of medical hospital admissions resulted in a prescription for one or more medications classified as "never" or "rarely appropriate" for older patients. The potential consequences of overprescribing include adverse drug events (ADEs), drug-drug interactions, duplication of drug therapy, decreased quality of life, and unnecessary costs.

The factors associated with inappropriate prescribing or overprescribing are listed in Table 10.1. Simply limiting the number of medications for a given patient, however, is not always possible or desirable. For example, a patient with heart failure may be appropriately treated with three or four drugs: a diuretic, an angiotensin-converting enzyme (ACE) inhibitor, a β-blocker, and perhaps digoxin. If this patient has hyperlipidemia and diabetes mellitus, another two or three medications could be required. Hence, such a

Table 10.1—Factors Associated With Inappropriate Prescribing or Overprescribing

Patient Factors

Advanced age

Female gender

Lower educational level

Rural residence

Belief in using "a pill for every ill"

Multiple health problems

Use of multiple medications

Use of multiple pharmacies

System Factors

Multiple prescribers for individual patient

Poor record keeping

Failure to review a patient's medication regimen at least annually

patient would be taking five to seven indicated medications for major medical conditions alone.

The underprescribing of medications to older adults is also of concern. Underprescribing may result from an effort to avoid overprescribing, a complex medication regimen, or adverse effects. It may also result from the thinking that older adults will not benefit from medications intended as primary or secondary prevention, or from aggressive management of chronic conditions, such as hypertension and diabetes mellitus.

Medications often cited as underprescribed in older adults include ACE inhibitors and β-blockers for heart failure and at discharge following an acute myocardial infarction (MI), aspirin within 24 hours and at discharge following an acute MI, warfarin for atrial fibrillation, HMG–CoA reductase inhibitors for primary prevention of cardiovascular events, gastroprotective agents for patients at high risk for NSAID-induced gastrointestinal bleeding, and narcotic analgesics for pain control.

Underprescribing was recognized by the Centers for Medicare and Medicaid Services (CMS), which implemented quality indicators in 1998 to measure the use of recommended medications prior to discharge for acute MI, stroke, and pneumonia in hospitalized patients with fee-for-service Medicare. Comparison of data from 1998–99 to 2000–2001 found that the percentage of patients receiving appropriate care had improved for the nation as a whole in the management of these conditions, but the prescribing of an ACE inhibitor in heart failure had declined. In spite of this overall improvement, between 16% and 29% of patients did not receive appropriate pharmacotherapy prior to discharge after their MI.

Investigators from the Assessing Care of Vulnerable Elders (ACOVE) project developed explicit medication quality indicators divided into four categories: prescribing indicated medications; avoiding inappropriate medications; education, continuity, and documentation; and medication monitoring. These indicators were applied to "vulnerable" older adults enrolled in two managed care organizations and the results were reported as the percentage of eligible patients who met the indicator or "pass rate." The prescribing of indicated medications category had an overall pass rate of 50% (range 11% to 94% for the 17 indicators); avoiding the prescription of inappropriate medications had an overall pass rate of 97% (range 79% to 100% avoidance across the 9 indicators). The overall pass rate for education, continuity, and documentation indicators was 81% (range 10% to 99% for the 8 indicators). The 9 indicators for medication monitoring had an overall pass rate of 64% (range 22% to 80%). These results suggest that the prescribing of inappropriate medications is less of a problem than the underprescribing of indicated medications and the failure to monitor medications, document information about medications, maintain continuity, and educate patients.

ADVERSE DRUG EVENTS

An ADE is defined as an injury resulting from the use of a drug. Preventable adverse drug events are among the most serious consequences of inappropriate drug prescribing among older adults. An adverse drug reaction (ADR) is a type of ADE; it refers to harm that is directly caused by a drug at usual doses. For a listing of risk factors for ADEs in older patients, see Table 10.2.

ADEs are estimated to be responsible for 5% to 28% of acute geriatric medical admissions; the estimated annual incidence rate is 26 per 1000 beds for hospitalized patients. It has been estimated that in the nursing home, for every dollar spent on medications, $1.33 in health care resources is consumed in the treatment of drug-related morbidity and mortality. A cohort study of all long-term-care residents in 18

Table 10.2—Risk Factors for Adverse Drug Events in Older Patients

- Age > 85 years
- Low body weight or body mass index
- ≥ 6 Concurrent chronic diagnoses
- An estimated creatinine clearance < 50 mL per minute
- ≥ 9 Medications
- ≥ 12 Doses of medications per day
- A prior adverse drug reaction

nursing homes in Massachusetts demonstrated that ADEs are common and often preventable in nursing homes. During the 28,839 resident-months of observations, 546 ADEs were identified. Overall, 51% of these adverse events were judged to have been preventable. Most of the errors occurred at the ordering and monitoring stages. A cohort study of residents of two long-term-care facilities found the overall rate of ADEs to be 9.8 per 100 resident months. Atypical antipsychotics, anticoagulants, and diuretics were the drug classes found to be most frequently associated with ADEs.

In the ambulatory setting, the ADE rate has been reported to be 50.1 per 1000 person-years, and the preventable ADE rate to be 13.8 per 1000 person-years. Cardiovascular drugs, diuretics, NSAIDs, hypoglycemics, and anticoagulants are the drug classes found to be most often associated with preventable ADEs. Again, errors occurred most often at the time of prescribing or were related to inadequate monitoring. The majority of ADEs (≥ 95%) experienced by older patients are considered to be predictable.

Lists of potentially inappropriate medications and medication-disease pairs have been published. One list that was developed by the consensus of experts in geriatric medicine and pharmacology (1997 Beers criteria) has been adapted by the CMS for identifying potentially inappropriate or unnecessary medication use by nursing-home residents. An updated version was published in late 2003 (see reference by Fick, 2003, in the list at the end of the chapter); however, CMS has not adopted this list as of the time of this writing. (For the current version, also see the most recent edition of *Geriatrics At Your Fingertips*, published annually by the American Geriatrics Society.)

A common pathway for ADEs and polypharmacy has been described as the "prescribing cascade." One form of this cascade occurs when a medication results in an ADE that is mistaken as a separate diagnosis and treated with more medications, which puts the patient at risk for additional ADEs and more medications. Examples that have been studied include metoclopramide-induced parkinsonism and the subsequent prescribing of antiparkinson medications, and calcium channel blockers that result in peripheral edema and the subsequent use of diuretics.

DRUG INTERACTIONS

A drug-drug interaction (DDI) is defined as the pharmacologic or clinical response to the administration of a drug combination that differs from that anticipated from the known effects of each of the two agents when given alone. Drug-drug interactions are important because they may lead to ADEs. The likelihood of DDIs increases as the number of medications a patient takes increases. Among prescription drugs, cardiovascular and psychotropic drugs are most commonly involved in DDIs. A positive correlation exists between the number of potential DDIs and the number of adverse effects experienced by hospitalized older patients. The most common adverse effects are neuropsychologic (primarily delirium), arterial hypotension, and acute kidney failure. Drug combinations that are reported to result in increased risk for hospitalization for older patients are shown in Table 10.3. Drugs commonly involved in DDIs in long-term care are listed in Table 10.4. Risk factors associated with DDIs include the use of multiple medications, receiving care from several prescribing clinicians, and using more than one pharmacy.

Drug interactions can take many forms. For example, absorption can be enhanced or diminished (as described above), drugs with similar or opposite pharmacologic effects can result in exaggerated or impaired effects, and drug metabolism may be inhibited or induced. Research focusing on the cytochrome P-450 system has proposed or studied in vivo or in vitro numerous DDIs involving the different P-450 isozymes. The effect of aging on the cytochrome P-450 system and the clinical implications for prescribing have not been completely determined. Cross-sectional data have shown that cytochrome P-450 content declines incrementally, once in the fourth decade and again after age 70. In vitro microsomal activity of cytochrome (CYP) 3A4 is not altered by aging, but in vivo age- and gender-related reductions in drug clearance have been found for CYP3A4 substrates erythromycin, prednisolone, verapamil, alprazolam, nifedipine, and diazepam. CYP3A4 accounts for 30% of the P-450 content in the liver and is also prominent in the intestinal tract. This isozyme is involved in the metabolism of more than 50% of drugs on the market and can be induced by drugs such as rifampin, phenytoin, and carbamazepine, and inhibited by many drugs, including the macrolide antibiotics, nefazodone, itraconazole, ketoconazole, as well as grapefruit juice. The isozyme CYP2D6 is involved in the metabolism of 25% to 30% of marketed drugs and has been associated with only minimal age-related changes. CYP2D6 is involved in the metabolism of many psychotropic drugs and can be inhibited by many agents. In addition, approximately 10% of white people are deficient in this isozyme and have reduced ability to clear and increased sensitivity to CYP2D6 substrates. Clinically, these patients and those taking CYP2D6 inhibitors (eg, quinidine, paroxetine, fluoxetine) cannot convert codeine and tramadol to their active metabolites and have a reduced analgesic response to these agents.

For DDIs involving herbal preparations, see "Complementary and Alternative Medicine" (p 80).

Table 10.3—Most Common Drug-Drug Adverse Effects Identified Upon Hospitalization

Combination	Risk
ACE inhibitor + diuretic	Hypotension; hyperkalemia
ACE inhibitor + potassium	Hyperkalemia
Antiarrhythmic + diuretic	Electrolyte imbalance; arrhythmias
Benzodiazepine + antidepressant	Confusion, sedation, falls
Benzodiazepine + antipsychotic	Confusion, sedation, falls
Benzodiazepine + benzodiazepine	Confusion, sedation, falls
Calcium channel blocker + diuretic	Hypotension
Calcium channel blocker + nitrate	Hypotension
Digitalis + antiarrhythmic	Bradycardia, arrhythmias
Diuretic + digitalis	Arrhythmias
Diuretic + diuretic	Dehydration, electrolyte imbalance
Diuretic + nitrate	Hypotension
Nitrate + vasodilator	Hypotension

NOTE: ACE = angiotensin-converting enzyme.
SOURCE: Data from Doucet J, Chassagne P, Trivalle C, et al. Drug-drug interactions related to hospital admissions in older adults: a prospective study of 1000 patients. *J Am Geriatr Soc.* 1996;44(8):944–948.

Table 10.4—Dangerous Drugs Involved in Drug-Drug Interactions in Long-Term Care

Medication	Interacting Medications
Angiotensin-converting enzyme inhibitors	Potassium supplements, potassium-sparing diuretics
Digoxin	Antiarrhythmics, verapamil
Quinolones	Theophylline, warfarin
Warfarin	Sulfa drugs, macrolides, quinolones, nonsteroidal anti-inflammatory drugs, phenytoin

SOURCE: Data from the American Society of Consultant Pharmacists. Multidisciplinary Medication Management Project. Top Ten Dangerous Drug Interactions in Long-Term Care. Available at http://www.scoup.net/M3Project/topten/#1 (accessed October 2005).

DRUG-DISEASE INTERACTIONS

Drug-disease combinations common in older patients can affect drug response and lead to adverse drug events. Obesity and ascites alter the volumes of distribution of lipophilic and hydrophilic drugs, respectively. Patients with dementia may have increased sensitivity or paradoxical reactions to drugs with central nervous system or anticholinergic activity. Patients with renal insufficiency or impaired hepatic function due to cirrhosis or hepatic congestion have impaired detoxification and excretion of drugs. (See reference by Fick, 2003, at the end of the chapter.)

PRINCIPLES OF PRESCRIBING

Principles of prescribing for older patients are shown in Table 10.5. This basic approach applies primarily to medications that will be used to treat chronic conditions for which an immediate, complete therapeutic response is not necessary. A dose adjustment may still be needed for medications used to treat conditions requiring an immediate response (eg, when prescribing antibiotics for a patient with impaired kidney function).

Overprescribing can be prevented by reviewing a patient's medications on a regular basis and each time a new medication is started or a dose is changed. The importance of maintaining accurate records of all medications taken by the patient cannot be overemphasized. Knowing what other prescribers have given the patient and what patients are self-prescribing, and documenting all of this in the patient's records is crucial. Many patients do not consider vitamins, herbal preparations, or over-the-counter medications (even aspirin) to be medications, so clinicians must be specific when they inquire about a patient's use of other medications. Medications that have been newly approved by the FDA should be used cautiously in treating older patients. Such drugs are likely to be more expensive, and information about their use in older patients is often limited.

It is best if the patient brings all medications to the review, including over-the-counter medications, vitamins, and any herbal preparations or other types of supplements (a "brown-bag" evaluation). Examining the containers and labels and asking what each medication is for and how and when it is taken can provide insight into the patient's understanding and adherence to his or her medication regimens. Discontinue any medications when there is no longer an indication for their continued use. Any new complaints or worsening of an existing condition should prompt the consideration of whether it could be drug-induced. When considering treatment for a new medical condition, always consider nonpharmacologic approaches first. If a drug therapy is still indicated, select within the class in order to minimize the risk of an ADE.

Table 10.5—Principles of Prescribing for Older Patients

The basics:

- Start with a low dose.
- Titrate the dose upward slowly, as tolerated by the patient.
- Try not to start two drugs at the same time.

Determine the following before prescribing a new medication:

- Is the medication necessary? Are there nonpharmacologic ways to treat the condition?
- What are the therapeutic end points and how will they be assessed?
- Do the benefits outweigh the risks of the medication?
- Is one medication being used to treat the adverse effects of another?
- Is there one medication that could be prescribed to treat two conditions?
- Are there potential drug-drug or drug-disease interactions?
- Will the new medication's administration times be the same as those of existing medications?
- Do the patient and caregiver understand what the medication is for, how to take it, how long to take it, when it should start to work, possible adverse effects that it might cause, and what to do if they occur?

At least annually:

- Ask the patient to bring in all medications (prescription, over-the-counter, supplements, and herbal preparations) to the office; for new patients, conduct a detailed medication history.
- For prescription medications, determine whether the label directions and dose match those in the patient's chart; ask the patient how each medication is being taken.
- Ask about medication side effects.
- Note who else is prescribing medications for the patient, and what the medications are and their indications.
- Look for medications with duplicate therapeutic, pharmacologic, or adverse effect profiles.
- Screen for drug-drug and drug-disease interactions.
- Eliminate unnecessary medications; confer with other prescribers if necessary.
- Simplify the medication regimen; use the fewest possible number of medications and doses per day.
- Always review any changes with the patient and caregiver; provide the changes in writing.

When initiating therapy, the basic principle should be to start low go and go slow. Though the FDA requires that labeling for new drugs regarding dosing in older patients not be extrapolated from another patient population (eg, patients with kidney impairment), it does not require that a drug be studied explicitly in older persons. Older persons are used in the studies of many new drugs for their phase I and II dose tolerability and their pharmacokinetic and pharmacodynamic actions, but the older persons chosen for these studies are usually healthy and free of concomitant illnesses. Much of what is known about medications and how to use them in sick older patients, particularly those who are frail, is learned only after a drug has been available for several years.

NONADHERENCE

Nonadherence and underadherence to medications is a huge and often unrecognized problem in drug treatment. It is estimated that nonadherence among elderly people may be as high as 50%. Patients may be reluctant to admit that they are not taking medications or not following directions. If nonadherence is suspected, the clinician needs to consider the patient's financial, cognitive, and functional status, as well as his or her beliefs about and understanding of medications and diseases.

Prescription drug costs have increased substantially, and supplemental prescription drug benefit plans are expensive. Some plans still may leave a patient with a copayment that he or she cannot afford or with only a fixed dollar amount for the year. Clinicians should avoid prescribing expensive new medications that have not been shown to be superior to less expensive generic alternatives.

Cognitive impairment may also cause nonadherence, as patients forget to take medications or confuse them. Simplifying the regimen and involving a caregiver to oversee medication management can be helpful approaches. Medication trays or drug calendars also may help with organization, and they are very useful for patients who have difficulty remembering when they last took a medication.

The older patient's ability to read labels, open containers, or pour medications or even a glass of water may be impaired, so functional assessment can be useful. Some patients may need additional education or reinforcement about the purpose of a medication, especially those used to treat conditions that are usually asymptomatic, such as diabetes mellitus and hypertension. Older patients also may need reassurance regarding the safety and possible adverse effects of certain medications, particularly newly prescribed medications or those associated with serious adverse events, such as warfarin.

ANNOTATED REFERENCES

- Fick DM, Cooper JW, Wade WE, et al. Updating the Beers criteria for potentially inappropriate medication use in older adults: results of a U.S. consensus panel of experts. *Arch Intern Med.* 2003;163(22):2716–2724.

  Recognizing that several of the drugs on the Beers criteria were no longer available or their use had declined substantially, the authors convened a group of experts in geriatrics and geriatric pharmacotherapy to revise and update the Beers criteria by the use of a modified Delphi method. The panel eliminated 15 medications or medication classes from the 1997 Beers criteria. The panel added 25 medications or medication classes independent of diagnosis and another 19 medications or medication classes considering diagnosis. This update has not been adopted by the Centers for Medicare and Medicaid Services, but it is a valuable tool for clinicians.

- Goulding MR. Inappropriate medication prescribing for elderly ambulatory care patients. *Arch Intern Med.* 2004;164(3):305–312.

  The author applies the 1997 Beers criteria and another modified version of the Beers criteria referred to as the Zhan list to the National Ambulatory Medical Care Survey and the National Hospital Ambulatory Medical Care Survey for the years 1995 to 2000. The findings show that over the 5-year period the prevalence of inappropriate prescribing did not change, that women were more likely and patients aged > 80 years were less likely to be prescribed an inappropriate medication. The odds of being prescribed an inappropriate medication increased with each prescription drug added to the patient's regimen. Propoxyphene, diazepam, amitriptyline, hydroxyzine, and oxybutynin were the most frequently prescribed inappropriate medications. Family and general practice physicians were more likely than other specialists to prescribe inappropriate medications.

- Gurwitz JH, Field TS, Harrold LR, et al. Incidence and preventability of adverse drug events among older persons in the ambulatory setting. *JAMA.* 2003;289(9):1107–1116.

  This cohort study was designed to determine the incidence and prevalence of adverse drug events in all ambulatory Medicare enrollees in a multispecialty practice. The frequency of adverse events was 50.1 per 1000 person-years; the rate of preventable adverse events was 13.8 per 1000 person-years. More than half of preventable events were due to errors in prescribing and monitoring. This study serves as evidence that a portion of adverse drug events are preventable.

- Murray MD, Callahan CM. Improving medication use for older adults: an integrated research agenda. *Ann Intern Med.* 2003;139(5 Pt 2):425–429.

  In this overview of the premarketing and postmarketing phases of drug development and study, the authors describe how pharmaceutical advances are an integral part of successful aging. Ways that medication use can be improved through a research agenda are discussed and include drug discovery and delivery, drug efficacy and safety, pharmacoepidemiology and drug policy, along with improved access to and use of drugs.

- Rollason V, Vogt N. Reduction of polypharmacy in the elderly: a systematic review of the role of the pharmacist. *Drugs Aging.* 2003;20(11):817–832.

This systematic review covers the definitions and prevalence of polypharmacy, its causes and consequences, and the impact of pharmacists on its reduction. Fourteen clinical trials were identified that included an intervention by a pharmacist. Interventions most often included a review of the patient's medication profile followed by the communication to the patient's prescriber of recommendations to reduce polypharmacy. Seven of the fourteen trials were shown to significantly reduce the number of medications taken by patients in the intervention groups. Other trials did not reduce the number of medications but improved overall care by eliminating unnecessary medications and adding medications for previously undiagnosed or undertreated conditions. The authors review the limitations of these trials and offer recommendations for further research on interventions to reduce polypharmacy.

Todd P. Semla, PharmD, MS
Paula A. Rochon, MD, MPH

CHAPTER 11—COMPLEMENTARY AND ALTERNATIVE MEDICINE

KEY POINTS

- The use of complementary and alternative medicine appears to be on the rise in all adult age groups, including the elderly population.

- Stress-reduction techniques may benefit many conditions prevalent among older patients, including falls, osteoporosis, osteoarthritis, high blood pressure, obesity, insomnia, depression, irritability related to the menopause, diabetes mellitus, and certain effects of cancer.

- Saw palmetto is commonly used to reduce the symptoms associated with benign prostatic hyperplasia, and in at least one well-conducted study it has been shown to exert effects similar to those of standard pharmacologic treatments.

- Though many herbal and biologic preparations offer promise, they are largely of unproven benefit and their contents are unregulated by government agencies, making their use very challenging to endorse and guide.

Complementary and alternative medicine (CAM), as currently defined by the National Center for Complementary and Alternative Medicine (NCCAM) of the National Institutes of Health, refers to "a group of diverse medical and health care systems, practices, and products that are not presently considered to be part of conventional medicine." Although some scientific evidence exists regarding certain CAM therapies, for most there are key questions that are yet to be answered through well-designed research studies— questions such as whether they are safe and whether they work for the diseases or medical conditions for which they are used.

NCCAM conceptualizes the diversity of CAM modalities as follows:

- Mind-body interventions, such as meditation, prayer, relaxation, and art, dance, and music therapies

- Biologically based therapies, such as herbal preparations, botanicals, and dietary supplements

- Manipulative and body-based methods, such as chiropractic, therapeutic massage, and osteopathic manipulation

- Energy therapies such as Reiki, therapeutic touch, and bioelectromagnetic-based therapies

- Whole medical systems, such as traditional Chinese medicine, Ayurvedic medicine, homeopathy, and naturopathic medicine, which incorporate many or all of the above-noted therapies.

The list of what is considered to be CAM is continually evolving, as therapies that are proved to be safe and effective become adopted into conventional health care and as new approaches to health care emerge.

The use of CAM is widespread. The National Health Interview Survey (NHIS) selected a nationally representative sample of over 31,000 U.S. adults. Sixty-two percent of those interviewed noted some use of 27 different CAM modalities during the previous 12 months when CAM was defined to include prayer for health reasons. Most CAM use is complementary, that is, in addition to mainstream interventions; only a minority of CAM use serves as an alternative to conventional treatment. Approximately 60% of CAM users in the United States do not discuss their use of CAM modalities with their health care providers. This is of particular concern in the care of older adults because of the increased risk for adverse interactions between conventional drugs and various CAM biologic agents. Moreover, aging impacts the metabolism of numerous prescription and over-the-counter medications, and possibly that of many herbal preparations, botanicals, and dietary supplements. Age-related alterations in hepatic and renal function contribute importantly to these phenomena, both in the absence and presence of disease.

HEALTH CARE FOR THE AGING POPULATION

The aging of the baby-boomer generation is contributing to the already established largest group of health care consumers—older adults. Among the most common health challenges in aged men are diseases of the circulatory, musculoskeletal, and connective tissue and of the genitourinary systems. In aging women, the most common health challenges are musculoskeletal, circulatory, and mental health disorders. Demographic considerations assure that the need of the expanding aging population for medical services will continue to increase, and it is logical to predict that specific interest in, and use of, CAM modalities will expand as well.

The use of CAM by older persons is beginning to be more closely studied, in part to help design safer and more efficacious treatments specific to the needs of those older than 65 years. In one small study, 30% of adults surveyed aged 65 and older (N = 311) reported using alternative medicine, and 19% visited an alternative medicine provider. The CAM modalities used most commonly by the older adults in this study were herbal preparations and chiropractic, both of which can cause problems in this population. Of note, CAM use can vary, depending on a particular geographic region as well as ethnic group.

In a study reported in 2003, which was conducted in three ethnically diverse groups of community-dwelling elderly persons (N = 525) in southern California, 251 respondents (47.8%) reported CAM use. The differences in predominant patterns of CAM use among the three groups—Asian, Hispanic, and white non-Hispanic—suggested that differing sociocultural beliefs influence the frequency and pattern of CAM use. Another such example can be found in the large variety of home remedies used by older black Americans, which can be related to regional customs in the United States. CAM use by black Americans is viewed as a combination of European, Native American, and African customs. In addition, Native American and black American groups also view spirituality as integral to the prevention of illness and maintenance of health. Knowledge of patients' spiritual beliefs can assist physicians to provide sensitive, culturally specific care. Recognition of the individual patient's cultural heritage may augment communication and trust between physicians and patients about CAM, resulting in improved, comprehensive health care. (See also "Cultural Aspects of Care," p 51.)

CURRENT ISSUES: SAFETY AND EFFICACY

Currently in the United States, a wide variety of CAM modalities are available from practitioners, or as self-care practices. These span the spectrum from indigenous health practices that are centuries old to CAM modalities that are licensed and provided by a trained practitioner. However, most CAM practices have not been regulated, and licensure and certification can vary among practices and by geographic location. There are numerous anecdotal reports or claims of the efficacy and safety of diverse CAM modalities, yet there is a general lack of product and practice standardization and a dearth of credible scientific information supporting these practices. There is substantial potential for adverse reactions with the use of herbal preparations and of botanical and dietary supplements in older adults (Table 11.1). Nonetheless, most consumers are satisfied, and few malpractice or wrongful injury lawsuits are filed.

CAM USE FOR MANAGING ILLNESS IN OLDER PERSONS

Musculoskeletal Disorders

The incidence of osteoporosis and nontraumatic fractures of the wrist, spine, and hip increase with age in women and men. Phytoestrogen and soy products are increasingly used to prevent or treat osteoporosis in postmenopausal women, although there is little evidence confirming their benefits. Dehydroepiandrosterone (DHEA), a widely used dietary supplement, is the most abundant adrenal steroid in humans. Circulating DHEA levels decline progressively with age. Small-scale trials of DHEA supplementation in older persons have produced conflicting results regarding its effects on bone density, and further studies are needed to determine its utility in preventing or treating osteoporosis in older people.

Osteoarthritis is one of the most common chronic diseases affecting older men and women. In one recent study, almost half (47%) of the patients with osteoarthritis aged 55 to 75 years reported using some CAM modality. Because the personal experience of pain can increase the levels of associated suffering, addressing any negative beliefs and emotions that the patient may be struggling with is as important as addressing the physical symptoms. CAM techniques specifically focused to provide stress relief, such as relaxation breathing and music therapy, may be of benefit as adjunctive therapy. Gentle movement and stretching techniques, such as those in yoga, Tai Chi, and warm-water aquatics, can provide an alternative to

Table 11.1—Safety Issues Related to Dietary Supplements Used by Older Adults

Supplement	Adverse Effects	Interacts With:
Coenzyme Q10	Infrequent nausea, emesis, epigastric pain, headaches > 300 mg/day linked to increased liver transaminase	Warfarin
Dehydroepiandrosterone (DHEA)	Women: weight gain, voice changes, facial hair, headaches Men: prostatic hypertrophy, possible increase in hormone-sensitive tumors	Calcium channel blockers, sildenafil
Echinacea	Allergic reactions, hepatitis, asthma, vertigo, anaphylaxis (rare)	Immunosuppressants
Ginkgo biloba	All rare: serious bleeding, seizures, headaches, dizziness, vertigo	Anticoagulants
Glucosamine	Nausea, diarrhea, heartburn	Hypoglycemic drugs (reduces effectiveness)
Omega-3 fatty acids	Belching, halitosis, blood glucose elevations	Antiplatelets, anticoagulants, antihypertensives
SAM-e	Nausea, vomiting, diarrhea, anxiety, restlessness	Tricyclics and selective serotonin-reuptake inhibitors
Saw palmetto	All rare: constipation, diarrhea, decreased libido, headaches, hypertension, urine retention	None described
St. John's wort	Nausea, allergic reactions, dizziness, headache, photosensitivity (rare)	Anticoagulants, antivirals, selective serotonin-reuptake inhibitors

more vigorous exercise regimens. Other CAM modalities that are chosen by osteoarthritis patients include acupuncture, massage, chiropractic manipulation, glucosamine supplements, Reiki, and prayer. Large multicenter trials are under way to assess the separate and combined effects of glucosamine, chondroitin sulphate, and acupuncture in the treatment of pain associated with osteoarthritis of the knee. Herbal preparations, including capsaicin cream and Phytodolor, may have limited but unproven efficacy in reducing pain and improving motility; they are thought to exert effects mechanistically in much the same way as conventional nonsteroidal anti-inflammatory treatments. (See also "Musculoskeletal Diseases and Disorders," p 430, and "Persistent Pain," p 140.)

Lower back pain is one of the most difficult health challenges for which CAM modalities are used, particularly, therapeutic massage, acupuncture, mind-body relaxation, and energy modalities. One study reported that the combined use of massage, self-care relaxation, and acupuncture may be more effective than the use of any of these modalities separately. (See also "Back and Neck Pain," p 445.) A meta-analysis of randomized trials of acupuncture for lower back pain found it to be superior to various control modalities, but a significant placebo effect was found.

Cardiovascular Disorders

Cardiovascular disease affects at least 60% to 70% of the population older than 65 years. Of particular relevance is the higher incidence of cardiovascular disease occurring in obese patients or those with type 2 diabetes mellitus. Increased individual and public health efforts to prevent disease and identify those older adults at risk of developing disease should contribute to decreases in morbidity and mortality.

Healthy diet and aerobic exercise are the first recommendations to manage high blood pressure and dyslipidemia. A heart-healthy diet includes limiting sodium intake, refined sugar, and saturated fat while increasing amounts of complex carbohydrates, fruits, and vegetables. In the Dietary Approach to Stop Hypertension (DASH) trial, nearly 70% of participants following the healthy diet decreased both systolic and diastolic blood-pressure measurements. In addition, recent studies suggest that diets including essential fatty acids may lower blood pressure, increase levels of high-density lipoproteins, and lower levels of triglycerides and low-density lipoproteins. Examples of essential fatty acids are omega-3 and omega-6 acids. The omega-3 fatty acids can be found in fresh deep-water fish and in flaxseed oil. Omega-6-linoleic acid is found in raw nuts and seeds. For further reduction of the risk of developing hypertension and obesity, aerobic exercise, such as swimming or brisk walking, is advised for at least 30 minutes three times a week. Recent reports suggest that even mild to moderate increases in physical activity, such as walking slowly or gardening, have beneficial cardiovascular effects. Increased blood pressure can also be associated with inadequate sleep. The use of stress-management techniques, such as relaxation breathing, music therapy, and meditation, may reduce blood pressure in hypertensive patients and improve sleep quality in aging patients. (See also "Hypertension," p 361; "Physical Activity," p 56; and "Sleep Problems," p 249.)

Neurologic and Emotional Disorders

Depression is one the most common and debilitating major public health problems, and its incidence increases with advancing age. Although depression is more common in women, increasing attention is focused on the issue of depression in men, in whom it is more often unrecognized or untreated. There is an alarming prevalence of depression and suicide in widowed men aged 70 years and over. CAM use by the aging patient may assist in the management of mild to moderate depression. However, adequate treatment of severe depression may involve psychotherapy and psychotropic medication to prevent further morbidity and mortality. Recent research suggests that depression is also a systemic disease and is associated with an increased incidence of sleep disorders, osteoporosis, obesity, insulin resistance, and immune dysfunction. The impact of CAM modalities on these outcomes is unclear.

A healthy diet can be one of the first recommendations to assist with improving mood. Dietary intake that includes complex carbohydrates can improve serotonin levels. Increasing essential fatty acids and protein intake may increase alertness and mood. Of equal importance is discontinuing excess alcohol, caffeine, and tobacco, which can contribute to depression and irritability.

Aerobic exercise is also prescribed as a treatment for mild to moderate depression in aged patients. Exercise in combination with antidepressants can yield faster, more lasting results than either alone.

The botanical known as St. John's wort has received considerable attention and remains widely used. A large multicenter study failed to show the efficacy of this agent in patients with major depression of mild to moderate degree. Whether St. John's wort will prove to be efficacious in patients with mild symptoms of depression, social phobia, and seasonal affective disorder remains to be determined. The adverse effects of St. John's wort include gastrointestinal upset, fatigue, dizziness, headache, dry mouth, and photosensitivity. St. John's wort interacts with the hepatic P-450 enzyme system that induces the metabolism of many drugs, thus causing clinically significant adverse interactions and potential therapeutic failure with various antiretroviral, anticoagulant, immunosuppressant, antidepressant, and chemotherapeutic drugs.

S-adenosylmethionine (SAM-e) is a naturally occurring compound that is necessary for the brain to adequately produce dopamine and serotonin. This compound is currently marketed as an antidepressant. In one promising study involving 195 patients, taking 400 mg of SAM-e daily was found to lessen depressive symptoms.

See also "Depression and Other Mood Disorders" (p 269).

Some studies have investigated the use of supplements for treatment of dementia from Alzheimer's disease and vascular insufficiency. *Ginkgo biloba* extract (EGb 761) has shown some benefit in improving cognitive ability and memory impairment in Alzheimer's patients, in some, but not all studies. Brain tissue studies and spinal fluid abnormalities in Alzheimer's patients also offer reasonable rationale for supplementing with various antioxidants, including vitamins A, C, and E and selenium, though evidence of their effect has yet to be demonstrated in clinical trials. (See also "Dementia," p 221.)

Studies have shown that Parkinson's disease patients have reduced brain levels of glutathione, an antioxidant involved in neuroprotective functions. Parkinson's patients also have deficiencies in coenzyme Q10. Supplementation with these two naturally occurring substances has been shown to slow the progression of disease and reduce the severity of symptoms in very small unblinded clinical trials. Patients with Parkinson's disease may also benefit from a combination of dietary food additions containing higher amounts of coenzyme Q10, as found in salmon, sardines, and mackerel. Acupuncture, music therapy, and physical therapy are used by Parkinson's patients to attempt to reduce disabilities and improve cognitive, emotional, and social functioning. (See also "Neurologic Diseases and Disorders," p 458.)

Sleep disorders are common in older persons, affecting both sleep quality and quantity. Studies suggest that abnormalities in slow-wave and rapid-eye-movement sleep may also be linked to psychologic, endocrine-metabolic, and immune system dysfunctions. Nutritional and exercise modifications are among the safest recommendations when working with the elderly patients. Milk contains tryptophan, which is a precursor of serotonin. Having warm milk before bedtime or eating other tryptophan-containing foods such as bananas, brown rice, and turkey may be helpful in relieving depression-associated sleep difficulties. Chamomile is an herbal tea that is also known for its relaxing properties. Evidence suggests that use of valerian root or melatonin may also promote improved sleep quality. Aerobic exercise in the early evening has been shown to contribute to improved sleep quality. However, exercise later in the evening can be too stimulating and counteract restful sleep. Other CAM modalities for improving sleep used by older patients include aromatherapy combined with a warm bath and relaxing music. (See also "Sleep Problems," p 249.)

Urogynecologic Disorders

Menopause is now seen more as a natural progression of aging than as a pathologic process. This perspective lends itself to the use of behavioral, nutritional, and exercise interventions as well as nonpharmacologic supplements to manage some of the symptoms associated with menopause. More than 30% of menopausal women report using one or more CAM modalities, such as acupuncture, natural and plant estrogens, and other herbal preparations, despite a lack of scientific evidence of efficacy. This number is likely to increase because of the expanding population of aged women and increasing concerns about the long-term safety of conventional estrogens. (See also the section on estrogen replacement therapy in "Endocrine and Metabolic Disorders," p 379.) Of particular importance is the necessity to use caution when recommending phytoestrogen to women with hormone-dependent cancers. Phytoestrogen has yet to be proven conclusively to be an agonist or antagonist of the estrogen receptor. Black cohosh is an herb that has shown some benefit for managing hot flushes, mood disturbances, and sleep disorders. Both aerobic exercise and mind-body relaxation techniques are also helpful in decreasing irritability, restlessness, and anxiety.

Symptomatic benign prostatic hyperplasia affects more than 40% of men aged 70 and older. During the past several years, men have increasingly begun to self-treat this condition with the herbal compound known as saw palmetto, which has become the fifth leading medicinal herb consumed in the United States. Saw palmetto and other supplements (eg, pygeum) have been studied and need further, more rigorous scientific investigation to confirm initial efficacy claims. In one study, older men averaging 65 years of age with moderate benign prostatic hyperplasia were evaluated for 3 months. The efficacy of saw palmetto was found to exceed that of placebo treatment and to be similar to that of standard pharmacologic treatment. (See also "Prostate Disease," p 423.)

Diabetes

Type 2 diabetes mellitus, a major public health problem, is associated with increased incidence of obesity, hypertension, dyslipidemia, and macro- and microvascular disease. Normal aging is associated with increased insulin resistance and glucose intolerances, and increased risk of developing type 2 diabetes. In one survey, approximately 50% to 60% of diabetic patients reported the use of CAM interventions, including folk remedies in ethnic populations. There is considerable interest in examining the potential benefit of using various CAM biologic agents (eg, chromium, vitamin C, other dietary antioxidants) or other modalities (eg, stress-reduction techniques) in combination with dietary modifications, exercise, and weight management. Acupuncture has shown some benefit in managing the pain associated with diabetic neuropathy. (See also "Diabetes Mellitus," p 382.)

Cancer

Approximately 30% to 50% of cancer patients in one survey noted that they were using CAM interventions to manage their specific cancer. Cancer CAM therapies purportedly can be used to strengthen the body's innate immune systems as well as to manage the adverse effects of conventional treatments, such as chemotherapy and radiation. One of the most important benefits for many cancer patients who use CAM modalities is the experience of being more empowered while dealing with the challenges of cancer. This has been substantiated by numerous studies examining various indices of health-related quality of life. The CAM therapies most frequently used are herbal preparations, exercise, and spiritual and energy modalities (such as qi gong, therapeutic touch, Reiki, polarity, healing touch, or Johrei).

Controversy remains regarding the role of diet as a possible risk factor for developing breast cancer. Of particular importance is the link between obesity and increased estrogen levels that may contribute to de novo breast cancer and recurrence after early-stage disease. High-fiber, low-fat diets with fruits, vegetables, whole grains, fish, and legumes are associated with a decreased risk of disease. Biologic agents, herbal preparations, and vitamins have all been tried by patients; however, most of these modalities have not had much scientific study. In addition, life-style changes to include exercise and stress management have been helpful with managing mood and energy changes associated with breast cancer.

Prostate cancer usually develops slowly in older men, and CAM use in combination with conventional treatment has been reported to reduce associated discomforts and improve the quality of life. Risk of death in this population is higher from heart disease than from prostate cancer per se. Until recently, the botanical mixture known as PC-SPES had been used as a CAM dietary supplement that in early small-scale trials was found to lead to decreases in serum prostate-specific antigen levels and pain, plus improved quality of life. However, in June 2002 several lots of PC-SPES were found to be adulterated with diethylstilbestrol, warfarin, and other undeclared prescription ingredients. As a result, PC-SPES was removed from the market. At present, exercise and healthy diet remain the safest CAM recommendations to assist with the management of side effects and improvement of quality of life in these patients. (See also "Prostate Disease," p 423.)

Lung cancer has been linked not only to smoking but also to excesses in dietary intake of dairy products, red meats, and saturated fats, though these associations have been questioned. In addition, preliminary research has suggested that ingestion of vitamin A by those who smoke may be harmful, whereas vitamin A intake in those who do not smoke may be beneficial. Dietary changes as well as mind-body interventions may assist lung cancer patients to manage emotional distress and the adverse effects of treatment. Cancer patients using relaxation and stress-management techniques have been able to manage cravings when pursuing tobacco cessation. These mind-body techniques are also effective in managing the emotional and physical distress associated with the adverse effects of treatment.

Currently, there are no herbal preparations or botanic supplements that appear to be useful in the prevention or management of patients with colon cancer. A fiber-rich diet has been postulated to possibly prevent the onset of colon cancer; however, studies are inconclusive. Lutein, which is present in broccoli, carrots, oranges, and spinach, was found in one study to be beneficial for colon cancer prevention.

See also "Oncology" (p 479).

SAFETY OF CAM MODALITIES

There are several important concerns regarding the safety of the use of CAM modalities by elderly persons. They often assume that the use of dietary supplements and related biologic products, which are among the most popular CAM therapies, are both safe and effective because these products are characterized as "natural." Under the Dietary Supplement Health and Education Act (DSHEA) of 1994, the U.S. Food and Drug Administration is not empowered to evaluate or regulate dietary supplements, and the industry is not required to prove that the advertised ingredients provide the health benefits or safety they claim. Multiple studies have found that dietary supplements often can contain little, none, or more of what the product labels claim, as well as contaminants or adulterants with unlisted products and prescription drugs.

There is little information related to possible differences in the pharmacokinetics and pharmacodynamics of various CAM biologic agents in elderly persons; as a result, proper dosage adjustments for these compounds are unknown. Coupled with the increased likelihood of elderly persons' use of multiple medications, there is an increased risk for adverse herbal-drug interactions in older persons. Without the knowledge of what these products contain in their entirety, or the consequences of their use, consumers and health care professionals must increase communication while continued research is conducted to provide accurate evaluations. It is imperative that practitioners ask patients specifically about their use of dietary supplements and biologic products and look at the ingredients in those supplements.

CAM use in the United States continues to increase in all age groups. The life stressors experienced by older adults, including depression, cognitive decline, chronic pain, musculoskeletal changes, and sleep disorders, may be ameliorated by CAM interventions. Given the particular concerns inherent in managing the health challenges of the aging population, more research to establish the safety and efficacy of CAM modalities commonly used by older persons is imperative.

ANNOTATED REFERENCES

■ Barnes PM, Powell-Griner E, McFann K, et al. Complementary and alternative medicine use among adults: United States, 2002. Advance data from the Vital and Health Statistics; No. 343. Hyattsville, MD: National Center for Health Statistics; 2004.

> The National Health Interview Survey (NHIS) provides the most comprehensive, current information describing the use of complementary and alternative medicine (CAM) in the U.S. adult population. By comparison with earlier surveys, the NHIS includes the most extensive list of CAM modalities and choices for specific health conditions. In-person interviews yielded a representative population of those with lower incomes and minorities who were previously excluded.

■ Fink S. International efforts spotlight traditional, complementary, and alternative medicine. *Am J Pub Health*. 2002; 92(11):1734–1739.

> This article highlights the gap between traditional and allopathic medicine in developing countries and the public health challenge that this presents in the United States and other countries because of regulation and treatment issues.

■ Foster DF, Phillips RS, Hamel MB, et al. Alternative medicine use in older Americans. *J Am Geriatr Soc*. 2000;48(12):1560–1565.

> This nationally representative, random telephone survey reported complementary and alternative medicine (CAM) use in a total of 2055 adults, 311 of whom were aged 65 and older. Thirty percent of adults aged 65 and older used at least one CAM modality, including chiropractic, herbal remedies, relaxation techniques, high-dose or megavitamins, and religious or spiritual healing by others. Six percent of older people were taking prescription drugs and herbal preparations, and 57% of overall CAM users did not discuss their use of the modalities with their health care provider.

■ Kaptchuk TJ. Acupuncture: theory, efficacy, and practice. *Ann Intern Med*. 2002;136(5):374–383.

This is an excellent review of acupuncture, with very useful summary tables of the evidence surrounding its use for various pain and nonpain conditions. The mechanisms of the effects of acupuncture are also explored.

■ Najm W, Reinsch S, Hoehler F, et al. Use of complementary and alternative medicine among the ethnic elderly. *Altern Ther Health Med.* 2003; 9(3):50–57.

This article discusses the results of a seven-page questionnaire that inquired about health status, current medical problems, and the use of complementary and alternative medicine (CAM) by older ethnic community-dwelling persons. In the 525-person convenience sample, Asian and Hispanic Americans were over-represented and white non-Hispanic Americans were under-represented. The questionnaire was translated into Spanish and Vietnamese and used as an interview tool by translators. In all, 47.8% of the elderly immigrants reported using CAM over the past year. Modalities and usage varied with the ethnicity of responders. Asians were higher users of acupuncture and Oriental medicine; Hispanics used more dietary supplements, home remedies, and curanderos; and white non-Hispanics were higher users of chiropractic, massage, and vitamins. Among the respondents, 62.4% reported that they did not discuss their use of CAM with their physicians.

■ Wertkin AD, Cizza G, Blackman MR. Complementary and alternative medicine in aging. In: Hazzard WR, Blass JP, Halter JB, et al., eds. *Principles of Geriatric Medicine and Gerontology.* 5th ed. New York: McGraw Hill; 2003:231–242.

This is a comprehensive chapter that highlights the use and misuse of complementary and alternative medicine, specifically focusing on common disorders of the older adult patient.

Barbara Moquin, PhD(c), MSN, APRN
Marc R. Blackman, MD

CHAPTER 12—ELDER MISTREATMENT

KEY POINTS

- Elder mistreatment affects almost 4% of adults aged 65 and over.

- Screening for elder mistreatment by clinicians is important and is most effective when conducted in a sensitive manner.

- Indicators of elder mistreatment range from dramatic (eg, bruising, fractures) to subtle (eg, withdrawn behavior, dehydration).

The term *elder mistreatment* (EM) as defined by the National Research Council in its report on elder mistreatment refers to "(a) intentional actions that cause harm or create a serious risk of harm (whether or not harm is intended) to a vulnerable elder by a caregiver or other person who stands in a trust relationship to the elder or (b) failure by a caregiver to satisfy the elder's basic needs or to protect the elder from harm." The authors of the American Medical Association (AMA) *Diagnostic and Treatment Guidelines on Elder Abuse and Neglect* describe EM as acts of omission or commission that result in harm or threatened harm to the health or welfare of an older adult. EM is a syndrome that may manifest itself in a variety of ways. It may take the form of physical abuse, emotional abuse, intentional or unintentional neglect, financial exploitation, or abandonment, or it may be a combination of these. Research suggests that the national incidence of EM is approximately 450,000 annually, with a prevalence range of 700,000 to 1.2 million older adults, accounting for approximately 4% of those aged 65 years or older. Given these estimates, routine screening for EM is an appropriate part of primary care for elderly people.

Research conducted in the context of a longitudinal aging cohort study sought to determine the mortality of EM. In a pooled logistic regression analysis that adjusted for demographics, chronic disease, functional status, social networks, cognitive status, and depressive symptoms, the risk of death was found to remain elevated for cohort members experiencing either EM or self-neglect. To date, no intervention studies have evaluated the impact of screening on health outcomes, and such studies are needed. However, screening for EM appears warranted, given the findings of case studies and longitudinal studies that document risk factors, as well as the information in the databases from the adult protective services organizations across the country.

RISK FACTORS AND PREVENTION

Risk factors for EM are known to include poverty, dependency of the elderly person for caregiving needs, age, race, functional disability, frailty, and cognitive impairment. Some factors may really be proxies for other variables. For example, lower socioeconomic status is often associated with fewer resources to meet caregiving demands.

Frail, debilitated older persons may need a level of care that at times exceeds caregiver ability. In particular, the demented person who exhibits disturbing behaviors, such as hitting, spitting, or screaming, poses immense challenges to caregivers. Caregiver stress may give way to any of the forms of EM, and a careful assessment of caregiver stress may identify opportunities to prevent EM. Table 12.1 lists factors that indicate a risk for the development of inadequate or abusive caregiving.

HISTORY

An interdisciplinary approach to assessment and care planning is optimal. Comprehensive interdisciplinary geriatric assessment (see "Assessment," p 49) that includes the physical, psychosocial, and financial domains of the older adult should detect potential or any alleged EM.

The EM history, provided by both the older person and caregiver(s), is conducted in privacy so that the patient and the caregiver(s) can speak freely and frankly. Studies suggest that the different cultures of racial and ethnic groups define abuse and neglect very differently; thus, cultural sensitivity is important (see "Cultural Aspects of Care," p 51). The older patient or caregiver from a different culture than the clinician's may be offended by some EM screening questions. Carefully worded EM questions will avoid alienating the patient or caregiver and closing down any further opportunity to help the patient and family.

If the patient's responses to EM questions indicate that mistreatment may be occurring, progressively focused follow-up questions are indicated. For example, the clinician might first ask, "Is there any difficult behavior in your family you would like to tell me about?" If the answer is positive, the questions to follow then might be, "Has anyone tried to hurt or hit you?" "Has anyone made you do things that you did not want to do?" "Has anyone taken your things?"

Table 12.1—Risk Factors for Inadequate or Abusive Caregiving

- Cognitive impairment in patient, caregiver, or both
- Dependency of the caregiver on the elderly patient, or vice versa
- Family conflict
- Family history of
  - abusive behavior
  - alcohol or drug misuse or abuse
  - mental illness
  - mental retardation
- Financial stress or lack of funds to meet new health demands
- Isolation of the patient or the caregiver, or both
- Living arrangements inadequate for the needs of the ill person
- Stressful events in the family, eg:
  - death of a loved one
  - loss of employment

Obtaining such information requires clinical interviewing skills similar to those needed when asking about sexual orientation, alcoholism, or substance abuse.

Private interviews with caregivers may detect not only abusive or neglectful behavior but also signs of stress, isolation, or depression in the caregiver, in which case help for the caregiver can also be provided. Caregivers may be reluctant to discuss their own problems in the presence of the person who depends on their care. Because caregivers may range from registered professionals to well-intended neighbors, it is important to know and to document the level of skill the caregiver has, as well as his or her understanding of the situation. The caregiver's level of understanding is an essential factor for evaluating the intentionality underlying any mistreatment of a dependent older person. For example, a registered nurse in a nursing home is held to a different level of accountability than a frail spouse providing care in the home setting.

Identification of shortcomings in the patient's care may be the most elusive aspect of a comprehensive assessment. The symptoms and signs of incomplete, inadequate, or neglectful caregiving may be subtle (eg, when a patient fails to do as well as expected on a given regimen) or attributable to the patient's physical or emotional disorders (eg, weight loss in a patient with a history of depression).

Effective assessment is that which detects EM without directing undue suspicion on well-meaning caregivers or undermining a family's ability to care for an elderly person with appropriate support and counseling.

Examples of symptoms and signs that indicate a particularly high level of risk for EM are listed in Table 12.2. A number of assessment instruments have been developed in order to help clinicians screen for and assess EM, though none have been fully validated yet, and research is ongoing.

PHYSICAL ASSESSMENT

Key signs of mistreatment are physical indicators that are incongruent with the patient's history; examples are bruises and welts in unusual places or in various stages of healing. Bilateral bruises on the upper torso are rarely the result of falls and warrant follow-up. Other indications of possible EM include frequent, unexplained, or inconsistently explained falls and injuries, multiple emergency department visits, delays in seeking treatment, inconsistent follow-up, or constant switching among doctors. The clinician needs to search for unusual patterns or marks, such as bruises on inner arms or thighs; cigarette, rope, chain, or chemical burns; lacerations and abrasions on the face, lips, and eyes; or marks occurring in areas of the body usually covered by clothes. The presence of head injuries, hair

Table 12.2—Screening for Elder Mistreatment: Key Indicators

General
  Clothing: inappropriate dress, soil or disrepair
  Hygiene
  Nutritional status
  Skin integrity

Abuse
  Anxiety, nervousness, esp. toward caregiver
  Bruising, in various healing stages, esp. bilateral or on inner arms
    or thighs
  Fractures, esp. in various healing stages
  Lacerations
  Repeated emergency department visits
  Repeated falls
  Signs of sexual abuse
  Statements about abuse by the patient

Neglect
  Contractures
  Dehydration
  Depression
  Diarrhea
  Failure to respond to warning of obvious disease
  Fecal impaction
  Malnutrition
  Medication under- or over use or otherwise inappropriate
  Poor hygiene
  Pressure ulcers
  Repeated falls
  Repeated hospital admissions
  Urine burns
  Statements about neglect by the patient

Exploitation
  Evidence of misuse of patient's assets
  Inability of patient to account for money and property or to pay
    for essential care
  Reports of demands for money or goods in exchange for
    caregiving or services
  Unexplained loss of Social Security, pension checks
  Statements about exploitation by the patient

Abandonment
  Evidence that patient is left alone unsafely
  Evidence of sudden withdrawal of care by caregiver
  Statements about abandonment by the patient

SOURCE: Data in part from Fulmer T. Elder abuse and neglect assessment. *Try This.* May 2002;2(15):2.

loss, or hemorrhages beneath the scalp as a consequence of hair pulling are significant markers. Cachectic states may be the result of malnutrition that is a consequence of neglect. Unusual discharges, bruising, bleeding, or trauma around the genitalia or rectum raise concern of possible sexual abuse, prompting gynecologic and rectal examination.

The behavior of the patient when in the presence of the suspected abuser may be significant. An EM victim may avoid eye contact, or dart his or her eyes continuously. He or she may sit a distance away from an abusive caregiver, cringe, back off, or startle easily as if expecting to be struck. The caregiver may be nervous and fearful, or quiet and passive. The patient may defer excessively to the caregiver, who may invariably answer for the patient or even try not to allow a private interview with or examination of the patient. Dubious explanations may be given to explain the patient's injuries.

The emergency department is an important setting for EM assessment. The emergency department may see elderly persons in crisis, and every effort should be made not to simply treat and release patients whose situation merits further assessment. Astute emergency personnel can identify cases where there may be serious safety problems in the caregiving situation.

PSYCHOLOGIC ASSESSMENT

EM is not invariably or entirely physical. Psychologic abuse or neglect is generally more difficult than outright physical abuse to detect and confirm, but it can be equally dangerous to the dependent older person. The behavior of both the patient and the caregiver may provide important clues about the quality of their relationship and of the care the older person is receiving. Factors that suggest a poor or deteriorating social and emotional situation are an important focus of assessment for EM.

Psychologic abuse includes taunting, name-calling, the promotion of regressive behaviors by infantilization, making painful jokes at the expense of the patient, or other activities that are demeaning. The caregiver's style of communication will provide important clues. Impatience, irritability, and demeaning statements may indicate a pattern of verbal abuse. However, psychologic neglect or mistreatment by the caregiver may take more subtle forms. For example, failing to provide social or emotional stimulation, or restricting or preventing the patient's normal activities may result in the patient's total social isolation.

The patient's demeanor and emotional status may suggest the presence of psychologic neglect or abuse. For example, ambivalence or high levels of anxiety, fearfulness, or anger toward the caregiver indicate the need for further assessment. Unexpected depression or uncharacteristic withdrawal also merits follow-up. Other high-risk behaviors include lack of adherence with treatment recommendations, frequent requests for sedating medication, or frequently canceled appointments.

Cognitive impairment, dementia, and depression have been shown to be prevalent in older adults referred for evaluation for possible EM. It is therefore appropriate to check any older adult presenting with cognitive impairment, dementia, or depression for symptoms and signs of neglect or mistreatment. Aggressive behaviors associated with dementia may trigger abusive responses in caregivers. (See also "Behavioral Problems in Dementia," p 231.)

FINANCIAL ASSESSMENT

Financial mistreatment includes unauthorized use of the older adult's funds, possessions, or property. Fiscal neglect consists of the failure to use the older adult's funds and resources for his or her needs. Signs that the elderly patient is being mistreated financially include:

- a recent marked disparity between the patient's living conditions or appearance and his or her assets,
- a sudden inability to pay for health care or other basic needs,
- an unusual interest on the part of caregivers in the patient's assets.

SELF-NEGLECT

For some elderly persons, especially those who live in isolation or who choose to accept and endure mistreatment, self-neglect may be an issue. Successful management in such cases will require an assessment of the patient's capacity to understand the risks and benefits of the situation, as well as consequences of allowing circumstances to persist. (See sections on decisional capacity in "Legal and Ethical Issues," p 23.) These are complex situations, but the patient's right to autonomy and self-determination must be honored. Paternalistic viewpoints regarding what the older person "should" do need to be avoided. In self-neglect cases, the clinician may need support when coming to terms with the requirement to respect the decisionally capable older person's wishes when this involves his or her choosing to continue in an abusive or neglectful situation. (The clinical dilemma resembles that confronting clinicians who treat battered women.) Intervention contrary to the decisionally capable patient's choice is generally inappropriate, although this may be uncomfortable for the clinician. (See also the section on autonomy versus protectionism in "Legal and Ethical Issues," p 29.)

THE ROLE OF THE OLDER PERSON

The relationship of the older person with caregivers can be very complex, and dysfunctional relations between a dependent older person and a caregiver may not be the fault entirely of the caregiver. To approach such situations with the idea that the older person is inevitably the victim infantilizes the person and is unfair to caregivers. Situations in which elderly persons are mistreated can be arrayed along a spectrum from victimization to mutual abusiveness to relationships where the older person can be viewed as a witting cause of the mistreatment. Moreover, there are cases where the older person and his or her caregivers are making the best of a tragic situation.

To determine the best possible approach for ameliorating if not solving a dysfunctional caregiving relationship, the clinician makes every effort to determine the facts in the situation and fathom the motives of the people involved. Consultation with social workers, psychologists, or psychiatrists may be useful. Legal reporting requirements are not limited in any way by these considerations. If an elderly man hits his son and the son strikes back, clinicians in most states are required to report the latter hitting.

INSTITUTIONAL MISTREATMENT

EM in the setting of home care by family or friends has been the focus of much of the discussion so far, but detecting and intervening to prevent EM in the institutional setting is also important. Several factors in this setting could aggravate the problem, including poor working conditions, low salaries, inadequate staff training and supervision resulting in poor motivation, and prejudiced attitudes. Disruptive or insulting behavior by the older adult may also be a factor; resident behaviors can at times be provocative.

The Omnibus Budget Reconciliation Act of 1987 set a new standard for care in nursing homes. (See "Nursing-Home Care," p 119.) The clinician who is alert to the possibility of abuse and neglect in any institutional setting plays an important role in protecting vulnerable older patients. Equally important is the clinician's readiness to use the resources available through the institution itself or through state regulatory agencies to investigate and intervene, where appropriate. In cases of suspected institutional EM, the challenge is to balance the rights of staff members with the rights of patients. State departments of public health are usually responsible for investigating nursing-home abuse and neglect cases.

INTERVENTION

The clinician who suspects EM can use the following questions to guide intervention:

- How safe is the patient if I send him or her back to the current setting, or does he or she need to be removed to a safe environment?
- What services or resources are available locally to support the care of this older person?
- Are there any caregivers who have health problems of their own that need attention?

- Does this situation need the expertise of others (eg, in medicine, nursing, social work), and if so, who would best serve the patient's needs?

Successful intervention in cases of EM can become complex. Among the factors governing the clinician's course of action are these:

- the exact nature and degree of the EM,
- whether the patient can or will cooperate with evaluation and intervention, and
- whether the caregiver(s) can or will cooperate with evaluation and intervention.

Procedures and interventions are laid out in two algorithms developed under AMA auspices (see the AMA guidelines listed in the references at the end of this chapter). Both algorithms take into account the issues highlighted above, especially the patient's safety, willingness to accept help, and capacity to understand and cooperate with the health care team.

Local resources in support of interventions for EM vary, but information is readily available. (See, eg, resources listed in the Appendix, p 504.) Consultation with the social work staff of the hospital, nursing home, or local health department may be a useful early step. Each state's Adult Protective Services (APS) will yield relevant information as well as direct assistance. In addition, the AMA Web site also provides a convenient starting point in the search for information and resources (http://www.ama-assn.org), as does the National Center on Elder Abuse (http://www.elderabusecenter.org).

THE MEDICAL-LEGAL INTERFACE

It is important to know state laws applicable to cases of EM; 46 states have a reporting mechanism for EM, either through APS or state agencies associated with aging. Clinicians need to be familiar with the reporting mandates that apply in their area. In some states, neglect by others must be reported, but reports of self-neglect are not required. Adult children can be charged with neglect of the elderly parent if a caregiving relationship can be proven and it can also be proven that care has been precipitously withdrawn without substitute services. In states where self-neglect is reportable, this is usually the largest intake category. Finally, states may mandate reports for self-neglect but may not provide any services unless the older adult agrees to accept them.

Clinicians are in a key position to assess and report suspected EM, and most states require such reporting. Although clinicians are appropriately wary of acting precipitously, they should be willing to enlist the help of government agencies and the courts when EM is clearly dangerous for an elderly patient. Penalties may be assessed against a nonreporter in some regions. Reports of EM are confidential, and, as is the case with child abuse reporting, the clinical reporter is protected from litigation unless it can be proven that the report was made maliciously. The home page for the National Center on Elder Abuse (cited above) provides one means for reporting information; in addition, published articles include tables that review all 50 states and the procedures expected in each (see the resources listed in the Appendix, p 504). The AMA guidelines also provide clinical algorithms for reporting suspected EM cases.

Especially when a case is to be reported, photographs and body charts may be required to document the findings on physical examination. Risk management personnel can provide guidance in documentation and assist the clinician when evidence suggests that there may be a need for police or court action. In any case where the clinician is called to court to discuss his or her findings, documentation is an important part of testimony. EM cases are often extremely complicated, and it is likely that experts in several fields will need to work with clinicians and administrators to avoid under- or over-reporting of EM and to provide the best outcomes for the victims of EM.

ANNOTATED REFERENCES

- Aravanis SC, Adelman RD, Breckman R, et al. *Diagnostic and Treatment Guidelines on Elder Abuse and Neglect.* Chicago, IL: American Medical Association; 1992.

    The purpose of these guidelines is to sensitize clinicians to elder mistreatment. The guidelines present what is known about elder mistreatment and its clinical manifestations and history, and they describe the barriers to properly identify and manage elder mistreatment. The authors outline an approach that the clinician can use to recognize elder mistreatment in various clinical settings, and they identify strategies for its management and prevention. They also discuss ethical, medical, and legal issues in detecting and reporting elder mistreatment. The guidelines are available online at http://www.ama-assn.org.

- Dyer CB, Pavlik VN, Murphy KP, et al. The high prevalence of depression and dementia in elder abuse or neglect. *J Am Geriatr Soc.* 2000;48(2):205–208.

    There is little information in the literature concerning the clinical profile of mistreated older people. The authors' objective was to describe the characteristics of abused or neglected patients and to compare the prevalence of depression and dementia in neglected patients with that of patients referred for other reasons. This is a case-control study with 47 older persons referred for neglect and 97 referred for other reasons. Using standard geriatric assessment tools, the authors found a statistically significant higher prevalence of depression (62% versus 12%) and dementia (51% versus 30%) in victims of self-neglect than in patients referred for other reasons. This was the first study using primary data that highlighted a high prevalence of depression as well as dementia in mistreated older people. Their findings indicate that it would be appropriate for clinicians to screen for neglect or abuse in their depressed or demented elderly patients.

■ Fulmer T, Guadagno L, Bitondo Dyer C, et al. Progress in elder abuse screening and assessment instruments. *J Am Geriatr Soc.* 2004;52(2):297–304.

This article reviews existing elder mistreatment screening and assessment instruments and analyzes their strengths and weaknesses. It is a comprehensive review with important clinical suggestions for assessment, depending on time and setting limitations. The information provided is useful for clinicians, teachers, and researchers.

■ Lachs MS, Williams CS, O'Brien S, et al. The mortality of elder mistreatment. *JAMA.* 1998;280(5):428–432.

Although elder mistreatment is suspected to be life threatening in some instances, little is known about the survival of elderly persons who have been mistreated. The authors observed a group of community-dwelling older adults with at least 9 years of follow-up. The study included 2812 community-dwelling adults who were older than 65 years in 1982, a subset of whom were referred to protective services for elderly persons. Their main outcome measure was an all-cause mortality among elderly persons for whom protective services were used for corroborated elder mistreatment (elder abuse, neglect, or exploitation), or elderly persons for whom protective services were used for self-neglect. In the first 9 years after the beginning of the study, 176 cohort members were seen by elderly protective services for verified allegations; 10 (5.7%) of these were for abuse, 30 (17.0%) for neglect, 8 (4.5%) for exploitation, and 128 (72.7%) for self-neglect. At the end of a 13-year follow-up period, group members seen for elder mistreatment at any time during the follow-up were found to have poorer survival (9%) than either those seen for self-neglect (17%) or other noninvestigated group members (40%) ($P < .001$). In a pooled logistic regression that adjusted for demographic characteristics, chronic diseases, functional status, social networks, cognitive status, and depressive symptoms, the risk of death remained elevated for cohort members experiencing either elder mistreatment (odds ratio, 3.1; 95% confidence interval, 1.4 to 6.7) or self-neglect (odds ratio, 1.7; 95% confidence interval, 1.2 to 2.5), when it was compared with that of other members of the cohort. The authors concluded that reported and corroborated elder mistreatment and self-neglect are associated with shorter survival after adjustments for other factors associated with increased mortality in older adults.

■ National Center on Elder Abuse at The American Public Human Services Association (Formerly the American Public Welfare Association) in Collaboration with Westat, Inc. *The National Elder Abuse Incidence Study; Final Report: September 1998.* Washington, DC: National Aging Information Center; 1998.

The National Elder Abuse Incidence Study research provides, for the first time, a national incidence estimate of elder abuse, which can serve as a baseline for future research and service interventions in this critical problem. Its findings confirm some widely held theories about elder abuse and neglect, notably, that officially reported cases of abuse are only a partial measure of a much larger, unidentified problem. The best national estimate is that a total of 449,924 elderly persons aged 60 and over experienced abuse or neglect, or both, in domestic settings in 1996. Of this total, 16% were reported to and substantiated by Adult Protective Services (APS), but the remaining 84% were not reported to APS. On the basis of these figures, the report concludes that more than five times as many new incidents of abuse and neglect went unreported and were not substantiated by the APS in 1996. The standard error suggests that nationwide, as many as 688,948 or as few as 210,000 elderly persons could have been victims of abuse and or neglect in domestic settings in 1996.

■ National Research Council. *Elder Mistreatment: Abuse, Neglect, and Exploitation in an Aging America.* Bonnie RJ, Wallace RB, eds. Washington, DC: National Academies Press; 2003.

This book resulted from the work of the Panel to Review Risk and Prevalence of Elder Abuse and Neglect convened by the National Research Council of the National Academies. It highlights the paucity of research on the subject and documents that fewer than 50 published scientific studies have addressed this problem. Concepts, definitions, and guidelines are presented, along with a new theoretical model for elder mistreatment. Measures and studies of elder mistreatment are catalogued with an analysis of definitions in the context of state laws.

Terry T. Fulmer, PhD, RN

CHAPTER 13—HOSPITAL CARE

KEY POINTS

- Persons aged 65 years or older make up 13% of the population and account for 36% of acute-care hospital admissions and nearly half of hospital expenditures for all adults.
- Older hospitalized patients should be routinely assessed for a limited number of common geriatric problems regardless of the admission diagnosis.
- Specific system changes in providing care to hospitalized older persons have resulted in improved patient outcomes.

Older people are at disproportionate risk of becoming seriously ill and requiring hospital care, whether it is in an emergency department, on a medical or surgical ward, or in a critical-care unit. Persons aged 65 years or older, who make up only 13% of the U.S. population, account for 36% of acute-care hospital admissions and nearly half of hospital expenditures for adults. The impact of older persons on acute hospital care will increase rapidly with the aging of the population: the proportion of the U.S. population aged 65 years or older is expected to increase to as much as 19% by 2025, with those aged 85 years or older increasing most rapidly.

Hospital use rates vary as much as threefold for Medicare beneficiaries with the same illnesses across different regions of the United States. There is no evidence that these differences in practice patterns are explained by differences in disease rates or severity. Hospital use and the use of hospital resources is much lower among patients enrolled in capitated insurance plans than among those enrolled in fee-for-service plans; this difference in resource use has not been systematically linked to differences in patient outcomes.

During hospitalization, older patients tend to receive less costly care than do younger patients. In the large Study to Understand Prognoses and Preferences for Outcomes and Risks of Treatments (SUPPORT), for example, seriously ill patients in their 80s were found to have received fewer invasive procedures and less resource-intensive, less costly hospital care than similar younger patients received. This preferential allocation of hospital services to younger patients was not based on differences in patients' severity of illness or general preferences for life-extending care and is consistent with evidence regarding outpatient care. Differences in the aggressiveness of care have not been shown to explain differences between older and younger patients in survival or other outcomes. The best guides to assessment and management in the care of any older hospitalized patient are the clinical circumstances and the patient's preferences, irrespective of the patient's age.

There is also wide variability among seriously ill older persons in preferences for life-sustaining treatments. On the basis of findings of SUPPORT, it has been recognized that even though fewer older patients prefer aggressive care than do younger patients, many older patients want cardiopulmonary resuscitation and care that is focused on life extension. Moreover, patients' families and physicians commonly underestimate older patients' desires for aggressive care. Thus, in providing care for acutely ill older persons, it is essential to determine individual preferences for the site of care and to define with the patient the goals of care.

ASSESSING AND MANAGING HOSPITALIZED OLDER PATIENTS

Many of the serious illnesses disproportionately experienced by older persons require hospital care for optimal management. The benefits of hospitalization can be remarkable: correcting serious physiologic de-

rangements, repairing vascular obstructions and broken bones, using highly technical biomedical advances in the treatment of life-threatening illnesses. The hospital can also be a place where older persons are exposed to unintended hazards: deteriorating functional status, adverse drug reactions, and cognitive decline. A systematic approach to assessing and managing older hospitalized patients offers the best chance of reducing the risk for and consequences of these common hazards.

An initial comprehensive assessment of the hospitalized older patient includes an evaluation of function at the level of the organ system, the whole person, and the person's environment. This assessment can identify needs for which targeted interventions may improve function or reduce risk for adverse outcomes. This approach complements the traditional medical assessment by highlighting problems that are common in hospitalized older persons, and it is similar in concept to comprehensive geriatric assessment conducted in other settings. (See "Assessment," p 45.)

Table 13.1 lists 10 hazards and opportunities that are commonly overlooked in elderly hospitalized patients. These problems are selected on the basis of their importance in relation to other clinical issues, the quality of relevant evidence, and their specificity to older persons. Other important problems (eg, prevention of deep-vein thrombosis, the effects of alcohol or tobacco use, ameliorating pain, and advance directives)

Table 13.1—Commonly Encountered Hazards and Opportunities to Address During an Elderly Patient's Hospital Stay

Problem	Possible Interventions
Functional impairments	Physical therapy, occupational therapy, assessment of social environment
Immobility and falls	Avoidance of restraints, encouragement of ambulation in hospital, physical therapy
Sensory impairment	Eyeglasses, hearing aids
Depression	Pharmacotherapy, cognitive therapy, or both
Cognitive impairment	Evaluation of dementia or delirium, assessment of social environment
Suboptimal pharmacotherapy	Modification of prescriptions
Atrial fibrillation	Warfarin or treatment to maintain sinus rhythm, or both
Nutrition	Supplementation of water, calories, protein; assessment of social environment
Mistreatment and social support	Early involvement of family and social services in discharge planning
Influenza, pneumonia vaccine	Vaccination against influenza, pneumococcus, or both

are not specific to older persons, and some problems specific to elderly persons (eg, age-related decline in renal function) are widely recognized. (See also "Alcohol and Drug Abuse," p 298, "Palliative Care," p 133, "Legal and Ethical Issues," p 22, "Kidney Diseases and Disorders," p 400, "Perioperative Care," p 99.) Table 13.2 shows where assessment for these common geriatric problems can be incorporated into the routine of a hospital admission history and physical examination.

Two types of evidence suggest that these interventions are a good use of physician time. First, for each problem, there is compelling evidence (cited below) supporting the proposed intervention, either because the efficacy of the intervention is well established (eg, warfarin to prevent stroke associated with atrial fibrillation), or because the associated problem is common, often overlooked, and ameliorable with a safe and inexpensive intervention. Second, systematic approaches to the evaluation and management of acutely ill older persons can improve patient outcomes and reduce hospital costs.

Functional Impairments

Once hospitalized, older patients are at high risk for loss of independence and institutionalization. Among hospitalized medical patients aged 70 years or older, ~15% decline during hospitalization in their ability to perform basic self-care activities of daily living (ADLs), another ~20% are discharged without recovering their baseline prehospitalization abilities, and 15% of those admitted from home are discharged to a nursing home. Loss of personal independence is often hastened by the combined effects of the acute illness that led to hospitalization and underlying chronic illnesses and impairments. In addition, many older patients have lost their "bounce"—their ability to adapt and maintain the homeostasis of their physiologic, psychologic, and social systems in the face of the acute insults to these systems by illness and hospitalization. Functional decline during hospitalization and failure to recover baseline function have been independently associated with increasing age, lower preadmission function in instrumental activities of daily living (IADLs), and several admission characteristics, including cognitive impairment, symptoms of depression, and malnutrition. Optimal care for the hospitalized older patient requires the physician to manage acute illness and simultaneously intervene where necessary to promote or maintain independent functioning.

The ability to perform ADLs and IADLs is necessary if the older person is to live independently, and functional dependence is associated with worse quality-of-life outcomes, shortened survival, and increased resource use. The older patient's ability to perform ADLs and IADLs, determined at the time of admission, will serve as a useful baseline. If functional dependence is uncovered, the causes can be explored (eg, dependence in IADLs is often associated with dementia), and strategies to maintain and improve functional capacity can be initiated (eg, physical and occupational therapy). These strategies may be best implemented effectively for many patients by ward staff without consultation or referral. Social work consultation and early involvement of family or other caregivers is often necessary to plan postdischarge care for those older patients who are functionally dependent. (See also "Rehabilitation," p 108; "Psychosocial Issues," p 16.)

Table 13.2—Systematic Assessment of the Older Patient at Admission to the Hospital

Step	Assessments to Include
Past medical history	■ Ask about vaccination history
Medications review	■ Assess indications for each drug, appropriateness of dosing, potential interactions ■ Determine patient's or caregiver's method for assuring adherence (eg, pill boxes)
Social history	■ Ask about help needed (and who provides) for ADLs and IADLs ■ Ask about social support ■ Ask if patient feels free and safe
Review of systems	■ Ask about weight loss in preceding 6 months ■ Ask about dietary change ■ Ask about anorexia, nausea, vomiting, diarrhea ■ Ask about problems with memory or confusion ■ Ask about falls or difficulty walking ■ Ask about difficulties with vision or hearing
Physical examination	■ Take pulse (confirm arrhythmias with electrocardiography) ■ Assess for loss of subcutaneous fat, muscle wasting, edema, ascites ■ Screen for cognitive function with Mini-Cog or MMSE* ■ Assess vision and hearing ■ Use a depression screen

NOTE: ADLs = activities of daily living; IADLs = instrumental activities of daily living; Mini-Cog = Mini-Cog Assessment Instrument for Dementia; MMSE = Mini–Mental State Examination.

* See Borson S, Scanlan J, Brush M, et al. The Mini-Cog: a cognitive "vital signs" measure for dementia screening in multi-lingual elderly. *Int J Geriatr Psychiatry.* 2000;15(11):1021–1027; and Folstein MF, Folstein SE, McHugh PR. Mini-Mental State Examination. Available at http://www.minimental.com (accessed October 2005). See also "Dementia," p 221.

Immobility and Falls

Walking facilitates the performance of virtually all ADLs and IADLs. The ability to walk briskly and the habit of regularly walking 1 mile or more daily are associated with prolonged survival. Immobility during hospitalization, however, leads rapidly to deconditioning and subsequent difficulty walking. The major risk for deconditioned hospital patients of walking is falling, which can lead to serious injury. Falls and fall-related injuries in hospitalized patients are associated with cognitive impairment, new medications and multiple medications, environmental factors in the hospital, and abnormalities of gait, balance, and lower-extremity strength, as well as with multiple chronic medical conditions and depression.

It is helpful to assess the patient's gait, balance, lower-extremity strength, ability to get up from bed, cognition, and mood during the initial physical examination. Persons able to walk independently should be encouraged to do so frequently during hospitalization. Those able to walk but unable to do so safely and independently can receive assistance from hospital staff while walking several times daily. Formal physical therapy may yield additional benefits. The initial physical examination is also a good time to assess a patient's risk for falls by inquiring about a history of falls and by a careful musculoskeletal and neurologic examination. Interventions that reduce falls in other settings may also prevent falls in the hospital. Prudent preventive strategies include avoiding restraints and tethers, providing walking assistance for those who walk with difficulty, and providing physical therapy for those with weakness or gait abnormalities. If significant soft-tissue and bony abnormalities of the feet are discovered, a referral for podiatric care is appropriate. (See "Falls," p 201; "Gait Impairment," p 195; "Physical Activity," p 56; "Rehabilitation," p 108; and "Diseases and Disorders of the Foot," p 451.)

Sensory Impairment

Most hospitalized elderly persons have impaired vision or hearing, and these sensory impairments are risk factors for falls, incontinence, delirium, and functional dependence. Although most visual and hearing impairments are readily corrected by eyeglasses or hearing aids, these appliances are often forgotten in the hospital.

Hospitalized older persons can be screened for sensory impairment by routinely asking if they have difficulty with seeing or hearing and whether they use eyeglasses or hearing aids. Physical examination including a test of visual acuity (eg, with a pocket card of the Jaeger eye test) and the whisper test of hearing, in which a short, easily answered question is whispered in each ear, is the next appropriate step in evaluation. For people with visual or hearing impairments, it is important to provide the appropriate assistive devices (eyeglasses or hearing aids brought from home), and staff may need to be instructed in the use of appliances to communicate more effectively. (See "Hearing Impairment," p 155, and "Visual Impairment," p 149.)

Depression

Depressive symptoms in hospitalized older persons are common, prognostically important, and potentially ameliorable. Major or minor depression occurs in roughly one third of hospitalized patients aged 65 years or older but is often undiagnosed. The presence of depressive symptoms is associated with increased risk for dependence in ADLs, nursing-home placement, and shortened long-term survival, even after controlling for baseline function and the severity of acute and chronic illness.

It is important to consider depression in all hospitalized older patients. Simply asking whether they feel down, depressed, or hopeless, or whether they have lost interest or pleasure in doing things, is a good place to start. A positive response to any one of these questions is likely sensitive to the diagnosis of depression (based on evidence from outpatients) and can be followed up by a formal assessment for an affective disorder. In hospitalized older persons, the presence of 3 or more of 11 depressive symptoms has been found to be 83% sensitive and 77% specific for a diagnosis of major depression.

Detection is the first and most important step in the management of depression. Psychotherapeutic interventions (environmental, behavioral, cognitive, and family) are safe and often effective in the initial management of patients with suspected depression. It is rarely necessary to begin pharmacotherapy during hospitalization for a medical or surgical condition, but follow-up shortly after discharge is critical. If pharmacotherapy is initiated, selective serotonin-reuptake inhibitors are often preferred because approximately 50% of older hospitalized patients have a contraindication to tricyclic antidepressants. (See "Depression and Other Mood Disorders," p 269.)

Cognitive Impairment

Delirium is present in 10% to 15% of hospitalized older persons on admission, and it develops in up to 30% during the course of hospitalization. Delirium arising during the course of hospitalization is a predictor of prolonged hospital stay. Delirium is also associated with increased rates of in-hospital death and nursing-home placement. Patients who develop delirium may experience a worsening of a chronic cognitive impairment. Symptoms of delirium commonly persist for months following hospital discharge. Roughly one third of cases of delirium can be prevented by managing six risk factors for delirium appropriately: cognitive impairment, sleep deprivation, immobility, visual impairment, hearing impairment, and dehydration. The diagnosis of delirium should be considered when any of the following is observed: fluctuation in mental status or behavior, inattention, disorganized thinking, and altered consciousness. The Confusion Assessment Method (CAM) is a useful screen for delirium. Prudent measures to prevent or ameliorate delirium include: avoiding medicines associated with delirium whenever possible; treating infection and fever; detecting and correcting metabolic abnormalities; frequently orienting patients with cognitive or sensory impairment; and avoiding excessive bed rest, room changes, and restraints. (See "Delirium," p 239.) Prevention is the best strategy: a recent randomized trial examined the effect of systematic assessment for established delirium in hospitalized elderly patients on a medical service, with multidisciplinary care provided to delirious patients. Patients in the intervention arm had no better outcomes than those assigned to usual care.

Underlying cognitive impairment consistent with dementia is present on admission in 20% to 40% of hospitalized older persons, and it commonly goes undetected. Preexisting cognitive impairment is a risk factor for delirium, falls, use of restraints, and nonadherence with therapy. Also, there is intrinsic value in identifying previously undiagnosed dementia so that appropriate evaluation and management strategies can be implemented after discharge. Cognitive function can be assessed by the use of an established test of cognitive function, such as the Mini–Mental State Examination (MMSE) or the Mini-Cog test. The diagnosis of dementia should be considered in those a score of 24 or less on the 30-point MMSE. When dementia is a possibility, it is important to exclude reversible causes and to identify those patients for whom pharmacologic therapy and family-oriented interventions are warranted. (See "Dementia," p 221.)

Suboptimal Pharmacotherapy

The number of drugs prescribed to hospitalized patients is directly proportional to their age. Moreover, hospitalization is a period of rapid turnover in drug therapies for older patients: One study found that 40% of drugs prescribed before admission were discontinued during hospitalization and 45% of drugs prescribed at discharge were started during hospitalization. Although older patients are at increased risk for inappropriate drug therapy, adverse drug effects, and drug-drug interactions, they may also be undertreated when effective therapies are not used or are used in inadequate doses. In one study 88% of older hospitalized patients were found to have had at least one or more clinically significant drug problem, and 22% had at least one potentially serious and life-threatening problem. Consultation by clinical pharmacists can improve appropriate prescribing and improve the older patient's adherence to prescribed therapy.

A hospital admission is an ideal time to completely review a patient's medication regimen and to discontinue those that are unnecessary or have low therapeutic value (eg, sedative hypnotics). During hospitalization and at discharge, a medication review is useful to identify prescribing errors in six common categories: inappropriate choice of therapy, incorrect dosage, incorrect schedule, drug-drug interactions, therapeutic duplication, and allergy. (See "Pharmacotherapy," p 72.)

Atrial Fibrillation

Nonvalvular atrial fibrillation is present in 5% or more of hospitalized older persons, often as an incidental finding. Consistent and compelling evidence from randomized trials shows that the risk of stroke in persons with atrial fibrillation can be reduced approximately two thirds by treatment with warfarin (eg, from 4.5% per year to 1.4% per year). Moreover, the beneficial effect of warfarin is maintained in persons aged 75 years or older and in those with other risk factors for stroke. Nonetheless, many older patients with atrial fibrillation are discharged from hospital without warfarin therapy, even when warfarin is indicated. Failure to prescribe warfarin is likely due to underestimation of the benefit of therapy, overestimation of its potential risk, and the difficulty of implementing, monitoring, and modifying therapy to minimize adverse effects.

In every hospitalized older patient, the history and physical examination can be targeted to identify the presence of chronic or paroxysmal atrial fibrillation. When atrial fibrillation is diagnosed, it is important to exclude valvular disease and hyperthyroidism as causes. In the absence of a strong contraindication, anticoagulation therapy is indicated to prevent stroke, usually with warfarin (see "Perioperative Care," p 99, and anticoagulation information in the Appendix, p 491). A large randomized trial compared the long-term effects of ventricular rate control and anticoagulation to rhythm control (in which an attempt is made to convert patients to and maintain them in normal sinus rhythm). Adverse drug effects were less frequent with rate control and anticoagulation, and mortality at 5 years was somewhat lower (23.8% versus 21.3%, $P = .08$). New joint guidelines from the American Academy of Family Physicians and the American College of Physicians recommend rate control with anticoagulation as the preferred strategy for most patients. (See also the section on atrial fibrillation in "Cardiovascular Diseases and Disorders," p 356.)

Nutrition

Serious deficiencies of macronutrients and micronutrients are common in hospitalized older patients. Key macronutrients are protein, calories, salt, water, and fiber. On admission, severe protein-calorie malnutrition is present in approximately 15% of patients aged 70 years or older, and moderate malnutrition is present in another 25%. Moreover, 25% of older patients suffer further nutritional depletion during hospitalization. Even after controlling for the underlying illness, its severity, and comorbid illnesses, malnutrition is associated with increased risk for death, dependence, and institutionalization.

In addition to other deficiencies of vitamins and electrolytes that may develop with protein-calorie malnutrition, vitamin-D deficiency is especially common among older hospitalized patients. In one large hospital, nearly two thirds of medical inpatients aged 65 years or older were found to be vitamin-D deficient; vitamin-D deficiency was nearly as common in inpatients without a risk factor for vitamin-D deficiency and in those taking multivitamins as in other patients. These data regarding the high prevalence of vitamin-D deficiency in hospitalized older persons complement evidence that vitamin D and calcium supplementation reduce by half the incidence of nonvertebral fractures in men and women aged 65 years or older. (See "Osteoporosis and Osteomalacia," p 210, and "Malnutrition," p 174.)

One review examined the evidence from randomized controlled trials of the benefits of oral nutritional supplements for older persons at risk of malnutrition. (Of the almost 2500 subjects included in the review, 22% were from studies of hospitalized patients.) Nutritional supplementation was found to be associated with reduced mortality and shortened length of hospital stay, although the reviewers call for additional research to substantiate these findings, as most of the studies included in their analysis were of poor quality. Beyond prescribing supplements, clinicians should assess malnourished older hospitalized patients for remediable factors such as difficulty chewing, or insufficient time or encouragement to eat. (See "Eating and Feeding Problems," p 181.)

The maintenance of water and electrolyte balance requires special attention in older persons during and after fluid administration because of their decreased capacity to achieve and maintain homeostasis. Initial efforts can be directed toward achieving normovolemia and correcting electrolyte abnormalities. Subsequent efforts to maintain fluid and electrolyte balance are based on estimates of daily metabolic requirements.

The intracellular volume is about 25% to 30% of body weight for men aged 65 to 85 years weighing between 40 and 80 kg (88 to 176 lb) and about 20% to 25% of body weight for women in the same age and weight ranges. The daily metabolic requirements, as a proportion of intracellular volume, can be estimated as follows: water in L, 10%; energy in 1000 kcal, 10%; protein in g, 0.3%; sodium in mol, 0.3%; and potassium in mol, 0.2%. Thus, for a 75-year-old woman weighing 60 kg (intracellular volume 12 to 15 L), the daily maintenance requirements are 1.2 to 1.5 L of water and nutrients providing 1200 to 1500 kcal, 36 to 45 mmol of sodium, and 24 to 30 mmol of potassium. Administration of fluids and electrolytes must be adjusted on the basis of daily physical examination and of serum values of electrolytes and renal function, as needed.

Mistreatment and Social Support

Hospitalization of older persons is sometimes precipitated by mistreatment, which includes physical or psychologic abuse, neglect, self-neglect, exploitation, and abandonment. Elder mistreatment was not recognized in the medical literature until 1975; it is now estimated to affect 700,000 to 1.2 million Americans annually. In a large prospective cohort study, the annual incidence of referral to protective services for mistreatment was found to be approximately 1% among persons aged 65 years or older. Those referred for abuse, neglect, or exploitation were found to have a lower rate of survival over 13 years of follow-up (9%) than those referred for self-neglect (17%) and those not referred (40%). Most older persons referred to protective services because of physical abuse have been seen in hospital emergency departments, and many emergency visits lead to hospitalization.

Universal screening for mistreatment has been recommended and can be implemented by asking each older patient, "Do you feel safe returning to where you live?" (The sensitivity and specificity of this and other screening approaches are unknown.) Further questions can explore the living situation and specific settings or aspects of mistreatment. It is important to consider the diagnosis of mistreatment when there are physical or psychologic stigmata, such as unexplained injury, dehydration, malnutrition, social withdrawal, or recalcitrant depression or anxiety. When mistreatment is suspected, most states require that Adult Protective Services or the equivalent state agency be contacted. (See "Elder Mistreatment," p 86.)

Influenza and Pneumococcus Vaccines

All persons aged 65 years or older should be asked at the time of admission to the hospital whether they have received influenza or pneumococcal vaccination. During the fall and winter months, influenza vaccination can be administered to those who have not already received it. Pneumococcal vaccination can be administered to older hospitalized patients who do not recall having received it in the past 10 years. (See also "Prevention," p 69.)

SYSTEMS OF CARE FOR OLDER HOSPITAL PATIENTS

Three systematic approaches have been demonstrated in controlled trials to improve hospital care of older persons. These approaches involve comprehensive multicomponent interventions, two of which were implemented on designated medical units.

Geriatric evaluation and management (GEM) units for elderly patients who have stabilized during an acute hospitalization were developed and pioneered in Veterans Affairs medical centers. These units incorporate comprehensive geriatric assessment (including screening for geriatric syndromes, and assessment for and treatment of functional, cognitive, affective, and nutritional problems) with interdisciplinary team-based care. A multicenter randomized trial demonstrated improved ADL function and physical performance, relative to usual hospital care, for veterans assigned to GEM units. Some measures of health-related quality of life were also superior for patients treated on GEM units. These units did not affect mortality and were cost-neutral after consideration of both initial hospitalization costs and the costs of care after discharge.

A second approach involves a system of care designed to help acutely ill older patients to maintain or achieve independence in ADLs and IADLs; this system has been called Acute Care for Elders (ACE). This approach has been adapted in many acute-care hospitals where acutely ill elderly patients are admitted to an ACE unit. The four components of this intervention are as follows:

- a prepared environment to promote mobility and orientation (eg, with carpeting, raised toilet seats, low beds, clocks, calendars, and pictures to promote orientation);
- patient-centered care with nursing-initiated protocols for independent self-care, nutrition, sleep hygiene, skin care, mood, and cognition;
- planning to go home, with early social work intervention to mobilize family and other resources at home; and
- medical care review to promote optimal prescribing.

In a randomized trial involving 651 medical patients aged 70 years or older in a university teaching hospital, ACE was found to be associated with greater independence in ADLs at discharge, less frequent nursing-home discharge, and somewhat shorter and less expensive hospitalization. In a second randomized trial involving 1531 community-dwelling persons aged 70 years or older in a community teaching hospital, ACE was found to be associated with substantial differences in the satisfaction of patients, family members, physicians, and nurses but with only modest differences ADL function. These findings demonstrate that ACE is a promising approach to improving outcomes and reducing hospital costs for acutely ill older general medical patients, but the effects of ACE on patient outcomes are likely sensitive to factors dependent on the function of the interdisciplinary team.

A third systematic approach (the Hospital Elder Life Program) involves a multicomponent intervention to prevent delirium in hospitalized older patients. The intervention consists of protocols to manage six risk factors for delirium: cognitive impairment, sleep deprivation, immobility, visual impairment, hearing impairment, and dehydration. Elderly patients receiving this intervention are not segregated on a special hospital ward or unit. In a prospective controlled study, the incidence of delirium was found to be reduced by one third, from 15.0% to 9.9%. The intervention was also associated with significant improvement in the degree of cognitive impairment among patients with cognitive impairment at admission and a reduction in the rate of use of sleep medications among all patients. Among the other risk factors, there were trends toward improvement in immobility, visual impairment, and hearing impairment. The intervention was not associated with a reduction in the severity, duration, or recurrence of delirium, and the effects of the intervention on other outcomes have not yet been reported. Nonetheless, these findings suggest that primary prevention of delirium is probably the most effective treatment strategy.

ALTERNATIVES TO AND TRANSITIONS FROM HOSPITAL CARE

It is often assumed that older persons would prefer to be treated for acute illness at home rather than in the hospital whenever possible. The safety and feasibility of this approach for acutely ill older persons who would usually be hospitalized has been demonstrated. This approach, sometimes called the *home hospital*, requires intensive resources for medical and nursing care at home that are not yet widely available.

Older persons' preferences for home rather than hospital care vary widely. In a study of community-dwelling older persons, virtually all preferred care in the site that would provide the higher probability of survival. When home care and hospital care provide equivalent probabilities of survival, roughly half of patients prefer care in each site, with those preferring home care being more likely to be white, better educated, living with a spouse, deeply religious, and dependent in two or more ADLs. The major difference perceived by older persons between home care and hospital care was feeling safer in the hospital than at home.

Almost one quarter of hospitalized patients aged 65 and older are discharged to another institution. Although it is labor-intensive, meticulous discharge planning may maximize the probability that patients maintain the clinical and functional benefits achieved by hospitalization, and probably reduces the risk of early readmission and the use of emergency services. Discharge planning ideally begins at hospital admission, with a projection of medical, nursing, rehabilitative, and functional support required by the patient at the time of discharge. The following items should be communicated to patients (or their caregivers) who are being discharged directly home: follow-up appointments; warning symptoms or signs to watch for with instructions on whom to contact; clinical disciplines (eg, nursing, physical therapy) contracted for provision in the home; and a reconciled medication list, with clarification of which prehospital medications are to be continued. Patients being discharged to other care venues should be oriented with respect to the nature of the institution, the identity of a new attending physician, and the expected frequency of physician visits. If the provider at the receiving institution differs from the hospital clinician, then clear and prompt communication is essential. Some items of information (critical but pending study results, nuances of goals of care or family dynamics) call for direct communication between sending and receiving clinicians. Otherwise, a pithy and prompt discharge summary containing the following will suffice: summary of hospital course with care provided; a list of problems and diagnoses; baseline physical functional status; baseline cognitive status; medication list (with termination dates for time-limited drugs such as antibiotics); allergies; tests results still outstanding; follow-up appointments; and information related to goals, preferences, and advance directives.

ANNOTATED REFERENCES

- Cohen HJ, Feussner JR, Weinberger M, et al. A controlled trial of inpatient and outpatient geriatric evaluation and management. *N Engl J Med.* 2002;346(12):905–912.

    Using a two-by-two factorial design, the authors performed a randomized study of both inpatient and outpatient geriatric evaluation and management (GEM) at 11 Veterans Affairs (VA) medical centers. Eleven VA sites were involved, and 1388 elderly veterans were enrolled and followed. Significant benefits were observed from the GEM unit (acute care) intervention in terms of subjects' physical performance and basic activities of daily living at hospital discharge. Subjects in the intervention arm also demonstrated higher ratings for health-related quality of life in physical functioning, bodily pain, energy, and general health.

- Coleman EA. Falling through the cracks: challenges and opportunities for improving transitional care for persons with continuous complex care needs. *J Am Geriatr Soc.* 2003;51(4):549–555.

    This article discusses the challenges of managing care transitions, provides statistics on numbers of elderly patients transferred from one care venue to another, lists characteristics of effective care transitions, and proposes a research agenda for this understudied area of geriatric medicine.

- Counsell SR, Holder CM, Liebenauer LL, et al. Effects of a multicomponent intervention on functional outcomes and process of care in hospitalized older patients: a randomized controlled trial of Acute Care for Elders (ACE) in a community hospital. *J Am Geriatr Soc.* 2000;48(12):1572–1581.

    This study reports the second large randomized trial of Acute Care for Elders (ACE), a multicomponent unit-based intervention designed to improve functional outcomes and the process of care for hospitalized older patients. In contrast to the first randomized trial, in this trial self-reported measures of function were not found to differ at discharge between the intervention and usual-care groups by intention-to-treat analysis. Nonetheless, the composite outcome of decline in activities of daily living from baseline or nursing-home placement occurred less in the intervention group at discharge (34% versus 40%; P = .027) and during the year following hospitalization (P = .022). Nursing care plans to promote independent function were more often implemented in the intervention group (79% versus 50%; P = .001), physical therapy consults were obtained more frequently (42% versus 36%; P = .027), and restraints were applied to fewer patients (2% versus 6%; P = .001). Satisfaction with care was higher for the intervention group than for the usual-care group among patients, caregivers, physicians, and nurses (P < .05 for each group). This study provides further evidence that ACE can improve the process of hospital care for acutely ill elderly patients but also demonstrates that ACE interventions will vary among hospitals and over time in their effects on patient outcomes.

- Milne AC, Potter J, Avenell A. Protein and energy supplementation in elderly people at risk from malnutrition (Cochrane Review). *The Cochrane Library.* Issue 1. Chichester, UK: John Wiley & Sons, Ltd; 2004.

    This review summarizes evidence from trials of oral nutritional supplementation in elderly patients. The authors selected randomized and quasi-randomized trials, and synthesized the findings of 31 trials including 2464 subjects. Most subjects were residents of long-term care or subacute wards, but 22% were hospitalized patients. Overall, nutritional supplementation appears to produce weight gain and may reduce mortality and shorten hospital stays. There was little evidence of benefit in terms of functional outcomes.

■ Walter LC, Brand RJ, Counsell SR, et al. Development and validation of a prognostic index for one-year mortality in older adults after hospitalization. *JAMA.* 2001;285(23):2987–2994.

> The authors developed a prognostic index in 1495 patients (mean age 81 years) discharged from the general medical service of a tertiary care hospital, then validated it in 1427 patients (mean age 79) from a community teaching hospital. The index employs a point system that assigns patients to one of four risk groups on the basis of six variables: gender, dependency in activities of daily living, presence of two comorbid conditions (heart failure or cancer), and two laboratory values drawn at admission (serum creatinine, serum albumin). The index demonstrated good discrimination and predictive ability.

William L. Lyons, MD
C. Seth Landefeld, MD

CHAPTER 14—PERIOPERATIVE CARE

KEY POINTS

- Operative therapy is an important option for many health problems that affect older persons.
- The overall complication rates of surgery on older persons are below 3%.
- Risk indices and practice guidelines for common cardiac, pulmonary, and neuropsychiatric problems assist in decision making and management of older surgical patients.
- Comprehensive preoperative assessment and attentive perioperative management can be helpful in minimizing complications of older persons with chronic medical problems and functional impairments.

OVERVIEW OF OPERATIVE THERAPY FOR OLDER PERSONS

Surgery is a common form of treatment for older persons; currently more than 55% of all operative procedures are done in patients aged 65 or over, and the proportion is expected to grow. Many of the chronic conditions that increase in prevalence with advancing age—cataracts, arthritis, vascular occlusions, and cancers—are amenable to surgery. Over half of all malignancies occur in patients aged 65 or over, and the primary treatment for many tumors is surgical. Advances in surgical, anesthetic, and medical care have lowered surgical risks and shifted the risk-benefit ratio to favor surgery in increasingly older patients with more complex conditions. Nevertheless, although older patients account for just over half of all surgical procedures, they suffer three quarters of the postoperative mortality and also the disproportionate majority of postoperative morbidity as well. For this reason, physicians are commonly asked to perform preoperative evaluations to reduce the risks of complications and death and to optimize patient outcomes.

Many of the changes of normal aging physiology impact the perioperative management of the elderly surgical patient. For example, altered body composition, diminished kidney function, and decreased liver blood flow and enzyme activity all contribute to changes in the pharmacokinetics of drugs. Cardiac and vascular stiffening complicate fluid management and optimization of intravascular volume. Both volume overload and volume depletion occur commonly and are poorly tolerated by many older persons. Stiffening of the thoracic cage and decrements in ciliary function contribute to decreases in pulmonary reserve and heightened risk of postoperative pneumonia. Because of decreased thermoregulation, the older surgical patient is at particular risk for perioperative hypothermia. Finally, by mechanisms that are not yet fully elucidated, changes in the brain that accompany aging make older individuals exquisitely susceptible to postoperative cognitive changes. The cumulative effect of multiple organ systems with limited physiologic reserve results in "homeostenosis," a condition that greatly increases the risk of iatrogenic events. (See "Biology," especially p 9.)

It is well recognized that the aging process is extremely variable from person to person and that within a person not all organ systems age at the same rate, producing dramatic heterogeneity even among healthy elderly persons. Older individuals may have accumulated several chronic conditions that may impact on the perioperative care, either directly or through the medications they use to treat those conditions. The heterogeneity in physiologic aging combined with the potential for multiple accumulated comorbidities means older patients require a more complex and individualized preoperative evaluation. They often benefit from a multidisciplinary approach to perioperative care and recovery.

Preoperative Assessment and Management

Cardiovascular System

It is estimated that 25% to 30% of postoperative deaths are from cardiac causes, and the rate of postoperative cardiac events is directly related to age. Cardiac risk assessment is the most fully developed and widely investigated portion of the preoperative medical assessment. Several schemes are available to help calculate cardiac risk, and decision trees have been well described to guide risk assessment and management. The American Society of Anesthesiologists (ASA) classification of patient physical status relies heavily on clinical judgment and is not specific for cardiovascular morbidity and mortality (see Table 14.1). This system has been used by anesthesiologists for years and has consistently been shown to be useful in predicting postoperative outcomes. An early cardiac risk index by Goldman and colleagues was published in the 1970s, a time when surgery on frail 80- and 90-year-olds was uncommon. The American College of Cardiology and the American Heart Association (ACC/AHA) Guideline for Perioperative Cardiovascular Evaluation for Noncardiac Surgery is widely employed to help stratify risk and direct management. This algorithm takes into account clinical predictors, functional status, and surgical risk and is available on the web at http://www.acc.org/clinical/guidelines/perio/update/periupdate_index.htm.

Because of increasing recognition of the benefit of medical therapy to reduce preoperative cardiac events in patients with clinical risk factors and mounting evidence of little benefit of noninvasive stress testing and invasive therapies to reduce preoperative cardiac events, the trend is now moving away from special preoperative cardiac testing and more toward treating with medical therapies on the basis of clinical judg-

ment. A coronary artery revascularization prophylaxis study demonstrated in a prospective and randomized controlled trial that in patients undergoing elective repair of abdominal aneurysm or surgical therapy for peripheral arterial disease who have coronary artery disease (CAD) amenable to revascularization, revascularization either by coronary artery bypass grafting (CABG) or angioplasty resulted in a delay until a proposed vascular surgery but otherwise no difference in postoperative death, myocardial infarction, stroke, dialysis, loss of limb, or survival up to 2.6 years in comparison with medical therapies, even in high-risk groups. It should be noted that patients with indications that have been shown to clearly benefit from CABG (ie, known left main disease, unstable angina, and multivessel disease with low ejection fraction) were excluded from randomization. Also, risk of perioperative myocardial infarction is markedly elevated when the surgical procedure is performed within the first 6 weeks after angioplasty and stenting. It seems clear that revascularization should not be performed simply to "get someone through a surgical procedure" and that this approach may be in fact harmful. The preoperative cardiac evaluation is therefore is quite simplified in the geriatric age group (see Figure 14.1).

The evidence base supporting the use of perioperative β-blockers, particularly in patients aged 65 or over with known CAD or risk factors for CAD, appears well established. This means the majority geriatric patients undergoing surgery are likely to derive benefit from perioperative β-blocker usage unless there is a clear contraindication to this. Growing interest in the use of both aspirin and so-called statin medications (HMG CoA reductase inhibitors) is based on evidence of benefit of these therapies from nonrandomized studies in high-risk patients. In a prospective but nonrandomized study of over 5000 patients undergoing CABG, those patients taking aspirin within 48 hours of their surgery had nearly a 50% reduced risk of myocardial infarction and stroke, almost three quarters the rate of kidney failure, and no increase in the risk of bleeding or gastritis. A case-control study of patients undergoing elective peripheral vascular surgery found that current users of statin medications had an 80% reduction in the odds of postoperative death in comparison with nonusers. Randomized trials of both of these therapies are needed to further investigate their utility in reducing postoperative cardiac complications.

The greatest risks associated with valvular heart disease include heart failure and endocarditis. Prophylactic antibiotics are recommended to prevent bacterial endocarditis in selected patients undergoing specific procedures. The highest risk for endocarditis is among patients with prosthetic cardiac valves, complex congenital heart disease, and surgically constructed

Table 14.1—ASA Classification of Physical Status

Class	Description
I or P1	A normal healthy patient
II or P2	A patient with mild systemic disease
III or P3	A patient with severe systemic disease
IV or P4	A patient with severe systemic disease that is a constant threat to life
V or P5	A moribund patient who is not expected to survive without surgery
VI or P6	A declared brain-dead patient whose organs are being harvested for donor purposes

NOTE: There is no additional information to help further define these categories.

SOURCE: Data from American Society of Anesthesiologists. ASA Physical Status Classification System. Available at http:/www.asahq.org/clinical/physicalstatus.htm (accessed October 2005).

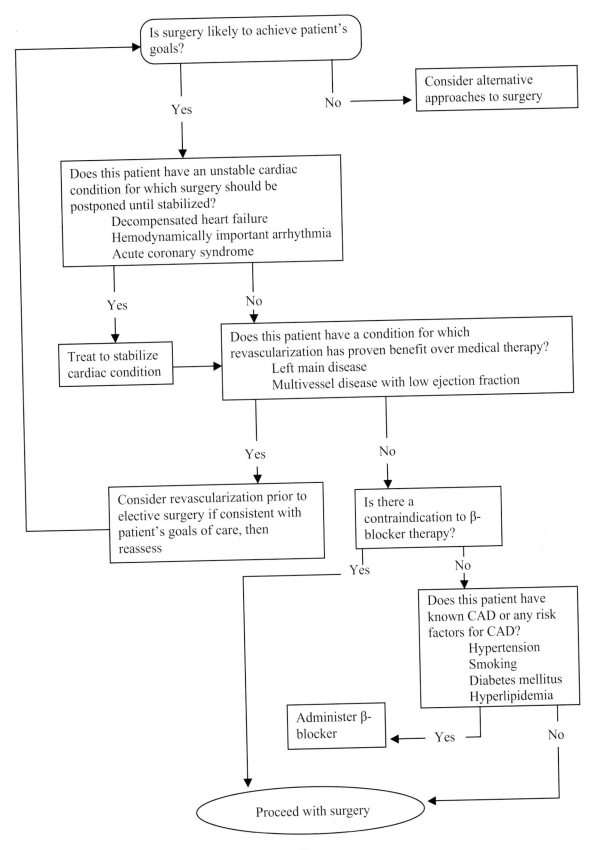

Figure 14.1—Approach to geriatric preoperative cardiac care.
CAD = coronary artery disease.

systemic-pulmonary shunts or conduits, or a previous history of endocarditis. Patients at moderate risk are those with other congenital cardiac malformations, acquired valvular dysfunction, hypertrophic cardio-myopathy, and mitral valve prolapse with regurgitation or thickened leaflets, or both. Endocarditis prophylaxis is recommended for patients undergoing procedures that involve the respiratory, biliary or intestinal mucosa, prostate surgery, cystoscopy, or urethral dilation. For the most recent guidelines of the American Heart Association, see their Web site: http://www.amhrt.org.

Respiratory System

Postoperative pulmonary complications have been reported to prolong the hospital stay by an average of 1 to 2 weeks in the elderly age group. The in-hospital mortality rate for those with postoperative respiratory failure is around 40%, versus 5% for those without respiratory failure. Possible patient-related factors for development of pulmonary complications postoperatively include smoking, general health status, age, obesity, chronic obstructive pulmonary disease (COPD), neurologic status, cardiovascular status, and intravascular volume shifts. Procedure-related risk factors include the site of the incision, length of the surgery, and type of anesthesia. The risk of pulmonary complications increases as the incision approaches the diaphragm; upper abdominal and thoracic procedures carry the greatest risk (10% to 40%).

A recent investigation of over 160,000 veterans undergoing noncardiac surgery established a clinical prediction model for postoperative pneumonia. Patients were assigned points based on the type of operation, age decile, functional status, and selected clinical conditions (weight loss, administration of general anesthesia, impaired sensorium, history of stroke, level of blood urea nitrogen, and transfusion of greater than 4 units of blood). Individual points were summed to create a score, and the study sample could be divided into five risk classes according to these scores. Pneumonia rates were 0.2% among those with 0 to 15 risk points, 1.2% for those with 16 to 25 risk points, 4.0% for those with 26 to 40 risk points, 9.4% for those with 41 to 55 risk points, and 15.3% for those with more than 55 risk points. As an example, an 82-year-old woman (17 points) with some functional limitations (6 points) who was undergoing an open cholecystectomy (10 points) under general anesthesia (4 points) would have a score of 37 points and fall into the category of those patients with 9.4% risk of postoperative pneumonia. This tool may be useful in guiding perioperative respiratory care, including encouragement of coughing, deep breathing exercises, incentive spirometry, and early mobility to reduce the risk of respiratory problems.

Whether age independently increases the risk of postoperative pulmonary complications is not clear. Chronologic age is less predictive of pulmonary complications following surgery than the presence of coexisting conditions. Patients with COPD have a threefold higher risk of postoperative pulmonary complications. Even among those with severe COPD, age has not been shown to be an independent risk factor for pulmonary complications. The use of perioperative pulmonary function tests in patients with known lung disease is largely discouraged but may be useful in evaluating dyspnea or wheezing when the diagnosis is unknown.

Thromboembolic complications, including pulmonary embolism, are common during the perioperative period. Since these complications can be serious and difficult to treat, attention is focused on prophylaxis. The most commonly used prophylactic regimens for patients over age 60 who are having general surgery are low-dose unfractionated heparin or low-molecular-weight heparin administered subcutaneously. More details regarding prophylactic anticoagulant regimens are found in the Appendix (p 491).

When a patient who is being treated with anticoagulants is being prepared for an operative intervention, the anticoagulants can be safely withheld for 5 doses preoperatively and then resumed the evening after surgery. This strategy may not be safe for those patients on warfarin therapy because of an artificial heart valve. In these high-risk patients, while warfarin is being withdrawn, intravenous heparin can be administered, holding it 6 hours before the operation and restarting postoperatively, continuing it until a therapeutic level of anticoagulation is achieved with warfarin. Low-molecular-weight heparins should be held for 12 hours before an operation and resumed 24 hours after the procedure, especially if spinal anesthesia is used. There is no standard for the management of antiplatelet agents. Traditionally, aspirin has been withheld for a week before surgery, but more recent data suggest that this practice is not needed to reduce bleeding complications. A large but nonrandomized study found dramatically lower rates of myocardial ischemia, gut ischemia, stroke, and kidney failure when aspirin is continued in the perioperative period in patients undergoing CABG. Importantly, in this study, the risk of bleeding and need for transfusions were not found to be increased in the patients who continued their aspirin. Randomized studies are needed to confirm the potential benefit of initiating or continuing aspirin in high-risk patients undergoing surgical procedures. For now, whether to continue, discontinue, or initiate aspirin is not clear.

Kidneys and Metabolism

As mentioned previously, renal and glomerular blood flow decreases with age. Concomitantly, there is a loss of muscle mass with age, such that an apparently normal serum creatinine may by misinterpreted as indicating normal kidney function. Glomerular filtration could be more accurately estimated by calculating the creatinine clearance using the Cockroft-Gault equation (see the section on elimination in "Pharmacotherapy," p 73) or relying on the MDRD (Modification of Diet in Renal Disease study) method that some laboratories use to automatically calculate glomerular filtration rate. Since many drugs administered during the perioperative period may require dosage adjustments with diminished renal function, accurate estimation of glomerular filtration rate is important.

Also, because of decrements in the ability of the kidney to appropriately retain salt or to maximally concentrate or dilute urine in response to intravascular volume, the use of intravenous fluids needs to be monitored very carefully. Volume resuscitation is best achieved with normal saline or blood (if appropriate), since half-normal saline or water are hypotonic and more readily diffuse to the extravascular tissues. The combination of pain in a patient who is receiving nothing by mouth and receiving intravenous D5 half-normal saline inevitably produces hyponatremia in this setting. See also the section on acute tubular necrosis in "Kidney Diseases and Disorders," p 405.)

Neuropsychiatric Concerns

Delirium is a common and morbid event in the postoperative period. The type of surgery appears to be an important determinant of delirium, with incidence rates ranging from about 4% or 5% in cataract or urologic procedures to rates reported to be as high as 50% or 60% in some series of patients with infrarenal abdominal aortic aneurysm repair or hip fracture surgery. Both preoperative and intraoperative factors have been evaluated as risk factors for delirium. Preoperative factors in patients undergoing noncardiac surgery that predispose to postoperative delirium include: age 70 years or over, cognitive impairment, limited physical function, a history of alcohol abuse, abnormal serum sodium, potassium or glucose, intrathoracic surgery, and abdominal aneurysm surgery. The most important intraoperative factor found to be associated with delirium is intraoperative blood loss. Patients with a postoperative hematocrit < 30% had an increased risk of delirium (odds ratio = 1.7, 95% confidence interval 1.1 to 2.7) irrespective of the presence or absence of preoperative risk factors. When preoperative risk factors are present, the physician can identify patients at greatest risk for developing delirium and can be especially vigilant about correcting fluid, electrolyte

and metabolic derangements, optimizing replacement of blood loss, maintaining circadian rhythms by getting patients out of bed during the day and minimizing sleep interruptions at night, and cautious drug prescribing. (See also the section on postoperative delirium in "Delirium," p 242.)

Avoiding Iatrogenic Complications

Untoward effects of well-intentioned interventions are common among older hospitalized persons. Some of the more common pitfalls to be avoided include restricting mobility, excessive use of catheters, inattention to nutrition and hydration status, and inappropriate use of medications. Few disease states benefit from bed rest. It is important to maintain mobility and function as much as possible by encouraging time out of bed and avoiding restraints. The risks of skin breakdown, muscle atrophy, joint stiffness, and bone loss can be reduced by preserving mobility. Although bladder catheters can sometimes be critical in accurately measuring urine output, there is a substantial risk of infection with prolonged use of an indwelling catheter. These can also contribute to restricted mobility and should be removed as soon as possible. Restricted diets and lack of access to water can contribute to compromise in nutrition and hydration. Conversely, continued administration of intravenous fluids after the patient is able to maintain hydration orally can result in volume overload and impaired oxygenation. A regular review of medication administration can avoid unnecessary drug use and inappropriate dosing.

POSTOPERATIVE MANAGEMENT OF SELECTED MEDICAL PROBLEMS

Surgery in elderly persons often results in destabilization of chronic, coexistent medical conditions. Additionally, because of the diminished physiologic reserve common in older persons, new medical problems may arise in the postoperative period. Some of the most common medical issues to contend with postoperatively are discussed here.

Cardiovascular Problems

The most common cardiovascular problems that arise in older persons after surgery are hypertension, rhythm disturbances, and heart failure. Postoperative hypertension should initially prompt a search for a noncardiovascular cause, such as pain or urinary retention. Next, it is important to assess volume status, review fluid administration records, and note whether antihypertensive medications were mistakenly omitted before the procedure. To treat uncontrolled essential hypertension, parenteral formulations are available in several classes of medications: β-blockers, calcium channel blockers, angiotensin-converting enzyme inhibitors, and drugs that block both α- and β-adrenergic receptors. Topical agents, such as topical nitroglycerine, could also be considered useful in this setting.

Cardiac rhythm disturbances are concerning because they can lead to myocardial ischemia and heart failure. Supraventricular tachycardia, commonly seen in older persons, is associated with a history of prior supraventricular dysrhythmias, asthma, heart failure, and premature atrial complexes on a preoperative electrocardiogram. This rhythm disturbance is also more common in patients who have had vascular, abdominal, or thoracic procedures. Early restoration of sinus rhythm, or at least controlling the ventricular rate, can be attempted with an infusion of adenosine, a β-blocker, or a calcium channel blocker. If the rhythm is atrial fibrillation, conversion to sinus rhythm can be attempted with electrical cardioversion or by an infusion of amiodarone. Since spontaneous reversion to sinus rhythm often occurs within 6 weeks of the operation, long-term use of an anti-dysrhythmic like amiodarone may not be necessary. Persistent atrial fibrillation beyond 24 to 48 hours is associated with an increased risk of thromboembolism, and consideration should be given to anticoagulation therapy to reduce the risk of stroke.

Cardiac reserve is often compromised among older persons, especially those with longstanding hypertension or CAD. Heart failure may develop as a result of excessive fluid administration, or new cardiac ischemia or a rhythm disturbance. It can be extremely challenging to ensure optimal ventricular filling pressures on the basis of the clinical assessment of volume status in older persons by physical examination and standard laboratory parameters alone. Although some have recommended the use of pulmonary artery catheters in high-risk patients, studies have not shown a mortality benefit for this intervention.

Kidney and Electrolyte Disorders

Impaired preoperative kidney function increases the risk of postoperative kidney failure. The impaired reserve makes the aging kidney more susceptible to the effects of even transient reduction of cardiac output or brief exposure to nephrotoxic medications. When kidney damage has been sustained, early clinical manifestations include oliguria, isosthenuria, and an increase in serum creatinine. When impaired renal blood flow is the cause, the urine sodium will typically be less than 40 mEq/L and the urine-to-plasma creatinine ratio will be greater than 10:1. In contrast, if acute tubular necrosis is the mechanism of injury, the urine sediment may have granular or epithelial cell casts, and the urine sodium will be greater than 40 mEq/L with a urine-to-plasma creatinine ratio of less than 10:1. When acute tubular necrosis is suspected, vigorous efforts should be made to preserve kidney function by holding all potentially nephrotoxic medications and meticulously maintaining a euvolemic state. The indications for dialysis are no different in the perioperative period and include hypervolemia, hyperkalemia, metabolic acidosis, or encephalopathy. Another important mechanism of postoperative kidney failure is obstructive nephropathy, especially in older men with prostatic hyperplasia. The partial outflow obstruction combined with immobility and exposure to medications with anticholinergic effects compromising detrusor function all conspire to precipitate acute urinary retention. In addition to oliguria and an increase in serum creatinine, the bladder will typically be palpable because of distention. Treatment consists of insertion of a bladder catheter to reduce the risk of hydronephrosis and impaired kidney function. (See also the section on acute tubular necrosis in "Kidney Diseases and Disorders," p 405.)

Gastrointestinal Concerns

Constipation is quite common postoperatively, as a consequence of the combined effects of altered diet, immobility, and usually narcotic and other constipating medication use. At times, ileus and obstipation may be severe and produce significant anorexia, nausea, and even vomiting. The role of postoperative iron therapy to treat anemia is unproven and likely also contributes. Given the common co-occurrence of these risk factors for constipation in the postoperative period, a reasonable approach is to simultaneously order a stool softener every time a narcotic prescription is ordered, particularly if the patient has a history of constipation or it is reasonably anticipated that mobility will be reduced for more than 1 day. Prunes or prune juice, applesauce, and bran can all also have promotility effects. Table 14.2 lists the many medications useful in preventing and managing constipation.

Postoperative diarrhea should raise concern for fecal impaction and antibiotic-associated or *Clostridium difficile* diarrhea in the setting of recent antibiotic use. Checking manually for fecal impaction and sending stool specimens for leukocytes and *C. difficile* toxin may be appropriate. Management must focus carefully on volume resuscitation and treating the underlying cause.

Finally, nausea is not uncommon in the postoperative period, often as a result of narcotic, anesthetic, and other medications or slowed gut motility. See the section on nausea in "Palliative Care" (p 136) for a discussion on approach to management.

Table 14.2—Medications That May Relieve Constipation

Medication	Onset of Action	Starting Dosage	Site and Mechanism of Action
Bulk laxatives			
Methylcellulose (Citrucel),* psyllium (Metamucil)*	12–24 h (up to 72 h)	1–2 rounded tsp or packets qd–tid with water or juice	Small and large intestine; holds water in feces; mechanical distention
Polycarbophil (FiberCon,* others)	12–24 h (up to 72 h)	1250 mg qd–qid	Small and large intestine; holds water in feces; mechanical distention
Osmotic laxatives			
Lactulose (Cephulac)	24–48 h	15–30 mL qd–bid	Colon; osmotic effect
Polyethylene glycol (MiraLax)	48–96 h	17 g pwd qd (~1 tbsp) dissolved in 8 oz water	Gastrointestinal tract tract; osmotic effect
Sorbitol 70%*	24–48 h	15–30 mL qd–bid	Colon; delivers osmotically active molecules to colon
Saline laxatives			
Magnesium citrate (Citroma*)	0.5–3 h	120–240 mL × 1	Small and large intestine; attracts, retains water in intestinal lumen
Magnesium hydroxide (Milk of Magnesia*)	30 min–3 h	30 mL qd–bid	Osmotic effect and increased peristalsis in colon
Sodium phosphate or biphosphate emollient enema (Fleet*)	2–15 min	14.5-oz enema × 1, repeat prn	Colon, osmotic effect; potential hyperphosphatemia in patients with renal insufficiency
Stimulant laxatives			
Bisacodyl tablet (Dulcolax*)	6–10 h	5–15 mg × 1	Colon; increases peristalsis
Bisacodyl suppository (Dulcolax*)	0.25–1 h	10 mg × 1	Colon; increases peristalsis
Senna (Senokot*)	6–10 h	2 tabs or 1 tsp qhs	Colon; direct action on intestine; stimulates myenteric plexus; alters water and electrolyte secretion
Surfactant laxative			
Docusate (Colace*)	24–72 h	100 mg qd–bid	Small and large intestine; detergent activity; facilitates admixture of fat and water to soften feces

* Over-the-counter medication.

NOTE: bid = twice a day; h = hour(s); min = minute(s); oz = ounces; prn = as needed; pwd = powder; qd = every day; qhs = each bedtime; qid = four times a day; tid = three times a day; tbsp = tablespoon; tsp = teaspoon.

Managing Common Endocrine Abnormalities

Type 2 diabetes mellitus is a common comorbid condition of many older persons undergoing surgery. Usually, given the long half-life of oral hypoglycemic agents and the nothing-by-mouth status for surgery, oral diabetes drugs are held the day of surgery. It may be especially important to hold metformin, given the potential additional risk of metabolic acidosis from this drug during a time of stress. To optimize glucose control, an intravenous solution containing glucose can be administered at a constant rate while blood glucose by finger stick assay is closely monitored, administering subcutaneous insulin as necessary to control glucose levels until the patient is able to resume eating. A type 2 insulin-using diabetic patient should have her insulin held on the day of surgery and receive sliding-scale insulin. Once the patient is able to advance her diet, usually half the outpatient dose of diabetes drugs are administered the first day of oral intake, with additional sliding-scale insulin coverage as needed, and then full doses are resumed as the patient consumes a usual diet. Notably, there is currently no evidence that rigorous control of blood glucose in the perioperative period provides benefit in terms of recovery of function, reduction of infections, or wound healing; thus, "permissive moderate hyperglycemia" may be prudent until adequate oral intake is ensured.

Patients taking supplemental corticosteroids require special consideration during the perioperative period. Those taking more than 20 to 30 mg of prednisone daily for more than a week or with known adrenal insufficiency should be given "stress doses" of steroids perioperatively. A single measure of cortisol, if elevated, is useful to assess the hypothalamic-pituitary axis (HPA) in patients who chronically use steroids when the function of the HPA is in question. If the cortisol level is not high, a 30-minute ACTH test may be useful. The dose of steroids to use is debated, but some authorities advise the equivalents of 25 mg of hydrocortisone the day of surgery only for minor procedures, 50 to 75 mg hydrocortisone equivalents daily (for example, hydrocortisone 20 mg intravenously every 8 hours) for 1 to 2 days for moderate surgical stress, and 100 to 150 mg hydrocortisone equivalents daily (for example, hydrocortisone 50 mg intravenously every 8 hours beginning within 2 hours of surgery) continuing for 2 to 3 days postoperatively, and then transitioned to the usual steroid regimen for high surgical stress. Other authorities simply recommend continuation of usual doses of steroids for elective, uncomplicated surgeries, or doubling or tripling the outpatient dose by giving hydrocortisone intravenously up to 100 to 150 mg daily for higher risk or anticipated complicated operations.

Delirium and Postoperative Cognitive Decline

Delirium is one of the most common postoperative complications, and certainly the one for which a geriatrician is most likely to be consulted. In a randomized study, a multicomponent intervention, focusing on reducing sleep interruptions, minimizing medications and immobility, enhancing sensory input, and reducing dehydration was found to reduce the rate of developing delirium by one third over standard care for hospitalized medical patients. This approach, though not specifically studied in the postoperative setting, is likely to be beneficial in the postoperative phase as well. See "Delirium" (p 239) for descriptions of risk factors for delirium and a reasonable approach to diagnosis, evaluation, and treatment. For the postoperative geriatric surgical patient, undertreated pain, constipation, electrolyte abnormalities, and perioperative myocardial infarction must be particularly considered.

Postoperative cognitive decline can be subtle or dramatic and is considered to be a syndrome distinct from delirium characterized by abnormalities in learning and memory. It has been reported most commonly after cardiac surgery but is experienced by patients undergoing procedures that do not involve extracorporal circulation. Although the symptoms are often short-lived, they persist for many months in 10% to 30% of patients. Efforts to define the cause of the syndrome have not yet been successful; studies have not been able to demonstrate links with hypotension, hypoxemia, or type of anesthesia. Lacking a better understanding of the pathophysiology, treatment efforts are supportive.

Pain Management

Management of postoperative pain remains a challenge, particularly in the patient with dementia, delirium, or both. The key points to the evaluation and management of acute pain are quite similar to those discussed in "Persistent Pain" (p 140), and Table 19.1, Common Pain Behaviors in Cognitively Impaired Elderly Persons (p 142), provides a useful guide to the tools to assist in assessment of postoperative pain in cognitively impaired patients. The oldest-old and cognitively impaired patients appear to be at highest risk for undertreatment of pain, so they deserve particular attention. Undertreatment of pain, at least in nondemented individuals, appears in fact to be a more powerful predictor of the development of postoperative delirium than narcotic use.

Most postsurgical pain will require therapy with narcotic analgesia. Cognitively intact patients may have improved pain relief and overall lower use of narcotics if drugs are administered by patient-controlled analgesia (PCA) pump. Individuals with less severe pain may be able to tolerate scheduled acetaminophen (not to exceed 4 g a day) with only as-needed use of narcotic analgesics, if they are able to ask for them. Patients who are unable to communicate effectively and have pain should be given standing orders for narcotic analgesics, with guidelines as to when to hold the medications, combined with frequent assessment of medication effect. Nonsteroidal anti-inflammatory medications are best avoided in this setting. Recall that narcotic analgesics may precipitate constipation; thus, concomitant use of stool softeners is generally advised. See the Web site for *Geriatrics At Your Fingertips* for comprehensive, up-to-date information on pain medications and dosing at http://www.geriatricsatyourfingertips.org.

Nonpharmacologic therapies, such as ice packs, heating pads, massage, and relaxation techniques, are also useful adjuncts to therapy.

Planning for Transitions

Geriatricians and internists can significantly aid patients by anticipating and planning for transitions in care. Well before the time of discharge, it is important to understand how the patient will get help if he or she returns home. Watching a patient transfer, walk, and perform activities of daily living will help guide choices about appropriate discharge destination and home services that would be required to maximize a safe transition.

The time of transition is also treacherous in terms of medication errors. Carefully review with the patient (or her caregiver) her diagnoses, the summary of her hospital course, what specific medications she should take at home, and which of her old medicines she should discontinue. Include any special instructions about dosing and timing of the medication; also assess whether she will be able to obtain and administer her medications appropriately. It is useful to make sure that she (or her caregiver) understands the basics about how to manage her disease and the treatments and the need for the follow-up appointments; it should also be clear who is responsible for scheduling these appointments. Because geriatric patients tend to be more complex, it may be useful to facilitate the transition by communicating directly with the next care provider, especially for those patients who are being discharged to another institutional setting.

ANNOTATED REFERENCES

■ Arozullah AM, Khuri SF, Henderson WG, et al. Development and validation of a multifactorial risk index for predicting postoperative pneumonia after major noncardiac surgery. *Ann Intern Med.* 2001;135(10):847–857.

This investigation used a database of more than 160,000 veterans to derive and validate a clinical prediction model for postoperative pneumonia in noncardiac surgical patients. Patients were divided into five risk classes by the use of risk index scores. Pneumonia rates were 0.2% among those with 0 to 15 risk points, 1.2% for those with 16 to 25 risk points, 4.0% for those with 26 to 40 risk points, 9.4% for those with 41 to 55 risk points, and 15.3% for those with more than 55 risk points. The postoperative pneumonia risk index evidently identified patients at risk for postoperative pneumonia and may therefore be useful in guiding perioperative respiratory care.

■ Eagle KA, Berger PB, Calkins H, et al. ACC/AHA guideline update for perioperative cardiovascular evaluation for noncardiac surgery—executive summary. *Circulation.* 2002;105(10):1257–1267. Also available at: http://www.acc.org and http://www.americanheart.org (both accessed October 2005).

This document is an update of the original evidence-based guidelines distributed from the American College of Cardiology and the American Heart Association in 1996. Recommendations for evaluation of preoperative cardiac risks and perioperative management of cardiac conditions are provided and graded on the level of supporting evidence found. This is a useful reference with a framework provided that is widely used by clinicians. The guidelines do not specifically pertain to geriatric patients, but to all adult patients. The authors conclude that preoperative testing should be limited given the lack of evidence that widespread use positively alters outcomes. The guidelines are reviewed and updated annually on the Web sites.

■ Geerts WH, Pineo GF, Heit JA, et al. Prevention of venous thromboembolism: the Seventh ACCP Conference on Antithrombotic and Thrombolytic Therapy. *Chest.* 2004;126(3 Suppl):338S–400S.

This is a comprehensive review of the evidence base for and guidelines for the use of antithrombotic and thrombolytic therapies for all indications. The sections on the use of these therapies to prevent deep-vein thrombosis in for patients planning various surgical procedures is particularly informative and is presented with a grading of the strength of the evidence base.

■ McFalls EO, Ward HB, Mortitz TE, et al. Coronary-artery revascularization before elective major vascular surgery. *N Engl J Med* 2004;351(27):2795–2804.

This prospective, randomized clinical trial entitled Coronary Artery Revascularization Prophylaxis (CARP) investigated coronary revascularization (either by angioplasty or bypass surgery) versus no revascularization before elective repair of either an expanding abdominal aortic aneurysm or of severe arterial occlusive disease of the legs. All patients had stable coronary artery disease and had coronary angiograms, and they were eligible for study if one or more major coronary artery had a stenosis of at least 70% suitable for revascularization. Patients were excluded if they had a left main occlusion greater than 50% and ejection fraction of less than 20%, or had severe aortic stenosis. There were no differences between the two groups in postoperative cardiac infarction, early postoperative death, hospital length of stay, or mortality for the 2.7 years of follow-up, and the revascularized group had a significant delay until the elective vascular surgery was performed. Thus, even in high-risk patients, preoperative revascularization should be reserved for patients with conditions that otherwise would warrant revascularization (unstable cardiac symptoms, significant left main disease, or multivessel disease with a low ejection fraction) regardless of the proposed surgery.

■ Marcantonio E, Flacker JM, Wright RJ, et al. Reducing delirium after hip fracture: a randomized trial. *J Am Geriatri Soc.* 2001;49(5):516–522.

This is a prospective randomized clinical trial involving 126 consenting and eligible patients admitted for acute hip fracture comparing "proactive" geriatrics consultation versus usual care. The intervention patients were seen by the geriatrician within 24 hours after surgery, though most were seen preoperatively. Orthopedics adherence with geriatrics recommendations was high (77%) and resulted in a one third reduction in the rate of developing delirium, though without impact on length of stay. This study demonstrated that collaborative and proactive efforts are effective in reducing postoperative delirium.

■ Smetana GW. Preoperative pulmonary evaluation. *N Engl J Med.* 1999;340(12):937–944.

This review article represents an excellent overview of the salient issues regarding the preoperative pulmonary evaluation in both young and old patients. This is a common source of consultation for internists. It is particularly important to understand the limitations of the current literature, main risk factors for postoperative pulmonary complications, and prudent postoperative maneuvers to minimize this particularly hazardous occurrence in the course of older patients' lives.

Colleen Christmas, MD
Peter Pompei, MD

CHAPTER 15—REHABILITATION

KEY POINTS

- The World Health Organization conceptual model of functioning and disability provides a useful framework for geriatric rehabilitation by taking into account the complex interactions of body functions and structures, health conditions, individual activities and participation in life situations, and environmental and personal factors.

- A Medicare-certified inpatient rehabilitation hospital program must demonstrate that a certain percentage of patients have at least one of thirteen conditions and receive 3 hours of therapy per day.

- Since rehabilitation treatments require active patient participation and long-term self-management, the patient and family are core members of the rehabilitation team.

- Factors that influence recovery after a hip fracture include prior mobility and functional status, comorbid conditions, cognitive status, and social support.

- Optimal rehabilitation outcomes depend on comprehensive assessment of the patient, coordinated interdisciplinary team management, multifaceted interventions, and access to appropriate and high-quality care.

OVERVIEW

Rehabilitation is a critical component of geriatric health care because disabling conditions in the elderly population are common. Although these conditions drastically influence quality of life, they often improve with treatment. Chronic disease almost always underlies disability in older adults; for example, stroke occurs most often in people with other vascular diseases, and hip fractures occur most often in people with osteoporosis and gait disorders. Worsening disability also occurs in progressive chronic diseases like osteoarthritis, Parkinson's disease, or amyotrophic lateral sclerosis or in the context of deconditioning from inactivity during acute illness. To provide the best functional recovery possible, those providing geriatric rehabilitation must

- use systematic approaches to assess the causes of disability,
- be familiar with the advantages and disadvantages of all potential sites of care,
- understand the role of multidisciplinary teams and care plans,
- adapt care to comorbidities and disabilities, and
- be familiar with the basic requirements for rehabilitation of common geriatric conditions.

This chapter is designed to provide an overview of these key issues.

CONCEPTUAL MODEL FOR GERIATRIC REHABILITATION

Geriatric rehabilitation services can be organized around a conceptual model of disability in order to assess the status and needs of the patient, match treatments with specific conditions, and evaluate rehabilitation outcomes. The recently revised World Health Organization (WHO) *International Classification of Functioning, Disability, and Health* (ICF) provides a useful framework. See the WHO Web site (available at http://www3.who.int/icf/beginners/bg.pdf) for an ICF guide and a discussion of the ICF model of disability (Figure 15.1). The ICF has two main domains: "Health Condition" and "Contextual Factors." Disability and functioning are viewed as outcomes of interactions between health conditions (diseases, disorders, injuries) and contextual factors, which range from a person's most immediate environment, like furniture in the room, to the more general environment, like access to public transportation. Personal factors include a person's age, race, gender, educational background, personality, fitness, and life style.

In the WHO model, interventions can be designed to modify a person's impairments, limitations in activities, and restrictions in participation. For example, a treatment plan may be developed to improve a person's strength (impairment level), but the significance of this intervention is due to its effect on his or her physical mobility (activity) and ultimately the person's ability to return to social or physical roles (participation). The effects of gains in strength and physical mobility on participation could be modified by the person's motivation or social support. For example, if a man improves in strength and balance but his family and friends continue to "do everything for him" and do not encourage independent function, he may remain dependent. The physical environment is another powerful modifier. Even the person who achieves improved function cannot regain prior work or household roles if physical barriers to access in the community are not removed or adapted by such means as

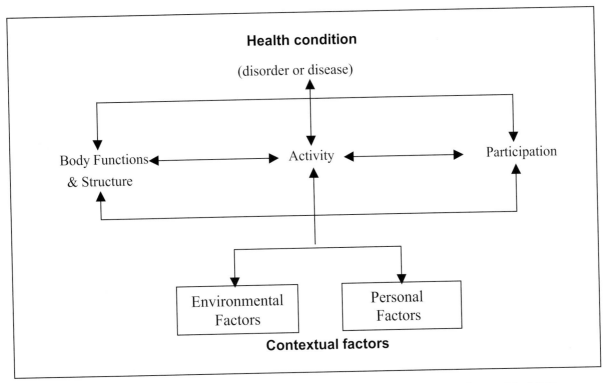

Figure 15.1—Current understanding of interactions among the components of the disability model of ICF.

The new edition of the International Classification of Functioning, Disability and Health (ICF) differs substantially from the 1980 version in its stress on health and functioning, rather than on disability. Previous models conceived of disability as beginning where health ended. The new model synthesizes the medical and social models of disability, providing a coherent view of its biological, individual, and social aspects.

SOURCE: World Health Organization, *Towards a Common Language for Disability and Health: ICF.* Geneva: World Health Organization; 2002:9. Reprinted with permission of the World Health Organization (WHO) and all rights are reserved by the Organization.

ramps or modified bathrooms. In summary, the interaction of disease and disability is particularly complex in older adults. The ICF model is useful for structuring comprehensive rehabilitation care for older patients.

SITES OF REHABILITATION CARE

Rehabilitation services are offered in both inpatient and community-based sites. Inpatient care may be provided in rehabilitation centers (freestanding hospitals or units attached to acute hospitals) or nursing facilities (Medicare skilled nursing facilities). Outpatient rehabilitation services can be provided in hospital-based or independent clinics, in day hospital settings, or in the home. The patient's eligibility, the particular services provided, and costs vary across sites of care. The balance of advantages and disadvantages for the individual patient are important factors for the clinician to consider in recommending a site or sites of rehabilitation care.

Sites of Care: Coverage and Services

A Medicare-certified inpatient rehabilitation hospital program must demonstrate that a certain percentage of their patients have at least one of thirteen conditions, and that at least a certain percentage of patients receive 3 hours of therapy per day. Patients must be seen by a physician on a daily basis, have 24-hour rehabilitation nursing care, and be managed by a interdisciplinary team of skilled nurses and therapists. Medicare prospective reimbursement is now based on case-mix groups using the Functional Independence Measure (FIM).

The Medicare-approved skilled nursing facility must provide 24-hour nursing care. Dietary, pharmaceutical, dental, and medical social services are also available. Physicians must supervise patient care and can visit the patient infrequently, but they must be available 24 hours a day on an emergency basis. Therapy services are available, but multidisciplinary coordination may not occur. In this setting, maintenance of function without progress may be the goal of care. Reimbursement is based on prospective payment according to the resource utilization groups (RUG III) classification, which is based on the Minimum Data Set (MDS 2).

Medicare provides home-health benefits to patients who require intermittent or part-time skilled nursing care and therapy services and who are homebound, defined flexibly to include individuals who "occasionally leave the home." These services must be prescribed and recertified every 60 days by a physician. There is no prior hospitalization requirement or limit on the number of visits a person may receive. Medicare provides care in 60-day episodes. As long as patients continue to remain eligible for home-health services, they may receive an unlimited number of medically necessary episodes of care. Home-health services provide skilled nursing and home-health aides, therapy services, medical social services, and supplies. Even though physicians must certify the patient for services, they are rarely involved in the supervision of care, and multidisciplinary coordination of care may not be available.

The escalating expenditures for Medicare's postacute care benefits from $2.5 billion in 1986 to more than $30 billion in 1996 led to the Balanced Budget Act (BBA) of 1997, which mandated prospective payment systems rather than fee-for-service reimbursement. In skilled nursing facilities, the BBA mandated the implementation of a per diem prospective payment system covering all costs (routine, ancillary, and capital) related to the services furnished to the patients under Part A of the Medicare program. Per diem payments for each admission are case-mix adjusted by the use of a resident classification system (RUG III) that is based on data from patient assessments (the MDS 2) and relative weights developed from staff time data. Home-health care reimbursement is now under a prospective payment system. Payment rates are based on relevant data from patient assessments conducted by clinicians using the Outcome and Assessment Information Set (OASIS). The OASIS was originally developed to assess quality of care in home health. The OASIS is lengthy, encompassing sociodemographic, environmental, support system, health status, and functional status attributes; it is required for reimbursement by Medicare for home-health services. For each 60-day episode of care, national payment rates vary, depending on the intensity of care required. Home-health agencies receive less than the full 60-day episode rate if they provide only a minimal number of visits to beneficiaries.

Sites of Care and Outcomes

The effect of site of care on rehabilitation outcomes is not well established. A study of outcomes among persons with stroke and hip fracture examined rates of discharge to home and recovery of function that were based on use of inpatient or nursing rehabilitation services. When controlling for case-mix differences, the researchers found that stroke but not hip fracture patients were more likely to be discharged home and to recover activities of daily living (ADLs) if treated in an inpatient rehabilitation setting. Nursing homes with high volumes of Medicare patients were found to influence stroke outcomes more than traditional nursing homes. Overall, there were no differences in outcomes for hip fracture patients by site of care. In another study, stroke patients treated under managed care were found to be more likely to receive rehabilitation in skilled nursing facilities than in inpatient rehabilitation hospitals. Patients in fee-for-service setting improved more in ADLs during the treatment phase, but there were no differences in ADLs between groups 1 year later. At 1 year, the patients in managed care were 2.4 times more likely to reside in nursing homes. On the other hand, a recent observational cohort study of the effect of rehabilitation site on recovery from stroke suggests that rehabilitation at inpatient facilities, in comparison with skilled nursing facilities, produces more rapid recovery and higher proportions of patients who achieve independence as measured by the Functional Independence Measure, even after accounting for baseline differences in patient populations between the sites of care.

The effect on outcomes of site of rehabilitation care for a more broad range of conditions has also been studied in a sample of consecutive patients enrolled from 52 hospitals in three cities with five targeted conditions (chronic obstructive pulmonary disease, heart failure, hip procedures, hip fractures, and stroke). Using case-mix adjustment models, these researchers found that patients who were discharged to nursing homes fared worst and those who were sent home with home-health or to rehabilitation hospitals did best. This type of observational study is vulnerable to bias, despite adjusting the analyses, since patient prognosis for recovery may influence discharge site; those with poor prognosis are more likely to go the nursing home, and those with better prognosis for recovery go to inpatient or home-health settings. Nevertheless, site of care may be an important factor in recovery.

The effect of prospective payment on postacute rehabilitation has been examined. Patients discharged from acute-care settings with one of five diagnoses that commonly use rehabilitation services were followed for patterns of postacute services before and after prospective payment. The transition to prospective payment appeared to result in an increase in the proportions of patients receiving no rehabilitation services, in a decrease in home-health services, and in stable or slightly increased inpatient services. This study found no consistent effects of these changes on clinical outcomes. Another study found decreases in intensity and duration of rehabilitation services in skilled facilities after prospective payment was initiated. The clinician who advocates for an appropriate site of rehabilitation care on the basis of severity of impairments, functional status, and social support might improve the outcomes of many patients.

Each site of care has advantages and disadvantages from the patient's perspective. Inpatient care is the most intense but may not be endurable for frail elderly patients, since it requires 3 hours per day of active (and fatiguing) therapy. Skilled nursing offers 24-hour care for those who cannot care for themselves or do not have a full-time caregiver. Outpatient services have clear advantages and disadvantages. Patients often prefer to return to their own homes but may not have the care support they need. Participation in day hospital or outpatient clinic requires transportation, which can be costly and time consuming.

In summary, clinicians must be familiar with the services provided in a wide range of rehabilitation settings and with the advantages and disadvantages of each. The clinician is responsible for recommending the best match between patient needs and program services. However, under certain insurance plans, decisions about location of services may be heavily influenced by costs. More systematic evaluation of rehabilitation outcomes that is based on the structures and processes of care offered by various settings is essential if we are to have more rational use of rehabilitation programs in the future. The Centers for Medicare and Medicaid Services (CMS) is currently monitoring the quality of patient care using information from the patient assessments. A research study of preventive rehabilitation ("Prehab") using a home-health approach in high-risk community-dwelling older adults demonstrated reduced frequency of functional decline.

TEAMS AND ROLES

Numerous health professionals are required to meet the rehabilitation needs of older adults. Coordinating this care is the function of the interdisciplinary care team; team members must be able to define roles, share tasks, and communicate within and outside the team. Team building and improving team function are important issues for geriatric rehabilitation service providers. All health professionals who work with older adults should have a basic understanding of the roles and functions of various team members. The primary goal of multidisciplinary team management is to ensure that patients receive comprehensive assessments and interventions for the disabling illness and associated comorbid conditions, as well as for the specific impair-

ments and environmental factors that may affect activities and participation. The team must establish common goals and a cohesive treatment plan.

The patient and the family are core members of the rehabilitation team; their expectations and preferences must be integrated into the care plan. Rehabilitation, unlike many other interventions, requires active patient participation. If the patient is the leader in decision making, he or she gains a sense of control and responsibility. Patient self-management is now an essential part of the effective management of chronic disease. Chronic disease self-management incorporates self-monitoring, knowledge about disease, and personal control over prevention and management practices.

IMPACT OF COMORBID CONDITIONS

In the elderly patient, comorbid diseases and conditions may interrupt or delay treatment and often require adaptations in the care plan. Many of the illnesses that can interfere with rehabilitation of the older adult are predictable in this high-risk population and are potentially preventable. A systematic approach to assessment, prevention, and management of comorbid conditions can improve the patient's chance of receiving maximal benefit from rehabilitation services. Table 15.1 highlights common causes in older patients of delayed or interrupted rehabilitation and describes measures that can be taken to reduce their impact on rehabilitation.

Older adults with reduced mobility are at high risk for skin breakdown, which can interfere with recovery and require extensive treatment. Immobility or altered weight bearing can precipitate pressure ulcers that heal poorly. Clinicians should monitor pressure and weight-bearing areas and be prepared to modify footwear, wheelchairs, and bedding as needed. (See also "Pressure Ulcers," p 259.) Since thromboembolic events are also common with reduced mobility, their prevention should be a routine part of care. (See also the discussions of thromboembolism in "Respiratory Diseases and Disorders," p 329, and "Perioperative Care," p 102.)

Incontinence is prevalent among older patients; causes include detrusor hyperactivity, obstruction, neurogenic bladder, immobility, and cognitive deficits. Indwelling catheters increase the risk of infection and are rarely appropriate. A structured approach to the assessment and treatment of bladder problems should be a basic component of any rehabilitation service. (See also "Urinary Incontinence," p 184.)

The risk of pneumonia is increased by inactivity and disordered swallowing, as well as underlying lung disease. The prevention of aspiration pneumonia involves difficult tradeoffs. Routine radiologic screening

Table 15.1—Methods to Reduce the Impact of Selected Comorbidities on Rehabilitation

Confusion
  Screening for toxic or metabolic contributors (eg, medications, hypoxia, electrolyte disturbance)
  Sensory aids
  Planned reassessment for improvement if confusion limits rehabilitation potential

Deep-vein thrombosis and pulmonary embolism
  Mobilization
  Hydration
  Compression stockings
  Intermittent pneumatic compression
  Coumadin
  Low-molecular-weight heparin

Depression or apathy
  Screening for depression
  Treatment with medications, counseling, support groups

Kidney or bladder infection
  Avoidance, removal of indwelling catheter
  Check of postvoid residual
  Frequent toileting
  Rarely helpful: prophylactic antibiotics

Pneumonia
  Mobilization
  Treatment of chronic obstructive pulmonary disease, as needed
  Influenza vaccination
  Incentive spirometry
  Screening, precautions for aspiration*

Seizures
  Prevention of recurrence with anticonvulsants, carbamazepine, or valproic acid

Skin breakdown
  Mobilization
  Positioning
  Pressure-relieving mattresses
  Early care with dressings

Spasticity
  Physical therapy to control
  Muscle relaxants
  Botulinum toxin (trials ongoing)

Upper gastrointestinal bleeding
  Avoidance of nonsteroidal anti-inflammatory drugs and use of acetaminophen for pain
  Hematocrit monitoring
  Consideration of prophylactic agents

* See text for controversies.

SOURCE: Data in part from Studenski SA, Duncan P, Maino JH. Principles of rehabilitation in older patients. In: Hazzard WR, Blass JP, Ettinger WH, et al., eds. *Principles of Geriatric Medicine and Gerontology.* 4th ed. New York: McGraw-Hill; 1999.

for aspiration has precipitated a marked increased awareness of this problem, but the clinical relevance of modest amounts of aspiration detected radiologically is unknown. Conservative measures such as changing food consistency with liquid thickeners and cohesive food substances and lowering head position while eating may help alleviate the problem. Sometimes aspiration risk is addressed by discontinuing all oral feeding and placing an enteral feeding tube. This approach eliminates the fundamental human pleasure of eating and may not be successful, since oral secretions or refluxed gastric contents can still be aspirated. (See also "Eating and Feeding Problems," p 181.) Upper gastrointestinal bleeds may occur during rehabilitation as a consequence of stress or medications and may not be preceded by typical symptoms. (See also "Gastrointestinal Diseases and Disorders," p 390.)

Mental functioning is critical for rehabilitation, which requires the ability to follow commands and learn. Since older adults who have been acutely ill are at increased risk for delirium, clinicians should assess mental status and screen for easily reversible causes in their older patients. (See also "Delirium," p 239.) Depression is endemic in newly disabled persons and can manifest as low motivation; formal screens for depression and early intervention are essential. (See also "Depression and Other Mood Disorders," p 269.) Seizures can develop after stroke, and spasticity can develop during stroke recovery. Interventions for spasticity such as physical therapy or muscle relaxants have offered only modest benefit; some trials of botulinum toxin have suggested promising results but others have had no effect. (See also the section in stroke in "Neurologic Diseases and Disorders," p 460.)

Certain comorbid conditions common in elderly patients, including diabetes mellitus, heart disease, peripheral vascular disease, musculoskeletal disorders, sensory impairments, and dementia, require ongoing adaptations in rehabilitation. Activity level is a powerful factor in glucose metabolism; diabetic patients are therefore likely to experience changes in glucose levels and medication requirements during rehabilitation. Increased caloric intake during recovery may also affect their medication needs. Therapy personnel should know how to assess diabetic control, use a glucometer, and intervene for hypoglycemia. (See also "Diabetes Mellitus," p 382.) Most abnormal gaits increase the energy requirements of walking; an abnormal gait in a patient with coronary artery disease may cause coronary symptoms to worsen. Persons with poor cardiac output may have extreme exercise limitations. Medication adjustments for heart diseases may be necessary but can cause adverse effects of their own, such as orthostatic hypotension. Patients with one vascular disease often have others; peripheral vascular disease is common, often associated with insensitive or painful feet and high risk of skin breakdown. Treatment of painful peripheral neuropathy may foster increased activity and avoid pressure ulcers. Musculoskeletal status should be monitored to avoid overuse syndromes involving increased demand on vulnerable joints. For those with vision and hearing impairment, corrections must be provided and teaching approaches adapted accordingly. In patients with dementia, rehabilitation progress is still possible, but carryover may be decreased and the need for supervision and cueing increased.

REHABILITATION APPROACHES AND INTERVENTIONS

The primary goals of rehabilitation treatment are restitution of function, compensation for and adaptation to functional losses, and prevention of secondary complications. Ultimately, rehabilitation should maximize the person's potential for participation in social, leisure, or work roles. Many strategies can be used to achieve these goals. Restitution of physical function usually depends on therapeutic exercises to improve flexibility, strength, motor control, and cardiovascular endurance. Although exercise has been shown to improve strength, endurance, and balance in well-defined populations of disabled older adults, there is still uncertainty about whether these gains translate into changes in mobility, ADLs, participation, or a reduction in falls. (See also "Physical Activity," p 56.) In stroke, speech and language therapy can be used to treat aphasia. Cognitive rehabilitation might improve alertness and attention. However, the research evidence is insufficient to demonstrate that speech and language therapy, or cognitive rehabilitation, improve functional deficits.

Therapeutic modalities such as massage, heat, cold, and ultrasound are used to decrease pain and muscle spasm. These and other pain management strategies may contribute to increased function and tolerance for further rehabilitation. There is little research evidence supporting objective benefits from modalities, but patients commonly report symptomatic relief. (See also "Persistent Pain," p 140.)

Equipment for mobility, dressing and bathing assistance, orthotic and prosthetic devices, and splints all can augment or replace the function of impaired body parts and thereby reduce limitations in activities and participation. For example, an ankle orthosis can prevent foot drop and improve safety and speed of walking. A wheelchair can provide mobility for community activities.

Repeated practice of task-specific activities such as bed mobility, transfers, and walking can improve functional mobility. Upper extremity function improves with specific functional training activities, such as grasps, reaches, and fine manipulations. Balance training may improve balance and reduce the risk of falls. Older adults may benefit from retraining in instrumental ADLs, such as cooking, managing finances, or driving a car.

Contextual factors, both environmental and personal, should be addressed to minimize restrictions on a person's activities and participation. For example, motivation may be addressed by collaborative goal setting, patient and family education, detection and management of depression, and use of support groups. Environmental modifications such as grab bars and raised toilet seats in the bathroom or curb cutouts on public streets can promote independent functioning.

To maintain function and enhance health status after rehabilitation, patients and families should assume responsibility for long-term self-management. Rehabilitation goals include a prevention program for worsening disability, including reintegration into social programs such as senior center programs, and health and wellness programs.

COMPREHENSIVE ASSESSMENT

Comprehensive assessment of rehabilitation patients is necessary for appropriate clinical management and for the evaluation of outcomes. The treatment plan should be guided by the results of the initial assessment. The primary components of any assessment include patient demographics, social support, place of residence prior to illness, medical comorbidities, severity of current illness, and the patient's prior functional status. Impairments such as deficits in range of motion and flexibility, strength, sensory functions, balance, cognition, and depression should always be assessed. In conditions such as stroke, there should be an evaluation of swallowing and language function. The patient's functional status is assessed with standardized measures of ADLs (eg, FIM, the Barthel ADL Index), and measures of instrumental ADLs. The patient's participation or quality of life is assessed with generic measures like the SF-36 Health Survey (available at http://www.sf-36.org) or disease-specific measures like the Stroke Impact Scale or the Harris Hip Questionnaire.

STROKE

Stroke is a major cause of mortality and morbidity in the United States, particularly among persons aged 55 years and over. Acute stroke occurs in more than 700,000 people each year, and 80% or more are likely to survive, many with residual neurologic difficulties. Stroke-related deficits are severe in approximately one third of the survivors. Many patients with mild and moderate stroke become independent in ADLs, but other more complex dimensions of health status may still be affected. As stroke survival continues to increase, the need for comprehensive stroke rehabilitation will rise. Rehabilitation programs must address a broad range of stroke-related disabilities, including those in basic ADLs, instrumental ADLs, participation, and integration into health and wellness programs.

Goals of Rehabilitation

The overall goals of rehabilitation for the elderly stroke patient include restitution of function, compensation for or adaptation to functional losses, and prevention of secondary complications. Specific objectives include:

- preventing or recognizing and managing comorbid illness and medical complications,
- assessing each patient comprehensively, using standardized assessments,
- matching the patient's needs to the program capabilities,
- training the patient to maximize independence in ADLs and instrumental ADLs,
- facilitating the patient's and family's psychosocial coping and adaptation,
- preventing recurrent stroke and other vascular conditions such as myocardial infarction, and
- assisting the patient in reintegrating into the community.

Rehabilitation for older adults with stroke is complex because of the heterogeneity of causes, symptoms, severity, and recovery. Stroke patients present with varying symptoms, depending on the site and size of the brain lesions. The most common type of neurologic deficit is hemiparesis, but other deficits may include sensory impairment, aphasia, dysarthria, cognitive impairment, motor incoordination, hemianopsia, visual-perceptual deficits, depression, dysphagia, and bowel and bladder incontinence. The degree of initial recovery and the time needed to reach maximal recovery is affected by the number of deficits. For example, individuals who have hemiparesis, hemianopsia, and sensory deficits are less likely to ambulate independently and require longer to regain skills than do those with hemiparesis only.

Stroke patients usually experience some degree of recovery. This recovery is most dramatic in the first 30 days but may continue more gradually for months. In the Framingham study, improvement in motor function and self-care was found to slow 3 months after stroke but to continue at a reduced pace throughout the first year. Language and visual-spatial function was recovered over 12 months, but cognitive function improved only during the first 3 months.

Approach to Management

Guidelines for rehabilitation following stroke have been updated by a team sponsored by the Department of Veterans Affairs and the Department of Defense (available at http://www.oqp.med.va.gov/cpg/STR/ STR_base.htm). The guidelines offer algorithms for initial assessment and rehabilitation referral, followed by management in inpatient or community settings. The guidelines assess the quality of evidence for a series of recommendations. Recommendations considered to have a "good" evidence base are highlighted. Many important issues in management have not yet been assessed in clinical trials and thus do not meet standards for a "good" evidence base. Yet, management recommendations may still be considered appropriate care, since a lack of evidence should not be considered to indicate a lack of benefit. The guidelines emphasize that better clinical outcomes are achieved when patients with acute stroke are treated in a setting that provides coordinated, multidisciplinary stroke-related evaluation and services. Recent studies have confirmed that adherence to guidelines promotes better outcomes. Coordinated care reduces 1-year mortality, improves functional independence, and increases satisfaction with care. Benefits are not restricted to any particular subgroup of patients. Stroke severity should be systematically assessed, using the NIH Stroke Scale (available at http://www.strokecenter.org/trials/ scales/nihss.html).

In general, therapy should be started early, but later supplementary interventions may also be beneficial. For persons who have completed acute poststroke rehabilitation, a structured, supervised, progressive therapeutic program in the home has been shown to produce gains in endurance, balance, and walking capacity, but no change in motor control. The benefits of this program are probably due to the aggressive intervention on deconditioning and mobility. There is less evidence to support specific therapeutic interventions for stroke.

There are several philosophical approaches to physical rehabilitation following stroke. Neurophysiologic approaches based on the theories of Bobath and Brunnstrom and on proprioceptive neuromuscular facilitation traditionally are used to restore motor control. These approaches consider the patient to be the recipient of therapy and the therapist to be the decision maker in charge of problem solving. There is no convincing evidence that any one specific technique is superior to another. New therapeutic interventions for restitution of motor function are in development. Constraint-induced movement therapy discourages the use of the unaffected extremity and encourages active use of the hemiparetic extremity, with a goal of improved motor recovery. Results in patients with chronic stroke impairment suggest potential gains beyond usual therapy. A large randomized clinical trial of constraint-induced therapy is now under way. Treadmill walking with partial body weight support using a harness connected to an overhead system may improve gait velocity, balance, and motor recovery. Speech and language therapy are often provided for stroke patients with aphasia. However, there is no universally accepted treatment. Although a recent Cochrane report states that the evidence does not support a finding of either clear effect or lack of effect, the Veterans Affairs guidelines support "good" evidence for follow-up evaluation and treatment by the speech language professional for long-term residual communication difficulties. The guidelines also support "good" evidence for cognitive retraining for attention or visual-spatial perceptual deficits and compensatory training for short-term memory deficits. The same guidelines find "good" evidence for medication treatment for depression and emotional lability. Spasticity can develop gradually after stroke and can inhibit function and interfere with hygiene. Most interventions have been disappointing, but investigational trials of botulinum toxin type A[OL] injection for hand spasticity have been encouraging.

The patient who has had a stroke is at high risk for recurrence: up to 7% to 10% annually. The rehabilitation phase is an appropriate time to ensure that assessment and treatment for stroke prevention has occurred. Assessments for significant carotid stenosis and for atrial fibrillation should be completed. Indications for carotid endarterectomy and anticoagulation with warfarin should be reviewed. Antiplatelet medications such as aspirin alone or in combination with dipyridamole or clopidogrel should be considered in many patients. Treatment with angiotensin-converting enzyme inhibitors[OL] and statins[OL] has also demonstrated reductions in risk of stroke. Other risk factors to be targeted include hypertension control and smoking.

In summary, the evidence for specific interventions for stroke rehabilitation is weak. The collective benefits of well-organized multidisciplinary care, including secondary prevention, are well established. (See also the section on cerebrovascular diseases in "Neurologic Diseases and Disorders," p 459.)

HIP FRACTURE

Epidemiology and Surgical Care

Each year in the United States, about 250,000 people have a hip fracture. The risk of fracture is higher in women, in nursing-home residents, and in persons with dementia. Mortality is about 5% during the initial hospitalization but nears 25% in the year following fracture. Recovery to the prior level of function occurs in about 75% of survivors, but their overall mobility will be more limited; up to half of those with recovery will still require an assistive device. About half of patients will have an initial decline requiring transient long-term care, and about 25% will still be in long-term care 1 year later.

For medically stable patients, surgical repair is recommended 24 to 72 hours after the fracture. This

early repair has been associated with a reduction in 1-year mortality as well as with lower incidence of complications like pressure ulcers and delirium. However, delay of surgery is warranted to allow a medically unstable patient to improve sufficiently to tolerate the procedure. The surgical approach is determined by the location of the fracture, the presence or absence of displacement, and the prefracture mobility. One third of hip fractures occur at the femoral neck, and the other two thirds are intertrochanteric, occurring lateral to the femoral neck. Prefracture mobility is used as a guide to determine the goal of surgical treatment and to allow the risks and benefits of each surgical procedure to be considered.

Femoral neck fractures without any displacement can be surgically corrected with simple screws. However, femoral neck fractures with any degree of displacement are at increased risk for nonunion or avascular necrosis and therefore are usually treated with a prosthetic femoral head (hemiarthroplasty). Patients with significant underlying boney acetabular disease and a displaced femoral neck fracture may benefit from complete hip arthroplasty. Patients are usually allowed to bear weight immediately after repair of a femoral neck fracture, no matter which technique has been used.

For intertrochanteric fractures, the treatment of choice is open reduction and internal fixation with a compression screw or similar device. Provided there is little or no displacement, immediate weight bearing is usually allowed. However, displaced or comminuted intertrochanteric fractures commonly remain unstable, even after surgical fixation. Therefore, full weight bearing is often not allowed for up to 6 weeks or until the stability of the fracture is assured. Factors that influence recovery should be assessed, including prior mobility and functional status, comorbid conditions, cognitive status, and social support. Other information includes type of injury and repair as well as pain status. Mobility performance can be systematically assessed with numerous instruments, including one developed specifically for hip fracture (Harris Hip Questionnaire).

See also "Perioperative Care" (p 99).

Rehabilitation of Hip Fracture

Rehabilitation of hip fracture includes pain management, mobilization, and prevention of complications, such as delirium and thromboembolic events. The most important factors influencing recovery appear to be how soon mobilization is initiated and how frequently therapy is provided. Delay in mobilization is often driven by surgical recommendation, with proper healing of the fracture taking precedence over mobility. Partial weight bearing is difficult for many older patients to achieve; they are either up on their feet or not. Prolonged inactivity is clearly associated with poorer functional outcomes, and early weight bearing has been shown to be associated with low rates of surgical failure. Accelerated rehabilitation with rapid mobilization, coordinated planning, early discharge, and community follow-up has been associated with a 17% reduction in costs and no detriment to rates of recovery. Intensity of service clearly affects outcome, as those who receive more than once-daily physical therapy during initial rehabilitation are more likely to be discharged directly to home than those who receive physical therapy once a day or less.

Prevention of Recurrence

Persons who have had a hip fracture often have other comorbidities, such as osteoporosis and balance problems, that place them at risk for further fractures. Efforts to diagnose and treat osteoporosis, improve balance, and reduce injury risk are a key part of treatment planning during rehabilitation. (See also "Osteoporosis and Osteomalacia," p 210.) The use of hip protectors has been extensively studied, with varying results. For those living in an institutional setting, there may be some benefit. For patients living in the community, hip protectors do not appear to decrease the incidence of hip fractures. As a recent study demonstrates, adherence remains a major issue. Only 38% of community-dwelling women in the study found the hip protectors to be acceptable and agreed to participate. At the end of 1 year, only about half the participants were still wearing the hip protectors daily.

TOTAL HIP AND KNEE ARTHROPLASTY

Natural History

In the United States, joint arthroplasty is the most common elective surgical procedure performed; approximately 280,000 are done annually. The primary indications for joint replacement are progressive pain and mobility limitation despite conservative care. The most common diagnosis associated with the need for joint replacement is osteoarthrosis, followed by rheumatoid arthritis. The long-term results of joint replacement have generally been excellent and include significant pain relief and improved function. Continued success rates in the 90% range are seen 10 to 15 years after joint replacement. The most common reason for failure of the hip or knee replacement is loosening of the implant. Joint infection is another major concern; infection affects 0.2% to 1.1% of total hip and 1% to 2% of total knee replacements. Deep infections often necessitate removal of the implant,

long-term antibiotics until there is no sign of infection, then ultimate replacement with another implant. (See also "Infectious Diseases," p 332, especially the section on prosthetic device infections, p 340.)

Assessment

Plain radiographs are the usual method for determining the severity of joint damage at both the hip and knee. Loss of cartilage is shown by joint-space narrowing, and often osteophyte formation is also present.

Management

Anticoagulation to prevent thromboembolism and good pain control are the major goals during the immediate postoperative period for both hip and knee arthroplasty. (See also "Perioperative Care," p 99, and anticoagulation information in the Appendix, p 491.) It is recognized that patients who have undergone a major orthopedic procedure like total hip or knee arthroplasty are at particularly high risk for both symptomatic and asymptomatic venous thromboembolism (VTE). Recent guidelines for the prevention of VTE suggest the routine use of low-molecular-weight heparin, fondaparinux, or adjusted-dose warfarin. Pain control in the initial postoperative period is often achieved with narcotics dispensed orally, intravenously, or by patient-controlled analgesia pumps. For both hip and knee arthroplasty, early mobilization is the standard of care, and weight bearing often begins on the second postoperative day. Patients at low risk can often be discharged from the acute care hospital within 5 days. For those at high risk, defined as being older than 70 years or having two or more comorbid conditions, early inpatient rehabilitation has been shown to improve functional outcomes and decrease total length of stay. Age alone should not be used as a criterion for eligibility for joint replacement, as even persons older than 80 years who are in good health with stable chronic conditions have excellent results.

To decrease the risk of dislocation after total hip arthroplasty, patients are taught to avoid motions such as deep squats and crossing their legs. To prevent excessive hip flexion, a raised toilet seat is recommended for the first few months after surgery. Rehabilitation focuses on strengthening especially the abductors, which are weakened by the surgical approach, as well as on progressive range-of-motion and gait training. Recently, orthopedic surgeons have been examining the use of a minimal incision, less than 10 centimeters, for total hip arthroplasty. This approach may lead to quicker recovery and return to function but is still being studied.

After total knee replacement, recovery of range of motion is the key to return of function and is often aided by the use of a continuous passive motion machine (CPM). Its use has been shown to decrease the need for postoperative manipulation and, combined with physical therapy, has increased active range of motion and shortened length of stay. Surgeons have also applied the concept of minimal incisions to the total knee replacement operation and with significantly more success. This operation, in the hands of an experienced surgeon, has been shown to decrease blood loss and length of stay. Postoperative swelling is common and interferes with regaining motion. However, thigh-high compression stockings, the CPM, and possibly cryotherapy can be used to manage swelling.

AMPUTATION

Epidemiology

More than 50,000 people undergo lower extremity amputation each year in the United States. Most of these people have systemic vascular disease, with or without diabetes mellitus. Those with diabetes often have other end-organ disease, such as blindness, end-stage renal disease, and peripheral neuropathy. Mortality in this group approaches 50% at 2 years and 70% at 5 years. For up to one fifth of patients, amputation of the contralateral extremity is needed within the first 2 years after the initial amputation. The majority of dysvascular amputees have such a burden of comorbid disease that the prosthesis is largely used for limited mobility, such as transfers and ambulation within the home.

Assessment

Key factors to assess include the patient's prior functional status, stability of comorbid conditions, cognition, and upper extremity use, as well as the condition of the stump and other lower extremity. Successful prosthetic ambulation is associated with independent prior ambulation, ability to bear weight on the contralateral leg, stable medical status, and ability to follow directions. Blindness and end-stage renal disease do not necessarily preclude rehabilitation. A systematic approach to monitoring amputee status has been incorporated into an instrument, the Prosthetic Profile of the Amputee.

Rehabilitation for Amputation

Rehabilitation starts in the preoperative stage, when the patient begins with strength and flexibility exercises and receives teaching about the recovery process.

OL Not approved by the U.S. Food and Drug Administration for this use.

Amputation surgery generally aims to preserve the knee, since the below-the-knee amputee has a much lower energy requirement of walking than does the above-the-knee amputee. This decision must be weighed against risks of poor wound healing with more distal amputation.

Postoperative rehabilitation includes efforts at early mobilization, prevention of contractures, wound healing, and shaping of the stump. Poor wound healing delays rehabilitation in about 25% of cases. Prostheses vary in weight, socket type, style of foot, and suspensions. The older amputee benefits from a prosthesis that is lightweight, stable, and easy to use. Prosthetic rehabilitation involves progressive ambulation, teaching about prosthesis and stump care, and monitoring for stump injury.

Last, phantom limb pain is common after amputation, with an estimated incidence of 60% to 80%, and pain management influences progress with rehabilitation. Treatment remains difficult, and clear evidence-based guidelines are lacking. As tricyclic antidepressants[OL] and sodium channel blockers[OL], like carbamazepine[OL], are generally effective for neuropathic pain, they are often used for phantom pain despite the lack of well-controlled trials. A number of other medication regimens, using such agents as opiates[OL] and anesthetic blocks[OL], have also had success in small trials. Two recent trials of memantine showed no benefit in the treatment of phantom limb pain.

MOBILITY AIDS, ORTHOTICS, ADAPTIVE METHODS, AND ENVIRONMENTAL MODIFICATIONS

Assistive devices, orthotics, adaptive methods, and environmental modifications are effective for elderly patients with disabilities and handicaps. It is important to identify the underlying causes of disability before prescribing a device or modification, because medical or surgical treatment for individual diseases and impairments may be more effective or may enhance the usefulness of these approaches.

Mobility Aids

Canes typically support 15% to 20% of the body weight and are to be used in the hand contralateral to the affected knee or hip. The tips, handles, materials, and lengths of canes vary. As the number of tips increases, the degree of support also increases, but the cane becomes heavier and more awkward to use. The cane tip is fitted with a 5-cm diameter rubber tip with a concentric ring to prevent slipping. The handle of the cane may be curved or have a pistol grip; the pistol grip offers more support but is less aesthetically pleasing to some people. Canes can be made of a variety of materials, but most are made of wood or lightweight aluminum. The length of the cane is important for stability. Some canes are adjustable, but wooden canes must be cut to size. One of three methods may be used to evaluate the proper cane length: measuring the distance from the distal wrist crease to the ground when the patient is standing erect, measuring the distance from the greater trochanter to the ground, or measuring the distance between the ground 15 cm in front of and to the side of the tip of the shoe and the elbow flexed at 30 degrees.

Crutches can support full body weight but are seldom recommended for older persons. Problems with crutches include the large amount of arm strength required, the risk of brachial plexus injury, and the necessity to use an unnatural gait pattern.

A walker is prescribed when a cane does not offer sufficient stability. A walker can completely support one lower extremity but cannot support full body weight. Walker types include pick-up and wheeled walkers. The pick-up walker is lifted and moved forward by the patient, who then advances before lifting the walker again; the result is a slow, staggering gait. It requires strength to repeatedly pick up the walker and cognitive ability to learn the necessary coordination. A wheeled walker allows for a smoother, coordinated, and faster gait and takes advantage of overlearned gait patterns. It is more likely to be correctly used by persons with cognitive impairment. The most commonly used type is the two-wheeled walker, which brakes automatically with increased downward pressure. Four-wheeled walkers are rarely used because they are less stable and more difficult to control, although they are occasionally useful for persons with Parkinson's disease. Three-wheeled walkers may offer some advantages in ease of turning but are not yet in common use. The Merry Walker Ambulation Device has a seat and bars all the way around. It is the same size as a wheelchair and is best reserved for those with severe balance problems. It is also useful for severely demented patients.

Patients who cannot safely use or are unable to ambulate with an assistive device will require a wheelchair. A wheelchair must be fitted according to the patient's body build, weight, disability, and prognosis. Incorrect fit may result in poor posture, joint deformity, reduced mobility, pressure ulcers, circulatory compromise, and discomfort. For the elderly patient with only one functional arm, the wheelchair may be lowered to allow for foot propulsion. Patients with lower extremity amputations may have the wheels set posteriorly to compensate for a change in the center of gravity. Motorized wheelchairs may be used by mentally alert persons with bilateral upper extremity weakness or severe cardiopulmonary disease who lack the endurance to push a wheelchair. Motorized scooters offer less trunk support than motorized wheelchairs but are more acceptable to some people. Motorized scooters and wheelchairs increase patients' mobility but increase their risk of deconditioning, as they might otherwise push a wheelchair or ambulate. The use of a wheelchair commonly requires home modifications, including ramps and widened doorways. Cars may need to be adapted with lifts.

Orthotics, Adaptive Methods, and Environmental Modifications

Orthotics are exoskeletons designed to assist, resist, align, and stimulate function. Orthotics are named by the use of letters for each joint that the device involves in its structure. Thus, an AFO is an ankle and foot orthotic device used to support weak calf or pretibial muscles (eg, for a stroke patient with lower extremity weakness).

Adaptations to facilitate dressing may be necessary for patients with problems such as frequent soiling or diminished flexibility, coordination, and endurance. Their clothing should be easy to clean, and tops should fit easily over the head or fasten in the front and allow for freedom of movement. Fastening clothes is commonly a problem for elderly persons. Hooks and loops or Velcro are usually easier to use than buttons, and they may be sewn on to replace buttons and zippers. When buttons are necessary, button hooks with customized grips may be used, or the buttons can be sewn on with elastic thread, which may eliminate the need to manipulate the buttons. Donning shoes and socks is particularly difficult for elderly persons with decreased agility. Longer, looser socks (eg, tubular socks) are easier to don. For patients who find that reaching the feet to put on shoes is a problem, a long-handled shoehorn may be useful. Elastic shoelaces eliminate the need for tying and untying.

Environmental modifications can have a major impact on the elderly person's ability to function independently or with minimal assistance at home. A variety of assistive devices, such as reachers, special utensils, and adapted telephones, can reduce the difficulty of performing daily tasks and have a significant impact on a person's quality of life.

The bathroom is a common place for falls. Any older person with impaired balance or lower extremity weakness should have bars installed near the toilet and tub or shower. Raised toilet seats and bathtub benches are available to assist those with lower extremity weakness. These are also useful for persons with arthritis of the hips or knees because they reduce biomechanical stress on the joint. Long-handled bath brushes, hand-held shower, and "soap on a rope" may be helpful for persons with upper extremity impairment.

ANNOTATED REFERENCES

■ Gill TM, Baker DI, Gottschalk M, et al. A program to prevent functional decline in physically frail, elderly persons who live at home. *N Engl J Med*. 2002; 347(14):1068–1074.

This is a randomized controlled trial of a restorative program called "Prehab" in 188 community-dwelling frail persons aged 75 or older. The Prehab program lasted up to 6 months and focused on physical therapy for mobility, balance, muscle strength, and transfers. The control group received education. The Prehab group was found to have less functional decline than the control group. Prehab was also found to have a beneficial effect among those with moderate but not severe frailty.

■ Gillespie WJ. Extracts from "clinical evidence": hip fracture. *BMJ*. 2001; 322(7292):968–975.

The author presents commonly asked questions, such as "What are the effects of specific surgical interventions in the treatment of hip fractures?" and provides answers based on evidence from randomized controlled trials. The benefits, harms, and a summary statement are given for each possible answer to the question. The topics that are included range from surgical management to common postoperative complications and rehabilitation after the fracture repair.

■ Hesse S, Werner C, von Frankenberg S, et al. Treadmill training with partial body weight support after stroke. *Phys Med Rehabil Clin N Am*. 2003;14 (1 Suppl):S111–S123.

This is a review of treadmill therapy with partial body weight support as an intervention for gait impairment after stroke. Chronic and acute patients have been studied. It was found that gait becomes more symmetric and efficient after treadmill training. Multicenter trials are under way.

■ Hoenig H, Duncan PW, Horner RD, et al. Structure, process, and outcomes in stroke rehabilitation. *Med Care*. 2002;40(11):1036–1047.

This prospective cohort study of 128 acute stroke patients in 11 Veterans Affairs medical centers examined the effect of the structure of stroke care on process of care that was based on Agency for Health Care Policy and Research (AHCPR) guidelines and outcome measured by Functional Independence Measure (FIM) motor score 6 months after discharge. Structural features such as systemic organization, staff expertise, and technological sophistication were found to predict adherence with guidelines. Guideline adherence was found to predict 6-month FIM scores.

■ Nikolajsen L, Jensen TS. Phantom limb pain. *Br J Anaesth*. 2001;87(1):107–116.

This review article presents the available literature on incidence and types of pain seen in persons after amputation. Possible mechanisms of phantom pain and other factors that influence phantom pain are described. Treatment options and timing for these options, either before or after the amputation, are presented.

■ Wells JL, Seabrook JA, Stolee P, et al. State of the art in geriatric rehabilitation: part II: clinical challenges. *Arch Phys Med Rehab*. 2003;84(6):898–903.

The authors present a review of the common clinical problems seen in geriatric rehabilitation, including rehabilitation for hip fracture and stroke. Information is provided, in a strength-of-evidence framework, about trials involving comorbidity and adverse outcomes, early rehabilitation after repair, and use of specialized orthopedic rehabilitation units.

Stephanie A. Studenski, MD, MPH
Cynthia J. Brown, MD, PT
Pamela W. Duncan, PhD

CHAPTER 16—NURSING-HOME CARE

KEY POINTS

■ Currently there are 17,000 U.S. nursing homes with 1.8 million beds, 1.6 million residents, and 2.4 million discharges each year.

■ The typical nursing-home physician is an internist or family physician who devotes 2 hours or less per week to nursing-home care.

■ The Omnibus Budget Reconciliation Act of 1987 requires a periodic comprehensive assessment of all nursing-home residents, sets minimum staffing requirements, and fosters residents' rights by limiting the use of restraints and psychoactive medications.

■ The care of nursing-home residents has become more complex over the past several years, commensurate with an increasing level of medical acuity in an environment constrained by lack of resources.

Nursing homes have evolved dramatically over the past several years, responding to a variety of government and market-driven forces. The almshouse, common at the turn of the century, has been transformed into a highly regulated institution for persons with severe physical and mental disabilities. Nursing homes, more than ever, present the clinician with a set of unique and complex care issues, many of which are best understood in the context of population needs, government policy, and reimbursement and staffing patterns.

THE NURSING-HOME POPULATION

The average nursing-home resident is characterized by significant impairments in physical and instrumental activities of daily living (ADLs). Overall, the level of disability in the nursing home has increased over the past decade and exceeds that found in persons receiving home care. Among nursing-home residents, 22.3% require assistance with one or two ADLs, and 74.9% require assistance with three or more. In addition to impairments of ADLs, 81% of nursing-home residents are impaired in their ability to make daily decisions; two thirds have orientation difficulties or memory problems, or both, and over half (54%) have either bowel or bladder incontinence. Hearing and visual impairments are found in 36% and 39% of residents, respectively. Dementia remains the most commonly occurring condition in the nursing home, with estimates ranging from 50% to 70%. Behavioral problems, understandably, are also common, occurring in at least one third of nursing-home residents. Such behaviors include verbal and physical abuse, social inappropriateness, resistance to care, and wandering. Communication problems are noted in 60% of residents; 44% have difficulty with both being understood and understanding others. Depression is diagnosed in 20% of nursing-home residents.

Almost half of all nursing-home residents are aged 85 years or over, with fewer than 9% under the age of 65. The majority are women (72%), white (89%), and unmarried (60% widowed) with limited social supports. The percentage of black residents in U.S. nursing homes has increased in recent years (9%), approaching national population norms. In fact, black Americans 65 to 74 years of age are more likely than white Americans to be admitted to a nursing home. Nonetheless, other nonwhite populations, such as Hispanic Americans, Asian Americans, and Native Americans, are underrepresented in nursing homes despite even higher disability rates in these groups. Older adults with developmental disabilities constitute another unique population that is requiring increasing nursing-home care as their elderly parents die. These persons often require specialized care that many nursing homes have difficulty providing (see "Mental Retardation," p 304).

NURSING-HOME AVAILABILITY AND FINANCING

Currently there are 17,000 U.S. nursing homes with 1.8 million beds, 1.6 million residents, and 2.4 million discharges (ie, to home, hospital, or secondary to death). Of these facilities, 65% are proprietary (for-profit), with voluntary nonprofit (25%) and government nursing homes (10%) accounting for the remainder. The average nursing home operates 107 beds, and a minority (8%) have more than 200 beds. A little more than half of all nursing homes (56%) are part of a chain.

By age 65 a person's risk of nursing-home admission before death is estimated at 46%; one third have lifetime risk of nursing-home stays of 90 days or less. The risk of nursing-home admission rises steeply with age; approximately 20% of persons aged 85 years and over reside in nursing homes versus 1.4% of those aged 65 to 74 years. Barring breakthroughs in the treatment of dementia, the number of persons 65 years and older using nursing homes will double by the year 2020. Interestingly, the occupancy rates in nursing homes nationally have declined over the past several years and now stand at 88%. This decline has generally been attributed to the availability of other long-term-care options, such as assisted living, but there are likely other causal social and financial variables that have yet to be articulated. The availability and use of home-care services for Medicare-eligible patients have not been found to consistently reduce nursing-home admissions.

Postacute care is increasingly being offered in nursing-home settings, a response to the higher care needs of older persons occurring in conjunction with declining lengths of hospital stays. Though the types of postacute services and programs vary significantly from one locale to another (ie, dialysis, orthopedic, ventilator, postoperative, rehabilitative, or wound care), they remain distinct from the standard nursing-home services by integrating the features of acute medical, long-term-care nursing, and rehabilitative settings. The challenge in postacute care is that of accommodating to patients with varying degrees of disease severity, functional dependence, and comorbidities. Some limited studies suggest that, for selected patient populations, postacute care in the nursing home achieves outcomes equal to or better than postacute care in acute hospitals. Definitions as to what constitutes postacute care, however, vary widely, as do regulatory standards, thus making comparison studies difficult.

Despite the significant disability associated with most nursing-home residents, the population remains quite heterogeneous. Short stayers (3 months or less) currently account for 25% of all nursing-home admissions, 50% will spend at least 1 year in the nursing home, and 21% will reside in the nursing home almost 5 years. Many short-stay residents are admitted for rehabilitation, and some enter nursing homes for terminal care. Interestingly, improvement in function for the longer-stay nursing-home residents is quite common, which reflects the heterogeneity of this population. The number of nursing-home admissions has risen since 1994, reflecting the dynamic nature of this sector of the long-term-care continuum.

Nursing-home expenditures currently total $90 billion and are projected to increase to $150 billion by 2007. Public expenditures constitute 62% of all nursing-home spending (Medicaid 48%, Medicare 12%, other 2%), with private spending constituting 38% of the total (31% out of pocket, 5% health insurance, 2% other private funds). On admission to a nursing home, almost one third of residents are eligible for Medicaid, and another third eventually qualify as financial resources are depleted. Under the new prospective payment system enacted as part of the Balanced Budget Act of 1997, Medicare payments to skilled nursing facilities are no longer cost-based, but are predicated on the person's functional needs and rehabilitative potential. Although the prospective payment system has not conclusively limited access to skilled nursing care for Medicare beneficiaries, it has definitely forced nursing homes to be more diligent with regard to their admission policies. Not unexpectedly, physical, occupational, and speech therapies are commonly prescribed in the nursing home, with half of all nursing-home admissions receiving at least 90 minutes of these rehabilitation services, according to one study. The prospective payment system requires nursing-home staff to carefully document gains in function to ensure reimbursement. Interestingly, declines in Medicare spending on home-health care since enactment of prospective payment may eventually force some individuals into nursing homes for lack of affordable home-care options. (See "Financing, Coverage, and Costs of Health Care," p 32.)

STAFFING PATTERNS

It is generally conceded that the current nursing-home population is "sicker" and more disabled than nursing-home residents were in the past. Studies have confirmed the correlation between the provision of quality care to total nursing hours and the ratio of professional nurses (ie, registered nurses) to nonprofessional nursing staff. An Institute of Medicine report in 2001 recommended increasing nurse staffing levels to enhance the quality of nursing-home care and has spurred Congress to debate the merits of mandatory minimum staffing ratios. The Centers for Medicare and Medicaid Services (CMS) has refused to institute regulatory changes that would be based on current evidence but has rather called for additional research in this area. Even if significantly higher staffing ratios eventually are mandated, the financial resources to achieve them remain elusive. Recruiting and retaining staff, particularly nursing assistants who constitute the bulk of the nursing-home workforce, also continues to

be difficult. Turnover rates for registered nurses and licensed practical nurses also are very high, at more than 50% per year. Turnover rates have been associated with increased rates of hospitalization for nursing-home residents and have been linked to the organizational culture within the nursing facility.

Staffing issues are also pertinent to physicians practicing in nursing homes. The typical nursing-home physician is a primary care internist or family physician who devotes 2 hours or less per week to nursing-home care. Many physicians avoid nursing-home practice because of perceptions of excessive regulations, paperwork, limited reimbursement, and aversion to the long-term-care environment. A paucity of credible role models for physicians in training has greatly contributed to this lack of interest and involvement in long-term-care issues. Closed staff models are thought to deliver a higher intensity and quality of care in part because of the integration of the physician into the nursing facility culture, which ultimately facilitates interdisciplinary communication and treatment. Limited evidence suggests that hospitalization rates for nursing-home residents may be lower in facilities that employ a limited number of committed physicians. One study has demonstrated that the quality of drug use in the nursing home is positively correlated with enhanced nurse-physician communication and with regular multidisciplinary team discussions.

FACTORS ASSOCIATED WITH NURSING-HOME PLACEMENT

Although there is a significant chance of being admitted to a nursing home with increasing age, other factors, such as low income, poor family supports (especially lack of spouse and children), and low social activity have been associated with institutionalization. Cognitive and functional impairments have also predicted nursing-home placement, often permanently. Interestingly, for patients with dementia, education and caregiver support have been shown to delay the need for nursing-home placement for up to 1 year. Not surprisingly, older adults with more positive attitudes toward nursing homes are more likely to use skilled nursing facilities than are adults with less favorable dispositions. The range of long-term-care services that are now available (ie, skilled nursing, home care, assisted living) further increases the complexity of placement decisions, as the relative value and merits of available options have not been empirically tested. The use of formal (ie, paid-for) community services does not necessarily reduce the likelihood of nursing-home placement for patients with severe disabilities.

THE INTERFACE OF ACUTE AND LONG-TERM CARE

The majority of nursing-home admissions derive from acute-care hospitals. Conversely, nursing-home residents have high rates of hospitalization, ranging upward of 549 admissions per 1000 nursing-home beds per year. A 2001 survey by the Centers for Disease Control and Prevention noted that nursing-home residents constitute 2% to 3% of all emergency department visits. Infection is the most common reason for transfer of nursing-home residents to short-stay hospitals, accounting for one quarter of all such admissions. Studies to date suggest that nurse practitioners and physician assistants, who act in concert with the primary care physician, provide more intensive care in the nursing home, enhance satisfaction with care, and often decrease hospitalization rates while maintaining cost neutrality. Unfortunately, the transition from acute to long-term care is often complicated by suboptimal information transfer. Illegible or nonexistent transfer summaries, omission of prescribed medications, and the lack of documentation of advanced directives, psychosocial information, and behavioral issues are but a few of the information gaps commonly reported. (See also the section on transitions from hospital care in "Hospital Care," p 97, and "Perioperative Care," p 106.)

QUALITY ISSUES

Extensive nursing-home reforms enacted in 1987 (in the Omnibus Budget Reconciliation Act of 1987) significantly changed the landscape of long-term care. In addition to setting training guidelines and minimum staffing requirements and bolstering residents' rights, including limiting the use of restraints and psychoactive medications, the law required a periodic comprehensive assessment of all nursing-home residents. This assessment, known as the Minimum Data Set (MDS), focuses specifically on clinical issues with relevance to quality care. If any real or potential problems are identified with any of these issues, the health care team must review accompanying resident assessment protocols that outline standard diagnostic and therapeutic approaches to the specific problems in question. The protocols are, in essence, practice guidelines that the team, including the primary care physician, is encouraged to use. In addition to comprehensive assessments, the physician must also clearly document the need for all medications, particularly psychoactive agents. Unnecessary drugs are defined as those that are given in excessive doses, for excessive periods of time, without adequate monitoring, without adequate indications for use, or in the presence of adverse consequences that indicate the need for dose reduction or discontinua-

tion. In addition to these generic instructions, specific types of drugs have been banned (ie, usage will warrant a citation from the state survey inspection team unless a clear rationale is documented in the chart) from use in the nursing home on the basis of criteria developed by a group of experts. Although some evidence exists to suggest that the 1987 act and subsequent mandates have resulted in a decreased prevalence of pressure ulcers and reduced use of restraints, their impact on the quality of care overall has been difficult to quantify. Interestingly, recent surveys indicate that only a minority of physicians ever review the MDS or related care plans. A new set of quality indicators based on MDS items has been instituted nationally in an effort to hasten efforts to improve quality. With this system, nursing facilities are able to compare their individual performance with regional and national norms to help guide their efforts to improve the quality of care (see http://www.cms.hhs.gov). Future versions of the MDS will likely include additional quality-of-life measures relating to personal preferences and activities.

A host of variables interact in nursing homes to determine the level of quality achieved. These include staffing levels, reimbursement rates, and processes of care extant in the nursing home. Although surveys of nursing facilities are mandated every 15 months, there is much debate as to whether the survey process can adequately identify quality practices and engender lasting improvements when deficiencies in care are found. The survey process, based on a deterrent regulatory paradigm, has been criticized for its inconsistencies, disassociation between outcome and process, surveyor subjectivity, and a failure to discriminate between trivial and important quality issues. The percentage of nursing-home residents receiving inadequate care or experiencing physical harm has declined to 20%, according to a recent General Accounting Office report. This figure, however, remains unacceptably high.

MEDICAL CARE ISSUES

The care of nursing-home residents has become more complex over the past several years, commensurate with an increasing level of medical acuity in an environment continually constrained by lack of adequate resources. Comprehensive, ongoing assessment within an interdisciplinary framework provides the practitioner the opportunity to restore function, whenever possible, and almost always to enhance quality of life.

Clinical challenges abound in the nursing home, created, in part, by the atypical and subtle presentation of illness so characteristic of patients with profound physical and psychologic frailty. In addition, limited access to biotechnology, frequent dependence on nonphysicians such as nurses and nurse assistants for patient evaluation, and the high prevalence of cognitive impairment in a setting of intense regulatory oversight all complicate the medical decision-making process. Families of nursing-home residents often remain an integral part of the overall care plan and may require specific educational and psychosocial supports. Ethical and legal concerns are also very common, particularly those regarding end-of-life, feeding, hydration, and resident rights issues. (See "Legal and Ethical Issues," p 22.) Finally, the heterogeneity among nursing-home residents precludes a uniform care plan, but rather demands an individualized, thoughtful, and reasoned approach to each person in the nursing-home setting.

Problems in nursing homes that commonly require unique diagnostic and treatment strategies include infections, falls, malnutrition, dehydration, incontinence, behavioral disturbances, the use of multiple medications, and prevention and screening. (See "Infectious Diseases," p 332; "Falls," p 201; "Malnutrition," p 174; "Urinary Incontinence," p 184; "Behavioral Problems in Dementia," p 231; "Pharmacotherapy," p 72; and "Prevention," p 64.) For example, determining the risks and benefits of tube feedings for frail nursing-home patients must be predicated not only on underlying illness but also on the resident's and the family's value system, the resources available in the nursing facility, and staff acceptance of the intervention. Given that the evidence for and against enteral feeding in nursing-home patients is controversial (ie, benefits are not well established, with up to one fourth of residents with chewing and swallowing problems able to have their feeding tubes removed), the practitioner must continue to individualize therapy. (See "Eating and Feeding Problems," p 181.) Many of the problems commonly encountered in the nursing home result when multiple comorbidities interact with a host of environmental factors, all of which may only be partially remediable. Unfortunately, expectations of family, as well as state regulators, often do not account for these complexities and commonly engender "risk-averse" behavior that is counter to autonomy and optimum quality of life.

PHYSICIAN PRACTICE IN THE NURSING HOME

Physicians have traditionally had limited involvement in nursing homes. Perceptions of excessive regulations, paperwork, and limited reimbursement raise further disincentives to nursing-home practice. In reality, the medical care of nursing-home residents is both challenging and fulfilling, requiring excellent clinical skills as well as sensitivity to a variety of ethical, legal, and interdisciplinary issues. Medical interventions, whether they be curative, preventive, or palliative, demand an individualized approach that recognizes the complex interplay among resident, family, and staff needs. Further, the evidence upon which to base treatment may be nonexistent.

The comorbidity present in most nursing-home residents commonly creates the need for multiple drug therapies, with attendant complications. Even though residents receiving more than nine medications (one third of all nursing-home residents) are flagged by state survey teams as reflecting potential quality concerns, the use of multiple medications cannot always be avoided. The most common health conditions found in the nursing home for persons aged 65 years and older, following dementia, are heart disease, hypertension, arthritis, and stroke. The approaches to these and other illnesses have evolved dramatically in recent years and complicate treatment decisions where cost-effectiveness is increasingly looked upon as a desirable goal. Clear documentation of the rationale for a given medication or intervention is the best way to protect against potential scrutiny; frequent discussion with the facility's consultant pharmacist is also helpful. (See "Pharmacotherapy," p 72.)

Physicians who schedule and structure their visits to the nursing home will benefit from the resultant efficiencies and secondarily will be more fully integrated into the health care team. Nurse practitioners and physician assistants have become increasingly involved in the primary care of nursing-home residents. Studies suggest that nurse practitioners and physician assistants who act in concert with the primary care physician as a coordinated team provide more intensive care to the nursing-home resident and may decrease hospitalization rates while maintaining cost neutrality. Information regarding physician responsibilities and Omnibus Budget Reconciliation Act mandates can be found at the Web site of the American Medical Directors Association (http://www.amda.com). Such responsibilities encompass ongoing comprehensive assessment and coordination of care in order to assure patient autonomy and safety as well as optimization of physical and psychosocial function. (See Table 16.1.)

Several studies have documented misdiagnoses, inappropriate interventions, and poor preventive care practices in nursing homes. In an often-cited study of Maryland nursing homes, for example, only 11% of patients with four common types of infection were found to have received even a minimal evaluation (eg, failure to obtain a urine sample when treated for a urinary tract infection). In a study of nursing-home patients with nonmalignant pain, 25% were found to be receiving no analgesics. Intensive research is currently being directed to understand the processes necessary to integrate validated care guidelines into nursing homes in an effort to improve quality of care.

Certain care strategies that have been developed may enhance care quality. The commonly employed

Table 16.1—The Physician's Responsibilities in the Nursing Home

- Comprehensive admission assessment, including history and physical examination, and review of available medical records.
- Development of a plan of care in concert with interdisciplinary team members, the resident, and the family that is consistent with the resident's needs and goals.
- Periodic monitoring of chronic health problems at appropriate intervals, using diagnostic testing, consultation, and pharmacologic and nonpharmacologic interventions as warranted.
- Prompt and thorough assessment of acute medical problems or change in function, instituting change in the medical treatment plan as indicated.
- Communication with interdisciplinary team members, the resident, and the family concerning new diagnoses and treatment plans.
- Periodic review, in concert with the consultant pharmacist, of all medications with regard to ongoing need, adverse effects, appropriate laboratory monitoring, and potential interactions.
- Optimization of quality of life and function, with special attention to cognition, mobility, falls, skin integrity, nutrition, and continence.
- Determination of each resident's decision-making capacity and assistance in establishing advance directives.
- Physical attendance to each resident, with documentation in the medical record in accordance with all state and federal guidelines.

special care units, though conceptually attractive, have not consistently been shown to enhance quality of care apart from the involvement of individual professionals. Specific consultation services in the nursing home, however, may improve care practices and patient outcomes, as shown by a randomized controlled trial of an effort to reduce falls in a group of Tennessee nursing-home residents. In addition, interactive educational programs for physicians and nursing staff may improve practice, as has been demonstrated in programs to promote appropriate psychoactive drug use.

Understanding each nursing-home resident's preference for care in the context of his or her underlying value system will undoubtedly improve overall quality. Interestingly, fewer than one in eight nursing-home residents have discussed preferences with their health care providers. In addition, there is often a lack of follow-up of do-not-resuscitate discussions in the hospital when the patient is subsequently admitted to the nursing home. Sixty percent of nursing-home residents have orders for cardiopulmonary resuscitation, and almost 90% desire hospitalization for acute illness. When ethical dilemmas do present themselves, the availability of institutional ethics committees can provide important guidance. The multidisciplinary nature of these committees ensures a spectrum of opinion and insight critical for nursing-home residents, and they are particularly relevant to end-of-life issues. (See also "Legal and Ethical Issues," p 22.)

THE ROLE OF THE MEDICAL DIRECTOR

The quality of physician practice in the nursing home is, in many ways, determined by the medical director. The medical director, in concert with the medical staff, sets quality standards for the nursing home and operationalizes these through specific policies and procedures. The medical director must ensure compliance with all relevant state and federal guidelines and work with the nursing-home administrator and director of nursing to foster effective team care and continuing staff education. The medical director of a nursing home works closely with all disciplines and must be constantly aware of the unique interplay between laws, regulations, organization, and delivery of medical care. Certification for medical directors following completion of a formal course is now offered through the American Medical Directors Association.

ANNOTATED REFERENCES

- Dimant J. Roles and responsibilities of attending physicians in skilled nursing facilities. *J Am Med Dir Assoc.* 2003;4(4):231–243.

- Dimant J. The role of the consultant in long-term care facilities. *J Am Med Dir Assoc.* 2003;4(5):274–280.

  The author describes the roles and responsibilities of both nursing-home attending physicians and consultants in great detail. Although these seem daunting and subject to countless rules and regulations, it is important for the physician not to lose sight of the primary goal in the nursing home—that of promoting the quality of care for each resident. An accompanying editorial (Katz PR. A silver lining. *J Am Med Dir Assoc.* 2003;4[4]:222) attempts to place the physician's role in realistic perspective.

- Kane RA. Definition, measurement, and correlates of quality of life in nursing homes: toward a reasonable practice, research, and policy agenda. *Gerontologist.* 2003;43(Spec No. 2):28–36.

  This seminal review challenges our current constructs of quality of life for nursing-home residents. Barriers to defining and measuring quality of life are clearly articulated; the centrality of the nursing-home residents' voice is emphasized. Several methodologic challenges in measuring quality of life are described, and potential solutions are offered.

- Katz PR, Mezey M, Kapp M, eds. Physician practice in long-term care: workforce shortages and implications for the future. In: *Advances in Long-Term Care.* Vol. 5. New York: Springer Publishing Co.; 2003.

  Continued concerns about the quality of care delivered in nursing homes have increased focus on staffing levels and competency. Although studies have generally affirmed the correlation between nurse staffing levels and quality, little if any research has systematically described the relationship between physician staffing patterns and relevant outcomes.

This chapter summarizes the extant literature on physician practice patterns in the nursing home and offers a research agenda for the future.

■ Saliba D, Kington R, Buchanan J, et al. Appropriateness of the decision to transfer nursing facility residents to the hospital. *J Am Geriatr Soc.* 2000;48(2):154–163.

The transfer of older patients between acute and long-term-care facilities is common, expensive, and fraught with potential morbidity. The dynamics underlying these transfers are complex, particularly those involving acutely ill nursing-home residents in need of acute care. The authors of this article make use of peer reviews of medical records in order to document the reasons underlying inappropriate transfers. This study, and the accompanying editorial, set the stage for future research in this arena.

■ Wunderlich GS, Kohler PO, eds. Strengthening the caregiving work force. In: *Improving Quality in Long-Term Care.* Washington, DC: National Academy Press; 2001.

This Institute of Medicine report profiles long-term care, both users and providers, with a primary focus on quality of care. Issues related to the measurement and monitoring of quality of care are clearly articulated. Approaches to strengthening the caregiving workforce are presented, as well as the means to improve care through the building of organizational capacity. Although quality of care has improved somewhat, this report highlights the many obstacles yet to be overcome.

Paul R. Katz, MD
Jurgis Karuza, PhD

CHAPTER 17—COMMUNITY-BASED CARE

KEY POINTS

■ Home care has changed dramatically since the introduction of prospective payment for services; a 20% decline in the number of recipients has occurred, and many home-health agencies have closed because of financial constraints, limiting access to home-care services in some areas.

■ Physicians and other providers often find home care rewarding; reimbursement charges for home visits has improved, making home visits more financially viable for clinicians.

■ Community-based services that do not require a change of residence (adult day care, day hospitals, home hospitals, PACE, telemedicine) may be a useful alternative to inpatient services. However, the availability of these services strongly depends on financial reimbursement.

■ Community-based services requiring a change of residence (assisted living, group homes, adult foster care, and continuing-care retirement communities) offer a wide range of services. These are regulated at the state level and vary considerably in availability, cost, and services provided.

HOME CARE

The 2000 U.S. census data revealed that almost 10 million older adults living in the community require help with activities of daily living (ADLs). For a large number of these people, home care has the potential to improve their quality of life and avoid unnecessary institutionalization.

Under a cost-based reimbursement system, home care grew rapidly in the 1980s and 1990s. This growth coincided with the initiation of the prospective payment system (diagnostic related groups or DRGs) for hospitals that resulted in patients' being discharged sooner from hospitals, which increased the need for home services. New technologies created the possibility of providing therapies in the home that were previously available only in hospitals or nursing homes. Because of an explosive increase in costs, Congress placed limits on Medicare spending as mandated in the 1997 Balanced Budget Act, which led to the development of a prospective payment system (PPS) for home-care services. Since enactment of the PPS, there has been more than a 20% decline in the number of recipients of home-care services and the number of visits for patients receiving home care. Many home-care agencies have adjusted to these changes and developed more efficient, targeted home care, but hundreds have closed because of the financial pressures. Rural agencies have closed at a higher rate than urban ones. The Outcome and Assessment Information Set (OASIS) is a tool meant to set fees for Home Health Related Groups (HHRGs). The OASIS instrument is completed by the home-health agency and tracks several domains of patients' functional status and medical needs. Like the DRGs, the HHRGs provide the basis for reimbursement to the agencies and are based on severity of the patient's illness, disabilities, and nursing needs; they include an adjustment for location in the United States. The instrument is also intended to provide a uniform means of measuring quality of care across all home-care agencies.

Like other sectors of our health care system, home-care agencies are charged with developing cost-effective high-quality care despite diminishing reimbursement. Another major challenge facing home-care agencies is recruiting and retaining qualified nurses and aides. Developing community-wide systems of care between hospitals, home care, nursing homes, and practitioners' offices may help meet these challenges and ensure that patients receive timely and appropriate care.

The Physician's Role in Home Care

The physician's role in home care is to serve as a member of an interdisciplinary team that is generally composed of nurses, therapists (speech, physical, occupational, and respiratory), social workers, personal care aides, home medical equipment suppliers, and, most importantly, informal caregivers. The physician is, by law, responsible for the patient's care plan. Physicians determine the patient's health care needs; develop, certify, and recertify the plan of care; and confer regularly with team members to address patient care issues and to handle documentation and other administrative matters. The change to a PPS makes it even more important for physicians to be attentive to the development, certification, and recertification of the plan of care. In particular, the PPS requires physicians to certify the level of need for individual therapy services; the amount of therapy services will partly determine the HHRG assignment. Patients requiring more than ten rehabilitation or therapy visits during a 60-day period will be assigned a higher HHRG level. Changes in patient condition within the 60-day episodic payment period will require recertification by the physician. The shift to prospective payment may encourage some home-health agencies to reduce services to lower costs. The advent of prospective payment makes it even more critical for the physician to certify that the patient requires services and to ensure that the appropriate quantity and quality of services are being provided.

Physicians are reimbursed for certification of the home-care plan and for oversight of complex cases in skilled home care and hospice. Table 17.1 lists the billing codes and requirements for these services. The documentation requirements for billing allow activities over multiple days in a month to be combined.

House calls can add an important dimension to the physician's knowledge of the patient's circumstances and environment. Home evaluation can identify additional problems not readily apparent in office-based assessment. Barriers to maximum functioning can be identified and addressed. House calls have the additional benefit of reducing the burden of transportation for patients who have difficulty getting outside of the home. Changes in Medicare have increased reimbursement for home visits, making home visits more financially feasible for clinicians.

Patient Assessment

Homebound patients have significant functional impairment. Comprehensive geriatric assessment is particularly valuable in this setting to establish a baseline, monitor the course of illness, and evaluate effects of intervention. However, assessment in the home has some important differences from office-based assessment.

During a home visit, an assessment of the patient's actual environment can be performed to determine

Table 17.1—Codes, Reimbursement, and Requirements in Home-Care Certification

Codes	Reimbursement*	Requirements**
G0179	$ 51.39	Physician recertification for Medicare-covered home-health services. This includes reviewing and signing Home Health Care Plan of Care (form 485), contacts with agency personnel, review of reports per 60-day certification period. Documentation (copy of form 485) must be present in patient medical record.
G0180	$ 66.44	Physician certification for Medicare-covered services. As above, the physician affirms the implementation of the care plan and affirms that it meets the patient's needs as documented in form 485, and a copy exists in patient record.
G0181	$112.25	Physician supervision of a patient receiving Medicare-covered services requiring complex and multidisciplinary care involving regular physician involvement or revision of care plans, review of subsequent reports of patient status, review of diagnostic tests, and discussions with family. This must be 30 minutes or more within a calendar month. Documentation must be present in the patient medical record or log.
G0182	$118.46	Same as G0180 but with a patient in a Medicare-approved hospice program.

* Reimbursement may vary with different health maintenance organizations and will change with continued enactment of the Balanced Budget Act.
** The patient is not present for these activities.

whether the home is safe and supportive, given the particular patient's abilities and disabilities. Performance-based functional assessment can focus on the practical aspects of performing ADLs by direct observation of the environment for bathing, dressing, and transferring. Difficulties can be identified, and the assessor can evaluate the caregiver's abilities to address the patient's needs. The caregiver's needs for counseling, training, support, and education can also be identified and addressed.

Environmental modifications can be recommended to improve function. For example, modifications of the bathtub, a hand-held shower, a shower seat, grab-bars, and a bedside commode can improve the patient's quality of life and functioning. Barriers to wheelchairs and walkers such as door sills can be identified and removed. Chair lifts and outdoor ramps can help patients circumvent stairs. Occupational therapy consultation can be particularly useful in identifying other personal care and assistive devices for performing ADLs and housekeeping chores. A number of home safety checklists are available to help a reviewer assess the home. Additional technological additions to improve home safety, including necklace or wrist radio devices to call for help, can be considered. Some types of emergency response systems require that a person push a button by a specified time each day to avoid triggering an emergency response or telephone call to check on the owner of the device.

Health care providers are finding that home diagnostics, including radiology and electrocardiography, are available in most areas, and hand-held laboratory devices are becoming more common. These home diagnostics allow for a much more comprehensive medical evaluation to take place in the home.

Developing an Office-Based House-Call Program

Medical care in the home may be provided as part of an ongoing office-based program, as an extension of hospitalization through a postacute care program, or as a freestanding entity. Regardless of the method chosen, it is important that the organization of the home-care program be well conceived to maximize effectiveness and efficiency and to remain financially viable. Current regulations allow house calls to be provided by physicians, nurse practitioners, and physician assistants. Regardless of the primary care medical provider, appropriate links to other providers of home-based services are necessary to develop an interdisciplinary team. Consistency and familiarity among all members of the interdisciplinary team are essential to a smoothly functioning house-call program.

Choosing the Right Patients

To qualify for Medicare home-care benefits, a patient must meet two criteria to establish homebound status. First, the patient must be absent from the home for reasons other than obtaining medical treatment infrequently (three times or fewer per month) or for short periods of time. Second, leaving home must require considerable and taxing effort on the part of the patient or the caregiver, or both—for example, if the patient is bedbound or has a severe mobility impairment.

Patients who are likely to be good candidates for house calls are those with mobility impairments that make transportation to the office difficult; those with disruptive behaviors; patients with terminal illnesses; and patients with multiple medical, psychiatric, and social problems. House calls are needed for some patients a limited amount of time, but others require house visits on an ongoing basis. Home visits may be particularly useful for patients who are either not responding to adequate therapy or responding inconsistently. A diagnostic home visit may reveal caregiver burnout, elder mistreatment, or the use of medications from other sources that may be interfering with the expected response. (See also "Pharmacotherapy," p 72; "Elder Mistreatment," p 86.)

Equipment for House Calls

Table 17.2 lists suggested equipment and drugs for house calls. A small bag with key equipment is particularly useful. A supply of forms needed for common diagnostic tests and orders, educational material for common problems, and community referral information are also useful.

Financial Considerations

House calls are now more financially feasible for clinicians; documentation remains the key to receiving requested remuneration. There are no specific restrictions on the number of visits as long as there is sufficient justification in the progress notes. As with most documentation, it is necessary that the primary care provider identify historical data, physical examination findings, diagnostic test results, and an assessment that reflects all the active diagnoses. Further, an evaluation of the patient's functioning, caregiver issues, and documentation of the medical plan of care are important elements to include in the house-call progress note. Physician assistants and nurse practitioners may also bill for home-care services under Medicare regulations adopted in January 1998. Table 17.3

Table 17.2—Suggested Equipment and Supplies for House Calls

Basic equipment and supplies

Cerumen curette	Sphygmomanometer
Cotton tip applicators	Stethoscope
Gloves	Stool guaiac cards and developer
Intravenous starting kit and fluid	Tape measure
Lubricating jelly	Toenail clippers
Oto-ophthalmoscope	Tongue depressors
Phlebotomy equipment	Tuning fork
Reflex hammer	Urine dipsticks
Snellen chart	Sharps container

Additional supplies

Emergency medications (protect from heat and cold)	Specimen cups
Foley and coudé catheter	Wound debridement kit
Genitourinary syringe	Wound dressing materials
Nasogastric tube	

Also consider

AudioScope	Portable oxygen
Glucometer with lancets in strips	Pulse oximeter
Portable electrocardiograph machine	Voice amplifier

lists codes and reimbursement for home visits. When visits become prolonged, time codes can be used that justify an enhanced reimbursement. Reimbursement can vary in different localities, particularly where health maintenance organizations act as intermediaries for Medicare.

Caregiver Support

Family caregivers provide most of the care received by patients in the community. In the United States, three out of four caregivers are women, either wives or daughters. Caregiving is often intense, time consuming, and stressful. The caregiver's physical and emotional health may be affected, resulting in depression and a worsening of his or her own health problems. Attention to caregiver support and issues are essential to help the patients continue to provide care. Caregiver support groups may be particularly helpful (see the resources listed in the Appendix, p 504).

For discussions of specific issues concerning caregiving, see "Psychosocial Issues" (p 18), "Dementia" (p 227), "Behavioral Problems in Dementia" (p 231), "Elder Mistreatment" (p 86), and "Depression and Other Mood Disorders" (p 269).

Limitations of Home Care

Most elderly persons would prefer to remain in their own home, but certain situations and conditions arise that make institutional care a more appropriate choice than in-home care. For example, caregivers may not be available to adequately address the needs of the patient. Relatively unstable medical situations requiring frequent laboratory testing, respiratory interventions, or intravenous medications may make institutional care a better choice than home care for some patients. Caregiver burnout and caregiver stress may prevent continued safe care for the patient in the home.

Further, the home environment itself may be a barrier to continuing in-home care. Unsafe neighborhoods, ongoing household social disruptions from

Table 17.3—Billing Codes and Reimbursement for Home Visits

New Patients		Established Patients		
Codes	Reimbursement	Codes	Reimbursement	Requirements
99341	$ 54.00	99347	$ 41.00	Problem-focused history and examination, straightforward medical decision making
99342	$ 81.00	99348	$ 69.00	Expanded problem-focused history and physical examination with medical decision making of low complexity. Generally 30 minutes spend with patient or family.
99343	$121.00	99349	$107.00	Detailed history and examination; medical decision making of moderate complexity. Typically about 45 minutes.
99344	$158.00	99350	$156.00	Comprehensive history and examination with medical decision making of moderate complexity. Time about 60 minutes.
99345	$193.12			Above plus medical decision making of high complexity. Time about 75 minutes.

SOURCE: Data from the 2005 American Medical Association Current Procedures and Terminology (CPT) booklet.

alcohol or drug use, and inadequate room for equipment or environmental modifications may make in-home care a poor or risky option.

Finally, home care may be prohibitively expensive for the patient. It is not always the least expensive alternative, and out-of-pocket expenses may make on-going home care unaffordable. Insurance coverage is more likely to cover care that is rendered in a nursing facility or other institutional setting.

Liability and Legal Issues

As elsewhere in the practice of medicine, clinicians offering home care are potentially liable for adverse outcomes; however, malpractice suits related to home care are relatively uncommon. It is important that appropriate documentation be maintained for medical purposes and also to support physician compensation; documentation is also necessary to support the request for payments to other providers of in-home services. In addition, physicians should be aware that inaccurate certificates of medical necessity could lead to charges of Medicare fraud. These forms should be reviewed carefully before they are signed.

It is important to be sensitive to potential conflicts of interest. Federal legislation prohibits physicians from receiving financial benefit, compensation, or rebate for referring a patient to a home-care provider. Further, physicians may not refer patients to home-care companies in which the physician or the physician's family has a "substantial" financial interest. In certain situations, there are exemptions to protect physicians in hospitals who are involved in "relatively innocuous or even beneficial arrangements." Seek legal advice if there is any question of a potential conflict of interest.

Ethics and Decisions About Institutionalization

Two ethical themes arise commonly in home care. The first is the balance between patient autonomy and patient safety. The second involves issues surrounding elder mistreatment and neglect.

Respect for patient autonomy often dictates that the patient remain in the home as a result of the patient's (or surrogate decision maker's) choice. Conflict arises when a patient's medical care or safety cannot be adequately maintained in the home, yet the patient insists on staying at home. It is difficult to balance respect for patient autonomy with the desire to prevent patient neglect. In some situations, the outcome is likely to be terminal, regardless of whether the patient is maintained at home or in an institution. In such situations, a hospice referral may help provide additional services in the home and support for both the patient and family. In situations where there is a clearly neglectful or abusive situation, Adult Protective Services should be contacted (see "Elder Mistreatment," p 86, and "Legal and Ethical Issues," p 22).

COMMUNITY-BASED SERVICES NOT REQUIRING A CHANGE IN RESIDENCE

Adult Day Care

Adult day care is a community-based option that provides a wide range of social and support services in a congregate setting. Adult day care has become increasingly common. Providers of adult day care may offer a variety of services, ranging from simple nonskilled custodial care to more advanced skilled services. The availability of a registered nurse allows for on-site health services, clinical assessment and monitoring, and assistance with medication management. Adult day care is used commonly for patients with dementia who need supervision and assistance with their ADLs while primary caregivers work. Adult day care may also serve as a form of respite for caregivers. Most adult day care centers are community based, either in churches or community centers. In general, custodial adult day care is not covered by Medicare, though some costs may be covered by Medicaid or other insurers.

Day Hospitals

Day hospitals provide a broad range of skilled nursing care services, including parenteral antibiotics, chemotherapy, and intensive rehabilitation. The majority of programs are housed in chronic care hospitals or rehabilitation centers. This arrangement allows for the provider to take advantage of in-house professional expertise and resources, while allowing the patient to return to his or her own home or alternative living site after day treatment is complete. Services are covered under Medicare, with similar requirements to those surrounding home-health care.

Day hospitals are most often used for two groups of patients: those needing multidisciplinary rehabilitation and those with psychiatric illnesses. A systematic review of day hospital care found that there are no significant differences between day hospitals and alternative sources of care with respect to death, disability, or use of health services, but that among those receiving care in a day hospital, there is a trend toward less functional decline and less hospital and institutional care.

Program of All-Inclusive Care for the Elderly

The Program of All-Inclusive Care for the Elderly (PACE) is a capitated model of care that pools funds from Medicare and Medicaid to provide acute and long-term care to frail older people. (See also "Financing, Coverage, and Costs of Health Care," p 39.) Participants in the PACE program must meet state-defined requirements regarding their need for a nursing-home level of care. The goal of the program is to keep the participant in the community for as long as it is medically, socially, and financially feasible. The system, designed to be seamless, uses an interdisciplinary team of health care providers who know the patient and caregivers well and who provide care across the spectrum of hospital, home, alternative living situations, and institutional care. Integrated financing allows the program to provide traditional coverage of acute, rehabilitative, home, and institutional care. It also allows for adult day care, respite care, transportation, medication coverage, rehabilitation including maintenance physical and occupational therapy, hearing aids, eyeglasses, and a variety of other benefits. The program, at the discretion of the interdisciplinary team, has the flexibility to pay for nonmedical costs in unusual circumstances (eg, paying a person's electric or gas bill). Care by the interdisciplinary team provides for the complex social as well as the medical needs of the participant. PACE has been described as one of the few truly integrated systems of care in the United States. Although the effectiveness of PACE has not been directly tested by a randomized controlled trial, research has shown that PACE provides high-quality care, albeit with significant site-to-site variation.

In 1997, legislation was passed that changed the status of PACE from a demonstration program to a permanent provider under Medicare. PACE is an optional program under state Medicaid. As of November 2003, 29 programs in 17 states were operational, and 50 more were in various stages of development. It is anticipated that the program will continue to expand.

Capitated financing for PACE is provided through Medicare and, in participating states, Medicaid. The Medicare rate-setting method for PACE has traditionally been based on the average cost of providing care to Medicare beneficiaries in a given geographic area, which is multiplied by a frailty adjuster. This method is likely to change in the near future. Each state determines the Medicaid rate of capitation.

Social Health Maintenance Organizations

The first generation Social Health Maintenance Organization (SHMO) project started in the middle 1980s with the intention of developing innovative, integrated, acute, and long-term care for Medicare beneficiaries. The four initial sites offered a variety of services and a system of care that focused on assessment and case management and that offered additional home and community-based services. Unlike the PACE program, the SHMOs serve not only low-income frail seniors but also healthier, more affluent, nondisabled Medicare recipients. The first round of the SHMO demonstration found that outcomes for participants were similar to those for control persons without any clear cost savings. One of the original four sites elected to drop out of the demonstration in 1994; an additional four sites for the second generation (SHMO II) were approved in 1996. It was hoped that SHMO II would provide a greater degree of effectiveness and integration through a variety of modifications to SHMO I, including more emphasis on personnel with geriatrics expertise, geriatric practice guidelines, and education of nongeriatrician practitioners on the essentials of geriatric care. Only one SHMO II, the Health Plan of Nevada, was actually implemented in the second phase of this program. A recent report from the Centers for Medicare and Medicaid Services concluded that there was no consistent evidence that SHMOs improved patient outcomes. There was evidence in a small subset of medically frail patients that hospital utilization was reduced. This begs the question of whether targeting a more frail population would result in the SHMOs' having a more positive impact on beneficiaries.

Telemedicine

The growth of telemedicine in home care has not paralleled the increasing availability and affordability of this type of technology. Although telemedicine has been used successfully in radiology, where it has been reimbursed, it has not been used to a great extent in other areas of medicine. Telemedicine has been used in some capitated health care programs in prisons and mental health centers. There are also a number of demonstration studies utilizing telemedicine in remote areas that include real-time physician-patient encounters and that store and forward recordings of patients which are later reviewed by a physician. Some home-health agencies are beginning to use telemedicine to monitor patients, as the PPS has created financial incentives to limit the number of home visits. Telemedicine may have particular applicability in rural settings and other areas where access to physicians and other health care providers is limited.

Telemedicine involves the transmission of data to the nurse or primary care provider, who can then evaluate and make decisions regarding the patient's health care. Systems vary considerably. For example, some systems are relatively disease specific. One example is an automated scale, blood-pressure cuff, and heart-rate monitor for patients with heart failure. More elaborate telemedicine systems allow for audio and video two-way communication, distance electrocardiography, distance auscultation through the use of an onsite stethoscope that can transmit breath, heart, and abdominal sounds, and camera lenses that allow for detailed examination of the skin and eyes. System costs vary considerably, ranging from approximately $1500 for simple audio and video systems to $20,000. In the future they are likely to become more affordable and useful, as broadband eliminates the need for expensive lines and allows for quicker transmission of data than do telephone connections. In certain situations telemedicine is Medicare reimbursable in rural areas. Some states are providing coverage through Medicaid.

Home Hospital

The home hospital focuses on providing more complex care at home to older people who would have been hospitalized for an acute-care need. Patients receiving home-hospital care have access to nurses and physicians on a regular basis and for episodic care through an on-call system that allows problems to be addressed promptly. The concept may be viewed as an evolution of home care, which it resembles, though it is more intense. Studies conducted outside of the United States suggest that care is comparable for selected patients and that patient satisfaction is high. (See also "Hospital Care," p 91.)

COMMUNITY-BASED SERVICES REQUIRING A CHANGE OF RESIDENCE

Assisted Living

More than 800,000 people live in assisted-living facilities, and the number is expected to grow rapidly as our population ages. Even though these facilities are based on a social (not medical) model, they are caring for more frail people with significant medical needs. The transitional nature of assisted living is suggested by the average length of residency, about 2 years in 2002. The most common reason for discharge is need for nursing-home care.

Assisted-living residences are characterized by some level of coordination or provision of personal care services, social activities, health-related services, and supervision, services that are provided in a home-like atmosphere that maximizes autonomy and privacy. The services provided under assisted living vary considerably, both within states and between states.

One national survey of assisted-living facilities found a range of privacy options, from private rooms to apartment units; about half would not admit residents with moderate to severe cognitive impairment; about two thirds did not have a registered nurse on staff but did provide 24-hour staff oversight, housekeeping, two meals, and personal assistance with ADLs. One example of the difference between state licensing requirements is in the area of medication administration. Depending on licensing requirements, medication administration and management may be directed by nonskilled, skilled, or fully licensed nursing staff.

In states where regulations do not require skilled care in assisted-living facilities, home-health skilled care is often provided as an external or independent service to the individual patient who happens to be living in an assisted-living facility. In this context, the boundary between assisted-living and skilled nursing facilities often becomes blurred. Since care in assisted living is generally less costly than in a nursing home, there has been a trend to use assisted living as a lower-cost alternative to nursing-home care. Part of the reason assisted-living care is usually less expensive is that there are fewer regulations governing assisted-living facilities. However, as these facilities have come to care for more people with increasing disability and more medical needs, there has been increasing pressure to regulate them.

Costs for assisted-living residences vary greatly and depend on the size of units, services provided, and location. A survey in 2001 found that 48% of residences charge an average between $1,000 and $2,000 in monthly rent and fees. Another 23% charge between $2,000 and $3,000, and 9% charge more than $3,000 each month; 16% of assisted-living facilities charge less than $1,000.

Assisted living is covered in a growing number of long-term-care insurance policies. The Health Insurance Association of America reports that all 11 of the leading insurance companies that sell long-term-care insurance offer assisted-living coverage. However, the majority of people in assisted-living residences or their families pay for care themselves because most elderly Americans do not carry long-term-care insurance.

Assisted living is not covered by Medicare, but certain services are paid under Supplementary Security Income and Social Services Block Grant programs. Thirty-eight states reimburse or plan to reimburse for assisted-living services as a Medicaid service. In addition, states have the option to pay for assisted living under Medicaid by including services in the state's Medicaid plan or petitioning the U.S. Department of Health and Human Services for a waiver.

See also the American Geriatrics Society position statement on assisted-living facilities in the Appendix (p 494).

Group Homes

Group homes (including domiciliary care, single-room occupancy residences, board-and-care homes, and some congregate living situations) are houses or apartments in which two or more unrelated people live together. Group homes vary in types of residents and often serve patients with chronic mental illness or dementia. Residents share a living room, dining room, and kitchen but usually have their own bedrooms. Advantages of this arrangement include a lower cost of living and socialization with peers. Independence and functional status are supported through the interdependence and relationships of the residents. Resident-to-staff ratios may be higher than in other supported-living environments. Opportunities for socialization are increased, reducing social isolation. Most group homes are run as for-profit businesses, and some states require licensing.

Adult Foster Care

Foster care homes generally provide room, board, and some assistance with ADLs by the sponsoring family or by paid caregivers, who customarily live on the premises. Perhaps the longest experience with adult foster care is in the state of Oregon, where it is used as an alternative to long-term care and institutionalization. Adult foster care has the advantages of maintaining frail elderly people in a more home-like environment. Regulations for foster care vary by state, and some states require licensing. Some states provide coverage of adult foster care through their Medicaid programs.

Sheltered Housing

Sheltered housing is funded through the Older Americans Act and is offered as an option for housing subsidized through section 8, Housing and Urban Development programs for seniors and disabled residents. Often these arrangements are sheltered homes offering personal care assistance, housekeeping services, and meals. Programs may be supplemented by social work services and activities coordinators. Charges to clients are based on a sliding scale, which may cost up to 30% of income.

Continuing-Care Retirement Communities

More affluent seniors may choose a continuing-care retirement community (CCRC). CCRCs usually have a variety of living options, ranging from apartments or condominiums, to assisted living, and skilled nursing-home care. Often, residents enter the more independent living areas and progress through assisted living and into skilled care as they age.

Three financial models are common: the all-inclusive model, which provides total health care coverage, including long-term care; the fee-for-service model in which payments match the level of care; and the modified coverage model, which covers long-term care to a predetermined maximum. Most CCRCs require an entry fee, which may or may not be refundable, plus a variable monthly fee to pay for rent and supportive services. Monthly fees vary, depending upon the level of care being provided. Funding is largely private, though some facilities have Medicare- or Medicaid-funded beds for skilled care.

See also "Financing, Coverage, and Costs of Health Care" (p 32).

ANNOTATED REFERENCES

■ Bodenheimer T. Long-term care for frail elderly people—the On Lok model. *N Engl J Med.* 1999;341(17):1324–1328.

> This article provides a brief overview of On Lok and the Program of All-Inclusive Care for the Elderly (PACE) projects. It is useful for those who would like a summary of the latter. Current issues surrounding the move to full provider status, expansion to other areas, and modifications of the program are discussed.

■ Boult C, Pacala JT. Integrating healthcare for older populations. *Am J Manag Care.* 1999;5(1):45–52.

> This general article provides an overview of PACE and the first and second Social Health Maintenance Organizations (SHMO I and SHMO II). The challenge of changing from a fragmented system of care to integrated systems that address the needs of older adults is discussed. The authors identify the financial issues that have driven the current system to fragmentation and discuss the benefits and limits of integrated financing.

■ Field MJ, Grigsby J. Telemedicine and remote patient monitoring. *JAMA.* 2002;288(4):423–425.

> This is a well-referenced review of the state of telemedicine in 2002. Several examples of the successful use of telemedicine are described, and the authors provide a thoughtful discussion of why this technology has had limited growth.

- Levine SA, Boal J, Boling PA. Home care. *JAMA.* 2003;290(9):1203–1207.

    This state-of-the-art paper provides an excellent review of home care. It provides up-to-date coding and financial information along with a history of how we got to where we are today in the field. The challenges and prospects of delivering quality home-care services in the present environment are also covered.

- Murkofsky RL, Phillips RS, McCarthy EP, et al. Length of stay in home care before and after the 1997 balanced budget act. *JAMA.* 2003;289(21):2841–2848.

    This cross-sectional study examines the effects of the prospective payment system (PPS) on the length of stay in home care. After the start of PPS in 1997, the median length of stay decreased by 16 days for all recipients of home care, and the decrease was even greater in for-profit home-care agencies. The probable reasons for these decreases and future ramifications for patients are discussed in detail.

- National Center for Health Statistics. *Health, United States, 2004, With Chartbook on Trends in the Health of Americans.* Hyattsville, MD: US Department of Health and Human Services, National Center for Health Statistics; September 2004. DHHS Pub. No. 2004-1232.

    This annual report on the health status of the nation is submitted by the Secretary of the Department of Health and Human Services to the President and Congress in compliance with Section 308 of the Public Health Service Act. The report presents national trends in health statistics; in each edition a chartbook focuses on a major health topic. Available at: http://www.cdc.gov/nchs/hus.htm (accessed October 2005).

- Tinetti ME, Baker D, Gallo WT, et al. Evaluation of restorative care vs usual care for older adults receiving an acute episode of home care. *JAMA.* 2002;287(16):2098–2105.

    This paper tested an innovative way to provide home care that reduces emergency department utilization and increases the likelihood of patients' remaining in their homes with less reported pain. A restorative care unit was compared with several other home-care offices. The unit reorganized the home-care staff in a way that provided more coordinated services, following the principles of geriatrics, rehabilitation, and nursing. The patient and family were made part of this process to set mutual goals with the health care team. The development and study of innovative models such as this one will be essential as we search for more cost-effective ways of delivering care.

Robert McCann, MD
G. Paul Eleazer, MD

CHAPTER 18—PALLIATIVE CARE

KEY POINTS

- For many older persons, dying is characterized by inadequately treated physical distress, fragmented care systems, poor to absent communication among doctors, patients, and families, and enormous strains on family caregiver and support systems.

- Geographic variations in practice patterns and services available, religious beliefs, economic status, medical differences, gender, and cognitive status all affect the experiences of the dying person.

- Pain assessment is especially challenging in patients with poor communication skills, and the clinician must be sensitive to nonverbal clues.

- Loss of appetite is almost a universal symptom at the end of life; often it is more distressing to loved ones than to the patient.

- The patient's self-report is the only reliable measure of dyspnea, one of the most distressing symptoms experienced by many dying persons.

In the United States the overwhelming majority of deaths occur among the elderly population. Older persons typically die slowly of chronic diseases, with multiple coexisting problems, progressive dependency on others, and heavy care needs that are met mostly by family members. Many of these deaths become protracted processes that must be negotiated by clinicians, patients, and family members, who must make difficult decisions about the use or discontinuation of life-prolonging treatments. There is abundant evidence that the quality of life during the dying process is often poor. For many older persons, dying is characterized by inadequately treated physical distress, fragmented care systems, poor to absent communication among doctors, patients, and families, and enormous strains on family caregiver and support systems.

Although most Americans spend the majority of their final months at home, in most parts of the country their deaths actually occur in the hospital or nursing home. The experience of dying, however, varies greatly from one part of the nation to another. In Portland, Oregon, for example, only 35% of adult deaths occur in hospitals, but in New York City more than 80% occur in hospitals, a difference associated in part with differences in regional hospital bed supply and the availability of community supports for the dying. Social and medical differences also account for some patterns. The need for institutionalization or paid caregivers in the last months of life is much higher among poor people and women. Similarly, elderly persons suffering from cognitive impairment and dementia are much more likely than cognitively intact elderly persons to spend their last days in a nursing home.

OVERALL CARE NEAR DEATH

The Hospitalized Elderly Longitudinal Project (HELP) attempted to characterize the last 6 months of life and dying in very old persons. It used a prospective study design, providing a retrospective characterization of the last 6 months of the lives of 1266 patients aged 80 and older. Results showed that patients tended to overestimate their chances of survival near the end of life. Patients who died within 1 year of enrollment had significant functional impairment in activities of daily living and expressed strong preferences for not being resuscitated and for comfort care. The number of patients reporting severe pain increased toward the end of life, with one in three reporting severe pain within 3 months of death. These results highlight the need for physicians to talk with their patients early about their preferences, as well as to provide better symptom control and palliative measures at the end of life.

Part of the challenge in providing excellent end-of-life care stems from the inability to adequately predict end of life. Through active research, we hope to be better able to predict death and thus better target efforts at palliation and facilitate setting of goals and expectations of care with patients and their families.

PALLIATIVE CARE AND HOSPICE

Palliative care, as defined here, seeks to prevent, relieve, reduce, or soothe the symptoms of disease or disorder without effecting cure. It attends closely to the emotional, spiritual, and practical needs and goals of patients and of those close to them. Palliative care is generally restricted to those who are at imminent risk of dying, as best as can be estimated, but is also important to those who are extremely ill or who are living with serious complications at the end stages of chronic disease.

Hospice as a Medicare health care benefit was established in 1982 by the federal government. Initially, hospice coverage was made available through an expanded Medicare benefit; now it is supported through a Medicare or Medicaid benefit, and it is also a benefit of most commercial insurances. The benefit is a highly regulated, fully capitated health care system, which is now implemented through more than 3000 hospice services, most nonprofit, and is dedicated to providing comprehensive palliative care for patients with all types of terminal illnesses and their families. Hospice is primarily a home-care program, with access to inpatient beds for the management of acute problems. Hospice receives one of four daily rates for reimbursement that are based on four levels of care: home care, inpatient level of care, continuous care, and respite care. The services hospice provides are summarized in Table 18.1.

Access to hospice is based on two conditions:

- A licensed physician must certify that he or she believes that the patient has a life expectancy of 6 months or less if the disease runs its expected course.

- The patient or proxy must elect hospice and thereby agree that the care plan with respect to the terminal illness will be managed by the hospice program.

The patient must be recertified on a regular basis. If the physician cannot state that life expectancy is still anticipated to be 6 months or less, then the patient must be discharged from hospice. The patient may revoke the hospice benefit at any time.

The referring physician must certify that the prognosis is 6 months or less and decide whether to remain the physician of record or refer the patient to the hospice medical director. If the referring physician remains the physician of record, he or she continues to direct the care of the patient, becomes part of the hospice interdisciplinary team, must coordinate treat-

Table 18.1—Hospice Services

- Care provided by an interdisciplinary team: nurse, social worker, chaplain, aides, volunteers, physical therapist, music therapist
- Case management by a hospice nurse
- Access to a hospice physician
- Drugs at no cost, as long as they are related to the terminal diagnosis and are palliative, as determined by the hospice plan of care
- Tests and other treatments at no cost, as long as they are related to the terminal diagnosis and are palliative, as determined by the hospice plan of care
- Durable medical equipment
- Bereavement services for 13 months after a death

ment decisions related to the terminal illness with the case manager (primary nurse), and may bill under Part B of Medicare or Medicaid.

See also "Financing, Coverage, and Costs of Health Care" (p 32).

COMMUNICATING BAD NEWS

The vast majority of Americans want to be told if they have a life-threatening illness. The ability to deliver bad news in an effective manner is an essential skill for physicians. However, physicians receive little formal training in communication skills, and as a result they may feel unprepared to deliver bad news. Others may fear that the news will adversely affect the patient and the family or the physician-patient relationship. A systematic approach to delivering bad news can foster collaboration among the patient, the family, and clinicians. Effective discussions can improve the patient's and the family's ability to plan for the future, set realistic goals, and support one another emotionally.

A six-step framework for communicating bad news can be used as a guide for these difficult conversations.

Step 1: Preparation

Discussions of bad news require careful preparation. Before delivering bad news to a patient, plan what will be discussed, ensure the medical facts, and ensure that all needed confirmation is available. Establishing the proper physical context is also important. Ideally, bad news should be delivered in person in a private area in which there will be no interruptions. Allot adequate time for discussions, minimize interruptions, and determine whether any support staff, family, or friends that the patient may want on hand are available.

Step 2: Establishing the Patient's Understanding

Begin the discussion by exploring the patient's knowledge of the illness. Patients with a thorough understanding of their illness require a different approach than an uninformed or less sophisticated patient. Useful questions to elicit this information include the following: "What do you understand about your illness?" "When you first had symptom x, what did you think it might be?" "What have other doctors told you about your condition or procedures that you have had?"

Step 3: What the Patient Wants to Know

Although the majority of Americans say they want to be fully informed about their illnesses, a substantial minority may not want to know the full details or may prefer to have another family member informed. Data suggests that this may be particularly true for certain ethnic groups. (See also "Cultural Aspects of Care," p 51.) Just as patients have the right to be told the truth, they also have the right to decline to learn unwanted information. Thus, it is crucial to establish how much each patient wants to know. Helpful questions to ask include the following: "If this condition turns out to be something serious, do you want to know?" "Would you like me to tell you the full details of your condition? If not, is there somebody else you would like me to talk to?"

Step 4: Telling the Patient

Once the physician has established the patient's understanding of the illness and willingness to hear bad news, it is time to tell the patient. Deliver information in a sensitive, straightforward manner, avoiding technical language or euphemisms. Frequently check for understanding and clarify difficult concepts and terms. Phrasing that includes a "warning shot" helps brace and prepare patients for the bad news. For example: "Mr. X, I feel bad to have to tell you this, but the growth turned out to be cancer." "The report is back, and it's not as we had hoped. It showed that there is cancer in your colon."

Step 5: Responding to Feelings

The responses of patients and families are both unpredictable and diverse. Active listening, encouraging the expression of emotion, and acknowledging patient's emotions are all important and helpful. Useful probes to help elicit an understanding of the patient's emotions include the following: "What does this news mean to you?" "What worries you the most?" "You appear angry. Can you tell me what you are feeling?" "Tell me more about how you are feeling about what I just said."

Step 6: Planning and Follow-Up

Finally, the physician should organize an immediate therapeutic plan that includes specific references to the patient's concerns and incorporates the patient's agenda. The plan should include an appointment for a follow-up visit; a discussion of additional tests, referrals, and sources of support; and information as to how you can be reached if additional questions arise. The physician also needs to ensure that the patient will be safe when he or she leaves the office.

PAIN

For assessing and treating pain, see "Persistent Pain" (p 140), which also includes a section on pain in cognitively impaired patients, and the section on postoperative pain management in 'Perioperative Care' (p 106).

PALLIATION OF NONPAIN SYMPTOMS

Constipation

Constipation is one of the most common and distressing symptoms seen in terminally ill patients. Constipation is a universal adverse effect of opioids, and it is exacerbated by the immobility and poor fluid intake that accompanies most serious and life-threatening illnesses. Other unwanted side effects of opioids generally diminish over time, but constipation can be expected to persist, requiring ongoing bowel management as long as opioid therapy is used. Patients on opioids should receive prophylactic laxatives consisting of a stool softener (eg, docusate sodium) and a bowel stimulant (eg, senna, bisacodyl) unless diarrhea has already been a problem. If these measures fail, then an osmotic laxative (eg, sorbitol, lactulose) should be added. Any time there has been no bowel movement within 4 or more days, an enema should be considered. Patients presenting with constipation should be evaluated for bowel obstruction or fecal impaction. If impaction is present, the patient should be disimpacted

manually or with enemas before laxative therapy is initiated. See also the section on postoperative gastrointestinal problems in "Perioperative Care" (p 104), especially Table 14.2.

Nausea and Vomiting

The incidence of nausea and vomiting is estimated to be between 40% and 70% in patients with advanced cancer. Symptoms may be caused by disease or its treatment, so it is first important to clarify the cause of the nausea and vomiting. Emesis is mediated centrally by the chemoreceptor trigger zone in the area postrema, in the floor of the fourth ventricle. Peripherally, emesis is mediated in the gut and in the vestibular apparatus. Various receptors are involved in the mediation of emesis (eg, serotonin [5-hydroxytryptamine or 5-HT], dopamine, histamine, acetylcholine), and the selection of an appropriate antiemetic agent should therefore seek to identify the likely cause, the pathway that is mediating symptoms, and the neurotransmitters involved (see Table 18.2).

Dopamine antagonists like haloperidol[OL], metoclopramide, or droperidol act primarily on the chemoreceptor trigger zone. Serotonin antagonists such as ondansetron or granisetron act in synergy with dopaminergic antagonists in the chemoreceptor trigger zone and additionally act peripherally in the gut. Muscarinic blockers such as scopolamine or meclizine are useful for patients with disturbed vestibular function. Prokinetic agents like metoclopramide can potentiate cholinergic activity in the gastrointestinal tract and are useful if the cause is gastroparesis. Antihistamines

Table 18.2—Treatment of Nausea and Vomiting

Site	Involved Receptors	Common Causes	Medications
Chemoreceptor trigger zone in the vomiting center	Dopamine Serotonin H_1	Drugs: opioids, digoxin, estrogen, cefotaxime Biochemical disorders: hypercalcemia, uremia Toxins: tumor-produced peptides, infection, radiotherapy, abnormal metabolites	Butyrophenones: eg, haloperidol[OL]; droperidol; phenothiazines: eg, prochlorperazine Prokinetic agents: eg, metoclopramide Serotonergic antagonists: eg, ondansetron, granisetron
Gut	Serotonin H_1	Gastric irritation (eg, drugs: alcohol, iron, mucolytics, expectorants; blood), tumors (external compression, intestinal obstruction), constipation, liver capsule stretch, peritoneal inflammation, gastric distension, stasis (eg, opioids), upper bowel, genitourinary, and biliary stasis	Serotonin antagonists, antihistamines, prokinetic agents
Vestibular apparatus	Muscarine Acetylcholine H_1	Toxic action of drugs: aspirin, opioids Motion sickness: Ménière's disease, labyrinthitis Local tumors: acoustic neuroma, brain tumors, bone metastases to base of skull	Antihistamines: eg, scopolamine, meclizine, hydrobromide
Cerebral cortex		Raised intracranial pressure	Dexamethasone

OL Not approved by the U.S. Food and Drug Administration for this use.

(eg, hydroxyzine[OL], dimenhydrinate) may be useful adjuvant agents when combined with either serotonergic or dopaminergic agents, although their side effects (eg, sedation, urinary retention, delirium) may limit their use in frail older adults. It is believed that these agents act on H_1 receptors in the vomiting center, vestibular afferents, and the gut. Serotonin-receptor blockers, including ondansetron, granisetron, and tropisetron, are very effective for radiotherapy- or chemotherapy-induced emesis. They do not reverse nausea mediated by dopamine pathways (eg, those that are opioid induced). Finally, corticosteroids possess intrinsic antiemetic properties and enhance the effect of other antiemetics. Corticosteroids are also useful for nausea and vomiting that is associated with increased intracranial pressure.

Diarrhea

Diarrhea, a relatively uncommon complaint of terminally ill patients, affects 7% to 10% of patients with cancer being admitted to hospice. Diarrhea is defined as the passage of more than three unformed stools within a 24-hour period. The clinician should be alert to the possibility of fecal impaction that presents as watery diarrhea, particularly in immobile older adults on opioids. Initiate the treatment of impaction with manual disimpaction and tapwater enemas, followed if unsuccessful by high colonic enemas. Laxatives should not be administered until the impaction is cleared because of the risk of bowel perforation. Untreated fecal impaction can be life threatening. Another common cause of diarrhea in palliative medicine is an excess of laxative therapy, especially after laxatives doses have been increased to clear an impaction. This will respond to temporary cessation of laxatives and reintroduction at a lower dosage. Radiotherapy involving the abdomen and pelvis causes diarrhea, peaking during the second or third week of therapy. This typically responds to cholestyramine 4 to 12 g three times a day. Diarrhea caused by fat malabsorption (eg, pancreatic insufficiency or small bowel disease) will respond to pancreatic enzymes such as pancreatin. Diarrhea following ileal resection also responds to cholestyramine.

Anorexia and Cachexia

Loss of appetite is almost a universal symptom of patients with serious and life-threatening illness. Anorexia in patients who are actively dying and who do not express a desire to eat should not be treated. Symptoms of dry mouth can be alleviated with ice chips, popsicles, moist compresses, or artificial saliva. Lemon glycerin swabs should not be used, because they irritate dry and cracked mucosa. Megestrol acetate and corticosteroids[OL] have been found to enhance appetite, cause weight gain (primarily fat), and improve quality of life in some patients with anorexia. These agents, however, have not been found to prolong survival, improve function, or improve treatment tolerance of cancer therapies and are associated with their own adverse effects. In general, patients should be encouraged to eat whatever is most appealing without regard to dietary restrictions.

Delirium

Delirium, agitation, and confusion are common in elderly terminally ill patients and are often distressing to both patients and family members. Initial efforts should be directed at identifying potentially reversible causes (eg, infection, impaction, uncontrolled pain, urinary retention, hypoxia). Antipsychotics like haloperidol[OL] or risperidone[OL] in low doses are effective treatments for both hypoactive and hyperactive delirium. Actively dying patients who are nonambulatory and who experience terminal delirium often appear less distressed with use of sedating antipsychotics, such as chlorpromazine. Because benzodiazepines are often associated with paradoxical agitation and a worsening of the delirium in older adults, their use should be carefully considered. (See also "Delirium," p 239.)

Depression

Depression is under-recognized and undertreated both in older adults and terminally ill patients. It may be underdiagnosed because of the clinician's mistaken belief that it is either a normal consequence of aging or appropriate in the context of a terminal illness. Because of the underlying illness, standard vegetative symptoms described in the fourth edition of the *Diagnostic and Statistical Manual of Mental Disorders* (insomnia, anorexia, weight change) are often not reliable indicators. Instead, the clinician should watch for change in mood, loss of interest, and suicidal ideation. Suicidal ideation should be openly discussed, including any symptoms that are contributing to the patient's suffering, which may be influencing his or her consideration of suicide. Aggressive treatment of symptoms, antidepressant therapy, and psychiatric consultation are all appropriate initial responses. Continued discussion with the patient about the wish to hasten death often reveals a change of mind as time passes.

Standard antidepressant therapy is effective, but most agents have a delayed onset of 2 to 6 weeks. Psychostimulants (methylphenidate[OL], dextroampheta-

---

[OL] Not approved by the U.S. Food and Drug Administration for this use.

mine[OL]) are well tolerated, safe, and effective treatments for medically ill depressed persons. Additionally, they have a rapid onset and beneficial effect on energy, mood, appetite, and mental alertness. Methylphenidate can be started at 2.5 mg in the early morning hours, can be given concurrently with standard antidepressants, and should be avoided in the evening hours. Finally, electroconvulsive therapy is an effective, safe method of rapidly treating depression and should be used for those who are severely depressed. The American Psychiatric Task Force Report states that electroconvulsive therapy be considered a first-line therapy when rapid response is needed. The presence of space-occupying central nervous system lesions is an important contraindication. (See also "Depression and Other Mood Disorders," p 277.)

Dyspnea

Dyspnea, the subjective experience of breathlessness, is one of the most distressing symptoms experienced by dying patients. Patient self-report is the only reliable measure of dyspnea, as respiratory rates and laboratory tests often do not correlate with breathlessness. Physicians may mistakenly fear that treating dyspnea in patients close to the end of life is associated with unacceptably high risks, leading some to withhold treatment and others to dose medications inadequately, which will not alleviate the patient's suffering.

There can be many causes of breathlessness (eg, anxiety, airway obstruction, bronchospasm, hypoxemia, pneumonia), so symptomatic management should begin immediately, while the underlying cause is being sought. Treatment should not be delayed in the pursuit of disease-modifying interventions. Like pain, dyspnea is mediated through the interaction of complex pathophysiologic processes with poorly defined psychologic factors. At a physiologic level, dyspnea results from the interplay of chemoreceptors in the respiratory tract and central nervous system, upper airway receptors that sense the mechanical effect of airflow or the temperature changes that accompany it, stretch receptors in chest wall skeletal muscles, irritant receptors in the airway epithelium, and C fibers located in the alveolar wall and blood vessels. The experience of dyspnea, however, depends on the modulation of these physiologic events by psychologic factors, and as a consequence, the patient's perception of dyspnea may not correlate well with objective signs, such as respiratory rate, pulmonary congestion, hypoxia, or hypercarbia.

The optimal therapy for dyspnea is to treat its underlying cause. When this is not possible, one of a number of agents that have been evaluated for the treatment of intractable dyspnea might be used. Oxygen is considered by many to be an important component of any regimen, although caution must be used for patients retaining carbon dioxide. Although oxygen is usually considered beneficial only when oxygen saturation falls below 90%, there are some circumstances when oxygen may reduce dyspnea when this saturation value is exceeded. Cool air moving across the face (eg, from fans or an open window) may also treat dyspnea by stimulating the second branch of the fifth cranial nerve (V2), which has a central inhibitory effect on the sensation of breathlessness.

In addition to oxygen, several centrally acting agents have been evaluated for the treatment of intractable dyspnea. Benzodiazepines may be beneficial in controlling the anxiety associated with dyspnea, but these agents have not been found to improve breathlessness in randomized controlled trials involving nonanxious persons with chronic obstructive pulmonary disease. The fact that respiratory depression can occur following the administration of benzodiazepines in normal adults suggests that these medications should be used only in breathless patients with an accompanying component of anxiety. Studies with phenothiazines, and the phenothiazine antihistamine promethazine, have shown mild improvement in dyspnea with their use. However, anticholinergic and sedative adverse effects may limit the use of these agents in elderly patients.

The most widely used centrally active agents for the treatment of dyspnea are opioids. Opioids are believed to act via a number of different mechanisms, although their predominant effect appears to be a reduction in the central respiratory responsiveness to carbon dioxide, resulting in a decrease in respiratory drive. The increase in Pco_2 that often accompanies this respiratory suppression can occasionally limit this approach in dyspnea management because of somnolence induced by the hypercarbia and by a decreased respiratory response to hypoxia. Opioids also appear to act centrally by decreasing the perception of dyspnea and peripherally on opioid receptors in the lung, perhaps by decreasing ventilatory response to, and oxygen cost of, exercise without affecting respiratory drive. Randomized controlled trials have shown both oral and parenteral formulations to be effective. Anecdotal evidence supports the use of nebulized morphine for intractable dyspnea, but studies supporting this approach are lacking. The advantages of nebulized morphine include the avoidance of systemic absorption and the resulting constipation, hypotension, sedation, respiratory depression, and hypercapnia; rapid and efficient absorption because of the large surface area of the lung parenchyma; and the ease of administration. Randomized controlled trials employing nebulized morphine have not demonstrated consistent benefit, and this

---

OL. Not approved by the U.S. Food and Drug Administration for this use.

route of administration should be reserved for patients who experience intolerable adverse effects from opioids administered by other routes.

Cough

Cough is a common symptom whose prevalence has been reported in the palliative care literature as ranging from 29% to 83%. Normal cough maintains the patency and cleanliness of the airways and thus should be treated only when distressing to the patient. Cough can be caused by the production of excessive amounts of fluids (eg, blood, mucus), inhalation of foreign material, or stimulation of irritant receptors in the airway. Additionally, patients with neuromuscular disorders may be unable to swallow saliva because of the involvement of bulbar cranial nerves, with the result that saliva causes coughing as it trickles into the larynx or trachea.

Underlying causes of cough should be sought and treated (eg, diuretics for heart failure, antibiotics for infection, anticholinergics for aspiration of saliva resulting from motor neuron disease); however, resolution of the underlying cause may be impossible. Opioids can be useful in these situations.

Dextromethorphan is structurally related to opioids and has central cough-suppressant action with few sedative effects. Codeine and dihydrocodeine, usually in the form of elixirs, are also good first-line choices. Methadone syrup may also be helpful when taken as a single dose because of its longer duration of action.

Cough due to an irritated pharynx because of local infection or malignancy may be helped by nebulized anesthetics. Nebulized lidocaine up to four times daily has been reported, anecdotally, to offer relief.

See also the section on intensive care for critically ill patients in "Respiratory Diseases and Disorders" (p 330).

ANNOTATED REFERENCES

- Buckman R. *How to Break Bad News: A Guide for Health Care Professionals.* Baltimore, MD: The John Hopkins University Press; 1992.

    This book provides a step-by-step guide for breaking bad news to patients and their family members. This readable and practical how-to manual describes the core skills required in order to communicate bad news.

- Doyle D, Hanks GWC, Macdonald N, eds. *Oxford Textbook of Palliative Medicine.* 2nd ed. Oxford, England: Oxford University Press; 1998.

    This is a comprehensive text of palliative care medicine. The *Oxford Textbook* summarizes approaches to pain and symptom management, addresses different delivery systems of palliative care, and summarizes other important topics in palliative care

(bereavement, communication, psychological distress). It is a core reference for anyone interested in palliative medicine.

- Field M.J, Cassel CK. *Approaching Death: Improving Care at the End of Life.* Washington, DC: National Academy Press for the Institute of Medicine; 1997.

    This report summarizes the status of palliative care in the United States and outlines a clinical, research, educational, and policy agenda to improve the care received by dying patients.

- Gloth FM 3rd. *Handbook of Pain Relief in Older Adults: An Evidence-Based Approach.* Totawa, NJ: Humana Press; 2003.

    This book is a useful introduction to pain management in the elderly patient. It covers pain assessment, management (including both pharmacotherapies as well as a somewhat limited discussion of behavioral modalities, such as rehabilitation), and some political issues that apply only to the United States. Informative chapters discuss the role of spirituality in the perception and treatment of pain and the use of neutriceuticals. It includes a detailed table of analgesic medications, including starting doses, maximum doses, and special considerations for the elderly patient.

- Gloth FM 3rd. Pain management in older adults: prevention and treatment. *J Am Geriatr Soc.* 2001; 49(2):188–199.

    This article summarizes the available literature about strategies for relieving pain in older persons. Pain scales designed for older persons, pharmacologic advances, alternative medicine, and progress in the identification of nonopioid pain receptors are addressed. The importance of clinician education about the appropriate use of assessment tools, therapeutic interventions, and hospice is emphasized.

- Jacox A, Carr DB, Payne R, et al. *Management of Cancer Pain. Clinical Practice Guideline No. 9.* Rockville, MD: US Department of Health and Human Services, Public Health Service, Agency for Health Care Policy and Research. March 1994. AHCPR Pub. No. 94-0592/3.

    This is an excellent overview and guideline for pain management in chronically ill patients. It provides an evidence-based approach to the assessment and management of pain in cancer patients. The guidelines can and should be used for the management of other chronic pain syndromes. Companion publications are available for patients.

- Morrison RS, Meier DE, eds. *Geriatric Palliative Care.* New York: Oxford University Press; 2003.

    This comprehensive text covers important management principles for treating a variety of disabling diseases as well as specific symptoms and includes discussion of cultural aspects of death and dying. The focus of the text is clinical, with emphasis on communication with patients and families to maximize patient-centered care. Clinicians who care for chronically ill patients will find this a useful reference.

- Phillips RS, Hamel MB, Covinsky KE, et al. Findings from SUPPORT and HELP: Study to Understand Prognoses and Preferences for Outcomes and Risks of Treatment; Hospitalized Elderly Longitudinal Project. *J Am Geriatr Soc.* 2000;48 (suppl 5):S1–S233.

This supplement focuses on findings from the SUPPORT and HELP studies and includes 29 articles with new analyses and conclusions concerning issues of end-of-life care directly related to older adults.

■ Standards and Accreditation Committee, Medical Guidelines Task Force. *Medical Guidelines for Determining Prognosis in Selected Non-Cancer Diseases.* 2nd ed. Arlington, VA: National Hospice Organization; 1996.

These guidelines were developed to help identify patients with nononcologic terminal illness who might benefit from hospice services. Guidelines for determining the prognosis in heart disease, pulmonary disease, dementia, human immunodeficiency virus, liver disease, renal disease, stroke and coma, and amyotrophic lateral sclerosis are offered.

■ SUPPORT Principal Investigators. A controlled trial to improve care for seriously ill hospitalized patients: The Study to Understand Prognoses and Preferences for Outcomes and Risks of Treatment (SUPPORT). *JAMA.* 1995;274(20):1591–1598.

This report summarizes the major finding from SUPPORT, a landmark study that examined the experience of dying in an American hospital for over 9000 adults with a serious and life-threatening illness. It describes the needs of patients living with a serious and life-threatening illness, identifies gaps in medical care, and suggests areas for improvement.

Stacie T. Pinderhughes, MD
R. Sean Morrison, MD

CHAPTER 19—PERSISTENT PAIN

KEY POINTS

■ Pain requires a thorough assessment to determine its source, severity, and impact on the functioning and well-being of the patient.

■ Multiple pain scales are available to help quantify the severity of pain. The selection of a pain scale is based on the cognitive and communication abilities of the patient.

■ A stepped approach to the treatment of pain is advised; local therapies, such as heat, cold, or massage, should be considered to alleviate the need for or reduce the amount of systemic therapies that have greater risk of toxicity.

■ Tolerance generally develops to the respiratory depression, fatigue, and sedation effects of opioid analgesics but not to the constipating effect.

Pain, defined as an unpleasant sensory and emotional experience, is common in older persons aged 65 and older. Studies have revealed that 25% to 50% of community-dwelling older adults and 45% to 80% of nursing-home residents have substantial pain. It is also believed to be commonly undertreated. This is due to several factors: some older adults tend to minimize or not report their symptoms, and others are unable to report their pain because of language or cognitive impairments. Also, clinicians may inadequately assess pain or undertreat it with ineffective therapies or encounter intolerable adverse effects with more effective therapies. This chapter describes the evaluation and treatment of persistent pain. Chronic or persistent pain,

in contrast to acute pain, is pain lasting 3 to 6 months or more after the original injury has healed, pain that is associated with a chronic medical condition, or pain that recurs at intervals of a month to years.

Persistent pain is complex, involving an amalgamation of physical, social, and psychologic factors. Untreated, it can result in difficulty performing activities of daily living, cognitive dysfunction, depression, anxiety, social isolation, appetite impairment, and sleep disorders. Lastly, patients with chronic pain accrue greater health care costs than do patients who are pain-free.

ASSESSMENT

A major barrier to effective pain treatment is inadequate assessment. A thorough assessment is necessary to formulate a plan to successfully treat persistent pain. This assessment should include an examination of physical, emotional, and social function, recognizing the considerable impact that each of these domains has on the experience of pain and suffering. Since there are no blood tests or imaging modalities to measure pain objectively, clinicians must rely on the patient's or caregiver's description of the pain and on the findings of a thorough physical examination. The goal of the assessment is to identify the source of the pain so that it can be treated with the most effective, targeted, and specific treatment known. The evaluation of older persons is complicated by several challenges, including under-reporting of symptoms by many older persons, the existence of multiple medical comorbidities exacerbating the pain and impairing the function of the patient, and the increased prevalence of cognitive impairment as people age.

Initial evaluation begins with a complete history of the pain, including inquiry about the character of the pain, the course of its onset, its duration, and its location. Patients should be asked what relieves and exacerbates their pain. The patient's functional status needs to be carefully evaluated to determine his or her ability to perform activities of daily living and instrumental activities of daily living. The patient's cognitive state, participation in social activities, mood, and quality of life are all components of a complete evaluation.

Pain intensity can be quantified using pain intensity scales. Three commonly used validated scales are the Numeric Rating Scale, the Faces Pain Scale, and the Verbal Descriptor Scale. These scales are referred to as unidimensional because they ask the patient to rate the intensity of a single characteristic of the symptom, in this case the intensity of the pain. The patient is asked to rate his or her pain by assigning a numerical value (with zero indicating no pain and 10 representing the worst pain imaginable), a verbal description ("no pain" to "pain as bad as it could be"), or a facial expression corresponding to the pain. The choice of scale depends on the presence of a particular language or sensory impairment. For example, if the patient does not speak English well, the faces scale may be the best choice because it relies on pictures rather than words or numbers. The same scale should be used at follow-up examinations to evaluate how the pain has changed since the initial assessment. Scales such as the McGill Pain Questionnaire and the Pain Disability Scale measure pain in a variety of domains, including the intensity, location, and affect. Although long, scales measuring multiple domains can provide a wealth of information about the patient's unique experience of pain.

Before the physical examination, the patient can describe the location of the pain using a drawing of a human figure, called a pain map. The patient is asked to indicate the locations on the figure that corresponds to their own pain. Pain maps can enhance patient-clinician communication. If the patient's pain pattern is erratic and diffuse and therefore nonsensical anatomically, referral to a mental health specialist may be appropriate.

The physical examination should include a careful examination of the reported site of the pain and any part of the body that may be a source of referred pain. Experts suggest that the initial evaluation should include a complete musculoskeletal examination, recognizing the common finding of a musculoskeletal disorder such as fibromyalgia, osteoarthritis, and myofascial pain as either the primary source of pain or an exacerbating process. Accurate diagnosis of these disorders is a critical part of formulating the correct therapeutic plan (see the section, below, on treatment). Fibromyalgia is an under-recognized but not uncommon disorder in older adults. It is typically characterized by multiple tender points, sleep disturbance, fatigue, generalized pain (often with a strong axial component), and morning stiffness. (See also the section on fibromyalgia in "Musculoskeletal Diseases and Disorders," p 432.) Myofascial pain is present in the vast majority of patients with persistent pain and is diagnosed by the presence of taut bands of muscles and trigger points (ie, pain that may radiate distally upon application of firm pressure to a muscle, as opposed to tender points, in which radiation of pain is absent).

Pain syndromes can be divided into at least three types: nociceptive, neuropathic, and mixed or unspecified. Nociceptive pain describes pain due to the activation of nociceptive sensory receptors by noxious stimuli resulting from inflammation, swelling, and injury to tissues. It can be defined further as either somatic or visceral pain. Somatic pain is well localized in skin, soft tissue, and bone. It is commonly described as throbbing, aching, and stabbing. Visceral pain, due to cardiac, gastrointestinal, and lung injury, is not well localized and difficult to describe. Patients describe visceral pain as crampy, tearing, dull, and aching. Neuropathic pain derives from the irritation of components of the central or peripheral nervous system. Patients typically report burning, numbness with "pins and needles" sensations, and shooting pains. Common causes of neuropathic pain include post-herpetic neuralgia, post-stroke central pain, and phantom limb pain experienced following amputation. Nociceptive pain is often adequately treated with common analgesics. Neuropathic pain responds unpredictably to opioid analgesia; it may respond well to nonopioid therapies such as anticonvulsants, tricyclic antidepressants (TCAs), and antiarrhythmic medications. Confusion between neuropathic pain and myofascial pain is possible, as patients may describe both as "burning." Careful physical examination will help to differentiate these disorders (ie, taut bands and trigger points with myofascial pain and allodynia or hyperalgesia with either disorder), although both may exist in the same patient. Mixed or unspecified pain is described as having characteristics of both nociceptive pain and neuropathic pain. An example of a mixed pain syndrome is chronic headaches of unknown causes. It may be necessary to treat these patients with trials of different medications or with combinations of medicines. Older adults often have mixed pain syndromes. Lower back pain, for example, is often a combination of spinal malalignment, myofascial pathology, and neurologic impingement.

Assessing and Treating Pain in Cognitively Impaired Persons

While they are able to speak, patients with mild to moderate dementia are often able to self-report pain and localize it. Patients with severe cognitive impairment who are unable to verbally express pain pose a challenge to the clinicians who care for them. Not only are they unable to describe the pain and request analgesia, but clinicians are hesitant to administer pain medications, fearing that drugs will worsen the patients' mental status. Clinicians must rely on observing the patient for possible pain-related behaviors as well as observations noted by the patient's caregivers. Table 19.1 lists common pain behaviors in cognitively impaired older adults. Validated scales such as the Hurley Discomfort Scale and the Checklist of Nonverbal Pain Indicators have been developed; however, these require trained evaluators to complete properly. Experts suggest providing empiric analgesic therapy during procedures and conditions known to be painful. Trials of analgesia should also be considered for patients exhibiting pain-related behaviors.

Table 19.1—Common Pain Behaviors in Cognitively Impaired Elderly Persons

Behavior	Examples
Facial expressions	Slight frown; sad, frightened face
	Grimacing, wrinkled forehead, closed or tightened eyes
	Any distorted expression
	Rapid blinking
Verbalizations, vocalizations	Sighing, moaning, groaning
	Grunting, chanting, calling out
	Noisy breathing
	Asking for help
	Verbal abusiveness
Body movements	Rigid, tense body posture, guarding
	Fidgeting
	Increased pacing, rocking
	Restricted movement
	Gait or mobility changes
Changes in interpersonal interactions	Aggressive, combative, resists care
	Decreased social interactions
	Socially inappropriate, disruptive
	Withdrawn
Changes in activity patterns or routines	Refusing food, appetite change
	Increase in rest periods
	Sleep, rest pattern changes
	Sudden cessation of common routines
	Increased wandering
Mental status changes	Crying or tears
	Increased confusion
	Irritability or distress

NOTE: Some patients demonstrate little or no specific behavior associated with severe pain.

SOURCE: AGS Panel on Persistent Pain in Older Persons. The management of persistent pain in older persons. *J Am Geriatr Soc.* 2002; 50(6 Suppl): S211. Reprinted with permission

Treatment

Fundamental Approaches to Pain Treatment

A comprehensive review of nonpharmacologic therapies for persistent pain is beyond the scope of this chapter; however, specific therapies are worth mentioning. Many of the strategies mentioned below are appropriate suggestions for all patients' treatment plans.

Patient education and involvement in treatment decisions are an important part of all treatment plans for persistent pain. Patients should be taught how to take medications properly and how to use assessment instruments. They can be given information on the use of nonpharmacologic treatments such as heat and cold application, massage therapy, and transcutaneous electrical nerve stimulation. Cognitive behavioral therapy may be particularly useful in helping patients learn to cope with the stresses of persistent pain. When possible, family members and caregivers should be included in the therapy.

Regular physical activity has been shown to improve mood, boost functional status, and stabilize gait. Referral to the Arthritis Foundation or community resources such as the YMCA for exercise classes can be considered for many patients. Others who are frail may require closely monitored rehabilitation services. The goals should include improvements in flexibility, strength, endurance, and function, with reduction in pain and improved quality of life.

Patients with persistent pain that do not respond to first-line treatment efforts should, if possible, be referred to a pain clinic that is geared toward interdisciplinary team treatment. Suboptimal treatment response should not be viewed as a permanent state, but as an opportunity for input from specialists who have additional expertise in treating these difficult problems.

See also "Complementary and Alternative Medicine" (p 80).

Pharmacologic Therapy

Individual analgesics, with their starting doses and common adverse effects, are listed in Table 19.2.

Pharmacologic therapy for patients with persistent pain should be viewed not as an end, but as a means to promote improved function and enhance adherence

Table 19.2—Systemic Pharmacotherapy for Persistent Pain Management

Drug	Starting Dose*	Usual Effective Dose (Maximum Dose)	Titration	Comments
NONOPIOIDS				
Acetaminophen (Tylenol)	325 mg q 4 h–500 mg q 6 h	2–4 g/24 h (4 g/24 h)	after 4–6 doses	Reduce maximum dose 50%–75% in patients with hepatic insufficiency, history of alcohol abuse
Anticonvulsants Carbamazepine[OL] (Tegretol)	100 mg qd	800–1200 mg/24 h (2400 mg/day)	after 3–5 days	Monitor liver enzymes, CBC, BUN/Creat., electrolytes. Approved only for trigeminal neuralgia and glossopharyngeal neuralgia; not approved for any other types of pain
Clonazepam[OL] (Klonopin)	0.25–0.5 mg hs	0.05–0.2 mg/kg/day (20 mg)	after 3–5 days	Monitor sedation, memory, CBC
Gabapentin[OL] (Neurontin)	100 mg hs	300–900 mg tid (3600 mg)	after 1–2 days	Monitor sedation, ataxia, edema. Approved for post-herpetic neuralgia; not approved for any other types of pain
Pregabalin (Lyrica)	25 mg tid	100 mg tid (200 mg tid)	may not be necessary; precise recommendations pending	Approved by FDA December 2004, made available September 2005; designated Schedule C-V. Dizziness and somnolence are the most troubling adverse effects. Use caution when CrCl < 30
Baclofen[OL] (Lioresal)	5 mg	5–20 mg bid–tid (200 mg)	after 3–5 days	Monitor muscle weakness, urinary function; avoid abrupt discontinuation because of CNS irritability
Choline magnesium trisalicylate (Tricosal, Trilisate)	500–750 mg q 8 h	2000–3000 mg/24 h (same)	after 4–6 doses	Long half-life may allow qd or bid dosing after steady state is reached. In frail patients or those with diminished hepatic or renal function, it may be important to check salicylate levels during dose titration and after steady state is reached
Corticosteroids (prednisone) (eg, Deltasone, Liquid Pred, Orasone)	5.0 mg qd	variable (NA)	after 2–3 doses	Use lowest possible dose to prevent chronic steroid effects; anticipate fluid retention and glycemic effects
Mexiletine[OL] (Mexitil)	150 mg	150 mg tid–qid (variable)	after 3–5 days	Avoid use in patients with conduction block, bradyarrhythmia; monitor ECG
Salsalate (eg, Disalcid, Mono-Gesic, Salflex)	500–750 mg q 12 h	1500–3000 mg/24 h (3000 mg/24h)	after 4–6 doses	In frail patients or those with diminished hepatic or renal function, it may be important to check salicylate levels during dose titration and after steady state is reached
Tricyclic antidepressants:** desipramine[OL] (Norpramin), nortriptyline[OL] (Aventyl, Pamelor)	10 mg hs	25–100 mg hs (variable)	after 3–5 days	Significant risk of adverse effects in older patients; anticholinergic effects

(table continued on next page)

[OL] Not approved by the U.S. Food and Drug Administration for this use.

Table 19.2—Systemic Pharmacotherapy for Persistent Pain Management (continued)

Drug	Starting Dose*	Usual Effective Dose (Maximum Dose)	Titration	Comments
		OPIOIDS		
Hydrocodone (eg, Lorcet, Lortab, Vicodin, Vicoprofen)	5 mg q 4–6 h	5–10 mg (see comments)	after 3–4 doses	Useful for acute recurrent, episodic, or breakthrough pain; daily dose limited by fixed-dose combinations with acetaminophen or NSAIDs
Hydromorphone (Dilaudid, Hydrostat)	2 mg q 3–4 h	variable (variable)	after 3–4 doses	For breakthrough pain or for around-the-clock dosing
Morphine, immediate release (eg, MSIR, Roxanol)	2.5–10 mg q 4 h	variable (variable)	after 1–2 doses	Oral liquid concentrate recommended for breakthrough pain
Morphine, sustained release (eg, MSContin, Kadian)	15 mg q 12 h	variable (variable)	after 3–5 days	Usually started after initial dose determined by effects of immediate-release opioid; toxic metabolites of morphine may limit usefulness in patients with renal insufficiency or when high-dose therapy is required; continuous-release formulations may require more frequent dosing if end-of-dose failure occurs regularly
Oxycodone, immediate release (OxyIR)	5 mg q 4–6 h	5–10 mg (see comments)	after 3–4 doses	Useful for acute recurrent, episodic, or breakthrough pain; daily dose limited by fixed-dose combinations with acetaminophen or NSAIDs
Oxycodone, sustained release (OxyContin)	10 mg q 12 h	variable (variable)	after 3–5 days	Usually started after initial dose determined by effects of immediate-release opioid
Tramadol (Ultram)	25 mg q 4–6 h	50–100 mg (300 mg/24 h)	after 4–6 doses	Mixed opioid and central neurotransmitter mechanism of action; monitor for opioid side effects, including drowsiness and nausea. Exert caution when used with another serotonergic drug, and observe for symptoms of serotonergic syndrome. Lowers seizure threshold.
Transdermal fentanyl (Duragesic)	25 µg/h patch q 72 h	variable (variable)	after 2–3 patch changes	Usually started after initial dose determined by effects of immediate-release opioid; currently available lowest dose patch (25 µg/h) recommended for patients who require 60 mg per 24-h oral morphine equivalents; peak effect of first dose takes 18–24 h. Duration of effect is usually 3 days, but may range from 48 h to 96 h

NOTE: ASA = acetylsalicylic acid; bid = twice daily; BUN = blood urea nitrogen; CBC = complete blood cell count; CNS = central nervous system; CrCl = creatinine clearance; Creat. = serum creatinine; CV = cardiovascular; DEA = U.S. Drug Enforcement Agency; ECG = electrocardiogram; FDA = U.S. Food and Drug Administration; GI = gastrointestinal; h = hour; hs = at bedtime; NA = not applicable; NSAIDs = nonsteroidal anti-inflammatory drugs; q = each, every; qd = daily; qid = four times daily; tid = three times daily.

* Oral dosing unless otherwise specified.

** Amitriptyline is not recommended.

SOURCE: Adapted from AGS Panel on Persistent Pain in Older Persons. The management of persistent pain in older persons. *J Am Geriatr Soc.* 2002; 50(6 Suppl): S214–S215. Reprinted with permission. For comprehensive, regularly updated information on drugs for pain, see the online version of *Geriatrics At Your Fingertips* at http://www.geriatricsatyourfingertips.org (accessed October 2005).

with rehabilitation efforts. When initiating pharmacologic therapy in older adults, it is important to consider the balance of risks and benefits of the treatment. If appropriate, nonsystemic therapies should be tried first. For example, patients that primarily have knee pain might respond to intra-articular corticosteroid injections, avoiding the need for systemic analgesics. Patients with myofascial pain often respond to local modalities such as massage, gentle stretching exercises, ultrasound, and trigger-point injections. Topical preparations such as capsaicin or ketamine gel[OL] or lidocaine patches might be effective as primary or adjunctive therapy in the treatment of patients with neuropathic or myofascial pain syndromes. If these modalities are ineffective and a decision is made to begin systemic therapy, patients will need to be monitored closely to ensure that the treatment is effective and adverse effects are minimized. Choice of initial dose and rate of titration depends on the individual patient's physiology, which varies considerably in older persons. As a general rule, when starting opioid therapy it is prudent to start with the lowest dose possible and to titrate slowly. That said, patients who are in a pain crisis should not have medications withheld. Rather, they need to be monitored closely to ensure that the dose can be safely and adequately escalated.

Mild to moderate pain can commonly be treated with acetaminophen or cautious use of nonsteroidal anti-inflammatory drugs (NSAIDs). Acetaminophen has been shown to provide adequate analgesia for many mild to moderate pain syndromes, particularly musculoskeletal pain. No more than 4 g of acetaminophen every 24 hours should be administered to patients with normal hepatic and renal function, given the risk of hepatotoxicity. Caution should be taken with treating patients at risk for liver dysfunction, particularly those who have a history of heavy alcohol intake. In these patients, the dose should be lowered by 50%, or acetaminophen should be avoided. Because acetaminophen is commonly contained in many over-the-counter and prescription products, knowledge of all medications that a patient is taking is critical to avoiding acetaminophen toxicity. NSAIDs are effective drugs for the treatment of mild to moderate pain and may be useful when acute exacerbations of pain are not controlled with acetaminophen. However, significant adverse effects, including renal dysfunction, gastrointestinal (GI) bleeding, platelet dysfunction, fluid retention, and precipitation of delirium limit their use in the treatment of older persons' chronic pain. COX-2 inhibitors were developed to decrease the risk of GI bleeding by acting on a more selective receptor, but the risk for renal complications, including hypertension, remains the same as with other NSAIDs, and the degree to which longer term GI toxicity is reduced is not clear. Several studies have confirmed high cardiovascular risks associated with COX-2 inhibitors, which is now believed to be a class effect. Though one is currently still on the market, the COX-2s certainly should be considered with caution if at all in older individuals. Misoprostol, a prostaglandin analog, or a proton-pump inhibitor may be used to reduce the risk of NSAID-induced GI bleeding, but this does not reduce the risks of renal disease, hypertension, fluid retention, or delirium. Alternatively, nonacetylated salicylates such as salsalate and trisalicylate may have less renal toxicity and antiplatelet activity than other NSAIDs and therefore may be preferable in older persons, though evidence supporting this theory is sparse.

Moderate to severe pain or pain that requires chronic treatment often requires opioid medications to provide sufficient relief. In general, continuous pain should be treated with 24-hour pain medications in long-acting or sustained-release formulations after opioid requirements are estimated on the basis of an initial trial of a short-acting agent. These may be combined with fast-onset medications with short half-lives to cover breakthrough pain. A typical patient requires approximately 5% to 15% the daily dose offered every 2 hours orally for breakthrough pain. In general, different opioids provide similar analgesic efficacy. Cost and route of delivery can help guide the choice of medication.

Opioids are metabolized by the liver and excreted by the kidney. In kidney failure, the active metabolites of morphine, including morphine-6-glucuronide and morphine-3-glucuronide, can accumulate, which places the patient at increased risk for prolonged sedation. The dosing intervals should be increased or the dose lowered to reduce this risk. Some experts and limited data suggest that oxycodone is safer in kidney failure because its metabolism results in fewer active metabolites, but this remains controversial.

Barriers to Using Opioids in Older Persons

Older persons may have concerns about addiction and tolerance that keep them from accepting adequate treatment for their pain. Patients may fear that taking opioid therapy for their current level of pain will result in the pain medicines' losing their effectiveness in the future when pain becomes more severe. They may fear addiction to the medicines. In fact, fear of addiction is a major obstacle to prescribing medications to older adults. A frank discussion of these concerns may help to alleviate these fears.

[OL] Not approved by the U.S. Food and Drug Administration for this use.

Physical dependence is an expected change in a patient's physiology that occurs while a patient is receiving chronic, continuous opioid medications. If opioids are discontinued suddenly, a patient who is physically dependent will experience a withdrawal syndrome that may include restlessness, tachycardia, hypertension, fever, tremors, and lacrimation. Symptoms of withdrawal can be avoided by tapering opioids carefully over days to weeks. *Tolerance* refers to a change in physiology resulting in the need to increase opioid medicines over time to achieve adequate analgesic effect. Experts note that tolerance to analgesia, as opposed to tolerance to sedation and respiratory depression, develops slowly in stable disease. If a rapid titration of medicines is required to reduce pain, the cause of the pain should be evaluated, including searching for new pathologies and exacerbation of known sources of pain, as well as consideration of nonphysical factors. Of note, there is limited cross-tolerance between different opioids. Therefore, when switching a patient from one opioid to another (eg, morphine to oxycodone), the clinician should reduce the dose to 50% to 65% of the equivalent dose.

Psychological *dependence*, or true *addiction*, refers to a psychiatric state defined by compulsive drug seeking and drug using with disregard for adverse social, physical, and economic consequences. It is very rare for patients who have chronic pain to become addicted to opioids. Addiction must be distinguished from *pseudo-addiction*, which refers to a patient with significant unrelieved pain who adopts behaviors similar to those of truly addicted patients while seeking relief from suffering, but generally with less prominent disregard for adverse social, physical, and economic consequences.

Adverse Effects of Opioids

The most common adverse effect of opioid treatment is constipation. Opioid-induced constipation is due to multiple mechanisms, including dehydration, decreased GI tract secretions, and decreased motility of the GI tract. Although tolerance develops fairly rapidly to other adverse effects of opioids, such as respiratory depression and sedation, constipation usually complicates opioid use for the duration of treatment. Therefore, education regarding the probable need for a laxative is recommended for all patients at the time opioid therapy is initiated. Many experts recommend starting therapy with a stimulant laxative (such as bisacodyl or senna); however, these should be avoided in any patient with signs or symptoms of bowel obstruction. Bulking agents such as fiber and psyllium should be avoided in patients who are inactive and who have poor oral intake, given the risk of causing stool impaction and obstruction. All patients should be encouraged to exercise, as they are able, and to stay well hydrated.

Nausea and vomiting are common side effects of opioids. They have a direct effect on the part of the brain associated with the sensation of vomiting called the *chemoreceptor trigger zone*. Other common causes of nausea and vomiting in patients taking opioids include gastroparesis, constipation, and metabolic disorders such as renal and hepatic failure. Although the nausea and vomiting is usually self-limited to the first few doses, some patients experience chronic nausea. After evaluation for reversible causes of nausea such as constipation, some patients benefit from changing to an alternative opioid. Others may need to be treated with chronic antiemetics, accepting the high prevalence of adverse effects in older adults treated with these medications, including drowsiness, delirium, and anticholinergic effects.

Older persons may experience sedation, fatigue, and mild cognitive impairment with opioid treatment. These changes commonly occur during dose adjustment. Patients commonly overcome the fatigue and sedation over days to weeks as they become tolerant to the medication. They need to be warned of the risks of increased falls and asked not to drive or operate heavy equipment when the medication is initiated. A small subset of patients treated with opioids experience incessant fatigue that limits their function significantly. A limited course of a stimulant such as low-dose methylphenidate could reasonably be tried in this situation. Rotation to a different opioid is an alternative strategy used to alleviate opioid-induced fatigue.

Respiratory depression is a feared complication of opioid therapy. Older persons and persons with a history of lung dysfunction are at particular risk when opioid doses are increased too rapidly. Naloxone, an opioid receptor antagonist, can reverse opioid-induced respiratory depression; however, when it is given to a patient who has been treated chronically with opioids, it can precipitate a pain crisis and acute withdrawal symptoms. Experts suggest withholding naloxone unless the patient's respiratory rate decreases to less than 8 breaths per minute or the oxygen saturation drops to below 90%. When it is needed, naloxone should be titrated carefully, using the lowest dose possible.

Nonopioid Medication to Treat Persistent Pain

Nonopioid or adjuvant medications can be used as the sole agent or in combination with opioids. These medications may be particularly useful in treating patients with neuropathic pain or mixed pain syndromes.

Tricyclic antidepressants (TCAs) are the most extensively studied medications for neuropathic pain, though none of the TCAs has been approved for the treatment of pain. Their efficacy in the treatment of post-herpetic neuralgia and diabetic neuropathy has been exhibited in numerous placebo-controlled studies. However, they are associated with significant anticholinergic adverse effects in older persons, including constipation, urinary retention, dry mouth, cognitive impairment, tachycardia, and blurred vision. Of note, desipramine[OL] and nortriptyline[OL] may have fewer adverse effects than amitriptyline[OL].

Clinical depression in patients with persistent pain requires treatment to effect optimal analgesia and quality of life. Other classes of antidepressants (eg, selective serotonin-reupake inhibitors) have generally been less studied than TCAs as analgesics, but older adults typically tolerate these agents better than TCAs when they are used in antidepressant doses. Duloxetine, an inhibitor of norepinephrine and serotonin uptake, is approved as both an antidepressant and for the treatment of pain from diabetic neuropathy.

Antiepileptic drugs such as carbamazepine (approved for some types of neuropathic pain), gabapentin, and clonazepam[OL] are commonly used as treatments for neuropathic pain. Gabapentin has demonstrated clinical efficacy in the treatment of post-herpetic neuralgia, and it has considerably fewer adverse effects than TCAs, though its cost is substantially more. The main side effects of gabapentin are sedation and dizziness, which frequently limit dose escalation.

Corticosteroids are useful adjuvants to treat pain associated with swelling, inflammation, and tissue infiltration, as well as neuropathic pain. In addition to their analgesic properties, they also may increase appetite and improve energy. Adverse effects occurring with short-term use of steroids include psychosis, fluid retention, hair loss, loss of skin integrity, hyperglycemia, and immunosuppression. Intravenous bisphosphonates may substantially reduce pain from malignant bone metastases.

Medications to Avoid in Older Persons

Several medications should not be administered to older persons. Propoxyphene (Darvon) is an older opioid medication used to treat mild to moderate pain. However, research and clinical experience has shown that the drug may accumulate in older persons and cause ataxia and dizziness as well as tremulousness and seizures. It has also never been shown to be more a more effective analgesic than placebo. Meperidine

(Demerol) is metabolized to normeperidine, a substance that has no analgesic properties but that can accumulate in patients with decreased kidney function and cause tremulousness, myoclonus, and seizures. Neither of these medications is recommended for use in older persons.

Tramadol (Ultram) has combined mechanisms of opioid-receptor binding and norepinephrine- and serotonin-reuptake inhibition. It can lower the seizure threshold and is therefore not recommended for patients with a history of seizures or taking other medications that could lower the seizure threshold. Caution should also be exercised in patients taking other medications with serotonergic properties to avoid serotonin syndrome (myoclonus, agitation, abdominal cramping, hyperpyrexia, hypertension, and potentially death).

Mixed agonist-antagonists such as nalbuphine and butorphanol also have the potential to cause restlessness and tremulousness and therefore should be avoided in older persons. Because of high risks of GI and renal toxicity and substantial risk of delirium in older individuals, NSAIDs should be used cautiously. As mentioned previously, COX-2 inhibitors have been shown to increase the risk of cardiovascular events, in addition to the risks associated with the nonselective NSAIDs.

ANNOTATED REFERENCES

■ AGS Panel on Persistent Pain in Older Persons. The management of persistent pain in older persons. *J Am Geriatr Soc.* 2002;50(6 Suppl): S205–S224.

> The American Geriatrics Society gathered a multidisciplinary panel of experts in the treatment of older persons' pain to create a thorough guideline describing the current standard of care. The contributors discuss the epidemiology, assessment, and treatment of pain in the geriatric population. This is a key resource for anyone who cares for geriatric patients.

■ Weiner DK, Herr K, Rudy TE. *Persistent Pain in Older Persons: An Interdisciplinary Guide for Treatment.* New York: Springer Publishing Company; 2002.

> This book is a valuable resource for clinicians of all disciplines who care for older patients. The sections describing the assessment and effects of pain are particularly comprehensive. The authors argue that the impact of pain, both physical and psychological, is greater in individuals who are already frail. Changes that can occur with aging such as cognitive decline, musculoskeletal disease, altered drug metabolism, and functional decline provide specific challenges to clinicians. The authors include effective and practical strategies to address and manage these issues relevant to the care of aging patients. Included in this book are sample questions for a pain interview and a helpful algorithm for the assessment of pain in elderly persons with severe cognitive impairment.

Jennifer M. Kapo, MD
Debra K. Weiner, MD

OL· Not approved by the U.S. Food and Drug Administration for this use.

SYNDROMES

CHAPTER 20—VISUAL IMPAIRMENT

KEY POINTS

- Visual impairment affects 20% to 30% of persons aged 75 and over.
- Cataracts and refractive error are common; both are correctable, and correction improves quality of life.
- Age-related macular degeneration (ARMD) is common; the wet form, the major complication of ARMD leading to blindness, may respond to laser surgery or intravitreal anti-angiogenesis injection. Antioxidant multivitamins may slow progression to the wet form.
- Glaucoma is common and no longer requires elevated intraocular pressure to meet diagnostic criteria. Screening for glaucoma should take place every 1 to 2 years after age 50, and more often in high-risk individuals.

Visual impairment, defined as visual acuity less than 20/40, increases exponentially with age such that 20% to 30% of the population aged 75 years or older is affected. Blindness, visual acuity of 20/200 or worse, affects 2% of the population aged 75 years and older. Those aged 65 and over make up 12% of the total U.S. population, but 50% of the blind population. Refractive error, cataract, age-related macular degeneration, diabetic retinopathy, and glaucoma are the most common causes of blindness. The respective order of importance varies according to the region and race surveyed. As the baby boomers age, the elderly population is expected to nearly double by the year 2030, and the prevalence of these conditions will surge.

Visual impairment has considerable impact on the medical system and the older age group. Chronic eye conditions represent one of the most common reasons for office-based visits to the physician among those aged 65 and over. Of all office visits by older persons, 14% are to ophthalmologists, one of the highest rates of all specialty visits. Falls and car crashes, each associated with impaired vision in elderly persons, consume considerable medical resources. Moreover, impaired vision has been linked to a significant deterioration in the quality of life and the activities of daily living of older persons.

The American Academy of Ophthalmology recommends a comprehensive eye examination every 1 to 2 years for persons aged 65 and over. The U.S. Preventive Services Task Force recommends annual vision testing. Prophylactic and therapeutic ocular management can effectively alter the course of various conditions causing visual impairment. About one third of all new cases of blindness can be avoided with effective use of available ophthalmologic services.

REFRACTIVE ERROR AND CATARACT

The leading cause of visual impairment worldwide is refractive error and cataract, for which eyeglasses and surgical cataract extraction, respectively, are mainstays of treatment. Despite the considerable successes of these therapeutic options, many populations do not receive adequate treatment for these problems.

Refractive error may be categorized as emmetropia (neutral refraction), ametropia, or presbyopia. Three forms of ametropia exist: myopia (nearsightedness), hyperopia (farsightedness), and astigmatism (distorted vision). Typically, older patients demonstrate increasing hyperopia, unless a cataract is present, which can induce a myopic shift. Although contact lens wear and laser refractive surgery are available for myopic and hyperopic refractive errors, these alternative forms of treatment traditionally have been used more by younger persons. After the age of approximately 40, emmetropic persons begin to develop progressive presbyopia, impaired ability to focus at near objects that is caused by gradual hardening of the lens and decreased muscular effectiveness of the ciliary body. Reading glasses or bifocal eyeglasses may be prescribed.

Approximately 20% of persons aged 65 years and over and 50% aged 75 years and over have a cataract, a vision-reducing lens opacity. Cataracts may be associated with increased glare, decreased contrast sensitivity, and decreased visual acuity. Several risk factors have been reported: decreased vitamin intake, light (ultraviolet B) exposure, smoking, alcohol use, long-term corticosteroid use, and diabetes mellitus. The most important risk factor is increased age.

Cataract extraction is one the most successful surgeries in medicine (90% of patients achieve vision of 20/40 or better). Approximately 1.5 million cataract procedures are performed each year in the United States alone. In inner cities and underdeveloped countries such as India, the demand for surgery has surpassed available resources.

Cataract extraction is safe and can be completed in less than 15 minutes under local or topical anesthesia. The surgery involves the sonographic breakdown and aspiration of the lens (phacoemulsification). An artificial implant (intraocular lens) is placed in the capsular bag that is the only remnant of the native lens retained. A secondary laser procedure (capsulotomy) may be necessary to ablate subsequent capsular opacification that may develop in 15% or more of patients.

AGE-RELATED MACULAR DEGENERATION

Age-related macular degeneration (ARMD) is the most common cause of blindness in older persons throughout the developed world. Increased age is the most important risk factor, although a genetic predisposition also contributes. Other risk factors include smoking and hypertension. Fair-skinned persons are at greater risk of developing this disease than those who are black, in whom pigment may serve as a protective element.

ARMD may be classified into two forms, dry and wet. The dry form is much more common and is characterized by deposits of drusen under the macula. Drusen, submacular yellow deposits composed of by-products of metabolism, do not typically cause vision loss but are a marker for the wet form of ARMD, which is characterized by angiogenesis or choroidal neovascularization (CNV). The presence of larger, more numerous drusen conveys the greatest risk for the development of CNV. The Age-Related Eye Disease Study found that the risk of development of CNV could be decreased by 25% when patients with high-risk drusen are treated with high-dose oral multivitamin therapy. Combination multivitamins containing beta-carotene 25,000 IU, vitamin E 400 IU, vitamin C 500 mg, and zinc 80 mg are available. This vitamin therapy, however, is contraindicated in smokers because of the risk of lung cancer in smokers who take beta-carotene supplements.

Patients with the dry form of ARMD should be examined periodically by an ophthalmologist. Patients who develop sudden distortion or vision loss, signaling the development of CNV, require urgent evaluation. Severe vision loss or central visual blindness is usually caused by the wet form of ARMD defined by the presence of CNV. Less commonly, geographic atrophy within the macular region may explain severe vision loss. CNV is marked by the presence of subretinal fluid and blood with or without a gray-green membrane (Figure 20.1). The natural history of CNV is progressive subfoveal growth and leakage with associated fibrotic scarring and central blindness.

Laser therapy for CNV has been beneficial, but only under very special circumstances, when membranes are well defined (ie, the margins of the lesion are clearly delineated) and extra- or juxtafoveal.

Figure 20.1—Choroidal neovascularization in a patient with the wet form of age-related macular degeneration demonstrating a gray-green membrane associated with subretinal hemorrhage.

Photodynamic therapy (PDT) using porphyrin-derived dyes has been shown to be useful in those patients with subfoveal CNV in whom conventional laser therapy will destroy the fovea. According to the Treatment of Age-Related Macular Degeneration with Photodynamic Therapy Study (TAP), 43% of patients receiving photodynamic therapy sustained moderate visual loss (> 15 letters from baseline) after 1 year of follow-up versus 57% of patients not receiving the photoactivated dye laser treatment. Moreover, 16% of those receiving photoactivated dye laser treatment sustained an improvement in visual acuity, but only 7% in the placebo group showed improvement. These benefits continued after 2 years of follow-up but required as many as five sessions of PDT. Although the benefits are not overwhelming, PDT is a relatively safe alternative that is the most effective procedure available for delaying visual loss in patients with wet ARMD and CNV that is not occult.

A great deal of excitement has been generated regarding angiogenesis inhibition. Specifically, various types of inhibitors to vascular endothelial growth factor (VEGF) have already been approved by the Food and Drug Administration (FDA) for treatment of diseases such as colorectal cancer and the wet form of ARMD; several additional indications await completion of the FDA review process. Serial intravitreal injections (9 per year) of pegaptanib sodium, an anti-VEGF aptamer or mRNA oligonucleotide that acts as an antagonist to VEGF, has been approved by the FDA for the treatment of all subtypes of wet ARMD. Similar to PDT, the injections do not typically improve vision but reduce the risk of vision loss. Another anti-angiogenesis inhibitor, ranibizumab, is a fragment antibody that exhibits broad-spectrum inhibition of VEGF and will likely be approved in the near future. This is another intravitreal pharmacotherapy that may require fewer injections than pegaptanib with equal or improved efficacy.

A concerted effort to find a candidate gene for ARMD has been for many years unsuccessful until recently, when multiple centers uncovered a 30% to 50% association of a mutation in the complement factor H (CFH) gene with various forms of ARMD. CFH is a regulator of complement activation, the mutation of which may lead to increased inflammation and leakage and the development of ARMD.

DIABETIC RETINOPATHY

Duration of disease and control of blood sugar are the most important variables in the development and progression of diabetic retinopathy. After 10 years, 70% of those with type 2 diabetes demonstrate some form of retinopathy, and nearly 10% show proliferative disease. Diet control, exercise, and proper glucose management with frequent daily glucose testing and the use of oral hypoglycemics or insulin, or both, are crucial in maintaining glycosylated hemoglobin levels lower than 7%. The Diabetic Control and Complications Trial demonstrated that tight blood-sugar control in those with type 1 diabetes results in a long-lasting decrease in the rate of development and progression of diabetic retinopathy. The United Kingdom Prospective Diabetes Study validated these results in an older population with type 2 diabetes. Tight blood-pressure control ($\leq$ 140/80) with either β-blockers or angiotensin-converting enzyme inhibitors was also found to be an important factor in decreasing microvascular complications, such as the need for retinal laser therapy. Other systemic risk factors, including kidney function and serum cholesterol, may also influence the course of diabetic retinopathy and should be optimized. Angiotensin-converting enzyme inhibitors have been found to decrease progressive nephropathy in diabetic patients and may have similar benefits to the retina.

Type 2 diabetic patients require baseline ophthalmologic screening at diagnosis of systemic disease. Subsequent follow-up will depend on the grade of retinopathy; however, even patients without retinopathy should be evaluated annually. Nonproliferative diabetic retinopathy, the earliest stage of retinopathy, may first be manifested by retinal microaneurysms. Intraretinal hemorrhages and exudates, with or without associated macular edema, may ensue. Progressive ischemia characterized by increasing hemorrhages, venous caliber changes or intraretinal microvascular abnormalities or both, and capillary nonperfusion on fluorescein angiography characterize the preproliferative stage of diabetic retinopathy. About 40% of patients with preproliferative retinopathy de-velop proliferative diabetic retinopathy (PDR) within 1 to 2 years, characterized by neovascularization or new blood vessel growth of the retina or disc, or both.

Visual loss in diabetic patients may occur as a result of macular nonperfusion or macular edema. The Early Treatment Diabetic Retinopathy Study demonstrated the benefit of focal or grid laser photocoagulation in stabilizing and improving vision in diabetic patients with clinically significant macular edema (Figure 20.2). Neovascularization (Figure 20.3) may cause severe visual loss or blindness in the setting of PDR as a result of vitreous hemorrhage or tractional retinal detachment. PDR is amenable to treatment by panretinal laser photocoagulation to inhibit the growth stimulus for neovascularization. The Diabetic Retinopathy Study demonstrated an 11% incidence of severe visual loss in patients treated with panretinal photocoagulation but a 26% incidence in those who did not receive laser during a 2-year follow-up. Nonclearing vitreous hemorrhage or tractional macular

Figure 20.2—Intraretinal edema and exudate in the superior macular region consistent with clinically significant macular edema in a patient with type 2 diabetes mellitus.

Figure 20.3—Florid neovascularization of the disc in a patient with high-risk proliferative diabetic retinopathy.

detachment may be addressed surgically by pars plana vitrectomy, membrane peeling, and endolaser.

GLAUCOMA

Glaucoma is the second most common cause of blindness worldwide and, in the United States, the most common cause of blindness in black Americans. It affects more than 2.25 million Americans aged 40 years or over and results in more than 3 million office visits each year. The financial burden is considerable because of the prevalence and chronicity of this disease and the debilitation that results. Federal costs are reported to reach as high as $1 billion for glaucoma-related Medicare and Medicaid payments and disability.

The definition of glaucoma, now defined as characteristic optic nerve head damage and visual field loss, has undergone a considerable evolution. Elevated intraocular pressure (IOP) is no longer considered an absolute criterion, although it is a very important risk factor. There are many different types of glaucoma, of which primary open-angle glaucoma (POAG) is the most common. Adults over age 50 should have screening for glaucoma every 1 to 2 years. Older adults with a positive family history of glaucoma, black origin, or other risk factors may need more frequent screening.

POAG is a chronic disease most commonly affecting older patients. Aqueous may access the filtration site, but the network is "clogged," resulting in impaired passage out of the angle. Slow aqueous drainage leads to chronically elevated IOPs. This is in contrast to acute angle-closure glaucoma, in which the entry site is suddenly blocked off, IOP rises precipitously, and the patient presents with considerable redness and pain with acute vision loss. Pain may be so severe as to cause headache, nausea, and vomiting. Emergent ophthalmologic referral is required to reverse the angle closure and reduce the IOP through the use of aqueous suppressants, miotics, and laser iridotomy. Conversely, the IOP rise in POAG is slow and much less severe. Patients with POAG are asymptomatic and may suffer substantial field loss before consulting an ophthalmologist, which underscores the importance of regular ophthalmologic screening of the older adult.

Development of POAG is most likely multifactorial and polygenic. Initial pedigrees were found to demonstrate linkage to the 1q locus. Subsequent investigations have more precisely defined the GLC1A gene that encodes for myocilin, the trabecular meshwork-induced glucocorticoid response protein. Several other chromosomal loci, including those mapped to chromosomes 2, 3, 7, and 10, have also been found to be associated with the development of glaucoma.

The management of POAG may be approached by the ophthalmologist in a stepwise manner. A variety of IOP-lowering medications, both local and systemic, exist. Mechanisms of action include decreased aqueous production or increased aqueous outflow (see Table 20.1). Various eyedrop formulations are available; prostaglandin analogs that increase uveal-scleral outflow and α_2-adrenergic agonists that decrease aqueous production are two relatively new and effective drugs. In the face of visual field progression despite maximal medications or intolerance to medications, argon laser trabeculoplasty (application of laser energy to the trabecular meshwork) can be effective in lowering IOP in approximately 50% of patients for 3 to 5 years after treatment. Intraocular surgery involves the creation of a fistula or filtration site to allow an alternative route of aqueous egress (trabeculectomy). Adjunctive antimetabolite use with 5-fluorouracil[OL] or mitomycin-C[OL] has increased the success of this procedure in those patients at high risk of failure because of fibrosis and scarring of the filtration site. Alternative surgeries for glaucoma include drainage devices or aqueous shunts. Drainage devices, which are made of a foreign material such as plastic, shunt fluid from the anterior chamber to the subconjunctival space. Ciliary body destructive procedures with cryotherapy or laser (cyclocryoablation or cyclophotocoagulation) may be used in eyes with a poor visual prognosis.

ANTERIOR ISCHEMIC OPTIC NEUROPATHY

Anterior ischemic optic neuropathy (Figure 20.4) may result in acute vision or field loss. Microvascular

Table 20.1—Adverse Effects of Selected Eyedrops for Glaucoma

Class	Adverse Effects
Aqueous suppressants:	
α-Agonists (eg, brimonidine)	Allergic conjunctivitis
β-Blockers (eg, timolol)	Bradycardia, dyspnea, asthma, heart failure exacerbations
Carbonic anhydrase inhibitors (eg, dorzolamide)	Blurriness
Aqueous outflow facilitators:	
Epinephrine (eg, dipivefrin)	Palpitations, angina, cystoid macular edema
Miotics (eg, pilocarpine)	Brow arch, blurriness, nyctalopia
Prostaglandins (eg, latanoprost)	Pain, redness, increased eyelashes, iris pigmentation, cystoid macular edema

[OL] Not approved by the U.S. Food and Drug Administration for this use.

Figure 20.4—Pallid swelling of the optic nerve head in a patient with anterior ischemic optic neuropathy.

occlusion of the blood supply to the optic nerve may be attributed to atherosclerotic vascular disease or inflammation in the setting of giant cell (temporal) arteritis. The former, the nonarteritic form, typically affects patients with vasculopathic risk factors such as diabetes mellitus and hypertension; the latter, the arteritic form, tends to occur in elderly patients with a history of myalgias, headaches, and weight loss. An elevated Westergren erythrocyte sedimentation rate and a positive temporal artery biopsy are diagnostic. Systemic corticosteroid treatment is crucial to avoid visual loss in the other eye.

MISCELLANEOUS

Red eye in elderly patients may be classified by cause, benign or malignant. Malignant causes are typically associated with significant pain and vision loss and include corneal ulceration identified by the presence of a white corneal infiltrate. Emergent corneal scraping by an ophthalmologist to exclude an infection and the need for fortified antibiotic treatment is indicated. The presence of a corneal abrasion in the absence of an infiltrate or ulcer is prognostically much more favorable and may be diagnosed with fluorescein staining and treated with patching. Anterior or posterior uveitis is relatively unusual in the older adult population. Suspicion should be aroused by the symptom of photophobia with vision loss; urgent ophthalmologic referral is required. Treatment may include corticosteroid eye drop therapy, which can be complicated by cataract and increased IOP, and which is best prescribed by an ophthalmologist. Systemic investigations to exclude autoimmune diseases, systemic infections, and occult malignancies may be necessary.

Benign causes of red eye may include blepharitis or dandruff of the eye lashes. Treatment includes lid hygiene, topical antibiotics, and gentle scrubbing with nontearing baby shampoo twice daily. Less commonly, viral conjunctivitis associated with mucus discharge and matting of the eyelids, especially in the morning, may be noted and may be treated supportively with warm compresses and education to limit spread of the infection to the other eye or to contacts.

Allergic conjunctivitis is a common benign condition affecting older adults and causing red, itchy eyes. Advise patients to avoid known precipitants (eg, pet dander). Management of allergic conjunctivitis includes systemic antihistamines, topical antihistamines or decongestants, and ophthalmic corticosteroids. Patients should be cautioned about side effects of topical ophthalmics.

The use of ophthalmic corticosteroids in older adults merits comment. Indications include inflammatory conditions of the eye; risks include secondary ocular infections, cataract formation, glaucoma, and corneal thinning. Because of the risks, the prescription of ophthalmic corticosteroids is best limited to practitioners with training and experience in their use.

Tears serve several important functions, including corneal lubrication, debris clearance, and immune protection. With age, tear production decreases, and older patients are prone to develop dry-eye syndrome or keratitis sicca, characterized by redness, foreign body sensation, and reflex tearing. Management includes tear replacement with artificial tears during the day and an ointment at bedtime. Temporary and permanent punctal plugs may be employed to retard tear egress through the nasolacrimal drainage system in more severe cases. Keratitis sicca may be associated with autoimmune disease; conditions such as Sjögren's syndrome should be excluded.

Lid abnormalities are a common problem for older persons. Because of the gradual loss of elasticity and tensile strength that develops with age, secondary degenerative changes may take place. Blepharochalasis (drooping of the brow) and blepharoptosis (drooping of the eyelid) may cause cosmetic deformity and, if severe, may impair vision. Lid ectropion or entropion, eversion and inversion of the lid margins, respectively, can disrupt the ocular surface and cause discomfort for the patient. Various surgical procedures are available to address these problems.

Herpes zoster ophthalmicus, or shingles, is a painful reactivation of varicella zoster virus that not uncommonly affects older persons. Dermatomal distribution of weeping vesicles affecting the ophthalmic division of the trigeminal nerve is the classic presentation. Ocular involvement may be signaled by lesions on the tip of the nose (Hutchinson's sign) and may include dendritic keratopathy or uveitis. Oral acyclovir may shorten the course of disease. Trifluridine eyedrops are indicated with herpetic, dendriform corneal ulcers. Post-herpetic neuralgia may be quite debilitating; various local ointments (eg, capsaicin, lidocaine[OL]) or systemic medications (eg, corticosteroids[OL], tricyclic antidepressants[OL]) may be helpful. (See also "Dermatologic Diseases and Disorders," p 309.)

LOW-VISION REHABILITATION

Despite considerable advancements in the medical treatment of ocular conditions, many patients, especially those with the wet form of ARMD, may ultimately sustain permanent visual loss. Visual training and the provision of visual aids are indispensable services available to the patient with low vision (visual acuity < 20/60).

Patients with low vision may develop useful adaptive skills with proper instruction. Eccentric viewing by ARMD patients with central macular pathology uses the principle of off-center fixation. The patient can benefit from formal training to find and use the most effective eccentric viewing points. Instruction in scanning and tracking and other skills may help the patient integrate his or her visual environment.

Various low-vision aids are available to improve one's ability to see both near and far. The fine detail required for reading is the most common indication for visual aids. Improved lighting is a simple modification that can enhance visualization of print. Selection of reading material using bold, enlarged fonts and accentuated black-on-white contrast may also be helpful. Magnification also is commonly employed. Various devices such as high-plus spectacles, hand-held magnifiers, stand magnifiers, and closed-circuit television can also enhance reading. Distance magnification may be achieved with the use of telescopic devices that can be hand-held for spot viewing or spectacle mounted for continuous viewing. Talking devices, which are computers used to create voice synthesis such as those used at stoplights, or Braille may be especially helpful for those who have lost vision altogether.

ANNOTATED REFERENCES

- Age-Related Eye Disease Study Group. A randomized, placebo-controlled, clinical trial of high-dose supplementation with vitamins C and E, beta carotene, and zinc for age-related macular degeneration and vision loss: AREDS report no. 8. *Arch Ophthalmol.* 2001;119(10):1417–1436.

    This landmark study prospectively randomized patients with various stages of the dry form of age-related macular degeneration in at least one eye and documented a 25% decreased risk of choroidal neovascularization development in those eyes at highest risk for this complication.

- Ferris FL 3rd, Davis MD, Aiello LM. Treatment of diabetic retinopathy. *N Engl J Med.* 1999;341(9):667–678.

    This review article summarizes the epidemiology, diagnosis, and laser management of diabetic retinopathy. Studies supporting optimal systemic control of various parameters, such as glucose, blood pressure, cholesterol, and kidney function, are also well represented.

- Gragoudas ES, Adamis AP, Cunningham ET Jr, et al. Pegaptanib for neovascular age-related macular degeneration. *N Engl J Med.* 2004;351(27):2805–2816.

    Anti-angiogenesis inhibitors may be serially injected into the eye, and this landmark study demonstrated a statistically significant decreased risk of vision loss in patients with all subtypes of subfoveal choroidal neovascularization (wet ARMD).

- Jain A, Sarraf D, Fong D. Preventing diabetic retinopathy through the control of systemic risk factors. *Curr Opin Ophthalmol.* 2003;14(6):389–394.

    This paper comprehensively reviews all of the systemic diabetic factors that possibly influence the development and progression of retinopathy and summarizes many of the studies that have investigated these associations. Optimization of control of the blood sugar and blood pressure is the most important systemic action that might favorably influence the course of retinopathy.

- Lee BL, Wilson MR. Ocular Hypertension Treatment Study (OHTS). Ocular Hypertension Treatment Study (OHTS) commentary. *Curr Opin Ophthalmol.* 2003;14(2):74–77.

    This article reviews the findings and recommendations of the Ocular Hypertension Treatment Study, a landmark prospective controlled trial which found that lowering the intraocular pressure in patients with elevated pressure but without glaucoma significantly decreases the risk of future transition to glaucoma.

- Treatment of Age-Related Macular Degeneration with Photodynamic Therapy (TAP) Study Group. Photodynamic therapy of subfoveal choroidal neovascularization in age-related macular degeneration with verteporfin: one-year results of 2 randomized clinical trials—TAP Report 1. *Arch Ophthalmol.* 1999; 117(10):1329–1345.

- Treatment of Age-Related Macular Degeneration with Photodynamic Therapy (TAP) Study Group. Photodynamic therapy of subfoveal choroidal neovascularization in age-related macular degeneration with verteporfin: two-year results of 2 randomized clinical trials—TAP Report 2. *Arch Ophthalmol.* 2001;119:198–207.

    The treatment of choroidal neovascularization in the setting of age-related maculopathy may be complicated by various factors, including the subfoveal presence of the new blood vessels. Photodynamic therapy uses a dye-activated laser to ablate the subretinal vessel complex that preferentially absorbs the laser energy; the overlying fovea remains relatively free of damage. The TAP study prospectively demonstrated the benefit of this treatment in delaying visual loss in patients with late age-related maculopathy.

[OL] Not approved by the U.S. Food and Drug Administration for this use.

■ U.K. Prospective Diabetes Study Group. Efficacy of atenolol and captopril in reducing risk of macrovascular and microvascular complications in type 2 diabetes: UKPDS 39. *BMJ.* 1998;317(7160):713–720.

The UKPDS validated the importance of tight blood-pressure control, either with β-blockers or angiotensin-converting enzyme inhibitors, in decreasing the rate of both microvascular and macrovascular complications of diabetes mellitus. The two classes of hypotensive drug were found to be equally effective.

■ U.K. Prospective Diabetes Study Group. Intensive blood glucose control with sulfonylureas or insulin compared with conventional treatment and risk of complications in patients with type 2 diabetes (UKPDS 33). *Lancet.* 1998; 352(9131):837–853.

Unlike the Diabetes Control and Complications Trial, which studied persons with type 1 diabetes, the UKPDS prospectively investigated those with type 2 diabetes but yielded similar conclusions. Tight blood-sugar control, aiming for a glycosylated hemoglobin level of less than 7%, decreases the rate of progression of microvascular complications, such as diabetic retinopathy.

David Sarraf, MD
Anne L. Coleman, MD, PhD

CHAPTER 21—HEARING IMPAIRMENT

KEY POINTS

■ Hearing loss is among the most common chronic diseases among older persons: 10% of persons aged 65 to 75 years and 25% of those older than 75 years have hearing loss.

■ Treatment of hearing loss and attention to communication strategies can improve the hearing-impaired person's quality of life.

■ Important issues when considering hearing aids for an older person with hearing loss are the nature and degree of hearing loss, the person's ability to manipulate the aid and adapt to its use, and the social support and financial resources available to him or her.

Hearing loss is the fourth most common chronic disease among elderly persons. Hearing impairment is often assumed to be benign, but it has been shown to have profound effects on quality of life. The psychologic effects of hearing loss include family discord, social isolation, loss of self-esteem, anger, and depression. Epidemiologic studies suggest an association between hearing loss and cognitive impairment, and between hearing loss and reduced mobility. Hearing loss can also affect an older person's interaction with clinicians, making history taking and patient education difficult. Treatment of hearing loss and attention to communication strategies can improve the hearing-impaired person's quality of life by facilitating interaction with family, friends, and caregivers. Studies indicate that hearing aid use can relieve symptoms of depression that are associated with hearing loss.

NORMAL HEARING AND AGE-RELATED CHANGES IN THE AUDITORY SYSTEM

The normal ear is an efficient transducer of sound energy into nerve impulses. Sound energy is transmitted through the external ear to the tympanic membrane and the auditory ossicles. The malleus, incus, and stapes in series transmit vibrations to the oval window of the cochlea. Fluid waves within the cochlea stimulate the outer hair cells of the scala tympani. These cells stimulate the inner hair cells, which generate sensory potential. In turn, an excitatory postsynaptic potential is generated. When threshold is reached, impulses are sent via cochlear neurons to the cochlear nuclei and then to auditory pathways elsewhere in the brain.

Age-related changes in the auditory system can interfere with its function. The walls of the external ear canal become thin. Cerumen becomes drier and more tenacious, increasing the likelihood of cerumen impaction. The eardrum becomes thicker and appears duller than in younger persons. Degenerative changes of the ossicular joints occur but generally do not interfere with sound transmission to the cochlea. Cochlear changes include loss of sensory hair cells and fibrocytes in the organ of Corti, stiffening of the basilar membrane, calcification of auditory structures, and cochlear neuronal loss. Changes in the stria vascularis include thickening of capillaries, decreased production of endolymph, and decreased Na+ K+ ATPase activity. These degenerative changes occur to varying degrees in different individuals. It currently is not possible to fully correlate the degree of hearing loss with histologic changes in the aging ear.

Changes in central auditory processing also occur with aging. One study found that when competing speech stimuli are presented to each ear, the right ear has a 5% to 10% advantage over the left ear in younger persons. (The effect of right- and left-handedness was not assessed; all the participants were right-handed.) In persons aged 80 to 89 years, this difference increases to more than 40%. This difference may be related to a loss of efficiency of interhemispheric transfer of auditory information through the corpus callosum.

EPIDEMIOLOGY OF HEARING LOSS

The prevalence of hearing loss increases with age. Ten percent of adults aged 65 to 75 years and 25% of those older than 75 years have hearing loss. In nursing homes, estimates of prevalence vary from 50% to 100%, depending on the criteria used to define hearing loss.

Hearing loss can be caused by pathology in the external ear canal, the middle ear, the inner ear, the auditory nerve, central auditory pathways, or a combination of these (see Figure 21.1 for typical audiograms for the forms of hearing loss).

Conductive hearing loss is due to disease in the external ear, such as ceruminosis, or foreign body in the canal, or to middle-ear pathology, such as otosclerosis, cholesteatoma, tympanic membrane perforation, or middle-ear effusion.

Sensorineural hearing loss is most often caused by cochlear disease. Noise is the most common factor in cochlear damage. Hearing loss is less common among persons in quiet rural environments than among people in industrialized communities. Other causes of hearing loss include ototoxic medications, genotype, vascular disease, and, rarely, occupational and environmental chemical exposures. Smokers have higher rates of hearing loss than nonsmokers. Autoimmune disease and auditory nerve tumors are rare causes of sensorineural hearing loss. Neuronal loss can affect the brain stem and cortical ascending auditory pathways, including the cochlear nuclei, superior olivary complex, lateral lemniscus, inferior colliculi, and medial geniculate complex. The resulting deficits in central auditory processing can affect perception of sound and the ability to understand speech.

PRESBYCUSIS

Most hearing loss in elderly persons is categorized as presbycusis (literally, "older hearing"). Presbycusis is a sensorineural, usually symmetrical hearing loss that may have central components. Presbycusis can be classified as sensory, neural, strial, cochlear conductive, combined, or indeterminate, depending on cochlear pathology. Many persons with presbycusis can be helped by amplification.

Sensory presbycusis results in a steeply sloping audiogram. It is often slowly progressive, beginning with the higher frequencies of 8000 Hz, 6000 Hz, and 4000 Hz. It may involve the 3000 and 2000 Hz range, which is the higher portion of the range of frequencies in human speech. (See Figure 21.2) Persons with this type of hearing loss often have trouble hearing in the presence of background noise but will be able to hear adequately in quiet settings. Amplification often helps these patients, since speech discrimination is satisfactory. This loss of auditory acuity can begin as early as the 20s but may not become clinically evident until later decades. Sensory presbycusis is attributed to a loss of sensory hair cells in the basal end of the cochlea.

Strial presbycusis is considered a metabolic form of hearing loss. The stria vascularis maintains high potassium concentrations in the endolymph. Strial presbycusis, pathologically defined as atrophy of 30% or more of the stria vascularis, is a form of cochlear dysfunction. This disorder typically begins between the ages of 20 and 60 and is characterized by mild to moderate hearing loss in most frequencies. Persons with strial presbycusis usually have good speech discrimination and do well with amplification.

Neural presbycusis is due to a cochlear neuronal loss of 50% or more compared with the normal number in neonates. Despite preserved pure-tone thresholds, which are not affected until more than 90% of cochlear neurons have been lost, patients with neural presbycusis show very poor speech discrimination. Successful use of amplification is difficult for this form of presbycusis.

Cochlear conductive presbycusis is caused by changes in cochlear mechanics produced by mass or stiffness changes or spiral ligament atrophy. It has a unique audiogram, which gradually descends over at least five octaves with no more than a 25-dB difference between any two adjacent frequencies. Speech discrimination may also be impaired. Pathologically, this form is defined by the absence of histologic changes seen in the other forms of presbycusis.

Most presbycusis is probably a mixture of these forms. The shape of the audiogram and speech discrimination scores depends on the extent of injury to various components of the cochlea.

DIAGNOSIS OF HEARING LOSS

Partly because of the slowly progressive nature of hearing loss, many older persons are unaware of their hearing deficit. In some cases, the stigma of wearing a hearing aid causes the patient to deny the problem. The hearing loss may be brought to medical attention by family members, who complain that the patient does not hear them or plays the television or radio too

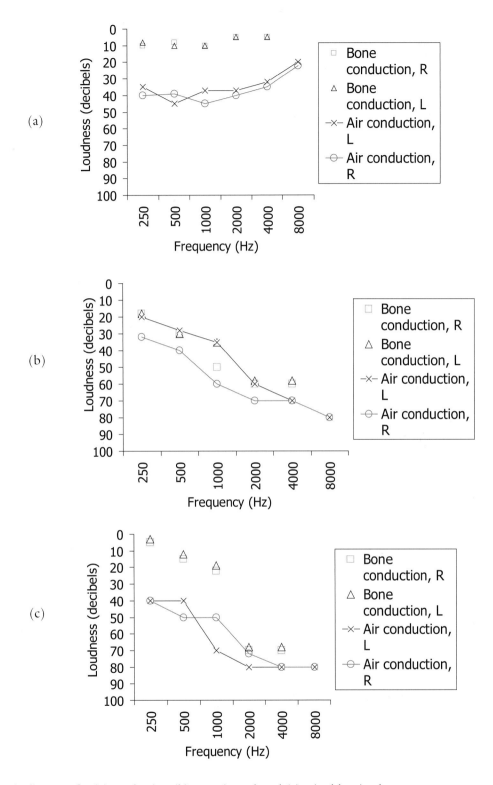

Figure 21.1—Audiograms for (a) conductive, (b) sensorineural, and (c) mixed hearing loss.

(a) Conductive hearing loss. Air conduction thresholds are greater than bone conduction thresholds, most likely because of middle-ear pathology.

(b) Sensorineural hearing loss. Air and bone conduction thresholds are the same, most likely because of inner-ear damage. The high-frequency pattern of this patient's hearing loss is typical for presbycusis.

(c) Mixed hearing loss. Air and bone conduction thresholds are abnormal, with the greatest difference seen for the left ear. This patient has pathology in both the middle and inner ears. Bone conduction thresholds for the left ear are measured by masking the right ear.

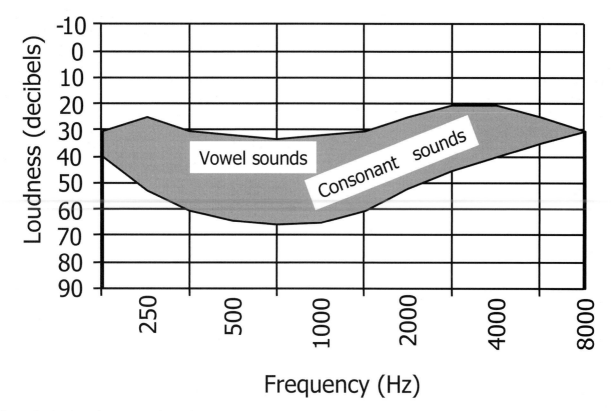

Figure 21.2—Speech range on the audiogram.

loud. Clinicians may notice that the patient does not respond when spoken to out of his or her field of view, or seems to misunderstand questions. Hearing loss can also be misunderstood as cognitive impairment. Caregivers and physicians may not recognize the presence of hearing loss or may assume it is a benign component of aging.

Screening programs to identify hearing loss are important. Fitting hearing aids early in the course of hearing loss may help the person adjust to their use, and treatment can reduce psychologic morbidity. A handheld otoscope with a tone generator can be used by primary care providers to screen for the presence of hearing loss at selected frequencies (0.5, 1, 2, and 4 KHz) and two loudness levels (25 and 40 dB HL). This device should be used in a quiet environment. When set at 40 dB HL, testing at 1 and 2 KHz has a sensitivity of 94% and a specificity between 82% and 90% for detecting hearing loss. The Hearing Handicap Inventory for the Elderly—Screening Version is a 10-item questionnaire that asks about difficulty with communication in various settings. It can be useful to determine the impact that hearing loss has on a patient's daily activities. When a screening test is consistent with hearing loss and the patient is willing and able to pay for a hearing aid, discuss referral to an audiologist. The patient's ear canals should be examined before referral to exclude the presence of obstruction. Cerumen impaction can cause a clinically significant hearing loss, as much as 40 dB.

The otolaryngologist will further evaluate the hearing loss and identify treatable causes. An asymmetrical hearing loss demands thorough investigation. Auditory nerve tumors are rare, but tumors of the posterior pharynx can obstruct the eustachian tube, causing a middle-ear effusion with conductive hearing loss.

The audiologist will assess hearing to determine the presence and the type of hearing loss. A comprehensive audiologic assessment consists of pure-tone thresholds for both air and bone conduction, speech-recognition thresholds, speech discrimination, and middle-ear function. This information, along with the medical evaluation, will be used to determine treatment for the patient. Audiologists recommend and fit hearing aids and provide auditory rehabilitation.

TREATMENT OF HEARING LOSS

Some causes of hearing loss are amenable to medical or surgical treatment. Paget's disease of the bone can affect the middle ear, causing conductive loss, or the inner ear, leading to sensorineural loss. This loss sometimes responds to bisphosphonates. Otosclerosis or tympanosclerosis may be correctable with surgery. Sudden hearing loss may be autoimmune in nature and sometimes responds to corticosteroids or immune-suppressant therapy. The majority of older persons with hearing loss are treated with communication strategies or amplification, or both. Hearing aids often improve ability to understand speech, particularly soft speech and conversational loud speech.

Strategies to Enhance Communication

Hearing-impaired persons should be encouraged to let others know about their hearing loss and to suggest strategies that will help them communicate more easily (Table 21.1). In addition to using these strategies, clinicians should provide options for patients with hearing loss, such as sign language interpreters, the use of pen and paper, or assistive devices. Office and hospital staff should be alerted to a patient's hearing loss. Background noise from the environment can interfere with hearing and should be reduced as much as possible.

Lipreading can be a useful adjunct to listening, but it requires thoughtfulness on the part of the speaker. When speaking to a hearing-impaired person who lip-reads, it is important to face him or her and obtain the person's attention before speaking; a gentle touch on the hand or arm will usually suffice. Speak each word clearly and distinctly. Shouting not only distorts lip movements so they are harder to read, but the speaker may sound angry even when not. Use complete sentences. Single words are hard to lip-read because the listener often needs cues from context to identify meaning. It is helpful to make certain the

person knows the topic of conversation. Use appropriate language for the listener's educational level. Unlike deaf persons who have been deaf all or most of their lives, most older persons with hearing loss do not know sign language. Sometimes amplification and lipreading are not enough. Gestures can aid communication even with cognitively impaired patients.

For patients with hearing impairment, it can also be helpful to write words down. For those with both hearing and visual impairment, large printing with a marker pen or a laptop computer screen with magnified print may be necessary. These patients may benefit from correction of the visual problem, if possible (eg, cataract removal or use of eyeglasses). In any case, providing written instructions to those who can read improves understanding and retention of important information.

Be alert to misunderstandings. If a reply does not make sense, try repeating what was said, using different words. Have the patient repeat what he or she heard, since misunderstandings are common.

Assistive Listening Devices

For some persons with hearing impairment, a personal amplifier may be more useful than hearing aids. These pocket-sized devices are considerably less expensive than hearing aids and are harder to misplace. Headphones stay on the head better than earbuds and provide sound to both ears. The volume and microphone placement of the amplifier should be adjusted to find the best combination for a given user. Every health care facility should have at least one or two of these devices available, as they are not personalized and can be used by different people.

Adaptive equipment can facilitate telephone use. State agencies for deaf and hard-of-hearing persons may provide amplified telephones, vibrating and flashing ringer alert devices, and text telephones (TTY) at no cost to hearing-impaired persons. This equipment is available from electronics and telephone equipment stores.

Many other assistive devices are available. Television listening devices can spare others from overly loud volume levels. FM loop systems can be used for groups of people with FM receivers or telecoil switches in their hearing aids. Wireless FM transmitters and receivers are also available for indoor or outdoor use. Infrared group listening devices are primarily useful indoors. Vibrating and flashing devices such as alarm clocks and timers, smoke alarms, doorbell alerts, and motion sensors can improve the hearing-impaired person's convenience and safety. These items can be purchased through the agencies mentioned above, or from catalog retailers of assistive listening devices.

Table 21.1—Strategies to Improve Communication with Hearing-Impaired Persons

- Obtain the listener's attention before speaking.
- Eliminate background noise as much as possible.
- Be sure the listener can see the speaker's lips; for example:

    Speak face-to-face in the same room.

    Do not obscure the lips with hands, mustaches, or other objects.

    Make certain that light shines directly on the speaker's face, not from behind the speaker.

- Speak slowly and clearly, but avoid shouting.
- Speak toward the better ear, if applicable.
- Change phrasing if the listener does not understand at first.
- Spell words out, use gestures, or write them down.
- Have the listener repeat back what he or she heard
- **Ask the listener what is the best way to communicate with him or her.**

Hearing Aids

Hearing aids are the most common form of amplification. Many factors need to be considered in deciding whether to fit the patient with a hearing aid. In addition to the nature and degree of hearing loss (Table 21.2), the patient's motivation and ability to adapt to its use and physically manipulate the aid (Table 21.3), the degree of his or social support, and his or her ability to afford the expense (Table 21.4) must be considered.

In general, two hearing aids are more beneficial than one. The first aid provides the most gain; the second one helps with speech discrimination and with localizing the source of sounds. However, the presence of asymmetrical hearing loss or significant difficulty in understanding competing speech stimuli may mean that the use of a single hearing aid is more appropriate.

Not everyone benefits from a hearing aid. The pattern of sensorineural damage may be such that speech discrimination is poor even with amplification. Some patients are unable to tolerate the presence of the hearing aid in the ear. Patients with dementia may remove and dispose of the aid. It is important to be sure that the aid can be returned during an initial trial period, usually 30 days, without having to pay the full cost. It is equally important not to give up on the aid too soon, since the audiologist often can adjust it to

Table 21.2—Effects and Rehabilitation of Hearing Loss, by Degree of Loss

Degree of Loss	Loss in db HL	Sounds Difficult to Hear	Effect on Communication	Amplification or Other Assistance Needed
Mild	25–40	Whisper	Difficulty understanding soft speech or normal speech in presence of background noise	Hearing aid needed in specific situations
Moderate	41–55	Conversational speech	Difficulty understanding any but loud speech	Frequent need for hearing aid
Severe	56–80	Shouting, vacuum cleaner	Can understand only amplified speech	Amplification needed for all communication
Profound	≥ 81	Hair dryer, heavy traffic, telephone ringer	Difficulty understanding amplified speech; may miss telephone calls	May need to supplement hearing aid with lip-reading, assistive listening devices, sign language

SOURCE: Data in part from *A Report on Hearing Aids: User Perspectives and Concerns.* Washington, DC: American Association of Retired Persons; 1993:2.

Table 21.3—Advantages and Disadvantages of Hearing Aid Styles

Style	Degree of Hearing Loss	Advantages	Disadvantages
CIC	Mild to moderate	Almost invisible Less occlusion of ear canal allows more natural sound Easier to use with headphones and telephone	Dexterity may be a problem Small size may limit available features May cost more than canal or ITE aids Shorter battery life
Canal	Mild to moderate	More cosmetic than larger aids Telecoil available in some models May be able to use with headphones	Dexterity may be a problem Small size may limit available features
ITE	Mild to severe	Ease of handling Comfortable fit Available options: telecoil, directional microphone More power than CIC or canal aid	More conspicuous than CIC or canal aid May be difficult to use with headphones
BTE	Mild to profound	Greatest power Available options: telecoil, direct audio input, directional microphone Earmold can be changed separately	More conspicuous May be more difficult to insert than ITE Difficult to use with headphones
Body aid	Severe to profound	Greatest separation of microphone from receiver reduces feedback	Most conspicuous Body-level microphone is subject to noise from clothing Microphone is on chest, but speech isusually directed at ear level
Bone conduction aid	Mild to severe	Bypasses middle ear; used if ear canal is unable to tolerate aid or earmold	Receiver causes pressure on the scalp, which can be uncomfortable; does not correct sensorineural loss

NOTE: BTE = behind the ear; CIC = completely in the canal; ITE = in the ear.

Table 21.4—Costs of Assistive Listening Devices and Hearing Aids

Type of Technology	Cost	Comments
Assistive listening devices (personal amplifiers, telephone amplifiers, television listening devices)	$150–$200	Useful for specific situations (see text for details)
Hearing aids		
Analog	$750–$1,100	Smaller aids are more expensive
Analog programmable	$1,150–$1,600	Smaller aids are more expensive
Digital, low end	$1,150–$1,500	Similar to analog aid, but with better sound quality
Digital, mid-range	$1,600–$2,300	Some sound processing included, eg, a second program, feedback control, telecoil
Digital, premium	$2,300–$3,000	Multiple features available, eg, background noise suppression, feedback management, multiple programs, telecoil
Bone conduction	$400–$900	Available as all-in-one headpiece or as body aid; used only if in-the-ear aid or earmold is not tolerated

NOTE: Assistive listening devices and hearing aids are not covered by Medicare.

improve comfort and sound quality. The audiologist should provide counseling for its optimum use.

Many different styles of hearing aids are available (Table 21.3). Behind-the-ear aids hang behind the ear and are connected directly to an earmold. The earmold is custom made to fit each patient's ear. Some behind-the-ear aids can be connected to assistive listening devices via a "boot," which fits over the end of the aid to provide direct audio input. Body aids are worn on the belt or in a pocket or a harness, and they are connected to a custom-made earmold by a wire. These are rarely used. All-in-the ear aids and canal aids have cases that are custom fit to the user. The smaller hearing aids may have remote controls. Selection of aid style for each individual depends on the degree of hearing loss, available features, and the person's dexterity and motivation.

The telecoil is an induction coupling coil that can be built into the hearing aid. It detects the magnetic field produced by telephones compatible with hearing aids. The telecoil is used to listen to the telephone with less distraction from noise in the same room. It can also be used with many assistive listening devices. The amount of coupling, and therefore the volume of the signal, depends on the angle of the telecoil with respect to the magnetic field. Users may need to experiment to find the right angle. Strongly magnetic devices such as computer monitors often produce interference, which is also dependent on the angle and the distance of the telecoil from the device. These drawbacks aside, the telecoil is a useful feature and can be added to hearing aids at a relatively small cost. Consumers with moderate to severe hearing loss should be encouraged to consider purchasing an aid with a telecoil.

The choice of analog or digital hearing aids depends on the individual consumer. Analog aids are less expensive than digital aids and may provide acceptable sound quality. However, newer digital technology has allowed improved sound quality, reduced size, and increased ability to customize the amplification of the aid to the needs of the user. Programmable aids are adjusted for each individual while he or she is wearing the aid. Often, two or more programs are available within a single aid. Using a computer, the audiologist makes adjustments to gain, response in different frequency ranges, and loudness balance for each program. One program may be most useful in the presence of background noise, whereas another works better in a quiet environment, and a third works with a telecoil. Persons with Ménière's disease can have their aids reprogrammed to accommodate fluctuating hearing loss. Some hearing aids automatically adjust the volume to increase amplification of soft sounds while avoiding uncomfortable loudness, reducing the need for the user to manipulate the aid. A study comparing different methods of limiting loudness suggested that consumers with mild to moderate hearing loss were more likely to prefer compression-limiting or wide dynamic range compression circuitry to peak-clipping circuitry, though the absolute differences in consumer preference and speech comprehension between these methods was small.

Background noise is a significant problem for hearing aid users. Traditional hearing aids amplify sound indiscriminately, so that noises from papers rattling or water running can be very distracting. The use of multiple microphones in the hearing aid, combined with digital signal processing, can decrease background noise. This can significantly improve the wearer's ability to understand speech and increase consumer satisfaction with the aid.

Unfortunately, the cost of hearing aids is often a significant barrier to their use and may affect the purchaser's choice of features (Table 21.4). Medicare and the majority of private health insurance companies typically do not pay for hearing aids, although they may provide coverage for audiometric evaluation for hearing aids. Medicaid may provide coverage for hearing aids, but the reimbursement may be below the provider's cost. Federal programs such as the Department of Veterans Affairs may pay for hearing aids, depending on the recipient's eligibility for services.

Cochlear Implants

For persons with severe to profound hearing loss who gain little or no benefit from hearing aids yet who are motivated to participate in the hearing world, cochlear implants can provide useful hearing. A cochlear implant is an electronic device that bypasses the function of damaged or absent cochlear hair cells by providing electrical stimulation to cochlear nerve fibers. A receiver-stimulator and an intracochlear electrode array are surgically implanted. A headset is worn behind the ear. The headset microphone transmits signals to the speech processor, which filters and digitizes the sound into coded signals. The coded signals are sent to the cochlear implant, which then stimulates auditory nerve fibers in the cochlea. Nerve signals are then sent through the auditory system to the brain. Patients must be able to tolerate general anesthesia and to participate in extensive pre-implant testing and post-implant training. The procedure is covered by most Medicare carriers and insurance companies. In general, outcomes of cochlear implantation in persons aged 65 and older have been comparable to those of younger adults, with patients obtaining excellent results by both audiologic and quality-of-life measures. Meningitis is a rare complication of cochlear implants.

ANNOTATED REFERENCES

■ American Academy of Audiology: Consumer Guides. Frequently asked questions about hearing aids. Available at: http://www.audiology.org/consumer/guides/hafaq. php (accessed October 2005).

> Consumers may be bewildered by the wide array of available hearing aids. Hearing aid selection is influenced by the shape of the ear, manual dexterity, external ear disease, and the nature of a person's hearing loss. Advanced features such as directional microphones, multichannel aids, and digital pro-

cessing add to the cost of hearing aids but may provide improved speech intelligibility. Consumers need to have realistic expectations of their hearing aids and to know how to manage problems such as feedback.

■ Department of Otolaryngology—Head and Neck Surgery, University of Washington Medical Center. Cochlear implants. Available at: http://depts.washington. edu/otoweb/patients/pts_specialties/pts_hear-n-bal/ pts_hear-n-bal_cochlear-implant.htm (accessed October 2005).

> The cochlear implant is a prosthetic replacement for the cochlea and is appropriate for people who receive minimal or no benefit from a conventional hearing aid, including selected older patients. Part of the device is surgically implanted in the skull behind the ear, and wires are inserted into the cochlea. The other part of the device is external and has a microphone and a speech processor to convert sound into electrical impulses. It is battery powered, adjustable, and expensive. The procedure requires extensive preoperative evaluation as well as postoperative fitting and training. Most people who had normal hearing at one time are able to understand sound without reading lips following a cochlear implant, although the degree of success varies.

■ Iezzoni LI, O'Day BL, Killeen M, et al. Communicating about health care: observations from persons who are deaf or hard of hearing. *Ann Intern Med*. 2004;140(5):356–362.

> Deaf and hard-of-hearing adults were interviewed about their experiences with health care. They reported that doctors commonly insist on inadequate communication methods and do not take the time to ensure that their patients understand everything that has been said, which can lead to medication and treatment errors. Participants offered numerous suggestions for improving health care communication, including recording and respecting patients' preferred method of communication.

■ Yueh B, Shapiro N, MacLean CH, et al. Screening and management of adult hearing loss in primary care: scientific review. *JAMA*. 2003;289(15):1976–1985.

> This article briefly discusses the physiology of hearing loss and reviews the utility of several screening tests for hearing disorder. The authors address treatment of hearing loss in the primary care setting and when to refer to a specialist (otolaryngologist or audiologist). This article contains the Hearing Handicap Inventory for the Elderly—Screening Version (HIEE-S). A companion article in this issue (pp 1986–1990) includes several case studies with clinical applications that illustrate ways in which primary care physicians can improve the detection, evaluation, and treatment of hearing loss.

Priscilla Faith Bade, MD, MS

CHAPTER 22—DIZZINESS

KEY POINTS

- The classification of dizziness into vertigo and nonvertiginous dizziness (presyncope, disequilibrium, and lightheadedness) may be useful in guiding the clinician in patient evaluation; however, precise classification is often difficult, and multiple causes of the same symptoms are common.

- Common causes of the spinning sensation of vertigo include benign positional vertigo, labyrinthitis, and Ménière's disease.

- Presyncope, the sensation of near fainting, implies impaired cerebral perfusion. Most older adults with presyncope have symptoms related to orthostatic blood-pressure changes or vagally mediated changes rather than cardiac causes.

- Multiple factors can contribute to disequilibrium, a feeling of unsteadiness: vestibulopathies, neuropathies, and visual and musculoskeletal problems. Nondescript lightheadedness may suggest depression, anxiety, or other emotional problems.

- Most dizziness resolves within days to several months. Despite the increased risk of falls, chronic or recurrent dizziness has not been found to be associated with increased mortality, hospitalization, or functional decline but is associated with syncope, depression, and worse self-rated health.

- Key physical examination steps include checking for orthostatic hypotension, performing the head-hanging (Dix-Hallpike) test, and observing gait. If the cause is not identified, a brief vestibular evaluation including other maneuvers for nystagmus is merited.

- Treatment options for dizziness vary with cause.

Dizziness accounts for an estimated 7 million clinic visits in the United States each year and is one of the most common symptoms of patients referred to neurology and otolaryngology practices. Among older persons, the reported prevalence ranges from 13% to 38%. Several factors make dizziness a challenging symptom to evaluate and manage. First, precise classification of the cause is often difficult. Second, patients and clinicians alike may worry about a serious cardiac or neurologic cause. Third, specific therapy is not available for many patients with dizziness. Fourth, like other geriatric syndromes such as delirium and falls, dizziness may be related to multiple potentially causative factors at least half of the time.

CLASSIFICATION

Drachman popularized a symptom-oriented approach, classifying dizziness as vertigo (rotational sensation), presyncope (impending faint), disequilibrium (loss of balance without head sensation), or lightheadedness (ill-defined, not otherwise classifiable). Although some sensations correspond more often than not to at least a general etiologic category (eg, vertigo suggests vestibular dysfunction at least 80% to 90% of the time), these four sensations remain nonspecific, occurring with many different disorders. Following is a brief delineation of the sensations and the most common corresponding causes.

Vertigo

The three most common specific peripheral vestibular disorders are benign positional vertigo (BPV), labyrinthitis, and Ménière's disease. BPV is episodic and aggravated or brought on by changes in position, such as turning, rolling over, getting in and out of bed, or bending over. BPV spells are often brief (5 to 15 seconds) and milder than the severe vertiginous attacks seen with disorders such as labyrinthitis and Ménière's disease. Labyrinthitis (sometimes called vestibular neuronitis) occurs acutely, lasts for several days, and resolves spontaneously. Ménière's disease is characterized by repeated episodes of tinnitus, fluctuating hearing loss, and severe vertigo accompanied eventually by a progressive sensorineural hearing loss. The frequency and severity of vertigo may improve as hearing impairment worsens.

Central vestibular disorders account for a minority of cases of vertigo; these include cerebrovascular disease, brain tumors, multiple sclerosis, and rarer central causes. In vertigo of vascular origin, dizziness has been reported as the presenting symptom less than 20% of the time. Much more commonly, it is preceded or accompanied by other neurologic deficits in the distribution of the posterior circulation. Indeed, verifying a transient ischemic attack as the cause of vertigo can be difficult in the absence of other neurologic deficits, since isolated vertigo is nonspecific and there is no good noninvasive diagnostic test of the vertebrobasilar circulation.

Tumors are found in less than 1% of dizzy patients and are slightly more prevalent (2% to 3%) among older patients referred to neurologists. The most common tumor associated with dizziness is an acoustic neuroma, for which cochlear symptoms (tinnitus and hearing loss) rather than dizziness predominate. Dizziness with unilateral cochlear symptoms suggests acoustic neuroma; bilateral symptoms in older persons typically represent presbycusis rather than a tumor.

Nonvertiginous Dizziness

Presyncope is the sensation of near fainting. This chapter does not deal with full loss of consciousness or syncope, which requires a different diagnostic approach. (See "Syncope," p 168.) Presyncope reflects diminished cerebral perfusion. Cardiac causes of presyncope can be electrical (tachy- or bradyarrhythmias) or structural (especially aortic outflow obstruction). Vascular causes of syncope are typically not ischemic events but are less serious, reversible conditions, such as orthostatic hypotension or temporary reactions due to vagal stimulation. Most presyncopal patients presenting with dizziness have symptoms attributable to postural change (with or without orthostatic hypotension) rather than more serious cardiac causes. Postural symptoms without orthostatic blood-pressure changes are particularly common in elderly persons. Likewise, orthostatic blood-pressure changes in the absence of symptoms are also quite common. Finally, certain stimuli (eg, micturition, defecation, coughing) can precipitate vagally mediated autonomic changes. Thus, the elderly man who rises to urinate in the middle of the night, the older person straining to have a bowel movement, or the pulmonary patient having paroxysms of coughing can experience lightheadedness or even frank syncope.

Disequilibrium is a sensation of being unsteady when standing or, in particular, walking. Balance depends not only on the vestibular system but also on the visual and somatosensory systems. Thus, multiple factors can contribute to imbalance, including chronic vestibulopathies, visual problems (eg, errors of refraction, cataract, loss of binocular vision, macular degeneration), musculoskeletal disorders (eg, arthritis, muscle weaknesses), and somatosensory or gait deficits (eg, neuropathies, previous strokes, cerebellar disease, Parkinson's disease, dementia).

Lightheadedness is a vaguer sensation best reserved as a descriptor for patients who do not experience one of the three more discrete types of dizziness sensations—vertigo, presyncope, or disequilibrium. In the vernacular of patients, these latter three sensations may be experienced as "spinning," "fainting," or "falling." Although any cause of dizziness may occasionally produce a nondescript "lightheaded" type of sensation, the two most prominent considerations are psychiatric (primarily depressive, anxiety, or somatoform disorders) or idiopathic causes, which together account for up to a third of all cases of dizziness.

Among other causes, prescription drug toxicity is an important contributing factor to dizziness in older patients. The use of at least three to five medications is a risk factor for dizziness among older adults, as are drugs that cause orthostatic hypotension, most commonly cardiovascular, antihypertensive, and psychotropic medications. Three purported causes particularly germane to elderly patients—cervical arthritis, visual disorders, and carotid sinus hypersensitivity—are seldom reported as causes in published series of dizzy patients. In part, this may be due to their common occurrence among older persons without dizziness as well as the fact that confirming these factors as the actual cause of dizziness can be difficult.

PROGNOSIS

Dizziness usually resolves within days to several months, but about one fourth of patients may experience chronic or recurrent symptoms. A 1-year prospective study of 102 patients found that dizziness due to psychiatric disorders, disequilibrium, or a vestibulopathy other than BPV or labyrinthitis was more likely to persist. Among 1087 community-dwelling older persons, chronic dizziness (ie, a month or longer) was reported by 24% and at 1-year follow-up was not associated with mortality, hospitalization, or functional status decline. Chronic dizziness, however, was associated with an increased risk of falling (relative risk of 1.4) and syncope (relative risk of 2.3), as well as worse self-rated health and depression.

EVALUATION

A brief, focused evaluation coupled with simple follow-up rather than initial diagnostic testing or referral is warranted in most patients. As mentioned, symptoms gradually improve in most patients. Moreover, specialized testing only occasionally reveals unsuspected diagnoses. More than 75% of the cases in which a diagnosis can be established are diagnosed by history and physical examination alone, with the history contributing most of these diagnoses.

History

As with many common symptoms, history is the single most useful part of the evaluation. The clinician must establish early on whether dizziness stems from a serious or benign cause. Although it is best to elicit the patient's own description of the event without prompting, four questions are particularly helpful:

- Is the dizziness characterized by one of three key sensations: spinning, fainting, or falling?
- Is there a positional effect on the dizziness and related symptoms? With BPV, the effect is almost always one of transient dizziness with change of head position, lying down, or sitting

up. The most common cause of presyncope is an orthostatic change in blood pressure, in which case the patient reports that dizziness occurs on assuming a more upright position (supine to sitting, or sitting to standing). Disequilibrium is manifested only when the patient is walking or standing.

- What associated symptoms are experienced along with the dizziness? Syncope is a particularly important symptom to inquire about, since actual loss of consciousness targets that very small subset of dizzy patients in whom early cardiac evaluation might be contemplated. Tinnitus or hearing changes, or both, are associated with certain vestibular disorders such as Ménière's disease or the rare acoustic neuroma. Nausea and, in particular, vomiting suggests vertigo rather than a nonvertiginous cause of dizziness. A central cause would not commonly present with isolated dizziness but instead would be expected to produce "neighboring" neurologic symptoms as well. Psychogenic causes, such as depression, anxiety, or somatoform disorders, typically have fatigue, insomnia, pain, or other physical and emotional symptoms in addition to dizziness.

- What medications is the patient taking? One should be particularly suspicious of new medications that were started around the time that symptoms of dizziness began.

Physical Examination

A focused physical examination would include the following steps.

- Measure the blood pressure and pulse while the patient is supine and again after standing for 2 to 3 minutes to detect orthostatic changes.

- Perform the head-hanging (Dix-Hallpike) test (described below).

- Perform a brief cardiovascular (murmurs, abnormal rhythm) and neurologic (cerebellar or focal deficits) examination.

- Observe the patient walk and turn (look for balance or gait difficulties).

Dizziness correlates best with postural hypotension when the latter is defined as a drop (eg, 20% decrease) in mean blood pressure, which is one third systolic plus two thirds diastolic, rather than a drop in systolic pressure only.

A screening vestibular examination is warranted in cases in which the cause of dizziness is not obvious. The four elements of a brief vestibular examination can be performed in about a minute and have in common the detection of nystagmus:

- **Primary position:** Have the patient look straight ahead and look for nystagmus.

- **Gaze-evoked:** Have the patient look to the right, left, up, and down, holding each position for 5 to 10 seconds. Deviations of 30 to 45 degrees of eye movement are sufficient to detect pathologic nystagmus; extreme gaze may accentuate physiologic nystagmus. More than three to five beats of nystagmus is abnormal.

- **Dix-Hallpike test:** With the patient seated on the examination table, help him or her lie down quickly with one ear turned toward the table. Help the patient up to a sitting position and repeat the maneuver with the other ear facing the table. Although hyperextending the patient's neck over the edge of the table has traditionally been recommended, this is not always possible and may not be necessary in many patients. The Dix-Hallpike test is positive in about half of patients with BPV—usually those with symptoms of recent onset. The occurrence of nystagmus (and often vertigo) that lasts 10 to 30 seconds after a few seconds of latency indicates a positive response.

- **Head-shaking:** Have the patient close his or her eyes, rapidly shake the head back and forth for 10 seconds, and then open his or her eyes. Look for nystagmus.

Nystagmus due to peripheral causes usually beats horizontally. Vertical nystagmus (ie, upward or downward beating) is uncommon and should prompt early evaluation (eg, neuroimaging, formal vestibular testing, neurology or otolaryngology referral) for central causes.

Diagnostic Testing

Simple laboratory tests, including complete blood cell counts, electrolytes, glucose level, serum creatinine, thyroid function, and serologic tests for syphilis, have a very low yield. Audiometry may be helpful in the patient with cochlear symptoms, such as tinnitus or asymmetric hearing loss. Abnormal audiograms may indicate Ménière's disease or, rarely, a cerebellopontine angle tumor such as acoustic neuroma. However, the most common abnormal audiometric finding in elderly patients is high-frequency hearing loss due to presbycusis; this represents a coincidental finding rather than a diagnostic explanation of dizziness.

Vestibular testing most commonly involves electronystagmography (ENG), which has important limitations. Sensitivity is variable, and it cannot readily distinguish between central and peripheral causes. In a community-based study of older persons, 80% of dizzy persons and 79% of persons in the control group were found to have at least two ENG abnormalities. Other tests include brain-stem auditory evoked responses, rotatory chair, and dynamic posturography. The latter two tests may substitute for or augment ENG in special situations, while testing for brain-stem auditory evoked responses is occasionally indicated if clinical evaluation, audiometry, or ENG suggest a central vestibulopathy.

Neuroimaging is occasionally warranted in the evaluation of the dizzy patient. This expensive and relatively low-yield testing should usually be reserved for patients with "red flags" (cerebellar or focal neurologic symptoms, vertical nystagmus). Although a computed tomography scan is the procedure of choice for strokes (because of cost and availability), magnetic resonance imaging (MRI) is better able to image posterior fossa structures. A community-based study of persons aged 65 and older found a similar prevalence of MRI abnormalities in the dizzy and nondizzy groups, prompting the authors to conclude that routine MRI is unlikely to identify a specific cause of dizziness. Neither electroencephalography nor lumbar puncture is typically useful in evaluating dizziness, and noninvasive carotid studies are warranted only if other neurologic symptoms suggest transient ischemic attacks.

An electrocardiogram is commonly obtained in older patients with cardiovascular risk factors but has a low diagnostic value in patients with a normal cardiac examination and nonsyncopal dizziness. Other tests helpful in evaluating syncope, ischemia, or valvular disease (Holter and event monitors, echocardiography, stress testing, tilt tables, and electrophysiologic studies) have not been shown to be useful in evaluating isolated dizziness.

Psychiatric disorders should be considered when the dizziness is nondescript (eg, lightheadedness), persistent and unexplained, or associated with multiple other somatic or emotional symptoms. Although brief case-finding instruments for depression are available, a single question about depressed mood has a sensitivity of 85% to 90% for detecting major depression. (See "Depression and Other Mood Disorders," p 269.)

MANAGEMENT

Although well-proven therapies for dizziness are limited, the natural history is nonetheless often favorable. In up to half of patients, dizziness spontaneously resolves or substantially improves within 2 weeks. In some cases, dizziness is an associated symptom of viral or other self-limited illnesses. Other times, it results from dehydration or a medication adverse effect. The two most common causes of peripheral vertigo—labyrinthitis and BPV—typically resolve within days or weeks, respectively. Types of dizziness for which specific management strategies may be helpful are discussed briefly below.

- **Acute vertigo attacks:** Attacks that occur with peripheral vestibular disorders such as labyrinthitis and Ménière's disease may benefit from meclizine and, if needed, a benzodiazepine. However, meclizine probably is overprescribed for chronic vestibulopathies and nonvertiginous dizziness.

- **Benign positional vertigo:** BPV usually can be treated with simple reassurance, since symptoms are typically mild and usually improve within weeks to several months. For severe or persistent symptoms, the patient may be educated about home habituation exercises or the canalolith repositioning (liberatory) maneuvers developed by Epley and Semont (see Figure 22.1).

- **Ménière's disease:** Attacks that are frequent or disabling may benefit from prophylactic treatment with salt restriction or diuretic therapy, or both. Occasional patients may require referral to otolaryngology for consideration of surgery.

- **Orthostatic hypotension:** Correct reversible causes.

- **Disequilibrium:** Advise the elderly patient with chronic disequilibrium to take measures to prevent falls, including the use of a cane, walker, or other assistive device, if necessary.

- **Psychogenic dizziness:** Psychogenic dizziness may be related to depressive or certain anxiety (eg, panic) disorders. Consider a trial of selective serotonin-reuptake inhibitors. In an open-label study involving 60 patients with dizziness, selective serotonin-reuptake inhibitors[OL] produced improvement in 63% of participants, many who had previously failed vestibular suppressants or benzodiazepines.

- **Chronic vestibulopathy:** Vestibular rehabilitation (a type of physical therapy exercise program) may be beneficial in persons with persistent dizziness.

Finally, when managing a patient with dizziness, it is important to remember that half of patients may have two or more potential causative or contributory factors for their symptoms. In community and clinic-based studies of older persons, Tinetti and col-

---

OL. Not approved by the U.S. Food and Drug Administration for this use.

Figure 22.1—Self-treatment of benign positional vertigo using the Epley's manuever.

Perform the maneuver three times a day until free of positional vertigo for 24 hours. Use the positions shown here when the right ear is affected. Reverse all positions (left instead of right) when the left ear is affected. The affected ear is the ear that when turned downward during the Dix-Hallpike maneuver triggers vertigo or nystagmus, or both.

Each maneuver consists of the following steps (numbered to match the illustration):

1. Sit on the bed with a pillow far enough behind you to be under your shoulders when you lie back. Turn your head 45 degrees to the left.

2. Holding your head in the turned position, lie back quickly so that your shoulders are supported on the pillow and your head is reclined on the bed. Hold this position for 30 seconds.

3. Remain prone on the bed and turn your head 90 degrees to the right. Hold this position 30 seconds.

4. Turn your head and body another 90 degrees to the right; you should now be looking down at the bed. Hold this position for 30 seconds.

5. Sit up, facing to the right.

SOURCE: Data from Radtke A, Neuhauser H, von Brevern M, et al. A modified Epley's procedure for self-treatment of benign paroxysmal positional vertigo. *Neurology* 1999;53(6):1358–1360.

leagues have found several factors associated with dizziness, including depressive or anxiety symptoms, impaired vision or hearing, the use of multiple medications, abnormal balance or gait, postural hypotension, diabetes mellitus, and past myocardial infarction. A multifactorial intervention targeting such factors might reduce the frequency or severity of dizziness in older patients. For example, an elderly patient may have a complex type of dizziness variably described as feeling faint when standing, unsteadiness when walking, and a nagging lightheadedness unrelated to position. Upon evaluation, the patient is found to have orthostatic hypotension related to one or more medications, depression, and disequilibrium due to a peripheral neuropathy and macular degeneration. Identifying potentially remediable factors, such as orthostasis and depression, may at least partially ameliorate the dizziness.

Annotated References

■ Colledge N, Lewis S, Mead G, et al. Magnetic resonance brain imaging in people with dizziness: a comparison with non-dizzy people. *J Neurol Neurosurg Psychiatry.* 2002;72(5):587–589.

This community-based case-control study examined magnetic resonance imaging (MRI) findings in persons aged 65 and over, comparing 125 dizzy individuals with 86 nondizzy individuals. Most MRI abnormalities (eg, white matter lesions, cortical atrophy) had a similar prevalence in both the dizzy and the nondizzy groups. The only finding significantly more common in the dizzy than in the nondizzy group was a white matter lesion in the midbrain (22% versus 4%); the clinical significance remains to be determined. The authors conclude that "routine" MRI is unlikely to reveal a specific cause for dizziness.

■ Hoffman R, Einstadter D, Kroenke K. Evaluating dizziness. *Am J Med.* 1999;107(5):468–478.

Studies were identified from MEDLINE searches (1966 through 1996), focusing on the causes and prognosis of dizziness as well as the performance of diagnostic tests. Peripheral vestibulopathies (35% to 55%) and psychiatric disorders (10% to 25%) were the most common causes for dizziness. Brain tumors (< 1%) and cerebrovascular disease (5%) were found infrequently. The history and physical examination led to a diagnosis in about 75% of cases, but at least 10% of dizzy patients eluded diagnosis. Symptoms are usually self-limited and not associated with an increased risk for mortality. Routine laboratory tests as well as cardiovascular and neurologic testing have a low yield in unselected dizzy patients. The role of specialized vestibular function tests such as electronystagmography remains inconclusive.

■ Kao AC, Nanda A, Williams CS, et al. Validation of dizziness as a possible geriatric syndrome. *J Am Geriatr Soc.* 2001;49(1):72–75.

A cross-sectional study of 262 consecutive patients (mean age, 78 years) attending a geriatric assessment center was conducted, involving 54 (21%) with dizziness and 208 without dizziness. Seven factors were found to be independently associated with dizziness, namely, depressive symptoms, cataracts, abnormal balance or gait, postural hypotension, diabetes mellitus, past myocardial infarction, and the use of three or more medications. The proportion of patients reporting dizziness was 0%, 6%, 12%, 26%, and 51% in the presence of 0, 1, 2, 3, and 4 or more risk factors, respectively. Similar

factors had been identified by the same investigators in a community-based sample (Tinetti ME, Williams CS, Gill TM, et al. Dizziness among older adults: a possible geriatric syndrome. *Ann Intern Med.* 2000;132[5]:337–344). A multifactorial intervention targeting these factors might reduce the frequency or severity of dizziness in older patients.

■ Parnes LS, Agrawal SK, Atlas J. Diagnosis and management of benign paroxysmal positional vertigo (BPPV). *Can Med Assoc J.* 2003;169(7):681–693.

Benign paroxysmal positional vertigo (BPPV) is the most common cause of vertigo and is a particularly common cause in older persons. This practical review covers the diagnosis and management of BPPV and provides both text and pictorial descriptions of several office maneuvers for treating BPPV.

■ Sloane PD, Coeytaux RR, Beck RS, et al. Dizziness: state of the science. *Ann Intern Med.* 2001;134(9 Pt 2):823–832.

This review covers several topics, including defining and classifying dizziness, its epidemiology, and selected issues in diagnosis and management. It also points out the gaps in our current knowledge.

■ Tinetti ME, Williams CS, Gill TM. Health, functional, and psychological outcomes among older persons with chronic dizziness. *J Am Geriatr Soc.* 2000;48(4):417–421.

In this probability sample of 1087 persons aged 72 or older and living in the community, 24% reported chronic dizziness. Over 1 year of follow-up, chronic dizziness was not found to be associated with mortality, hospitalization, or functional status, but was associated with risk of falling (relative risk [RR] of 1.4) and syncope (RR of 2.3) as well as worse self-rated health and depression. The authors conclude that the goals of care for chronic dizziness in older patients should be redirected from solely identifying and treating discrete diseases—an often expensive and unrewarding task—toward reducing the symptoms and disability associated with chronic dizziness.

Kurt Kroenke, MD

CHAPTER 23—SYNCOPE

KEY POINTS

- The incidence of syncope increases with age.

- In older adults, the cause of syncope is often multifactorial. In nearly one in five cases, the cause of syncope is not determined, but these cases generally have a favorable prognosis.

- Though many diagnostic procedures are available to search for the cause of syncope, most of them are expensive and have a low yield unless findings from the history or physical examination suggest a particular cause.

- The absence of cardiac disease strongly suggests that the cause of syncope is not cardiac.

- Bradycardia is the single most common cardiac cause of syncope.

- The treatment of syncope focuses on treating the underlying disorder and often with geriatric patients requires treatment of multiple possible underlying causes.

Syncope—a sudden, transient loss of postural tone and consciousness not due to trauma and with spontaneous full recovery—is common. Annually it accounts for approximately 3% of emergency department visits and 2% to 6% of hospital admissions. The incidence of syncope doubles among those aged 70 and older, and rates among those 80 and older is three to four times that seen among younger persons. Approximately 80% of the patients hospitalized for syncope are aged 65 or older. Syncope is a clinically important condition that is commonly difficult to evaluate. Its potential causes range from those that are benign and self-limited to those that are life threatening. In the older adult, the cause of syncope may also be multifactorial, adding to the diagnostic difficulty. Because it encompasses a wide range of potential causes (see Table 23.1 for the most common causes), the diagnostic evaluation of syncope can be complex and expensive. Although a wide variety of diagnostic tools can be employed, in many cases the patient's history provides the best clues to the cause and help direct the work-up.

NATURAL HISTORY

Syncope is generally caused by a reduction in cerebral perfusion. Hemodynamic disturbances that can decrease cerebral perfusion include alterations in systemic blood pressure or an increase in cerebral vascular resistance. Common causes of transient decreases in blood pressure include the following:

- Cardiac arrhythmias, such as atrial fibrillation with a rapid ventricular response, ventricular tachycardia, sick sinus syndrome with sinus pauses, and atrioventricular block
- Alterations in the peripheral vasculature due to arterial vasodilation or increased venous pooling
- Cardiopulmonary obstruction, such as that due to pulmonary emboli, aortic stenosis, hypertrophic obstructive cardiomyopathy, and atrial myxoma

Syncope can also occur as a consequence of an increase in cerebrovascular resistance. In hyperventilation syndrome and panic attacks, cerebrovascular vasoconstriction can occur without a change in systemic vascular resistance. In this situation, syncope can occur as a result of the relative decrease in cerebral blood flow without systemic hypotension. In rare instances, localized atherosclerotic disease can predispose a person to syncope by decreasing cerebral perfusion without a decrease in systemic blood pressure (vertebral basilar insufficiency and subclavian steal).

Syncope occurs most commonly while a person is standing. The effects of gravity cause up to a third of the blood volume to pool in the lower extremities when a person assumes the standing position. Unopposed, this reduces cardiac output by reducing venous return and decreases cerebral blood pressure. A number of reflex pathways involving the autonomic and endocrine systems are responsible for rapid compensation of the gravitational effects of standing. The baroreceptor reflex is triggered by carotid and aortic baroreceptors, which act to increase autonomic sympathetic tone, resulting in peripheral vasoconstriction and an increase in heart rate. Increased sympathetic activity of the renal nerve leads to stimulation of renin release from the juxtaglomerular apparatus. The activation of the renin-angiotensin system leads to direct vasoconstriction by the action of angiotensin II and the secretion of aldosterone from the adrenal cortex to retain sodium, thereby raising the extracelluar fluid volume. A postural change to a standing position also rapidly reduces the level of atrial natriuretic factor, which is a vasodilator and inhibitor of the renin-angiotensin system. The reduction in atrial natriuretic factor facilitates vasoconstriction, and the activity of the volume effects of the renin-angiotensin contributes to vasoconstriction.

In aging, many of these reflex mechanisms are less responsive. The cardiac response to β-adrenergic stimulation (cardiac acceleration and increased contractility) decreases with advancing age. As a result of this and perhaps other mechanisms, the baroreflex (increasing heart rate and vasoconstriction) is also less effective with advancing age. In addition, comorbid conditions that can affect postural responses, such as diabetes mellitus, are prevalent among elderly persons. Medications such as α-blockers, β-blockers, and tricyclic antidepressants may also impair postural reflexes. The effects of age-related decline in adaptive reflexes, comorbid conditions, and medications may combine, becoming factors in syncopal events in the elderly person. Because older persons have a decreased ability to increase heart rate in response to sympathetic stimulation, blood volume maintenance and vasoconstriction become more important in maintaining postural blood pressure. Thus, the elderly person may be particularly sensitive to the effects of dehydration and vasodilator drugs.

Table 23.1—Common Causes of Syncope in Elderly Persons

Arrhythmia

Aortic stenosis

Carotid sinus hypersensitivity

Hypoglycemia

Myocardial infarction

Orthostatic hypotension

Postprandial hypotension

Psychogenic causes

Pulmonary embolism (large)

Vasovagal faint

The prognosis of syncope depends on the underlying cause. The major issue is whether a cardiac cause is responsible. The 1-year mortality for patients with cardiac causes for syncope averages 18% to 33% (deaths are due to underlying disease, not syncope), whereas syncope due to noncardiac causes has a much more favorable prognosis, a 1-year mortality of approximately 6%. In one third to one half of syncopal patients, no cause can be found. The prognosis for these patients is intermediate but generally favorable.

EVALUATION OF THE PATIENT WITH SYNCOPE

History

The clinical history obtained from the patient and, if possible, from witnesses to the event may provide a diagnosis in up to 50% of cases in which a diagnosis can be established. First, it is important to establish whether the patient suffered a true syncopal event, as opposed to dizziness (disequilibrium) or lightheadedness. Key elements to obtain from the history follow:

- Was there a precipitant? Could the patient's activities around the time of the event have triggered it? Such activities include eating, urinating, coughing, using medication, and experiencing emotional stress. Syncope occurring during physical exertion should raise the possibility of myocardial ischemia or aortic stenosis. A history of syncope after turning motions of the head should raise the possibility of carotid sinus hypersensitivity.

- Were there prodromal symptoms before the event? Symptoms of chest pain, palpitations, or shortness of breath suggest a cardiac or pulmonary cause. Diaphoresis, presyncope, and gastrointestinal symptoms, such as nausea or vomiting, can be associated with vasovagal syncope. Sudden onset of syncope with less than 5 seconds of warning is characteristic of syncope due to a cardiac arrhythmia.

- What medications are being used? It is important to establish how medications were taken with relationship to meals and other activities, and whether there have been recent changes in the medication regimen. Specifics about dosage times should be obtained.

- What did witnesses observe? They should be queried about the duration of the event and the appearance of the patient during the event. Patients with cardiac causes of syncope are generally flaccid in tone and motionless while unconscious, unless the event lasts for more than 15 seconds, when myoclonic jerks and truncal extension may be seen. In contrast, increased body motion, tone, and head turning to one side with loss of consciousness are more common with seizure activity.

- Are there significant comorbid conditions? A history of coronary artery disease or its associated symptoms is particularly important. Approximately 5% of myocardial infarctions present as syncope. Sustained ventricular tachycardia resulting in syncope is most common in patients with prior myocardial infarction. Patients with diabetes mellitus are at increased risk for coronary atherosclerosis as well as autonomic dysfunction predisposing to syncope.

Table 23.2 summarizes the characteristics of three classes of syncope.

Physical Examination

A physical examination should focus on elements raised by the history. It is estimated that of those patients in whom a cause of syncope can be established, 20% are identified by features found during physical examination. The blood pressure should be measured in both arms, as well as postural changes in the blood pressure. The pulse should be taken with the patient in the supine and standing positions. Blood pressure with the patient in the standing position should be obtained after 1 minute of standing and repeated after the patient has been standing for 3 minutes. Although any definition of postural hypotension is arbitrary, a decrease in systolic blood pressure of more than 20 mm Hg is the definition used most frequently.

The character of the carotid pulse should also be assessed for the delayed upstroke and low volume characteristic of significant aortic stenosis. The presence of a carotid bruit, a history of cerebrovascular disease, and recent myocardial infarction are relative contraindications to carotid sinus massage. Even in the absence of contraindications, carotid sinus massage should be performed only under continuous electrocardiographic monitoring (to detect induced atrioventricular [AV] block or other arrhythmias) in a setting where resuscitation equipment is available.

The physical examination of the patient with syncope should include cardiac examination for evidence of murmurs characteristic of valvular abnormalities or extra heart sounds suggestive of cardiomyopathy. Examination of the stool for occult blood and neurologic examination for focal deficits are also important.

An electrocardiogram (ECG) is indicated for all patients presenting with syncope. Though ECG estab-

Table 23.2—Characteristics of Three Classes of Syncope

Phase	Cardiac Arrhythmia	Vasovagal	Seizure
Prior to event	Occurs in any position	Aborted if person lies flat	Any position
	Less than 5 seconds' warning	Seconds' to minutes' warning	No warning or prodrome
	Precipitant absent	Precipitant present	—
	Palpitations rare	—	—
	—	Nausea, diaphoresis common	—
	—	Visual changes	—
During event	Flaccid tone	Motionless, relaxed tone	Rigid tone
	Pulse absent, faint	Slow, faint pulse	Rapid pulse, elevated blood pressure
	Blue, ashen	Pale color	—
	Incontinence rare	—	—
	—	Dilated, reactive pupils	Tonic eye deviation common
	—	—	Frothing at mouth
Recovery	Rapid and complete	Fatigue common after event	Slow, incomplete recovery
	—	No retrograde amnesia	Disorientation
	—	Diaphoresis and nausea common	—
	—	—	Focal neurologic findings

lishes a diagnosis in only 5% of those with syncope, approximately 50% have an abnormal ECG. Abnormalities on an ECG may provide clues for further cardiovascular evaluation; a normal ECG is associated with a more favorable prognosis. Key features to assess on an ECG include evidence of acute or remote myocardial infarction. Conduction abnormalities, especially block in the AV node or below, and pre-excitation, such as Wolff-Parkinson-White, may be detected as well; inappropriate sinus bradycardia may also be found. A prolonged QT interval can predispose a person to ventricular arrhythmias, including torsade de pointes.

Ambulatory Electrocardiographic Monitoring

An ambulatory ECG recording can establish or exclude many causes of syncope if the patient experiences syncopal or presyncopal symptoms during the recording. Unfortunately, the occurrence of symptoms during ambulatory ECG monitoring is relatively rare in most patients with syncope that remains unexplained after a history, physical examination, and ECG. On average, studies examining the diagnostic yield of ambulatory ECG report an arrhythmia correlating with symptoms in approximately 4% of patients. In another 15% of patients studied, an arrhythmia was excluded by the presence of symptoms during the recording, but without evidence of an arrhythmia; in approximately 14% of patients, arrhythmias were found to be present but without concomitant symptoms. These patients may

represent a diagnostic dilemma. However, certain arrhythmias, even asymptomatic ones, such as nonsustained ventricular tachycardia, second- and third-degree AV block, and sinus pauses in excess of 3 seconds, are rare in persons without heart disease. Their presence, even if asymptomatic, in a patient with a history of syncope indicates the need for further evaluation.

Ambulatory loop recorders that may be worn for a many days or weeks at a time are commonly used to capture ECG recordings of symptoms that occur infrequently. These devices constantly record an ECG tracing on a 5- to 10-minute loop; the patient presses a button to stop the recording after an event has occurred and then transmits this by telephone to a monitoring center. Among patients who are able operate the recorder, the diagnostic yield is approximately 25%. However, many elderly patients are unable or unwilling to capture and transmit these recordings.

Implantable Loop Recorders

Subcutaneous implantable loop recorders have been developed; these devices are placed in the prepectoral region under local anesthesia. The devices have long-term memories and a battery life of approximately 14 to 18 months. Generally, no patient intervention is required for the device to store recordings, but the patient can also trigger the device to record and retain an ECG if symptoms occur. Implantable loop recorders have recently been shown to be efficient and cost-effective in establishing a cause in selected patients with an ejection fraction > 35% and symptoms not consistent with a neural cause of syncope.

Echocardiography

Two-dimensional echocardiography has a low yield in the absence of features suggestive of heart disease by history, physical examination, or ECG. It is most useful in confirming a specific diagnosis suspected by other assessment. However, unsuspected findings on echocardiography are reported in approximately 5% to 10% of unselected patients. Thus, echocardiography has been advocated for the evaluation of syncope. Occult coronary artery disease is also prevalent among elderly persons, and stress testing is often employed to screen for this. In some patients, particularly those with the suggestion of structural cardiac abnormalities and ischemia by history, physical examination, or ECG, it is efficient to perform stress echocardiography as a single procedure.

Tilt-Table Testing

Head-up tilt-table testing results in pooling of blood in the lower extremities and, in susceptible individuals, may trigger syncope mediated by neurocardiogenic mechanisms. Tilt-table testing is useful for patients suspected of having vasovagal syncope and those with unexplained syncope who are not suspected of having a cardiac cause. In tilt-table testing, the patient reclines on a table that then slowly rotates the patient from supine to head up slowly and passively. The patient is secured on the surface, usually with straps and a foot rest, to minimize muscle contraction and maximize venous pooling in the extremities. The patient is continuously monitored for symptoms and with an electrocardiograph and blood-pressure monitor. The test is considered positive if the patient has a cardioinhibitory or vasodepressor response to tilting, or both. Various protocols are available for this testing, and some may include administration of intravenous medications. The sensitivity and specificity of tilt-table testing vary considerably, depending on the protocol used and the patient population. A positive tilt-table result occurs in approximately 11% of normal elderly persons. Thus, a positive tilt-table result alone does not ensure that a vasovagal event is the cause. It is generally recommended that men over the age of 45 and women over the age of 55 have stress testing prior to tilt-table testing so that a positive result on a tilt-table test does not delay diagnosis of coronary ischemia when that is the true culprit.

Responses to tilt testing performed for syncope evaluation tend to differ by age among persons without significant structural heart disease. Those aged 65 and older tend to have far higher rates of symptoms due to pure vasodilatation without significant change in heart rate than do individuals aged 35 or younger. In contrast, individuals aged 35 or younger tend to have more profound cardioinhibitory responses characterized by profound bradycardia or asystole induced by tilt testing than do those aged 65 and older. The different pattern of responses induced by tilt studies between younger and older persons suggests that different mechanisms for neurocardiogenic syncope predominate at different ages. Exaggerated autonomic response is common in younger persons, whereas attenuated autonomic responses become predominant with advancing age.

Electrophysiologic Studies

Guidelines suggest that invasive electrophysiologic (EP) testing should be employed in the evaluation of patients with structural heart disease with unexplained syncope. There is also agreement that EP testing should not be employed in situations where the results of the test would not influence subsequent treatment or in which a cause of the syncope has been established. The role of EP testing in patients with recurrent syncope with no structural heart disease and negative tilt-table studies remains undefined. EP testing is most sensitive for detecting ventricular arrhythmias in the setting of ischemic heart disease and is less sensitive for the detection of ventricular arrhythmias in dilated nonischemic cardiomyopathies. The sensitivity of EP testing for detecting most bradyarrhythmias is also low.

Neurologic Testing

Neurologic testing, including imaging of the head by computed tomography or magnetic resonance imaging and electroencephalographic recording, is appropriate in situations when focal neurologic signs or symptoms are present or when the history suggests seizure.

TREATMENT

The treatment of syncope depends on the underlying cause. When a single underlying cause is established, that is where therapeutic interventions should be concentrated. This is particularly important for cardiac causes. Myocardial ischemia causing syncope may require revascularization (percutaneous or surgical) or aggressive medical therapy. Valvular heart disease causing syncope, particularly aortic stenosis, is typically managed surgically. Treatment of symptomatic supraventricular tachyarrhythmias, such as atrial flutter or fibrillation, may involve antiarrhythmic drug therapy or electrophysiology ablation procedures. Significant ventricular tachyarrhythmias are often treated with implanted defibrillators or antiarrhythmic drugs. Most bradyarrhythmias causing syncope require pacemakers, unless drug side effects or metabolic disturbances are the principal factors.

Orthostatic hypotension is common among older adults and often responds to modifications in drug regimens. In particular, avoidance of vasodilator drugs may help. An important measure is to ensure that patients have adequate volume by reducing or discontinuing diuretics and, if necessary, liberalizing salt intake. Other nonpharmacologic measures that may help include the use of waist-high compression stockings, squatting, and sleeping in a head-up position. Avoidance of excessively warm environment and activities associated with straining (Valsalva) may also be beneficial. If autonomic dysfunction is present and hypertension, heart failure, and hypokalemia are not concerns, then low-dose fludrocortisone may be effective.

When vasovagal syncope occurs as the result of a specific trigger (eg, sights, smells), avoidance is best if this is feasible. A number of pharmacologic therapies have been proposed, including β-blockers, clonidine, paroxetine, midodrine, and others. The pharmacologic approach to the treatment of vasovagal syncope remains somewhat controversial and may require sequential trials of several agents.

Carotid sinus hypersensitivity is best treated by avoiding stimulating factors (tight collars or rapid neck motions). If these measures are ineffective, pacemaker implantation may be useful.

Postprandial hypotension may be improved by avoidance of alcohol and large carbohydrate meals. Caffeine consumption and remaining recumbent following meals may also help.

When syncope in the geriatric patient has several causes, addressing a single factor in isolation may be only partially effective, and a broader approach addressing several contributing causes is required. Careful review of medications, as well as discontinuation of medications that increase the risk of syncope, is always an early step.

For patients with recurrent syncope without an identifiable cause, care must be taken to help them avoid harming themselves or others if they remain at risk for syncope. The issue of driving may need to be addressed. Guidelines from the American Heart Association recommend that driving be restricted for several months and that, if the patient remains recurrence free, driving be resumed. However, physicians should be aware that many states have laws regarding driving with a history of syncope.

ANNOTATED REFERENCES

■ Garcia-Civera R, Ruiz-Granell R, Morell-Cabedo S, et al. Selective use of diagnostic tests inpatients with syncope of unknown cause. *J Am Coll Cardiol.* 2003;41(5):787–790.

This study evaluated the diagnostic yield of cardiac testing in patients clinically identified to have high or low risk of cardiac arrhythmia but no established diagnosis after an initial history, physical, and laboratory examination. Patients believed to be at high risk were sent directly to electrophysiologic study (EPS) and had any of the following clinical characteristics: structural heart disease, family history of sudden death, abnormal electrocardiogram, arrhythmia on Holter, or palpitations prior to onset of syncope. The EPS was abnormal in 44% of patients with these clinical characteristics, and the most common diagnoses were paroxysmal atrioventricular block, ventricular tachycardia, supraventricular tachycardia, and sinus node dysfunction. Among the 56% with negative EPS, tilt-table tests (TTT) were performed and were abnormal in 58% of patients, resulting in an overall diagnostic yield of 74%. In contrast, patients without features suggestive of cardiac arrhythmia were referred directly for TTT, which was abnormal in 71% of that population. The patients judged to be at increased risk for cardiac arrhythmia were significantly older than the lower-risk group (59 + 14 years versus 51 + 18 years, *P* = .002).

■ Kurbaan AS, Bowker TJ, Wijesekara N, et al. Age and hemodynamic responses to tilt testing in those with syncope of unknown origin. *J Am Coll Cardiol.* 2003;41(6):1004–1007.

This was a study of tilt-table responses in 472 patients without evidence of symptomatic structural heart disease referred for evaluation of syncope of unknown cause. The patients older than 65 years were more likely to have a pure vasodepressor response (hypotension without change in heart rate; odds radio 29.5, *P* < .0001) and less likely to have a severe cardioinhibitory response (marked bradycardia or asystole; odds ratio 0.18, *P* < .0001) when compared with those younger than 35 years.

■ Soteriades ES, Evans JC, Larson MG, et al. Incidence and prognosis of syncope. *N Engl J Med.* 2002;347(12):878–885.

Of 7814 participants in the Framingham Heart Study, 822 reported syncope. The rate of syncope was fairly constant between the ages of 20 and 69, between 2.6 and 5.7 per 1000 person years. A sharp increase in syncope was present in those aged 70 to 79 (11.1 per 1000 person years) and aged 80 and older (16.9 to 19.5 per 1000 person years). The most commonly identified causes of syncope were vasovagal (21.2%), cardiac (9.5%), and orthostatic (9.4%). Patients with cardiac syncope were older than patients with neurologic, vasovagal, or unknown syncope. In comparison with persons without syncope, in those with syncope the hazard ratio for all-cause mortality was 1.31. Syncope due to cardiac causes was associated with the highest all-cause mortality, hazard ratio 2.01 compared with 1.54 and 1.32 for those with neurologic and unknown causes, respectively. The mortality among those with and without vasovagal syncope did not differ.

David Bush, MD

CHAPTER 24—MALNUTRITION

KEY POINTS

- Aging is associated with changes in body composition such that well-standardized nutrient requirements for younger or middle-aged adults cannot be generalized to older persons.

- The Mini-Nutritional Assessment—Short Form is a brief and simple instrument useful for nutritional screening in geriatric patients.

- Identification of the presence of protein-energy undernutrition or obesity can be facilitated by determining a patient's body mass index.

- Many drugs have anorexia as a major adverse effect or can reduce nutrient availability in the older adult.

- Various appetite stimulants and trophic agents are being used in older patients and are the focus of intensive investigation.

Older persons suffer a burden of malnutrition that spans the spectrum from under- to overnutrition. Nutritional problems accompany many of the chronic disease processes that afflict older persons. Moreover, age-related changes in physiology, metabolism, and function may alter the older person's nutritional requirements. Better understanding among clinicians of the aging process and of nutritional screening, assessment, and interventions could potentially improve the health and independence of older persons.

AGE-RELATED CHANGES

Body Composition

Aging is associated with notable changes in body composition: bone mass, lean mass, and water content all decrease, while fat mass increases. The increase in total body fat is commonly accompanied by greater intra-abdominal fat stores. The consequence of these changes in body composition is that well-standardized nutrient requirements for younger or middle-aged adults cannot be generalized to older persons. The aging process also affects organ functions, although the degree of change observed is highly variable among individuals. Decline in organ functions may affect nutritional assessment and intervention.

Energy Requirements

Reduced basal metabolic rate in older persons reflects loss of muscle mass. The basal metabolic rate is the

principal determinant of total energy expenditure; energy expenditure in relation to physical activity is the most variable component. The Harris-Benedict equations may be used to predict basal energy expenditure. A simple method for estimating the total daily energy needs of the older patient is based on body weight alone (Table 24.1). In any determination of energy needs for older persons, care must be taken to avoid overfeeding while still meeting basal requirements.

Macronutrient Needs

Modified food guide pyramids for older persons based upon the U.S. Department of Agriculture food guide pyramid have been released (Russell RM, Rasmussen H, Lichtenstein AH. Modified food guide pyramid for people over seventy years of age. *J Nutr.* 1999;129:751–753. See also http://nutrition.tufts. edu/consumer/pyramid.html). The food selections are more relevant to the target audience, and appropriate intakes of water, fiber, and supplements of calcium, vitamin D, and vitamin B_{12} are highlighted. The new USDA food pyramid (http://www.mypyramid.gov) released in 2005 may offer opportunity to further tailor recommendations for older persons.

The Food and Nutrition Board of the Institute of Medicine has released macronutrient guidelines that recommend a prudent diet, with 20% to 35% calories as fat and reduced intakes of cholesterol, saturated fat, and trans-fatty acids. Carbohydrates should constitute 45% to 65% of total calories; complex carbohydrates are the preferred fiber source. More specifically, the

---

Table 24.1—Nutritional Requirement Calculations

Estimation of energy needs on basis of body weight

25–30 kcal/kg body weight /day

For the obese individual, use a reduced compromise body weight that approximates 120% of ideal.

Estimation of energy needs using the Harris-Benedict equation for basal energy expenditure (BEE)

Male BEE = 66 + (13.7 × weight in kg) + (5 × height in cm) − (6.8 × age)

Female BEE = 655 + (9.6 × weight in kg) + (1.8 × height in cm) − (4.7 × age)

Adjust BEE with empiric stress factors (1.00 for nonstressed and 1.5 for stressed) to estimate total energy expenditure of ill elderly patients.

Estimation of protein needs on basis of body weight

Protein = (0.8 to 1.5) g / kg body weight / day

For the obese individual, use ideal body weight.

NOTE: 1 lb = 0.453 kg; 1 in = 2.54 cm.

recommended fiber intake for those aged 60 years and over is 30 g for men and 21 g for women. Protein intake is recommended at 0.8 g per kg of body weight per day at approximately 10% to 35% of total calories. With stress or injury, protein requirements are typically estimated at 1.5 g per kg of body weight per day, but underlying renal or hepatic insufficiency may warrant protein restriction (Table 24.1).

Micronutrient Requirements

Revisions of the Dietary Reference Intakes include recommended dietary allowances (RDAs) with more specific guidelines for older persons; those for the group aged 71 years and older are shown in Table 24.2.

Fluid Needs

Dehydration is the most common fluid or electrolyte disturbance in older persons. Normal aging is associated with a decreased perception of thirst, impaired response to serum osmolarity, and reduced ability to concentrate urine following fluid deprivation. A decline in fluid intake can also result from disease states that cause a reduction in mental or physical ability to recognize or express thirst, or that result in decreased access to water. In general, fluid needs of older persons can be met with 30 mL per kg of body weight per day or 1 mL per kcal ingested. Fluid needs may be altered during episodes of fever or infection, as well as with diuretic or laxative therapy. Common signs of dehydration are decreased urine output, elevated body temperature, constipation, mucosal dryness, skin turgor changes, and confusion. Altered fluid status (overhydration or underhydration) may affect anthropometric and biochemical measures, resulting in inaccurate assessments.

NUTRITION SCREENING AND ASSESSMENT

Anthropometrics

Anthropometric measurements are a mainstay of nutritional assessment of older persons. An unintended weight loss of 10 pounds in the preceding 6 months is a useful indicator of morbidity. This degree of weight loss is predictive of functional limitations, health care charges, and need for hospitalization. The Minimum Data Set (MDS) used by Medicare-certified nursing homes defines weight loss as 5% or more in the past month or 10% or more in the past 6 months. Body mass index (BMI)—weight in kilograms / (height in meters)^2—has received increasing attention. National Institutes of Health guidelines regarding body size classification have been released (Table 24.3). BMI is a useful measure of body size and indirect measure of body fatness that does not require the use of a reference table of ideal weights. The risk threshold for low BMI is set at 18.5. Other anthropometric tools include skin-fold and circumference measurements, but these have had limited practical application because of the difficulty of training personnel to achieve acceptable reliability.

Table 24.2—Micronutrients: Recommended Dietary Allowances for Persons Aged 71 and Older

Nutrient	Men	Women
Calcium (mg)*	1200	1200
Phosphorus (mg)	700	700
Magnesium (mg)	420	320
Vitamin D (μg)*	15	15
Fluoride (mg)*	4	3
Thiamin (mg)	1.2	1.1
Riboflavin (mg)	1.3	1.1
Niacin (mg)	16	14
Vitamin B$_6$ (mg)	1.7	1.5
Folate (μg)	400	400
Vitamin B$_{12}$ (μg)	2.4	2.4
Pantothenic acid (mg)*	5	5
Biotin (μg)*	30	30
Choline (mg)*	550	425
Vitamin C (mg)	90	75
α-Tocopherol (mg)	15	15
Selenium (μg)	55	55

*Adequate intakes, not recommended dietary allowances.

SOURCES: Data from: Standing Committee on the Scientific Evaluation of Dietary Reference Intakes, Food and Nutrition Board, Institute of Medicine, *Dietary Reference Intakes for Calcium, Phosphorus, Magnesium, Vitamin D, and Fluoride*. Washington, DC: National Academy Press; 1997. Standing Committee on the Scientific Evaluation of Dietary Reference Intakes, Institute of Medicine, *Dietary Reference Intakes for Thiamin, Riboflavin, Niacin, Vitamin B6, Folate, Vitamin B12, Pantothenic Acid, Biotin, and Choline*. Washington, DC: National Academy Press; 1999. Standing Committee on the Scientific Evaluation of Dietary Reference Intakes, Food and Nutrition Board, *Dietary Reference Intakes for Vitamin C, Vitamin E, Selenium, and Beta Carotene, and Other Carotenoids*. Washington, DC: National Academy Press; 2000. Available at http://www.nal.usda.gov/fnic/etext/000105.html (accessed October 2005).

Table 24.3—Body Size Classification

Body Size	Body Mass Index (kg/m^2)
Underweight	< 18.5
Normal weight	18.5–24.9
Overweight	25–29.9
Obesity	≥ 30
Extreme obesity	≥ 40

NOTE: 1 lb = 0.453 kg; 1 in = 2.54 cm.

SOURCE: Data from: NHLBI Obesity Education Initiative Expert Panel. *Clinical Guidelines on the Identification, Evaluation, and Treatment of Overweight and Obesity in Adults: The Evidence Report*. Bethesda, MD: National Institutes of Health, National Heart, Lung and Blood Institute; September 1998: xiv. Pub. No. 98-4083.

Nutritional Intake

Generally, inadequate nutritional intake has been defined as average or usual intake of servings of food groups, nutrients, or energy below a threshold level of the RDA. The limited reliability of accurately assessing dietary intake measures is well known, so thresholds of 25% to 50% below the RDA have generally been selected. A study found reduced energy intake (less than 50% of calculated maintenance energy requirements) in 21% of a sample of hospitalized older persons. This subset of patients had higher rates of in-hospital mortality and 90-day mortality than did those above the threshold of energy intake. The MDS uses a different measure: intake of less than 75% of food provided is the threshold to trigger nutrition assessment in nursing homes. Surveys of nutritional status conducted among chronically institutionalized older persons suggest that 5% to 18% of nursing-home residents have energy intakes below their recommended average energy expenditure.

Energy intakes of men and women aged 65 to 98 years have been estimated in a nationwide food consumption survey. Investigators report that 37% to 40% of the men and women studied had energy intakes lower than two thirds of the RDA, and many reported skipping at least one meal each day. Estimated intakes by consumption surveys, however, may be unreliable because some studies suggest that older persons under-report energy intakes by 20% to 30%.

Food security issues are prevalent contributors to inadequate nutritional intakes among older persons. It is important to ascertain whether limitations in resources, transportation, or functionality may limit access to food or ability to prepare food.

Laboratory Tests: Albumin, Prealbumin, Cholesterol

Serum albumin has been recognized as a risk indicator for morbidity and mortality. Hypoalbuminemia lacks specificity and sensitivity as an indicator of malnutrition; however, it may be associated with injury, disease, or inflammatory conditions. As a negative acute phase reactant, it is subject to cytokine-mediated decline in synthesis and to increased degradation and transcapillary leakage. It is thought that albumin synthesis does not decrease with age; however, longitudinal studies of serum albumin suggest a modest decline in levels with aging that may be independent of disease. The prognostic value of hypoalbuminemia may be largely due to its utility as a proxy measure for injury, disease, or inflammation. In the community setting, hypoalbuminemia has been associated with functional limitation, sarcopenia, increased health care use, and mortality. In the hospital setting, it has also been associated with increased length of hospital stay, complications, readmissions, and mortality. Other protein markers of nutritional status are being investigated. Prealbumin has received the most attention, as it has a considerably shorter half-life than albumin and may therefore more adequately reflect short-term changes in protein status. Unfortunately, prealbumin otherwise appears to suffer the same limitations as albumin as an indicator of nutritional status.

Serum cholesterol has also been linked to nutritional status. Low cholesterol levels (< 160 mg/dL) are often detected in persons with serious underlying disease, such as malignancy. Poor clinical outcomes have been observed among hospitalized and institutionalized older persons with hypocholesterolemia. A study of community-dwelling older persons found that those in the lowest quartile of serum cholesterol did not differ from others in their nutrient intakes. It appears likely, again, that acquired hypocholesterolemia is a nonspecific feature of poor health status that is independent of nutrient or energy intakes, and that it may better reflect a proinflammatory condition. Of interest is the observation that community-dwelling older persons with both hypoalbuminemia and hypocholesterolemia exhibit the highest rates for adverse functional and mortality outcomes in comparison with those with hypoalbuminemia or hypocholesterolemia alone.

Drug-Nutrient Interactions

Drugs may modify the nutrient needs and metabolism of older persons. Certain drugs, such as digoxin and phenytoin, even at therapeutic levels, can cause anorexia in the older person. Additional agents that have anorexia as a major potential adverse effect include selective serotonin-reuptake inhibitors, calcium channel blockers (dihydropyridines), H_2 receptor antagonists, proton-pump inhibitors, narcotic analgesics, furosemide, potassium supplement, ipratropium bromide, and theophylline. Many drugs are known to interfere with taste and smell (see "Oral Diseases and Disorders," Table 42.2, p 324) and others may reduce the availability of specific nutrients (Table 24.4).

Multi-Item Tools for Nutrition Screening

The nutritional status of the older person can be influenced by a variety of factors (Table 24.5). The absence of single assessment measures that are valid indicators of comprehensive nutritional status has prompted the development of multi-item tools. Older persons in acute- or chronic-care facilities have been extensively studied to identify indicators and predictors

Table 24.4—Drug-Nutrient Interactions

Drug	Reduced Nutrient Availability
Alcohol	Zinc, vitamins A, B_1, B_2, B_6, folate, vitamin B_{12}
Antacids	Vitamin B_{12}, folate, iron, total kcal
Antibiotics, broad-spectrum	Vitamin K
Colchicine	Vitamin B_{12}
Digoxin	Zinc, total kcal (via anorexia)
Diuretics	Zinc, magnesium, vitamin B_6, potassium, copper
Isoniazid	Vitamin B_6, niacin
Levodopa	Vitamin B_6
Laxatives	Calcium, vitamins A, B_2, B_{12}, D, E, K
Lipid-binding resins	Vitamins A, D, E, K
Metformin	Vitamin B_{12}, total kcal
Mineral oil	Vitamins A, D, E, K
Phenytoin	Vitamin D, folate
Salicylates	Vitamin C, folate
SSRIs	Total kcal (via anorexia)
Theophylline	Total kcal (via anorexia)
Trimethoprim	Folate

NOTE: SSRI = selective serotonin-reuptake inhibitor.

SOURCE: Modified from Silver AJ. Malnutrition. In: Beck JC, ed. *Geriatric Review Syllabus: A Core Curriculum in Geriatric Medicine.* 1st ed. New York: American Geriatrics Society; 1989:100.

Table 24.5—Risk Factors for Poor Nutritional Status

Alcohol or substance abuse

Cognitive dysfunction

Decreased exercise

Depression, poor mental health

Functional limitations

Inadequate funds

Limited education

Limited mobility, transportation

Medical problems, chronic diseases

Medications

Poor dentition

Restricted diet, poor eating habits

Social isolation

of nutritional status, but those in the community setting have been subject to less investigation. Nutrition screening tools for older persons have been widely disseminated, and health professionals are beginning to use such tools for a variety of purposes. Their effectiveness remains to be demonstrated; specifically, we need to learn whether these tools can identify undernour-

ished individuals whose problems are amenable to intervention.

The Nutrition Screening Initiative is a collaborative effort of the American Dietetic Association, the American Academy of Family Practitioners, and the National Council on Aging, Inc. Three interdisciplinary tools to screen for nutrition risk were developed by the Nutrition Screening Initiative to aid in the evaluation of the nutritional status of older persons. The DETERMINE checklist was created to raise public awareness about the importance of nutrition to the health of older persons (see the Appendix, p 501 and http://www.aafp.org/nsi.xml). This self-report questionnaire is composed of 10 items and is intended to identify potential risks, but not to diagnose malnutrition. The Level I screen, intended for use by health care professionals, incorporates additional assessment items regarding dietary habits, functional status, living environment, and weight change, as well as measures of height and weight. The Level II screen, for use by more highly trained medical and nutrition professionals and suggested for use in the diagnosis of malnutrition, contains all the items from Level I with additional biochemical and anthropometric measures, as well as provision for more detailed evaluation of depression and mental status, as indicated (see http://www.aafp.org/nsi.xml).

The Mini-Nutritional Assessment tool was developed to evaluate the risk of malnutrition among frail older persons and identify those who may benefit from early intervention. More extensive cross-validation studies among healthy older persons have since been completed. This assessment tool requires administration by a trained professional and is composed of 18 items. The assessment includes questions about BMI, mid-arm and calf circumferences, weight loss, living environment, medications use, dietary habits, clinical global assessment, and self-perception of health and nutrition status. A shortened screening version that contains only six items, the short form Mini-Nutritional Assessment (MNA-SF), is now available (see http://www.mna-elderly.com/clinical-practice.htm and reference by Rubenstein, 2001, at the end of the chapter).

NUTRITION SYNDROMES

Undernutrition

Attempts to subdivide the group of nutritional syndromes characterized by loss of weight have been challenging. The nomenclature used implies that these syndromes are distinct, when in practice it is often quite difficult to distinguish one from another, and the syndromes commonly overlap. The presence (cachexia) or absence (wasting) of cytokine-mediated response to injury or disease is at times used, but in examples such as the weight loss from AIDS, there appears that some, but not all, of the loss is the result of inflammation. Some authors note that with cachexia, resting energy expenditure is increased whereas with wasting it is decreased, but this measure is not generally available to most practicing clinicians. Even more confusing are the terms *semi-starvation* and *protein-energy undernutrition*, both of which imply that nutritional interventions would be the appropriate correction of the underlying problem, but as will be discussed in the following section, data to support this implication are weak.

Obesity

The growing prevalence of obesity in America extends to older persons in their 60s and 70s. According to National Health and Nutrition Examination Surveys (NHANES), the prevalence of obesity (BMI ≥ 30) has climbed from 14% to 31% between the years 1976 and 2000. Trends were similar for all age, gender, and racial or ethnic groups (see Table 24.6 and reference by Flegal, 2002, at the end of the chapter).

Excess body weight and modest weight gain (≥ 5 kg or greater) in middle age may be associated with medical comorbidities in later life that include hypertension, diabetes mellitus, cardiovascular disease, and osteoarthritis. Adverse outcomes associated with obesity include impaired functional status, increased health care resource use, and increased mortality. A BMI of 35 or greater is associated with increased risk for functional decline among older persons. Many homebound older persons are now found to be obese. Of interest, poor diet quality and micronutrient deficiencies are relatively common among obese older persons, especially obese older women living alone. Change (increase or decrease) in body weight may be even more strongly correlated with mortality and comorbid conditions like cardiovascular disease or functional limitation. The National Institutes of Health has suggested: "Age alone should not preclude weight loss treatment for older adults. A careful evaluation of potential risks and benefits in the individual patient should guide management." The focus must be on achieving a more healthful weight to promote improved health, function, and quality of life. A combination of prudent diet, behavior modification, and activity or exercise may be appropriate for selected candidates. For obese older persons with frailty, the emphasis may better be placed not upon weight reduction, but upon preservation of strength and flexibility.

NUTRITIONAL INTERVENTIONS

Oral Nutrition and Supplements

Preventing undernutrition is much easier than treating it. Food intake can be enhanced by catering to food preferences as much as possible and avoiding therapeutic diets unless their clinical value is certain. Patients should be prepared for meals with appropriate hand and mouth care, and they should be comfortably situated for eating. Those needing assistance with eating should be helped. Placing two or more patients together for meals can increase sociability and food intake. Foods should be of appropriate consistency, prepared with attention to color, texture, temperature, and arrangement. The use of herbs, spices, and hot foods helps to compensate for loss of the sense of taste and smell often accompanying old age and to avoid the excessive use of salt and sugar (see "Oral Diseases and Disorders," p 319). Hard-to-open individual packages should be avoided. Adequate time should be taken for leisurely meals. Title III C of the Older Americans Act has provided for congregate and home-delivered meals for older persons, regardless of economic status. This service is available in most parts of the country, although in some locations there is a waiting list. Adequate access to nutritious and appetizing food should be assured to patients of various cultural backgrounds and in all settings.

Dietary supplements have been widely used in an effort to enhance nutrient intake. Food intake is often decreased by the use of such supplements, but there is usually an increase in overall nutritional intake owing to the nutrient quality and density of the supplements. Standard supplements contain macro- and

Table 24.6—Prevalence of Overweight and Obesity Among Older Persons: NHANES 1976–80, 1988–94, and 1999–2000

Age (*years*) and Gender	Overweight (%)			Obese (%)		
	1976–80	1988–94	1999–2000	1976–80	1988–94	1999–2000
Men 65–74	54.2	68.5	77.2	13.2	24.1	33.4
Men ≥ 75	—	56.5	66.4	—	13.2	20.4
Women 65–74	59.5	60.3	70.1	21.5	26.9	38.8
Women ≥ 75	—	52.3	59.6	—	19.2	25.1

SOURCE: Data from National Center for Health Statistics, *Health, United States, 2002* (Hyattsville, MD: Centers for Disease Control and Prevention, National Center for Health Statistics; 2002), table 70.

micronutrients and are available in liquid and bar forms. They are selected on the basis of the patient's preference and chewing ability and on their cost.

There is also growing interest in the use of micronutrient supplements in health promotion. A wide variety of vitamin and mineral supplements are now commonly available in supermarkets and drugstores. New recommendations for older persons include higher intake of calcium and vitamin D to prevent osteoporosis (see Table 24.2). Folic acid, B_6, and B_{12} can lower homocysteine levels, possibly reducing the risk of coronary artery disease and helping to prevent decline in cognitive function. Immune function may be improved by supplementation of protein, vitamin E, zinc, and other micronutrients. Whether the effects of antioxidants are beneficial is the subject of controversy; it has been suggested that they may help in preventing age-related cataracts and macular degeneration and that naturally occurring dietary antioxidants may reduce cardiovascular disease and mortality. Vitamin E supplementation has not been shown to slow the progression of Alzheimer's disease or prevent cardiovascular disease and may be associated with higher risk of hemorrhagic stroke. DNA damage from micronutrient deficiencies may be factors in cancer promotion. Since approximately 50% of older persons may also take self-prescribed dietary supplements, it is imperative that the clinician obtain information about the older patient's use of all supplements. The appropriateness and safety of each supplement should be evaluated, since consumers are often unaware of potential risks and adverse effects of many over-the-counter supplements, and solid evidence in favor of these purported benefits are currently lacking.

Drug Treatment for Undernutrition Syndromes

A number of agents have been suggested to promote increased appetite or to serve as anabolic aids. Appetite stimulants include the antidepressant mirtazapine[OL], an atypical serotonin enhancer, which antagonizes the 5-HT_3 receptor, possibly stimulating appetite by that mechanism, but proof of this effect is lacking. Dosing is at 3.75 to 45 mg orally at bedtime, with cautious dose escalation for older persons and reduced dosing for hepatic or renal insufficiency. Cyproheptadine[OL], a serotonin and histamine antagonist, may also enhance appetite. It is given at a dose of 2 to 4 mg orally with meals, with attention for potential confusion in elderly patients. Megestrol[OL] is a progestin that stimulates appetite and is given in a daily dose of 320 to 800 mg orally in four divided doses. Improvements in appetite

---

[OL] Not approved by the U.S. Food and Drug Administration for this use.

and usually gain in weight have been demonstrated with megestrol acetate; however, it is believed that this weight gain is primarily fat, and clinical benefits to the patient have not been demonstrated. Megestrol acetate in nursing-home populations has been shown to be associated with a higher risk of deep-vein thrombosis. Dronabinol[OL], a cannabinoid, may stimulate appetite at 5 to 15 mg per m^2 per day orally, but it is associated with somnolence and dysphoria in older persons.

Cytokine-modulating agents are experimental. They include anti–tumor-necrosis factor, consisting of antibodies that may inhibit cytokine-mediated inflammation; thalidomide, which may decrease levels of tumor-necrosis factor; and n-3 fatty acids and antioxidants, which may modulate cytokine production.

Trophic agents include human growth hormone[OL], which induces preferential utilization of carbohydrates and fats while preserving proteins and increasing muscle mass. Dosing is 0.125 mg per kg per day intramuscularly, divided in three doses daily. Increased muscle strength and functional capacity, however, are dependent on exercise rehabilitation. Growth hormone is contraindicated in cancer states. Hyperglycemia and fluid retention may be observed. Testosterone[OL] is an anabolic androgen that promotes increased muscle protein synthesis with decreased catabolism. Testosterone dosing schemes include 100 to 600 mg intramuscularly every 3 weeks, or 5 mg topical patch or gel daily. Virilizing side effects are expected. Oxandrolone[OL] is another anabolic steroid that increases muscle protein synthesis; it is given at 5 to 20 mg per day orally. Research on all of these trophic agents has failed to demonstrate clinically meaningful benefits to date, but little research has been done.

ETHICAL AND LEGAL ISSUES

In the nursing home, unacceptable weight loss, as defined by the Omnibus Budget Reconciliation Act of 1987, is any loss greater than or equal to 5% in the past month or 10% in the past 6 months. The MDS is a functionally based assessment tool performed on admissions to long-term-care facilities that are receiving payments from the Centers for Medicare and Medicaid Services. Sections of the MDS that are related to nutritional status include those assessing cognitive function, mood and behavior, physical function, health condition, oral and nutritional status, dental status, skin condition, and special treatments and procedures, including restorative care for eating and swallowing. Resident Assessment Protocols ensure prompt identification of problems focused on by the MDS. Standards of care dictate that:

- a resident maintain acceptable parameters of nutritional status such as body weight and protein levels, unless the resident's clinical condition demonstrates that this is not possible, and
- a resident receive a therapeutic diet when there is a problem.

Adequate nutrition and hydration should always be provided to the elderly patient unless:

- a fully competent older person refuses invasive nutritional support after having been fully apprised of the potential consequences and states this in written form with witnesses, or
- the terminally ill older person has executed a legally binding living will or medical directive that precludes artificial feeding in the event of terminal illness or impending death.

Standards of care and ethical principles also maintain that artificial feeding may be withheld or terminated in accordance with a patient's advance directive (known as *advance care plan* in some contexts), with careful consideration of additional comorbidities and futility. Appropriate counseling of the patient and surrogate regarding the consequences of withholding feeding is obligatory. After total cessation of nutrition, several weeks may ensue before death. In this setting, palliative care, including emotional support, is extremely important and complex (see "Palliative Care," p 133, "Legal and Ethical Issues," p 22; "Eating and Feeding Problems," p 181).

ANNOTATED REFERENCES

- Flegal, KM, Carroll MD, Ogden CL, et al. Prevalence and trends in obesity among US adults, 1999–2000. *JAMA*. 2002;288(14):1723–1727.

  The prevalence of obesity continues to grow among American adults, according to this latest examination of National Health and Nutrition Examination Survey data from 1999–2000. Increases occurred for men and women in all age groups and for non-Hispanic whites, non-Hispanic blacks, and Mexican Americans. Of particular note, these increases extended into the older age categories.

- Institute of Medicine, Food and Nutrition Board. *Dietary Reference Intakes for Energy, Carbohydrate, Fiber, Fat, Fatty Acids, Cholesterol, Protein, and Amino Acids (Macronutrients)*. Washington, DC: National Academy Press; 2002.

  The latest macronutrient guidelines from the Food and Nutrition Board for the first time specifically address the needs of older persons.

- Jensen GL, McGee M, Binkley J. Nutrition in the elderly. *Gastroenterol Clin North Am*. 2001;30(2):313–334.

  This comprehensive review of nutrition in the elderly age group provides many of the original references used in this chapter. Topics include changes with aging, nutrient requirements, screening and assessment, nutrition syndromes, and nutritional interventions.

- Millen BE, Silliman RA, Cantey-Kisler J, et al. Nutritional risk in an urban homebound older population. The nutrition and healthy aging project. *J Nutr Health Aging*. 2001;5(4):269–277.

  Nutritional status of homebound older persons is poor, particularly those of advanced age with comorbid disease. Poor diet quality is nearly universal; more than half of the subjects deviate from recommended standard intakes for at least 13 of the 24 nutritional guidelines. Of interest, fully one third of the homebound older persons studied were obese, with body mass index > 30.

- Powers JS. Facilitated feeding in disabled elderly. *Curr Opin Clin Nutr Metab Care*. 2002;5(3):315–319.

  This is a review of diseases of undernutrition and their treatment. Changes in physiology, metabolism, and function accompanying aging result in altered nutritional requirements. Designing nutrition therapy to treat malnutrition associated with illness in older patients requires an understanding of the aging processes, a careful setting of treatment goals, and multidisciplinary collaboration.

- Rubenstein LZ, Harker JO, Salva A, et al. Screening for undernutrition in geriatric practice: developing the short-form mini-nutritional assessment (MNA-SF). *J Gerontol A Biol Sci Med Sci*. 2001;56(6):M366–M372.

  A shortened version of the Mini-Nutritional Assessment, the MNA-SF has 6 questions instead of 18 and can be administered in approximately 3 minutes. The MNA-SF has high diagnostic accuracy relative to clinical nutritional status. Authors recommend that the MNA-SF be administered to patients undergoing comprehensive geriatric assessment or periodic health-risk appraisal as the first step in nutritional screening. The screen is available at http://www.mna-elderly.com/clinical-practice.htm (accessed October 2005).

Gordon L. Jensen, MD, PhD
James S. Powers, MD

CHAPTER 25—EATING AND FEEDING PROBLEMS

KEY POINTS

- Several age-related changes in older persons contribute to a slowed ability to swallow.

- Dementia is the most common cause of oral dysphagia.

- Most healthy people aspirate without any important clinical consequences.

- Aspiration pneumonia is believed to occur when contaminated oral secretions arrive in the lungs in a high enough inoculum to overcome host defenses.

- No studies demonstrate that feeding tubes reduce the occurrence of aspiration, but rather, many studies identify feeding tubes as major risk factors for aspiration.

- The assessment of swallowing function is controversial. Data correlating specific findings from any type of swallowing examination with clinically meaningful outcomes are lacking.

Swallowing is an important and complex task that can be affected by both normal aging and by diseases that are common in older persons. Treatment of eating and feeding problems varies, depending on the identified cause or causes and contributing factors.

SWALLOWING IN HEALTH AND DISEASE

Swallowing and Aging

Swallowing can be divided into three phases on the basis of anatomy. First is the preparatory or oral phase, which includes the complex activities of mastication and propelling the food bolus to the back of the mouth toward the pharynx. This stage is under voluntary control. The second or pharyngeal phase is involuntary and involves the initiation of the swallow reflex with propulsion of the food bolus past the laryngeal vestibule and into the esophagus. Execution of the oral and pharyngeal phases of swallowing requires the complex coordination of five cranial nerves and a large number of small muscles in the head and neck, with regulation from cortical input to the medullary swallow center, all in the appropriate sequence, usually within 1 second. The third stage of swallowing is the esophageal phase, during which food is propelled down the esophagus by the action of skeletal muscle proximally and smooth muscle distally; this phase is regulated by its own intrinsic innervation.

Normal aging is associated with several alterations in eating. With advanced age, there is a diminution of the taste sensation, but not of taste discrimination (an older person may be able to distinguish sweet from salty but may need to add more salt to food to taste it sufficiently). Further, olfactory function declines with advancing age, further impairing taste sensation. Salivary function is not clearly reduced with aging, but xerostomia is a common complaint of older persons, usually owing to the adverse effects of medication. Loss of teeth greatly reduces chewing efficiency (ie, the need to chew for a longer period of time and with more chewing strokes to achieve the same level of food maceration), which is only partly ameliorated with dental prostheses. Sarcopenia, or age-related loss of lean muscle mass, may contribute to loss in chewing efficiency and to pharyngeal muscle weakness demonstrated on videofluoroscopic deglutition examination of asymptomatic older persons. Whether aging alone contributes to esophageal dysmotility (so-called *presbyesophagus*) remains a subject of debate. Esophageal function is probably well preserved, except, perhaps, in very advanced age. In total, these changes with age result in a prolonged duration of each swallow. Further, many diseases that produce dysphagia are more common in older persons.

Dysphagia

Dysphagia, or difficulty swallowing, can occur when a disease affects any level of swallowing function. Dysphagia is usually classified as oral, pharyngeal, or esophageal. Oral dysphagia occurs when there is difficulty with the voluntary transfer of food from the mouth to the pharynx. This might be diagnosed, for example, when scrambled eggs are discovered in the cheeks of a demented patient shortly before lunch. The most common cause of oral dysphagia is dementia.

In pharyngeal dysphagia, reflexive transfer of the food bolus from the pharynx to initiate the involuntary esophageal phase of swallowing while simultaneously protecting the airway from misdirection of food is difficult. The affected person may notice coughing, choking, or nasal regurgitation while eating and localize the symptoms to the throat. The most common cause of pharyngeal dysphagia is stroke, but any disease that impairs the swallowing center in the brain stem or the cranial nerves involved (eg, Parkinson's disease, central nervous system tumor), the oropharyngeal striated muscle (eg, myasthenia gravis, amyotrophic lateral sclerosis), or the local structures involved (eg, retropharyngeal abscess, tumor) may lead to pharyngeal dysphagia. Treatment of both oral and pharyngeal dysphagia involves treatment of the underlying disorder and devising an individualized, often labor-intensive, feeding program.

Esophageal dysphagia presents with the sensation that food has gotten "stuck" after a swallow. Dysphagia for both solids and liquids suggests an esophageal motility disorder (eg, achalasia, scleroderma), whereas progressive dysphagia for solids suggests a mechanical obstruction (eg, cancer, esophageal ring, stricture from mucosal irritation). None of these diseases is unique to the geriatric population, though older persons tend to take more medications and are therefore more likely to experience medication-induced esophagitis (which manifests initially as odynophagia, followed by dysphagia). Common causes of medication-induced esophagitis in older persons are potassium, nonsteroidal anti-inflammatory agents, alendronate, and tetracycline-related antibiotics. (See also the section on dysphagia in "Gastrointestinal Diseases and Disorders," p 390.)

Aspiration

The misdirection of pharyngeal contents into the airway is termed *aspiration*. Generally, there are two major sources of aspiration: oropharyngeal flora or gastric contents. Despite this relatively straightforward definition, however, controversy persists over the definition of *aspiration pneumonia*. Aspiration pneumonia is believed to occur when bacteria arrive in the lungs from the pharynx in a large enough inoculum to overcome host defenses. Pneumococcal pneumonia arises from aspiration of this organism from a colonized oropharynx, however, and is usually not considered an aspiration pneumonia. Aspiration of gastric contents, or Mendelson's syndrome, usually results in a chemical pneumonitis, and the usefulness of antibiotics in this situation is questionable. Most often, local host defense mechanisms clear the lung of the offending aspirate, without serious clinical impact. It is well established that many healthy individuals episodically aspirate without any important clinical consequences.

Neither aspiration of contaminated oral contents nor of gastric contents is prevented by placement of a feeding tube. Tube feeding is universally cited as a risk factor for major aspiration, and some patients who have never previously aspirated begin to do so after placement of a feeding tube. A 1996 review found no evidence that tube feeding of any sort would reduce the risk of aspiration pneumonia. A common misconception is that jejunostomy tube feeding has lower rates of associated aspiration of gastric contents than gastrostomy does; however, there is no evidence to support this misconception. A single nonrandomized prospective comparison of hand with tube feeding in patients with oropharyngeal aspiration found that hand feeding (personal assistance with oral intake) results in lower rates of pneumonia. No prospective randomized trials comparing hand with tube feeding to reduce aspiration have been published. An active area of clinical research is focused on the role of substance P in swallowing and aspiration and the potential benefit of angiotensin-converting enzyme inhibitors (which prevent the breakdown of substance P) in patients who aspirate, but to date this research is inconclusive.

Assessment of Oropharyngeal Dysphagia

Several tools may be used to assess swallowing function when oropharyngeal dysphagia is clinically suspected. The most common are the full bedside evaluation, of which there are many variations, and the videofluoroscopic deglutition examination (VDE), a variant of the modified barium swallow. There is considerable controversy regarding the relative efficacy of these tools.

VDE is usually performed by a speech-language pathologist who videotapes the patient swallowing several consistencies of barium-impregnated foods while the patient maintains various head positions. This may permit identification of the food consistency or compensatory mechanisms that minimize fluoroscopic evidence of aspiration. Depending on the results of the VDE, the therapist may recommend swallow therapy or diet modifications, or both. Swallow therapy may be compensatory (eg, turn head toward weaker side while swallowing), indirect (eg, exercises to improve the strength of the involved muscles), or direct (ie, exercises to perform while swallowing, such as swallowing multiple times per bolus). Dietary recommendations generally consist of altering bolus size or consistency of food or of restricting foods of certain consistencies.

Data conflict regarding the usefulness of VDE and subsequent treatment recommendations and derive from small, historically controlled studies rather than larger prospective randomized trials. A systematic review of studies of dysphagia secondary to stroke published by the Agency for Health Care Policy and Research (now the Agency for Healthcare Research and Quality) concluded that evidence was insufficient to recommend one type of swallowing study over another and that data correlating specific findings from any type of examination with clinically meaningful outcomes are lacking.

FEEDING

When an older person experiences difficulty eating, the two main therapeutic approaches are careful feeding by hand or tube. The first requires extraordinary patience and is labor intensive; the latter is an invasive intervention associated with its own risks. Data about either approach are limited, and randomized comparisons have not been done. The role of dietary supplements, if any, in augmenting the caloric intake of hand-fed persons has not been clearly defined. One systematic review suggested a mortality benefit to the use of oral protein and energy supplements in acutely hospitalized or community-dwelling persons older than age 65 years, though the quality of the studies reviewed was not optimal. Functional status does not appear to be improved with oral nutritional supplements in any of the studies evaluating this outcome. (See Table 25.1 for details about the composition of specific feeding solutions.)

The number of percutaneous endoscopic gastrostomy (PEG) feeding tubes placed in patients aged 65 years and older has grown at an astonishing rate over the past decade. Low procedure-related complication rates are often cited; however, long-term studies reveal substantial mortality among tube-fed patients. Despite the popularity of feeding tubes, a review of the literature from 1966 to 1999 found no studies demonstrating improved survival, reduced incidence of pneumonia or other infections, improved symptoms or function, or reduced pressure ulcers with the use of feeding tubes of any type in demented persons who have eating difficulties. Median survival after placement of a feeding tube is well under a year, but it is unknown whether this results from tube feeding or if the need for tube feeding is a marker that death is near.

Complications described with feeding tubes are numerous and include an increased risk of aspiration pneumonia, metabolic disturbances, diarrhea, and local cellulitis. Monitoring for these complications should be meticulous. A study employing a large administrative data set found that 1-year mortality was higher in 5266 nursing-home residents with chewing or swallowing difficulties who were fed with a tube than in those who were not, even when statistically accounting for potential confounding variables. A second study by the same authors of 1386 nursing-home residents with

recent progression to severe cognitive impairment found no improvement in 2-year survival in the group who were tube fed, again adjusting for potential confounders. No prospective randomized studies comparing tube and hand feeding have been published, and information on quality-of-life outcomes is sorely needed.

Placement of a PEG or jejunostomy bypasses the oropharynx and the esophagus and allows nutrients and medications to be instilled directly into the stomach or the jejunum and be absorbed by a functioning gut. There is little evidence to support the use of feeding tubes in most debilitating chronic diseases, and in particular the wealth of data demonstrate that their use has no clinical benefit in patients with oropharyngeal dysphagia from dementia. It is clear that neither gastrostomy nor jejunostomy feeding tubes reduce aspiration in comparison with a program of hand feeding, but no randomized trials comparing these interventions have been published. The only disease for which feeding tubes have been shown to be of clinical benefit to the patient is esophageal obstruction, such as from malignancy. For most other disease states, their utility remains unproved.

Contraindications to gastrostomy include the inability to pass an endoscope into the stomach, uncorrectable coagulopathy, massive ascites, peritonitis, and bowel obstruction. After successful placement of a gastrostomy, tube feedings of commercially available canned nutritional supplements can be initiated either as slow gravity boluses over 30 to 60 minutes or as a continuous drip. The feeding tube should be flushed with water before and after each feeding or at least four times a day in cases of continuous feedings.

Consideration of feeding tube placement requires careful examination of the data, with a focus on whether there is evidence of clinical benefit to support this invasive and potentially burdensome approach.

Not all feeding problems, of course, are related to dysphagia, and many contributing factors are quite amenable to therapy. Other approaches to consider in older persons who demonstrate eating or feeding

Table 25.1—Composition of Commonly Used Tube-Feeding Solutions

Trade Name	Calories (kCal/mL)	Protein (g/L)	Carbohydrate (g/L)	Sodium (mEq/L)	Osmolarity (mOsm/kg)	Comments
Ensure HP	0.95	50	150	53	610	Useful when caloric requirements are less
Ensure Plus HN	1.50	63	199	52	650	Useful for fluid-restricted patients
Jevity Plus	1.20	56	175	59	450	Good source of fiber
Nepro	2.00	70	215		635	Designed for patients with renal failure
Osmolite	1.06	37	151	28	300	Standard feeding solution
Pulmocare	1.50	63	106	57	475	Designed to reduce CO_2 production
Two Cal HN	2.00	84	217	57	690	Useful for fluid-restricted patients

problems are evaluation for depression, elimination of unduly restrictive diets, consideration of individual food preferences, consideration of the environment in which the person eats to improve socialization and reduce disruptive stimuli, examination of the condition of the oral cavity, determination of the needs for personal assistance with feeding, and reduction or elimination of medications that may cause inattention, xerostomia, movement disorders, or anorexia. Small studies have documented improved clinical outcomes in nursing-home residents with the use of flavor enhancers, increased food variety, and attention to the meal ambiance.

ANNOTATED REFERENCES

- Finucane TE, Christmas C, Travis K. Tube feeding in patients with advanced dementia. *JAMA*. 1999;282(14): 1365–1370.

    This is a thorough review of published studies from 1966 to March 1999 relevant to the topic. Evidence to support the purported benefits of tube feeding to prevent pneumonia or other infections, prolong survival, reduce the risk of pressure ulcers, improve function or quality of life, and provide palliation were sought. No randomized trials comparing hand feeding with tube feeding in this population were found. No data were identified that supported the use of tube feeding in patients with advanced dementia for any of these clinical indications.

- Marik PE, Kaplan D. Aspiration pneumonia and dysphagia in the elderly. *Chest*. 2003;124(1):328–336.

    This is a comprehensive review of the pathophysiology and evaluation of aspiration in older patients, with some suggestions for treatment. This review does encourage the use of instrumental assessment of swallowing function; however, this is not supported either by data linking the outcomes from these tests to clinical outcomes or by the consensus of experts.

- Milne AC, Potter J, Avenell A. Protein and energy supplementation in elderly people at risk from malnutrition. *Cochrane Database Syst Rev*. 2002;(3):CD003288.

    This is a systematic review of randomized trials, though of variable quality, that concluded that oral nutritional supplementation reduces mortality but does not impact functional status or quality of life in hospitalized or community-dwelling people over the age of 65 years.

- Mitchell SL, Kiely DK, Lipsitz LA. Does artificial enteral nutrition prolong the survival of institutionalized elders with chewing and swallowing problems? *J Gerontol A Biol Sci Med Sci*. 1998;53(3):M207–M213.

    A large prospective cohort of nursing-home residents with chewing or swallowing problems was studied for 1 year. Of these 5266 residents, 10.5% had a feeding tube. Of those tube-fed persons who survived 1 year, 25% were able to discontinue tube feeding. The study found that the risk of death (relative risk 1.44) was higher in residents who were tube fed than in those who were not, even after statistical adjustment for potential confounding covariables.

Colleen Christmas, MD

CHAPTER 26—URINARY INCONTINENCE

KEY POINTS

- Of persons aged 65 years and over, 15% to 30% in the community and at least 50% in long-term care are incontinent.

- Especially in older persons, incontinence may not reflect abnormal micturition physiology. Continence also depends on the ability to toilet oneself and the absence of medical conditions, medications, or other factors that cause or contribute to lower urinary tract dysfunction or affect volume status and urine excretion.

- The multifactorial nature of urinary incontinence requires a comprehensive diagnostic evaluation with a careful search for all possible causes and precipitants beyond the genitourinary tract.

- Correction of medical illnesses, medications, and other precipitating factors are crucial for improving continence.

Urinary incontinence (UI) is a multifactorial syndrome produced by a combination of genitourinary pathology, age-related changes, and comorbid conditions that impair normal micturition or the functional ability to toilet oneself, or both.

PREVALENCE AND IMPACT

The prevalence of UI increases with age and affects women more than men (2:1) until age 80, after which men and women are equally affected. Of persons aged 65 years and over, 15% to 30% in the community and at least 50% in long-term care are incontinent. UI may cause morbidity, including cellulitis, pressure ulcers, urinary tract infections, falls with fractures, sleep deprivation, social withdrawal, depression, and sexual dysfunction. UI is not associated with increased mortality. UI impairs quality of life, affecting the older person's emotional well-being, social function, and general health. Incontinent persons often manage to maintain their activities, but with an increased burden of coping, embarrassment, and poor self-perception. Caregiver burden is higher with incontinent older persons, which can contribute to decisions to institutionalize. Estimated annual UI-related costs total more than $26 billion.

THE PATHOPHYSIOLOGY OF INCONTINENCE

Normal Micturition

The detrusor contracts via parasympathetic nerves from spinal cord levels S2 to S4 (sacral micturition center). Urethral sphincter mechanisms include proximal urethral smooth muscle (which contracts by sympathetic stimulation from spinal levels T11 to L2), distal urethral striated muscle (which contracts via cholinergic somatic stimulation from the sacral micturition center), and musculofascial urethral supports. In women, these tissues form a two-layered "hammock" that supports and compresses the urethra when abdominal pressure increases. Micturition is coordinated by the central nervous system: Parietal lobes and thalamus receive and coordinate detrusor afferent stimuli; frontal lobes and basal ganglia provide signals to inhibit voiding; and the pontine micturition center integrates these inputs into socially appropriate voiding with coordinated urethral relaxation and detrusor contraction until the bladder is empty. Urine storage is under sympathetic control (inhibiting detrusor contraction and increasing sphincter tone), and voiding is parasympathetic (detrusor contraction and relaxation of sphincter tone).

Incontinence in Older Persons

Especially in older persons, incontinence may not reflect abnormal micturition physiology. Continence also depends on the ability to toilet oneself—requiring physical function, cognition, motivation, and toilet availability—and the absence of medical conditions, medications, or other factors that affect lower urinary tract function, volume status, and urine excretion. Table 26.1 and Table 26.2 list the mechanisms by which these conditions may impair continence. Evaluation and correction of these factors are crucial in the care of older persons with UI.

Age-related changes in the lower urinary tract (Table 26.3) are found in both continent and incontinent older persons. Why some older persons develop UI and others do not remains unclear; differences in lower urinary tract and other compensatory mechanisms may play a role.

Table 26.1—Medications Commonly Associated With Incontinence

Medication	Effect on Continence
Alcohol	Frequency, urgency, sedation, delirium, immobility
α-Adrenergic agonists	Outlet obstruction (men)
α-Adrenergic blockers	Stress leakage (women)
Angiotensin-converting enzyme inhibitors	Associated cough with stress or stress-induced urge leakage
Anticholinergics: Antiarrhythmics (Norpace) Antidiarrheals (Lomotil) Antihistamines Antiparkinsonian (Artane) Antispasmodics (Bentyl)	Impaired emptying, retention, delirium, fecal impaction
Antidepressants	Anticholinergic effects, sedation
Antipsychotics	Anticholinergic effects, sedation, immobility, rigidity
Calcium channel blockers	Impaired detrusor contractility, retention, pedal edema causing nocturnal diuresis (dihydropyridine agents)
Loop diuretics	Polyuria, frequency, urgency
Narcotic analgesics	Urinary retention, fecal impaction, sedation, delirium
Nonsteroidal anti-inflammatory drugs	Pedal edema causing nocturnal enuresis
Sedative hypnotics	Sedation, delirium, immobility
Thiazolidinediones	Pedal edema causing nocturnal enuresis

SOURCE: Data from Dubeau CE. Interpreting the effect of common medical conditions on voiding dysfunction in the elderly. *Urol Clin North Am.* 1996;23(1):11–18.

Table 26.2—Comorbidities Commonly Associated With Incontinence

Comorbidity	Effect on Continence
Cardiovascular disease	
Arteriovascular disease	Detrusor underactivity or areflexia from ischemic myopathy or neuropathy
Heart failure	Nocturnal diuresis
Metabolic disease	
Diabetes mellitus	Detrusor underactivity due to neuropathy, DO, osmotic diuresis; altered mental status from hyper- or hypoglycemia; retention and overflow from constipation
Hypercalcemia	Diuresis, altered mental status
Vitamin-B$_{12}$ deficiency	Impaired bladder sensation and detrusor underactivity from peripheral neuropathy
Neurologic disease	
Cerebrovascular disease, stroke	DO from damage to upper motor neurons; impaired sensation to void from interruption of subcortical pathways; impaired function and cognition
Delirium	Impaired function and cognition
Dementia	DO from damage to upper motor neurons; impaired function and cognition
Multiple sclerosis	DO, areflexia, or sphincter dyssynergia (dependent on level of spinal cord involvement)
Normal-pressure hydrocephalus	DO from compression of frontal inhibitory centers; impaired function and cognition
Parkinson's disease	DO from loss of inhibitory inputs to pontine micturition center; impaired function and cognition; retention and overflow from constipation
Spinal cord injury	DO, areflexia, or sphincter dyssynergia (dependent on level of injury)
Spinal stenosis	DO from damage to detrusor upper motor neurons (cervical stenosis); DO or areflexia (lumbar stenosis)
Psychiatric disease	
Affective and anxiety disorders	Decreased motivation
Alcoholism	Functional and cognitive impairment; rapid diuresis and retention in acute intoxication
Psychosis	Functional and cognitive impairment; decreased motivation
Other organ system diseases	
Gastrointestinal disease	Retention and overflow UI from constipation; fecal and urinary incontinence commonly coexist
Musculoskeletal disease	Mobility impairment; DO from cervical myelopathy in rheumatoid arthritis and osteoarthritis
Peripheral venous insufficiency	Nocturnal diuresis
Pulmonary disease	Exacerbation of stress UI by chronic cough

NOTE: DO = detrusor overactivity; UI = urinary incontinence.

SOURCE: Data from Dubeau CE. Interpreting the effect of common medical conditions on voiding dysfunction in the elderly. *Urol Clin North Am.* 1996;23(1):11–18.

Table 26.3—Age-Related Changes Potentially Resulting in Urinary Incontinence

Change	Predisposition	Type of Urinary Incontinence
Atrophic vaginitis and urethritis	Decreased urethral mucosal seal, irritation, UTI	Urge and stress UI
Benign prostatic hyperplasia	Prostatic hyperplasia or outlet obstruction or both with frequency, urgency, nocturia, DO	Urge or "overflow" UI
Decreased ability to postpone voiding	Frequency, urgency, nocturia	New or worsening urge, stress, mixed UI
Decreased detrusor contractility	Decreased flow rate, elevated postvoid residual, hesitancy	"Overflow" UI, DHIC
Decreased total bladder capacity	Frequency, urgency, nocturia	New or worsening urge, stress, mixed UI
DO (~20% of healthy, continent persons)	Frequency, urgency, nocturia	Urge and mixed UI, DHIC
Increased postvoid residual (< 50 mL)	Frequency, nocturia	New or worsening urge, stress, mixed UI
More urine output later in the day	Nocturia	Nocturnal UI

NOTE: DHIC = detrusor hyperactivity with impaired contractility; DO = detrusor overactivity; UI = urinary incontinence; UTI = urinary tract infection.

Risk Factors

Risk factors in community-dwelling older persons include advanced age, parity, depression, transient ischemic attacks and stroke, heart failure, fecal incontinence and constipation, obesity, chronic obstructive lung disease, chronic cough, diabetes mellitus, impaired mobility, and impaired activities of daily living. Among institutionalized older persons, UI is associated with impaired mobility, depression, stroke, diabetes mellitus, and Parkinson's disease; at least one third have multiple conditions. Although moderate to severe dementia is associated with UI, even severely demented persons remain continent if they have mobility for transfers. Thus, UI in demented persons may not be caused by dementia but may be a multifactorial epiphenomenon with treatable causes.

Urge Incontinence

Urge UI is the most common type in older persons. It is characterized by abrupt urgency, frequency, and nocturia; the volume of leakage may be small or large. Urge UI is associated with uninhibited bladder contractions—detrusor overactivity (DO)—that may be age related, idiopathic, secondary to lesions in central inhibitory pathways (eg, stroke, cervical stenosis), or due to local bladder irritation (infection, bladder stones, inflammation, tumors). Because DO is found in healthy, continent older persons, failure of lower urinary tract and functional compensatory mechanisms may play an important role in urge UI. Distinctions between neurogenic DO (due to central nervous system lesions) and idiopathic DO are commonly blurred in the older person with comorbidity. Less common causes of urge UI are interstitial cystitis (urge UI with otherwise unexplained pelvic pain) and spinal cord injury, which results in impaired detrusor compliance (excessive pressure response to filling), detrusor-sphincter dyssynergia, or both. Stress maneuvers may trigger DO; with such stress-related urge UI, leakage occurs after a several-second delay following the stress maneuver.

DO may coexist with impaired detrusor contractility (detrusor hyperactivity with impaired contractility, or DHIC), characterized by urge UI with an elevated postvoid residual (PVR) volume in the absence of outlet obstruction. DHIC accounts for most established UI in frail older persons. Women with DHIC can be misdiagnosed with stress UI if weak DHIC contractions are not detected, and men misdiagnosed with outlet obstruction because of the similarity of the symptoms (urgency, frequency, weak flow rate, and elevated PVR).

Stress Incontinence

Stress UI, the second most common type of UI in older women, results from failure of the sphincter mechanisms to preserve outlet closure during bladder filling. Leakage is due to impaired pelvic supports or, less commonly, failure of urethral closure. The latter occurs with trauma, scarring from anti-incontinence surgery, severe urethral atrophy in women, and post-prostatectomy in men. Unlike the episodic leakage of "genuine" stress UI, this leakage is typically continual and can occur while the person is sitting or standing quietly. Many women may have mixed UI, with both stress and urge symptoms.

Bladder Outlet Obstruction and Detrusor Underactivity

So-called "overflow" UI results from detrusor underactivity (impaired contractility), bladder outlet obstruction, or both. Leakage is typically small in volume but continual. The PVR volume is high, and symptoms may include dribbling, weak urinary stream, intermittency, hesitancy, frequency, and nocturia. Associated urge and stress UI may occur. Rarely, continual leakage is due to extraurethral incontinence (eg, vesicovaginal fistula).

Outlet obstruction is the second most common cause of UI in older men; most obstructed men, however, are not incontinent. Causes include benign prostatic hyperplasia, prostate cancer, and urethral stricture. In women, obstruction is uncommon and usually due to previous anti-incontinence surgery or a large cystocele that kinks the urethra.

Detrusor underactivity causing urinary retention and UI occurs in only 5% to 10% of older persons. Intrinsic causes are replacement of detrusor smooth muscle by fibrosis and connective tissue (eg, from chronic outlet obstruction). Neurologic causes include peripheral neuropathy (diabetes mellitus, vitamin B_{12} deficiency, alcoholism) or damage to the spinal detrusor afferents by disc herniation, spinal stenosis, tumor, or degenerative neurologic disease.

ASSESSMENT AND MANAGEMENT

UI is like many geriatric syndromes, in that its multifactorial nature requires a comprehensive diagnostic evaluation, with a careful search for all possible causes and precipitants beyond the genitourinary tract. UI management is similar to that for other chronic conditions, using a stepped approach over time. Table 26.4 provides a framework for evaluating and managing common types of UI over several visits. The sections below describe techniques.

Table 26.4—Stepped Approach to Urinary Incontinence Evaluation and Management

Measures to Take	Comments, Examples
Visit 1: Initial screening and behavioral interventions	
Screen for UI in all adult patients	Ask "Have you had any problems with bladder or urine control?" If yes, then ask: "Do you leak urine when you lift something, cough, or sneeze?" "Do you have sudden urge to urinate and then leak urine before you can reach the bathroom?" "Do you ever leak urine with any physical activity or warning?"
Conduct brief UI history, pertinent past medical history, and review of systems	Review lower urinary tract symptoms. Target system review at medical conditions and functional impairments associated with UI. Review all medications and fluid intake. Ask about UI impact on quality of life
Evaluate for any pathologic conditions (eg, UTI, malignancy)	Ask about bleeding, pelvic pain, dysuria, sudden UI onset. Screen for neurologic syptoms
Perform physical examination	Assess patient's mobility, volume status (including checking for pedal edema). Perform rectal examination—note sphincter strength with voluntary contraction. Perform pelvic examination and note any signficant pelvic organ prolapse (consider gynecology referral if past the introitus); check pelvic muscle contraction during manual examination. Perform clinic stress test, if possible. Include PVR, if time allows (see visit 2)
Urinalysis	Flags: hematuria, glycosuria (see text, p 189, regarding pyuria and bacteriuria)
General management and behavioral therapy	Physical therapy for patients with impaired mobility; bedside commode. Volume management (eg, adjust intake, diuretics, compression hose, foot elevation). See text (p 190) for behavioral therapies
Medication review	See Table 26.1
Ask patient to complete a 2- to 3-day bladder diary	For sample bladder diary see http://www.healthinaging.org/public_education/bladder_control.php
Visit 2 (4–8 weeks): Detailed evaluation and treatment	
Review completed bladder diary	See text (p 189)
Re-review UI and lower urinary tract symptoms	Review fluid intake for volume and caffeine, which can contribute to UI. Assess response to therapy aimed at transient factors
Evaluate further	Ideally, PVR should be assessed in all patients; it should always be done in men and in persons with diabetes mellitus, neurologic disorders, significant pelvic prolapse, or taking medications that impair detrusor contractility; may be done by catheterization or ultrasound by provider or referral. Perform clinical stress test, if possible and not done previously
Refine treatment	Review and reinforce general management and behavioral therapy. Consider antimuscarinic medication for patients with urge UI (see text, p 000)
Consider referral for further evaluation and treatment	Referral for biofeedback- or electrical stimulation-assisted pelvic muscle exercises for women with mixed or stress UI. Other indications: persistent pelvic pain, hematuria, urinary retention, elevated PVR (> 200–300 mL, possibly lower in men); persistent postprostatectomy UI; bothersome pelvic prolapse (or try pessary); patient requests surgical consultation for stress UI or possible bladder outlet obstruction; diagnosis remains uncertain
Visit 3 (4–6 weeks after visit 2): Treatment evaluation and referral	
Evaluate response to therapy	Review behavioral management and response to medications. Titrate medications on basis of UI, adverse effects, and (especially if UI has worsened) PVR
Consider referral for further evaluation and treatment	Indications: same as above, plus failure to respond to empirical therapy

NOTE: PVR = postvoid residual; UI = urinary incontinence; UTI = urinary tract infection.

SOURCE: Adapted with permission from: American Geriatrics Society Urinary Incontinence Education Initiative Editorial Board: Goode PS, Chair, Brown J, DuBeau C, et al. Evaluating and treating older adult urinary incontinence: a step-wise approach for primary care providers. See http://www.americangeriatrics.org/jasper_test/education/ui_index.shtml (accessed October 2005).

History

The clinician must ask the patient about UI symptoms because 50% of affected persons do not volunteer UI symptoms. Sudden, compelling urgency suggests DO, and leakage with cough, for example, is sensitive for stress UI. Leakage with minimal maneuvers or continual urine dripping suggests intrinsic sphincter damage. Frequency, nocturia, slow urine stream, hesitancy, interrupted voiding, straining, and terminal dribbling are common with DO, DHIC, bladder outlet obstruction, detrusor underactivity, many medical conditions, and volume overload. Symptom scores (eg, the American Urological Association symptom score for benign prostatic hyperplasia) are useful as severity measures but lack specificity. Assess UI characteristics such as frequency, volume, timing, and precipitants (eg, medications, caffeine, alcohol, physical activity, cough), and associated factors (bowel and sexual function, medical conditions and medications with temporal relation to UI). Inquire how patient and caregiver quality of life are affected with respect to activities of daily living, social role, emotional and interpersonal (eg, sexual) relations, self-concept, general health perception, and the most bothersome aspect.

Physical Examination

The general examination must include cognition and functional status. Cardiovascular examination focuses on volume status (peripheral edema, heart failure). Abdominal palpation for bladder distension is insensitive. Neurologic evaluation should include cervical signs (limited lateral rotation and lateral flexion, interossei wasting, and Hoffman's or Babinski's sign). Assess rectum for masses, prostate nodules or firmness, and tone (at rest and volitional, tightening around examiner's finger). Prostate sizing by digital examination is inaccurate (see "Prostate Disease," p 423). Check sacral root integrity by perineal sensation, anal "wink" (lightly scratch the perianal area and look for anal sphincter contraction), and bulbocavernosus reflex (lightly touch the clitoris or glans and look for rectal contraction). Assess vaginal mucosa and pelvic support (see "Gynecologic Diseases and Disorders," p 410). Check uncircumcised men for phimosis, paraphimosis, and balanitis.

Testing

Laboratory tests include renal function and urinalysis. Pyuria and bacteriuria on urinalysis may represent asymptomatic bacteriuria (see the section on urinary tract infection in "Infectious Diseases," p 337). Urine cytology and cystoscopy are indicated if hematuria or pelvic pain is present. Tests for glucose, calcium, and vitamin B_{12} levels are optional.

A bladder diary provides baseline UI severity, the timing and circumstances of UI and typical voided volume, voiding frequency, and the total day and nocturnal urine output (for a sample diary see http://www.healthinaging.org/public_education/bladder_control.php). In institutions, have staff record the patient's continence status (dry, damp, soaked) every 2 hours. If nocturnal diuresis occurs, seek causes (eg, pedal edema, heart failure, or use of an alcohol "nightcap"). UI occurrence at a typical time of day suggests an association with medication, beverages, or activity.

Postvoiding residual volume (PVR) measurement is recommended. Men with a PVR volume > 200 should be screened for hydronephrosis.

A clinical stress test is best done with the bladder full, the patient relaxed, and using a single vigorous cough. It is specific for stress UI if leakage is instantaneous but insensitive if the patient cannot cooperate, is inhibited, or if bladder volume is low. If results are negative, consider repeating the test with the patient standing. On urine flow rate testing (if available), a peak flow $\geq$ 12 mL/sec with voided volume $\geq$ 150 mL excludes bladder outlet obstruction. Routine urodynamic testing is usually not needed. Precise diagnosis is most important when surgical treatment is being considered for stress UI or outlet obstruction, because surgery is ineffective for DO, DHIC, and detrusor weakness that present with similar symptoms. Geriatric UI is multifactorial, and lower urinary tract pathology is rarely the only cause. A focus on urodynamic diagnosis detracts from more relevant precipitants. Moreover, some treatments are effective for several types of UI (see the section, below, on specific treatment strategies). Urodynamics also should be considered if the diagnosis is unclear or if empiric therapy has failed. Cystometry measures bladder proprioception, capacity, detrusor stability, and contractility; carbon dioxide cystometry may be unreliable. Simultaneous measurement of abdominal pressure is necessary to exclude abdominal straining and detect DHIC. Fluoroscopic monitoring, abdominal leak-point pressure, or profilometry tests detect and quantify stress UI. Pressure-flow studies are the criterion standard for obstruction.

Management

Correction of medical illnesses, medications, and other precipitating factors alone often improves continence. Relieving the most bothersome aspects of UI for the patient is key. A stepped strategy moving from the least to more invasive treatments should be used, with behavioral methods tried before medication, and both tried before surgery. Treatment that simply decreases the number of UI episodes may not be sufficient for persons most bothered by the timing of UI, nocturia, or leakage with exercise. Cure often requires multiple visits. Evidence for the efficacy of UI treatment is summarized in Table 26.5, Table 26.6, and Table 26.7.

General management suggestions include avoiding high fluid intake (> 2L/day), caffeinated beverages, and alcohol, and minimizing evening intake if nocturnal UI is bothersome. Constipation should be reduced. If pads and protective garments are used, they should be chosen on the basis of the patient's gender and the type and volume of UI. Because these products are expensive, some patients may not change pads frequently enough. Medical supply companies and patient advocacy groups publish illustrated catalogs for product selection.

SPECIFIC TREATMENT STRATEGIES

Urge Incontinence

Behavioral treatment for urge UI employs two principles: frequent voluntary voiding to keep bladder volume low, and retraining of central nervous system and pelvic mechanisms to inhibit detrusor contractions and leakage. Cognitively intact persons can use bladder retraining, with timed voiding while awake and suppression of urgency by relaxation techniques (for patient handouts see http://www.healthinaging.org/public_education/bladder_control.php). The initial toileting frequency can be every 2 hours or based on a

Table 26.5—Efficacy of Behavioral and Pharmacologic Treatments for Urge Incontinence

Treatment	Target Population	Efficacy	Evidence*
Behavioral			
Bladder training	Cognitively intact	≥ 35% decrease in UI episodes over controls; patient's perception of cure at 6 months RR 1.69 [1.21 to 2.34]	A
Prompted voiding	Dependent, cognitively impaired	Average reduction 0.8–1.8 episodes daily; cure rare	A
Habit training	Able to complete voiding record	≥ 25% decrease in episodes in one third of patients	B
Scheduled toileting	Unable to toilet independently	30%–80% decrease in episodes, study quality fair	C
Pelvic muscle exercises	Women	Up to 80% decrease in episodes; motivated patients	A
Pharmacologic			
All antimuscarinics	Unresponsive to behavioral treatment alone	WMD in daily UI episodes 0.6 (95% CI, 0.4 to 0.8); RR dry mouth 2.56 (95% CI, 2.24 to 2.92)	A
Darifenacin	Unresponsive to behavioral treatment alone	7.5 or 15 mg daily: 68% and 73% respectively, median reduction in weekly UI episodes (vs 56% with placebo), dry mouth 19% and 31% respectively, constipation 14% (both doses)	
Oxybutynin	Unresponsive to behavioral treatment alone	ER: 71% mean reduction weekly UI episodes, cure rate 23%, dry mouth 30%	A
Solifenacin	Unresponsive to behavioral treatment alone	5 or 10 mg daily: 61% and 52% respectively, mean reduction daily UI episodes (vs 28% with placebo), dry mouth 8% and 23% respectively, constipation 4% and 9% respectively	
Tolterodine	Unresponsive to behavioral treatment alone	ER: 69% mean reduction weekly UI episodes, cure rate 17%, dry mouth 22%	A
Trospium	Unresponsive to behavioral treatment alone	20 mg bid: 59% mean reduction daily urge UI episodes (vs 44% with placebo), cure rate 21%, dry mouth 22%, constipation 10%	

* Evidence strength: A = randomized controlled studies; B = case-control studies; C = case descriptions or expert opinion.

NOTE: CI = confidence interval; ER = extended release; RR = relative risk; UI = urinary incontinence; WMD = weighted mean difference.

SOURCES: Data from Fantl JA, Newman DK, Colling J, et al. *Urinary Incontinence in Adults: Acute and Chronic Management.* Clinical Practice Guideline No. 2, 1996 Update. Rockville, MD: US Department of Health and Human Services, Public Health Service, Agency for Health Care Policy and Research; March 1996. AHCPR Pub. No. 96-0682; Abrams P, Cardozo L, Khoury S, et al., eds. *2nd International Consultation on Incontinence.* Plymouth, UK: Health Publication Ltd; 2002; Cochrane Library (accessed July 2003); Diokno A, Appell RA, Sand PK, et al. Prospective, randomized, double-blind study of the efficacy and tolerability of the extended-release formulations of oxybutynin and tolterodine for overactive bladder: results of the OPERA trail. *Mayo Clin Proc.* 2003;78:687–695; Zinner N, Gittelman M, Harris R, et al. Trospium chloride improves overactive bladder symptoms: a multicenter phase III trial. *J Urol.* 2004;171:2311–2315; Cardoza L, Lisec M, Millard R, et al. Randomized, double-blind placebo controlled trial of the once daily antimuscarinic agent solifenacin succinate in patients with overactive bladder. *J Urol.* 2004;172:1919–1924; Haab F, Stewart L, Dwyer P. Darifenacin, an M3 selective receptor antagonist, is an effective and well-tolerated once-daily treatment for overactive bladder. *Eur Urol.* 2004;45:420–429.

Table 26.6—Efficacy of Behavioral and Pharmacologic Treatments for Stress and for Mixed Urge and Stress Incontinence

Treatment	Target Population	Efficacy	Evidence*
Behavioral			
PME	Women	56%–95% decrease in episodes	A
PME and biofeedback	Women	50%–87% improvement	A
	Men, postprostatectomy	RR for continued UI vs no treatment 0.74 [0.6 to 0.93]	A–C
PME and vaginal cones	Women	No data in postmenopausal women	—
Electrical stimulation	Women, stress ± urge UI	No marginal benefit over behavioral therapy alone	A
Bladder retraining	Mixed UI, cognitively intact	≥ 50% decrease in episodes in 75% of patients	A
Prompted voiding	Mixed UI, dependent, cognitively impaired	Average reduction 0.8–1.8 episodes daily	A
Habit training	Mixed UI, voiding record available	≥ 25% decrease in episodes in one third of patients	B
Scheduled toileting	Mixed UI, unable to toilet independently	30%–80% decrease in episodes	C
Pharmacologic			
Duloxetine[OL]	Women	All UI episodes reduced 64% versus 41% with placebo	A
Estrogens	Women	Oral ineffective, especially when combined with a progestin; scant data on topical forms	A–B

* Evidence strength: A = randomized controlled studies; B = case-control studies; C = case descriptions or expert opinion.

NOTE: PME = pelvic muscle exercises; UI = urinary incontinence.

SOURCES: Data from Fantl JA, Newman DK, Colling J, et al. *Urinary Incontinence in Adults: Acute and Chronic Management.* Clinical Practice Guideline No. 2, 1996 Update. Rockville, MD: US Department of Health and Human Services, Public Health Service, Agency for Health Care Policy and Research; March 1996. AHCPR Pub. No. 96-0682; Abrams P, Cardozo L, Khoury S, et al., eds. *2nd International Consultation on Incontinence.* Plymouth, UK: Health Publication Ltd; 2002; Cochrane Library (accessed July 2003); Goode PS, Burgio KL, Locher JL, et al. Effect of behavioral training with or without pelvic floor electrical stimulation on stress incontinence in women. *JAMA.* 2003;290:345–352.

bladder diary (using the shortest interval between voids). When the urgency occurs, the patient is instructed to stand still or sit down, contract the pelvic muscles, and concentrate on making the urgency decrease and pass: to take a deep breath and let it out slowly, or to visualize the urgency as a wave that peaks and then falls. Once in control of the urgency, the patient should walk slowly to a bathroom and void. After 2 days without leakage, the time between scheduled voids is increased by 30 to 60 minutes until the person voids every 3 to 4 hours without leakage. Although marginal benefit is unproven, many experts believe biofeedback can improve teaching and outcomes. Successful bladder retraining usually takes several weeks; patients need reassurance to proceed despite any initial failure.

For cognitively impaired patients, behavioral methods include habit training (timed voiding, with the interval based on a person's usual voiding schedule), scheduled voiding (timed voiding usually every 2 to 3 hours), and prompted voiding. Prompted voiding has three components: regular monitoring with encouragement to report continence status, prompting to toilet on a scheduled basis, and praise and positive feedback when the person is continent and attempts to toilet.

Persons most likely to respond to prompted voiding are those with who void four or fewer times in 12 daytime hours and who toilet correctly over 75% of the time in an initial trial. These methods require training, motivation, and continued effort by patients and caregivers; special attention and staff reinforcement are needed in institutionalized settings to ensure continued treatment success.

When behavioral methods alone are not sufficient, bladder-suppressant medications can be added. The combination of behavioral and drug therapy has higher efficacy than either alone. There are now five available antimuscarinic agents. The oxybutynin (immediate-release 2.5 to 5mg mg two to four times daily; extended-release 5 to 20 mg once daily; topical patch 3.9 mg applied to abdomen, thighs, or buttocks twice weekly); tolterodine (immediate-release 1 to 2 mg twice daily, extended-release 2 to 4 mg once daily); trospium 20 mg twice daily; darifenacin 7.5 to 15 mg once daily; and solifenacin 10 to 20 mg once daily. Overall, they have similar efficacy, with some variation in adverse events (See Table 26.5). Lack of response to one agent does not preclude response to another.

Anticholinergic side effects can be bothersome (eg, constipation and compensatory fluid intake for xerostomia may exacerbate UI) but also potentially dangerous. Chronic xerostomia predisposes the patient

---

[OL] Not approved by the U.S. Food and Drug Administration for this use.

Table 26.7—Efficacy of Surgical Treatments for Stress Incontinence

Treatment	Target Population	Efficacy	Evidence*
Retropubic suspension	Women	Short term cure 69%-88%, 5 years 70%; cure or improvement 84%;** complications 18% (range 6%–57%)	A–B
Needle suspension	Women	More likely to fail than open suspension (29% failed vs 16%, RR 2.00 [95% CI, 1.47 to 2.72]), with no differences in complications (23% vs 16%) if first UI surgery. May be as effective as anterior vaginal repair (36% failed vs 39%, RR 0.93 [0.68 to 1.26]). Limited data comparing with suburethral slings.	A
Anterior vaginal repair (colporrhaphy)	Women	Less effective than open suspension (year 1 failure rate 29% vs 14%; long-term 41% vs 17%), with more repeat operations (23% vs 2%, RR 8.87 [95% CI, 3.28 to 23.9])	A–B
Vaginal sling	Women with stress UI, ISD, hypermobility	Short term-cure rates with TVT similar to open abdominal retropubic suspension; complications 9%. Gore-Tex slings may have higher complications than rectus fascia slings. Limited long-term results	B–C
Marshall-Marchetti-Krantz (open suspension)	Women	Scant data in older or frail women; in younger women up to 88% success rate	C
Periurethral bulking injections	Women with ISD	Cure 50% (range 8%–100%), cure or improvement 67%	B
	Men with ISD	Cure 20% (range 0%–66%), cure or improvement 42%	B
Artificial sphincter	Women with ISD	Cure 77%, cure or improvement 80%; revision rate 40%–50%; less data than with men	B
	Men with ISD	Cure 66% (range 33%–88%), cure or improvement 85% (range 75%–95%); revision rate 40%–50%	B

* Evidence strength: A = randomized controlled studies; B = case-control studies; C = case descriptions or expert opinion.

** Subjective cure may be less because of persistent or de novo urge incontinence or voiding difficulty.

NOTE: CI = confidence interval; ISD = intrinsic sphincter deficiency; RR = relative risk; TVT = tension-free vaginal tape; UI = urinary incontinence.

SOURCES: Data from Fantl JA, Newman DK, Colling J, et al. *Urinary Incontinence in Adults: Acute and Chronic Management.* Clinical Practice Guideline No. 2, 1996 Update. Rockville, MD: US Department of Health and Human Services, Public Health Service, Agency for Health Care Policy and Research; March 1996. AHCPR Pub. No. 96-0682; Abrams P, Cardozo L, Khoury S, et al., eds. *2nd International Consultation on Incontinence.* Plymouth, UK: Health Publication Ltd; 2002; Cochrane Library (accessed July 2003).

to caries and tooth loss. Visual changes and cognitive impairment present safety issues. Although there are a growing number of case reports regarding cognitive effects, outcome studies of cognitive impairment from these agents are still under way. The PVR should be monitored if UI worsens; if high, then UI may improve when the dose is lowered. Patients with DHIC may tolerate bladder-suppressant medications if initial dose is low and titration is slow and based on symptom response; the PVR should be monitored.

These agents also differ in metabolism, drug interactions, and ease of use. Trospium should be given once daily in persons with renal insufficiency, and it needs to be taken on an empty stomach. Tolterodine is metabolized by the cytochrome P-450 pathways and interacts with drugs that induce 2D6 (eg, fluoxetine) or are metabolized by 3A4 (eg, erythromycin, ketoconazole). There are case reports of interactions between bladder relaxants and cholinesterase inhibitors, and caution should be used if drugs in the two classes are to be used together.

Other agents (propantheline, dicyclomine, imipramine, hyoscyamine, calcium channel blockers,

and nonsteroidal anti-inflammatories) have scant efficacy data. Flavoxate is ineffective. Vasopressin was found to decrease nocturnal voids in a small randomized trial in healthy older persons, yet its expense and risk of heart failure and hyponatremia argue against routine use.

Sacral nerve neuromodulation by an implanted S3 electrode may decrease severe refractory DO, but reimplantation is required in one third of patients. Augmentation cystoplasty surgery has high morbidity and is reserved for patients with profound DO (usually younger persons with poorly compliant bladders from neurologic disease).

Stress Incontinence

Pelvic muscle exercises (PME) strengthen the muscular components of urethral support and are the cornerstone of noninvasive treatment for stress UI. PME, like strength training, employ a small number of isometric repetitions at maximal exertion. Unfortunately, professional and lay misinformation about PME abounds; persons who report failing PME trials may have used inadequate methods. PME requires motivated patients and instruction and monitoring by health professionals, although simple instruction booklets alone have been shown to have moderate benefit. PME instruction should focus on isolation of pelvic muscles; avoidance of buttock, abdomen, or thigh muscle contraction; moderate repetitions of a strong, slow-velocity contraction sustained for 6 to 8 seconds, performed in sets of 8 to 12 contractions three or four times a week and continued for at least 15 to 20 weeks (the patient handout at http://www.healthinaging.org/public_education/bladder_control.php should be amended to decrease initial contraction frequency). The marginal benefit of adding biofeedback or weighted vaginal cones is uncertain, yet many experts feel that biofeedback helps instruction. Adjunctive electrical stimulation does not increase efficacy.

Pessaries may benefit women with stress UI exacerbated by bladder or uterine prolapse. (See "Gynecologic Diseases and Disorders," p 413.)

In numerous epidemiologic and intervention studies, oral estrogen was not found to be effective for the treatment of stress or mixed UI, especially when combined with progestins. Further studies are needed to evaluate topical estrogen (cream, vaginal tablet, or slow-release ring). α-Adrenergic agonists stimulate urethral smooth muscle contraction, but no pure α-agonists are currently available. The α-agonist and anticholinergic actions of imipramine[OL] have been used for mixed UI, yet efficacy data are scant and anticholinergic effects are marked. Duloxetine[OL] is a novel norepinephrine- and serotonin-reuptake inhibitor that increases sphincter contraction; early short-term data suggest efficacy for both stress and mixed UI. However, the dose for incontinence is twice the dose used to treat depression and neuropathic pain, with concomitant higher rates of adverse effects such as nausea. (The manufacturer has put the application for this indication in the United States on hold. The drug does have approval for this indication in Europe and is approved in the United States for depression and pain.)

Surgery provides the highest cure rates for stress UI in women, yet there are few data to assist in procedure and patient selection for older women, especially if they have mixed UI, poor detrusor contractility, prior failed anti-incontinence surgery, and comorbidity. The standard procedure has been bladder neck suspension (eg, transvaginal colposuspension). Suburethral slings and tension-free vaginal tape (synthetic sling inserted at midurethra without tension) are increasingly used; complication rates can exceed 10%. Periurethral injection of collagen, Teflon, or autologous fat is a short-term (≤ 1 year) alternative, usually requiring a series of injections. Anterior colpor-

rhaphy and needle suspensions are less effective and not recommended. Artificial sphincters are used for severe sphincter damage (eg, from surgical scarring).

Postprostatectomy stress UI is more common in older men. Overall, UI rates decline over 6 to 12 months, regardless of PME therapy. Although preoperative PME improves early postoperative UI rates, there is no difference from controls at 1 year. No drugs are known to be effective. Artificial sphincter replacement can be effective but requires manual dexterity and cognition, and it has high revision rates (up to 40%); urodynamics should assist patient selection, as outcomes are worse with severe DO and poor detrusor compliance. Early short-term reports suggest that suburethral sling placement may offer benefit.

Bladder Outlet Obstruction

A range of medical and surgical alternatives are available for prostatic obstruction (see "Prostate Disease," p 423). Obstruction should be considered as a diagnosis in women with previous vaginal or urethral surgery; treatment by unilateral suture removal or urethrolysis (remobilization of adhesions) may restore continence. Pessaries may improve urethral kinking due to pelvic organ prolapse; otherwise, prolapse repair surgery can be considered.

Detrusor Underactivity

Treatment is supportive. Drugs that impair detrusor contractility and increase urethral tone should be decreased or stopped, and constipation should be treated. Bethanechol chloride is ineffective except possibly for patients with overflow UI who must remain on anticholinergic agents (eg, antidepressant or antipsychotic medications). Intermittent clean catheterization is effective for willing and able patients. Sterile intermittent catheterization is preferred for frailer patients and those in institutionalized settings. In some cases bladder emptying may improve with double voiding or simply unhurried voiding.

Catheters and Catheter Care

Indwelling catheters cause significant morbidity, including polymicrobial bacteriuria (universal by 30 days), febrile episodes (1 per 100 patient days), nephrolithiasis, bladder stones, epididymitis, chronic renal inflammation and pyelonephritis, and meatal damage. External collection devices also cause bacteriuria, infection, penile cellulitis and necrosis, and urinary retention and hydronephrosis if the condom twists or its external band is too tight.

[OL] Not approved by the U.S. Food and Drug Administration for this use.

Indwelling catheters should be reserved for the following situations: short-term decompression of acute retention; chronic retention that cannot be managed surgically or medically; wounds that need protection from urine; a terminally ill or severely impaired patient who cannot tolerate garment changes, or when there is persistent patient preference for catheter management despite risks. The passage of the 1990 Omnibus Budget Reconciliation Act has resulted in more appropriate and decreased catheter use in long-term care but with an increased prevalence of UI.

Several general principles guide safe and effective catheter care. Bacteriuria and infection are reduced by closed drainage systems. Topical meatal antimicrobials, catheters with antimicrobial coating, collection bag disinfectants, and antimicrobial irrigation are not effective. Although antibiotics decrease bacteriuria and infection, routine use induces resistant organisms and secondary infections such as *Clostridium difficile* colitis. Bacteriuria is universal in catheterized patients and should not be treated unless there are clear symptoms. Routine cultures should not be done because of the changing flora and failure to predict infection. In symptomatic patients, cultures should be done after the old catheter is removed and a new catheter is placed. Institutionalized patients with catheters should be kept in separate rooms to decrease cross-infection.

With acute urinary retention, decompression should continue at least 7 days, followed by a voiding trial after catheter removal (never clamping). Prophylactic antibiotics are recommended only with short-term catheterization in high-risk patients (eg, those with prosthetic heart valves). For men with chronic obstruction, suprapubic catheters can avoid meatal and penile trauma, and intraurethral stents, if available, may be another alternative (but sometimes at a cost of increased urgency and frequency).

Risk factors for catheter blockage include alkaline urine, female gender, poor mobility, calciuria, proteinuria, copious mucin, *Proteus* colonization, and preexistent bladder stones. Changing the catheter every 7 to 10 days may decrease blockage in such patients. In the absence of risk factors, catheters need not be changed routinely as long as monitoring is adequate. If patients cannot be monitored, changing catheters every 30 days is reasonable. Persistent leakage around the catheter can be caused by irritation by a large Foley balloon, catheter diameter that is too large, bacteriuria, constipation or impaction, improper catheter positioning, or catheter materials.

Clean intermittent catheterization is an alternative for willing patients with sufficient dexterity. Strict sterility is not necessary, although good handwashing and regular decontamination of the catheters is needed. Bacteriuria can be minimized by a frequency of catheterization that keeps bladder volume < 400 mL. Stiffer catheters are easier to insert.

Resources, including Web site addresses, of use to clinicians treating patients with UI are listed in the Appendix (p 514).

ANNOTATED REFERENCES

■ Carlson KV, Nitti VW. Prevention and management of incontinence following radical prostatectomy. *Urol Clin North Am.* 2001;28(3):595–612.

This review covers behavioral treatment, injection therapy, and the use of artificial sphincters for post-prostatectomy incontinence, which is predominantly stress urinary incontinence with intrinsic sphincter deficiency. Case series are now emerging about the potential use of urethral "sling" operations for this condition (analogous to sling or tension-free transvaginal tape procedures for women with stress incontinence).

■ Diokno A, Appell RA, Sand PK, et al. Prospective, randomized, double-blind study of the efficacy and tolerability of the extended-release formulations of oxybutynin and tolterodine for overactive bladder: results of the OPERA trial. *Mayo Clin Proc.* 2003;78(6):687–695.

This is the first prospective randomized, controlled, double-blind multicenter trial comparing extended-release oxybutynin 10 mg per day versus extended-release tolterodine 4 mg per day in women. Subjects were 790 women (mean age 60, 39% at least 65 years, 15% at least 75 years) who had moderate to severe overactive bladder with at least 21 urge urinary incontinence episodes weekly and a mean frequency of 10 voids per day; 47% had previously taken antimuscarinic medication for incontinence. At 12 weeks, reduction in weekly urge incontinence episodes was similar. Cure rate with oxybutynin was 23%, versus 17% with tolterodine ($P = .03$). Dry mouth was more common with oxybutynin (30% versus 22%, $P = .02$), though study withdrawal rates were similar. These results may aid clinicians in making initial drug choices for similar patients, balancing efficacy and tolerability on the basis of the individual patient's needs.

■ Goode PS, Burgio KL, Locher JL, et al. Effect of behavioral training with or without pelvic floor electrical stimulation on stress incontinence in women. *JAMA.* 2003; 290(3):345–352.

This prospective, randomized, controlled, double-blind trial compared behavioral training (BT) with and without adjunctive home pelvic floor electrical stimulation (PFES) with a self-administered behavioral therapy instruction booklet in treating 200 healthy, community-based women (mean age 56.2 [9.8]) with stress or stress-predominant mixed urinary incontinence (UI). Total UI frequency was reduced 69% with BT alone, 72% with BT plus PFES, and 53% with the instruction booklet ($P = .60$ BT versus BT plus PFES, $P = .002$ active therapy versus instruction book). Rates of patient-defined "much better" outcome was highest with BT plus PFES (77%, versus 57% BT alone [$P = .048$] and 30% with booklet [$P < .001$]). Quality-of-life improvement, determined by using the Incontinence Impact Questionnaire, did not differ between the groups. These results emphasize the discordance between objective and patient-based outcomes of UI interventions. PFES would be cost-effective by subjective but not objective or quality-of-life outcomes—an interesting dilemma for providers and payers. The results with the self-instruction booklet show that modest but real improvement is possible without intense intervention.

■ Schnelle JF, Kapur K, Alessi C, et al. Does an exercise and incontinence intervention save healthcare costs in a nursing home population? *J Am Geriatr Soc.* 2003, 51(2):161–168.

■ Wagner TH. Subak LL. Evaluating an incontinence intervention in nursing home resident [editorial]. *J Amer Geriatr Soc.* 2003, 51(2):275–276.

This randomized controlled trial examined the effect of low-intensity, functionally oriented exercise program on physical inactivity, urinary incontinence, immobility, and costs in 190 incontinent residents in four nursing homes. The program, based on federal and clinical practice guidelines, was provided every 2 hours during 8 daytime hours, 5 days a week for 8 months. The program group had significantly better functional outcomes (strength, mobility endurance, urinary and fecal incontinence), but there was no difference in prevalence or cost of acute health conditions. The authors conclude that the cost of implementing such labor-intensive interventions in nursing homes will have to be justified on the basis of functional and quality-of-life outcomes, as they are unlikely to be offset by savings in medical care costs. In the accompanying editorial, Wagner and Subak emphasize the importance of and need for cost-effectiveness analysis to support the use of such interventions in nursing homes.

■ Schnelle JF, Smith RL. Quality indicators for the management of urinary incontinence in vulnerable community-dwelling elders. *Ann Intern Med.* 2001;135(8 Pt 2):752–758.

Quality indicators based on evidence and expert opinion were developed as part of the Assessing Care of the Vulnerable Elderly project (see *Ann Intern Med.* 2001;135[8], Part 2). The target population is community-based frail elderly persons. The ten indicators are in the domains of evaluation, documentation, patient education, and treatment.

■ Walters MD, Daneshgari F. Surgical management of stress urinary incontinence. *Clin Obstet Gynecol.* 2004;47(1):93–103.

Stress urinary incontinence is the most common form of incontinence in women and surgery is held as the mainstay of therapy. This is a review of the various surgical approaches for the management of stress urinary incontinence. The authors recommend specific surgical approaches for patients with various characteristics, on the basis of evidence.

Catherine E. DuBeau, MD

CHAPTER 27—GAIT IMPAIRMENT

KEY POINTS

- Gait disorders are common in older adults and are a predictor of functional decline.
- The cause of gait impairment in older adults is usually multifactorial; a full assessment must therefore consider a number of different causes, as determined from a detailed physical examination as well as functional performance evaluation.
- Interventions, ranging from medical to surgical to exercise, are effective and reduce the extent of the disorder, although residual impairment is often present.

Gait disorders are commonly associated with falls and disability in older adults. This chapter reviews the epidemiology of gait impairments, comorbidities that contribute to these disorders, and office-based clinical assessments and interventions to reduce their functional impact.

EPIDEMIOLOGY

Limitations in walking increase with age. At least 20% of noninstitutionalized older adults admit to difficulty with walking or require the assistance of another person or special equipment to walk. In some samples of noninstitutionalized older adults aged 85 and over, the incidence of limitation in walking can be over 54%. Age-related gait changes such as decrease in speed are most apparent past age 75 or 80, but the majority of gait disorders appear in connection with underlying diseases, particularly as disease severity increases. For example, advanced age (> 85 years), three or more chronic conditions at baseline, and the occurrence of stroke, hip fracture, or cancer predict catastrophic loss of walking ability.

Determining that a gait is disordered is difficult because there are no clearly accepted general standards of normal gait for older adults. Some believe that slowed gait speed suggests a disorder; others believe that deviations in smoothness, symmetry, and synchrony of movement patterns suggest a disorder.

Longitudinal studies suggest that certain gait-related mobility disorders progress with age and that this progression is associated with morbidity and mortality. Gait or postural disorders, as measured by the Unified Parkinson's Disease Rating Scale (UPDRS) (including abnormalities in rising from a chair and turning), increased variably in most (79%) of a sample of nondemented Catholic clergy (mean age 75) who were followed for up to 7 years. This increase was more common in the older age groups and was associated with a higher mortality rate. The increased UPDRS score may represent increased parkinsonian-like signs with age but likely also represents an increasing burden of associated disease and inactivity.

CONDITIONS THAT CONTRIBUTE TO GAIT IMPAIRMENT

Impaired gait may not be an inevitable consequence of aging but rather a reflection of the increased prevalence and severity of age-associated diseases. These diseases, both neurologic and non-neurologic, are the major contributors to impaired gait. In addition, attributing a gait disorder to one disease in an older adult is particularly difficult because similar gait abnormalities are common to many diseases. (For a glossary of gait abnormalities, see Table 27.1.)

Patients in primary care consider pain, stiffness, dizziness, numbness, weakness, and sensations of abnormal movement to be the most common contributors to their walking difficulties. The most common conditions found in primary care that are thought to contribute to gait disorders are degenerative joint disease, acquired musculoskeletal deformities, intermittent claudication, impairments following orthopedic surgery and stroke, and postural hypotension. Usually, more than one contributing condition is found. In a

group of community-dwelling adults older than age 88, joint pain was by far the most common contributor, followed by multiple causes such as stroke and visual loss. Factors such as dementia and fear of falling also contribute to gait disorders. The disorders found in a neurologic referral population include frontal gait disorders (usually related to normal-pressure hydrocephalus and cerebrovascular processes), sensory disorders (also involving vestibular and visual function), myelopathy, previously undiagnosed Parkinson's disease or parkinsonian syndromes, and cerebellar disease. Known conditions causing severe gait impairment, such as hemiplegia and severe hip or knee disease, are commonly not mentioned in these neurologic referral populations. Thus, many gait disorders, particularly those that are classical and discrete (eg, those related to stroke and osteoarthritis) and those that are mild or may relate to irreversible disease (eg, vascular dementia), are presumably diagnosed in primary care and treated without a referral to a neurologist. Other less common contributors to gait disorders include metabolic disorders (related to renal or hepatic disease), central nervous system tumors or subdural hematoma, depression, and psychotropic medications. Case reports also document reversible gait disorders due to clinically overt hypo- or hyperthyroidism and B_{12} and folate deficiency.

Factors that contribute to slowed gait speed are also considered contributors to gait disorders. These factors are commonly disease associated (eg, cardiopulmonary or musculoskeletal disease) and include reductions in leg strength, vision, aerobic function, standing balance, and decreased physical activity, as well as joint impairment, previous falls, and fear of falling. Combining these factors may result in an effect greater than the sum of the single impairments (as when combining balance and strength impairments). Furthermore, the effect of improved strength and aerobic capacity on gait speed may be nonlinear, that is, for very impaired individuals, small improvements in strength or aerobic capacity yield relatively larger gains in gait speed, whereas these small improvements yield little gait speed change in healthy older persons.

Although older adults may maintain a relatively normal gait pattern well into their 80s, some slowing occurs, and decreased stride length thus becomes a common feature in descriptions of gait disorders of older adults. Some authors have proposed the emergence of an age-related gait disorder without accompanying clinical abnormalities, that is, essential "senile" gait disorder. This gait pattern is described as broad-based with small steps, diminished arm swing, stooped posture, decreased flexion of the hips and knees, uncertainty and stiffness in turning, occasional difficulty initiating steps, and a tendency toward falling. These and other nonspecific findings (such as the

Table 27.1—Glossary of Gait Abnormalities

Term	Description
Circumduction	Outward swing of leg in semicircle from the hip
Equinovarus	Excessive plantar flexion and inversion of the ankle
Festination	Acceleration of gait
Foot drop	Loss of ankle dorsiflexion secondary to weakness of ankle dorsiflexors
Foot slap	Early, frequent audible foot-floor contact with steppage gait compensation
Genu recurvatum	Hyperextension of the knee
Propulsion	Falling forward
Retropulsion	Falling backward
Scissoring	Hip adduction such that the knees cross in front of each other with each step
Steppage gait	Exaggerated hip flexion, knee extension, and foot lifting
Trendelenburg gait	Shift of the trunk over the affected hip, which drops because of hip abductor weakness
Turn en bloc	Moving the whole body while turning

inability to perform tandem gait) are similar to gait patterns found in a number of other diseases, and yet the clinical abnormalities are insufficient to make a specific diagnosis. This "disorder" may be a precursor to an as-yet-undiagnosed disease (eg, related to subtle extrapyramidal signs) and is likely to be a manifestation of concurrent, progressive cognitive impairment (eg, Alzheimer's disease or vascular dementia). "Senile" gait disorder thus may reflect a number of potential diseases and is generally not useful in labeling gait disorders in older adults.

Subclinical as well as clinically evident cerebrovascular disease is increasingly recognized as a major contributor to gait disorders (see the section below on assessment). Nondemented persons with clinically abnormal gait (particularly unsteady, frontal, or hemiparetic gait) followed for approximately 7 years were found to be at higher risk of developing non-Alzheimer's, particularly vascular, dementia. Of note, those with abnormal gait at baseline may not have met criteria for dementia but already had abnormalities in neuropsychologic function, such as in visual-perceptual processing and language skills. Gait disorders with no apparent cause (also termed *idiopathic* or *senile* gait disorder) are associated with a higher mortality rate, primarily from cardiovascular causes. These cardiovascular causes are likely linked to concomitant, possibly undetected, cerebrovascular disease.

ASSESSMENT

A potentially useful approach to assessing contributors to a gait impairment (see Table 27.2) categorizes these deficits according to the sensorimotor levels that are affected.

Disorders that are the result of pathology of the low sensorimotor level can be divided into peripheral sensory and peripheral motor dysfunction, including myopathic or neuropathic disorders that cause weakness and musculoskeletal diseases. These disorders are generally distal to the central nervous system. With peripheral sensory impairment, unsteady and tentative gait is commonly caused by vestibular disorders, peripheral neuropathy, posterior column (proprioceptive) deficits, or visual impairment. With peripheral motor impairment, a number of classical gait patterns emerge. Examples of these patterns include Trendelenburg gait (weight shifts over the weak hip, which drops because of hip abductor weakness), antalgic gait (avoidance of weight bearing and shortening of stance on one side because of pain), and foot drop (due to ankle dorsiflexor weakness, early, frequently audible foot-floor contact with steppage gait compensation, ie, excessive hip flexion). These gait impairments are the result of body segment and joint deformities, pain, and

focal myopathic and neuropathic weakness. Note that if the gait disorder is limited to this low sensorimotor level (ie, the central nervous system is intact), the person adapts well to the gait disorder, compensating with an assistive device or learning to negotiate the environment safely.

At the middle level, the execution of centrally selected postural and locomotor responses is faulty, and the sensory and motor modulation of gait is disrupted. Gait may be initiated normally but stepping patterns are abnormal. Diseases causing spasticity (eg, those related to myelopathy, B_{12} deficiency, and stroke), parkinsonism (idiopathic as well as drug induced), and cerebellar disease (eg, alcohol induced) are examples of those that cause this type of impairment. Gait abnormalities appear when the spasticity is sufficient to cause leg circumduction and fixed deformities (eg, equinovarus), when the Parkinson's produces shuffling steps and reduced arm swing, and when the cerebellar ataxia increases trunk sway sufficiently to require a broad base of gait support.

At the high or central level the gait impairments become more nonspecific. Lesions in the frontal lobe account for most of the gait abnormalities at this level. The severity of the frontal-related disorders runs a spectrum from gait ignition failure (ie, difficulty with initiation) to frontal disequilibrium, where unsupported stance is not possible. Cerebrovascular insults to the cortex, as well as to the basal ganglia and their interconnections, may contribute to gait ignition failure and apraxia.

Dementia and depression are also thought to contribute to an abnormal gait at this level. With increasing severity of the dementia, particularly in patients with Alzheimer's disease, frontal-related symptoms also increase. Gait impairments in this category have been given a number of overlapping descriptions, including *gait apraxia*, *marche à petits pas*, and *arteriosclerotic parkinsonism*.

There is likely to be more than one disease or impairment present that contributes to a gait disorder; one example is the longstanding diabetic patient with peripheral neuropathy and a recent stroke who is now very fearful of falls. Certain disorders may actually involve multiple parts of the nervous system, such as Parkinson's disease affecting cortical and subcortical structures. Drug and metabolic causes (eg, from sedatives, tranquilizers, and anticonvulsants) may involve both central and peripheral nervous systems; phenothiazines, for example, can cause central sedation and extrapyramidal effects.

History and Physical Examination

A careful medical history will help elucidate the multiple factors contributing to the older patient's gait

Table 27.2—Abnormalities of Gait and Associated Findings, by Sensorimotor Level

Sensorimotor Level	Type of Impairment	Condition or Disease	Physical Findings	Gait Abnormality*
Low	Peripheral sensory dysfunction	Peripheral neuropathy, proprioceptive deficits	Loss of position sense, touch	Possible steppage gait
		Vestibular disorders		May weave, fall to one side
		Visual impairment	Visual loss	Tentative, uncertain, uncoordinated
	Peripheral motor dysfunction	Extremity (body segment and joint) deformities Pain Focal myopathic, neuropathic weakness	Pain-related avoidance of weight bearing on affected side Limited flexion in painful extremity (especially knee) and may lead to loss of joint range and contracture Decreased lumbar lordosis	Shortened stance phase on affected side Trendelenburg gait Painful limb may buckle with weight bearing Unequal leg length can produce trunk and pelvic motion abnormalities (including Trendelenburg gait)
			Stooped posture Pelvic or hip girdle weakness	Pelvic girdle weakness can lead to exaggerated lumbar lordosis and lateral trunk flexion (Trendelenburg and waddling gait)
			Proximal muscle weakness Distal muscle weakness	Proximal weakness can produce waddling gait Weak ankle dorsiflexors result in foot drop or slap or steppage gait
Middle	Postural and locomotor impairment	Cerebellar ataxia	Poor trunk control, incoordination or other cerebellar signs	Wide-based with increased trunk sway, irregular stepping, staggering, especially on turns
		Parkinsonism	Rigidity Bradykinesia Trunk flexion	Small shuffling steps, hesitation, festination, propulsion, retropulsion, turning en bloc, absent arm swing
		Hemiplegia or hemiparesis	Arm and leg weakness, spasticity Equinovarus Genu recurvatum	Leg circumduction Loss of arm swing Foot drag or scrape
		Paraplegia or paraparesis	Leg weakness, spasticity	Bilateral leg circumduction, scraping feet, possibly also scissoring
High	Central nervous system (esp frontal) disorder	Cautious gait Mild Alzheimer's disease	May have fear of falling	Normal to widened base, shortened stride, decreased velocity, en bloc turns
		Cerebrovascular disease Normal-pressure hydrocephalus	May have evidence of other atherosclerotic disease, cognitive impairment, weakness and spasticity, and urinary incontinence	Range of findings may include difficulty initiating gait and shuffling gait, preservation of upright posture and arm swing, leg apraxia (can imitate gait movements in non-weight-bearing position), freezing (especially with attention diversion)

NOTE: For descriptions of gait abnormalities, see Table 27.1.

impairment. A brief systemic evaluation for evidence of subacute metabolic disease (eg, thyroid disorders), acute cardiopulmonary disorders (eg, myocardial infarction), or other acute illness (eg, sepsis) is warranted because an acute gait disorder may be the presenting feature of acute systemic decompensation in an older adult. The physical examination should include an attempt to identify motion-related factors, for example, by provoking both vestibular and orthostatic responses. Blood pressure should be measured with the patient both supine and standing to exclude orthostatic hypotension. Vision screening, at least for acuity, is essential. The neck, spine, extremities, and feet should be evaluated for pain, deformities, and limitations in range of motion, particularly regarding subtle hip or knee contractures. Leg-length discrepancies such as may occur with a hip prosthesis and either as an antecedent or subsequent to lower back pain can be measured simply as the distance from the anterior superior iliac spine to the medial malleolus. A formal neurologic assessment is critical, to include assessment of strength and tone, sensation (including proprioception), coordination (including cerebellar function), station, and gait. The Romberg test screens for simple postural control and whether the proprioceptive and vestibular systems are functional. Some investigators have proposed one-legged stance time less than 5 seconds as a risk factor for injurious falls, although even relatively healthy adults aged 70 and older may have difficulty with one-legged stance. Given the importance of cognition as a risk factor, assessing cognitive function is also indicated.

Laboratory and Imaging Assessments

Depending upon the history and physical examination, further laboratory and diagnostic imaging evaluation may be warranted. Complete blood cell count, chemistries, and other metabolic studies may be useful only where systemic disease is suspected. Head or spine imaging, including radiography, computed tomography, or magnetic resonance imaging (MRI) are not indicated unless there are neurologic abnormalities by history and physical examination, either preceding or of recent onset, that are related to the gait disorder. However, cerebral white matter changes, often considered to be vascular (termed *leukoaraiosis*), have been increasingly associated with nonspecific gait disorders. Periventricular high signal measurements on MRI as well as increased ventricular volume, even in apparently healthy older adults, are associated with gait slowing. White matter hyperintensities on MRI correlate with longitudinal changes in balance, and the periventricular frontal and occipitoparietal regions appear to be most affected. Age-specific guidelines for and the sensitivity, specificity, and cost-effectiveness of these work-ups remain to be determined.

Performance-Based Functional Assessment

Technologically oriented assessments involving formal kinematic and kinetic analyses have not been applied widely in clinical assessments of balance and gait disorders in older adults. Comfortable gait speed and a related measure, distance walked (as measured by the 6-minute walk test), are powerful predictors of a number of important outcomes, such as disability, institutionalization, and mortality. Gait speed is faster in individuals who are taller, who have a lower disease burden, and who are more active and less functionally

disabled. It has been suggested that slow (impaired) walkers can be defined as those who walk at a speed < 0.6 m/sec and fast walkers (unimpaired) walkers walk at > 1.0 m/sec. A number of timed and semiquantitative balance and gait scales have been proposed as a means to detect and quantify abnormalities and to direct interventions. Fall risk, for example, may be increased with more abnormal gait and balance scale scores. Perhaps the simplest battery in the clinical setting is the Timed Get Up and Go (TUG), a timed sequence of rising from a chair, walking 3 meters, turning, and returning to sit in the chair. One study suggests a TUG score of 14 seconds or higher as an indicator for fall risk. Other investigators have found limitations in TUG in the presence of cognitive impairment and difficulty in completing the test due to immobility, safety concerns, or refusal. Another functional approach that may be useful clinically is the Functional Ambulation Classification scale, which rates the use of assistive devices, the degree of human assistance (either manual or verbal), the distance the patient can walk, and the types of surfaces the patient can negotiate.

INTERVENTIONS TO REDUCE GAIT DISORDERS

Even if a diagnosable condition is found on evaluation, many conditions causing a gait disorder are, at best, only partially treatable. Functional improvement becomes the treatment goal. Achievement of premorbid gait patterns may be unrealistic, but improvement in measures such as gait speed is reasonable as long as gait remains safe. Comorbidity, disease severity, and overall health status tend to strongly influence treatment outcome.

Many of the older reports dealing with treatment and rehabilitation of gait disorders in older adults are retrospective chart reviews and case studies. Gait disorders presumably secondary to B_{12} deficiency, folate deficiency, hypothyroidism, hyperthyroidism, knee osteoarthritis, Parkinson's disease, and inflammatory polyneuropathy show improvement as a result of medical therapy. A variety of modes of physical therapy for diseases such as knee osteoarthritis and stroke also result in modest improvements in function but continued residual disability. For example, a combined aerobic, strength, and functionally based group exercise program was found to increase gait speed approximately 5% in patients with knee osteoarthritis. The focus is on strengthening the extensor groups (especially knee and hip) and stretching commonly shortened muscles (such as the hip flexors). A recent review suggests that the effects of conventional physical therapy in the treatment of Parkinson's gait disorders are unclear, but that cueing, specifically audio and visual, can improve gait speed. Other studies suggest an incremental reduction of gait impairment with the use of a body-weight support and a treadmill to provide task-specific gait training following total hip arthroplasty, in Parkinson's disease, and particularly in hemiparetic stroke patients. However, a Cochrane review found no statistically significant effect favoring treadmill training with or without body support over conventional training to improve gait speed or disability in stroke patients. Note that the Cochrane review found a small but clinically important trend (an improvement of 0.24 m/sec in the body-weight support plus treadmill group) in those who could walk independently.

A few studies of group exercise have demonstrated improvements in gait parameters such as gait speed. Generally, the most consistent effects are with varied types of exercise provided in the same program. A 12-week combined program of leg resistance, standing balance, and flexibility exercises was found to increase usual gait speed 8% in minimally impaired life-care community residents. A similar varied 16-week format with more intensive individual support and prompting in selected demented older adults (mean MMSE 15) resulted in a 23% improvement in gait speed. A number of these studies note improvement in functional, gait-oriented measures (although not strictly gait "disorder" measures), such as the distance walked in 6 minutes by knee osteoarthritis patients undergoing either an aerobic or resistance training program.

Modest improvement and residual disability are also the result of surgical treatment for compressive cervical myelopathy, lumbar stenosis, and normal-pressure hydrocephalus. Few controlled prospective studies and virtually no randomized studies address the outcome of surgical versus nonsurgical treatment for these disorders. A number of problems plague the available series: outcomes such as pain and walking disability are not reported separately, the source of the outcome rating is not clearly identified or blinded, the criteria for classifying outcomes differ, the outcomes may be subjective and subject to interpretation, the follow-up intervals are variable, the subjects who are reported in follow-up may be a highly select group, the selection factors for conservative versus surgical treatment between studies differ or are unspecified, and there is publication bias (only positive results are published). Many of the surgical series include all ages, although the mean age is usually above 60 years old. A few studies document equivalent surgical outcomes with conservative, nonsurgical treatment.

Many older adults with lumbar stenosis have reduction in pain and improvement in maximal walking distance following laminectomies and lumbar fusion surgery, although they have continued residual disability. In a somewhat younger cohort (mean age 69) and after an average of 8 years of follow-up after surgery for lumbar stenosis, approximately half reported that they were unable to walk two blocks and many of them attributed their decreased walking ability to their back problem. Part of the problem in determining long-term lumbar stenosis surgical outcomes are other mobility-influencing comorbidities, such as cardiovascular or musculoskeletal disease. Nevertheless, some improvement can be found in selected patients older than 75 (mean age 78); one uncontrolled study found that the 45% of patients with preoperative "severe" limitation of ambulatory ability wound up with either "minimal" or "moderate" limitation postoperatively after an average of 1.5 years of follow-up. Studies involving cervical stenosis gait outcomes in older adults are limited, although significant improvement in walking speed following cervical myelopathy decompression can be expected in most patients.

In a noncontrolled study post-shunt for normal-pressure hydrocephalus (follow-up interval not specified), walking speed was found to have increased more than 10% in 75% of the patients and more than 25% in over 57% of the patients. Although there may be initial improvement following shunt placement, long-term results are often disappointing (eg, 65% of post-shunt patients have initial improvement in their gait disorder, but only 26% maintain this improvement by 3-year follow-up). The poor long-term outcomes may be related to concurrent cerebrovascular and cardiovascular disease, a common cause of mortality in these cohorts. Post-shunt gait outcomes may be better in those in whom the gait disturbance precedes cognitive impairment and in those who respond with improvement in gait speed following a trial of cerebrospinal fluid removal.

Outcomes for hip and knee replacement surgery for osteoarthritis are better, although some of the same methodologic problems exist. Sizable gains in pain relief, gait speed, and joint motion occur, although residual walking disability continues for a number of reasons, including residual pathology on the operated side and symptoms on the nonoperated side. For total knee replacements, despite rehabilitation postoperatively, some residual weakness, stiffness, and slowed or altered gait may remain. Simple function may be maintained following knee replacement, such as maintaining the ability to safely clear an obstacle, but usually at the expense of additional compensation by the ipsilateral hip and foot.

Finally, the use of orthoses and other mobility aids will help reduce the gait disorder. Although there are few data supporting their use, lifts (either internal or external) to correct for limb length inequality may be provided in a conservative, gradually progressive manner. Other ankle braces, shoe inserts, shoe body and sole modifications, and their subsequent adjustments are part of standard care for foot and ankle weakness, deformities, and pain but are beyond the scope of this review. In general, well-fitting walking shoes with low heels, relatively thin firm soles, and, if feasible, high, fixed heel collar support are recommended to maximize balance and improve gait. Mobility aids such as canes and walkers reduce load on a painful joint and increase stability. Note that light touching of any firm surface like walls or "furniture surfing" provides feedback and enhances balance. (See also "Rehabilitation," p 108, and "Diseases and Disorders of the Foot," p 451.)

ANNOTATED REFERENCES

■ Alexander NB. Gait disorders in older adults. *J Am Geriatr Soc.* 1996;44(4):434–451.

This review examines the factors underlying changes in gait as a function of aging and of underlying disease. An approach to gait evaluation and an evaluation of various interventions to reduce gait disorders are also included.

■ Liston R, Mickelborough J, Bene J, et al. A new classification of higher level gait disorders in patients with cerebral multi-infarct states. *Age Ageing.* 2003;32(3):252–258.

The authors' hypothesis is that there are three main types of higher level gait disorders: ignition apraxia, equilibrium apraxia, and mixed gait apraxia. Patients with ignition apraxia may have problems with internal cueing that are caused by

lesions in the supplementary motor area, whereas patients with equilibrium apraxia may have dysfunction predominantly in the pre-motor area.

■ Nutt JG. Classification of gait and balance disorders. In: Ruzicka E, Hallet M, Jankovic J, eds. *Gait Disorders. Advances in Neurology, Vol. 87.* Philadelphia: Lippincott, Williams and Wilkins; 2001.

This review (and other chapters in this volume) focus on the neurologic and neuroanatomic basis for the assessment of gait disorders.

■ Studenski S, Perera S, Wallace D, et al. Physical performance measures in the clinical setting. *J Am Geriatr Soc.* 2003;51(3):314–322.

In older adults in a primary care setting, gait speed or measures of lower extremity performance were found to be better than self-report functional measures in predicting outcomes such as hospitalization and functional decline. Using gait speed criteria, this study excluded the extremely fit or fragile (> 1.3 m/sec or < 0.2 m/sec) and utilized values of < 0.6 m/sec and > 1.0 m/sec as slow (impaired) and fast (unimpaired) walker status.

■ Van Hook FW, Demonbreun D, Weiss BD. Ambulatory devices for chronic gait disorders in the elderly. *Am Fam Physician.* 2003;67(8):1717–1724.

This article provides an overview of the ambulatory devices such as canes, crutches, and walkers that are useful for patients with chronic gait disorders.

■ Verghese J, Lipton RB, Hall CB, et al. Abnormality of gait as a predictor of non-Alzheimer's dementia. *N Engl J Med.* 2002;347(22):1761–1768.

In this study, nondemented patients with clinically abnormal gait were found to be at higher risk of developing non-Alzheimer's dementia, particularly vascular dementia.

Neil B. Alexander, MD

CHAPTER 28—FALLS

KEY POINTS

- A fall is one of the most common events threatening the independence of older adults. Complications resulting from falls are the leading cause of death from injury in men and women aged 65 and older.

- The causes of a fall often involve a complex interaction among factors intrinsic to the individual (age-related declines, chronic disease, acute illness, medications), challenges to postural control (environment, changing position, normal activities), and mediating

factors (risk-taking behaviors, underlying mobility level).

- For patients presenting with a fall, important components of the history include the activity of the faller at the time of the incident, the occurrence of prodromal symptoms (lightheadedness, imbalance, and dizziness), the location of the fall, and the time of the fall.

- A systematic review of interventions to reduce the incidence of falls by elderly persons revealed several that were likely to be effective.

PREVALENCE AND MORBIDITY

A fall is one of the most common events threatening the independence of older persons. A fall is considered to have occurred when a person comes to rest inadvertently on the ground or a lower level. Most discussions in the literature of falls by older persons do not include falls associated with loss of consciousness (eg, syncope, seizure) or with overwhelming trauma. The majority of falls are not associated with syncope.

The incidence of falls increases with age and varies according to living status. Each year, between 30% and 40% of community-dwelling persons aged 65 years and older fall. Among those with a history of a fall in the previous year, the annual incidence of falls is close to 60%. In the long-term-care setting each year, about half of all persons fall.

Complications resulting from falls are the leading cause of death from injury in men and women aged 65 and older. The death rate attributable to falls increases with age, with white men aged 85 years and older having the highest death rate (> 180 deaths per 100,000 population). Most falls result in an injury of some type, usually minor soft-tissue injuries, such as bruises and scrapes; however, 10% to 15% result in fracture or other serious injury. In general, falls are associated with subsequent declines in functional status, greater likelihood of nursing-home placement, increased use of medical services, and the development of a fear of falling. Of those elderly persons who fall, only half are able to get up without help, thus experiencing the "long lie." Long lies are associated with lasting declines in functional status.

The true cost of falls in health care dollars is difficult to ascertain. It has been estimated that in the United States the lifetime costs of fall-related injuries for persons aged 65 and older is $12.6 billion. Since many falls result in injury, there is a significant use of emergency department facilities among fallers. Studies from the early 1990s indicate that each year almost 8% of persons aged 70 and older go to emergency departments because of a fall-related injury, and close to a third of these people are admitted to the hospital for a median length of stay of 8 days.

CAUSES

Falls, incontinence, delirium, and other geriatric syndromes result from the accumulated effects of impairments in multiple domains. The falls of older people are rarely due to a single cause. Rather, there is often a complex interaction among factors intrinsic to the individual (age-related declines, chronic disease, acute illness, medications), challenges to postural control (environment, changing positions, normal activities), and mediating factors (risk-taking behaviors, underlying mobility level).

Multiple prospective cohort studies of risk factors for falls have been published over the past decade. Across these studies, many risk factors were found to be consistently associated with falls. These included age, cognitive impairment, female gender, past history of a fall, lower extremity weakness, gait problems, foot disorders, balance problems, hypovitaminosis D, psychotropic drug use, arthritis, and Parkinson's disease. These studies differed significantly in the types of risk factors evaluated, the types of population studied (eg, past fall history was sometimes an entry criterion), and the outcome (one fall, two or more falls, injurious falls). The multiple risk factors found across the studies highlights the multifactorial nature of falls and suggests that there may also be unique circumstances surrounding falls that are not accounted for in the studies. In general, the risk of falling increases with the number of risk factors, although some persons with no risk factors experience falls.

Successful prevention of falls begins with a knowledge of the age-related changes that increase the risk of falls. Thus, with aging, there are declines in the visual, proprioceptive, and vestibular systems. For example, the visual system demonstrates reductions in visual acuity, depth perception, contrast sensitivity, and dark adaptation. The proprioceptive system loses sensitivity in the lower extremities. The vestibular system demonstrates a loss of labyrinthine hair cells, vestibular ganglion cells, and nerve fibers.

Despite these age-related changes in sensory systems, it has been difficult to quantify the age-related changes in postural control that are independent of disease. In general, when postural stability is tested in young and old persons with no apparent musculoskeletal or neurologic impairment, age-related differences in measured sway are found to be most pronounced when moderately severe perturbations of stance are administered, such as changing the support surface, changing body position, altering the visual input, or moving the support surface horizontally or rotationally. This occurs because these perturbations stress the redundancy of the sensory systems in their ability to maintain postural stability. In addition, there may be other age-related changes in the central nervous system that affect postural control, including the loss of neurons and dendrites, and the depletion of neurotransmitters, such as dopamine, within the basal ganglia.

Since it is difficult to find elderly persons without at least subtle neurologic findings, studies have been unable to determine whether some of the young-old differences may be due to these factors. Some of the most striking postural control differences between young and old persons relate to the order or grouping of muscle activation patterns. Thus, in response to perturbations of the support surface, older persons tend to activate the proximal muscles, such as the quadriceps, before the more distal muscles, such as the tibialis anterior. This strategy may not be an efficient way to maintain postural stability. Similarly, in the elderly person there may be greater co-contraction of antagonistic muscles, and the onset of the muscle activation and associated joint torque may be delayed. Finally, the ability to recover balance upon a postural disturbance may be compromised by an age-related decline in the ability to rapidly develop joint torque by using muscles of the lower extremity. All of these strategies potentially impair maintenance of upright posture.

Another important physiologic contributor to the successful maintenance of upright posture is the regulation of systemic blood pressure. The failure to perfuse the brain, which accompanies hypotension, increases the risk of a fall, usually in association with syncope. In addition to the age-related declines in baroreflex sensitivity to hypotensive stimuli manifested as a failure to cardio-accelerate, everyday stresses such as changing posture, eating a meal, or suffering an acute illness may result in hypotension. Since many elderly persons have a resting cerebral perfusion that is compromised by vascular disease, even slight reductions in blood pressure may produce cerebral ischemic symptoms, such as falls. Finally, with aging, there is a reduction in total body water, which places older persons at increased risk of dehydration with acute illness, diuretic use, or hot weather. Since there is a progressive decrease in basal and stimulated renin levels, as well as a decrease in aldosterone production with aging, dehydrating stresses may lead to orthostatic hypotension and a fall.

A number of age-related chronic conditions deserve special mention because of their association with fall risk. Parkinson's disease, in particular, increases the risk of falls through several mechanisms, including the rigidity of lower extremity musculature, the inability to correct sway trajectory because of the slowness in initiating movement, hypotensive drug effects, and, in some cases, cognitive impairment. Another common disease contributing to falls is osteoarthritis. When present in the knee, osteoarthritis may affect mobility, the ability to step over objects and maneuver, and the tendency to avoid complete weight bearing on a painful joint.

One of the most easily modified risk factors for falls that has been repeatedly demonstrated in observational studies is medication use. Individual classes of medications, such as the benzodiazepines, antidepressants (including selective serotonin-reuptake inhibitors), and antipsychotic drugs, have been associated with an increased risk of hip fracture. An increased risk of falling has also been found to be associated with recent changes in the dose of a medication and the total number of prescriptions.

The relative importance of environmental factors to the risk of falling appears to be much less than intrinsic factors in the individual; however, the interaction between environmental factors and intrinsic factors has not been well quantified. Well-designed intervention studies have focused on improving the risk-factor profile of the person or have combined individual interventions with environmental manipulation, making it difficult to isolate the contributions of the environmental factors. Nevertheless, attention to safety hazards in the home environment would appear to be worthwhile, and one intervention study targeting environmental factors was successful in reducing falls.

DIAGNOSTIC APPROACH

The evaluation and management of falls in the geriatric patient may differ according to the clinical setting (home, hospital, nursing home). Table 28.1 highlights some of the differences that might be considered according to setting.

History and Physical Examination

Many falls never come to clinical attention for a variety of reasons: The patient may never mention the event, there is no injury at the time of the fall, the clinician may fail to ask the patient about a history of falls, or the patient or the clinician may make the invalid assumption that falls are an inevitable part of the aging process. In institutional settings, despite attention to falls and even incident reporting, not all falls come to the attention of the nursing staff. The treatment of injuries resulting from falls commonly fails to include an investigation of the cause of the fall.

In the clinical evaluation of the noninstitutionalized geriatric patient who is not specifically being seen for a problem with falling, it is still important that an assessment of fall risk be integrated into the history and physical examination. (See Figure 28.1 for an overview of falls assessment and management in all older persons.) The most important point in the history is the previous history of a fall, since this is a strong risk factor for future falls. For patients presenting with a fall, important components of the history include the activity of the faller at the time of the incident, the occurrence of prodromal symptoms (lightheadedness, imbalance, dizziness), the location of the fall, and the time of the fall. Loss of consciousness

Table 28.1—The Role of Setting in the Assessment and Management of Falls Risk

Characteristic	Home	Hospital	Nursing Home
How falls come to clinical attention	Patient or family reports or clinician queries patient	Nurse, other staff witnesses fall or finds patient on floor	Nurse, other staff witnesses fall or finds resident on floor
Assessment of falls risk	Age Past history of fall Cognitive impairment Female gender Lower extremity weakness Gait problems, foot disorders Balance problems Hypovitaminosis D Psychotropic drug use Arthritis Parkinson's disease	Age Past history of a fall Impaired mental status Special toileting needs Impaired mobility Visual impairment	Using MDS data: Age ≥87 years Past history of fall Male gender Unsteady gait Wandering Walking aid ADLs deterioration Transfer independence Wheelchair independence
Management	Muscle strengthening or balance training individual prescribed by clinician Tai Chi Home hazard assessment prescribed for those with history of falls Multidisciplinary, multifactorial health and environmental risk-factor screening or intervention programs for: ■ unselected community-dwelling older people ■ older people with a history of falling ■ older people selected because of known risk factors	No proven interventions have been reported Many risk assessments have reasonable sensitivity and specificity to be of potential value in targeting high-risk patients if a proven intervention is developed	No proven interventions have been reported Since nursing-home residents are a very high-risk population, applying universal precautions may be more appropriate than relying on individual assessments

NOTE: ADL = activities of daily living; MDS = Minimum Data Set.

is associated with injurious falls and should raise important considerations, such as orthostatic hypotension or cardiac or neurologic disease. (See "Syncope," p 168.) Information on previous falls should be collected to identify patterns that may help target strategies to reduce risk factors. A complete medication history should focus specifically on the use of vasodilators, diuretics, and sedative hypnotics because these agents have been associated with increased risk of falls. In addition to inquiring about the circumstances surrounding the fall, the clinician taking the history should attempt to identify environmental factors that may have contributed. Thus, information on lighting, floor covering, door thresholds, railings, and furniture may add important clues.

The physical examination of the person who has fallen should focus on risk factors. Much of the examination duplicates that of a gait assessment (see "Gait Impairment," p 197.) Footwear may also be an important factor to consider. In one small study to test the effect of various shoe types on balance in older men, shoes with thin, hard soles were found to produce the best results, even though they were perceived as less comfortable than thick, soft, mid-soled shoes, such as running shoes.

Probably the most important part of the physical examination is an assessment of integrated musculoskeletal function, which can be accomplished by performing one or more of the following tests of postural stability.

A simple maneuver called the *functional reach test* is a practical way to test the integrated neuromuscular base of support and has predictive validity for falls by elderly men. This test is performed with a leveled yardstick secured to a wall at the height of the acromion. The person being tested assumes a comfortable stance without shoes or socks and stands so that his or her shoulders are perpendicular to the yardstick. He or she makes a fist and extends the arm forward as far as possible along the wall without taking a step or losing balance. The total reach is measured along the yardstick and recorded. Inability to reach 6 inches or

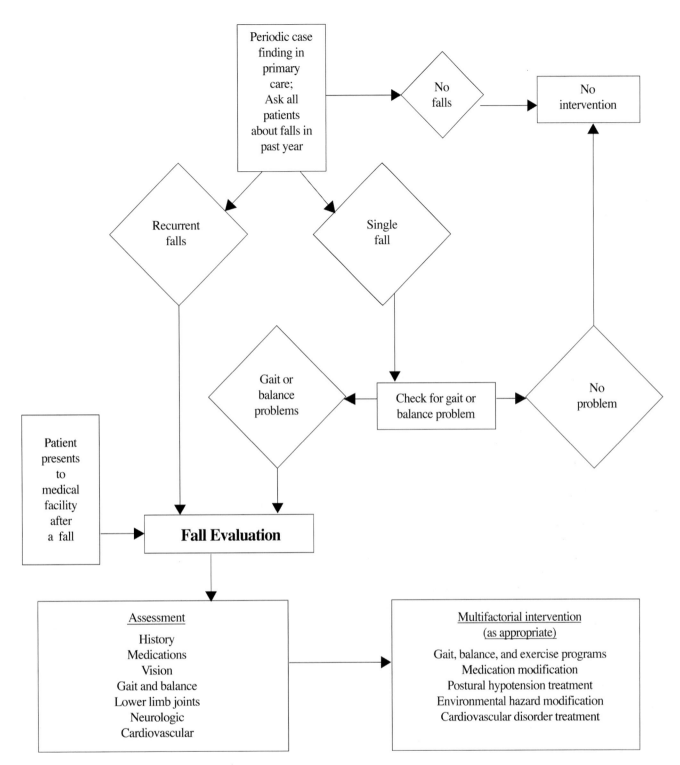

Figure 28.1—The assessment and management of falls.

SOURCE: American Geriatrics Society, British Geriatrics Society, and American Academy of Orthopaedic Surgeons Panel on Falls Prevention. Guideline for the prevention of falls in older persons. *J Am Geriatr Soc.* 2001;49(5):666. Reprinted by permission of Blackwell Science, Inc.

more is cause for concern and merits further evaluation. In its initial description, the functional reach correlated with other physical performance measures, such as walking speed (r = 0.71), tandem walk using an ordinal scale (r = 0.67), and standing on one foot measured as number of seconds that a one-footed stance could be maintained (r = 0.64).

Another useful test of integrated strength and balance is the Get Up and Go test, which can be performed with or without timing. It consists of observation of an individual standing up from a chair without using the arms to push against the chair, walking across a room, turning around, walking back, and sitting down without using the arms. This test can demonstrate muscle weakness, balance problems, and gait abnormalities.

Laboratory and Diagnostic Tests

There is no standard diagnostic evaluation of a person with a history of falls or with a high risk of falling. Obviously, laboratory tests for hemoglobin, serum urea nitrogen, creatinine, or glucose levels can help to exclude such causes of falling as anemia, dehydration, or hyperglycemia with hyperosmolar dehydration. There is no proven value of routinely performing Holter monitoring of persons who have fallen. Because data demonstrate that carotid sinus hypersensitivity contributes to falls and even hip fracture, some have advocated performing carotid sinus massage with continuous heart rate and phasic blood-pressure measurement in persons with unexplained falls. Similarly, the decision to perform echocardiography, brain imaging, or radiographic studies of the spine should be driven by the findings of the history and physical examination. Echocardiography should be reserved for those with cardiac conditions believed to contribute to the maintenance of blood flow to the brain. Spine radiographs or magnetic resonance imaging may be useful in patients with gait disorders, abnormalities on neurologic examination, lower extremity spasticity, or hyperreflexia to exclude cervical spondylosis or lumbar stenosis as a cause of falls.

TREATMENT AND PREVENTION

Multiple studies of preventive interventions have been conducted over the past decade, including programs to improve strength or balance, educational programs, optimization of medications, and environmental modifications in homes or institutions. Some interventions have targeted single risk factors; others have attempted to address multiple factors.

A Cochrane Collaboration systematic review of interventions to reduce the incidence of falling in elderly persons was performed. This review considered only studies that included elderly persons of either sex who were living in the community or in institutional care, randomized to an intervention versus control or into one of two interventions. As of the February 2005 update of this systematic review, 62 individual trials meeting the inclusion criteria were identified. Of the 62 studies, 47 reported the effect of interventions in persons living in the community, eight were set in long-term-care institutions or in nursing homes, and four studies were in rehabilitation or geriatric assessment wards in hospitals. Three further studies included participants with specific conditions from a range of residential settings. Interventions were grouped into ten groups:

- Exercise or physical therapy
- Modification of home hazards
- Cognitive-behavioral intervention
- Medication withdrawal or adjustment
- Nutritional or vitamin supplementation
- Hormonal and other pharmacologic therapies
- Referral for correction of visual deficiency
- Cardiac pacemaker insertion for syncope-associated falls
- Multidisciplinary, multifactorial, health, and environmental risk-factor screening and intervention
- System modifications to prevent falls in high-risk hospital patients

Results from this systematic review suggested interventions that were likely to be beneficial:

- A program of muscle strengthening and balance training, individually prescribed at home by a trained health professional (three trials, 566 participants, pooled relative risk [RR] 0.80, 95% confidence interval [CI], 0.66 to 0.98)
- A 15-week Tai Chi group exercise intervention (one trial, 200 participants, risk ratio 0.51, 95% CI, 0.36 to 0.74)
- Assessment and modification of home hazards that is professionally prescribed for older people with a history of falling (three trials, 374 participants, relative hazard 0.66, 95% CI, 0.54 to 0.81)
- Multidisciplinary, multifactorial, health and environmental risk factor screening or intervention programs, both for unselected community-dwelling older people (data pooled from four trials, 1651 participants, pooled RR

0.73, 95% CI, 0.63 to 0.85), and for older people with a history of falling or selected because of known risk factors (data pooled from five trials, 1176 participants, pooled RR 0.86, 95% CI, 0.76 to 0.98)

- Withdrawal of psychotropic medications (1 trial, 93 participants, relative hazard 0.34, 95% CI, 0.16 to 0.74)
- Cardiac pacing for fallers with cardioinhibitory carotid sinus hypersensitivity (1 trial, 175 participants, weighted mean difference −5.20, 95% CI, −9.40 to −1.00)

In contrast, many interventions were reviewed as being of unknown effectiveness:

- Group-delivered exercise interventions (nine trials, 2177 participants)
- Nutritional supplementation (one trial, 50 participants)
- Vitamin D supplementation, with or without calcium (three trials, 679 participants)
- Modification of home hazards in association with advice on optimizing medication (one trial, 658 participants) or in association with an education package on exercise and reducing fall risk (one trial, 3182 participants)
- Pharmacologic therapy with raubasine-dihydroergocristine, a European drug not listed in U.S. formularies (one trial, 95 participants)
- Falls prevention programs in institutional settings
- Interventions using a cognitive-behavioral approach alone (two trials, 145 participants)
- Modification of home hazards for older people without a history of falling (one trial, 530 participants)
- Hormone replacement therapy (one trial, 116 participants)
- Individual lower limb strength training (one trial, 222 participants)
- Correction of visual deficiency (one trial, 276 participants)

More data are needed to confirm whether strategies apparently effective in significantly reducing the number of older people sustaining falls are also effective in reducing more serious sequelae of falls, such as fractures or other injuries.

Interventions that target risk factors for falls in three domains—medications, mobility, and medical conditions—constitute a practical approach for clinicians who are treating older patients with a high risk for or a history of falling (see Table 28.2).

HIP PROTECTORS

Many geriatricians are beginning to consider the use of hip protectors to reduce fall-related hip fractures. Systematic reviews of the topic have concluded that there is no evidence that hip protectors are effective in reducing hip fractures in studies in which randomization was by individual patient within an institution or among patients living at home. Earlier studies that found benefits with hip protectors randomly assigned groups of patients to an intervention based on setting (such as by ward in a nursing home) and were potentially susceptible to bias on this basis; more recent studies have randomized individual patients, which is less susceptible to bias. This suggests that there may be unintended "co-interventions" that occur when whole units or facilities participate in trials and are allocated to use hip protectors, and that these co-interventions may benefit residents of these facilities. In addition, the apparent lack of efficacy of hip protectors may be due in part to low adherence rates.

At least a dozen types of hip protectors are commercially available. Many of these hip protectors have not been tested in either the laboratory or in clinical trials, yet they are being promoted by manufacturers. Despite these concerns, until the results from studies with higher rates of adherence are available, it is not unreasonable for clinicians to consider the use of hip protectors in patients at high risk of hip fractures who are willing to use them. Most of the published trials used Safe Hip.

CLINICAL GUIDELINES

For elderly patients who have sustained a fall, a multifactorial approach that is based on data about risk factors and a multidimensional assessment of the patient and that targets interventions on the basis of these findings is appropriate. For elderly persons who have no history of falling, it is reasonable to use traditional multidimensional geriatric assessment with targeted interventions as risk factors are identified. For a summary of the recommendations of the expert panel on falls prevention assembled by the American Geriatrics Society, the British Geriatrics Society, and the American Academy of Orthopaedic Surgeons, see the Appendix (p 497).

Table 28.2—Preventing Falls: Selected Risk Factors and Suggested Interventions

Factors	Suggested Interventions
Medication-related factors	
Benzodiazepines, sedative-hypnotics, or antipsychotics, antidepressants	Taper and discontinue medications, as possible Address sleep and mood problems with nonpharmacologic interventions (see "Sleep Problems," p 249) Educate regarding appropriate use of medications and monitoring for adverse effects
Recent change in dose or number of prescription medications or use of ≥ 4 prescription medications or use of other medications associated with fall risk	Review medication profile and modify, as possible Monitor response to medications and to dose changes
Mobility-related factors	
Presence of environmental hazards (eg, improper bed height, cluttered walking surfaces, lack of railings, poor lighting)	Improve lighting, especially at night Remove floor barriers (eg, loose carpeting) Replace existing furniture with safer furniture (eg, correct height, more stable) Install support structures (eg, railings and grab bars, esp. in bathroom) Use nonslip bath mats
Impaired gait, balance, or transfer skills	Refer to physical therapy for comprehensive evaluation and rehabilitation Gait training Balance or strengthening exercises If able to perform semi-tandem stance, refer for Tai Chi, yoga, or postural awareness Provide training in transfer skills Prescribe appropriate assistive devices Recommend protective hip padding Install environmental changes (eg, grab bars, raised toilet seats) Recommend appropriate footwear (eg, good fit, nonslip)
Impaired leg or arm strength or range of motion, or proprioception	Strengthening exercises (eg, use of resistive rubber bands, putty) Resistance training 2–3 times/wk to 10 repetitions with full range of motion, then increase resistance Tai Chi Physical therapy
Medical factors	
Parkinson's disease, osteoarthritis, depressive symptoms, impaired cognition, other conditions associated with increased falls	Optimize medical therapy Monitor for disease progression and impact on mobility and impairments Determine need for assistive devices Use bedside commode if frequent nighttime urination
Postural hypotension: drop in systolic blood pressure ≥ 20 mm Hg (or ≥ 20%) with or without symptoms, either immediately or within 3 min of standing	Review medications potentially contributing and adjust dosing or switch to less hypotensive agents; avoid vasodilators and diuretics if possible Educate on activities to decrease effect (eg, slow rising, ankle pumps, hand clenching, elevation of head of bed) and slow rising from recumbent or seated position Prescribe pressure stockings (eg, Jobst) Liberalize salt intake if appropriate Caffeinated coffee (1 cup) or caffeine 100 mg with meals for postprandial hypotension Consider medication to increase pressure (if hypertension, heart failure, and hypokalemia not serious): ■ midodrine 2.5–5 mg three times a day ■ fludrocortisone 0.1 mg once to three times a day
Vision or hearing impairment	Refraction Cataract extraction Good lighting Home safety evaluation Mobility training for visually impaired Cerumen removal Audiological evaluation with hearing aid, if appropriate

SOURCE: Adapted from Reuben DB, Herr KA, Pacala JT, et al. *Geriatrics At Your Fingertips, 2006*, 8th ed. New York: American Geriatrics Society; 2006: Table 39. Reprinted with permission.

Annotated References

- American Geriatrics Society, British Geriatrics Society, and American Academy of Orthopaedic Surgeons Panel on Falls Prevention. Guideline for the prevention of falls in older persons. *J Am Geriatr Soc.* 2001;49(5):664–672.

    The aim of this publication is to guide clinicians in assessing fall risk and managing older patients at risk of falling or who have fallen. A review of the literature was performed to allow recommendations to be evidence based, wherever possible. Grades, based on the quality of the evidence and potential effect of the intervention, are provided for each recommendation. The recommendations cover the following areas: Approach to assessing older persons as part of routine care, not presenting with a fall; approach to assessing older persons with one or more falls, or who report recurrent falls or abnormalities of gait or balance; multifactorial interventions for the management of falls by older persons in various settings; and single interventions for managing falls by older persons. See the Appendix, p 497, for a summary of specific recommendations of the panel.

- Bischoff-Ferrari HA, Dawson-Hughes B, Willett WC, et al. Effect of Vitamin D on falls: a meta-analysis. *JAMA.* 2004;291(16):1999–2006.

    Vitamin D supplementation appears to reduce the risk of falls among ambulatory or institutionalized older individuals with stable health by more than 20%.

- Fletcher PC, Hirdes JP. Risk factors for falling among community-based seniors using home care services. *J Gerontol A Biol Sci Med Sci.* 2002;57(8):M504–M510.

    This study and the Kron study (see below) focus on the use of easy-to-administer instruments to assess fall risk, one for nursing-home residents, and one for seniors using home care. There are no surprising results here, but the sample sizes are quite large and the findings quite compatible with previously recognized fall risk factors. Application of these instruments to the appropriate populations might better operationalize the targeting of interventions to those at greatest risk of falls.

- Gillespie L, Gillespie W, Robertson M, et al. Interventions for preventing falls in elderly people. *Cochrane Database Syst Rev.* 2003;4:CD00340; 2005 update.

    The Cochrane Library of systematic review is a valuable resource for evaluating clinical trials of various therapeutic interventions. Since few such reviews specifically focus on older persons, it is particularly notable that this systematic review, first published in 1995, has now been updated to 2003. This most recent update reviews the growing number of clinical trials in the area of falls prevention. The results of this systematic review demonstrated which interventions are likely to be beneficial: multidisciplinary, multifactorial, health and environmental risk-factor screening or intervention programs; Tai Chi, muscle strengthening, and balance training by trained professionals; home hazard assessment and modification that is professionally prescribed for elderly persons with a history of falling; and withdrawal of psychotropic medication.

- Kron M, Loy S, Sturm E, et al. Risk indicators for falls in institutionalized frail elderly. *Am J Epidemiol.* 2003;158(7):645–653.

    This is a 1-year prospective observational study of risk factors for falls in a sample of institutional frail elderly persons residing in German long-term-care facilities. The value of the study is that the authors used variables derived from the Minimum Data Set, thus permitting clinical application to nursing-home assessments commonly performed in the United States. In addition, the study identified five modifiable risks (urinary incontinence, cognitive impairment, use of restraints, depression, and transfer difficulties) that might be targeted to reduce the risk of falls in the nursing home.

- Parker MJ, Gillespie LD, Gillespie WJ. Hip protectors for preventing hip fractures in the elderly. *Cochrane Database Syst Rev.* 2004;3:CD001255.

    This outstanding systematic review from the Cochrane Collaboration highlights the controversy surrounding the randomized trials of hip protectors. The finding that hip protectors conferred a benefit in reducing hip fractures when considering studies that randomized facilities or units within facilities but not when considering studies that randomized individuals suggests that the hip protectors studied may not be effective. Alternatively, by being in a study, seniors wearing hip protectors may be "protected" by other safeguards used by staff within a facility housing seniors who are wearing these garments.

- Robertson MC, Devlin N, Gardner MM, et al. Effectiveness of economic evaluation of a nurse delivered home exercise programme to prevent falls. 1: randomised controlled trial. *BMJ.* 2001;322(7288):697–701.

    The authors used a randomized controlled trial to study the impact of a nurse-delivered home exercise program on 240 men and women aged 75 years and older. Outcome measures included number of falls, number of resultant injuries, program costs, and hospital costs associated with falls. Total falls, serious injuries, and hospitalizations due to falls were all reduced. Cost-effectiveness was demonstrated for participants 80 years and older.

Douglas P. Kiel, MD, MPH

CHAPTER 29—OSTEOPOROSIS AND OSTEOMALACIA

KEY POINTS

- Osteoporosis is a common, preventable, and treatable disorder in older adults. Osteomalacia, though less common, is also treatable and preventable; it should be considered in older adults with myalgias, fatigue, proximal muscle weakness, and fractures.

- Measurement of bone mineral density is recommended routinely in women aged 65 and over, and in others with risk factors for osteoporosis.

- Secondary osteoporosis should be excluded in men and women with osteoporosis. Common causes of secondary osteoporosis include medications, hypogonadism, hyperthyroidism, hyperparathyroidism, and osteomalacia.

- Prevention of osteoporosis includes adequate calcium and vitamin D intake, weight-bearing exercise, and consideration of bisphosphonates, which continue to be first-line pharmacologic treatment. Consider raloxifene for high-risk patients.

- Because osteoporosis is a result of unbalanced bone formation and resorption, and associated fractures usually involve a fall, optimal prevention and treatment also include strategies to minimize bone resorption and to reduce falls, as well as measures to reduce risk factors, especially smoking, low physical activity, and poor diet.

DEFINITION OF OSTEOPOROSIS

Osteoporosis was defined previously by a consensus panel as a "disease characterized by low bone mass and microarchitectural deterioration of bone tissue leading to enhanced bone fragility and a consequent increase in fracture incidence." According to this definition, the diagnosis of osteoporosis requires the presence of a fracture. The World Health Organization now defines osteoporosis by bone mineral density (BMD) measurement, which allows diagnosis and treatment of osteoporosis prior to incident fracture. If a woman has a BMD measurement at any site < 2.5 standard deviations below the young adult standard (a T score of < −2.5), the diagnosis of osteoporosis can be made. Further, women with osteopenia (low bone mass, with a T score of ≥ −2.5 but < −1) and normal bone mass (with a T score of ≥ −1) can also be identified. Thus, the clinician can make the diagnosis of osteoporosis and begin the appropriate therapy

before fracture in the older adult occurs. In addition, women with osteopenia can be placed on a preventive regimen and then followed carefully for further bone loss. Specific standards for definitions of osteoporosis have not been established for men or for racial and ethnic groups other than white persons, although it appears that similar standards apply to men and to Hispanic women.

EPIDEMIOLOGY AND IMPACT OF OSTEOPOROSIS

In 1990 more than 1.25 million hip fractures were reported worldwide in women, and 500,000 in men. In the United States the estimated numbers of hip and vertebral fractures in women annually are more than 250,000 and 500,000, respectively. To this number must be added fragility fractures in men, which occur at about one third the rate seen in women. Thus, approximately 1 million Americans suffer fragility fractures each year, at a cost of more than $14 billion. The consequences of osteoporosis include diminished quality of life, decreased independence, and increased morbidity and mortality. The pain and kyphosis, height loss, and other changes in body habitus that occur as a result of vertebral compression fractures erode quality of life for both women and men. In addition, the functional status of patients who have had vertebral crush fractures may also decrease. These patients may be unable to bathe, dress, or walk independently. Increased mortality is related primarily to hip fractures; 20% excess mortality occurs in older persons in the year following hip fracture. In addition, approximately 50% of women with hip fracture do not fully recover prior function. Thus, in older adults, it is important to prevent as many fractures as possible.

BONE REMODELING AND BONE LOSS IN AGING

Bone is able to repair itself by actively remodeling, a coupled process (also called *bone turnover*) of bone resorption followed by bone formation; bone remodeling continues throughout life. Local signals, not yet fully understood, bring osteoclasts to specific areas of bone where resorption is initiated and resorption cavities are formed. Once osteoclasts have completed the resorption process, osteoblasts move into the area and begin to lay down osteoid and, later, to calcify the matrix. Under optimal conditions, once bone remodeling is completed in a specific area, the resorption spaces are completely filled with new bone. However, after menopause in women, and with aging in men and women, the remodeling cycle becomes unbalanced, and bone resorption increases more than formation does, resulting in net bone loss. The majority of treatments for osteoporosis act to inhibit bone resorption rather than to increase bone formation.

Bone mass changes over the life span of an individual. In women, bone mass increases rapidly from the time of puberty until approximately the mid-20s to mid-30s, at which time peak bone mass is reached. Once women reach peak bone mass, a few years of stability are followed by a slow rate of bone loss, beginning well before the onset of menopause. After menopause, the rate of bone loss is quite rapid—as much as 7% per year—for up to 7 years, as a consequence of estrogen deficiency. In later life, bone loss continues, albeit at a slower rate, generally 1% to 2% per year; however, some older women may lose bone density at a higher rate. Data strongly suggest that terminating bone loss at any time will decrease fracture risk. It has been estimated that a 14% increase in bone density in 80-year-old women would halve the hip fracture risk. This 14% increase would also be realized if bone loss were prevented in 70-year-old women.

Although studies thus far have focused mostly on women, it is well documented that men lose bone with age. Cross-sectional studies have detected a slower rate of bone loss in men than in women, but in a longitudinal study the rates of bone loss in men were found to equal those of older women, although men start from a higher bone mass. It is estimated that men aged 30 to 90 years lose approximately 1% per year in the radius and spine; some men with risk factors lose as much as 6% per year. These data suggest that older men lose bone at rates similar to those of older women; however, vertebral fracture rates in men are lower.

Both men and women lose predominantly cancellous bone, which is concentrated in the vertebral spine. Cortical bone accounts for 45% to 75% of the mechanical resistance to compression of the vertebral spine, and men actually gain cortical bone through periosteal bone deposition. Men also increase the cross-sectional area of their vertebrae by 15% to 20%, increasing maximum load levels until the age of 75. The increased bone strength seems to be reversed by thinning of the cortical ring by age 75, the age at which men begin to present with vertebral fractures. Although bone loss at the hip has not been extensively studied in men, in cross-sectional analyses healthy men were found to lose 40% of femoral neck BMD between the ages of 20 and 90 years.

PATHOGENESIS OF OSTEOPOROSIS

Estrogen Deficiency in Women

The pathogenesis of osteoporosis in women is complex. Factors that affect the level of peak bone mass, the rate of bone resorption, and the rate of bone formation need to be considered. Peak bone mass appears to be 75% to 80% genetically determined, although which genes are involved is not clear. A number of candidate genes that may be important to osteoporosis are being explored currently: vitamin D receptor, estrogen receptor, transforming growth factor, interleukin-6, interleukin-1 receptor 2, type I collagen genes, and collagenases. Several factors may work to increase bone resorption in older women. After menopause, and with estrogen deficiency, a variety of factors that act locally on bone may lead to increased bone resorption. Factors thought to play a role in the bone loss of estrogen deficiency include interleukin-1, interleukin-1 receptor antagonist, interleukin-6, and tumor necrosis factor, as well as their binding proteins and receptors.

Calcium Deficiency and Secondary Hyperparathyroidism

The mechanism by which older men and women continue to lose bone is likely related to calcium deficiency, which produces secondary hyperparathyroidism. Parathyroid hormone (PTH) is a potent stimulator of bone resorption when chronically elevated. Aging skin and decreased exposure to sunlight reduce the conversion of 7-dehydrocholesterol to cholecalciferol (vitamin D_3) by ultraviolet light, and the result is vitamin-D insufficiency in older adults. Vitamin-D insufficiency, in turn, reduces the absorption of calcium. Further, older adults tend to ingest inadequate amounts of vitamin D and calcium. As a result of decreased serum levels of calcium, PTH—acting to maintain serum levels of calcium—increases, which leads to increased bone resorption. In one study, older women (mean age 79 years) hospitalized with a hip fracture were found to have lower 25(OH)D levels and higher PTH, higher bone resorption, and lower bone formation than women in the control group (mean age 77 years). Further, data from the Study of Osteoporotic Fractures indicate that women with low fractional absorption of calcium are at increased risk for hip fracture. (See also "Endocrine and Metabolic Disorders," p 373, for more on disorders of calcium metabolism.)

Androgens in Men

Androgens are important determinants for peak bone mass in men. Bone accretion is closely related to sexual maturity, and men who have abnormal puberty or delayed puberty have reduced bone mass. In addition, men with estrogen deficiency or resistance have decreased bone mass and failure of epiphyseal closure. Several studies have demonstrated that late-onset hypogonadism can also play a role in osteoporosis in men. Although it is evident that severe male hypogonadism can cause osteoporosis, the effect of moderate decreases in testosterone levels in aging men on rates of bone loss is uncertain. One study found that more than 60% of men presenting with hip fracture had low testosterone levels, compared with about 20% of those in the control group.

Changes in Bone Formation

In men and women, osteoblast activity appears to decrease with aging, compounding the bone loss that results from increased resorption seen with aging and, for women, with menopause. Growth factors, such as transforming growth factor B and insulin-like growth factor 1, may be impaired with estrogen deficiency or with aging, resulting in decreased osteoblast function.

DIAGNOSIS OF OSTEOPOROSIS AND PREDICTION OF FRACTURE

Risk Factors

Risk factors for osteoporosis and osteoporotic fracture have been identified and have been used to determine who should be placed on preventive or therapeutic regimens. Risk factors, however, are mediocre predictors of low bone density and fractures, and it is more useful to identify modifiable risk factors and to implement change as part of a treatment or preventive program. Table 29.1 lists modifications of risk factors of osteoporosis; all of these risk factors should be addressed by the clinician as part of the routine care of an older adult. Risk factors can also be used to identify women younger than 65 years of age who should have BMD screening.

Secondary Causes

The diagnosis of idiopathic or primary osteoporosis is made by bone density measurement prior to fracture or by incident fracture. Exclusion of other diseases that may present as fracture or with low bone mass is important in the evaluation of women and men with osteoporosis, since different treatment would be re-

quired. The major secondary causes of osteoporosis are listed in Table 29.2, along with laboratory tests used to exclude each disease. These laboratory tests should be considered for persons who present with acute compression fracture or who present with a diagnosis of osteoporosis by BMD measurement. The most common causes of secondary osteoporosis in women are primary hyperparathyroidism and glucocorticoid use. Men are more likely to have a secondary cause of osteoporosis than women; as many as 50% of osteoporotic men may have a secondary cause. The most commonly reported secondary causes of osteoporosis in men are hypogonadism and malabsorption syndromes, including gastrectomy. Medications that might have a detrimental effect on bone should be given with adjusted doses or discontinued. Medications that have been shown to adversely affect BMD include glucocorticoids, excess thyroid supplement, anticonvulsants, methotrexate, cyclosporine, and heparin. In older adults, glucocorticoids and thyroid hormone are used quite commonly; accordingly, clini-

---

Table 29.1—Modifications to Reduce the Risk of Osteoporosis

Exercise: Encourage regular, weight-bearing exercise

Nutrition: Encourage

- adequate intake of calcium and vitamin D
- lower intake of animal protein

Medications that may increase risk of osteoporosis—use with caution:

- anticonvulsants
- cyclosporine
- glucocorticoids
- long-term heparin
- methotrexate
- thyroid hormone replacement (dose dependent)

Smoking cessation

Table 29.2—Screening for Secondary Osteoporosis*

Disease	Recommended Laboratory Tests
Cushing's disease	**Electrolytes**, 24-hour urinary cortisol
Hyperthyroidism	**Thyroid-stimulating hormone**, thyroxine levels
Hypogonadism (men only)	**Bioavailable testosterone**
Multiple myeloma	**Complete blood cell count, serum electrophoresis**, urine electrophoresis
Osteomalacia	**Alkaline phosphatase**, 25(OH)D
Paget's disease	**Alkaline phosphatase**
Primary hyperparathyroidism	**Calcium**, parathyroid hormone levels

* Bolded items are recommended routinely.

cians should consider the effects these medications may have on the already increased risk of fracture when prescribing them for older adults.

Glucocorticoids result in bone loss primarily through the direct suppression of bone formation, although they also further reduce sex hormone levels and cause secondary hyperparathyroidism through their effects on intestinal calcium absorption. The prevalence of vertebral fractures in persons taking glucocorticoids for 1 year is estimated to be 11%. The rate of trabecular bone loss is dose dependent and generally occurs in the first 6 months of therapy. Although inhaled corticosteroids have not been as well studied, high doses of high-potency inhaled steroids may also result in bone loss. The best strategy for older persons who require long-term glucocorticoid therapy is to maximize bone health by a variety of interventions. It is important to use the lowest possible dose of glucocorticoids, to assure adequate calcium and vitamin D intake (see the treatment section, below). Further, alendronate[OL], risedronate, and intermittent etidronate[OL] have been shown to successfully prevent bone loss that is due to glucocorticoid therapy when they are initiated at the same time as the steroids (see the treatment section, below).

Bone Density Measurement

BMD, or bone mass measurement, is the best predictor of fracture. The relative risk of fracture is 10 times greater in women in the lowest quartile of BMD than in women whose BMD is in the highest quartile.

Bone density of the hip, spine, wrist, or calcaneus may be measured by a variety of techniques. The preferred method of BMD measurement is dual-energy radiographic absorptiometry (DXA). BMD of the hip, anterior-posterior spine, lateral spine, and wrist can be measured with this technology. There are several other methods of measuring BMD, including quantitative computed tomography, ultrasonography of the calcaneus, single radiographic absorptiometry of the calcaneus, and radiographic absorptiometry. Quantitative DXA is the best predictor of hip fracture and is equal to the wrist in predicting fractures at other sites; the relative risk of fracture for each one–standard deviation decrease in BMD is 2.6. In the Study of Osteoporotic Fractures, heel ultrasonography was found to be slightly worse that DXA of the hip in predicting hip fracture in women 65 years and older. In a large study (> 200,000) of postmenopausal women aged 50 years and over, baseline T scores were for the heel (ultrasound or single radiographic absorptiometry), forearm (DXA), and finger (DXA). After 1 year of follow-up, women with T scores less

than −2.5 by any measure had an adjusted relative risk for all fractures of 2.74 (confidence interval [CI], 2.4 to 3.1). These measures were not compared with DXA of the hip, and information on performance by age group or risk factors was not provided.

The National Osteoporosis Foundation, in conjunction with numerous specialty organizations including the U.S. Preventive Services Task Force, recommends BMD testing for all women aged 65 years and over, regardless of risk-factor status; there are no data to determine the frequency of screening or the age to stop screening for osteoporosis in women. For women between 60 and 64 years of age, the presence of additional risk factors, particularly low body weight and no estrogen replacement therapy, makes their risk of osteoporosis and fracture comparable to that of women over 65 years. Indications for BMD testing are listed in Table 29.3. Interpretation of BMD involves evaluating the quality of the DXA as well as the T scores. As previously stated, osteoporosis is defined as 2.5 or more standard deviations below the young adult mean (also known as the T score). The BMD of the individual patient is compared with that of young women (25 to 35 years of age) who are considered to be at or near peak bone mass. For every standard deviation below the young adult mean (or decrease in 1 unit T score), fracture risk at the spine and hip approximately doubles. For example, if a woman has a T score of −2, her risk of fracture is four times that of a woman with normal bone density (controlled for height and weight). When evaluating the spine BMD over time, several considerations are important. Vertebral or arterial or lymph node calcification or any scoliosis may falsely increase BMD of the posteroanterior spine DXA. Thus, a woman with osteoporosis of the spine may have a DXA T score that is higher than −2.5. Usually, one can see these changes on the DXA report if the picture of the scan is included in the report. It is important to evaluate BMD of lumbar vertebrae 1–4 when making a decision about therapeutic intervention. Because these changes in and around the spine are common in older adults,

Table 29.3—Indications for Bone Mineral Density Testing*

Postmenopausal women with multiple risk factors** for osteoporosis

Postmenopausal women who present with fractures

Men with conditions† indicating high risk for osteoporosis

Women and men with osteoporosis who have been on treatment for prolonged periods

All women ≥ 65 years old

* In persons who would consider treatment for osteoporosis.

** Early menopause, white or Asian race, low body weight, no current use of estrogen therapy, sedentary, smoking, alcohol abuse, primary hyperparathyroidism, hyperthyroidism, glucocorticoid use.

† Hypogonadism and glucocorticoid use are the two most common.

OL Not approved by the U.S. Food and Drug Administration for this use.

hip BMD tends to be the more reliable site for estimating fracture risk. Another important issue when using DXA over time is the measurement variability. The DXA equipment is stable over time, but regular testing will allow detection of any drift. More importantly, one needs to be assured that patient positioning is consistent over time. With the founding of the International Society of Clinical Densitometry, standardized training courses are now available for technicians and also for physicians interpreting the results. The cost for DXA testing is between $200 and $300, and Medicare and Medicaid will cover the cost if indications for its use (eg, estrogen deficiency) are met.

BMD testing may also be used to establish the diagnosis and severity of osteoporosis in men, and it should be considered for men with low-trauma fractures, radiographic criteria consistent with low bone mass, or diseases known to place a person at risk for osteoporosis. Data relating BMD to fracture risk are derived from studies of women, but data suggest that similar associations may be valid for men. Data from several studies indicate that patients with hip fractures are often not evaluated and treated for osteoporosis. It is important to consider the diagnosis of osteoporosis in any older person with a fracture, and evaluation is indicated if treatment would be considered for the individual patient.

Biochemical Markers of Bone Turnover

Serum and urine biochemical markers can estimate the rate of bone turnover (remodeling) and may provide additional information to assist the clinician. A number of markers have been developed that reflect collagen breakdown (or bone resorption) and bone formation. Several markers have been associated with increased hip fracture risk, decreased bone density, and bone loss in older adults. In addition, markers of bone resorption and formation decrease in response to antiresorptive treatment. The use of markers in clinical practice, however, is controversial because of the substantial overlap of marker values in women with high and low bone density or rate of bone loss. Further, few studies have compared the response of a particular marker (or combination of markers) and bone density with therapy in order to determine the magnitude of decrease of a biochemical marker necessary to prevent bone loss or, more importantly, fracture. Two markers of bone resorption, deoxypyridinoline cross-links and cross-linked N-telopeptides of type I collagen, and one formation marker, bone alkaline phosphatase, may be used in clinical practice to provide an early assessment of treatment efficacy. A decrease from baseline levels in the level of these markers after 3 to 6 months of therapy would indicate successful treatment.

PREVENTION AND TREATMENT OF OSTEOPOROSIS

The Role of Exercise

Exercise is an important component of osteoporosis treatment and prevention, although exercise alone is not adequate to prevent the rapid bone loss associated with estrogen deficiency in early menopause. Among exercisers in the Rancho Bernardo cohort, those who reported strenuous or moderate exercise had higher BMD at the hip than did those who reported mild or less-than-mild exercise. Similar associations were seen for lifelong regular exercisers and hip BMD. In a randomized study of women ≥ 10 years postmenopausal, the group receiving calcium supplementation plus exercise had less bone loss at the hip than did those assigned to calcium alone. Further, the effectiveness of high-intensity strength training in maintaining femoral neck BMD as well as in improving muscle mass, strength, and balance in postmenopausal women has been demonstrated, suggesting that resistance training would be useful to help maintain BMD and to reduce the risk of falls among older adults.

Marked decrease in physical activity or immobilization results in a decline in bone mass; accordingly, it is important to encourage older adults to be as active as possible. Weight-bearing exercise, such as walking, can be recommended for all adults. Older persons should be encouraged to start slowly and gradually increase both the number of days as well as the time spent walking each day. (See "Physical Activity," p 56.)

Calcium and Vitamin D

Calcium and vitamin D are required for bone health at all ages. In order to maintain a positive calcium balance, the current recommendations for calcium intake for postmenopausal women and men aged 65 years and older is at least 1200 mg per day of elemental calcium. The amount of vitamin D required is between 400 and 800 IU per day. In older adults, regardless of climate or exposure to sunlight, a daily supplement of ≥ 400 IU per day of vitamin D is recommended because skin changes that occur with aging result in less efficient use of ultraviolet light by the skin to synthesize vitamin-D precursors. Calcium plus vitamin D at different doses have been shown to increase or maintain bone density in postmenopausal women and to prevent hip as well as all nonvertebral fractures in older adults. The dietary intake of calcium for postmenopausal women in the United States averages 500 to 700 mg per day; thus, most American women require calcium supplementation to ensure adequate intake. (See Table 29.4 for information on the calcium contained in selected foods.)

Table 29.4—Calcium-Containing Foods

Food	Serving Size	Calcium (mg) per serving
Dairy Products		
Milk	1 cup	290–300
Yogurt	1 cup	240–400
Swiss cheese	1 ounce (1 slice)	250–270
American cheese	1 ounce (1 slice)	165–200
Ice cream	½ cup	90–100
Cottage cheese	½ cup	80–100
Parmesan cheese	1 tablespoon	70
Powdered non-fat milk	1 teaspoon	50
Other		
Sardines in oil with bones	3 ounces	370
Calcium-fortified orange juice	1 cup	300
Canned salmon with bones	3 ounces	170–210
Broccoli	1 cup	160–180
Tofu (soybean curd)	4 ounces	145–155
Turnip greens	½ cup, cooked	100–125
Kale	½ cup, cooked	90–100
Cornbread	2 ½-inch square	80–90
Egg	1 medium	55
Other fortified foods (bread, cereal, fruit juices)	1 serving	Varies: read label

Pharmacologic Options

The dosing, relative costs, and special considerations for the medications used to prevent and treat osteoporosis are provided in Table 29.5.

Bisphosphonates

Alendronate has been approved for osteoporosis prevention (women) and treatment (men and women). Women with osteoporosis who were treated with alendronate and compared with women on placebo were found to have increased bone density of the spine and hip, as well as decreased vertebral fracture rate. The Fracture Intervention Trial examined the effect of alendronate on postmenopausal women with severe osteoporosis, with or without vertebral fracture at baseline. Regardless of the presence of vertebral fractures at baseline, alendronate was found to decrease the vertebral fracture rate. In addition, alendronate resulted in a 50% reduction in hip fractures. A study in women aged 60 to 85 years indicated that an even lower dose of alendronate might be effective in older women. Further, data indicate that once-weekly dosing with alendronate (70 mg) is as effective in increasing spine BMD over 1 year as is daily dosing (10 mg) in postmenopausal women with osteoporosis (age range 42 to 95 years). Alendronate has also been approved for the prevention of osteoporosis in early postmenopausal women. The daily dose for prevention is lower—5 mg—than that given for the treatment of osteoporosis—10 mg. If treatment with alendronate alone is not effective (bone loss of > 4% or fracture within 3 months of initiation), combining raloxifene or estrogen replacement therapy with alendronate, which has an additive effect on bone density, may be indicated. In women with lesser degrees of osteoporosis, alendronate has not been shown to prevent hip fracture. Alendronate has now been approved to treat osteoporosis in men and in glucocorticoid-induced osteoporosis. The optimal duration of treatment with bisphosphonates is unclear; however, one study indicated that the greatest increase in vertebral bone mass occurred during the first 5 years of treatment, and benefit was maintained for 10 years without undue risk.

The major adverse effects of alendronate are gastrointestinal, including abdominal pain, dyspepsia, esophagitis, nausea, vomiting, and diarrhea. Musculoskeletal pain may also occur. Esophagitis, particularly erosive esophagitis, may be seen most commonly in patients who do not take the medication properly. The absorption of oral bisphosphonates is very poor; thus, it is extremely important to provide specific and detailed instructions for patients receiving any bisphosphonate therapy (Table 29.6).

Table 29.5—Medications Used to Prevent and Treat Osteoporosis

Medication	Dosage	Cost	Special Considerations
Bisphosphonates			
Alendronate	10 mg/d or 70 mg/week; 5 mg/d for prevention	$$$$$	Adherence to dosing instructions required (Table 29.6); used in men and women to prevent glucocorticoid-induced osteoporosis
Etidronate	400 mg/day for 2 weeks every 3 months	$$	May be used in men and women to prevent glucocorticoid-induced osteoporosis; use for idiopathic osteoporosis only if all other treatments are not tolerated or effective
Ibandronate	150 mg/month	$$$$$	Must be taken fasting with water, standing upright and taking nothing by mouth for at least 60 minutes after taking; do not use if creatinine clearance is less than 30 mL/minute
Risedronate	5 mg/d	$$$$$	Adherence to dosing instructions required (see Table 29.6)
Selective estrogen receptor modulator			
Raloxifene	60 mg/d	$$$$$	May prevent breast cancer
Calcitonin			
Nasal spray	200 IU/d	$$$$$	Metered spray; 1 spray gives daily dose; alternate nostrils each day to reduce side effects
Injectable (subcutaneously or intramuscularly)	50–100 IU 3 to 5 times/week	$$$$	Injectable still useful, depending on patient
Estrogen	See text	$	Not recommended as first-line choice
Parathyroid hormone (teriparatide)	20 µg/d (injection)	$$$$$	For use in patients who cannot tolerate other approved treatments for osteoporosis

NOTE: $ = approximately $10 per month.

Table 29.6—Instructions for Administration of Bisphosphonates

- Take first thing in the morning before eating or drinking anything else
- Take with at least 8 ounces of plain tap water
- Take while upright in a chair or standing, and remain upright after ingestion
- Do not eat or drink anything for 1 half-hour after taking the medication

Risedronate, another bisphosphonate, has been approved for osteoporosis prevention and treatment (women only). In a 3-year study of postmenopausal women with ≥ 1 vertebral fracture at baseline, the cumulative incidence of new vertebral fractures was reduced by 41% (95% CI, 18% to 58%) in the group receiving risedronate (5 mg per day) rather than placebo. In addition, the incidence of nonvertebral fractures also decreased by 39% (95% CI, 6% to 61%) in the treatment group. BMD of the hip and spine increased significantly in the risedronate group. In the same study, 2.5 mg per day of risedronate was found to be ineffective and was discontinued after the first year of the study. Withdrawals because of side effects and any upper gastrointestinal adverse events were similar in the risedronate and placebo groups. In older women (70 to 79 years) with osteoporosis, risedronate was found to decrease the risk of hip fracture by 40% in comparison with placebo (all participants received adequate calcium and vitamin D) with a relative risk of 0.6 (95% CI, 0.4 to 0.9). In women at least 80 years of age, risedronate was not found to significantly reduce hip fracture incidence; however, these women were selected primarily on the basis of clinical risk factors rather than BMD criteria. This study demonstrates that even in older women, BMD measurement and assessment of previous vertebral fractures are needed to identify those for whom the treatment will be the most effective.

Etidronate was shown to increase spinal bone mass and decrease vertebral fractures in two studies in the early 1990s, and a 5-year follow-up study demonstrated continued benefit. Etidronate was given intermittently—400 mg per day orally for 14 days, and then stopped for 2.5 months—in these studies because continuous high doses can impair mineralization and produce osteomalacia. However, etidronate is not approved for use in treating osteoporosis because the data supporting fracture reduction were not sufficient. A separate study indicated a role for etidronate in preventing bone loss in patients who require long-term glucocorticoids.

Selective Estrogen Receptor Modulators

The selective estrogen receptor modulators are agents that act as estrogen agonists in bone and heart but act as estrogen antagonists in breast and uterine tissue. These medications have the potential to prevent osteoporosis or cardiovascular disease without the increased risk of breast or uterine cancer. Tamoxifen, an agent used to treat breast cancer, has beneficial effects on bone, as reported in several studies, but it also has stimulatory effects on the uterus. Thus, tamoxifen is not indicated for osteoporosis treatment or prevention.

Raloxifene has been approved for the treatment and prevention of osteoporosis in postmenopausal women. Comparison of raloxifene with placebo in postmenopausal women with osteoporosis found that raloxifene decreases bone turnover and maintains hip and total body bone density. There were no differences between groups in breast abnormalities or endometrial thickness. Most importantly, data demonstrate that raloxifene (60 mg per day) reduces incident vertebral fractures by about 60%, despite only modest increases in bone density. In this study raloxifene was not found to significantly reduce nonvertebral, hip, or wrist fractures. Reported adverse effects with raloxifene include flu-like symptoms, hot flushes, leg cramps, and peripheral edema.

Another important finding with raloxifene was a reduction in breast cancer risk in women who participated in the Multiple Outcomes of Raloxifene Trial. When women receiving raloxifene were compared with women receiving placebo, the relative risk for women receiving raloxifene of developing breast cancer was found to be 0.24 (95% CI, 0.13 to 0.44). In the same study, raloxifene was not found to increase the risk of endometrial cancer but was found to increase the risk of venous thromboembolic disease. In other studies, raloxifene was found to decrease total and low-density lipoprotein cholesterol and lipoprotein (a) levels without affecting high-density lipoprotein cholesterol or triglyceride levels. Thus, in clinical trials to date, raloxifene appears to be beneficial to several organ systems, although further study is required with regard to cardiovascular diseases and breast cancer prevention.

Calcitonin

Calcitonin is a hormonal inhibitor of bone resorption that is approved for the treatment of osteoporosis in women. It is available as a subcutaneous injection and as a nasal spray. The nasal spray has fewer reported side effects and greater patient acceptance, but it may be less effective. Calcitonin has been shown to increase bone density in the spine and reduce vertebral fractures. In epidemiologic studies, calcitonin has been shown to reduce the incidence of hip fractures, although in clinical trials, hip bone density has not been found to increase. Results of a 5-year study demonstrated that the incidence of vertebral fractures in women receiving 200 IU per day of nasal spray calcitonin was lower than that of women on placebo. The reduction in hip fracture incidence was not statistically significant in the group receiving calcitonin in comparison with the placebo group. Doses of 100 and 400 IU per day were studied as well, but they did not reduce incidence of vertebral fractures. In the same study, BMD changes at 3 years and changes in markers of bone turnover in the treatment and placebo groups were found not to be significantly different. Although there are no direct comparisons, calcitonin appears to be less effective than other antiresorptive drugs. There is some evidence that calcitonin produces an analgesic effect in some women with painful vertebral compression fractures.

Estrogen Replacement Therapy

Estrogen replacement therapy (ERT) is an option for osteoporosis prevention (approved by the Food and Drug Administration; indication withdrawn as a treatment); however, it is not recommended as a first-line choice. In case-control and cohort studies, ERT has been found to be associated with a 30% to 70% reduction in hip fracture incidence. Multiple studies have demonstrated that postmenopausal estrogen use prevents bone loss at the hip and spine when initiated within 10 years of menopause. However, in a cross-sectional study, BMD in women who initiated hormone replacement therapy (HRT) after age 60 years was found not to be significantly different from women who initiated HRT within 2 years of menopause. In the Postmenopausal Estrogen/Progestin Intervention trial, older women, women with low initial BMD, and women who had not previously used HRT were found to gain more bone than did young women, women with higher baseline BMD, and those who had previously used HRT. Decreased incident vertebral fractures were seen in a small study of postmenopausal women using a transdermal estradiol preparation. Recent prospective data from the Women's Health Initiative (WHI) also demonstrated that postmenopausal women who took hormone replacement therapy for approximately 7 years had a decreased hip fracture risk; however, the dose and preparation of hormone therapy used also increased the risk of breast cancer, heart disease, stroke, and deep-vein thrombosis. Given the WHI findings, recent U.S. Preventive Services Task Force guidelines advise against the routine use of estrogen plus progesterone for the prevention of chronic conditions in postmenopausal women. The estrogen-only arm of WHI was also stopped 1 year ahead of schedule and demonstrated an increased risk of stroke but not of coronary heart disease or breast cancer. Estrogen alone decreased hip fracture risk (relative risk 0.61 [95% CI, 0.41 to 0.91]). Previously, HRT was recommended for prevention of osteoporosis; however, given the results of the WHI and the availability of other effective medications for osteoporosis prevention and treatment, the Food and Drug Administration changed its indication for estrogen and estrogen-progestin products. "When these products are being prescribed solely for the prevention of postmenopausal osteoporosis, approved non-estrogen treatments should be carefully considered. Estrogens and combined estrogen-progestin products should only be considered for women with significant risk of osteoporosis that outweighs the risks of the drug."

Other data suggest that lower-than-usual doses of estrogen, when given with adequate calcium and vitamin D, are effective in reducing bone turnover and bone loss in older women. In a randomized controlled study, women treated with 0.3 mg per day of conjugated equine estrogen plus 2.5 mg per day of medroxyprogesterone acetate were found to gain spine and hip BMD, whereas women treated with placebo showed no change. A more recent study compared 0.25 mg per day of 17β-estradiol with placebo and determined that this dose increases BMD at all sites and decreases bone turnover in older women, with minimal side effects. The effect of lower-dose estrogen on fracture incidence and other health outcomes is unknown at this time.

See also the section on hormone replacement therapy in "Endocrine and Metabolic Disorders" (p 379).

Parathyroid Hormone

PTH (teriparatide), although leading to increased bone resorption when continuously elevated, can increase bone mass, trabecular connectivity, and mechanical strength when administered intermittently. PTH is approved for the treatment of osteoporosis in men and women. It has been shown to increase spinal BMD in osteoporotic men and women. In a 3-year randomized study of postmenopausal women with osteoporosis, the group receiving estrogen plus intermittent PTH was found to have continuous increase in spinal bone mass over the study period, as well as decreased vertebral fracture rate. Bone mass of the hip and total body also increased significantly in the estrogen-plus-PTH group, in comparison with the group on estrogen alone. Recent studies have also demonstrated the effectiveness of PTH in reducing vertebral and nonvertebral fractures in postmenopausal women. In men with primary or hypogonadal osteoporosis, PTH also increased BMD at all sites. The combination of alendronate and PTH does have a synergistic effect on bone; in fact, it appears that alendronate attenuates the anabolic effect

of PTH in both men and women. PTH, which is given subcutaneously, is approved for men and women who are at risk for osteoporotic fracture and who are unable to tolerate other approved agents. PTH was found to increase the incidence of osteosarcomas in male and female rats; the relevance of these findings to humans is unknown. PTH should not be used as a first-line therapy for osteoporosis.

Investigational Agents

Other bisphosphonates currently under investigation for the treatment and prevention of osteoporosis include pamidronate, zoledronate, and tiludronate. New selective estrogen receptor modulators are also being tested for use in osteoporosis treatment.

Zoledronate has been shown to decrease bone turnover and increase BMD of the hip and spine, in comparison with placebo, in doses given one, two, or four times per year. All women in this study were postmenopausal with spine BMD T score ≤ -2 at baseline. The change in bone turnover parameters and bone density were similar in magnitude to those achieved with oral bisphosphonates that have already been approved for prevention and treatment of osteoporosis.

The use of fluoride to treat osteoporosis is appealing because fluoride results in a large increase in spine bone density; however, the increase in BMD has not been found to be consistently associated with a decrease in vertebral fractures. In fact, in one study, the group receiving fluoride therapy was found to have a higher rate of appendicular fractures. Slow-release fluoride therapy has been found to be associated with an increase in spine BMD, as well as decreased incidence of vertebral fractures. Further studies are required before slow-release fluoride can be recommended for the treatment of osteoporosis.

The use of 3-hydroxy-3-methylglutaryl coenzyme A reductase inhibitors (statins) may also affect bone. This class of medication is commonly prescribed for the management of hypercholesterolemia and has been shown to stimulate bone formation in animals. Preliminary epidemiologic data suggest that the use of statins is associated with decreased incidence of fracture. However, recent data from the WHI Observational Study indicated that neither fracture risk nor BMD is altered by statin use.

Strontium ranelate increases bone formation and decreases bone resorption in animals. A randomized, placebo-controlled study in postmenopausal women with osteoporosis (at least one vertebral fracture plus lumbar spine T score < -2.5) at baseline demonstrated that strontium ranelate increases BMD and decreases the incidence of vertebral fractures at the highest dose tested (2 g per day). At this dose, bone alkaline phosphatase increases and urinary excretion of N-telopeptides of type I collagen decreases.

WORKING WITH THE PATIENT

Establishing and maintaining an optimal regimen usually requires considerable discussion with individual patients and is much easier if patients are well informed. The use of educational materials can be quite helpful, as can the efforts of a nurse or other office personnel. Effective prevention and treatment of osteoporosis is possible if the patient and clinician work together in a sustained fashion.

The osteoporosis patient's adherence to the medication regimen is important. Baseline and follow-up BMD measurements (every 1 to 2 years) are important to assess response to therapy; these measurements may also improve adherence by providing visual information regarding the effectiveness of the therapy. Another way to inform patients about their response to therapy is to measure markers of bone resorption. In particular, adequate estrogen and bisphosphonate therapy will almost certainly decrease the levels of urine or serum markers of bone resorption within 3 to 6 months.

MANAGEMENT OF VERTEBRAL FRACTURES

Most vertebral fractures are asymptomatic and are diagnosed by spinal radiographs. Over time, one may notice decreased height, increased kyphosis, or simply the fact that clothes no longer fit the person properly. Many older adults have chronic back pain due to the changes in the spine that occur with vertebral compression. In the case of symptomatic vertebral compression fractures, adequate pain control is essential. The pain usually lasts 2 to 4 weeks and can be quite debilitating. Nonsteroidal anti-inflammatory drugs and calcitonin can be tried; narcotics are commonly required to control the pain. Physical therapy is an important part of osteoporosis treatment programs for the management of acute and chronic pain, as well as for patient education. The physical therapist can provide postural exercises, alternative modalities for pain reduction, and information on changes in body mechanics that may help prevent future fractures. (See also "Persistent Pain," p 140.) Support groups for patients with osteoporosis are also important. Newer treatments for vertebral fractures involve the injection of bone cement into the collapsed vertebra (vertebroplasty) or use of a balloon tamp into the fractured vertebrae (kyphoplasty). Although these methods have not been studied in randomized controlled studies, case reports suggest that they decrease pain and improve quality of life and function. Long-term benefits and complications have not yet been demonstrated; therefore, further study is required before these procedures are used routinely.

OSTEOMALACIA

Osteomalacia, an impairment of bone mineralization, is much less common than osteoporosis and can be definitively diagnosed only by bone biopsy. The clinical syndrome associated with osteomalacia consists of pain, myopathy, and fracture. The most common cause of osteomalacia in older adults is vitamin-D deficiency as a result of inadequate intake. In addition, excessive use of phosphate-binding antacids, chronic use of anticonvulsants, chronic kidney failure, hepatobiliary disease, and malabsorption syndromes may also result in osteomalacia. The use of high-dose etidronate and fluoride may cause osteomalacia, albeit rarely. The symptoms of osteomalacia may be subtle, and thus the diagnosis may be delayed. Patients typically complain of diffuse bone pain and tenderness, proximal muscle weakness, and generalized fatigue. A characteristic waddling gait may result from the hip pain and thigh weakness. Laboratory studies typically demonstrate an elevated alkaline phosphatase, low phosphate, low or normal calcium, and low 25(OH)D levels. Plain radiographic films may show osteopenia or characteristic pseudofractures, most commonly seen in the proximal femur.

Osteomalacia is managed by treating the underlying cause. If vitamin-D deficiency is diagnosed, repletion can be accomplished with oral vitamin D, 1000 IU per day. Hypophosphatemia is corrected by the use of neutral phosphate salts, 500 mg four times daily. Patients on long-term anticonvulsant therapy may be supplemented with 400 to 800 IU of vitamin D daily. Osteomalacia due to hepatobiliary disease or chronic kidney failure is managed with supplemental 25(OH)D and 1,25(OH)$_2$D, respectively.

ANNOTATED REFERENCES

■ Bauer DC, Ettinger B, Nevitt MC, et al. Risk for fracture in women with low serum levels of thyroid-stimulating hormone. *Ann Intern Med.* 2001; 134(7):561–568.

This study evaluated the association between low levels of thyroid-stimulating hormone (TSH) and fracture in older women in case-cohort sampling from the Study of Osteoporotic Fractures (postmenopausal women > 65 years). Baseline calcaneal bone mineral density was measured, lateral spine films taken, and serum collected in all participants. Baseline serum samples were randomly selected from women with hip fracture (N = 148) and women with incident vertebral fracture (N = 149), and 398 women were randomly selected from the original cohort to be controls. TSH levels were then measured on archived serum in the case-cohort sample. The risk for hip and vertebral fractures was found to be higher in women with low TSH (≤ 0.1 mIU/L) after adjustment for age, history of previous hyperthyroidism, self-rated health, and use of estrogen and thyroid hormone. Previous history of hyperthyroidism, but not use of thyroid hormone itself, was associated with a higher risk of hip fracture. The authors concluded that women aged 65 years and older with low TSH levels are at increased risk for hip and vertebral fractures.

■ Cauley JA, Robbins J, Chen Z, et al. Effects of estrogen plus progestin on risk of fracture and bone mineral density: the Women's Health Initiative randomized trial. *JAMA.* 2003; 290(13):1729–1738.

This is a randomized controlled trial of more than 16,000 women with an intact uterus aged 50 to 79 years. They were assigned either to placebo or to conjugated equine estrogen 0.625 mg with medroxyprogesterone acetate 2.5 mg. The main outcome measure was confirmed osteoporotic fractures; bone mineral density (BMD) was measured in a subset of women. The study also evaluated a global index, which summarizes the risk and benefits of therapy, across tertiles of fracture risk. Estrogen plus progestin reduced hip fracture risk by 33% (hazard ratio: 0.67 [0.47 to 0.96 unadjusted and 0.41 to 1.10 adjusted]). The reduction in incident hip fracture was greater in women who took more that 1200 mg calcium per day. The risk of hip fracture was similarly reduced with estrogen-progestin therapy across age, smoking, falls, previous fracture history, past use of hormone replacement therapy, years since menopause, and summary fracture-risk score. BMD of the spine and hip was found to increase over time in the women receiving estrogen-progestin therapy, in comparison with placebo. Using the global index, the researchers found no evidence of a net benefit to estrogen-progestin, even in women at high risk of fracture. The authors conclude that although estrogen-progestin decreases hip fracture risk and increases BMD measurements, the overall risk-benefit ratio does not support the use of hormone therapy except in women with vasomotor symptoms.

■ Finklestein JS, Hayes A, Hunzelman JL, et al. The effects of parathyroid hormone, alendronate or both in men with osteoporosis. *N Engl J Med.* 2003;349(13):1216–1226.

This study examined the effect on bone of combining alendronate, an antiresorptive agent, with parathyroid hormone (PTH), an agent that increases both bone resorption and bone formation. Men (46 to 85 years) were randomly assigned to receive alendronate (10 mg per day), PTH (40 μg per day), or both. Bone mineral density (BMD) of the spine was the primary outcome; hip, radius, and total body BMD were also measured. Overall, PTH alone was found to increase spine (posterior-anterior and lateral) and femoral neck BMD and trabecular bone mineral density (measured by quantitative computed tomography) more than combination therapy or alendronate monotherapy. Total hip BMD was found to increase in the group receiving PTH in comparison with the alendronate group, and radial shaft BMD was found to increase slightly in the alendronate and combination group but to decrease slightly in the PTH group. In addition, serum alkaline phosphatase, a marker of bone formation, increased in the group receiving PTH alone in comparison with the other groups. The authors concluded that alendronate impairs the ability of PTH to stimulate new bone formation and to increase BMD of the spine and hip. This study suggests that the anabolic effects of PTH are dependent on the ability of PTH to stimulate bone resorption.

■ McClung MR, Geusens P, Miller PD, et al. Effect of risedronate on the risk of hip fracture in elderly women. *N Engl J Med.* 2001;344(5):333–340.

This study examined the effect of risedronate on hip fractures in two groups of older women: women aged 70 to 79 years with osteoporosis and women aged 80 and older with at least one nonskeletal risk factor for hip fracture or low femoral neck bone mass. Women in each age group were randomly assigned to receive risedronate (2.5 or 5.0 mg) or placebo. The primary endpoint was hip fracture incidence over 3 years. Overall, risedronate was found to decrease the incidence of hip fractures (relative risk 0.7 [0.6 to 0.9]). In the group with osteoporosis (70 to 79 years), the relative risk was 0.6 (0.4 to 0.9) but in the group selected in the basis of risk factors, hip fracture risk did not decrease with treatment in comparison with placebo. The adverse-event profile was similar in the treatment and placebo groups. The authors concluded that risedronate can reduce hip fractures in older women with osteoporosis but not in older women selected on risk factors other than low bone mass. These data demonstrate the importance of bone mineral density measurement in identifying older women who will benefit from pharmacologic treatment.

■ Orwoll E, Ettinger M, Weiss S, et al. Alendronate for the treatment of osteoporosis in men. *N Engl J Med.* 2000;343(9):604–610.

A 2-year double-blind, placebo-controlled trial of 10 mg of alendronate daily was carried out in 241 men with osteoporosis who were aged 31 to 87. Men with secondary causes of osteoporosis except for low serum testosterone were excluded from the study; 36% of the men studied had a low testosterone level. After 2 years, men in the alendronate group showed a 7.1% increase in bone density at the lumbar spine, but those in the placebo group showed a 1.8% increase. Comparison also showed significant increases in bone marrow density of the hip, trochanter, and femoral neck in the experimental group over the placebo group. On follow-up radiographs, 7.1% of the men in the placebo group were found to have sustained a vertebral fracture, whereas 0.8% in the alendronate group had a fracture (number needed to treat to prevent one fracture = 16). These results are comparable to the effects of alendronate observed in women and in persons with glucocorticoid-induced osteoporosis.

■ Prestwood KM, Kenny AM, Kleppinger A, et al. Ultralow-dose micronized 17β-estradiol and bone density and bone metabolism in older women: a randomized controlled trial. *JAMA.* 2003;290(8):1042–1048.

This was 3-year placebo-controlled study examining the effect of 17β-estradiol on bone density and bone metabolism in older women (mean age 75 years). Older women were randomly assigned to receive 17β-estradiol (0.25 mg) or placebo daily; all women received for 1300 mg of elemental calcium plus 1000 IU of vitamin D per day. Women with an intact uterus received micronized progesterone 100 mg per day for 2 weeks every 6 months. This dose of estrogen significantly increased bone mineral density at the hip, spine, total body, and wrist in comparison with placebo. Bone alkaline phosphatase and N-telopeptides of type I collagen, markers of bone turnover, were found to significantly decrease in the treatment group in comparison with placebo. The adverse-event profiles of the two groups were similar. The authors concluded that ultralow-dose estrogen is beneficial to bone with minimal adverse effects and recommended a study to determine the effect of ultralow-dose estrogen on fractures.

■ Van Schoor NM, Smit JH, Twisk JWR, et al. Prevention of hip fractures by external hip protectors: a randomized controlled trial. *JAMA.* 2003;289(15):1957–1962.

This is a randomized controlled study to determine the effectiveness of hip protectors in preventing hip fracture in a group of persons at high risk for hip fracture. All persons were older than 70 years and had low bone density (as determined by broadband ultrasound measurement of the calcaneus) or a high risk for falling, or both. The primary outcome was time to first hip fracture, determined by using survival analysis. The overall incidence of hip fracture in the control group was 7%. Overall, there was no significant difference between the intervention and the control group with regard to time to first hip fracture. Eighteen hip fractures occurred in the hip protector group and 20 in the control group; the fracture rate was 5/100 in both groups. The authors concluded that hip protectors are not effective in preventing hip fractures in a high-risk population, possibly because adherence was good during the day but not at night.

Karen M. Prestwood, MD

CHAPTER 30—DEMENTIA

KEY POINTS

- Alzheimer's disease, vascular dementia, and dementia with Lewy bodies are the most common forms of degenerative dementias seen in late life.

- Cholinesterase inhibitors and N-methyl-d-aspartate antagonists may be modestly helpful in reducing the rate of decline in Alzheimer's dementia.

- Behavioral symptoms may occur with any type of dementia and tend to respond best to a combination of environmental modifications and symptomatic medication management.

Dementia is a general term used to describe a series of disorders that cause significant decline in two or more areas of cognitive functioning. One of these areas must be severe enough to cause functional decline. Of those who suffer from dementia, most have Alzheimer's disease (AD), which affects an estimated 4 million people in the United States. The pain and anguish of the disorder also afflicts millions more caregivers and relatives, who must cope with the patient's progressive and irreversible decline in cognition, functioning, and behavior. Both caregivers and patients may misinterpret the initial symptoms of dementia as normal age-related cognitive losses, and physicians may not recognize early signs or may misdiagnose them. However, dementia and aging are not synonymous. As people age, they usually experience such memory changes as slowing in information processing, but these kinds of changes are benign. By contrast, dementia is progressive and disabling and not an inherent aspect of aging.

Diagnostic and treatment advances have benefited many patients. Early and accurate diagnosis of dementia and its cause may minimize costly use of medical resources and give patients and their relatives time to anticipate future medical, financial, and legal needs. Sustained reversal of the progressive cognitive decline of dementia is not currently possible, but psychosocial and pharmacologic treatments may improve such associated conditions as depression, psychosis, and agitation. (See also "Psychosocial Issues," p 16, "Legal and Ethical Issues," p 22, "Financing, Coverage, and Costs of Health Care," p 32.)

EPIDEMIOLOGY AND SOCIETAL IMPACT

Dementia is a disease of late life, generally beginning after age 60 years. AD represents the most common type of dementia, accounting for approximately two thirds of all cases and affecting 6% to 8% of those aged 65 and over. The disease prevalence doubles every 5 years after age 60; an estimated 30% or more of those who are aged 85 or older have AD. Vascular dementia is thought to be the second most common, causing an estimated 15% to 25% of cases. In recent years, dementia associated with Lewy bodies has received increased attention, and although the exact prevalence is not known, estimates suggest that it may be as common as vascular dementia. Frontotemporal dementia is also a more recent diagnostic category of dementia and represents a smaller percentage of cases, with a younger age of onset than other dementias. Neurodegenerative diseases such as Huntington's disease, Parkinson's disease, or other metabolic causes such as head injury and alcoholism account for other dementia syndromes.

Dementia has a major impact on society. The total costs approach $100 billion annually if the costs of medical and long-term care, home care, and lost productivity for caregivers are included. Medicare, Medicaid, and private insurance pay much of the direct cost, but families caring for patients with dementia must bear the greatest burden of expense.

The financial costs of dementia are only one aspect of the total burden. The emotional toll is immense for both patients and their families. Nearly half of primary caregivers of patients with dementia experience psychologic distress, particularly depression. An accurate economic assessment of the problem underestimates the true cost of the disease to society unless the quality of life of both patients and caregivers is included in the analysis.

RISK FACTORS AND PREVENTION

The two greatest risk factors for AD are age and family history. Studies that account for death from other causes suggest that by age 90 years, nearly half of persons with first-degree relatives (ie, parents, siblings) with AD develop the disease themselves. Rare forms of familial AD beginning before age 60 have been associated with genetic mutations on chromosomes 1, 14, and 21. Most commonly, AD begins late in life; for such late-onset cases, the apolipoprotein E gene (*APOE*) on chromosome 19 influences risk.

The *APOE* gene has three alleles, *APOE*2*, *APOE*3*, and *APOE*4*. Everyone inherits one allele from each parent, so that six common genotypes are possible (2/2, 2/3, 3/3, 2/4, 3/4, and 4/4). Approximately 3% of the general population has the 4/4 genotype, 20% has the 3/4 genotype, and most persons have the 3/3 genotype. The *APOE*4* allele increases risk and decreases age of onset in a dose-related fashion, whereas the *APOE*2* allele may have a protective effect. Thus, the 2/3 genotype has a lower risk for AD than the 3/4 genotype; the AD risk is higher for the 3/4 genotype, and highest for the 4/4 genotype. The *APOE*4* allele may be less common in black Americans.

Using *APOE* genotyping as a prognostic test for asymptomatic persons is not recommended until results from further studies are available. *APOE*4* is neither necessary nor sufficient to cause AD, and cognitively normal centenarians who are homozygous for *APOE*4* have been reported. The asymptomatic person who learns that his or her genotype is 3/3 or 2/3 may be falsely reassured, whereas the person who learns that his or her genotype is 3/4 may be falsely alarmed. *APOE* genotyping may be useful only in increasing the diagnostic confidence for AD if a patient already has dementia.

Other possible risk factors include a previous head injury, female sex, and fewer years of educational achievement. Head trauma is thought to disrupt neuronal synapses. Research suggests that education may delay the onset of dementia, which may represent a confounding variable of socioeconomic status or a factor that truly provides protection by supplying a cognitive "reserve." Risk factors for vascular dementia include hypertension, hyperlipidemia, diabetes mellitus, smoking, age, male sex, and perhaps homocysteine levels. These factors are thought to increase risk by predisposing individuals to impairment in cognition through ischemic mechanisms, although there is new evidence linking some vascular risk factors to Alzheimer's pathology.

The prevention of dementia, especially AD, has been the subject of recent research. Drugs associated with reduced risk in epidemiologic studies include nonsteroidal anti-inflammatory drugs, statins, and possibly antioxidants. Research in normal elderly persons shows a possible protective effect of physical and intellectual activity on the risk for cognitive decline. The onset of dementia may also be delayed by the treatment of hypertension. Table 30.1 lists both risk and protective factors for dementia.

ASSESSMENT METHODS

Most cases of dementia can be diagnosed on the basis of a general medical and psychiatric evaluation. It is important for primary care physicians to be alert to the early symptoms, as dementia is often undetected until severe symptoms or an adverse event flags its presence. If a patient or family member expresses concerns about cognitive decline, a mental status assessment and probably a dementia evaluation are indicated. There are now consensus guidelines available for the clinical diagnosis and treatment of most types of dementia.

The informant interview and office-based clinical assessment are the most important diagnostic tools for dementia. Both the patient and a reliable informant should be interviewed to determine the patient's current condition, medical and medication history, patterns of alcohol use, and living arrangements. Useful informant-based instruments, such as the Functional Activities Questionnaire, can help determine whether lapses in memory or language use have occurred and

Table 30.1—Risk Factors and Protective Factors for Alzheimer's Disease

Definite	
Protective Factors	Risk Factors
Unknown	Age
	Family history
	*APOE*4* allele
	Down syndrome
Possible	
Protective Factors	Risk Factors
Nonsteroidal anti-inflammatory drugs	Other genes
Antioxidants	Head trauma
Intellectual activity	Lower educational achievement
Physical activity	Late-onset depression
Statins	

assess the patient's ability to learn and retain new information, handle complex tasks, and demonstrate sound judgment. Any changes are best determined by comparing present with previous performance, since functional decline and multiple cognitive deficits confirm the diagnosis.

A comprehensive physical examination includes a brief neurologic and mental status evaluation. Brief quantified screening tests of cognitive function, such as the Folstein Mini–Mental State Examination or the Mini-Cog Assessment Instrument for Dementia, may be useful, particularly if they demonstrate change over a 6-month or 1-year follow-up period. A laboratory evaluation, generally including a complete blood cell count, blood chemistries, liver function test, rapid plasma reagent test, and thyrotropin stimulating hormone and vitamin B_{12} levels, is also recommended. In addition, the history or physical examination may indicate the need for other laboratory tests. It is important to conduct cognitive and functional assessments in the patient's native language, if at all possible. In the face of cognitive decline, it is common for dementia patients to retain the greatest fluency in their language of origin.

Although brain imaging studies are optional, specialists may recommend them. They may be considered if:

- onset occurs at an age below 65 years;

- the condition is postacute, that is, symptoms have occurred for less than 2 years;

- there is evidence of focal or asymmetrical neurologic deficits;

- the clinical picture suggests normal-pressure hydrocephalus (ie, onset has occurred within 1 year, gait disorder is present, unexplained incontinence is present); or

- there is a history of a recent fall or other head trauma.

In general, a noncontrast computed tomography head scan is adequate to exclude intracranial bleeding, space-occupying lesions, and hydrocephalus. If vascular dementia is suspected, magnetic resonance imaging (MRI) is often performed, but white matter changes revealed by T2 weighted MRI images generally are not related to dementia and should not be overinterpreted. In cases of unclear diagnosis, a repeat assessment in 6 months will confirm the presence or absence of progressive cognitive decline. Functional brain imaging studies such as positron emission tomography often show the characteristic parietal and temporal deficits in AD or the widespread irregular deficits in vascular dementia and may be useful when the diagnosis is uncertain after routine testing.

Cognitive tests are influenced by educational level. Affected patients with more years of education may have normal scores while patients with less education may have low scores and no decline in function. In addition, it has been shown that tests that are most sensitive to language performance may have cultural differences that lead to an overinterpretation of dementia in minority patients. Poor performance on cognitive tests may result in an increased rate of dementia diagnoses among patients in ethnic minority groups, even though the actual rate of dementia determined in systematic cross-cultural studies does not appear to be different across populations. One way to improve the accuracy of assessment is to evaluate changes in everyday memory function by evaluating a person's performance of daily living skills, either by direct observation or obtaining information from reliable family members.

The practical utility of cognitive measures is that they provide a quantitative baseline against which to compare future assessments. Neuropsychologic testing is helpful in distinguishing normal aging from dementia, as well as identifying deficits that point to a specific diagnosis, and it is recommended when the diagnosis is unclear. In general, the diagnosis of dementia is a clinical one, and laboratory assessment is used to identify uncommon treatable causes and common treatable comorbid conditions.

DIFFERENTIAL DIAGNOSIS OF DEMENTIA

Dementia can be defined as an acquired syndrome of decline in memory and other cognitive functions sufficient to affect daily life in an alert patient. Diagnosis then requires further investigation to identify the cause of the dementia by determining chronology of symptoms along with the pattern and extent of deficits. A general discussion of the most common dementias is provided below, and an overview of diagnostic features is provided in Table 30.2.

Cognition in aging is now understood to be a continuum ranging from mild changes in normal aging to the significant impairments that define dementia. Although studies are not conclusive, it appears that normal aging involves some mild decline in memory, usually requiring more effort and time to recall new information. However, this decline does not impair functioning and is usually well compensated with lists, calendars, and other memory supports.

With early identification of cognitive deficits, a disorder now referred to as *mild cognitive impairment* has been identified. These patients do not have dementia but do have significant impairment in memory without deficits in other cognitive domains and no overt functional impairment. Some research

Table 30.2—Diagnostic Features of Dementia Syndromes

Feature	Mild Cognitive Impairment	Alzheimer's Disease	Vascular Dementia	Lewy Body Dementia	Fronto-temporal Dementia
Onset	Gradual	Gradual	May be sudden or stepwise	Gradual	Gradual, age < 60
Cognitive domains, symptoms	Primarily memory	Memory, language, visuospatial	Depends on anatomy of ischemia	Memory, visuospatial, hallucinations, fluctuating symptoms	Executive: disinhibition, apathy, language, +/- memory
Motor symptoms	Rare	Rare early, apraxia later	Correlates with ischemia	Parkinsonism	None
Progression	Unknown, 12% per year proceed to AD	Gradual, over 8 to 10 years	Stepwise with further ischemia	Gradual, but faster than AD	Gradual, but faster than AD
Laboratory tests	Normal	Normal	Normal	Normal	Normal
Imaging	Possible global atrophy, small hippocampal volumes	Possible global atrophy, small hippocampal volumes	Cortical or subcortical changes on MRI	Possible global atrophy	Atrophy in frontal and temporal lobes

NOTE: AD = Alzheimer's disease; MRI = magnetic resonance imaging.

suggests that these individuals convert to AD at a rate of about 12% per year. There is disagreement among experts if this is a unique disorder or merely an early prodrome to AD that has been identified with earlier diagnosis of memory impairments. Studies are under way to determine what if any interventions may be beneficial in this condition.

AD is characterized by gradual onset and progressive decline in cognitive functioning; motor and sensory functions are spared until late stages. Memory impairment is a core symptom of any dementia, and in AD it is present in the earliest stages. Typically, AD patients demonstrate difficulty learning new information and retaining it for more than a few minutes. In later disease stages their ability to learn shows even greater compromise, and patients are unable to access older, more distant memories. Aphasia, apraxia, disorientation, visuospatial dysfunction, and impaired judgment and executive functioning are also present. The initial stages of AD are characterized by normal motor, sensory, and cerebellar functioning. If focal motor or sensory signs, except fluent aphasia and apraxia, are present, a diagnosis of vascular dementia or mixed vascular dementia with AD is likely.

Vascular dementia refers to cognitive deficits most often associated with vascular damage in the brain. Cognitive and neurologic impairments should correlate anatomically with the areas of ischemia, although the often diffuse nature of vascular disease may make this correlation difficult to identify. A history of "small strokes," unless accompanied by a clear demonstration of focal signs of motor or sensory impairment, may not necessarily constitute vascular dementia. Cerebrovascular disease, however, does appear to contribute to the severity of cognitive symptoms in AD.

In recent years dementia with Lewy bodies has received increased attention. For a diagnosis of dementia with Lewy bodies, both dementia and at least one of the following must be present: detailed visual hallucinations, parkinsonian signs, and alterations of alertness or attention. The diagnosis may overlap with AD and the dementia associated with Parkinson's disease. Poor visuospatial abilities are also often out of proportion to other cognitive deficits. The chronology of symptoms and pattern of cognitive deficits allow differentiation between dementia with Lewy bodies and AD or the dementia associated with Parkinson's disease. Parkinsonian signs, particularly a "pill rolling" tremor that develops prior to cognitive impairment, generally indicate Parkinson's disease rather than AD. When parkinsonian rigidity and bradykinesia are present during the onset of dementia, a diagnosis of dementia with Lewy bodies should be considered.

Frontotemporal dementia is a disease often seen in patients with younger onset of cognitive symptoms; these patients present most often with executive and language dysfunction and significant behavioral changes. These include disinhibition and hyperorality, and they often have had a profound effect on the patient's social functioning. Memory deficits are often not as pronounced in these patients in the early stages as they are in patients with other dementias. The language impairments in frontotemporal dementia may be detected in neuropsychologic tests such as the Boston Naming Test and may progress even early in the course of illness in excess of other cognitive impairments. It is important to recognize the difference between frontotemporal dementia and AD with "frontal" symptoms. The latter refers to social disinhibition and behavioral impulsivity that may occur with AD. In these patients the behavioral problems occur much later in the course of illness, after a memory problem is already clearly evident. In contrast, the patient with frontotemporal dementia will display social disinhibition prior to prominent memory decline.

Common to all types of dementia, cognitive impairment eventually has a profound effect on the patient's daily life. Difficulties in planning meals, managing finances or medications, using a telephone, and driving without getting lost are not uncommon. Such functional impairments may first alert others that a problem is emerging. Numerous functions are maintained in patients with dementia of mild to moderate severity, including such activities of daily living as eating, bathing, and grooming. Many patients remain socially appropriate during the early disease stages.

Behavior and mood changes are common, including personality alterations, irritability, anxiety, or depression. During the middle and late stages of the disease, delusions, hallucinations, aggression, and wandering may develop. These behaviors are extremely troubling to caregivers and often result in family distress and nursing-home placement. Although the course of dementia is variable, the progression of dementia often follows a sequential clinical and functional pattern of decline (see Table 30.3).

Dementia recognition may be complicated by the presence of either delirium or depression. Delirium has been defined as an acquired impairment of attention, alertness, and perception. Delirium and dementia are in some ways similar: both are characterized by global cognitive impairment. Delirium can be distinguished by an acute onset, cognitive fluctuations throughout the course of a day, impaired consciousness and attention, and altered sleep cycles. In hospitalized patients, delirium and dementia often occur together. The presence of dementia increases the risk for delirium and accounts in part for the high rate of delirium in elderly patients. A delirium episode in an older person, therefore, should alert the clinician to search for dementia once the delirium clears. (See also "Delirium," p 239.)

Symptoms of depression and dementia often overlap, presenting additional diagnostic challenges. Patients with primary dementia commonly experience symptoms of depression, and such patients may minimize cognitive losses. By contrast, patients with primary depression may demonstrate decreased motivation during the cognitive examination and express cognitive complaints that exceed objectively measured deficits. Patients with primary depression, moreover, usually have intact language and motor skills, whereas patients with primary dementia may show impairment in these domains. As many as half of elderly patients who present with reversible dementia and depression become progressively demented within 5 years. (See also "Depression and Other Mood Disorders," p 269.)

TREATMENT AND MANAGEMENT

The primary treatment goals for patients with dementia are to enhance quality of life and maximize functional performance by improving cognition, mood, and behavior. Both pharmacologic and nonpharmacologic treatments are available, and the latter should be emphasized. Patients with dementia often develop significant behavioral symptoms that are a challenge to both family and professional caregivers. Any acute change requires an evaluation for undiagnosed medical problems, pain, depression, anxiety, sleep loss, or delirium. Other factors that may contribute to behavioral symptoms include interpersonal or emotional issues. Addressing such issues, treating underlying medical conditions, providing reassurance, and attending to the possible need for changes in the patient's environment may reduce agitation. (See "Behavioral Problems in Dementia," p 231.) The use of pharmacologic treatments for behavioral problems is recommended only after nonpharmacologic ones prove ineffective, or there is an emergent need for them (eg, risk of danger, extreme patient distress).

Nonpharmacologic Treatment

Cognitive Enhancement

Reality orientation and memory retraining have been proposed as possible psychotherapeutic techniques to restore cognitive impairment. Although memory retraining may provide modest, transient benefit, it can also cause frustration for both patients and caregivers. Given that new learning is a skill lost very early in the course of AD, an overemphasis on quizzing or retraining may lead to anxiety and self-depreciation. In general, a preferred approach is to provide support to accommodate lost skills.

Individual and Group Therapy

Emotion-oriented psychotherapy, such as "pleasant events" and "reminiscence" therapy, and stimulation-oriented treatment, including art and other expressive recreational or social therapies, exercise, and dance, are examples of psychosocial treatments that may influence depressive symptoms. Patient support groups may be helpful, but only when patients are mildly impaired. Well-controlled trials have not demonstrated efficacy for these approaches, but preliminary studies and clinical experience suggest their usefulness for some behavioral and mood symptoms in patients and family members.

Table 30.3—The General Progression of Dementia

Stage 1: No cognitive impairment

Unimpaired individuals experience no memory problems, and none are evident to a health care professional during a medical interview.

Stage 2: Very mild cognitive decline

Individuals at this stage feel as if they have memory lapses, especially in forgetting familiar words or names or the location of keys, eyeglasses, or other everyday objects. However, these problems are not evident during a medical examination or apparent to friends, family, or coworkers.

Stage 3: Mild cognitive decline

Early-stage Alzheimer's can be diagnosed in some, but not all, individuals with these symptoms.

Friends, family, or coworkers begin to notice deficiencies. Problems with memory or concentration may be measurable in clinical testing or discernible during a detailed medical interview. Common difficulties include:

- Word- or name-finding problems noticeable to family or close associates
- Decreased ability to remember names when introduced to new people
- Performance issues in social or work settings noticeable to family, friends, or coworkers
- Reading a passage and retaining little material
- Losing or misplacing a valuable object
- Decline in ability to plan or organize

Stage 4: Moderate cognitive decline (mild or early-stage Alzheimer's disease)

At this stage, a careful medical interview detects clear-cut deficiencies in the following areas:

- Decreased knowledge of recent occasions or current events
- Impaired ability to perform challenging mental arithmetic—for example, to count backward from 100 by 7s
- Decreased capacity to perform complex tasks, such as marketing, planning dinner for guests, or paying bills and managing finances
- Reduced memory of personal history

The affected individual may seem subdued and withdrawn, especially in socially or mentally challenging situations.

Stage 5: Moderately severe cognitive decline (moderate or mid-stage Alzheimer's disease)

Major gaps in memory and deficits in cognitive function emerge. Some assistance with day-to-day activities becomes essential. At this stage, individuals may:

- Be unable during a medical interview to recall such important details as their current address, their telephone number, or the name of the college or high school from which they graduated
- Become confused about where they are or about the date, day of the week, or season
- Have trouble with less challenging mental arithmetic; for example, counting backward from 40 by 4s or from 20 by 2s
- Need help choosing proper clothing for the season or the occasion
- Usually retain substantial knowledge about themselves and know their own name and the names of their spouse or children
- Usually require no assistance with eating or using the toilet

Stage 6: Severe cognitive decline (moderately severe or mid-stage Alzheimer's disease)

Memory difficulties continue to worsen, significant personality changes may emerge, and affected individuals need extensive help with customary daily activities. At this stage, individuals may:

- Lose most awareness of recent experiences and events as well as of their surroundings
- Recollect their personal history imperfectly, although they generally recall their own name
- Occasionally forget the name of their spouse or primary caregiver but generally can distinguish familiar from unfamiliar faces
- Need help getting dressed properly; without supervision, may make such errors as putting pajamas over daytime clothes or shoes on wrong feet
- Experience disruption of their normal sleep-waking cycle
- Need help with handling details of toileting (flushing toilet, wiping, and disposing of tissue properly)
- Have increasing episodes of urinary or fecal incontinence
- Experience significant personality changes and behavioral symptoms, including suspiciousness and delusions (for example, believing that their caregiver is an impostor); hallucinations (seeing or hearing things that are not really there); or compulsive, repetitive behaviors such as hand wringing or tissue shredding
- Tend to wander and become lost

Stage 7: Very severe cognitive decline (severe or late-stage Alzheimer's disease)

This is the final stage of the disease when individuals lose the ability to respond to their environment, the ability to speak, and, ultimately, the ability to control movement.

- Frequently individuals lose their capacity for recognizable speech, although words or phrases may occasionally be uttered.
- Individuals need help with eating and toileting, and there is general incontinence of urine.
- Individuals lose the ability to walk without assistance, then the ability to sit without support, the ability to smile, and the ability to hold their head up. Reflexes become abnormal and muscles grow rigid. Swallowing is impaired.

SOURCE: Excerpted from http://www.alz.org/AboutAD/Stages.asp and reproduced with permission of the Alzheimer's Association. Copyright 2004 Alzheimer's Association, www.alz.org, 800.272.3900.

Regular Appointments

One approach to ensuring optimal health care for patients with dementia is to schedule regular patient surveillance and health maintenance visits every 3 to 6 months. During such visits the physician should address and treat comorbid conditions, evaluate ongoing medications, and consider initiating drug-free periods. In addition, it is useful to check for sleep and behavioral disturbances and provide guidance on proper sleep hygiene. Caregiver well-being should also be regularly assessed.

Communication With Family and Caregivers

Working closely with family members and caregivers will help establish a therapeutic alliance. Education of family and caregivers about diagnosis, clinical course, treatment options, and management strategies is critical. Information about community resources as well as strategies for managing challenging behavioral symptoms can allow families to cope more effectively. Relatives are often helpful sources of information about cognitive and behavioral changes, and generally they take the primary responsibility for implementing and monitoring treatment. Often they are responsible for medical and legal assistance as well. However, early identification of dementia can allow the affected individual to participate in treatment decision and future planning. Subjects to pursue with family include medical and legal advance directives (also called *advance care plans* in some contexts). It is often best for a trusted relative to cosign important financial transactions and attend to paying bills. (See "Legal and Ethical Issues," p 22.)

Discussion about long-term-care placement options should be initiated early rather than late, to provide the individual or family members time to complete the arrangements and begin to adjust emotionally. Eventually, almost 75% of patients with dementia need admission to a long-term-care facility and remain for a long time. Caregivers often express concern about their own memory lapses, which should be addressed with counseling or neuropsychologic assessment. Caregiver distress is often reduced with support-group participation, which may relieve common feelings of anger, frustration, and guilt. Respite care is another community resource that offers caregivers relief. Psychosocial support may enhance quality of life for patients and family and even delay nursing-home placement. (See the resources section in the Appendix, p 504.)

Environmental Modification

Patients with dementia can be extremely sensitive to their environment; in general, a moderate level of stimulation is best. When they experience overstimulation, increased confusion or agitation may result, whereas too little stimulation may cause withdrawal. Familiar surroundings will maximize existing cognitive functions, and predictability through daily routines is often reassuring. Other helpful orientation and memory measures include conspicuous displays of clocks, calendars, and to-do lists. Links to the outside world through newspapers, radios, and televisions may benefit some mildly impaired patients. Simple sentence structure and repeated reminders about conversation content also may enhance communication.

Attention to Safety

Door locks or electronic guards prevent wandering, and many families benefit from registering with Safe Return through the Alzheimer's Association. (See the resources section in the Appendix, p 504.) Patient name tags and medical-alert bracelets will assist in locating lost patients.

Cognitive impairment affects driving skills, and the visuospatial and planning disabilities of many even mildly demented patients may make them unsafe drivers. Discussions about driving are best initiated early in treatment. In California and some other states, physicians must report patients with dementia to the health department, which forwards the information to the motor vehicle department for further assessment. Patients with advanced dementia definitely should not drive, but clinicians disagree about driving by mildly demented patients. Referral for an independent driving assessment is recommended if there is any concern regarding safety. Certainly, when a patient has a history of traffic accidents or significant spatial and executive dysfunction, driving abilities should be carefully scrutinized. (See also the section on the elderly driver in "Assessment," p 49.)

Pharmacologic Treatment

General Issues

When prescribing medications for older patients with dementia, the clinician should consider several factors. Patients in the upper age groups vary in their response, so that treatments need to be individualized. In addition, age is associated with decreased renal clearance and slowed hepatic metabolism. Older patients often take several medications simultaneously, so drug interactions and side effects are likely. Drugs with anticholinergic effects present a particular problem for patients with dementia because they may worsen cognitive impairment and lead to delirium. Another group of problem drugs that may worsen cognition include those causing central nervous system sedation. The best strategy, in light of such factors, is to start with low doses and increase dosing gradually ("start low and go slow"). The goal is to identify the lowest effective dose, thus minimizing side effects, and still avoid subtherapeutic dosing. Before initiating any treatment, conduct a thorough medical examination to identify and treat any underlying medical conditions that might impair cognition.

Cholinesterase Inhibitors

The primary treatments available for stabilizing cognitive function in AD are cholinesterase inhibitors. Currently, four cholinesterase inhibitors approved by the U.S. Food and Drug Administration (FDA) are available: tacrine (rarely prescribed because of its side effects), donepezil, rivastigmine, and galantamine. By slowing the breakdown of the neurotransmitter acetylcholine, these medications are thought to facilitate memory function because of the association of acetylcholine and memory. Clinical trials show that these drugs may modestly improve cognition and activities of daily living in patients with AD of mild to moderate severity. Studies of patients with dementing disorders other than AD are also becoming available. Data indicate that cholinesterase inhibitors may be helpful in managing the hallucinations associated with dementia with Lewy bodies, and preliminary data indicates a potential role in vascular dementia as well. There appears to be no role for cholinesterase inhibitors in treating frontotemporal dementia.

Donepezil is the most widely prescribed cholinesterase inhibitor. The recommended starting dosage is 5 mg per day; after 4 to 6 weeks of treatment, an increase to 10 mg daily is recommended. For patients experiencing gastrointestinal side effects such as nausea and diarrhea, a slower titration may reduce side effects. Rivastigmine is started at 1.5 mg by mouth twice daily for 2 weeks and then doubled no faster than every 2 weeks, to a maximum of 6 mg twice daily. Galantamine is prescribed in initial doses of 4 mg by mouth twice daily for at least 4 weeks, then 8 mg twice daily for at least 4 weeks, and then increased to a maximum of 12 mg twice daily. An extended-release formulation is also now available that permits the option of once-daily dosing. Although the higher doses are more efficacious for all agents, they are more likely to cause such cholinergic effects as nausea, diarrhea, and insomnia, especially if the dose is increased too rapidly. Such adverse effects also may worsen the patient's behavior. Other cholinesterase inhibitors and cholinergic receptor antagonists are currently under development. Direct comparisons among them have not been conducted.

Memantine

Memantine, an N-methyl-d-aspartate antagonist, has been used in Europe for many years. This drug is thought to have neuroprotective effects by reducing glutamate-mediated excitotoxicity. Recently completed clinical trials in the United States support the efficacy of this medication in moderate to severe stages of AD. Memantine now has FDA approval for the treatment of moderate to severe AD. The recommended dosing for memantine in the management of Alzheimer's type dementia involves 5 mg by mouth once daily, which may then be increased on a weekly basis in 5-mg increments to 10 mg per day, dosed as 5 mg by mouth twice daily, then up to 15 mg per day dosed as 5 mg by mouth in the morning then 10 mg by mouth in the evening, and finally arriving at a target dose of 20 mg per day dosed as 10 mg twice daily after a 4-week titration period. The most common side effects noted with memantine are constipation, dizziness, and headache. Memantine has been used safely in conjunction with cholinesterase inhibitors, and one study in 2004 has suggested additional benefits, but this area awaits further research.

Other Cognitive Enhancers

Ongoing studies are assessing a variety of other agents in AD, including antioxidants and Ginkgo biloba extract. In a trial including over 300 patients with moderately severe AD, treatment with vitamin E (α-tocopherol) or the selective monoamine oxidase-B inhibitor selegiline (approved for Parkinson's disease treatment) was found to lower rates of functional decline. The use of these agents, however, was not associated with evidence of cognitive improvement, but this study involved patients with moderate to severe dementia, so effects on cognition earlier in the illness remain unknown. Results from a randomized placebo-controlled trial of the use of vitamin E and donepezil in mild cognitive impairment showed some short-term benefit from donepezil in delaying conversion to AD but no effect of vitamin E. High-dose vitamin E supplementation was associated with increased mortality in a meta-analysis and should be prescribed with caution.

Extract from the leaf of the ginkgo tree has been promoted primarily in Europe for peripheral vascular disease as well as "cerebral insufficiency." Other studies in Europe and the United States have explored its use in AD. One 52-week double-blind, placebo-controlled study of ginkgo leaf extract in treating AD seemed to show small but statistically significant improvement in some cognitive measures. However, global measures did not improve in the small, limited study. Uncommonly, *G. biloba* has been linked to an increase of bleeding. More research is needed before ginkgo can be recommended.

Many patients also use over-the-counter preparations for cognitive enhancement. A complete review of medications includes questions about over-the-counter medications being used.

Antidepressants

Antidepressant drug treatment is generally considered for AD patients with depressive symptoms, including depressed mood, appetite loss, insomnia, fatigue, irritability, and agitation. (See "Depression and Other Mood Disorders," p 273.) Anecdotal evidence exists that selective serotonin-reuptake inhibitors may be helpful in managing the disinhibitions and compulsive behaviors associated with frontotemporal dementia.

Psychoactive Medications

Behavioral symptoms of dementia—paranoia, agitation, and irritability—are best managed by nonpharmacologic strategies, such as reducing overstimulation. However, when medications are required, identify the target symptoms and select therapy accordingly. Cholinesterase inhibitors have been demonstrated to have modest effects on controlling behavioral symptoms. Antipsychotics can be used to manage delusions, hallucinations, and paranoia as well as some of the irritability associated with dementia. The antipsychotics have been associated with extrapyramidal (eg, rigidity, tremor) symptoms in dementia with Lewy bodies, and only very small doses of atypical antipsychotic medications should be considered for treating these patients. However, the FDA recently issued a "black box" warning that atypical antipsychotics have been associated with an increase in mortality among elderly patients with dementia who are being treated for behavioral disorders. This warning arose from an analysis of placebo-controlled trials performed with olanzapine, aripiprazole, risperidone, or quetiapine in elderly dementia patients with behavioral disorders. These trials showed a 1.6- to 1.7-fold increase in mortality in the drug-treated groups over that in the placebo-treated patients. Specific causes of death revealed that most were due either to heart-related events (eg, heart failure, sudden death) or infections (mostly pneumonia). More information is available at: http://www.fda.gov/cder/drug/infopage/ antipsychotics/default.htm. Data on the use of drugs such as carbamazapine and valproic acid in managing irritability and agitation suggest that they may be included as options for drug therapy. Avoid the use of benzodiazepines and medications with anticholinergic effects. Finally, antidepressants with sedating effects such as mirtazapine and trazodone can be considered in the management of insomnia.

Other Resources

Most primary care physicians successfully treat and manage most patients with dementia, but referral to a specialist is sometimes necessary. When the presentation or history is atypical or complex, particularly when the onset begins before age 60, consultation with a specialist in treating dementia patients (eg, geriatric psychiatrist, neurologist) can be useful. Geriatric specialists with psychology or psychiatry training can assist with behavioral management, particularly when patients are agitated, psychotic, or violent. They are also helpful when patients are suicidal or suffer from major depression or when individual or family therapy is indicated for patients or caregivers.

A neurologist can be helpful for patients with parkinsonism, focal neurologic signs, unusually rapid progression, or abnormal neuroimaging findings. Neuropsychologic consultation may clarify diagnostically complex cases, and clinical psychologists can provide psychotherapy, especially for caregivers. Social workers may provide counseling and contact with community resources. Guidance on physical and group activity can be sought from physical therapists, and occupational therapists can assess the patient's functional level and suggest approaches to maximize functioning. Nurses can make management suggestions and guide behavior management, feeding, and other care issues. Wills, conservatorships, estate planning, and other legal matters are best addressed with the assistance of an attorney. Because most dementias are progressive, patients with early dementia should be offered an opportunity to plan for future incapacity and illness. (See "Legal and Ethical Issues," p 22.)

Community support can be informal, when neighbors or friends help out, or formal, such as home-care or family service agencies, the aging or mental health networks, or adult day care centers. Available specialized services include adult day care and respite care, home-health agencies that can provide skilled nursing, help lines of the Alzheimer's Association, and outreach services offered by Area Agencies on Aging and Councils on Aging, which are mandated and funded under the federal Older Americans Act. Food services for the homebound are available from meals-on-wheels, and many senior citizens' centers, church and community groups, and hospitals offer transportation options.

Organizations providing information and referral for dementia patients and families are listed in the resources section of the Appendix (p 504).

ANNOTATED REFERENCES

■ Borson S, Scanlan J, Brush M, et al. The mini-cog: a cognitive 'vital signs' measure for dementia screening in multi-lingual elderly. *Int J Geriatr Psychiatry.* 2000;15(11):1021–1027.

> The Mini-Cog is a 3-minute instrument to screen for cognitive impairment in older adults in the primary care setting. It consists of a three-item recall task to assess memory as well as a clock-drawing task to help clarify when the memory score is equivocal. The Mini-Cog was designed as a brief test for distinguishing dementia in a community sample of older adults. The Mini-Cog has been shown to be an effective and useful screening test for dementia particularly for the busy clinical practice, as it may be conducted more expediently than the Mini–Mental State Examination and can detect a variety of different dementias.

■ Doody RS, Stevens JC, Beck C, et al. Practice parameter: management of dementia (an evidence-based review). Report of the Quality Standards Subcommittee of the American Academy of Neurology. *Neurology.* 2001;56(9):1154–66.

> This is a review of studies to make literature-based treatment recommendations about pharmacotherapy for cognitive and noncognitive symptoms of dementia, education interventions for patients and caregivers, and other nonpharmacologic interventions. Cholinesterase inhibitors may benefit patients with Alzheimer's disease, and vitamin E may delay time to clinical worsening; however, further study is needed of antioxidants, selegiline, and nonsteroidal anti-inflammatory drugs. Educational programs should be offered and may improve caregiver satisfaction and delay nursing-home placement. Nonpharmacologic therapies such as scheduled toileting and behavior modification are also recommended.

■ Geldmacher DS, ed. Dementia update: overview from the first annual dementia congress. *J Am Geriatr Soc.* 2003;51(5 Suppl):S281–S326.

> This overview provides information on the pathophysiology and current approaches to the management of Alzheimer's disease and other dementias. It includes review articles about early diagnosis of Alzheimer's disease, current pharmacotherapy for Alzheimer's disease, diagnosis and management of vascular dementia, medical management of advanced dementia, and an update on new developments in treating Alzheimer's disease.

■ Knopman DS, Dekosky ST, Cummings JL, et al. Practice parameter: diagnosis of dementia (an evidence-based review). Report of the Quality Standards Subcommittee of the American Academy of Neurology. *Neurology.* 2001;56(9):1143–1153.

> This is a review of studies to determine criteria for the diagnosis of dementia and appropriate work-up. Results were an update to the 1994 practice guidelines developed by the American Academy of Neurology. Diagnostic criteria for Alzheimer's disease and Creutzfeldt-Jakob disease were found to be reliable and valid, whereas those for vascular dementia, dementia with Lewy bodies, and frontotemporal dementia may be of use, though their reliability and validity are not well established.

■ Newman MF, Kirchner JL, Phillips-Bute B, et al. Longitudinal assessment of neurocognitive function after coronary artery bypass surgery. *N Engl J Med.* 2001:344(6):395–402.

> This article describes changes in neurocognitive function among 261 patients undergoing coronary artery bypass graft surgery. A detailed neurocognitive battery was administered prior to surgery, at the time of hospital discharge, 6 weeks, 6 months, and 5 years after discharge. Decline was defined as a one–standard deviation drop (approximately 20%) in the scores of tests in any one or more of four cognitive domains. Delirium itself was not assessed. Among the patients studied, the incidence of cognitive decline was 53% at discharge, 36% at 6 weeks, 24% at 6 months, and 42% at 5 years. Cognitive dysfunction at discharge was a significant predictor of long-term dysfunction ($P < .001$). This article brings attention to the magnitude of cognitive dysfunction after cardiac surgery and raises provocative questions as to the nature of the "late decline" following surgery.

■ Peterson RC, Stevens JC, Ganguli M, et al. Practice parameter: early detection of dementia: mild cognitive impairment (an evidence-based review). Report of the Quality Standards Subcommittee of the American Academy of Neurology. *Neurology.* 2001;56(9):1133–1142.

> This is a review of epidemiologic studies of aging and dementia to determine whether screening elderly persons in a general or specialty practice would be beneficial in detecting dementia. There were sufficient data to recommend the evaluation and clinical monitoring of persons with mild cognitive impairment. Screening instruments, neuropsychologic batteries, brief focused cognitive instruments, and structured interview were found to be useful.

■ Sink KM, Holden KF, Yaffe K. Pharmacological treatment of neuropsychiatric symptoms of dementia: a review of the evidence. *JAMA.* 2005;293(5):596–607.

> This article describes a systematic review of 29 articles published between 1966 and 2004 describing randomized controlled trials or meta-analyses of any drug therapy for patients with dementia that included neuropsychiatric outcomes. Results indicated that pharmacologic therapies were not very effective for managing neuropsychiatric symptoms of dementia. Of agents reviewed, atypical antipsychotics had the best evidence for efficacy; however, effects were modest and complicated by increased risk of stroke.

■ Trinh NH, Hoblyn J, Mohanty S, et al. Efficacy of cholinesterase inhibitors in the treatment of neuropsychiatric symptoms and functional impairment in Alzheimer's disease: a meta-analysis. *JAMA.* 2003;289(2):210–216.

> This is a review of trials of cholinesterase inhibitors published between 1966 and 2002 for effects on neuropsychiatric and functional outcomes in patients with mild to moderate Alzheimer's disease. Results indicated that cholinesterase inhibitors have a modest beneficial impact on neuropsychiatric and functional outcomes for patients with Alzheimer's.

Cynthia Barton, RN, MSN
Gary W. Small, MD
Kristine Yaffe, MD

CHAPTER 31—BEHAVIORAL PROBLEMS IN DEMENTIA

KEY POINTS

- The need to express basic needs such as hunger, thirst, or fatigue, which the patient cannot adequately communicate in dementia, may precipitate a behavioral disturbance.

- Delirium secondary to an underlying condition such as dehydration, urinary tract infection, or medication toxicity is a common cause of abrupt behavioral disturbances in patients with dementia.

- Medication effects on behavioral disturbances in dementia tend to be modest and should be implemented only after environmental and nonpharmacologic techniques have been employed.

- Antipsychotic medications may reduce agitation, and antidepressants may be helpful if symptoms of depression are evident in the patient with a behavioral disturbance.

Most dementias are associated with a range of neuropsychiatric and behavioral disturbances, with as many as 80% to 90% of patients developing at least one distressing symptom over the course of their illness. The development of behavioral disturbances or psychotic symptoms in dementia often precipitates nursing-home placement. These disturbances are potentially treatable, and it is vital that clinicians anticipate and recognize them early. If these symptoms become apparent, it is essential to perform a thorough evaluation of contributing factors, identify the target symptoms of treatment, and implement appropriate interventions for the patient and caregiver.

Research that compares different treatment strategies for the behavioral and psychologic symptoms of dementia is growing in response to the great need for evidence-based treatment guidelines. It is possible to draw some conclusions from randomized controlled trials of studies of medications for the treatment of depression and psychosis, but this area is still lacking rigorous studies of elderly adults with dementia. Interventions using behavioral treatment modalities have also been studied, but often in small samples and using varying methods. These studies have allowed for recommendations in many areas; however, many aspects of treatment must still draw on case reports and clinical experience.

CLINICAL FEATURES

Particularly as the dementia progresses, psychiatric symptoms may develop that take on a variety of characteristics resembling discrete mental disorders such as depression or mania; however, the course and features are more difficult to predict, and treatments are less reliably effective than when these disorders occur in younger adults without dementia. Depressive symptoms are common and often manifest as apathy or a lack of interest in previously enjoyable activities. This depressive syndrome may also include a loss of interest in self-care, eating, or interacting with peers. A propensity for irritability and impulsivity may also occur. If these features become progressive, overt hostility or violence may ensue. It is at this juncture that patients may be characterized as "agitated," reflecting a loss of the ability to modulate their behavior in a socially acceptable way. This may involve verbal outbursts, physical aggression, resistance to bathing or other care needs, and restless motor activity such as pacing or rocking. This type of overlap across symptoms, where some are associated with a depressive disorder but others such as hostility are considered atypical, often creates a significant challenge in diagnostic labeling. In this situation, the fairly nonspecific term *agitation* is commonly employed to describe the patient, but it may best be accompanied by additional description as to whether the problem is accompanied by simple irritability, vocal or physical aggression, or motor disturbances.

In many cases the presence of agitation may occur concomitantly with evidence of paranoia or delusional thinking, such as a false belief that caregivers are plotting to steal one's possessions or incur harm. When delusions occur, the patient is then characterized as suffering from "psychotic" symptoms. False perceptions such as hallucinations are another type of psychotic symptom that may accompany episodes of agitated behavior. One way to conceptualize this complex condition is to consider the term *agitation* as a descriptor for the presence of abnormal behavior such as aggression, while the presence of psychosis (eg, paranoid delusions) reflects the abnormal perceptions and beliefs that may lead to the agitated behavior. Depending on the degree of communication deficits in a given patient, the ability to discern the presence of psychosis is variable, and in many cases agitated behaviors may occur in the absence of clear evidence as to whether delusions or other psychoses may be precipitating the disturbance. Antipsychotic medications are commonly used in the management of agitated behaviors, with the presumption that disturbed perceptions may be underlying the problem.

Occasionally a behavioral syndrome occurs that includes features of hyperactivity, euphoric mood, and grandiose beliefs that resemble a manic episode associated with bipolar affective disorder. The features of this "manic-like" syndrome are described later in this chapter, and much like other mood symptoms in dementia, the features are similar but less predictable than those seen in younger adults and treatment strategies are more challenging. One key feature of the manic-like syndromes seen in dementia patients is the tendency to develop additional symptoms outside the typical course of a bipolar manic episode, such as agitated behaviors, defiance, and confusion.

Among the behavioral complications of dementia, the most severe disruptions in caregiving occur when patients develop physical behaviors such as hitting or wandering, or develop paranoid delusions that lead to hostility and altercations with the caregiver. Caregivers, both professional and family, may use the word *agitation* to describe a variety of behaviors and psychologic symptoms. The clinician must consider agitation to be a nonspecific complaint and pursue further history of the problem, including a description of specific behaviors and the time course, frequency, and severity with which they occur. Environmental precipitants such as excessive stimuli or a change in the environment such as a new roommate may induce behavioral problems. The presenting complaint may relate to internal cues such as pain, hunger, thirst, or other needs that the patient is not able to express.

The complaints from family caregivers and professional caregivers in a nursing home or assisted-living facility often arise from behavioral complications occurring during daily care that involve a resistance to bathing, dressing, or other routines. Family members may feel more overwhelmed than professional caregivers do and may consequently attribute more overall distress to these episodes. This type of overt resistance to care is most often seen in later stages of dementia, but it is important to note that behavioral problems may also be a first sign of an incipient cognitive decline in earlier stages as well. Neuropsychiatric symptoms such as apathy, poor self-care, or paranoia may be the first indication of dementia before cognitive decline is recognized, such that an evaluation for dementia in any older patient who presents with new behavioral or emotional symptoms may reveal a previously undetected dementia syndrome.

ASSESSMENT AND DIFFERENTIAL DIAGNOSIS

Comprehensive assessment includes a history both from the patient and from an informant or other source. The information should include a clear description of the behavior: its temporal onset, course, associated circumstances, and its relationship to key environmental factors, such as caregiver status and recent stressors. The problem behaviors and symptoms should be then considered in the context of the patient's family, past, personal, social, and medical history.

A differential diagnosis of the disturbance should proceed on the basis of findings from a comprehensive geriatric evaluation. The first step is to decide whether the disturbance is a symptom of a new or a preexisting medical condition or a medication adverse effect. Disturbances that are new, acute in onset, or evolving rapidly are most often due to a medical condition or medication toxicity. An isolated behavioral disturbance in a demented patient can be the *sole* presenting symptom for acute conditions such as pneumonia, urinary tract infection, arthritis, pain, angina, constipation, or poorly controlled diabetes mellitus. Additionally, the need to satisfy basic physical needs, such as hunger, sleepiness, thirst, boredom, or fatigue, which the patient cannot adequately communicate, may precipitate a behavioral disturbance. Medication toxicity due to new or existing medications might also present as behavioral symptoms alone. Treatment or stabilization of the medical or physical cause is often sufficient to resolve the disturbance. Older adults with dementia may require several weeks longer to recover from routine medical problems than those who are cognitively intact.

The second step is to consider whether the behavioral disturbance is related to an environmental precipitant. These include disruptions in routine, time change (eg, with daylight savings time or travel across time zones), changes in the caregiving environment, new caregivers, a new roommate, or a life stressor (eg, death of a spouse or family member). Other common environmental precipitants include overstimulation (eg, too much noise, crowded rooms, close contact with too many people), understimulation (eg, relative absence of people, spending much time alone, use of television as a companion), and the disruptive behavior of other patients. For many disturbances, correcting an environmental precipitant or removing the stressor commonly improves the symptoms.

Another consideration is whether the disturbance results from stress in the patient-caregiver relationship. Caring for dementia patients is difficult and requires a degree of perseverance that most caregivers are capable of learning if proper guidance and support is provided. Inexperienced caregivers, domineering caregivers, or caregivers who themselves are impaired by medical or psychiatric disturbances may exacerbate or cause a behavioral disturbance. Caregiver burden may be a problem both in community settings and in nursing homes. It is important for the clinician to assess the level of stress and burden on the caregiver as part of the evaluation of behavioral disturbances. Interventions to improve the patient-caregiver relationship and provide caregiver education and support are a vital part of treatment of behavioral disturbances in dementia. Providing resources to caregivers such as referral to support groups and respite services is often very helpful. (See the list of resources in the Appendix, p 504.)

After medical, environmental, and caregiving causes are excluded, it might be concluded that the behavioral problem is a manifestation of the dementia and may not be amenable to a pharmacologic intervention. Such disturbances that are closely linked to the dementia syndrome take on the form of a catastrophic reaction. A catastrophic reaction is an acute behavioral, physical, or verbal reaction to environmental stressors that result from an inability to make routine adjustments in daily life. The reaction might include anger, emotional lability, or aggression when the patient is confronted with a deficit, such as the inability to find a word, or confusion about where she is or what she is supposed to do. Catastrophic reactions are best treated by identifying and avoiding their precipitants, by providing structured routines and activities, and by recognizing early signs of the impending catastrophic reaction so that the patient can be distracted and supported before reacting.

If the disturbance is not related to an identifiable cause or environmental precipitant, it may be a consequence of the brain deterioration that occurs during the course of dementia. Disturbances with a more insidious onset or that are persistent are more likely to be symptoms of the underlying disease. Epidemiologic and clinical studies suggest that such disturbances fall into three groups: mood symptoms, psychosis, and specific behaviors. The overlap in the symptoms of these groups can make treatment choices difficult. One approach for the clinician is to decide whether the predominant symptom of a polysymptomatic disturbance is psychosis (delusions or hallucinations), mood symptoms (dysphoria, sadness, irritability, lability), aggression, or agitation, and then target treatment toward the prevailing feature.

Behavioral disturbances may occur in all types of dementias, including Alzheimer's type, vascular, and mixed. Frontotemporal dementia (Pick's disease) is a less common type of dementia often associated with prominent disinhibition, compulsive behaviors, and social impairment due to more advanced frontal lobe degeneration. In severe cases, a syndrome of hyperphagia, hyperactivity, and hypersexuality may occur that is related to bilateral temporal lobe atrophy. Another dementia associated with prominent psychiatric symptoms and behavioral disturbances is dementia with Lewy bodies (DLB). This form of dementia may be more common than previously thought. It is characterized by cognitive deterioration and parkinsonian features with prominent psychosis characterized by visual hallucinations. Patients with DLB often suffer from distressing hallucinations and a fluctuating clinical course. These patients are extremely sensitive to the extrapyramidal side effects of antipsychotic medications (such as muscle rigidity and tremor) and often cannot tolerate even low doses of atypical agents.

TREATMENT: BASIC APPROACH

The treatment of the psychiatric and behavioral disturbances in dementia is complex and may require several interventions applied as part of a comprehensive plan of care. Specialists should be consulted in refractory cases. In general, treatment begins with appropriate environmental and caregiver interventions. Nonpharmacologic interventions should always be used as a first-line treatment in the management of disruptive, aggressive, or agitated behavior. Table 31.1 provides a list of key behavioral interventions that might ameliorate behavioral symptoms in patients with dementia. The implementation of a daily routine and introduction of meaningful activities is vital. Patients with dementia may display a reduction in behavioral disturbances with the use of music, particularly during meals and bathing, and with light physical exercise or walking. Massage, pet therapy, white noise, videotapes of family, and cognitive stimulation programs may also

Table 31.1—Behavioral Interventions for Dementia Care

- Treat underlying medical precipitants
- Correct sensory deficits; replace poorly fitting hearing aids, eyeglasses, and dentures
- Remove offending medications, particularly anticholinergic agents
- Keep the environment comfortable, calm, and homelike with use of familiar possessions
- Provide regular daily activities and structure; refer patient to adult day care programs, if needed
- Monitor for new medical problems
- Attend to patient's sleep and eating patterns
- Install safety measures to prevent accidents
- Ensure that the caregiver has adequate respite
- Educate caregivers about practical aspects of dementia care and about behavioral disturbances
- Teach caregivers the skills of caregiving: communication skills, avoiding confrontational behavior management, techniques of ADL support, activities for dementia care
- Simplify bathing and dressing with the use of adaptive clothing and assistive devices if needed
- Provide access to experienced professionals and community resources
- Refer family and patient to local Alzheimer's Association
- Consult with caregiving professionals, such as geriatric case managers

NOTE: ADL = activity of daily living.

be helpful. If the disturbances persist despite best efforts, pharmacologic interventions for specific target symptoms are often necessary. Their disorder-specific use, in conjunction with nonbiologic therapies, is discussed in the next section.

TREATMENTS FOR SPECIFIC DISTURBANCES

At the core of treatment is the identification of any possible underlying cause of the behavior change, with the recognition that multiple causes may be operating concurrently. First and foremost, managing pain, dehydration, hunger, and thirst is paramount. Consider the possibilities of positional discomforts or nausea secondary to medication effects, as these are common possible culprits. Environmental modifications can improve patient orientation. Good lighting, one-on-one attention, supportive care, and attention to personal needs and wants are also important aspects of treatment. If there is sleep-wake cycle disturbance, efforts should be made to stabilize the sleep cycle by maintaining a stable routine, using bright lights, or prescribing short-term use of medications (see the sleep disturbances section, below).

Mood Disturbances in Patients with Dementia

In dementia patients experiencing mood symptoms, procedures similar to those used with other behavior disturbances should be employed, that is, optimize the environment by reducing adversive stimuli and assess physical health comprehensively. Recreation programs and activity therapies have demonstrated positive results in improving mood in depressive symptoms in dementia. Criteria for the diagnosis of depression in Alzheimer's dementia have been proposed that note common features of irritability and social isolation or withdrawal. The waxing and waning course of mood symptoms in dementia is attributed to the cognitive loss and reduction in communication skills related to the dementia. Depression of 2 weeks' duration resulting in significant distress should likely receive a trial of an antidepressant medication. Similarly, sustained depressive features lasting more than 2 months following the initiation of behavioral interventions warrants treatment with antidepressant medications.

First-line agents are the selective serotonin-reuptake inhibitors, preferred for their favorable side-effect profiles. Studies of depression in patients with dementia have demonstrated the efficacy of sertraline and citalopram in comparison with placebo,

but other studies using the same medications as well as paroxetine and fluoxetine have been inconclusive. Table 31.2 lists the antidepressants most commonly used to treat depressive symptoms in dementia.

The treatment of depression in dementia requires persistence. If a first agent has failed an adequate therapeutic dose for 8 to 12 weeks, an alternative agent should be tried. Venlafaxine, bupropion, mirtazapine, and the tricyclic agents desipramine and nortriptyline might be considered. Tricyclics should be avoided if a bundle branch block or other significant cardiac conduction disturbance is present. For patients who are partial responders to an antidepressant, augmentation strategies might be considered. The addition of a stimulant such as methylphenidate[OL] (2.5 to 10 mg per day) may be helpful in some cases, but there is some risk of increasing psychotic symptoms if the patient has a tendency to be suspicious or delusional. Also, the addition of stimulants such as methylphenidate to augment bupropion should be avoided, as bupropion already possesses stimulant effects. If the patient does not improve, the agents should be discontinued. If a patient continues to be significantly depressed after several antidepressant trials and is in danger because of serious weight loss or suicidal ideas, electroconvulsive therapy might be considered. This is the most efficacious and rapidly effective treatment for severe major depression and has a favorable safety profile even in mild dementia.

Manic-like Behavioral Syndromes in Dementia Patients

Occasionally mood syndromes may develop in dementia patients that are characterized by pressured speech, disinhibition, elevated mood, intrusiveness, hyperactivity, and reduced sleep. These syndromes therefore resemble manic episodes observed in the context of bipolar affective disorder in younger adults, although they are generally considered to be secondary to the dementing disorder. The important distinction in the dementia patient is the frequent co-occurrence with confusional states and a tendency to have more of a fluctuating mood, that is, the patient's mood may be irritable or hostile as opposed to euphoric. The appearance of hypersexual behaviors may be observed in this clinical scenario, although sexual disinhibition frequently occurs with dementia as a consequence of reduced frontal-executive functioning and may not necessarily be part of a manic syndrome. Treatment of manic-like states, emotional lability, disinhibition, or irritability typically begins with the use of mood-stabilizing agents such as divalproex sodium[OL] (see Table 31.3). The sustained-release preparation divalproex sodium is commonly recommended. In dementia patients, a typical starting dose of divalproex

Table 31.2—Drugs to Treat Depressive Features of Behavioral Disturbances in Dementia

Medication	Daily Dose	Uses	Precautions
Selective serotonin-reuptake inhibitors			
Citalopram	10–40 mg	Depression, anxiety[OL]	Gastrointestinal upset, nausea, insomnia
Escitalopram	5–20 mg	Depression, anxiety	
Fluoxetine	10–40 mg	Depression, anxiety	
Paroxetine	10–40 mg	Depression, anxiety	Inhibits the cytochrome P-450 system
Sertraline	25–100 mg	Depression, anxiety	
Trazodone	25–150 mg	When sedation is desirable	Sedation, falls, hypotension
Serotonin norepinephrine-reuptake inhibitors			
Duloxetine	20–60 mg	Depression, diabetic neuropathy	Nausea, dry mouth, dizziness
Mirtazapine	7.5–30 mg	Useful for depression with insomnia	Sedation, hypotension
Venlafaxine	25–150 mg	Useful in severe depression	Hypertension may be a problem, insomnia
Tricyclic antidepressants			
Desipramine	10–100 mg	Depression, anxiety	Anticholinergic effects, hypotension, sedation, cardiac arrhythmias
Nortriptyline	10–75 mg	High efficacy for depression if side effects are tolerable; therapeutic range 50–150 ng/dL	Anticholinergic effects, hypotension, sedation, cardiac arrhythmias
Other			
Bupropion	75–225 mg	More activating, lack of cardiac effects	Irritability, insomnia

Table 31.3—Mood Stabilizers for Behavioral Disturbances in Dementia With Manic Features

Drug	Geriatric Dosage	Adverse Effects	Comments
Carbamazepine[OL]*	200–1000 mg/day (therapeutic level 4–12 µg/mL)	Nausea, fatigue, ataxia, blurred vision, hyponatremia	Poor tolerability in older adults; must monitor CBC, LFTs, electrolytes q 2 weeks for first 2 months, then q 3 months
Lithium[OL]*	150–1000 mg/day (therapeutic level 0.5–0.8 mEq/L)	Nausea, vomiting, tremor, confusion, leukocytosis	Poor tolerability in older adults; toxicity at low serum levels; monitor thyroid and renal function
Divalproex sodium[OL]*	250–2000 mg/day (therapeutic level 40–100 µg/mL)	Nausea, GI upset, ataxia, sedation	Requires monitoring of CBC, platelets, LFTs at baseline and q 6 months; better tolerated than other mood stabilizers in older patients

* Approved by the Food and Drug Administration for the treatment of bipolar disorder.

NOTE: CBC = complete blood cell count; GI = gastrointestinal; LFTs = liver function tests; q = every.

is 125 mg twice a day. The dose should be titrated upward slowly while the patient is monitored for sedation, ataxia, and falls. Blood levels in the range of 40 to 100 µg/dL have been shown to be effective, but individual variability in dose and response is great. Because of the potential adverse effects on the liver and thrombocytopenia, transaminase levels and a complete blood cell count (CBC) should be taken before therapy is initiated, rechecked with each dose increase, and repeated at least every 6 months while the patient remains on the drug. Alternatives to divalproex sodium are carbamazepine[OL], lamotrigine[OL], or lithium[OL].

Carbamazepine starting at 100 mg twice a day (with monitoring of liver enzymes and CBC) is an acceptable alternative for manic-like states, mood lability, or irritability in dementia. Leukopenia is of concern with carbamazepine, and monitoring the CBC with every dose increase and at least every 3 months while the patient remains on the drug is needed. Lamotrigine has been used in the treatment of mania, but no geriatric trials have been conducted. Lithium is valuable as a mood stabilizer, but its use may be a problem in the elderly patient because of enhanced sensitivity to adverse effects. Elevated lithium levels may occur in the context of reduced renal function and dehydration, resulting in ataxia, tremor, gastrointestinal distress, and confusion.

[OL] Not approved by the U.S. Food and Drug Administration for this use.

Psychosis in Dementia: Delusions and Hallucinations

Delusions (paranoid or unfounded ideas) or hallucinations (false perceptions), whether occurring independently or in association with mood syndromes, typically require specific pharmacologic treatment if the patient is disturbed by these experiences, or if the experiences lead to disruptions in the patient's environment that cannot otherwise be controlled. Clinical criteria for the diagnosis of Alzheimer's dementia with psychosis specifies that the presence of delusions or hallucinations occur for at least 1 month, at least intermittently, and must cause distress for the patient. Antipsychotic drugs are listed in Table 31.4, along with dosing information. The atypical agents risperidone[OL], olanzapine[OL], quetiapine[OL], and aripiprazole[OL] are being used more commonly than older agents such as haloperidol[OL]. The older agents are more likely to cause extrapyramidal side effects, such as parkinsonism and tardive dyskinesia. Sedation, hypotension, and falls are common adverse effects among all antipsychotic agents. As these medications are more widely used, differences in side-effect profile are emerging. An increased risk of cerebrovascular events in patients with dementia has been identified with use of risperidone, olanzapine, and aripiprazole. The U.S. Food and Drug Administration (FDA) has required that warnings re-

garding diabetes mellitus, hyperglycemia, ketoacidosis, and hyperosmolar states be included as a risk of therapy with all of the atypical antipsychotic agents. Quetiapine is the most sedating of the atypical agents. Clozapine[OL], the first atypical agent introduced, is difficult to use because of the need for weekly CBC monitoring, adverse effects of sedation and orthostatic hypotension, and the risk of agranulocytosis. Clozapine is still helpful in a small group of patients with psychosis associated with Parkinson's dementia and those with DLB who are unable to tolerate the extrapyramidal adverse effects of other agents. It is clear that more information on side effects of all atypical agents will become available and should be considered by the clinician before prescribing them.

Although antipsychotic agents have demonstrated efficacy in large controlled trials in the treatment of dementia with psychosis and aggression, it is important to note that the overall positive effects have been relatively modest. Controlled studies of geriatric patients have had notorious difficulty with very high placebo responses. Although 45% to 55% of patients have been found to improve on antipsychotic medications, the response to placebo ranged from 30% to 50% across studies. Antipsychotic agents clearly play an important role in the treatment of delusions, hallucinations, and aggression in dementia, but they must be

Table 31.4—Antipsychotic Agents for the Treatment of Psychosis (Hallucinations and Delusions) in Dementia

Drug	Daily Dose	Adverse Effects	Comments	Formulations
Aripiprazole[OL]	5–15 mg	Mild sedation, mild hypotension	Warning about increased cerebrovascular events in dementia, possible hyperglycemia	Tablet, liquid concentrate
Clozapine[OL]	12.5–200 mg	Sedation, hypotension, anticholinergic effects, agranulocytosis	Weekly CBCs required, poorly tolerated by older adults, reserved for treatment of refractory cases, warning about hyperglycemia	Tablet, rapidly dissolving tablet
Olanzapine[OL]	2.5–10 mg	Sedation, falls, gait disturbance	Warning about hyperglycemia and cerebrovascular events in patients with dementia	Tablet, rapidly dissolving tablet, IM injection
Quetiapine[OL]	25–200 mg	Sedation, hypotension	Warning about hyperglycemia, ophthalmologic exam recommended every 6 months	Tablet
Risperidone[OL]	0.5–2 mg	Sedation, hypotension, EPS with doses > 1 mg/day	Warning about cerebrovascular events in patients with dementia, hyperglycemia warning	Tablet, rapidly dissolving tablet, liquid concentrate, depot IM injection
Ziprasidone[OL]	40–160 mg	Higher risk of QTc prolongation	Warning regarding increased QTc prolongation, possible hyperglycemia. Little published information on use in older adults	Capsule, IM injection

NOTE: CBCs = complete blood cell counts; EPS = extrapyramidal symptoms; IM = intramuscular.

[OL] Not approved by the U.S. Food and Drug Administration for this use.

part of a comprehensive treatment plan. The FDA has requested that the manufacturers of aripiprazole[OL], olanzapine[OL], quetiapine[OL], risperidone[OL], clozapine[OL], and ziprasidone[OL] add a boxed warning to their labeling describing an increased risk of mortality that has been observed in 17 placebo-controlled studies. In these studies, the rate of death for patients with dementia was approximately 1.6 to 1.7 times that of placebo. In most cases the cause of death appeared to be heart related or from infections (eg, pneumonia). More information on this warning is available at http://www.fda.gov/cder/drug/infopage/antipsychotics/default.htm.

There is some evidence that cholinomimetic agents such as donepezil or galantamine may reduce the psychosis and behavioral disturbances of Alzheimer's disease. Studies comparing these agents with placebo in patients with mild to moderate Alzheimer's disease have suggested that they may reduce the rate of emergence of behavioral disturbances and psychosis. One area where cholinesterase inhibitors may be likely to improve psychosis is in the case of DLB; reduced visual hallucinations have been reported with cholinesterase inhibitors. Galantamine in dosages of 16 to 24 mg per day may be useful in the treatment of patients with DLB, who are uniquely sensitive to the extrapyramidal adverse effects of antipsychotic agents.

Disturbances of Sleep

Treatment of insomnia and sleep-wake cycle disturbance should begin with improvement of sleep hygiene (see Table 31.5). This consists of efforts to get the patient to go to sleep later every day, around 10:00 or 11:00 PM, while keeping the environment calm, comfortable, and conducive to sleep, into the next morning. If the sleep disturbance is associated with depression, suspiciousness, or delusions, those conditions should be treated.

For primary sleep disturbances when good sleep hygiene and increasing daytime activity level are not successful, trazodone[OL] (25 to 150 mg at bedtime) or mirtazapine[OL] (7.5 to 15 mg at bedtime) might be used. Benzodiazepines or antihistamines, such as diphenhydramine, should be avoided, since they carry a high risk for falls, hip fractures, disinhibition, and cognitive disturbance when prescribed for patients with dementia. (See also "Sleep Problems," p 249.)

Zolpidem[OL] and zaleplon[OL] are short-acting nonbenzodiazepine sedative hypnotics that may be helpful for sleep disturbances in the elderly patient, although there have been no controlled trials for their use in sleep disturbances secondary to dementia. Zolpidem has been studied in elderly patients without

---

OL Not approved by the U.S. Food and Drug Administration for this use.

Table 31.5—Behavioral Management of Insomnia

- Establish a stable routine for going to bed and awakening
- Optimize sleep environment (attention to noise, light, temperature)
- Increase daytime activity and light exercise
- Reduce or eliminate caffeine, nicotine, alcohol
- Reduce evening fluid consumption to minimize nocturia
- Give activating medications early in the day if patient unable to eliminate
- Control nighttime pain
- Limit daytime napping to brief periods of 20 to 30 minutes
- Use relaxation, stress management, breathing techniques to promote natural sleep

dementia and appears to be effective in improving sleep onset, although it does not improve sleep duration because of its short half-life. The recommended dose of zolpidem in the elderly person is 5 mg, as an increased risk of adverse effects appears to be dose related. Zaleplon has been less extensively studied in the older patient but appears to have similar properties.

Aggression and Hypersexuality

If hypersexuality occurs in association with another recognizable syndrome such as a mania-like state, treatment of the specific syndrome should be attempted. In men with dementia who are dangerously hypersexual or aggressive, a trial of an antiandrogen might be attempted to reduce the sexual drive. Patients may be tried on progesterone[OL] 5 mg orally once daily at first. The dose should be adjusted to suppress serum testosterone well below normal. If the patient responds well behaviorally, 10 mg of depot intramuscular progesterone may be given weekly to maintain a reduction of sexual drive. An alternative treatment to reduce sexual drive is leuprolide acetate[OL] (5 to 10 mg intramuscularly every month), also an antiandrogen. The use of antipsychotic medications is often adopted clinically, given the seriousness of hypersexual behaviors in institutionalized setting such as nursing homes; however, there are no controlled studies supporting this use. Presumably, the medication may enhance the cognitive focus of the individual's perceptions by reducing any psychotic thinking that may in some way be contributing to hypersexual behavior. Additional studies are needed for this problem.

Intermittent Aggression or Agitation

When disruptive behavior occurs intermittently or episodically, such as once per week or less, behavioral interventions focusing on identifying the antecedents of the behavior and avoiding the triggers are often most useful. Behavior modification using positive reinforcement of desirable behavior has been shown to be helpful, and it also helps encourage the caregiver to focus on times when behavior is not a problem. Reminiscence, validation therapy, aromatherapy, and environmental modifications of light, sound, and space may all help promote positive behavior. Distraction techniques, activity therapies, and exercise also show promise in reducing troublesome behaviors.

Physical restraint in any form should be avoided if at all possible. If restraining measures are necessary, careful supportive care should be provided to the patient. Over time, it is usually possible to reduce or eliminate the amount of restraint. (See also the section on quality issues in "Nursing-Home Care," p 122, and the section on restraints in the nursing home in "Legal and Ethical Issues," p 30.)

ANNOTATED REFERENCES

- American Psychiatric Association. Practice guideline for the treatment of Alzheimer's disease and other dementias of later life. *Am J Psychiatry*. 1997; 154(5 Suppl):1–39.

   This practice guideline by the American Psychiatric Association remains the standard reference for evidence-based treatment of Alzheimer's dementia. It discusses in depth the evidence for and against various therapies for Alzheimer's disease and related conditions. This small supplement to a main issue of the journal provides a ready reference for clinicians.

- Doody RS, Stevens JC, Beck C, et al. Practice parameter: management of dementia (an evidence-based review). Report of the quality standards subcommittee of the American Academy of Neurology. *Neurology*. 2001;56(9): 1154–1166.

   This standard of care provided by a consensus committee of the American Academy of Neurology covers all aspects of dementia care, including interdisciplinary assessment and care planning and caregiver support. This is a well-balanced review that assigns a level of recommendation for each treatment (standard, guideline, or option) on the basis of the type of evidence provided (ranging from meta-analyses of randomized controlled trials, observational studies, and expert opinions to case series and studies).

- Lyketsos CG, Sheppard JM, Steele CD, et al. Randomized, placebo-controlled, double-blind clinical trial of sertraline in the treatment of depression complicating Alzheimer's disease: initial results for the Depression in Alzheimer's Disease study. *Am J Psychiatry*. 2000;157(10):1686–1689.

   This is the first randomized controlled trial of antidepressant efficacy in persons with Alzheimer's disease and major depression. It demonstrates benefits similar to those seen in persons with major depression and no dementia.

- Snowden M, Sato K, Roy-Byrne P. Assessment and treatment of nursing home residents with depression or behavioral symptoms associated with dementia: a review of the literature. *J Am Geriatr Soc*. 2003;51(9):1305–1317.

   This comprehensive review critically assesses all studies from 1970 to the present of the treatment of behavioral and psychologic symptoms of dementia in the nursing home. Neither pharmacologic nor behavioral interventions eliminate problem symptoms, but both offer a reduction in intensity and severity. This thorough review provides a basis upon which to begin an evidenced-based approach to the treatment of behavioral symptoms in dementia, and it highlights studies by strength of design.

- Steinberg M, Sheppard JM, Tschanz JT, et al. The incidence of mental and behavioral disturbances in dementia: the Cache County study. *J Neuropsychiatry Clin Neurosci*. 2003;15(3):340–345.

   This paper provides longitudinal data on the new and cumulative incidence of mental and behavioral symptoms in a sample of patients with dementia followed over an 18-month period. The cumulative prevalence of all symptoms approached 90%; delusions were most common (28%), followed by apathy (21%) and aberrant motor behavior (21%). This well-conducted study reveals both the high incidence rate of behavioral and psychologic disturbances (61%) and suggests that all patients with dementia be assessed for the presence of behavior symptoms as part of routine evaluation.

- Tariot PN, Ryan JM, Porsteinsson AP, et al. Pharmacologic therapy for behavioral symptoms of Alzheimer's disease. *Clin Geriatri Med*. 2001;17(2):359–376.

   This practical review offers the clinician an approach to the use of psychotropic medications for specific target symptoms in dementia. The monitoring of side effects and the use of clinical outcome measures are discussed.

- Weiner MF, Lipton AM, eds. *The Dementias Diagnosis Treatment and Research*. 3rd ed. Washington DC: American Psychiatric Press, Inc.; 2003.

   This thorough text serves as both a reference and clinical guide to all aspects of dementia care. This book provides an update on dementias of all types, including Alzheimer's, vascular, fronto-temporal, and Lewy body. Recommendations for clinical management and evidenced-based guidelines are provided. It includes rating scales, assessment tools, and resources for the practitioner and caregiver.

Melinda S. Lantz, MD
Constantine G. Lyketsos, MD, MHS

CHAPTER 32—DELIRIUM

KEY POINTS

- Delirium is under-recognized and often inappropriately evaluated and managed. Approximately one third of patients aged 70 or older admitted to the general medical service experience delirium.

- The Confusion Assessment Method is the most clinically useful diagnostic tool.

- Most of the treatable causes of delirium lie outside the central nervous system, and these should be investigated first.

- The management of delirium requires an interdisciplinary effort by physicians, nurses, family members, and others involved in the care of the patient. A multifactorial approach is the most successful since many factors contribute to delirium.

Delirium has been described in the medical literature for more than two thousand years. Despite this, it remains under-recognized and often inappropriately evaluated and managed. Clinicians call delirium by many different names: up to 30 synonyms exist in the peer-reviewed literature, and far more in common medical parlance. *Acute confusional state* is the most common synonym, and the term still preferred today by many neurologists. Other synonyms for delirium range from the frequently used *acute mental status change*, *altered mental status*, *organic brain syndrome*, *reversible dementia*, and *toxic* or *metabolic encephalopathy* to the arcane *dysergastic reaction* and *subacute befuddlement*.

INCIDENCE AND PROGNOSIS

Delirium is common and associated with substantial morbidity. Approximately one third of patients aged 70 or older admitted to a general medical service experience delirium: one half of these are delirious on admission to the hospital; the other half develop delirium in the hospital. Among those admitted to intensive care units, the prevalence of delirium is much higher, and when rates for delirium are combined with those for stupor and coma, prevalence rates may exceed 75%. One third of older patients presenting to the emergency department are delirious. In postacute skilled nursing facilities, 16% of new admissions meet the full criteria for delirium, and an additional 49% have subsyndromal delirium. The prevalence of delirium among older patients discharged from the hospital into the community remains unknown.

Although delirium is traditionally viewed as a transient phenomenon, there is growing evidence that it may persist for weeks to months in a substantial portion of affected persons. A study of very old hospitalized medical and surgical patients found that approximately one third of those with incident delirium still met full criteria 3 and 6 months later. Subsequent studies performed in somewhat younger groups have found slightly lower but substantial persistence rates weeks to months after acute hospitalization. Risk factors for delirium persistence are starting to be defined—very elderly patients and those with preexisting cognitive impairment seem to be at highest risk for prolonged or permanent cognitive decline after the acute onset.

There is mounting evidence that delirium is strongly and independently associated with poor patient outcomes. Delirium has been associated with a tenfold increased risk of death in the hospital and three- to fivefold increased risk of nosocomial complications, prolonged hospital length of stay, and greater need for postacute nursing-home placement. Studies that have incorporated postdischarge follow-up have found that delirium is associated with poor functional recovery and increased risk of death up to 2 years after hospital discharge. Most of these associations persist after adjustment for factors such as patient age, preexisting dementia, and severity of illness. There is evidence that patients with persistent delirium have worse functional recovery than those whose delirium clears, suggesting that persistence of delirium may play an important role in poor long-term outcomes.

DIAGNOSIS AND DIFFERENTIAL DIAGNOSIS

Under-recognition of delirium is a major problem. The criteria of the 4th edition of the *Diagnostic and Statistical Manual of Mental Disorders* (*DSM-IV*), although precise, may be difficult to apply in clinical practice. More clinically useful is the Confusion Assessment Method (CAM), which was derived from *DSM-III-R* but is equally compatible with *DSM-IV*. (See Table 32.1 for a comparison of the *DSM-IV* and CAM criteria for delirium.) By judging the presence or absence of the four key CAM features shown in the table, the clinician can establish the diagnosis of delirium with better than 95% sensitivity and specificity. The CAM is a diagnostic algorithm, not a patient interview, and therefore the assessment done prior to its application is not specified. Although the CAM can be completed by using observations from routine care,

Table 32.1—A Comparison of the *DSM-IV* Diagnostic Criteria for Delirium and the Confusion Assessment Method

DSM-IV Criteria	Confusion Assessment Method
■ Disturbance of consciousness (ie, reduced clarity of awareness of the environment) with reduced ability to focus, sustain, or shift attention	1. Acute change in mental status and fluctuating course —Is there evidence of an acute change in cognition from the patient's baseline? —Does the abnormal behavior fluctuate during the day, ie, tend to come and go, or increase and decrease in severity?
■ A change in cognition (such as memory deficit, disorientation, language disturbance) or the development of a perceptual disturbance that is not better accounted for by a preexisting, established, or evolving dementia	2. Inattention —Does the patient have difficulty focusing attention, eg, being easily distractible, or having difficulty keeping track of what is being said?
■ The disturbance develops over a short period of time (usually hours to days) and tends to fluctuate during the course of the day	3. Disorganized thinking Is the patient's thinking disorganized or incoherent, eg, rambling or irrelevant conversation, unclear or illogical flow of ideas, or unpredictable switching from subject to subject?
■ There is evidence from the history, physical examination, or laboratory findings that the disturbance is caused by the direct physiologic consequences of a general medical condition or a drug, or both	4. Altered level of consciousness —Is the patient's mental status anything besides alert, ie, vigilant (hyperalert), lethargic (drowsy, easily aroused), stuporous (difficult to arouse), or comatose (unarousable)?
	The diagnosis of delirium requires the presence of features 1 and 2 and either 3 or 4

SOURCES: Data from (1) *Diagnostic and Statistical Manual of Mental Disorders.* 4th ed. Washington, DC: American Psychiatric Association; 1994 and (2) Inouye SK, van Dyck CH, Alessi CA, et al. Clarifying confusion: the Confusion Assessment Method: a new method for detection of delirium. *Ann Intern Med.* 1990;113(12):941–948.

recent evidence suggests that the use of a formal mental status evaluation is superior. In fact, one study examining nurses' application of the CAM using observations from routine care found a sensitivity of only 19% when compared with a formal mental status assessment by trained research staff. Factors associated with nonrecognition included hypoactive delirium, preexisting cognitive impairment, advanced age, and visual impairment. A brief formal cognitive assessment such as the Mini–Mental State Examination, with supplemental attentional testing, is recommended prior to using the CAM. Table 32.2 shows some commonly used tests of attention. In the absence of a formal evaluation or when there is doubt, any older patient with acute change in mental status should be considered delirious, and evaluated and managed as described below.

Until recently, application of the CAM has required a conversant patient. The Confusion Assessment Method for the Intensive Care Unit (CAM-ICU) is a variant of the CAM that does not require verbal responses from the patient. Although it was designed for ventilated patients in the ICU, it can be used more generally for patients who are unable to speak. It uses the same four features as the CAM diagnostic algorithm but uses mental status testing that requires only yes-no answers that can be indicated by a nod or raised finger. Attention is tested using the Attention Screening Examination, in which patients are required to immediately recall simple pictures. Disorganized thinking is tested by answers to a series of simple yes-no questions (eg, "Does 1 pound weigh more than 2 pounds?").

The differential diagnosis of delirium includes dementia, depression, and acute psychiatric syndromes. In many cases, it is not truly a "differential" diagnosis, since these syndromes can coexist and indeed are risk factors for one another. Instead, it is better thought of as a series of independent questions: Does this patient have delirium? . . . dementia? . . . depression? The most common diagnostic issue is whether a newly presenting confused patient has dementia, delirium, or both. To make this determination, the physician must know the patient's baseline status. In the absence of baseline data, information from family members, caregivers, or others who know the patient is essential. An acute change in mental status from baseline is not consistent with dementia and suggests delirium. In

Table 32.2—Commonly Used Tests of Attention

Test	Patient Is Asked To:	Comments
Digit span	Repeat random sequence of numbers Repeat sequence of numbers in reverse order	Should be able to do at least 5 forward, 4 backward
Days, months	Recite the days of the week backward Recite the months of the year backward	Advantage: not much affected by poor memory, hearing, education, knowledge of English
Continuous performance task	Raise hand whenever he or she hears a certain letter or number in a list	Does not require a verbal response
Attention screening examination	Show 5 pictures; ask patient to remember them and to recall them out of a series of 10 pictures shown subsequently	Used in the CAM-ICU Does not require a verbal response
MMSE items	Subtract 7 from 100, then subtract 7 from each remainder ("serial sevens")	Requires ability to calculate
	Spell *world* backward	Requires knowledge of English

NOTE: CAM-ICU = Confusion Assessment Method for the Intensive Care Unit; MMSE = Folstein's Mini–Mental State Examination.

addition, a rapidly fluctuating course (over minutes to hours) and an abnormal level of consciousness are also highly suggestive of delirium. Depression may also be confused with hypoactive delirium. In one study, one third of psychiatric consultations for depression in the acute-care setting actually had hypoactive delirium. Finally, certain acute psychiatric syndromes, such as mania, can present similarly to hyperactive delirium. In the absence of known bipolar disease, it is best initially to evaluate and manage hyperactive patients as if they have delirium rather than attributing the presentation to psychiatric disease and missing a serious underlying medical disorder.

THE SPECTRUM OF DELIRIUM

The classic presentation of delirium is thought to be the wildly agitated patient. However, studies have demonstrated that agitated or hyperactive delirium represents only 25% of all cases. More common is hypoactive or "quiet" delirium, or delirium with mixed features. Hypoactive delirium has no better prognosis than hyperactive delirium; it is recognized and appropriately treated less frequently. Special case-finding efforts are necessary to detect quiet delirium among high-risk elderly patients. If agitation is present, behavioral control measures may be necessary (see below), but such measures alone are not adequate treatment for delirium, and in some cases they may exacerbate or prolong the delirium.

Though we often speak of delirium as being either present or absent, it is important to recognize that the number and severity of symptoms vary widely. To more completely describe delirium, several severity scales have been validated and published: the Memorial Delirium Assessment Scale and the Delirium Rating Scale are among these. The Delirium Index is a severity measure based on the CAM and may be used in conjunction with it. When patients with delirium are stratified according to these scales, it is found that those with severe delirium have worse outcomes than those with mild delirium. Moreover, patients who do not fulfill all CAM or *DSM* criteria for delirium but who still demonstrate significant delirium symptoms have worse outcomes than patients with no symptoms of delirium. There is a gradient of worsening outcomes over the spectrum of delirium.

THE NEUROPATHOPHYSIOLOGY OF DELIRIUM

Research into the neuropathophysiology of delirium is in its infancy, but it suggests that different underlying mechanisms may pertain in different situations. Our understanding of the pathophysiology of delirium has not yet progressed to the point that it has an impact on the management of most delirious patients. One of the best-documented mechanisms for delirium is cholinergic deficiency. This is seen classically in overdoses of anticholinergic drugs such as atropine, which in severe cases can be reversed by the administration of physostigmine. In addition, many drugs not classified as anticholinergic (antihistamines, certain opioids, and antidepressants) have substantial anticholinergic activity and may also precipitate delirium. Delirium has been associated with increased serum anticholinergic activity measured by bioassay in both medical and surgical patients. Moreover, significant anticholinergic activity has been found in the serum of patients who were taking no drugs with anticholinergic properties, which suggests that there may be endogenous activity predisposing certain patients to the development of delirium.

A second potential mechanism for delirium is an alteration in the ratio of amino acids important in neurotransmitter production. Serotonin, a key central nervous system neurotransmitter, is dependent on the transport of tryptophan across the blood-brain barrier. Tryptophan competes with other large neutral amino acids, most notably phenylalanine, for transport into the central nervous system. Alterations in the tryptophan-to-phenylalanine ratio may result in serotonin excess or deficiency, which in turn may result in delirium. In fact, high levels of phenylalanine (common in postoperative or posttraumatic catabolic states) and low tryptophan-to-phenylalanine ratios have been associated with delirium in several medical and surgical cohorts.

Other mechanisms for delirium may be important in other settings. In patients with infections or cancer, delirium may be mediated through cytokines, particularly interleukin-2 and tumor necrosis factor. Other neurotransmitter systems, including γ-aminobutyric acid and dopamine, are also involved in some cases of delirium. The evidence for most of these mechanisms is based on cross-sectional comparisons of patients with and without delirium. Obtaining better longitudinal data, in which blood samples are examined at several time points in the same patient, is a crucial next step. In addition, more research is necessary to determine what mechanisms are most important in which patient populations, to begin to design targeted, pathophysiologically based preventive or treatment strategies.

RISK FACTORS

In the absence of a clear neuropathophysiologic basis for delirium, the cornerstone of its management focuses on the assessment and treatment of modifiable risk factors. Fortunately, research has identified several consistent risk factors for delirium. These risk factors classify into two groups: baseline factors that predispose patients to delirium, and acute factors that precipitate delirium. Among the predisposing factors, advanced age, preexisting dementia, preexisting functional impairment in activities of daily living, and high medical comorbidity are consistent risk factors. Male gender, sensory impairment (poor vision and hearing), and history of alcohol abuse have also been reported by some studies. Among acute precipitating factors, medications, especially those that are sedating or highly anticholinergic, uncontrolled pain, low hematocrit level, bed rest, and use of certain indwelling devices and restraints have been associated with the development of delirium. A useful model suggests that delirium is precipitated when the sum of predisposing and precipitating factors crosses a certain threshold. In such a model, the greater the predisposing factors, the fewer precipitating factors are required to initiate delirium. This would explain why older, frail persons develop delirium in the face of stressors that are much less severe than those that can cause delirium in younger, healthy persons. A mnemonic for reversible risk factors for delirium is presented in Table 32.3.

POSTOPERATIVE DELIRIUM

Delirium may be the most common complication after surgery in older persons. There is a 15% incidence after elective noncardiac surgery, and the incidence may exceed 50% after emergency procedures such as hip fracture repair. A prospectively validated clinical prediction rule for delirium after elective noncardiac surgery described seven risk factors that can be identified preoperatively: advanced age, cognitive impairment, physical functional impairment, history of alcohol abuse, markedly abnormal serum chemistries, intrathoracic surgery, and aortic aneurysm surgery. Patients

Table 32.3—Mnemonic for Reversible Causes of Delirium

Drugs	Any new additions, increased doses, or interactions Consider over-the-counter drugs and alcohol Consider esp. high-risk drugs (see Table 32.5)
Electrolyte disturbances	Especially dehydration, sodium imbalance Thyroid abnormalities
Lack of drugs	Withdrawals from chronically used sedatives, including alcohol and sleeping pills Poorly controlled pain (lack of analgesia)
Infection	Especially urinary and respiratory tract infections
Reduced sensory input	Poor vision, poor hearing
Intracranial	Infection, hemorrhage, stroke, tumor Rare: consider only if new focal neurologic findings, suggestive history, or work-up otherwise negative
Urinary, fecal	Urinary retention: "cystocerebral syndrome" Fecal impaction
Myocardial, pulmonary	Myocardial infarction, arrhythmia, exacerbation of heart failure, exacerbation of chronic obstructive pulmonary disease, hypoxia

with none of these risk factors had a 2% risk of delirium, those with one or two risk factors had a 10% risk, and those with three or more risk factors had a 50% risk.

In addition to baseline risk factors, postoperative management plays an important role in the development of delirium. Contrary to popular belief, the peak incidence of delirium is not immediately upon emergence from anesthesia, but on the second postoperative day. The stresses of surgery and anesthesia are not likely to be the sole precipitants of most cases of postoperative delirium.

Several studies have demonstrated that the route of intraoperative anesthesia, whether general, spinal, epidural, or other, has little impact on the risk of delirium. Postoperative medication management plays a much more important role. Postoperative use of benzodiazepines and certain opioids, especially meperidine, is strongly associated with the development of delirium. Although pain medications can cause delirium, adequate pain management is also important, because high levels of postoperative pain have also been associated with delirium. Strategies to provide adequate analgesia with minimal doses of opioids should be employed. These include the use of scheduled rather than as-needed dosing, patient-controlled or regional analgesia, and opioid-sparing analgesics such as acetaminophen or nonpharmacologic approaches, such as ice packs. Low postoperative hematocrit level (< 30%) has also been associated with postoperative delirium. Appropriate transfusion of high-risk patients should be considered, especially after elective procedures for which autologous blood is available, though transfusions have not yet been shown to reduce delirium.

In recent years, several studies have documented the high incidence of cognitive dysfunction in patients who have undergone coronary artery bypass graft surgery (CABG). Although the exact nature and frequency of this dysfunction remains an area of active study, one large longitudinal study showed a 53% incidence of cognitive decline at hospital discharge, 36% at 6 weeks, and 24% at 6 months. Although post-CABG cognitive dysfunction is sometimes referred to as "pump head," studies have failed to find significant differences in cognitive outcomes of those undergoing on-pump as opposed to off-pump surgery, a finding that belies this name. None of the existing studies of cognitive outcomes after CABG have explicitly assessed for delirium, so the interplay between delirium and these more global measures of cognitive dysfunction remains unknown.

EVALUATION

All patients with newly diagnosed delirium require a careful history, physical examination, and targeted laboratory testing. Most of the treatable causes for delirium lie outside the central nervous system, and these should be investigated first. Moreover, multiple contributing factors are often present, so the work-up should not be terminated because a single "cause" is identified. Key steps in the evaluation and management of delirium are summarized in Table 32.4.

The history should focus on the time course of the changes in mental status and their association with other symptoms or events (eg, fever, shortness of breath, medication change). Because medications are the most common and treatable cause of delirium, a careful medication history, using the nursing administration sheets in the hospital or a "brown-bag" review in the outpatient setting, is imperative. In the outpatient setting, it is also important to review the patient's use of over-the-counter drugs and alcohol. The physical examination should include vital signs and oxygen saturation, a careful general medical examination, and a neurologic and mental status examination. The emphasis should be on identifying acute medical problems or exacerbations of chronic medical problems that might be contributing to delirium. Laboratory tests should be selected on the basis of history and examination findings. Most patients require at least a complete blood cell count, electrolytes, and kidney function tests. Urinalysis, tests for liver function, serum drug levels, and arterial blood gases, as well as chest radiograms, electrocardiogram, and appropriate cultures are helpful in selected situations. Cerebral imaging is often performed but is rarely helpful, except in cases of head trauma or new focal neurologic findings. In the absence of seizure activity or signs of meningitis, electroencephalograms and cerebrospinal fluid analysis rarely yield helpful results.

MANAGEMENT

Delirious hospitalized patients are particularly vulnerable to complications and poor outcomes and must be given special care. This requires an interdisciplinary effort by physicians, nurses, family members, and others involved in the care of the patient. A multifactorial approach is the most successful since many factors contribute to delirium; thus, multiple interventions, even if individually small, may yield marked clinical improvement (See Table 32.4). Failure to diagnose and manage delirium properly may result in costly and life-threatening complications and long-term loss of function.

Modifying the risk factors that contribute to delirium is critically important. Some factors, such as age and prior cognitive impairment, cannot be modified. However, even some predisposing factors, such as sensory impairment, may be modifiable through proper use of eyeglasses and hearing aids. Drugs are the most

Table 32.4—Management of Delirium

Step	Key Issues	Proposed Treatment
1. Identify and treat reversible contributors	Medications	Reduce or eliminate offending medications, or substitute less psychoactive medications
	Infections	Treat common infections: urinary, respiratory, soft-tissue
	Fluid balance disorders	Assess and treat dehydration, heart failure, electrolyte disorders
	Impaired CNS oxygenation	Treat severe anemia (transfusion), hypoxia, hypotension
	Severe pain	Assess and treat; use local measures and scheduled pain regimens that minimize opioids Avoid meperidine
	Sensory deprivation	Use eyeglasses, hearing aid, portable amplifier
	Elimination problems	Assess and treat urinary retention and fecal impaction
2. Maintain behavioral control	Behavioral interventions	Teach hospital staff appropriate interaction with delirious patients Encourage family visitation
	Pharmacologic interventions	If necessary, use low-dose high-potency antipsychotics (see Table 32.6)
3. Anticipate and prevent or manage complications	Urinary incontinence	Implement scheduled toileting program
	Immobility and falls	Avoid physical restraints; mobilize with assistance; employ physical therapy
	Pressure ulcers	Mobilize Reposition immobilized patient frequently and monitor pressure points
	Sleep disturbance	Implement a nonpharmacologic sleep hygiene program, including a nighttime sleep protocol Avoid sedatives
	Feeding disorders	Assist with feeding; use aspiration precautions; provide nutritional supplementation as necessary
4. Restore function in delirious patients	Hospital environment	Reduce clutter and noise (esp. at night); provide adequate lighting; have familiar objects brought from home
	Cognitive reconditioning	Have staff reorient patient to time, place, person at least three times daily
	Ability to perform ADLs	As delirium clears, match performance to capacity
	Family education, support, and participation	Provide education about delirium, its causes, its reversibility, how to interact, and family's role in restoration of function
	Discharge	As delirium may persist, provide for increased ADLs support; follow mental status changes as "barometer" of recovery

NOTE: ADLs = activities of daily living; CNS = central nervous system.

common reversible causes of delirium. Anticholinergics, H_2-blockers, benzodiazepines, opioids, and antipsychotic medications should be replaced with drugs that have no central effects. For example, H_2-blockers may be replaced by antacids or proton-pump inhibitors, and regular dosing of 1 g of acetaminophen three to four times daily may reduce or eliminate the need for opioids in many patients (see Table 32.5).

The delirious patient is susceptible to a wide range of iatrogenic complications, and careful surveillance is critical. Bowel and bladder function should be monitored closely, but urinary catheters, which can lead to urinary tract infection, are to be avoided unless absolutely required for monitoring fluids or treating urinary retention. Bowel stimulants and stool softeners can be used to prevent obstipation, particularly in those who are concomitantly using opioids. Complete bed rest should be avoided, as it may lead to increasing disability through disuse of muscles and the development of pressure ulcers and atelectasis in the lungs. Exercise and ambulation prevent the deconditioning often associated with hospitalization. Malnutrition can be avoided through the use of nutritional supplements and careful attention to intake of food and fluids. Some delirious patients may need assistance in feeding.

Managing behavioral problems while ensuring both the comfort and safety of the patient can be challenging. The patient should be placed in a room near the nursing station for close observation. Nonpharmacologic behavioral measures provide orientation and a feeling of safety. Orienting items such as

Table 32.5—Drugs to Reduce or Eliminate in the Management of Delirium

Agent	Adverse Effects	Possible Substitutes	Comments
Alcohol	CNS sedation and withdrawal	If history of heavy intake, careful monitoring and benzodiazepines if withdrawal symptoms	Alcohol history is imperative
Anticholinergics (oxybutynin, benztropine)	Anticholinergic toxicity	A lower dose, behavioral measures	Rare at low doses
Anticonvulsants (esp. primidone, phenobarbital, phenytoin)	CNS sedation and withdrawal	Alternative agent or none	Toxic reactions can occur despite "therapeutic" drug levels
Antidepressants, esp. tertiary amine tricyclic agents (amitriptyline, imipramine, doxepin)	Anticholinergic toxicity	Secondary amine tricyclics (nortriptyline, desipramine) SSRIs or other agents	Secondary amines as good as tertiary for adjuvant treatment of chronic pain
Antihistamines (including diphenhydramine)	Anticholinergic toxicity	Nonpharmacologic protocol for sleep; pseudoephedrine for colds	Must take OTC medication history
Antiparkinsonian agents (levodopa-carbidopa, dopamine agonists, amantadine)	Dopaminergic toxicity	A lower dose; adjusted dosing schedule	Usually with end-stage disease and high doses
Antipsychotics, esp. low-potency anticholinergic agents and atypical agents (clozapine)	Anticholinergic toxicity; CNS sedation	No agents or, if necessary, low-dose high-potency agents	See note to Table 32.6 for warnings about atypical antipsychotics
Barbiturates	CNS sedation; severe withdrawal syndrome	Gradual discontinuation or benzodiazepine	In most cases, should no longer be prescribed; avoid inadvertent or abrupt discontinuation
Benzodiazepines, esp. long-acting (including diazepam, flurazepam, chlordiazepoxide)	CNS sedation	Nonpharmacologic sleep management; intermediate agents (lorazepam, temazepam)	Associated with delirium in medical and surgical patients
Benzodiazepines: ultra short-acting (including triazolam, alprazolam)	CNS sedation and withdrawal	Nonpharmacologic sleep management; intermediate agents (lorazepam, temazepam)	Associated with delirium in case reports and series
Chloral hydrate	CNS sedation	Nonpharmacologic sleep protocol	No better for delirium than benzodiazepines
H_2-blocking agents	Possible anticholinergic toxicity	A lower dosage; antacids or proton-pump inhibitors	Most common with high-dose intravenous infusions
Nonbenzodiazepine hypnotics (eg, zolpidem)	CNS sedation and withdrawal	Nonpharmacologic sleep protocol	Like other sedatives, can cause delirium
Opioid analgesics (esp. meperidine)	Anticholinergic toxicity, CNS sedation, fecal impaction	Local measures and nonpsychoactive pain medications around the clock; opioids only for breakthrough and severe pain	Higher risk in patients with renal insufficiency; must titrate risks from drugs versus risks from pain
Almost any medication if time course is appropriate			**Consider risks and benefits of all medications in the elderly patient**

NOTE: CNS = central nervous system; OTC = over-the-counter; SSRI = selective serotonin-reuptake inhibitor.

clocks, calendars, and even a window view should be made available. Patients should be encouraged to wear their eyeglasses and hearing aids. Although physical restraint use has not been well studied in the hospital, evidence from the long-term-care setting suggests that such restraints probably do not decrease the rate of falls by confused ambulatory patients, and they may actually increase the risk of fall-related injury. Restraints, though objectionable, may be required be-cause of violent behavior or to prevent the removal of important devices, such as endotracheal tubes, intra-arterial devices, and catheters. Even for persons with these devices, the calm reassurance provided by a sitter or family member may be much more effective than the use of physical restraints or drugs. Whenever restraints are used, the indicators for use should be frequently reassessed, and the restraints should be removed as soon as possible.

When drugs are used as restraints to "save staff time," they extract a costly toll in accidents, adverse effects, and loss of mobility, and they should be avoided if possible. Chemical intervention may be necessary for symptoms such as delusions or hallucinations that are frightening to the patient when verbal comfort and reassurance are not successful. Some delirious patients display behavior that is dangerous to themselves or others and cannot be calmed by the provision of a sitter or family companionship. However, the mere presence of delirium is not an indication for pharmacologic intervention. Indications for such interventions should be clearly identified, documented, and constantly reassessed.

When medications are used, high-potency antipsychotics are preferred because of their low anticholinergic potency and minimal hypotensive effects. However, these medications must be used cautiously, as they may actually prolong delirium and may increase the risk of complications by converting a hyperactive, confused patient into a stuporous one whose risk of a fall or aspiration is increased. In older patients with mild delirium, low doses of haloperidol[OL]

(0.5 to 1 mg orally or 0.25 to 0.5 mg parenterally) should be used initially, with careful reassessment prior to additional dosing. In more severe delirium, somewhat higher doses may be used initially (0.5 to 2 mg parenterally), with additional dosing every 60 minutes as required for symptom management. One must be careful to assess for akathisia (motor restlessness), which may be an adverse effect of high-potency antipsychotic medications and can be confused with worsening delirium. The treatment for akathisia is less, not more antipsychotic medication. Because of extrapyramidal effects, haloperidol should be avoided in older persons with parkinsonism, and a benzodiazepine such as lorazepam[OL] may be substituted. Low doses of atypical antipsychotic agents may be effective in delirium, as well. (The atypical antipsychotics have been found to be associated with increased risk of stoke and mortality, primarily in long-term use for agitation in dementia.) The pharmacologic management of agitated delirium is summarized in Table 32.6.

High-dose intravenous haloperidol may be the drug of choice for critically ill patients in intensive care.

Table 32.6—Pharmacologic Therapy of Agitated Delirium

Agent	Mechanism of Action	Dosage	Benefits	Adverse Effects	Comments
Haloperidol[OL]	Antipsychotic	0.25–1.0 mg po or IV q 4 h prn agitation	Relatively nonsedating; few hemodynamic effects	EPS, esp. if > 3 mg per day	Usually, agent of choice*
Lorazepam[OL]	Sedative	0.25–1.0 mg po or IV tid prn agitation	Use in sedative and alcohol withdrawal, Parkinson's, Lewy body disease, and history of neuroleptic malignant syndrome	More paradoxical excitation, respiratory depression than haloperidol	Second-line agent, except in specific cases noted
Olanzapine[OL]	Antipsychotic	2.5–10 mg po qd	Fewer EPS than haloperidol	More sedating than haloperidol	Small case series only**
		dissolving tablet: 2.5–10 mg po qd			Oral formulations are less effective for acute management
		IV or IM: 2.5–10 mg qd			
Quetiapine[OL]	Antipsychotic	25–50 mg po bid	Fewer EPS than haloperidol	Hypotension	Small case series**
Risperidone[OL]	Antipsychotic	0.25–1.0 mg po or IV q 4 h prn agitation	Similar to haloperidol	Might have slightly fewer EPS	Case series only**

NOTE: bid = twice a day; EPS = extrapyramidal symptoms; h = hour; IM = intramuscularly; IV = intravenously; prn = as needed; po = by mouth; q = each; qd = each day; tid = three times a day.

* In a randomized trial comparing haloperidol, chlorpromazine, and lorazepam in the treatment of agitated delirium in young patients with AIDS, all were found to be equally effective, but haloperidol had the fewest side effects or adverse sequelae.

** The U.S. Food and Drug Administration has attached warnings to the atypical antipsychotics because of the increased risk of stroke and mortality that as been found to be associated with their long-term use, primarily for agitation in dementia.

[OL] Not approved by the U.S. Food and Drug Administration for this use.

For such patients, the risk-benefit ratio of medication adverse effects versus the removal of lines and devices often favors pharmacologic treatment. Such therapy must be used with special caution in older persons. In addition to extrapyramidal effects, the potential for QT interval prolongation and torsades de pointes, neuroleptic malignant syndrome, and withdrawal dyskinesias are important concerns. As with physical restraints, in all cases where pharmacologic restraints are used, the health care team must clearly identify the target symptoms necessitating their use, frequently review the efficacy of the sedative or antipsychotic in controlling the target symptoms, and assess the patient for adverse effects and complications.

It is important to stress to family members that delirium is usually not a permanent condition, but rather that it improves over time. Unfortunately, the persistence of delirium is common. Thus, when counseling families, it is important to point out that many cognitive deficits associated with the delirium syndrome can continue, abating only weeks and even months following the illness. Advanced age (85 years or older), preexisting cognitive impairment, and severe illness are risk factors for slow recovery of cognitive function. Careful monitoring of mental status and provision of adequate functional supports during this period are necessary to give the patient the maximum chance of returning to his or her baseline level. Family members can play an important role in the hospital and postacute setting by providing appropriate orientation, support, and functional assistance. Hospitals are increasingly making provisions for family members to sleep overnight with relatives who are already delirious or at high risk for developing delirium. While symptoms of delirium may persist, acute exacerbation of cognitive dysfunction is not expected during the convalescent period and therefore likely heralds a new medical problem. Families should be counseled to seek prompt medical attention if patient's mental status acutely worsens.

PREVENTION

Finally, it should be stated that the most effective way to manage delirium is to prevent it from developing in the first place. A study demonstrated that a unit-based proactive multifactorial intervention can reduce the incidence of delirium among older hospitalized patients aged 70 or older by more than one third (adjusted odds ratio = 0.60, 95% confidence interval, 0.39 to 0.92). Six intervention components were used selectively on the basis of patient-specific risk factors determined at an admission assessment. These included interventions for cognitive impairment, sleep deprivation, immobility, visual impairment, hearing impair-

ment, and dehydration. Among these, the most creative and successful was a nonpharmacologic sleep protocol that involved trained volunteers offering patients warm milk, back rubs, and soothing music at bedtime; this intervention substantially reduced the use of sedative-hypnotic medication. Similar programs to prevent delirium should be developed and implemented in hospitals and other settings that care for acutely ill elderly patients. One example of such programs is the Hospital Elder Life Program (HELP), which is currently being disseminated to hospitals (see http://elderlife.med.yale.edu/public/public-main.php?pageid=01.00.00).

Although a unit-based intervention can be highly successful, it may be difficult to apply in all settings, especially in surgical patients. A randomized trial demonstrated that proactive geriatrics consultation can reduce the incidence of delirium in elderly patients undergoing hip fracture repair. Consultation began in most cases preoperatively and continued throughout the duration of hospitalization. Daily recommendations were based on a structured protocol that covered key elements in delirium prevention, such as limitation of psychoactive medications; 77% adherence was achieved. The geriatrics consultation group achieved a reduction in the incidence of delirium (32% versus 50% usual care, $P < .05$) of similar magnitude to the unit-based protocol described above. Geriatrics consultation, if performed proactively and intensively, may be an important strategy for preventing delirium in high-risk surgical patients.

Even though multifactorial intervention is effective in preventing delirium, existing data suggest that it may be less effective in treating established delirium. The two studies cited above failed to show an effect on delirium once it developed. Moreover, a recent study randomized 227 patients with prevalent or incident delirium on a general medical unit to either geriatric specialist consultation and follow-up care by an intervention nurse, or usual care. No differences were found in the rate of improvement of delirium symptoms, functional recovery, or discharge to the community between the two groups. This study provides a sobering reminder of the need for more research on how to optimally manage the delirious patient and the development of novel approaches based on a better understanding of the pathophysiology of this common, morbid, and costly syndrome.

ANNOTATED REFERENCES

■ Cole MG, McCusker J, Bellevance F, et al. Systematic detection and multidisciplinary care of delirium in older medical inpatients: a randomized trial. *CMAJ*. 2002; 167(7):753–759.

This article describes the results of a randomized trial for the management of established delirium in general medical patients. A total of 227 hospitalized patients aged 65 or older were randomized to geriatric specialist consultation versus usual care. Consultation patients were followed by an intervention nurse for up to 8 weeks or until hospital discharge. Overall, 48% of those in the intervention group and 45% of those in the control group met the criteria for improvement. There were no significant differences between the two groups in improvement of delirium symptoms, functional recovery, length of stay, discharge to the community, or survival. There was a trend toward benefit from consultation among those without preexisting dementia and those with less comorbidity. This article questions the adequacy of the current paradigms for the management of established delirium and suggests that further research is needed to develop new, more effective approaches.

- Ely EW, Inouye SK, Bernard GR, et al. Delirium in mechanically ventilated patients: validity and reliability of the Confusion Assessment Method for the intensive care unit (CAM-ICU). *JAMA*. 2001;286(21):2703–2710.

    This article describes the development of the Confusion Assessment Method for the Intensive Care Unit (CAM-ICU). The CAM-ICU assesses the same four features as the original Confusion Assessment Method (CAM) but does not require verbal responses from the patient and therefore can be used in mechanically ventilated patients. The CAM assesses attention using the Attention Screening Examination, in which patients are required to remember and recognize simple pictures. Disorganized thinking is tested by responses to a series of simple yes-no questions (eg, "Does 1 pound weigh more than 2 pounds?"). When used by trained study nurses, the CAM-ICU had better than 95% sensitivity and specificity in comparison with the reference standard (diagnosis by a geriatric psychiatrist or geriatrician), and high inter-rater reliability. Delirium occurred in 83% of patients during their ICU stay and persisted in 10% of patients at the time of hospital discharge.

- Inouye SK, Bogardus ST Jr, Charpentier PA, et al. A multicomponent intervention to prevent delirium in hospitalized older patients. *N Engl J Med*. 1999;340(9):669–676.

    This seminal article describes the results of a multicomponent acute hospital unit–based intervention to prevent delirium. The intervention consisted of standardized protocols for the management of six risk factors for delirium: cognitive impairment, sleep deprivation, immobility, visual impairment, hearing impairment, and dehydration. The overall rate of adherence to the intervention was very high, at 87%. Delirium developed in 9.9% of the intervention group, compared with 15% of the usual-care group (matched odds ratio 0.60, 95% confidence interval, 0.39 to 0.92). Among the targeted risk factors, the intervention was associated with significant improvement in the degree of cognitive impairment among patients with cognitive impairment on admission, and a significant reduction in the use of sleep medications among all patients. Interestingly, the severity of delirium and recurrence rates was not different in the two groups, suggesting that the primary prevention of delirium is probably the most effective treatment strategy.

- Inouye SK, Foreman MD, Mion LC, et al. Nurses' recognition of delirium and its symptoms. *Arch Intern Med*. 2001;161(20):2467–2473.

    This article compares the detection of delirium using the CAM as applied by trained primary care nurses using observations from clinical care and by trained research staff using observations from formal mental status assessment. In comparison with that of the research staff, the sensitivity of nursing assessments was poor: 19% per assessment and 31% over the entire hospitalization. Significant risk factors for the nonrecognition of delirium by the nursing staff included hypoactive ("quiet") delirium, preexisting dementia, advanced age, and visual impairment. These findings confirm the importance of formal mental status assessment prior to the application of the CAM algorithm, even when done by clinical staff presumably familiar with the patient.

- Inouye SK, van Dyck CH, Alessi CA, et al. Clarifying confusion: the Confusion Assessment Method: a new method for detection of delirium. *Ann Intern Med*. 1990;113(12):941–948.

    This is the original prospective study validating the Confusion Assessment Method (CAM) as a tool to enable clinicians to quickly and accurately detect delirium. It was found to be highly sensitive and specific, with both high positive and negative predictive accuracy. The interobserver reliability of the CAM was also high.

- Kiely DK, Bergmann MA, Murphy KM, et al. Delirium among newly admitted post-acute facility patients: prevalence, symptoms, and severity. *J Gerontol A Biol Sci Med Sci*. 2003; 58(5): M441–M445.

    This article describes the prevalence of delirium among 2158 elderly patients admitted to seven postacute skilled nursing facilities. Of these, 16% met full CAM criteria for delirium, and an additional 49% met the criteria for subsyndromal delirium (one or more key CAM features). All individual symptoms of delirium were more common among the delirious patients, except for sleep-wake cycle disturbance, which was equally common in the nondelirious group. This study points out the high prevalence of delirium and delirium symptoms in the postacute setting. Efforts are under way to improve the awareness of delirium among postacute facility staff. Persistent delirium has been included among the newly published quality indicators for postacute care by the Centers for Medicare and Medicaid Services.

- Trzepacz P, Breitbart W, Franklin J, et al. Practice guideline for the treatment of patients with delirium. Web site of the American Psychiatric Association; 1999. Available at http://www.psych.org/psych_pract/treatg/pg/pg_delirium.cfm (accessed October 2005).

    This Web site, developed by the American Psychiatric Association in 1999, is a thorough, detailed, evidence-based document on the causes, natural history, diagnosis, management, and treatment of delirium. It contains insightful recommendations on how to help the patient, medical team, and family understand the illness. It is written primarily for psychiatrists, but it is full of important and well-researched information for physicians of any specialty. The authors state that the document is to be updated every 3 to 5 years.

Edward R. Marcantonio, MD, SM

CHAPTER 33—SLEEP PROBLEMS

KEY POINTS

- Studies show an association between sleep complaints and risk factors for sleep disturbance (eg, chronic illness, mood disturbance, less physical activity, and physical disability) but little association with older age, suggesting that these risk factors rather than aging itself account for insomnia in the majority of those studied.

- Notable age-related changes in sleep structure as measured by polysomnography include a decrease in stage 3 and stage 4 sleep (the deeper stages of sleep) with an increase or maintenance of stages 1 and 2 (the lighter stages of sleep).

- Insomnia is usually due to psychiatric, medical, or neurologic illness; excessive daytime sleepiness is usually due to a primary sleep disorder, such as sleep apnea.

- The appropriate treatment of sleep problems must be guided by knowledge of likely causes and potential contributing factors. Trials have shown that nonpharmacologic interventions can be quite effective in improving sleep in older adults.

EPIDEMIOLOGY

Several studies have documented a high prevalence of sleeping problems among older people. In one representative sample, the most common sleeping complaints among community-dwelling older people were found to be difficulty falling asleep (37% of the sample), nighttime awakening (29%), and early morning awakening (19%). Daytime sleepiness is also common, with 20% of noninstitutionalized Americans reporting that they are "usually sleepy in the daytime." As a result of such complaints, at least one half of community-dwelling older people use either over-the-counter or prescription sleeping medications.

Three large epidemiologic studies of older people found an association between sleep complaints and risk factors for sleep disturbance (eg, chronic illness, mood disturbance, less physical activity, and physical disability) but little association with older age, suggesting that these risk factors, rather than aging per se, account for insomnia in the majority of those studied. However, some primary sleep disorders, such as sleep apnea and periodic limb movements in sleep, increase in prevalence with age. Although some studies have shown an increased risk of sleep complaints in women, others have not. Studies have shown that self-reported sleeping difficulties are more common in older black Americans, particularly women and those with depression and chronic illness.

Unfortunately, late-life insomnia is commonly a chronic problem. A study of older people in Britain found that 36% of those with insomnia at baseline reported severely disrupted sleep 4 years later. Of those who reported the use of prescription hypnotics at baseline, 32% were still using these agents 4 years later. Another study of a volunteer sample of urban women aged 85 years and older found that all had health problems and sleeping difficulties, and the majority regularly used alcohol, an over-the-counter sleeping medication, or both, in an effort to improve their sleep. Previous research has suggested that insomnia is a predictor of death and nursing-home placement in older men, but not in older women.

CHANGES IN SLEEP WITH AGING

Older people have a decreased sleep efficiency (time asleep divided by time in bed), a stable or decreased total sleep time, and an increased sleep latency (time to fall asleep). Older people also report an earlier bedtime and earlier morning awakening, more arousals during the night, and more daytime napping. Notable age-related changes in sleep structure as measured by polysomnography include a decrease in stage 3 and stage 4 sleep (the deeper stages of sleep). Stages 1 and 2 (the lighter stages of sleep) increase or remain the same. The decline in deep sleep seems to begin in early adulthood and progresses throughout life. In persons over age 90 years, stages 3 and 4 may disappear completely. Other common findings include an earlier onset of rapid-eye-movement (REM) sleep in the night and decreased total REM sleep but no change or a decrease in percentage of REM sleep. Older people have more equal distribution of REM sleep throughout the night, whereas younger people have longer periods of REM sleep as the night progresses. Older persons also have a decrease in sleep spindles and K complexes on electroencephalogram during sleep.

The significance of these changes in sleep is unclear. Most experts believe that the decreased sleep in older people is due to a decreased *ability* to sleep, rather than a decreased *need* for sleep. However, some research has shown that after a period of sleep deprivation older people show less daytime sleepiness, less evidence of decline in performance measures, and a quicker recovery of normal sleep structure than younger people. Older people have more sleep disturbance with jet lag and shift work, which may reflect physiologic changes in circadian rhythm with age. In addition, it is not clear to what extent changes in sleep are due to changes of normal aging or to pathologic changes from other processes. In studies comparing good sleepers with poor sleepers, poor sleepers were found to take more medications, make more physician visits, and have poorer self-ratings of health. In addition, as noted above, chronologic age per se does not seem to correlate with higher prevalence of poor sleep.

EVALUATION OF SLEEP

To aid in screening older patients for sleep problems, several years ago the National Institutes of Health Consensus Statement on the Treatment of Sleep Disorders of Older People suggested that clinicians ask three simple questions:

- Is the person satisfied with his or her sleep?
- Does sleep or fatigue interfere with daytime activities?
- Does the bed partner or others complain of unusual behavior during sleep, such as snoring, interrupted breathing, or leg movements?

These, or similar screening questions, can be quite useful to identify sleep complaints in the older patient. Transient sleep problems (eg, those lasting less than 2 to 3 weeks) are usually situational; persistent sleep problems are likely to require more detailed evaluation.

The initial and subsequent office evaluations of a patient with persistent sleep complaints can be rather lengthy. To obtain a careful description of the sleep complaint, it may be helpful to have the patient keep a sleep log, recording each morning the time spent in bed, the estimated amount of sleep, the number of awakenings, the time of morning awakening, and any symptoms that occurred during the night. This should be supplemented by information from the bed partner, or others who may have observed unusual symptoms during the night. Several validated sleep questionnaires are available in the literature (see the annotated references at the end of the chapter). The focused physical examination depends on evidence from the history. For example, reports of painful joints should be followed by a careful examination of the affected areas. Reports of nocturia that disrupts sleep should be followed by evaluation for cardiac, renal, or prostatic disease, or diabetes mellitus. Careful mental status testing is also indicated. The findings of the history and physical examination should guide laboratory testing.

Polysomnography is indicated when the clinician suspects a primary sleep disorder, such as sleep apnea, periodic limb movement disorder, or violent or other unusual behaviors during sleep. Objective methods to measure sleep other than traditional polysomnography in a sleep laboratory have been developed and are being used more extensively in studies of sleep. Portable monitoring systems for use in the home have been developed and are used primarily to screen for sleep apnea. These systems generally measure pulse oximetry, heart rate, respiration, and nasal airflow. Although they are used extensively, research testing the validity of these systems is ongoing. Another methodology is a wrist-activity monitor, which estimates sleep versus wakefulness on the basis of the person's wrist activity. Some studies have demonstrated that the wrist monitor is sensitive enough to assess the efficacy of treatment for insomnia in older people. Observational measures for detecting sleep problems and sleep-related breathing disorders have been used for research in nursing-home residents.

COMMON SLEEP DISORDERS

Insomnia (ie, difficulty in initiating or maintaining sleep) is usually due to psychiatric, medical, or neurologic illness; excessive daytime sleepiness is usually due to a primary sleep disorder, such as sleep apnea. However, there is significant overlap among these symptoms. In one large study of patients of all ages referred to sleep disorders centers, insomnia was found to be most commonly due to psychiatric illness, psychophysiologic problems, drug or alcohol dependence, and restless legs syndrome; excessive daytime sleepiness was found to be most commonly due to sleep apnea, periodic limb movement disorder, or narcolepsy. However, patients referred to sleep centers are a select population, and the most common causes of excessive sleepiness in the community are probably chronic insufficient sleep (either voluntarily or because of work schedules), medical problems, or sleep-disruptive environmental conditions. Thus, the clinician should not exclude a primary sleep disorder in the patient presenting with insomnia and likewise should probably not refer every patient with daytime sleepiness to a sleep laboratory.

Psychiatric Disorders and Psychosocial Problems

Many studies report that psychiatric disorders are the cause of sleep problems in more than half of all patients presenting with insomnia. Depression is a particularly common cause. Early morning awakening is a common pattern, although increased sleep latency and more nighttime wakefulness are also seen. However, these changes may not be present or may be less marked in depressed persons who do not seek medical care. Conversely, sleep disturbance in older people who are not currently depressed may be an important predictor of future depression. In depressed older patients with sleep disturbance, treatment of depression may also improve the sleep abnormalities. Several studies using electroencephalography have found that antidepressant medications alter sleep architecture, suggesting that antidepressant drug efficacy may depend to some extent on regulation of sleep and changes in REM-sleep regulation. (See also "Depression and Other Mood Disorders," p 269.)

Bereavement can also affect sleep. Bereavement without major depression is not associated with significant changes in sleep measures, but people with bereavement and depression and those with major depression have identical sleep patterns. These sleep abnormalities improve with treatment of depression. Anxiety and stress can also be associated with sleeping difficulty, usually difficulty with initiating sleep or perhaps early awakening. Patients may have difficulty falling asleep because of excessive worrying at bedtime. (See also "Anxiety Disorders," p 281.) Research has found that older caregivers report more sleep complaints than do similarly aged noncaregivers. In one study, nearly 40% of older women who were family caregivers of adults with dementia reported using a sleeping medication for themselves in the past month. (See also the sections on caregiving in "Psychosocial Issues," p 18; "Community-Based Care," p 128; and "Elder Mistreatment," p 89.)

Drug and Alcohol Dependency

Drug and alcohol use account for 10% to 15% of cases of insomnia. Chronic use of sedatives may cause light, fragmented sleep. Many sleeping medications, when used chronically, lead to tolerance and the potential for increasing doses. When chronic hypnotic use is suddenly stopped, rebound insomnia may occur, and the person may start taking the medication again.

Alcohol abuse is often associated with lighter sleep of shorter duration. In addition, some persons try to treat their sleeping difficulties with alcohol. Older persons with poor sleep should be instructed to avoid nighttime alcohol because although alcohol causes an initial drowsiness, it can impair sleep later in the night. Finally, it is important to remember that sedatives and alcohol can worsen sleep apnea; the use of these respiratory depressants should be avoided in older persons with documented or suspected untreated sleep apnea. (See also "Alcohol and Drug Abuse," p 298.)

Medical Problems

Examples of treatable medical problems that may contribute to sleep difficulty in older people include pain from arthritis and other conditions, paresthesias, cough, dyspnea from cardiac or pulmonary illness, gastroesophageal reflux, and nighttime urination. In patients with sleeping difficulties who describe pain at night, assessment and management of the painful condition is the appropriate approach (see "Persistent Pain," p 140). Nighttime urination may be associated with sleep disorder, poorer quality of sleep, nighttime thirst, and increased fatigue in the daytime.

Sleep can be impaired by diuretics or stimulating agents (eg, caffeine, sympathomimetics, and bronchodilators) taken near bedtime. Some antidepressants, antiparkinson agents, and antihypertensives (eg, propranolol) can induce nightmares and impair sleep. Required medications that are sedating (eg, sedating antidepressants) should be given at bedtime if possible.

Sleep Apnea

Sleep apnea is a disorder of periodic reductions in ventilation during sleep. Various terms have been used for this syndrome (eg, *sleep-related breathing disorder*, *sleep-disordered breathing*), but *sleep apnea* remains the term used by most clinicians. Patients with obstructive sleep apnea usually present with excessive daytime sleepiness and are typically unaware of their frequent arousals at night that are associated with reductions in ventilation. Patients are often obese and may have morning headache, personality changes, poor memory, confusion, and irritability. A bed partner may report loud snoring, cessation of breathing, and choking sounds during sleep.

The reported prevalence of sleep apnea among older persons varies from 20% to 70%, depending on the population studied. The prevalence of sleep apnea increases with age. Sleep apnea is very common among patients referred to sleep centers for evaluation of daytime sleepiness, reportedly occurring in 70% of such patients. The most important predictor of obstructive sleep apnea is large body mass. Other reported predictors identified in community-dwelling elderly persons include falling asleep at inappropriate times, male gender, and napping. The classic sleep apnea patient is the obese, sleepy snorer with hypertension. Large neck circumference has also been reported as a marker for sleep apnea.

Alcoholism is an important risk factor for sleep apnea, and sleep-disordered breathing is a significant contributor to sleep disturbance in men over age 40 with a history of alcoholism. Finally, there appears to be an association between sleep apnea and dementia. One nursing-home study found that sleep apnea is associated with dementia, and the sleep disorder was found to be positively correlated with the severity of dementia. However, another study concluded that sleep-disordered breathing in Alzheimer's patients is mild and not associated with mental status or behavioral changes.

The importance of mild degrees of sleep-disordered breathing in elderly persons is unclear. One study found no association between mild or moderate sleep-disordered breathing and subjective sleep-wake disturbance. The long-term consequences of asymptomatic sleep-disordered breathing are also unclear.

Patients suspected of having sleep apnea should be referred to a sleep laboratory for evaluation and, if the diagnosis is documented, a trial of treatment. Home-based diagnostic systems are also available, but the validity of such systems (in comparison with polysomnography in a sleep laboratory) is not clear. There is conflicting evidence whether older patients tolerate the main treatment of obstructive sleep apnea, nasal continuous positive airway pressure (CPAP), as well as middle-aged patients. Careful efforts to use devices that improve comfort may improve adherence with CPAP. Unfortunately, there may be prejudice among clinicians against the use of nasal CPAP in older patients, perhaps because they assume that the treatment will not be tolerated or successful in this population. Oral appliances are an alternative treatment in some patients. Several upper airway surgical approaches have also been used.

Periodic Limb Movements During Sleep and Restless Legs Syndrome

Periodic limb movements during sleep (PLMS) is a condition of debilitating, repetitive, stereotypic leg movements that occur in non-REM sleep. The leg movements occur every 20 to 40 seconds and can last hours or even much of the night, and each movement may be associated with an arousal. The occurrence of PLMS increases with age. One study found evidence of PLMS in over one third of community-dwelling older persons. Correlates of PLMS included dissatisfaction with sleep, sleeping alone, and reported kicking at night. Some authors have suggested that the high prevalence of PLMS with age is associated with delayed motor and sensory latencies noted on nerve conduction testing. PLMS may present as difficulty maintaining sleep or excessive daytime sleepiness. A bed partner may be aware of the leg movements, or these movements may remain occult until identified in a sleep laboratory. When PLMS is associated with sleep complaints that are not explained by another sleep disorder, this is called periodic limb movement disorder (PLMD). Polysomnography is required to establish a diagnosis of PLMD.

The restless legs syndrome is a condition of an uncontrollable urge to move one's legs at night. The symptoms occur while the person is awake, and symptoms can also involve the arms. The diagnosis is based on the patient's description of symptoms, and the patient's complaint is usually of nighttime leg discomfort or difficulty in initiating sleep. Polysomnography is not required to make this diagnosis. There may be a family history of the condition and, in some cases, an underlying medical disorder (eg, anemia, or renal or neurologic disease). The prevalence of restless legs syndrome also increases with age. Many patients with the condition also have PLMS. In older patients with PLMD or restless legs syndrome, dopaminergic agents are the initial agent of choice. An evening dose of a dopamine agonist (eg, pramipexole[OL] or ropinirole) are commonly used for patients with frequent (eg, nightly) symptoms. A nighttime dose of carbidopa-levodopa[OL] can be used for patients who need medication infrequently (ie, for as-needed use). Some patients may describe a shift of their symptoms to daytime hours with successful treatment of symptoms at night. There is some evidence that patients with restless legs syndrome and a low serum ferritin level may improve with iron-replacement therapy. Benzodiazepines, anticonvulsants, and narcotics have also been used for restless leg syndrome but likely have more adverse effects in older people than the dopaminergic agents.

Disturbances in the Sleep-Wake Cycle

Disturbances in the sleep-wake cycle may be transient, as in jet lag, or associated with an obvious cause (eg, shift work). Some patients have persistent disturbance, with either a delayed sleep phase (fall asleep late and awaken late) or an advanced sleep phase (fall asleep early and awaken early). The advanced sleep phase is particularly common in older people. Some patients have persistent sleep-phase disturbance, in which circadian rhythms and sleeping period have become completely desynchronized (eg, persons who are always asleep during the day and awake at night), or sleep-wake cycles are irregular and sleep habits are very disjointed. It is unclear to what degree, if any, changes in sleep pattern in older people (such as increased daytime napping and disrupted nighttime sleep) are due to alterations in the circadian rhythm. Although results are mixed, several studies have shown age-related decreases in hormonal levels and evidence of earlier circadian rises in certain hormones, suggesting the existence of age-related alteration in circadian rhythm. Problems related to an advanced sleep phase may respond to appropriately timed exposure to bright light (see the section on nonpharmacologic interventions, p 255). Patients with a significant sleep-phase cycle disturbance should be referred to a sleep laboratory for evaluation. Dementia and delirium may also

[OL] Not approved by the U.S. Food and Drug Administration for this use.

cause sleep-wake disturbance, frequent nighttime awakenings, nighttime wandering, and nighttime agitation.

REM Sleep Behavior Disorder

REM sleep behavior disorder is characterized by excessive motor activities during sleep and a pathologic absence of the normal muscle atonia during REM sleep. The presenting symptoms are usually vigorous sleep behaviors associated with vivid dreams. These behaviors may result in injury (to the patient or bed partner). The condition may be acute or chronic, and it is more common in older men. There may be a family predisposition. Transient REM sleep behavior disorder has been associated with toxic-metabolic abnormalities, primarily drug or alcohol withdrawal or intoxication. The chronic form of the disorder is usually idiopathic or associated with a neurologic abnormality (eg, drug intoxication, vascular disease, tumor, infection, neurodegeneration disorders such as Parkinson's disease, or trauma). Several psychiatric medications have been associated with this disorder, including tricyclic antidepressants, monoamine oxidase inhibitors, fluoxetine, venlafaxine, cholinesterase inhibitors, and other agents. Polysomnography is recommended to establish the diagnosis. Removal of the offending agent is indicated for drug-induced REM sleep behavior disorder. Clonazepam[OL] is reported to be effective for the treatment of REM sleep behavior disorder, with little evidence of tolerance or abuse over long periods of treatment, but some patients may have adverse effects from this agent. There is some evidence for the use of melatonin in the treatment of REM sleep behavior disorder in patients with coexisting neurodegenerative disorders (eg, Parkinson's disease, dementia with Lewy bodies). Environmental safety interventions are also indicated, such as removing dangerous objects from the bedroom, putting cushions on the floor around the bed, protecting windows, and, in some cases, putting the mattress on the floor.

CHANGES IN SLEEP WITH DEMENTIA

Most studies of sleep in dementia have focused on Alzheimer's disease. Unfortunately, the baseline slowing of electroencephalographic activity often seen with dementia can cloud the distinction between sleep and wakefulness and between the various stages of non-REM sleep in the sleep laboratory. Older patients with dementia have more sleep disruption and arousals, lower sleep efficiency, a higher percentage of stage 1 sleep, and decreases in stage 3 and 4 sleep than do nondemented older people. Some authors have noted a decreased percentage of sleep spent in REM, but this has not been reported in all studies. Of interest, some studies suggest that older persons with dementia have less sleep disturbance than older depressed persons. Disturbances of the sleep-wake cycle are common with dementia, resulting in daytime sleep and nighttime wakefulness.

SLEEP DISTURBANCES IN THE HOSPITAL

Acute hospitalization is commonly cited as one of the stressors that can precipitate transient or short-term insomnia. This insomnia is likely multifactorial in origin and related to illness, medications, change from usual nighttime routines at home, and a sleep-disruptive hospital environment. For example, high noise levels have been documented in the acute hospital setting. Some nursing-based nonpharmacologic interventions to improve sleep have been tested. One small uncontrolled study described increased nighttime melatonin levels in hospitalized older patients treated with daytime bright-light exposure. Another small study implemented "flexible medication times" that allowed inpatients to sleep longer in the morning, and their resulting in-hospital sleeping patterns were more similar to their at-home sleeping patterns. However, adherence with nonpharmacologic interventions may be difficult to achieve in the acute hospital. For example, one large clinical trial of nonpharmacologic interventions to prevent delirium in hospitalized older people reported only a 10% adherence rate for the sleep protocol portion of the intervention.

Sleeping medications are commonly prescribed in hospitalized older people. A large Belgian study of consecutively admitted patients at a university hospital found that 45% of patients took a sleeping medication in hospital, with greater use among patients aged 60 years or older. In this sample, over 15% of patients who were newly prescribed a sleeping pill while in the hospital reported that they planned to use the medication after discharge to home. Another study of hospitalized older people in India found that among those prescribed a benzodiazepine agonist for sleep during their acute hospitalization, over half were not taking a sleeping pill prior to their admission. This study reported that the use of sleeping pills in the hospital did not increase the use of these agents after discharge home.

There is little research comparing the use of different sleeping medications in this setting. Benzodiazepine receptor agonists are very commonly used. Because of increased sensitivity in elderly patients, smaller doses may be effective as well as safer. Sedating antihistamines (eg, diphenhydramine) should

---

OL Not approved by the U.S. Food and Drug Administration for this use.

not be used as a sleep aid in hospitalized older people because of possible complications related to anticholinergic adverse effects (eg, delirium, urinary retention, and constipation).

It is important to keep in mind that sleep-related breathing disorders may be common in hospitalized adults, particularly among those with cardiac illness and stroke. A large random sample of older men on medicine wards in a Veterans Affairs hospital found a shorter survival among patients with heart failure with central sleep apnea than among heart failure patients without evidence of this disorder. An English study found that nearly one fourth of hospitalized patients (mean age 74 years) with an acute stroke who had normal oxygen levels during the daytime had 30 minutes or more of "unexpected" nocturnal hypoxia. A small study in Hong Kong found significant sleep-disordered breathing in nearly half of patients (mean age 64 years) hospitalized with an acute stroke. Another study found that one third of severely obese (body mass index $[kg/m^2] \geq 35$) hospitalized people had unexplained hypoventilation (mean $Paco_2$ 52 mm Hg), which was associated with more reported sleepiness and excess morbidity and mortality than was found in severely obese persons without hypoventilation. The implications of these findings for the recognition and treatment of sleep-disordered breathing in the acute hospital setting are unknown.

SLEEP IN THE NURSING HOME

Studies of sleep in nursing-home residents have demonstrated marked sleep disruptions and frequent nighttime arousals. In addition, sleep-related problems are a common reason for institutionalization. For example, up to 70% of caregivers report that nighttime difficulties played a significant role in their decision to institutionalize the older person, often because the sleep of the caregiver was being disrupted. Once in the nursing home, many residents nap on and off throughout the day and have frequent awakenings during the night. One study found that 65% of residents reported problems with their sleep and that the use of hypnotic medications was common, but no association was found between the use of sedative hypnotics and the presence, absence, or change in sleep complaints after 6 months of follow-up. Another study found the average duration of sleep episodes during the night in nursing-home residents to be only 20 minutes. Common conditions in nursing-home residents that may contribute to these sleep difficulties include multiple physical illnesses, the use of psychoactive medications, debility and inactivity, increased prevalence of sleep disorders, as well as environmental factors such as nighttime noise, light, and disruptive nursing care. The lack of exposure to bright light during the day may also be a factor.

MANAGEMENT OF SLEEP PROBLEMS

The appropriate treatment of sleep problems must be guided by knowledge of likely causes and potential contributing factors. It is not appropriate to start an older patient with persistent sleep complaints on a sedative hypnotic agent without a careful clinical assessment to identify the cause. Sedative hypnotics have a documented association with falls, hip fracture, and daytime carryover symptoms in older people. If the initial history and physical examination do not suggest a serious underlying cause for the sleep problem, a trial of improved sleep habits is usually the best first approach (see Table 33.1). If the patient takes daytime naps, it is important to determine whether these are needed rest periods or due to inactivity, boredom, or sedating medications. It is important to explain to the person that daytime naps will decrease nighttime sleep.

Short-term hypnotic therapy may be appropriate in conjunction with improved sleep habits in cases of transient, situational insomnia, particularly during bereavement, acute hospitalization, and other periods of

---

Table 33.1—Measures to Improve Sleep Hygiene

- Maintain a regular rising time.
- Maintain a regular bed time, but do not go to bed unless sleepy.
- Decrease or eliminate naps, unless necessary part of sleeping schedule.
- Exercise daily, but not immediately before bedtime.
- Do not use bed for reading or watching television.
- Relax mentally before going to sleep; do not use bedtime as worry time.
- If hungry, have a light snack (except with symptoms of gastroesophageal reflux or medical contraindications), but avoid heavy meals at bedtime.
- Limit or eliminate alcohol, caffeine, and nicotine, especially before bedtime.
- Wind down before bedtime, and maintain a routine period of preparation for bed (eg, washing up, going to the bathroom).
- Control the nighttime environment with comfortable cool temperature, quiet, and darkness.
- Try a familiar background noise (eg, a fan or other "white noise" machine).
- Wear comfortable bed clothing.
- If unable to fall asleep within 30 minutes, get out of bed and perform soothing activity such as listening to soft music or light reading (but avoid exposure to bright light).
- Get adequate exposure to bright light during the day.

temporary acute stress. The clinician should not withhold sedative hypnotic medication treatment in situations where it is clearly indicated. People generally do not feel well if they do not sleep well. However, in the older patient with chronic insomnia, sedative hypnotic agents should be used cautiously because of the complications associated with their long-term use (see the section on chronic hypnotic use, p 257). The chronic use of benzodiazepines can lead to dependence or cognitive impairment. It must be noted that there is increasing debate among sleep experts on the risks and benefits of long-term use of sleeping medications in adults of all ages. However, there is good evidence of increased risk of confusion, falls, and fracture with chronic sedative use by older people. Regardless, in chronic insomnia, it is imperative that the clinician exclude primary sleep disorders and review medications and other medical conditions that may be contributory.

Nonpharmacologic Interventions

Trials have shown that nonpharmacologic interventions can be quite effective in improving sleep in older people (see Table 33.2 for a summary of such interventions). A review of more than 12 studies of behavioral interventions in community-dwelling older people with insomnia concluded that these interventions produce reliable and durable therapeutic benefits, including improved sleep efficiency, sleep continuity, and satisfaction with sleep; treatment is also helpful in reducing chronic hypnotic use. Stimulus control and sleep restriction, which focus on poor sleep habits,

seem to be especially helpful for older persons with insomnia. Cognitive and educational interventions are also important in changing inaccurate beliefs and attitudes about sleep. However, relaxation-based interventions seem less effective for older persons. One large randomized trial of insomniacs with a mean age of 65 years compared cognitive behavior therapy (stimulus control, sleep restriction, sleep hygiene, and cognitive therapy), pharmacotherapy (with temazepam), both cognitive behavioral therapy and pharmacotherapy, and placebo. All three active treatments were found to be effective in short-term follow-up in improving sleep, as indicated by sleep diaries and polysomnography. However, people reported more satisfaction with the cognitive behavioral therapy, and sleep improvements were found to be better sustained over time (up to 2 years) with behavioral treatment.

Several small studies have also tested the effectiveness of exposure to bright light (either natural sunlight or with commercially available light boxes) on the sleep of older persons with insomnia. Positive effects on sleep have been demonstrated with light exposure of various intensities for various durations and at various times during the day. Evening exposure seems to be particularly useful in the older person with an advanced sleep phase. One author recommends that older persons with sleep-maintenance insomnia be treated with 2 hours of bright-light exposure equal to the amount of outdoor light found at mid-day or artificial bright light of at least 2500 lux. However, even short durations of bright light in the morning have been

Table 33.2—Examples of Nonpharmacologic Interventions to Improve Sleep

Intervention	Goal	Description
Stimulus control	To recondition maladaptive sleep-related behaviors	Patient is instructed to go to bed only when sleepy, not use the bed for eating or watching television, get out of bed if unable to fall asleep, return to bed only when sleepy, get up at the same time each morning, not take naps during the day.
Sleep restriction	To improve sleep efficiency (time asleep over time in bed) by causing sleep deprivation	Patient first collects a 2-week sleep diary to determine average total daily sleep time, then stays in bed only that duration plus 15 minutes, gets up at same time each morning, takes no naps in the daytime, gradually increases time allowed in bed as sleep efficiency improves.
Cognitive interventions	To change misunderstandings and false beliefs regarding sleep	Patient's dysfunctional beliefs and attitudes about sleep are identified; patient is educated to change these false beliefs and attitudes, including normal changes in sleep with increased age and changes that are pathologic.
Relaxation techniques	To recognize and relieve tension and anxiety	In progressive muscle relaxation, patient is taught to tense and relax each muscle group. In electromyographic biofeedback, the patient is given feedback regarding muscle tension and learns techniques to relieve it. Meditation or imagery techniques are taught to relieve racing thoughts or anxiety.
Bright light	To correct circadian rhythm causes of sleeping difficulty (ie, sleep-phase problems)	The patient is exposed to sunlight or a light box. Best evidence is from treatment of seasonal affective disorder (from 2500 lux for 2 hours/day to 10,000 lux for 30 minutes/day). For delayed sleep phase, 2 hours early morning light at 2500 lux. For advanced sleep phase, 2 hours evening light at 2500 lux. Shorter durations may be as effective. Routine eye examination is recommended before treatment; avoid light boxes with ultraviolet exposure.

shown to improve sleep complaints in healthy older people. Beneficial effects have been reported in older people using a visor that provided 2000 lux to each eye and was worn for only 30 minutes in the evening.

Bathing before sleep has been demonstrated to enhance the quality of sleep in older people, perhaps related to changes in body temperature with bathing. Moderate-intensity exercise has also been shown to improve sleep in healthy, sedentary people aged 50 and older who reported moderate sleep complaints at baseline. However, strenuous exercise should not be performed immediately before bedtime.

Nonpharmacologic interventions have also been studied in institutional settings. A study of institutionalized demented residents with sleep and behavior problems found morning exposure to bright light to be associated with better nighttime sleep and less daytime agitation. Another study of residents with dementia and behavioral problems found that a program of social interaction with nurses was effective in reducing behavioral problems and sleep-wake rhythm disorders in 30% of the residents. Another small trial of incontinent nursing-home residents demonstrated increased nighttime sleep and less agitation among those randomized to receive a combined daytime physical activity program plus nighttime intervention to decrease noise and light disruption. Another trial combined an enforced schedule of structured social and physical activity for 2 weeks in a small sample of assisted-living residents and found that treated residents had enhanced slow-wave sleep and improved performance in memory-oriented tasks. A large trial of nonpharmacologic interventions on sleep in nursing-home residents was most successful in decreasing daytime sleeping.

Nonpharmacologic interventions may also be important in the acute hospital. A large study testing the feasibility of a nonpharmacologic sleep protocol for hospitalized older patients (consisting of a back rub, warm drink, and relaxation tapes) administered by nurses was successful in reducing sedative hypnotic drug use; the sleep protocol was found to have a stronger association than sedative-hypnotic drugs with improved quality of sleep.

Pharmacotherapy

Short-acting agents are recommended for patients with problems initiating sleep, and intermediate-acting agents are recommended for problems with sleep maintenance. Short-acting agents have lower associations with falls and hip fractures. However, agents with rapid elimination in general also produce the most pronounced rebound and withdrawal syndromes after

discontinuation. Rebound insomnia after cessation of short-acting agents is dose dependent and can be reduced by tapering the dosage prior to discontinuing the drug. Triazolam is a short-acting benzodiazepine that is not listed in Table 33.3 because it has been associated with nocturnal amnesia and confusion and is generally not recommended for older persons.

Zolpidem, zaleplon, and eszopiclone are nonbenzodiazepine hypnotics. These agents are structurally unrelated to the benzodiazepines, but they share some of the pharmacologic properties of benzodiazepines and have been shown to interact with the central nervous system γ-aminobutyric acid (GABA) receptor complex at benzodiazepine (GABA-BZ) receptors. The selectivity of these newer agents to the GABA-BZ receptor may account for their decreased muscle-relaxant, anxiolytic, and anticonvulsant effects in comparison with benzodiazepines in some studies. Zolpidem is a nonbenzodiazepine imidazopyridine that has been studied in older persons with insomnia. In older patients, studies suggest that zolpidem does not produce rebound insomnia, agitation, or anxiety with cessation; does not seem to produce impaired daytime performance on cognitive and psychomotor performance tests; and may have a therapeutic effect that outlasts the period of drug treatment. Zaleplon is a nonbenzodiazepine hypnotic from the pyrazolopyrimidine class, which has also been studied for short-term use by older persons with insomnia. Because of their rapid onset of action, zolpidem and zaleplon should be taken only immediately before bedtime or after the patient has gone to bed and has been unable to fall asleep. Eszopiclone has been approved by the Food and Drug Administration for use in the United States. There is some evidence that it is effective in long-term management of insomnia. Guidelines recommend that zolpidem or zaleplon, like benzodiazepines, be used only for a short term (2 or 3 weeks) and that, if used longer, these agents be used no more than 2 or 3 nights per week. Concerns remain regarding the risks of confusion, falls, and fracture with chronic use of these medications in older people, and caution is warranted even with these newer agents.

Low doses of sedating antidepressants such as trazodone[OL] or mirtazapine[OL] at bedtime may be used as a sleeping aid, particularly for patients with depression. These agents have been suggested for use as a nighttime adjuvant for sleep in depressed patients receiving another antidepressant at therapeutic doses during the daytime. Other indications may be patients with a history of psychoactive substance use problems, failure with other sleeping medications, suspected untreated sleep apnea (where further respiratory depression is a concern), and fibromyalgia (where there is some evidence for antidepressant medication treatment

---

OL- Not approved by the U.S. Food and Drug Administration for this use.

Table 33.3—Prescription Medications Commonly Used for Insomnia in Older People

Class, Drug	Starting Dose	Usual Dose	Half-Life (hours)	Comments
Intermediate-acting benzodiazepines				
Temazepam	7.5 mg	7.5–30 mg	8.8	Psychomotor impairment, increases risk of falls
Short-acting nonbenzodiazepines				
Eszopiclone	1 mg	1–2 mg	6	Reportedly effective for long-term use in selected individuals; may be associated with unpleasant taste, headache; avoid administration with high-fat meal.
Zaleplon (a pyrazolopyrimidine)	5 mg	5–10 mg	1 (reported unchanged in elderly persons)	Reportedly little daytime carryover, tolerance, or rebound insomnia
Zolpidem (an imidazopyridine)	5 mg	5–10 mg	1.5–4.5 (3 in elderly persons, 10 in hepatic cirrhosis)	Reportedly little daytime carryover, tolerance, or rebound insomnia
Sedating antidepressants				
Mirtazapine[OL]	15 mg	5–45 mg	31–39 in older adults; 13–34 in younger adults; mean = 21	Increased appetite, weight gain, headache, dizziness, daytime carryover; used for insomnia with depression
Trazodone[OL]	25–50 mg	25–150 mg	Reportedly 6 ± 2; prolonged in elderly and obese persons	Moderate orthostatic effects; reportedly effective for insomnia with depression; administration after food minimizes sedation and postural hypotension

effect). However, the adverse effects of sedating antide-pressants may limit their usefulness.

Chronic Hypnotic Use

European studies have reported the prevalence of regular (eg, daily) benzodiazepine use in older people to be at least 5%, with greater use among older women than among older men. One Finnish study found chronic use of these agents to be even higher, with habitual use reported by 8% of older men and 25% of older women; the prevalence of use increased with age for both genders. There is strong epidemiologic evidence for increased morbidity and mortality with chronic use of prescription sleeping pills; however, much of this evidence predates the availability of newer, nonbenzodiazepine hypnotics. It has been reported that the nightly use of prescription sleeping pills is associated with an increased mortality that is similar to the mortality hazard of smoking one to two packs of cigarettes per day. In addition, after tolerance to hypnotics develops, long-term use of these agents may actually make sleep worse. In data reported from a longitudinal study of older people in Germany, those who took sleeping medications had a higher rate of sleep-related complaints than those who did not take a medication for sleep. Additional research is needed to help clarify the consequences of long-term use of the newer, nonbenzodiazepine hypnotics in older people.

Several studies have shown that the bulk of pre-scription sleeping medication use is occurring among chronic users, and not those with transient sleeping difficulties. A cross-sectional study in Spain found that 88% of prescription hypnotic users reported daily use of the drug, and 72% of people reported use for more than 3 months. Long-term use was two to three times more common in older people than in middle-aged respondents. Likewise, studies in Canada and France have shown that sleep-promoting medications were prescribed for a year or longer in more than two thirds of people who were taking these medications. Studies in the United States have also demonstrated more benzodiazepine use by older persons and by women, with chronic use being more common in older people. The association between long-acting benzodiazepines and falls in older people has been known for some time. A prospective, population-based Finnish study found this association to be particularly true in older people with physical disability, but not in independent older people.

Methods to help older chronic hypnotic users reduce or eliminate their use of these agents have been reported. One small controlled trial in older women found that decreasing the hypnotic dose by one half for 2 weeks, followed by full withdrawal (perhaps with the use of a substitute pill to maintain the ritual of nightly pill taking) was effective (over short-term follow-up) in eliminating hypnotic use without adverse effects on nighttime sleep, depressive symptoms, or daytime sleepiness. Another small controlled trial in-

---

[OL] Not approved by the U.S. Food and Drug Administration for this use.

volving tapering benzodiazepine use to complete withdrawal over as many as 6 weeks found better success in those persons randomized to receive a nightly dose of 2 mg of controlled-release melatonin rather than placebo. At follow-up 6 months later, nearly 80% of persons who successfully discontinued benzodiazepines continued to report good sleep quality.

Nonprescription Sleeping Agents

Nearly half of older people report using nonprescription sleeping products. The most commonly used products are sedating antihistamines, acetaminophen, alcohol, and melatonin. Sedating antihistamines (eg, diphenhydramine) are common ingredients in over-the-counter sleeping agents as well as in combination analgesic–sleeping agents that are marketed for nighttime use. Diphenhydramine has potent anticholinergic effects, and tolerance to its sedating effects develops after several weeks, so it is generally not recommended for older people. Patients with mild discomfort and sleeping difficulties may have adequate relief with a simple pain reliever (eg, acetaminophen) at bedtime and thus avoid risking the adverse effects of the combination agent. Although alcohol causes some initial drowsiness, it can interfere with sleep later in the night and may actually worsen sleeping difficulties. Evidence is mixed regarding the effectiveness of melatonin as a treatment for insomnia. There is some evidence in older people with insomnia that melatonin administration decreases sleep latency (time to fall asleep) and wake time after sleep onset, and increases sleep efficiency (time asleep over time in bed). There is some intriguing evidence on the use of melatonin in blind people with an impaired sleep-wake cycle. However, a small trial in which persons aged 55 years and older with sleep-maintenance insomnia were treated with either 0.5 mg of transbuccal melatonin or placebo for 4 days at a time did not find polysomnographic evidence of improved sleep. Because of these mixed results and the lack of regulative control in the currently available melatonin products, it is difficult for the clinician to recommend use of these products. The exception may be chronic hypnotic users, for whom there is some evidence for success in withdrawal of the hypnotic with concomitant use of melatonin. Valerian is an herbal product with mild sedative action that has been marketed for insomnia. The mechanism of action of valerian is uncertain, and it contains several potentially active compounds. Given this information, its use is not recommended.

ANNOTATED REFERENCES

■ Alessi CA, Martin JL, Webber AP, et al. Randomized, controlled trial of a nonpharmacological intervention to improve abnormal sleep/wake patterns in nursing home residents. *J Am Geriatr Soc.* 2005;53(5):803–810.

> This article reports results of a randomized controlled trial of a multicomponent nonpharmacologic intervention to improve sleep-wake patterns in nursing-home residents (N = 118) with excessive daytime sleeping and nighttime sleep disruption. The intervention combined efforts to decrease daytime in-bed time, 30 minutes or more of daily sunlight exposure, increased physical activity, a structured bedtime routine, and efforts to decrease nighttime noise and light. The only effect on nighttime sleep was a modest decrease in mean duration of nighttime awakenings, but there was a significant decrease in daytime sleeping with the intervention. Intervention participants also had increased participation in social and physical activities and social conversation, which may translate to an improvement in quality of life.

■ Ancoli-Israel S, Martin JL, Kripke DF, et al. Effect of light treatment on sleep and circadian rhythms in demented nursing home patients. *J Am Geriatr Soc.* 2002;50(2):282–289.

> This article reports on findings from a randomized controlled trial involving testing the effects of four treatments (evening bright light, morning bright light, daytime sleep restriction, or evening dim red light) on fragmented sleep patterns in 77 nursing-home residents. Although there were no improvements in nighttime sleep or daytime alertness with any of the treatment groups, participants randomized to morning bright-light therapy had more robust circadian rhythm activity patterns than the other groups. This provides some preliminary evidence of modest, but potentially important, effects of bright-light exposure on circadian activity rhythms in nursing-home residents.

■ Baskett JJ, Broad JB, Wood PC, et al. Does melatonin improve sleep in older people? a randomized crossover trial. *Age Ageing.* 2003;32(2):164–170.

> This study was a double blind, randomized, placebo-controlled cross-over trial in 20 normal and 20 problem sleepers aged 65 years or older. Melatonin 5 mg or placebo was taken at bedtime for 4 weeks, separated by a 4-week washout period. Melatonin did not significantly improve any of the sleep parameters measured in either normal or problem sleepers.

■ Cohen-Zion M, Stepnowsky C, Marler M, et al. Changes in cognitive function associated with sleep disordered breathing in older people. *J Am Geriatr Soc.* 2001;49(12):1622–1627.

> This was a population-based longitudinal study of community-dwelling people aged 65 years and older with high risk for sleep-disordered breathing. In-home interviews and home sleep recordings were reported for 46 participants, with longitudinal follow-up. Increases in cognitive impairment were found to be associated with increases in respiratory disturbance index (a measure of sleep-disordered breathing) and increases in daytime sleepiness. In regression analysis, increases in cognitive impairment were found to be associated with daytime sleepiness, suggesting that the potential relationship between sleep-disordered breathing and cognitive function may be mediated by daytime sleepiness.

■ Foley D, Monjan A, Masaki K, et al. Daytime sleepiness is associated with 3-year incident dementia and cognitive decline in older Japanese-American men. *J Am Geriatr Soc.* 2001;49(12):1628–1632.

This community-based longitudinal cohort study reports findings from 2346 Japanese-American men aged 71 to 93 years who screened negative for dementia at baseline and were screened again for dementia in a 3-year follow-up examination. After adjusting for age and other factors, researchers found that participants with self-reported excessive daytime sleepiness at baseline were more likely to develop dementia and more likely to have worsened cognitive testing scores (on the Cognitive Abilities Screening Instrument) at follow-up. Symptoms of insomnia (trouble falling asleep or early morning awakening) were not found to be associated with cognitive decline or development of dementia. The authors suggest that these findings indicate that daytime sleepiness in older adults may be an early indicator of decline in cognition and onset of dementia.

■ Kripke DF. Chronic hypnotic use: deadly risks, doubtful benefit. *Sleep Med Rev.* 2000;4(1):5–20.

This review article describes the prevalence and consequences of chronic hypnotic use. In the United States approximately two thirds of all hypnotic prescriptions go to chronic users, who have taken hypnotics for an average of 5 years or more. Epidemiologic studies have shown that the use of prescription sleeping pills (in particular, use 30 times in the past month) is associated with an increased mortality, which is similar to the mortality hazard of smoking one to two packs of cigarettes per day. Furthermore, after tolerance to hypnotics develops,

long-term use may make sleep worse. The author concludes with practice recommendations for avoiding chronic hypnotic use and for gradually withdrawing medication in chronic users, possibly with the addition of cognitive-behavioral therapy.

■ Moul DE, Hall M, Pilkonis PA, et al. Self-report measures of insomnia in adults: rationales, choices, and needs. *Sleep Med Rev.* 2004;8(3):177–198.

This article reviews questionnaire criteria and attributes, including the use of questionnaires in aging studies of insomnia. The document includes an extensive table of currently available questionnaires.

■ Russo-Magno P, O'Brien A, Panciera T, et al. Compliance with CPAP therapy in older men with obstructive sleep apnea. *J Am Geriatr Soc.* 2001;49(9):1205–1211.

This study was a retrospective chart review of men aged 65 years and older (N = 33) who were prescribed continuous positive airway pressure (CPAP) therapy for obstructive sleep apnea over an 8-year period at a Veterans Affairs medical center. Twenty patients were adherent with their CPAP, and factors associated with nonadherence included cigarette smoking, nocturia, and benign prostatic hyperplasia. Patient who were adherent with CPAP were more likely to have attended a patient CPAP education and support group.

Cathy A. Alessi, MD

CHAPTER 34—PRESSURE ULCERS

KEY POINTS

■ A pressure ulcer is defined as damage caused to skin and underlying soft tissue by unrelieved pressure when the tissue is compressed between a bony prominence and external surface over a prolonged period of time.

■ Three main factors are believed to play a role in pressure-ulcer formation: pressure, friction, and shear forces. Intrinsic and extrinsic factors determine the tolerance of soft tissue to the adverse effects of pressure.

■ Risk assessment and preventive strategies are required to decrease the incidence of pressure ulcers.

■ The stage of an ulcer determines the appropriate treatment plan.

Pressure ulcers are a serious and common problem for older persons, affecting approximately 1 million adults in the United States. As the population ages, pressure ulcers will continue to be a major health care problem. The surgeon general's Healthy People 2010 document

has identified pressure ulcers as a national health issue for long-term care, and the Centers for Medicare and Medicaid Services (CMS) has designated pressure ulcers as one of the three primary markers of quality of care in the long-term-care setting. The prevention and healing of pressure ulcers requires the cooperation and skills of the entire multidisciplinary health care team.

EPIDEMIOLOGY

A pressure ulcer is defined as damage caused to skin and underlying soft tissue by unrelieved pressure when the tissue is compressed between a bony prominence and external surface over a prolonged period of time. Because pressure is the major physiologic factor that leads to soft-tissue destruction, the term *pressure ulcer* is most widely used and preferred over *decubitus ulcer* or *bedsore*.

The causes of pressure ulcers are still not fully understood. Most research into the causes of pressure ulcers has been done in animal models. Three main factors are believed to play a role in pressure-ulcer formation: pressure, friction, and shear forces. It appears that the amount of pressure, friction, or shear force needed to create a pressure ulcer depends on the quality of tissue, the blood flow, and the amount of pressure applied. Hence, for patients with poor-quality tissue (ie, tissue with inadequate blood perfusion), it may take less sustained pressure over a shorter period of time to develop a pressure ulcer. Conversely, patients with good-quality tissue may be able to sustain higher loads of pressure over a longer period of time before an ulcer develops. Ulcers caused by shearing forces tend to develop deep in the fascia, whereas ulcers caused by friction tend to be quite superficial, starting in the epidermal and dermal layers. With aging, local blood supply to the skin decreases, epithelial layers flatten and thin, subcutaneous fat decreases, and collagen fibers lose elasticity. These changes in aging skin and the resultant lowered tolerance to hypoxia may predispose the older person to pressure-ulcer development.

The incidence and prevalence of pressure ulcers vary greatly, depending on the setting. In the hospital, incidence rates have ranged from 0.4% to 38%. Higher rates are noted in intensive care units, where patients are less mobile and have severe systemic illnesses. The Fourth National Pressure Ulcer Prevalence Survey found an annual hospital prevalence rate of 10.1%. In the long-term-care setting, incidence and prevalence rates have ranged from 3% to 30%. Less is known about pressure ulcers in home care, but studies have reported incidence rates of 4% to 17% and prevalence rates of 5% to 15%.

The incidence of pressure ulcers not only differs by health care setting but also by stage of ulceration. The stage I pressure ulcer (persistent erythema) occurs most commonly, accounting for 47% of all pressure ulcers. The stage II pressure ulcers (partial thickness loss involving only the epidermal and dermal layers) are second, at 33%. Stage III (full-thickness skin loss involving subcutaneous tissue) and stage IV (full thickness involving muscle or bone or supporting structures) pressure ulcers make up the remaining 20%. Several studies have noted that the incidence rates of pressure ulcers among black Americans and white Americans may differ; blacks tend to have a greater incidence of stage III and stage IV pressure ulcers than whites have. Whether this can be attributed to structural skin changes or socioeconomic factors is unknown because of the paucity of pressure-ulcer research among patients in U.S. minority groups.

RISK FACTORS AND RISK-ASSESSMENT SCALES

The literature abounds with lists of risk factors associated with pressure-ulcer development. However, any disease process that renders an elderly person immobile for an extended period of time will increase the risk for pressure-ulcer development. There are intrinsic and extrinsic factors that determine the tolerance of soft tissue to the adverse effects of pressure. Intrinsic risk factors are physiologic factors or disease states that increase the risk for pressure-ulcer development, for example, age, poor nutritional status, and decreased arteriolar blood pressure. Extrinsic factors are external factors that damage the skin, for example, friction and shear, moisture, and urinary or fecal incontinence or both. Variables that appear to be predictors of pressure-ulcer development include age of 70 years or older, impaired mobility, current smoking history, low body mass index, altered mental status (eg, confusion), urinary and fecal incontinence, malnutrition, restraints, malignancy, diabetes mellitus, stroke, pneumonia, heart failure, fever, sepsis, hypotension, kidney failure, dry and scaly skin, history of pressure ulcers, anemia, lymphopenia, and hypoalbuminemia. Some physiologic risk factors (eg, diabetes mellitus, cerebral vascular accident) have been associated with microcirculatory impairment, thus leading to neural and endothelial compromise and increasing the risk of ulceration.

Because of the myriad of risk factors associated with pressure-ulcer development, various scales have been developed to quantify a person's risk by identifying the presence of factors in several categories. The Braden Scale (http://www.bradenscale.com/bradenscale.htm) and the Norton Scale (http://www.woundcarehelpline.com/NortonScale.pdf) are probably the most widely used tools for identifying elderly patients who are at risk for developing pressure ulcers and have been validated. Both tools are recommended by the Agency for Healthcare Research and Quality (AHRQ). The Braden Scale has a sensitivity of 83% to 100% and a specificity of 64% to 77%; the Norton Scale has a sensitivity of 73% to 92% and a specificity of 61% to 94%.

The AHRQ guidelines for preventing pressure ulcers recommend that bed- and chairbound patients or those with impaired ability to be repositioned should be assessed upon admission to the hospital or the nursing home for additional factors that increase the risk for developing pressure ulcers. Pressure-ulcer risk should also be reassessed at periodic intervals and when there is a change in level of activity or mobility. Studies have demonstrated that the incorporation of systematic risk-assessment tools has significantly reduced the incidence of pressure ulcers. To date, the Braden Scale is the only tool to be validated in nonwhite populations. It is important to note that the use of risk-assessment tools will not guarantee that all elderly persons at risk for pressure ulcers will be identified.

PREVENTION

The AHRQ sponsored the development of recommendations for the prevention of pressure ulcers in adults. These clinical practice guidelines (*Pressure Ulcers in Adults: Prediction and Prevention,* published in May 1992) provide an excellent approach to evidenced-based pressure-ulcer prevention (available at http://www.guideline.gov/summary/summary.aspx?doc_id=2601&nbr=1827&string=pressure+ulcers).

Skin Care

There is limited evidence on the role of skin care in pressure-ulcer prevention. Most recommendations are based on expert opinions. After identification of the older person at risk for pressure ulcers, the goal of skin care is to maintain and improve tissue tolerance to pressure in order to prevent injury.

All older persons at risk should have a systematic skin inspection at least once a day, with emphasis on the bony prominences. The skin should be cleansed with warm water and a mild cleansing agent to minimize irritation and dryness of the skin. Every effort should be made to minimize environmental factors leading to skin drying, such as low humidity (less than 40%) and exposure to cold. Decreased skin hydration has been found to result in decreased pliability, and severely dry skin has been noted to damage the stratum corneum. Dry skin should be managed with moisturizers.

Massaging over bony prominences should be avoided. Previously, it was believed that massaging the bony prominences promoted circulation. However, postmortem biopsies found degenerated tissue in those areas exposed to massage but no degenerated tissue on those areas that were not massaged. All efforts should be made to avoid exposing the skin to perspiration, wound drainage, or urine and fecal matter resulting from incontinence. When disposable briefs are used to manage incontinence, the patient must be checked and changed frequently, since perineal dermatitis can develop quickly. The use of disposable underpads to control excessive moisture and perspiration may help wick moisture away from skin. The use of moisturizers and moisture barriers should also be considered to protect the skin.

Nutrition

An association has been observed between pressure-ulcer development and malnutrition; several studies have identified malnutrition as a risk factor for pressure-ulcer formation. Ensuring an adequate diet to prevent malnutrition that is compatible with an individual's ability to eat and goals of care is a reasonable strategy to reduce the risk of ulcer formation.

Mechanical Loading

Minimizing friction and shear is also important. This can be accomplished through proper repositioning, transferring, and turning techniques. The use of lubricants (eg, cornstarch and creams), protective films (eg, transparent film dressings and skin sealants), protective dressings (eg, hydrocolloids), and protective padding may be used to reduce the possibility of friction and shear. Older persons who are at risk for developing pressure ulcers should be repositioned at least every 2 hours. Bed-positioning devices such as pillows or foam wedges should be used to keep bony prominences from direct contact with one another. The head of the bed should be at the lowest degree of elevation consistent with medical conditions. The use of lifting devices, such as trapezes or bed linen, to move the person in bed will also decrease the potential for friction and shear forces. The heel is quite vulnerable to pressure-ulcer development; studies suggest that approximately 20% of all pressure-ulcer development occurs at the heels. This may be attributed to the limited amount of soft tissue over the heel. Specific clinical interventions to prevent heel pressure ulcers have been developed (see Table 34.1).

Patients seated in a chair should be assessed for good postural alignment, distribution of weight, and balance. They should be taught or reminded to shift weight every 15 minutes. The use of doughnuts as seating cushions is contraindicated because they increase pressure over the area of contact and may actually cause pressure ulcers.

Table 34.1—Prevention of Heel Pressure Ulcers

- Assess the heels of patients at high risk for pressure ulcers every day.
- Use moisturizer on the heels twice a day; do not massage.
- Apply transparent film dressings to the heels of older persons prone to friction problems (eg, stroke patients).
- Apply hydrocolloid dressing (either single or extra-thick) to the heels of older persons with reactive hyperemia (pre-stage I).
- Have older persons wear socks to help prevent friction; remove at bedtime.
- Have older persons in wheelchairs wear properly fitting padded sneakers or shoes.
- Place pillow vertically under the person's legs (without hyperextending them) to support heels off the bed surface.
- Turn the person every 2 hours, repositioning heels.

Mobility

Maintaining or improving mobility is also extremely important. It is one of the most effective ways to decrease pressure on bony prominences. For bedbound patients there are benefits of both active and passive range-of-motion exercises. Those patients not confined to bed should be encouraged to move from bed to chair to standing to ambulating to minimize the risk of developing pressure ulcers.

Support Surfaces

Any elderly person identified as being at risk for developing pressure ulcers should be placed on a pressure-reducing device. Two types exist: static (foam, static air, gel or water, or a combination) and dynamic (alternating air, low air loss, or air fluidized). Most static devices are less expensive than dynamic surfaces. Table 34.2 provides details about the various types of support surfaces that can guide selection for particular situations. Most experts would agree that for pressure-ulcer prevention, the use of static devices is appropriate. Two conditions warrant consideration of a dynamic surface:

- bottoming-out occurs (the static surface is compressed to less than 1 inch), or
- the patient is at high risk for pressure ulcers and reactive hyperemia is noted on a bony prominence despite the use of a static support surface.

Although effective at reducing pressure, dynamic airflow beds have several potential adverse effects, including dehydration, sensory deprivation, loss of muscle strength, and difficulty with mobilization.

MANAGEMENT

The AHRQ developed evidence-based guidelines on the management of pressure ulcers. This guideline, *Treatment of Pressure Ulcers*, published in December 1994, reviews the foundation for providing evidence-based pressure-ulcer management (available at http://www.guideline.gov/summary/summary.aspx?doc_id=810).

Assessment

A pressure ulcer will not heal unless underlying causes are identified and effective interventions are implemented. When a pressure ulcer has developed, a systematic evaluation is necessary. Table 34.3 presents an approach to assessment and documentation when a pressure ulcer develops.

There is no universal agreement on a single system for classifying pressure ulcers. Most experts do agree that the stage of an ulcer determines the appropriate treatment plan. It should be noted that staging alone does not determine the seriousness of the ulcer. Most systems use four stages to classify ulceration. Table 34.4 describes one staging system. When eschar, a thick brown or black devitalized tissue, is covering the ulcer, the ulcer cannot be accurately staged.

The challenge for most staging systems occurs in the definition of the stage I pressure ulcer. There is more variability in attempts to classify the first stage of ulcer development than in any other stage. Most systems define the stage I pressure ulcer as nonblanchable erythema of intact skin; both the AHRQ prediction and prevention guidelines and the Minimum Data Set (required by CMS for all patients in long-term-care facilities) refer to stage I pressure ulcer in these terms. However, it is difficult (at best) to blanch the skin of persons with darkly pigmented skin. To address this

Table 34.2—Support Surfaces for Persons at Risk for Pressure Ulcers

Type	Examples	Support Area	Low Moisture Retention	Reduced Heat Accumulation	Shear Reduction	Pressure Reduction	Cost per Day
Static surfaces	Foam	Yes	No	No	No	Yes	Low
	Standard mattress	No	No	No	No	No	Low
	Static flotation—air or water	Yes	No	No	Yes	Yes	Low
Dynamic surfaces	Air fluidized	Yes	Yes	Yes	Yes	Yes	High
	Low-air-loss	Yes	Yes	Yes	?	Yes	High
	Alternating air	Yes	No	No	Yes	Yes	Moderate

SOURCE: Adapted from Bergstrom N, Bennett MA, Carlson CE, et al. *Treatment of Pressure Ulcers. Clinical Practice Guideline No. 15.* Rockville, MD: US Department of Health and Human Services, Public Health Service, Agency for Health Care Policy and Research. December 1994:38. AHCPR Pub. No. 95-0652.

Table 34.3—A Systematic Approach to the Management of Pressure Ulcers

Evaluate and Document:	Consider These Strategies:
Location	Examine high-risk sites.
	Develop targeted pressure-relieving strategies (eg, positioning and repositioning, padding, seat cushions, and heel elevation).
	Limit shearing forces by special attention to positioning when the head of bed is elevated.
	Lift rather than slide the patient.
	Cleanse and dry regularly if wetted frequently.
Stage	Differentiate between minor stage I lesions (nonblanchable erythema related to extravasation of red blood cells into the interstitium) and deep tissue injuries that can progress to full-thickness lesions.
	Discuss with caregivers and families the possibility of significant pressure-ulcer development when deep tissue injury is identified.
Area	Record diameter for circular lesions.
	Record lengths of largest perpendiculars for irregular lesions.
Depth	Measure depth from plane of skin.
	Probe and measure extent of undermining or depth of sinus tracts.
Drainage	Estimate amount.
	Identify degree of odor and purulence.
	Monitor hematocrit if more than minor blood loss with dressing changes occurs.
	Monitor serum albumin if volume of ulcer drainage is large.
Necrosis	Consider simple blunt debridement of small amounts of necrotic tissue.
	Involve general or plastic surgeons for extensive debridement.
	Monitor damage to healthy tissue whenever using blunt, enzymatic, or wet-to-dry dressings for debridement.
	Monitor use of pressure dressings (which can cause necrosis) after blunt debridement.
Granulation	Identify granulation as an indication that wound healing is occurring.
	Look for regression when other infections (eg, urinary tract infection or pneumonia) occur.
	Develop strategies to protect and enhance growth of granulation tissue (eg, nourishment, vitamins, and minerals; use of dressings to ensure moist wound surfaces).
	Avoid damage with dressing changes.
Cellulitis	Differentiate from a thin rim of erythema surrounding most healing wounds.
	Look for tender, warmth, redness, particularly if there is progression.
	Consider treatment with systemic antibiotics active against gram-positive cocci.

SOURCE: Bennett RG. Pressure ulcers. In: Cobbs EL, Duthie EH Jr, Murphy JB. *Geriatrics Review Syllabus: A Core Curriculum in Geriatric Medicine*, 4th ed. Dubuque, IA: Kendall Hunt Publishing Company for the American Geriatrics Society; 1996:155.

Table 34.4—Staging System for Pressure Ulcers

Stage I	Persistent nonblanchable erythema of intact skin.*
Stage II	Partial-thickness skin loss involving epidermis or dermis, or both. The ulcer is superficial and presents clinically as an abrasion, blister, or shallow crater.
Stage III	Full-thickness skin loss involving damage or necrosis of subcutaneous tissue that may extend down to, but not through, underlying fascia.
Stage IV	Full-thickness skin loss with extensive destruction, tissue necrosis, or damage to muscle, bone, or supporting structures (eg, tendon or joint capsule). Undermining and sinus tracts may also be associated with stage IV pressure ulcers.

* The National Pressure Ulcer Advisory Panel further expands this definition as follows: A Stage I pressure ulcer is an observable pressure-related alteration of intact skin whose indicators as compared with the adjacent or opposite area on the body may include changes in one or more of the following: skin temperature (warmth or coolness), tissue consistency (firm or boggy feel), and/or sensation (pain, itching). The ulcer appears as a defined area of persistent redness in lightly pigmented skin, whereas in darker skin tones, the ulcer may appear with persistent red, blue, or purple hues.

SOURCE: Adapted from definitions by the Agency for Health Care Policy and Research. See Bergstrom N, Bennett MA, Carlson CE, et al. *Treatment of Pressure Ulcers. Clinical Practice Guideline No. 15.* Rockville, MD: US Department of Health and Human Services, Public Health Service, Agency for Health Care Policy and Research. December 1994:47–49. AHCPR Pub. No. 95-0652.

concern, the National Pressure Ulcer Advisory Panel (NPUAP) revised its definition of a stage I pressure ulcer to encompass the skin alterations that might be seen in stage I pressure ulcers regardless of skin pigmentation. This system defines a stage I ulcer as an observable pressure-related alteration of intact skin whose indicators, as compared with an adjacent or opposite area on the body, may include changes in one or more of the following: skin temperature (warmth or coolness), tissue consistency (firm or boggy feel), or sensation (pain, itching). The NPUAP definition further states that the pressure ulcer appears as a defined area of persistent redness in lightly pigmented skin, whereas in darker skin tones, the pressure ulcer may appear with persistent erythema, or blue or purple hues. Although this definition is cumbersome, it is the only definition that includes patients with darkly pigmented skin.

Treatment

Debridement

Debridement is necessary when there is necrotic, devitalized tissue within the wound. Such tissue supports the growth of pathologic organisms and prevents healing. There are four major types of debridement methods: mechanical, enzymatic, autolytic, and sharp (Table 34.5) used in the United States. It should be noted that biosurgery (maggot or larva therapy), which is used widely in Europe, is another potential debridement option. The debridement method should be selected on the basis of the patient's health condition, the ulcer presentation, the presence or absence of infection, and the patient's ability to tolerate the procedure.

Dressings

Numerous dressings are used in the healing of pressure ulcers. The use of gauze wet-to-dry has been discouraged by experts; it is actually a debriding technique that can damage the tissue matrix and prolong healing. Many experts advocate the use of hydrocolloid dressings. These dressings, when compared with gauze, have been found to significantly speed the healing process. This is most likely because hydrocolloids require fewer dressing changes (inflicting less trauma), block bacteria from penetrating the wound bed, and maintain a moist wound environment (facilitating increases in the growth factors needed in the healing process). Moreover, studies have demonstrated that the use of hydrocolloids, when compared with the use of gauze, decreases direct and indirect institutional costs. It is essential to select an appropriate dressing, not on the basis of the stage of the pressure ulcer, but rather on the amount of wound exudate. Table 34.6 identifies some of the most common dressings and the indications for their use.

Surgical Repair

The use of surgical repair of a pressure ulcer remains a viable option for stage III and stage IV pressure ulcers. However, because many stage III and stage IV pressure ulcers eventually heal over a long period of time with the use of modern wound-healing principles and the rate of recurrence of surgically closed pressure ulcers is high, the practitioner must carefully weigh the benefits of the surgery. When the surgical option is exercised, the most common type of surgical repairs are direct closure, skin grafting, skin flaps, musculocutaneous flaps, and free flaps.

Table 34.5—Methods of Debridement

Type	Description	Advantages, Disadvantages
Mechanical	Use of physical forces to remove devitalized tissues; methods include wet-to-dry irrigation (using 19-gauge needle with 35-cc syringe), hydrotherapy, and dextranomer	May remove both devitalized and vitalized tissues; may cause pain
Surgical, Sharp	Use of scalpel, scissors, and forceps to remove the devitalized tissue; laser debridement is also under this category	Quick, effective if performed by skilled professional; should be used when infection is suspected; pain management is needed
Enzymatic	Use of topical debriding agent to dissolve the devitalized tissue (chemical force)	Appropriate when there are no signs or symptoms of local infection; some may damage surrounding skin
Autolytic	Use of synthetic dressings to allow the devitalized tissue to self-digest from the enzymes found in the ulcer fluids (natural force)	Recommended when the older person cannot tolerate other forms of debridement and when infection is not suspected; may take a long time to be effective
Biosurgery	Use of larvae to digest devitalized tissue	Quick, effective; good option when older person cannot tolerate surgical debridement

SOURCE: Data from Bergstrom N, Bennett MA, Carlson CE, et al. *Treatment of Pressure Ulcers. Clinical Practice Guideline No. 15.* Rockville, MD: US Department of Health and Human Services, Public Health Service, Agency for Health Care Policy and Research. December 1994:47–49. AHCPR Pub. No. 95-0652.

Table 34.6—Common Dressings for Treating Pressure Ulcers

Dressing	Indications	Contraindications	Example	Comments
Transparent film	Stage I, II Protection from friction Superficial scrape	Draining ulcers Suspected skin infection or fungus	Bioclusive Tegaderm Op-site	Apply skin prep to intact skin to protect from adhesive
Foam island	Stage II, III Low to moderate exudate Can apply as window to secure transparent film	Excessive exudate Dry, crusted wound	Allevyn Lyofoam	
Hydrocolloids	Stage II, III Low to moderate drainage Good peri-wound skin integrity Autolytic debridement of necrotic tissue	Poor skin integrity Infected ulcers Wound needs packing	DuoDERM Extra thin film DuoDERM Tegasorb RepliCare Comfeel Nu-derm	Left in place 3–5 days Can apply as window to secure transparent film Can apply over alginate to control drainage Must control maceration Apply skin prep to intact skin to protect from adhesive
Alginate	Stage III, IV Excessive drainage	Dry or minimally draining wound Superficial wounds with maceration	Sorbsan Kaltostat Algosteril AlgiDERM	Apply dressing within wound borders Requires secondary dressing Must use skin prep Must control for maceration
Hydrogel (amorphous gels)	Stage II, III, IV	Macerated areas Wounds with excess exudate	IntraSite gel SoloSite gel Restore gel	Needs to be combined with gauze dressing Stays moist longer than saline gauze Changed 1–2 times/day Used as alternative to saline gauze for packing deep wounds with tunnels, undermining Reduces adherence of gauze to wound Must control for maceration
(gel sheet)	Stage II	Macerated areas Wounds with moderate to heavy exudate	Vigilon Restore Impregnated Gauze	Needs to be held in place with topper dressing
Gauze packing (moistened with saline)	Stage III, IV Wounds with depth, especially those with tunnels, undermining		square 2 × 2s, 4 × 4s Fluffed Kerlix Plain NuGauze	Must be remoistened often to maintain moist wound environment
Silver dressings (silver with alginates, gels, charcoal)	Malodorous wounds High level of exudates Wound highly suspicious for critical bacterial load Peri-wound with signs of inflammation Slow-healing wound	Systemic infection Cellulitis Signs of systemic side effects, esp. erythema multiforme Fungal proliferation Sensitivity of skin to sun Interstitial nephritis Leukopenia Skin necrosis Concurrent use with proteolytic enzymes	Silvercel Silvadene Aquacel Ag Acticoat	

SOURCE: Copyright © 2006 by Rita Frantz. Reprinted from Reuben DB, Herr K, Pacala JT, et al. *Geriatrics At Your Fingertips. 2006.* 8th ed. New York: American Geriatrics Society; 2006:187. Reprinted with permission.

Diet and Nutritional Supplements

If a patient with a pressure ulcer is malnourished, the importance of diet and dietary supplements is controversial. The AHRQ treatment guideline rates the strength of the evidence as "C," the weakest rating, for nutritional support that achieves approximately 30 to 35 calories per kg per day and 1.25 to 1.50 g of protein per kg per day. Evidence to support the use of supplemental vitamins and minerals is equally weak.

New or Unproven Therapies

Throughout the years a number of treatments have been advocated for the healing of pressure ulcers without sufficient data to support their various claims. Data on the therapeutic efficacy of hyperbaric oxygen, low-energy laser irradiation, and therapeutic ultrasound have not been established. However, areas of great promise include the use of recombinant platelet-derived growth factors to stimulate healing and skin equivalents that may prove to heal stage III and stage IV pressure ulcers. Preliminary data on the uses of electrical stimulation, vacuum-assisted closures, and warm-up therapy, which increases the basal temperature of the ulcer to promote healing, are promising.

Monitoring Healing

Monitoring the healing of pressure ulcers can pose a challenge to the practitioner. The accurate measurements of a pressure ulcer can inform the practitioner about the effectiveness of ulcer treatment. However, the use of traditional measurements (rulers and tracing paper) produces highly variable results among raters. In the past 8 years, two instruments to measure healing of pressure ulcers with some level of validity and reliability have been developed. The Pressure Sore Status Tool and the Pressure Ulcer Scale for Healing (http://www.npuap.org/push3-0.html) are excellent tools for monitoring pressure-ulcer healing. The use of high-frequency portable ultrasound to measure wound healing has been introduced. The use of this technology, which can capture three-dimensional measurements, has been shown to be quite beneficial in objectively monitoring healing. Moreover, because ultrasound is "color blind," it can detect stage I pressure ulcers in darkly pigmented skin.

There has been considerable debate regarding the use of reverse staging of pressure ulcers to monitor healing. Staging of pressure ulcers is appropriate only for defining the maximum anatomic depth of tissue damage. Since pressure ulcers heal to a progressively more shallow depth, they do not replace lost muscle, subcutaneous fat, or dermis before they re-epithelialize. Instead, pressure ulcers are filled with granulation

(scar) tissue composed primarily of endothelial cells, fibroblasts, collagen, and extracellular matrix. A stage IV pressure ulcer cannot become a stage III, stage II, and then stage I; reverse staging does not accurately characterize what is physiologically occurring as the pressure ulcer heals. When a stage IV pressure ulcer has healed, it should be classified as a healed stage IV pressure ulcer, not a stage 0. The progress of healing can be documented only by describing ulcer characteristics or measuring wound characteristics with a validated tool.

Ulcer care should be evaluated for healing progress on a weekly basis. There are no standard healing rates for pressure ulcers. Review of the literature suggests that a majority of stage I pressure ulcers heal within 1 day to 1 week; stage II, within 5 days to 3 months; stage III, within 1 month to 6 months; and stage IV, within 6 months to 1 year. Clearly, some full-thickness pressure ulcers may never heal, depending on comorbidity; however, no clear guidelines exist to determine when a pressure ulcer can be truly defined as recalcitrant or what characteristics must be present to predict that an ulcer will never heal.

Control of Infections

All pressure ulcers become colonized with both aerobic and anaerobic bacteria, and superficial swab cultures of the wounds have not been shown to be helpful in determining which organism may be causing the infection. Therefore, routine swab cultures are not recommended. However, there is some evidence to suggest that quantitative tissue swab cultures can be used to determine the wound bioburden. Wound cleansing and dressing changes are two of the most important methods for minimizing the amount of bacterial colonization. Increasing the frequency of wound cleansing and dressing changes is an important first step when purulent or foul-smelling drainage is observed on the ulcer. When ulcers are not healing or have persistent exudate after 2 weeks of optimal cleansing and dressing changes, it is reasonable to consider the use of antimicrobials.

The use of topical antimicrobials has been shown to decrease the bioburden in pressure ulcers. The use of antimicrobials such as silver sulfadiazine and mupirocin ointment can be applied up to three times a day for 1 to 2 weeks, with careful monitoring for allergic reactions. Because prolonged use of these antimicrobials may result in resistant organisms, they should not be used indefinitely. In the past several years, the uses of silver-impregnated dressings to decrease the bioburden has become quite popular. Although the exact mechanism of how silver kills the infection remains unknown, it is hypothesized that it stops the enzyme that feeds the proliferation of bacteria, viruses, and fungi. These dressings (Aquacel Ag, Acticoat, Actisorb, and Arglaes) control bacterial load and ideally control odor caused by the bacteria. The dressing selected determines how the silver is delivered, the length of treatment, the amount of exudate absorption, the incidence of maceration, the ease of dressing removal, and the pain intensity at dressing changes. It is important to select a dressing that meets the needs of the patient and the staff.

Because most topical antibiotics do not penetrate the wound bed, they are not effective for control of infections. When ulcers fail to heal despite the treatments described above, it is reasonable to consider the possibility of cellulitis or osteomyelitis. Biopsy of the ulcer for quantitative bacterial cultures or of the underlying bone can be used to establish these diagnoses. Cellulitis, osteomyelitis, bacteremia, and sepsis are all indications for the use of systemic antibiotics.

The use of topical antiseptics (eg, povidone iodine, iodophor, sodium hypochlorite, hydrogen peroxide, and acetic acid) is not recommended because of their tissue toxicity. There is some new literature suggesting that diluted povidone iodine ($< 5\%$) is not cytotoxic to healthy granulation tissue.

COMPLICATIONS FROM PRESSURE ULCERS

The development of pressure ulcers can lead to several complications. Probably the most serious complication is sepsis. When a pressure ulcer is present and there is aerobic or anaerobic bacteremia, or both, the pressure ulcer is most often the primary source of the infection. Additional complications of pressure ulcers include localized infection, cellulitis, and osteomyelitis. Quite often, a nonhealing pressure ulcer may indicate underlying osteomyelitis. Mortality can also be associated with pressure-ulcer development. Several studies have noted the association of pressure-ulcer development and mortality in both the hospital and nursing-home settings. In fact, the mortality rate has been noted to be as high as 60% for those older persons who develop a pressure ulcer within 1 year of hospital discharge. Thus, careful assessment of a pressure ulcer is essential. Finally, other complications of pressure ulcers include pain and depression. Both pain and depression have been associated with decreased wound healing.

ANNOTATED REFERENCES

■ Allman RM, Goode PS, Patrick MM, et al. Pressure ulcer risk factors among hospitalized patients with activity limitation. *JAMA* 1995;273(11):865–870.

This prospective inception cohort study examined demographic, medical, functional status, and nutritional characteris-

tics that predicted stage II or greater pressure ulcers in a cohort of bed- or chairbound patients. The main outcome measure was time to in-hospital pressure-ulcer development of a stage II or greater pressure ulcer. The study found that the total cumulative incidence of pressure ulcers was 12.9%, with a median time of 9 days. This study also found that nonblanchable erythema, lymphopenia, immobility, dry skin, and decreased weight were all independent and significant risk factors for pressure-ulcer development in hospitals.

■ Berlowitz DR, Bezerra HQ, Brandeis GH, et al. Are we improving the quality of nursing home care: the case of pressure ulcers. *J Am Geriatr Soc.* 2000;48(1):59–62.

This is a retrospective study using the Minimum Data Set to examine the National Health Care Corporation nursing homes from 1991 through 1995. Risk-adjusted rates of pressure-ulcer development that were based on 144,379 observations from 30,150 residents in 107 nursing homes were determined. The study found that between 1991 and 1995, there was a significant ($P < .05$) decrease of 25% in pressure-ulcer development. Moreover, the rate of stage III and stage IV pressure ulcers significantly decreased, from 30% to 2.2% ($P < .01$).

■ Lyder CH, Preston J, Grady JN, et al. Quality of care for hospitalized Medicare patients at risk for pressure ulcers. *Arch Intern Med.* 2001;161(12):1549–1554.

This is a multicenter retrospective cohort study using medical record abstraction to obtain a total of 2425 patients aged 65 years and older discharged from acute-care hospitals after treatment for pneumonia, cerebrovascular disease, or heart failure. Six processes of care for prevention of pressure ulcers in hospitals were evaluated. The national estimates of compliance with process of care were as follows: use of daily skin assessment, 94%; use of pressure-reducing device, 7.5%; documentation of being at risk, 22.6%; repositioning for a minimum of 2 hours, 66.2%; nutritional consultation, 34.3%; stage I pressure ulcer staged, 20.2%; and stage II or greater ulcer staged, 30.9%. These results suggest that U.S. hospitals and physicians have numerous opportunities to improve care that is related to pressure-ulcer prediction and prevention. More importantly, this study suggests that the timing of preventive interventions may be associated with the likelihood of pressure-ulcer development.

■ Lyder CH, Shannon R, Empleo-Frazier O, et al. A comprehensive program to prevent pressure ulcers in long-term care: exploring costs and outcomes. *Ostomy Wound Manage.* 2002;48(4):52–62.

This study examined the use of a comprehensive approach to pressure-ulcer prevention in two long-term-care facilities. Implementation of the comprehensive prevention program resulted in an 87% decrease in pressure-ulcer incidence in facility A (from 13.2% to 1.7% per month, $P = .02$) and a 76% decrease in facility B (from 15% to 3.5% per month, $P = .02$). The average monthly cost of prevention for a high-risk resident was $519.73 (plus a one-time cost of $277 for mattress and chair overlays). More than half ($277.15) of the monthly costs relates to labor; the most expensive item cost is for support surfaces.

■ Stotts NA, Rodeheaver GT, Thomas DR, et al. An instrument to measure healing in pressure ulcers: development and validation of the Pressure Ulcer Scale for Healing (PUSH). *J Gerontol A Biol Sci Med Sci.* 2001;56(12):M795–M799.

The purpose of this retrospective study was to determine the validity of the Pressure Ulcer Scale for Healing (PUSH) tool to monitor healing of stage II–IV pressure ulcers. Two studies were conducted to determine the PUSH tool's validity. Results revealed that the PUSH tool accounted for 58% to 74% of the wound-healing variance over a 10-week period in Study 1 and 40% to 57% of the wound-healing variance over a 12-week period in Study 2. Multiple regression analysis revealed that the PUSH tool accounted for 39% of the variance in 6 weeks and 31% of the variance over 12 weeks ($P < .001$; Studies 1 and 2, respectively). Thus, it was concluded that PUSH tool is clinically valid for measuring pressure-ulcer healing.

Courtney H. Lyder, ND, GNP

PSYCHIATRY

CHAPTER 35—DEPRESSION AND OTHER MOOD DISORDERS

KEY POINTS

- Symptoms of depression below the threshold for a diagnosis of major depression are common in late life and may incur disability, therefore warranting an intervention.

- Selective serotonin-reuptake inhibitors (SSRIs) such as sertraline and citalopram are most commonly used as first-line agents for older adults with depression.

- Treatment of depression may require up to 12 weeks before a response to medication is noted; trials of more than one antidepressant may be required before a satisfactory response is achieved.

- The side-effect profile and propensity to interact with other medications are key factors to consider in selecting an antidepressant for an older patient.

EPIDEMIOLOGY

Prevalence studies of community residents demonstrate surprisingly low rates of depressive disorders among those aged 65 years and older. Only 1% to 2% of women and fewer than 1% of men interviewed with standardized instruments meet diagnostic criteria for major depression. Both current and lifetime prevalence rates for older persons are lower than those for middle-aged persons; furthermore, these relatively low rates persist after accounting for possible premature death and institutionalization, both of which may be associated with depression. Similarly, the incidence of first-episode major depression decreases after age 65. Data demonstrating that older persons are less likely to recognize depression and to endorse depressed mood offer one explanation for the lower prevalence and incidence of depressive syndromes among older community residents.

However, the prevalence of depressive symptoms that do not meet the threshold for a clinical diagnosis is substantial in seniors, with most studies reporting rates in the range of 15%. These subsyndromal states are not inconsequential. "Minor" or subsyndromal depression has been associated with increased use of health services, excess disability, and poor health outcomes, including higher mortality rates.

The prevalence rates of both major and subsyndromal depression are related to the setting in which older persons are seen and methods used to identify cases. Thus, major depression has been identified in 6% to 10% of older persons in primary care clinics and 12% to 20% of nursing-home residents. More varied rates of 11% up to 45% have been reported among elderly patients requiring inpatient medical care. The reported prevalence rates of minor depression in outpatient medical settings have been varied as well, with rates from 8% to over 40% reported. Studies that count symptoms due to physical illness toward a diagnosis of depression may inflate prevalence rates among medical patients because of symptom overlap. In the psychiatric clinic setting, major depression is the most common disorder seen among elderly patients and accounts for more than 40% of outpatient caseloads and inpatient psychiatry admissions.

CLINICAL PRESENTATION AND DIAGNOSIS

The Geriatric Syndrome of Late-Life Depression

Symptoms used to diagnose major depression are listed in Table 35.1, which summarizes the criteria for major depression from the fourth edition of the *Diagnostic and Statistical Manual of Mental Disorders* (*DSM-IV*). Although aging does not markedly affect the overall phenomenology of major depression, some differences between younger and older depressed patients have been reported. Older patients are more preoccupied with somatic symptoms and less frequently report depressed mood and guilty preoccupations. Among patients who do not acknowledge sustained feelings of sadness, the demonstration of the second core symptom, a persistent loss of pleasure and interest in previously enjoyable activities (*anhedonia*), is necessary for a diagnosis of major depression. Thus, one need not exhibit depressed mood to meet criteria for major depressive disorder. The core symptoms are particularly important to detect in primary care settings and have been found to identify most medically ill patients who also meet full diagnostic criteria. Furthermore, these core symptoms are less likely to overlap with those of a medical illness.

The diagnosis of major depression in older persons is complicated by the overlap among symptoms of major depression with those of physical illness. Patients

Table 35.1—*DSM-IV* Diagnostic Criteria for Major Depression

Depressed mood*

Loss of interest or pleasure*

Appetite change or weight loss

Insomnia or hypersomnia

Psychomotor agitation or retardation

Loss of energy

Feelings of worthlessness or guilt

Difficulties with concentration or decision making

Recurrent thoughts of death or suicide

* "Gateway" (or "core") symptoms, at least one of which must be present for a diagnosis of major depression.

NOTE: The diagnosis requires that the patient have at least one gateway or core symptom and that five or more symptoms have occurred nearly every day for most of the day for at least 2 weeks. Also, the symptoms must be causing significant distress or impaired functioning and must not be due to a direct physiologic cause.

SOURCE: Data from the American Psychiatric Association. *Diagnostic and Statistical Manual of Mental Disorders.* 4th ed. Washington, DC: American Psychiatric Association; 1994.

with serious medical illness may be preoccupied with thoughts about death or feel worthless because of concomitant disability. The *DSM-IV* criteria require that the depressive symptoms are not a direct effect of a general medical condition or medication used to treat it, but this distinction based on cause may be difficult to make reliably. Alternative diagnostic criteria have been suggested for medical patients, including an inclusive approach that counts all symptoms regardless of cause. Inclusive approaches result in the highest prevalence rates. Furthermore, a depressed person's thoughts of death and worthlessness appear to differ from those of a patient with a serious medical illness. In depression, these thoughts are not based on a realistic assessment of prognosis or overall self-worth. The perspective of depressed patients is influenced by the feelings of sadness or guilt that accompany the disordered mood. The alternative diagnosis of mood disorder due to a general medical condition should be used for patients with depression that appears to result directly from a specific medical condition (eg, hypothyroidism).

The recognition of psychotic depression has particular relevance to primary care clinicians. Patients with psychotic depression have sustained irrational beliefs (delusions) in association with their depression, and these beliefs not infrequently focus on physical or medical preoccupations, such as the belief that one's bowels are "blocked with cancer." Psychotic depression may be suspected when the irrational belief focuses on somatic symptoms or around fears of a serious physical condition such as cancer when there is no medical source identified to support the belief.

Screening for mood symptoms is an important part of a comprehensive assessment of all older patients regardless of socioeconomic or ethnic status, although cultural variation may influence how emotional states are expressed. Since the diagnosis of depression hinges on a qualitative change from a patient's normal mood state, it is essential to obtain information from involved family members or caregivers to determine whether a clinically meaningful syndrome has developed. Recent large-scale studies of mental health in the elderly age group (eg, the Primary Care Research in Substance Abuse and Mental Health for the Elderly, PRISM-E) have shown that among older persons with depression, there is a preponderance of women and ethnic minorities. This suggests that a higher degree of vigilance for mood disorders is warranted in these groups.

Bipolar Disorder

A diagnosis of mania requires a distinct period of persistently elevated mood lasting for 1 or more weeks and three additional symptoms that may include inflated self-esteem or grandiosity, hypersexuality, increased activity, decreased need for sleep, pressured speech, racing thoughts or flight of ideas, and distractibility. Grandiose or paranoid delusions may be present. Although the criteria for diagnosing bipolar disorder in younger and older patients are identical, some differences in phenomenology have been noted. Elderly patients with bipolar disorder are more likely to have a mixture of depression and marked irritability. Pressured speech that tends to go off on tangents is common, although the severity of thinking disturbance is less pronounced than in young adults and flight of ideas is less common. Hypersexuality and grandiosity may be present but are less prominent, as well. Manic-like syndromes in late life are also distinguished by a greater likelihood of confusion, often a reflection of an underlying cognitive disturbance, such as an incipient dementia.

DIFFERENTIAL DIAGNOSIS

Approximately 30% to 50% of patients with late-life depression are experiencing a recurrence of episodes that began in early adulthood. Despite the associations between late-onset depression and chronic medical illness, disability, and psychosocial stresses, most episodes develop without an identifiable precipitant. Because late-onset depression is less likely than typical recurrent depression to be familial, a positive family history is less useful for establishing a diagnosis.

Differentiation From Medical Illness

Medical disorders that may imitate depression are particularly important to consider in elderly patients because of the increased vulnerability of this population to physical illnesses. Hyperthyroidism merits special consideration, because older hyperthyroid patients may present with apathy and diminished energy that mimics depression. Although apathy may be commonly associated with the core depressive symptom of anhedonia, apathy may also occur in persons who retain a reactive capacity for experiencing pleasure. The distinction of apathy from true depression becomes particularly important among patients with Parkinson's disease, carcinoma of the pancreas, and dementia, because depressive syndromes that occur commonly in these disorders are responsive to antidepressant medications.

Depression Associated With Structural Brain Disease

Major depression may be a prodrome of dementia such as Alzheimer's disease or may develop after the onset of cognitive decline. Differentiation may be confounded because depression is commonly accompanied by symptoms of impaired concentration, indecisiveness, and lack of motivation that are also associated with dementia. An older person with depression may both report memory loss and poor concentration and be unable to perform simple cognitive tests without having dementia. Differentiation from dementia requires evidence that the cognitive impairment, developed concurrently with the onset of depression, and reverses with improvement in mood. Conversely, patients with true dementia may have symptoms that imitate depression. These include loss of interest, apathy, psychomotor retardation, and disrupted sleep. A diagnosis of major depression requires the presence of at least one core symptom and the persistence of symptoms for at least 2 weeks; approximately 20% of patients with early Alzheimer's disease meet these criteria.

Studies have described a syndrome of "vascular" depression that is associated commonly with anhedonia, executive dysfunction, and the absence of guilty preoccupations. The syndrome is thought to result from prefrontal and subcortical lesions due to microinfarcts. These patients tend to have a late age of onset, risk factors for vascular disease, prefrontal or subcortical white matter hyperintensities on T2 weighted magnetic resonance imaging, and evidence of non-amnestic neuropsychologic deficits in tasks requiring initiation, persistence, and self-monitoring. Execution of tasks requiring planning and shifting between cognitive sets is impaired. Depressed patients with such defects in executive function may experience a remission of disturbed mood in response to standard pharmacotherapies but remain substantially disabled because of the cognitive dysfunction.

Bereavement

Bereavement is common among older persons. Feelings of sadness, disturbed sleep, and diminished appetite are common among bereaved persons but are generally time limited and resolve within a few months. Up to 14% of bereaved adults develop a major depression within 2 years of the loss, which occurs with a lower frequency among bereaved elderly persons. Bereavement that has evolved into a major depression is characterized by morbid preoccupations with guilt or suicidal ideas beyond transient thoughts of joining the deceased that would be expected in association with the loss. Also, bereavement is not associated with sustained functional impairment, so a marked decline in self-care may be a sign of a depressive syndrome.

COURSE

Major depression is often a recurrent disorder in both younger and older adults. Evidence from observational studies in which treatment was not provided systematically indicate that up to one third of patients run a chronic course and another third have partial recovery with residual disability. Patients who suffer their first episode in later life take longer to recover. Depressed elderly persons also use health services, including outpatient visits, specialist consultations, and laboratory assessments, more than nondepressed elderly persons do.

Comorbid medical illness is associated with more refractory mood symptoms, and medical morbidity and mortality are themselves increased in patients who have suffered a depressive episode. The relationship between depression and increased mortality rates from cardiovascular causes is particularly striking. Depressed patients have an increased risk of cardiovascular mortality generally, and the development of depression in patients following a myocardial infarction, heart failure, or cardiac bypass surgery increases mortality from cardiovascular events.

Old age is associated with an increased risk for suicide. Persons aged 65 and over represent less than 13% of the population but account for 25% of suicides. The likelihood that an attempt will be lethal approximates 25%, a rate far greater than in young adults. "Psychologic autopsy" studies that use interviews with relatives and physicians to reconstruct a suicide victim's premorbid mental state have demonstrated that as many as 75% of older adults who commit suicide were suffering from depression. The vast majority had seen a primary care physician within the previous month. In addition to depression, risk factors for late-life suicide include a comorbid physical illness, living alone, male gender, and alcoholism. Older men and women commit suicide violently; firearms and hanging are the methods most commonly employed.

TREATMENT

Overview

The course of treatment for major depression can be conceptualized as follows: acute treatment to reverse the current episode, continuation treatment to prevent relapse, and maintenance treatment to prevent recurrence. Continuation treatment to stabilize the recovery involves ongoing antidepressant therapy for an additional 6 months. Maintenance treatment (3 years or longer) is provided to patients with a history of recurrent depression. The duration of maintenance therapy should be based on the frequency and severity of previous episodes. Recurrent episodes complicated by suicidal ideas or attempts warrant lifelong treatment. Psychotherapy, antidepressants, and electroconvulsive therapy (ECT) are empirically proven treatments for depression in older persons.

Initiatives have been developed to increase the likelihood that patients with major depression treated in primary care settings will receive antidepressant treatment that is adequate in dose and duration. The increased attention to this problem results from findings that most elderly patients prefer being treated for depression by their primary care physicians. Studies have shown that the majority of patients who are prescribed antidepressants by their primary care physicians do not obtain refills of their initial prescription. Educational programs and the use of depression nurse specialists have been developed to increase recognition and treatment intensity.

Psychotherapy

Table 35.2 lists the variety and characteristics of psychotherapies advocated for older adults. Research demonstrating the efficacy of psychotherapy for major depression in older adults has included cognitive-behavioral therapy, interpersonal psychotherapy, and problem-solving therapy. Problem-solving therapy involves working with the patient to identify practical life difficulties that are causing distress and providing guidance to help the patient identify solutions. The treatment is delivered generally in six to eight meetings spaced 1 to 2 weeks apart. Cognitive and interpersonal psychotherapy are also time-limited but less highly structured. Psychotherapy for minor depression has been promising, with efficacy demonstrated particularly in persons who have suffered a loss. Also, caregivers of older persons may develop minor or major depressive syndromes that benefit from psychotherapy. Psychotherapy may be combined with an antidepressant, and the combination has been associated with a longer period of remission following recovery from the acute episode. Psychotherapy combined with antidepressant medication is recommended for all patients with severe or suicidal depression.

Table 35.2—Psychotherapy for the Geriatric Syndrome of Late-Life Depression

Therapy	Distinguishing Characteristics
Cognitive-behavioral	Directive, symptom focused Techniques practiced outside of therapy Counters negativistic misperceptions and mistaken pessimistic beliefs
Interpersonal	Exploratory but not open ended Focused on interpersonal conflict, role change, role deficits
Short-term psychodynamic	Problem focused Transference not examined
Life review, reminiscence	Recall of personal history to master one's present and future
Problem solving	Brief, focused on patient-defined solutions Accepts that some problems cannot be changed May be useful to counter executive deficits
Supportive	Meant to maintain present level of function or symptom control
Dementia caregiver counseling	Focused on the caregiver role and activities Combines elements of cognitive-behavioral, problem-solving, and interpersonal therapy
Bereavement therapy	Restructuring (not restoration) the experience of the lost loved one through review of both positive and negative aspects of the relationship
Behavioral	Educational, pragmatic Directed at reducing negative and increasing positive experiences
Dialectical-behavioral therapy	Focused on reduction of counterproductive behaviors Emphasis on acceptance of affect and the inevitability of conflict

Choice of Antidepressants: First Considerations

The choice of agent depends on the patient's comorbid medical conditions, the side-effect profile of the antidepressant, and the individual patient's sensitivity to these effects. Potential interactions with other medications also should be considered. Prominent complaints of sleep disturbance, anxiety, or psychomotor retardation will direct the practitioner toward agents that are, respectively, more sedative or more activating. And because the SSRIs are now the mainstay of antidepressant prescribing, a hierarchy of choices is available in published protocols designed for either primary care or older patient practices. Sertraline and citalopram are often preferred because adverse effects and drug interactions may be less likely than with some other SSRIs, such as fluoxetine and paroxetine.

A number of researchers have explored various strategies to optimally manage depressive syndromes in older persons, recognizing that a systematic approach is often helpful. One such treatment strategy, developed by Steffans and colleagues at Duke University, is called the Duke Somatic Treatment Algorithm for Geriatric Depression. The graded approach in this algorithm begins with a 6- to 12-week trial of the SSRI sertraline for the older depressed patient who has not previously been treated. The only stipulation at this point is that the patient's illness not be severe enough to warrant an intervention such as ECT (eg, an imminent risk of suicide, life-threatening food refusal, psychosis). For an initial SSRI trial, it is recommended that the dose be gradually titrated upward at weekly intervals for the first 3 weeks, as tolerated. If the SSRI is not well tolerated, the clinician may proceed to the venlafaxine trial described below. For patients who have had a previous successful response to an antidepressant, that particular agent would be the medication of choice.

If, after 6 to 12 weeks, a satisfactory response is not evident, then a trial of sustained-release venlafaxine is recommended at a dosage of 150 mg daily for 6 to 12 weeks. If the symptoms do not remit with venlafaxine, other options may be considered at this point, such as augmentation with another medication. For example, if there is a partial response to the SSRI but with residual low energy and low interest, then the SSRI may be augmented with sustained-release bupropion for an additional 6 weeks. Other options in the context of incomplete response may include augmenting with lithium carbonate or switching to a tricyclic antidepressant or monoamine oxidase inhibitor (MAOI). However, at this juncture it might be helpful to obtain consultation from a psychiatrist or other mental health professional.

Selective Serotonin-Reuptake Inhibitors

SSRIs and tricyclic antidepressants are comparably effective for treating mild to moderate major depression, but SSRIs are often better tolerated. Table 35.3 provides a detailed summary of dosing, formulations, precautions, and advantages of the individual SSRIs. Controversy continues about whether the most severe melancholic form of depression that generally requires treatment in a psychiatric hospital responds better to a tricyclic antidepressant. Melancholic patients typically suffer from marked appetite and weight loss, diurnal mood variation that is worse in the morning, early morning awakening, and either retardation of motor movement or agitation.

Although the SSRIs are generally free of severe side effects, a small proportion of elderly patients develop hyponatremia that is due to the syndrome of inappropriate antidiuretic hormone secretion during SSRI treatment, particularly at higher doses. Rare patients are unable to tolerate SSRIs because of induced anxiety, sleep disturbance, or agitation. This reaction appears to be more common in older persons and may in some cases be related to the inhibition of the metabolism of other medications, discussed later in this section. Beginning at lower doses may reduce the incidence of anxiety with activating SSRIs such as fluoxetine and may decrease the gastrointestinal adverse effects of nausea or diarrhea that occur with SSRIs. Sexual side effects occur commonly with all SSRIs, and many patients may not wish to continue SSRI treatment because of them, so inquiring about sexual function is an important part of follow-up care. Although SSRIs have been associated with mild weight loss initially, long-term use with many of these medications has been associated with weight gain. Pseudoparkinsonism and other movement disorders may occur, particularly if these medications are used in combination with other drugs that block dopamine (eg, metoclopramide).

SSRIs inhibit various P-450 hepatic cytochrome isoenzymes that metabolize most medications. Fluoxetine and paroxetine are potent inhibitors of the P-450 2D6 isoenzyme responsible for the metabolism of most psychiatric medications, as well as dextromethorphan, codeine, tricyclic antidepressants, and metoprolol. Sertraline is a weak inhibitor of both the 2D6 and 3A4 isoenzymes. Inhibition of 2D6 can decrease the analgesic effects of codeine (and related compounds) and tramadol by preventing their conversion to their active metabolites, morphine and O-desmethyltramadol. Fluoxetine's active metabolite, norfluoxetine, also inhibits the 3A4 isozymes. The SSRI fluvoxamine inhibits the 3A4, 2D6, and 1A2 systems. Because P-450 1A2 is required to metabolize theophylline, olanzapine, and phenacetin, concurrent

Table 35.3—Selective Serotonin-Reuptake Inhibitors for Older Adults

Generic (Trade) Name	Initial Dosage	Final Dosage	Sedative Potential	Precautions	Advantages
Citalopram (Celexa)	10 mg am	20–40 mg am	Low	Side effects include nausea, tremor, dizziness, sweating, agitation	Few drug interactions, well tolerated
Escitalopram (Lexapro)	10 mg am	10–20 mg am	Low	Nausea, tremor, dizziness, sweating, agitation	May have fewer side effects than citalopram, well tolerated
Fluoxetine (Prozac)	10 mg am	20–40 mg am	Low	Nausea, tremor, dizziness, sweating, agitation, prolonged half-life, insomnia, drug interactions	Liquid preparation available
Paroxetine (Paxil)	10 mg hs	20–40 mg hs	Low	Nausea, tremor, dizziness, sweating, agitation, drug interactions, anticholinergic effects	Mild sedative effect
Sertraline (Zoloft)	25 mg am	100–200 mg am	Low	Nausea, tremor, dizziness, sweating, agitation	Few drug interactions, well tolerated

NOTE: am = *ante meridiem* or before noon; hs = *hora somni* or at bedtime.

use of fluvoxamine may result in markedly increased concentrations of these medications. Given its potential for multiple interactions, the use of fluvoxamine in older patients is best limited unless monitored very closely.

SSRIs may increase the anticoagulant effects of medications such as warfarin, potentially through cytochrome isoenzyme inhibition or the inhibition of platelet activity. Careful monitoring of prothrombin times or another suitable index of blood clotting is indicated following the introduction of an SSRI to patients being treated with warfarin.

SSRIs have been considered particularly safe for older persons because these antidepressants do not cause orthostatic hypotension, arrhythmias, or marked sedation. However, evidence indicates that nursing-home residents treated with SSRIs are at increased risk for falling and suffering hip fractures. It is not clear whether these findings are due to patient selection in that patients considered at greatest risk for falling may be treated with SSRIs preferentially. Alternatively, SSRIs may contribute to falls by causing a subtle balance disturbance or pseudoparkinsonism in vulnerable patients. Or depression itself may be a risk factor.

With the introduction of serotonergic reuptake inhibitors, reports emerged of a serotonergic withdrawal syndrome following discontinuation lasting 2 to 3 weeks and characterized by lightheadedness, insomnia, agitation, nausea, headache, and sensory disturbances. Mood disturbance may also occur. The shorter-acting SSRIs (sertraline, paroxetine) appear to induce this syndrome, but venlafaxine and other SSRIs have also been implicated. Therefore, these agents should be tapered rather than stopped abruptly.

Tricyclic Antidepressants

The tricyclic antidepressants nortriptyline and desipramine are the most appropriate for use in older persons. Table 35.4 provides a detailed summary of dosing, formulations, precautions, and advantages of these agents. They are effective in the most severe forms of depression but are associated with anticholinergic side effects that may be problems in older patients. For nortriptyline, therapeutic response is associated with blood levels between 50 and 150 ng/mL and for desipramine, levels above 120 ng/mL. Over 60% of patients with nonpsychotic major depression or with depression that is not associated with dementia respond within 6 weeks to levels in these ranges. Although 5% of the population requires lower dosing because of the absence of the enzyme required to metabolize secondary amine tricyclics, most patients achieve target concentrations at dosages of 50 to 75 mg per day of nortriptyline and 100 to 150 mg per day of desipramine.

The potential for side effects that are due to the anticholinergic and sedative properties of tricyclics limits their use in older patients. These medications are particularly inappropriate for patients who are sensitive to constipation or vulnerable to orthostatic hypotension and for men with benign prostatic hyperplasia. Also, tricyclic antidepressants have a quinidine-like effect that delays ventricular conduction. Among patients with a pretreatment first-degree heart block, 10% may develop a second-degree block during treatment. Patients with bundle branch block or prolonged QT_c interval are at risk for developing a ventricular arrhythmia.

Table 35.4—Tricyclic Antidepressants for Older Adults

Generic (Trade) Name	Initial Dosage	Final Dosage	Sedative Potential	Precautions	Advantages
Desipramine (Norpramin)	10–25 mg hs	25–150 mg hs	Low	May be fatal in overdose May exacerbate glaucoma, anticholinergic effects	Therapeutic plasma level 115–200 ng/mL May have stimulant properties
Nortriptyline (Pamelor, Aventyl)	10–25 mg hs	25–100 mg hs	Moderate	Lower final dose May be fatal in overdose May exacerbate glaucoma, anticholinergic effects	Therapeutic window for plasma levels of 50–150 ng/mL

NOTE: hs = *hora somni* or at bedtime.

Other Antidepressants

Table 35.5 provides a detailed summary of dosing, formulations, precautions, and advantages of other antidepressants, including a stimulant. Bupropion is generally safe, free of sexual side effects, and well tolerated when used at recommended doses. Bupropion has been associated with a 0.4% risk of seizures, which is much higher when recommended doses are exceeded, and is contraindicated in persons with a seizure disorder. Bupropion appears to act by increasing the activity of dopamine and norepinephrine and therefore has stimulant-like qualities. Because of the activating property of bupropion, dosing of the short-acting form in the morning and mid-afternoon may help to avoid insomnia. Long-acting bupropion has a smaller seizure risk and is less likely to cause insomnia. Doses are increased gradually by the use of a twice-a-day regimen to achieve target doses of 150 to 300 mg per day of the short-acting form. The dosage range of sustained-release bupropion is 150 to 300 mg per day given as a single daily dose.

Venlafaxine acts as an SSRI at lower doses while also inhibiting the reuptake of norepinephrine at the high end of the therapeutic range of 75 to 225 mg per day. Venlafaxine is effective for both generalized anxiety and major depression and may treat both effectively at dosages of 75 to 150 mg per day. A dose-response relationship for severe depression has been demonstrated, and patients with melancholia may require dosages of 225 mg per day or greater. Initial dosing should use gradual increases to minimize the early side effect of nausea. The noradrenergic properties of higher doses may explain the association between doses of 225 mg and higher with hypertension. Patients requiring doses at the high end of the therapeutic range should have blood-pressure monitoring. This side effect does not occur in patients with hypertension controlled by a β-blocker. Venlafaxine should also be discontinued several days prior to ECT to avoid hypertension during ECT. Venlafaxine, like other SSRIs, has been associated with decreased sexual functioning. Venlafaxine should be discontinued by gradual tapering to avoid the risk of flu-like discontinuation symptoms.

Duloxetine is a new antidepressant medication that has been approved for the treatment of both depression and neuropathic pain secondary to diabetes mellitus. Duloxetine is a serotonin- and norepinephrine-reuptake inhibitor, and its pharmacodynamic characteristics are generally like those of venlafaxine, although it is structurally unique. Because of its effects of increasing neural sphincter activity and bladder capacity, it has also been approved for the treatment of urinary incontinence and has been shown to reduce stress incontinence in women. These features may make duloxetine advantageous for the older patient.

Mirtazapine is a norepinephrine, 5-HT$_2$, and 5-HT$_3$ antagonist. The total daily dosage is 15 to 45 mg. Mirtazapine is given as a single bedtime dose to capitalize on its sedative properties and is available in rapidly dissolving form for patients who have difficulty swallowing pills. Mirtazapine is also associated with increased appetite and weight gain. This side-effect profile has contributed to the use of mirtazapine before bed in nursing-home residents with depression and dementia who demonstrate nighttime agitation and weight loss. Mirtazapine is also free of sexual side effects.

The MAOIs are effective antidepressants that have been in use for nearly half a century. Orthostatic hypotension is a common adverse effect of MAOIs and in older patients may increase the risk of falling. Concomitant ingestion of a food product rich in tyramine (eg, cheese) or of pseudoephedrine or pressor amines can cause a life-threatening hypertensive crisis. The use of MAOIs with an SSRI or meperidine can cause a fatal serotonin syndrome associated with delirium and hyperthermia.

Although methylphenidate and other stimulants have been used for decades to treat major depression, controlled data demonstrating their efficacy are limited. However, these agents may have a role in reversing the apathy and lack of energy seen in some patients with

Table 35.5—Other Antidepressants, Including Stimulants, for Older Adults

Generic (Trade) Name	Initial Dosage	Final Dosage	Sedative Potential	Precautions	Advantages
Other Antidepressants					
Bupropion (Wellbutrin SR)	SR: 75 mg qd	SR: 150–300 mg qd	Low	Dopaminergic, noradrenergic, agitation, insomnia, seizures Dose should be divided	May help apathetic depression Sustained-release form available
Duloxetine (Cymbalta)	20 mg	30–60 mg	Low	Drug interactions (CYP 1A2, 2D6 substrate)	Equally SSRI and SNRI, narrow dose range FDA approved for neuropathic pain
Hypericum perforatum, or St. John's wort	300 mg bid	900 mg tid	Low	Use standardized, freeze-dried extract, 0.3% hypericin Drug interactions with other antidepressants	Low side-effect profile, OTC
Mirtazapine (Remeron, Sol-tabs)	7.5 mg hs	15–45 mg hs	Moderate	Prolonged half-life, renal clearance Dry mouth, weight gain Serotonergic and noradrenergic	Sedative effects may improve sleep
Trazodone (Desyrel)	25–50 mg hs	100–200 mg hs	High	Very sedative	For sleep disturbance
Venlafaxine (Effexor, Effexor XR)	37.5 mg bid XR: 75 mg qd	75–225 mg qd	Low	Headache, nausea, vomiting Hypertension, withdrawal syndrome	Fewer drug interactions Extended-release preparation available, may be more effective than SSRIs
Stimulants					
Methylphenidate (Ritalin)	5 mg am	20 mg bid	Low	Side effects include anorexia, insomnia Daytime use only	Quick results For frail and apathetic patients
Modafinil (Provigil)	200 mg am	400 mg am	Low	Little used in elderly patients	Once-daily dosing, reverses daytime sedation sometimes observed with SSRIs

NOTE: am = *ante meridiem* or before noon; bid = *bis in die* or twice a day; FDA = U.S. Food and Drug Administration; hs = *hora somni* or at bedtime; OTC = over-the-counter; qd = *quaque die* or every day; SR = sustained release; SNRI = serotonin-norepinephrine reuptake inhibitor; SSRI = selective serotonin-reuptake inhibitor; TCA = tricyclic antidepressant; tid = *ter in die* or three times a day; XR = extended release.

dementia or disabling medical conditions. Benzodiazepines may be useful temporary adjuncts to treat anxiety and sleep disturbance associated with a major depression, but older persons are particularly sensitive to the adverse effects of these medications on cognition and gait stability.

Management of Partial Response and Nonresponse: Optimize, Switch, or Augment

Approximately 50% of patients with major depression demonstrate a robust response to treatment within 6 weeks. An additional 15% to 25% who have begun to improve achieve remission if treatment is continued for an additional 4 to 6 weeks. Some published studies using SSRIs have reported 6-week response rates of 40% that increases to more than 60% when treatment extends to 12 weeks. However, noticeable improvement within the first 2 weeks of treatment predicts the likelihood of successful recovery with the initial medication. The admonition to "start low, go slow" in treating the older patient is too often interpreted as "start low, stay low," which can lead to mistaken labeling of the patient as a nonresponder. A less than 30% reduction in symptom severity by the sixth week of treatment at the indicated dose defines nonresponse. A 50% reduction in symptom severity indicates partial response. In either case the dose should be "optimized" by increasing to the upper limit of the final recommended dose range, depending on patient tolerance. Patients with a genuine nonresponse should be switched from an SSRI to a non-SSRI. Patients experiencing a partial response to an SSRI may receive augmentation (combination) therapy with a non-SSRI.

The options of switching to an antidepressant from another class or consulting a psychiatrist are more appropriate than initiating unfamiliar combination treatments.

Electroconvulsive Therapy for Psychotic Depression

Psychotic depression is often resistant to standard antidepressant regimens. Aggressive pharmacotherapy is required, with best results obtained in young adults when high doses of antidepressants and antipsychotic medications are combined. However, the effectiveness of combination treatment for older patients with psychotic depression remains uncertain. Available evidence suggests that most elderly patients who have depression with pronounced psychotic features either cannot tolerate adequate doses of conventional medications or do not respond to them. Therefore, ECT has become the standard treatment for late-life psychotic depression.

MANAGEMENT OF BIPOLAR DISORDER

Most persons with bipolar disorder have a history of episodes in early adulthood and often receive chronic treatment with an anti-manic medication. Occasionally this regimen may need adjustment if a new episode of mania emerges. Evidence to support an array of medications for mania has increased substantially in the past decade (see Table 35.6). In addition to lithium and established mood stabilizers for mania, newer antipsychotic and anticonvulsant medications are used in managing manic symptoms, although controlled trials in elderly patients are lacking.

Lithium Carbonate

Lithium carbonate is highly effective for the acute and maintenance treatment of classical manic episodes. It is important to recognize that much lower plasma levels are recommended for older patients than for younger patients. For example, plasma ranges of 0.8 to 1.2 mEq/L are used to treat acute mania in younger adults, and levels of 0.6 to 0.8 mEq/L are used for mania prophylaxis. The use of lithium for treating elderly patients is complicated by the 30% decrease in renal functioning that accompanies normal aging and the increased sensitivity of older persons to neurologic side effects from this medication, particularly if structural brain disease is present.

The decreased renal clearance of lithium in the older patient is addressed simply by reducing the total daily dose. Furthermore, lower concentrations may be adequate in older adults; some patients respond acutely to levels in the range of 0.6 to 0.8 mEq/L or less. Levels of 0.4 to 0.6 mEq/L may provide effective prophylaxis. Also, older persons develop neurologic

side effects at concentrations that are well tolerated in young adults. A fine resting tremor, diarrhea, myoclonus, an intention tremor, or pseudo-parkinsonism may develop with levels in the standard therapeutic range. Sensitivity to these effects and to increased confusion is increased among patients with dementia and when lithium is coadministered with an antipsychotic medication. Clinicians are advised to balance the therapeutic effects of a concentration at the low end of the usual target range against side effects that develop in a particular patient. Consideration should be given to a time lag of 1 to 2 weeks that may occur between achieving a steady-state dose and either therapeutic efficacy or the development of neurologic side effects.

Drugs that inhibit lithium excretion may raise concentrations by up to 50% and result in toxicity if the lithium dose is not decreased. Many of the nonsteroidal anti-inflammatory agents, including ibuprofen, have this effect. Thiazide and potassium-sparing diuretics, angiotensin-converting enzyme inhibitors, and angiotensin-receptor blockers raise lithium levels as well. The effect of furosemide is less clear, but lithium levels should be checked a few days after this diuretic is added in an older patient receiving lithium. Both dehydration and salt depletion are known to raise lithium levels. With adequate monitoring, bipolar patients who have benefited from lithium need not be deprived of this medication because of advanced age.

Anticonvulsants

Valproic acid (valproate, divalproex) has been approved for the treatment of bipolar disorder and is comparable in efficacy to lithium. Target concentrations of 50 to 100 µg/mL used to treat seizure disorders appear to be appropriate. Divalproex has been used effectively to treat agitation in patients with dementia and may be particularly useful for the treatment of behavioral disturbance associated with mood lability. However, upward titration in the frail elderly person must be carried out carefully because dementia patients may be particularly vulnerable to developing excessive sedation during valproic acid treatment. As with other anticonvulsants used to treat mania, valproic acid is associated with allergic skin rashes in 5% to 10% of patients. Decreased platelet counts occur at higher doses, and platelet functioning may be diminished. Patients with hepatic disease may develop liver toxicity during valproic acid treatment. Patients with low albumin concentrations will also have a higher proportion of free drug in their blood and are at greater risk for toxicity.

Carbamazepine[OL] is another antiepileptic medication that has been used to treat mania. Leukopenia and

---

[OL] Not approved by the U.S. Food and Drug Administration for this use.

Table 35.6—Agents Used to Stabilize Mania and Manic-Like Symptoms

Generic (Trade) Name	Initial Dosage	Final Dosage	Sedative Potential	Precautions	Advantages
Anticonvulsants					
Divalproex sodium (Depakote, Depakote ER)	250 mg bid; ER: 500 mg hs	1000 mg bid; ER: 1000 mg hs	Moderate	Delayed onset of action, drug interactions GI upset, tremor, weight gain, edema, thrombocytopenia Inhibits hepatic enzymes; increases other drug levels Hepatoxicity, pancreatitis	Better tolerated than carbamazepine Therapeutic level 50–100 µg/mL
Carbamazepine (Tegretol, Epitol)	100 mg bid	400 mg bid	Moderate	Delayed onset of action, drug interactions Dizziness, unsteady gait, rare agranulocytosis Enhances cytochrome P-450 activity and decreases other drug levels Not FDA approved for bipolar disorder	Therapeutic level 4–12 µg/mL Available as a liquid
Antipsychotics					
Olanzapine (Zyprexa, Zyprexa Zydis [oral dissolving])	2.5 mg qd	5–15 mg qd	Moderate	Anticholinergic as dose increases Cost Weight gain, hyperglycemia	FDA approved for acute mania and maintenance monotherapy for bipolar I disorder but not for bipolar depression
Quetiapine (Seroquel)	25 mg bid	100 mg bid	More than moderate	Slit-lamp examination for cataracts	Sedative, not anticholinergic, fewer EPS, less TD FDA approved for mania
Risperidone (Risperdal, Risperdal Consta [injectable])	0.25 mg qd Inj: 25 mg q 2 weeks	6 mg qd Inj: 50 mg q 2 weeks	Moderate	EPS likely at doses above 2 mg, high potency, cost, reports of stroke	Available in liquid form FDA approved for acute mania
Benzodiazepine					
Clonazepam (Klonopin)	0.5 mg bid	5 mg bid	Moderate	Long half-life Fall risk limits use in elderly patients May exacerbate confusion in dementia Not FDA approved for bipolar disorder	Calming, sedation
Lithium					
Lithium carbonate (Eskalith, Eskalith CR)	300 mg qd; CR: 450 mg qd	300 mg tid; CR: 450 mg bid	Low	Renal clearance is sole route of elimination Toxicity may appear below therapeutic range Nausea, vomiting are signs of toxicity Risk of hypothyroidism with long-term use Drug interactions	Patient preference, otherwise, none Therapeutic level 0.4–1.0 mEq/mL

NOTE: bid = *bis in die* or twice a day; CBC = complete blood cell count; CR = controlled release; EPS = extrapyramidal symptoms; ER = extended release; FDA = U.S. Food and Drug Administration; GI = gastrointestinal; hs = *hora somni* or at bedtime; q = *quaque* or every; qd = *quaque die* or every day; TD = tardive dyskinesia; tid = *ter in die* or three times a day.

thrombocytopenia occurs in 5% to 10% of patients within the first 2 weeks of treatment. However, life-threatening agranulocytosis and aplastic anemia occur rarely.

Lamotrigine is a newer anticonvulsant that has been approved for the treatment of depression in the context of bipolar affective disorder, although trials specifically in elderly patients are not available. Titration should be conducted very carefully in patients who may also be taking hepatic cytochrome isoenzyme-inducing drugs or valproic acid. In the absence of these, titration begins at 25 mg per day for 2 weeks, then 50 mg per day for 2 weeks, then 100 mg per day for 1 week, then 200 mg per day for usual maintenance. As with most of the anticonvulsants, for patients with moderate liver dysfunction the doses should be reduced by approximately 50%, and with more severe dysfunction the doses should be reduced by approximately 75%.

For patients in whom ECT is anticipated, anticonvulsants agents should be tapered and discontinued if at all possible because of the likelihood of interfering with an adequate seizure duration during the course of treatments.

Antipsychotics

Most antipsychotic medications are observed clinically to exert some anti-manic effects; however, olanzapine has been approved by the U.S. Food and Drug Administration for the acute treatment of mania. Concerns about olanzapine-associated metabolic syndrome need to be considered. Mania in late life may be associated with confusion and cognitive dysfunction; the anticholinergic effects of olanzapine may exacerbate these symptoms. Risperidone and quetiapine are also FDA approved for the acute treatment of mania.

Electroconvulsive Therapy

ECT is highly effective for the treatment of major depression and mania, with response rates exceeding 70% in older adults. ECT is the first-line treatment for patients at serious risk for suicide or life-threatening poor intake due to a major depression. Patients with delusional depression may demonstrate paranoia about their food or caregivers, precluding pharmacologic treatment because of the unreliable oral intake. Also, delusional depression is less responsive to standard medication regimens. Therefore, ECT is generally the first-line treatment for these patients and is associated with response rates that approximate 80%.

The cognitive side effects of ECT are the principal factor limiting its acceptance. Anterograde amnesia or the inability to learn new information may be pronounced initially, particularly during bilateral ECT, but it improves rapidly following completion of treatment. Retrograde amnesia is more persistent, and the recall of events that immediately preceded ECT may be lost permanently. Although patients may complain that ECT has had a long-term effect on their memory, longitudinal studies have failed to demonstrate lasting cognitive effects; furthermore, improved memory, perhaps owing to recovery from depression, has been reported. There are few absolute medical contraindications other than the presence of increased intracranial pressure or unstable angina. Patients with coronary artery disease or cerebral vascular disease may be administered ECT safely by the use of appropriate pharmacologic management of the autonomic responses that may occur during treatment. Nevertheless, a recent myocardial infarction or cerebral vascular event and unstable coronary artery disease increase the risk of complications. Right unilateral treatment produces fewer cognitive side effects than bilateral treatment but is less effective unless doses markedly exceeding a patient's seizure threshold are used.

The selection of ECT over aggressive pharmacotherapy is generally made by weighing the risk of waiting for a medication to work against the burden of hospital treatment, any medical conditions that may complicate general anesthesia, and patient biases against this treatment. After a course of ECT, patients should be treated with continuation pharmacotherapy following recovery. Patients who have failed intensive antidepressant treatment before receiving ECT have lower acute response rates and are more likely to relapse subsequently, even when antidepressant continuation treatment with a new medication is provided. Although maintenance ECT is sometimes used to prevent relapse, the burden that maintenance ECT places on patients and their families may limit its usefulness for the long-term management of late-life major depression.

ANNOTATED REFERENCES

■ Alexopoulos GS, Meyers BS, Young RC, et al. Executive dysfunction and long-term outcomes of geriatric depression. *Arch Gen Psychiatry.* 2000;57(3):285–290.

This study assessed relapse and recurrence rates among elderly patients with major depression during 16 weeks of continuation treatment with therapeutic concentrations of nortriptyline and during up to 2 years of maintenance treatment with nortriptyline or placebo. All patients had achieved remission with nortriptyline. Patients who demonstrated abnormal initiation and perseveration scores indicative of executive dysfunction had significantly higher relapse rates during continuation treatment and higher recurrence rates during either nortriptyline or placebo maintenance. Memory impairment did not affect the course of remission. The data are consistent with the hypothesis that disruption of prefrontal pathways worsens the treatment response and course of geriatric depression.

■ Denihan A, Kirby M, Bruce I, et al. Three-year prognosis of depression in the community-dwelling elderly. *Br J Psychiatry*. 2000;176(5):453–457.

This study builds on prognostic research of clinical samples of elderly persons with major depression by investigating community residents at baseline and 3 years later to determine their course of illness. Late-life depression was found to be associated with higher-than-expected mortality rates and persistent impairment. Poor physical health was found to be associated with a poor outcome, and having been treated with antidepressants was found to significantly improve the prognosis.

■ Fava M, Rush AJ, Trivedi MH, et al. Background and rationale for the Sequenced Treatment Alternatives to Relieve Depression (STAR*D) study. *Psychiatr Clin N Am*. 2003;26(2):457–494.

Results from the Sequenced Treatment Alternatives to Relieve Depression (STAR*D) study, once complete, will provide evidence to guide both switch and augmentation strategies. The study is being conducted in both primary care and specialty practices in public and private settings. Citalopram is the first choice, followed by switching to either sertraline, bupropion, or venlafaxine. Cognitive-behavioral therapy is also an option with or without medications. The first choice for augmentation includes bupropion sustained release, cognitive therapy, or addition of the antianxiety agent buspirone. Additional steps in treatment include mirtazapine or nortriptyline as well as augmentation strategies. STAR*D will provide data on the "switch or augment" strategy by anticipating partial responses and genuine treatment resistance.

■ Kennedy GJ, Marcus P. Use of antidepressants in older patients with co-morbid medical conditions: guidance from studies of depression in somatic illness. *Drugs Aging*. 2005;22(4):273–287.

In this review the authors survey the antidepressant literature for the eight most common disabling somatic illnesses in late life. They observe that the increasing number of antidepressants and adjunctive medications have increased the practitioner's perplexity when confronted with a very old, very depressed patient. However, a growing body of evidence from antidepressant studies in the context of age-related somatic illnesses allows reasonable inferences to guide the diagnosis and treatment of depression in the oldest-old patient. They advise practitioners to assess the benefits of prescribed medication within the first days rather than first weeks of treatment and to escalate the antidepressant to the established therapeutic range rather than seek the lowest effective dose. Patients who experience no benefit whatsoever within the first weeks of treatment despite being within the therapeutic range should be prescribed an alternative.

■ Mulsant BH, Alexopoulos GS, Reyolds CF 3rd, et al. Pharmacologic treatment of depression in older primary care patients: the PROSPECT algorithm. *Int J Geriatr Psychiatry*. 2001;16(6):585–592.

The Prevention of Suicide in Primary Care Elderly: Collaborative Trial (PROSPECT) algorithm adapted existing treatment guidelines for depression in older adults to primary care settings. The aim of the study was to prevent suicide through aggressive treatment of late-life depression in primary care patients. Strict definitions for nonresponse and partial response were linked to unambiguous options. Augmentation is preferred for partial responders, switch for nonresponders. Citalopram is the first choice, but if the patient is taking another antidepressant at substandard dose or duration, that medication should be "optimized" to the recommended dose for 12 weeks before choosing switch or augmentation. Psychotherapy is included as augmentation for partial responders or as sole therapy for those who prefer drug-free treatment. Psychotherapy as augmentation is also recommended at the outset for severe depression. Nonresponders may be switched to nortriptyline. Lithium and nortriptyline as well as the newer antidepressants may be used to augment the treatment of partial responders.

■ Steffens DC, McQuoid DR, Krishnan KR. The Duke Somatic Treatment Algorithm for Geriatric Depression (STAGED) approach. *Psychopharmacol Bull*. 2002; 36(2):58–68.

The Duke Somatic Treatment Algorithm for Geriatric Depression (STAGED) offers five stages of treatment that are based on the patient's past experience with antidepressants. Nearly 90% of patients achieved partial remission and nearly two thirds full recovery, as defined by predetermined symptom assessment measures. For persons with either a partial response or no response, the choices included both switch and augmentation. Through stage 4 the newer antidepressants were employed before nortriptyline singly or combined with either lithium or a selective serotonin-reuptake inhibitor was prescribed. Cumulative response rates took 9 months to plateau, but ranged from 95% (stage 1) to 81% (stage 5). The authors acknowledge that their practice site is a university-based psychiatric research setting with access to laboratory and diagnostic procedures as well as an inpatient unit, resources that are not available to every primary care site. Indeed, nearly one quarter of patients studied received electroconvulsive therapy. In summary, as applied by expert practitioners in an ideal setting with aggressive follow-through, STAGED gets nearly every patient better and almost two thirds well.

Gary J. Kennedy, MD

CHAPTER 36—ANXIETY DISORDERS

KEY POINTS

- Late-life anxiety is often a comorbid condition with other problems such as cognitive decline and depression.

- Comorbid medical problems that commonly lead to anxiety include cardiovascular and pulmonary disorders.

- Selective serotonin-reuptake inhibitor medications such as sertraline are often used as first-line treatment for anxiety in late life.

- Nonpharmacologic therapies such as relaxation training may be helpful, particularly for generalized anxiety and anxiety secondary to medical conditions.

Older adults suffer from the entire range of anxiety disorders. The clinician treating older persons therefore needs to be familiar with the hallmarks and available treatments for each type of anxiety disorder. Since the published literature on anxiety in elderly patients is relatively sparse, some of the characterizations and treatment strategies described here are based on research carried out in younger populations. They have been modified to take into account the physiologic and psychologic differences between older and younger adults.

Familiarity with the various diagnostic criteria, along with the skill to conduct a thorough psychologic assessment, is crucial in determining the most appropriate treatment for anxiety. Clinicians need to be aware of difficulties in proper assessment of geriatric anxiety; these include medical comorbidity, the difficulty of differentiating anxiety from depression, falsely high scores on anxiety rating scales resulting from overemphasis of cardiac and respiratory problems, and the tendency of older patients to resist psychiatric evaluation.

Anxiety assessment begins with a clinical interview to determine the course and nature of symptoms, along with the nature of the patient's mental status and external support. Supplemental rating scales, which aid in comparing a patient's level of difficulties with that of others and assessing difficulties over time, along with laboratory investigations, can result in an accurate clinical picture and the ability to formulate an effective management plan. Even though discrete anxiety disorders such as panic disorders are less prevalent among older than among younger adults, anxiety as a symptom is a common problem. The ability to recognize and effectively treat anxiety in older persons is important, given the debilitating effects that an unhealthy level of anxiety can have in this vulnerable population.

CLASSES OF ANXIETY DISORDERS

The types of anxiety disorders as currently defined in the fourth edition of the *Diagnostic and Statistical Manual of Mental Disorders* (*DSM-IV*) are listed in Table 36.1.

Panic Disorder

Panic attacks are acute, discrete episodes of intense anxiety that result as a reaction to some perceived threat (eg, emotional, environmental). The term *panic attack* is used when a person experiences an intense and acute reaction to an internal or external cue; it lasts between a few minutes and a half hour. The physiologic symptoms may include trembling, accelerated heart rate, sweating, shortness of breath, chest pain, dizziness, nausea, and the sense that one is somehow detached from the surroundings. For example, a person might have a fear of being trapped on an elevator and report feeling dizzy and nauseated when entering one. Another might report high levels of acute anxiety at the mere sight of elevator doors. A clinically significant degree of panic symptoms exists if a review of the patient's history reveals that recurrent and unpredictable panic attacks have occurred for at least 1 month and time is being spent in worried

Table 36.1—Types of Anxiety Disorders Defined in *DSM-IV*

Panic disorder without agoraphobia

Panic disorder with agoraphobia

Agoraphobia without history of panic disorder

Specific phobias

    Animal type

    Natural environment type

    Blood-injection-injury type

    Situational type

    Other type

Social phobia

Obsessive-compulsive disorder

Posttraumatic stress disorder

Acute stress disorder

Generalized anxiety disorder

Anxiety disorder due to a general medical condition

Substance-induced anxiety disorder

Anxiety disorder not otherwise specified

SOURCE: Data from *Diagnostic and Statistical Manual of Mental Disorders.* 4th ed. Washington, DC: American Psychiatric Association; 1994.

anticipation of possible reoccurrence. Diagnostically, one needs also to consider whether agoraphobia related to the panic attacks is present. In such cases, agoraphobia involves the persistent fear of situations that result in a panic attack, as when a patient reports remaining at home in order to avoid an attack. Common examples of feared situations include being caught in a crowd or trapped in traffic. Comparison of young and older adults with panic disorder indicates that age of onset can affect the clinical presentation. Patients with late-onset panic disorder (at or after age 55) report fewer panic symptoms and less avoidance, and they score lower on somatization measures than do those with early-onset panic disorder. Also, earlier-onset panic more commonly persists into old age.

Phobic Disorders

Phobias include several distinct disorders, categorized as specific phobia and social phobia. A specific phobia involves a distinct trigger, such as a specific person, animal, place, object, event, or situation that results in symptoms of anxiety. Commonly, the patient's anxiety level increases instantly when the feared trigger is encountered. Interestingly, he or she is able to identify this fear as unrealistic and unsupported, even though the cognitive and physiologic responses persist. Specific phobias often involve a great amount of anticipatory anxiety (thoughts of just the possibility of encountering the feared stimulus), and avoidance behaviors are likely to be reported. The consequence of such a clinical profile is that the person experiences a variety of personal difficulties as a result of the anxiety. These behaviors interfere with work and daily routines, and they decrease the person's opportunities to experience pleasurable situations (for fear that a trigger might be present). They may also contribute to secondary symptoms, such as frustration, hopelessness, and a sense that one lacks control in one's life. The level of anxiety or fear usually varies as a function of both the degree of proximity to the phobic stimuli and the degree to which escape is limited. Examples of common phobias include fear of specific animals, closed spaces, flying, or heights. Frequently, specific phobias occur with panic disorder, with or without agoraphobia. Among elderly persons, especially in urban settings, fear of crime seems to be particularly prevalent. Phobic disorders tend to be chronic and persist into old age. However, fear of falling is a specific phobia that is increasingly recognized to have an onset in later life.

Persons with social phobia suffer from fears that they will behave in a manner that is inept or embarrassing. Commonly, the fear is that of trembling, blushing, or sweating profusely in social situations. Other common feared situations involve giving public speeches, going on dates, or simply socializing with others at a function or party. Again, as with specific phobias, social phobia is often accompanied with a significant degree of anticipatory anxiety or avoidance, or both. Though systematic studies of this disorder in elderly persons are lacking, epidemiologic data indicate that this disorder is chronic and persistent in old age. Common manifestations in old age include the inability to eat food in the presence of strangers, and, especially in men, being unable to urinate in public lavatories.

Obsessive-Compulsive Disorder

Obsessive-compulsive disorder involves persistent thoughts (obsessions) and behaviors (compulsions) that are performed in an effort to decrease the anxiety experienced as a result of the thoughts. Obsessions are thoughts or ideas that come to a person's mind, commonly while completing a specific task or during a particular type of situation. For example, a person may wash his hands repeatedly, for hours at a time, after shaking a stranger's hand; the unwanted thought is that he may have exposed himself to a serious disease. The act of washing in this example is the compulsion. Obsessive-compulsive disorder is chronic and often disabling. Depression and other symptoms of anxiety may also be comorbid in an older population. A new occurrence of obsessive-compulsive disorder in late life is unlikely. More commonly, symptoms of obsessions occur along with a depressive syndrome or early dementia. For example, obsessions about paying bills on time may occur in the context of difficulty in estimating time and planning.

Posttraumatic Stress Disorder

The distinctive feature of posttraumatic stress disorder is that the person has experienced, either as a witness or a victim, a traumatic event to which he or she has reacted with feelings of fear and helplessness. Examples of such events include those that involve actual or threatened death or serious injury, other threats to one's integrity, witnessing an event that involves death or serious injury of another, or even hearing about death or serious injury to a family member or close associate. Commonly observed symptoms include the re-experiencing of the traumatic event, avoidance (both cognitively and behaviorally) of stimuli associated with the event, psychologic numbing, and increased physiologic arousal. Symptoms of hyperarousal include difficulty falling or staying asleep, hypervigilance, and exaggerated startle response. Disorders often found to occur with posttraumatic stress disorder include depression, panic disorder, and substance-use disorders. Symptoms must be present for at least 1 month and cause clinically significant distress or impairment in social, occupational, or other important areas of functioning. In the short term, that is, between 2 days and 1 month after the traumatic event, a diagnosis of acute stress disorder is given; thereafter, one must consider a diagnosis of posttraumatic stress disorder.

Generalized Anxiety Disorder

The distinctive symptoms of generalized anxiety disorder include feeling easily tired and experiencing other physical symptoms, such as muscle tension, having trouble sleeping through the night, difficulty concentrating on a task, and feeling irritable or on edge. These symptoms need to have occurred for at least 6 months and must be accompanied by the sense that one cannot control the feelings of anxiety. In addition, these feelings of intense worry must be a result of more than one stressor. For example, intense worry over financial matters or a medical illness alone, even with all the associated symptoms, in and of itself does not qualify a person for a diagnosis of generalized anxiety disorder. Because many elderly patients with this disorder also present with features of depression, the clinician may try to distinguish between the two diagnoses. Commonly the overlap is sufficiently extensive to preclude this distinction, as described below.

COMORBIDITY

Mixed Anxiety and Depression

Mixed anxiety and depression is a presentation that is included in the *DSM-IV* "Criteria for Further Study." The essential features of this proposed disorder are dysphoric mood for at least 1 month that is composed of at least four anxious or depressive symptoms, such as irritability, worry, sleep disturbance, anticipating the worst, concentration or memory difficulties, and hopelessness. Clinicians working with elderly persons have long observed the significant overlap in symptoms of anxiety and depression. In fact, it is quite common to see individuals with a combination of anxiety and depression, although one or both disorders might be present only at subsyndromal levels.

Anxiety and Agitation in Dementia

Patients with dementia, whether living at home or in a long-term-care institution, commonly display behaviors described as agitation. Agitation takes the form of verbal or motor activity that is either appropriate behavior but repeated frequently or inappropriate behavior that suggests lack of judgment. As many as 85% of dementia patients eventually develop disruptive, agitated behavior. Early identification of triggers, in-

cluding environmental stimuli, medication side effects, and uncommunicated internal needs, can result in effective treatment and relief for already overburdened caregivers. See "Dementia" (p 221) and "Behavioral Problems in Dementia" (p 231) for details on diagnosing and managing disruptive, agitated behavior.

Anxiety and Medical Disorders

It is common to encounter patients with comorbid anxiety and medical disorders. This could be due to longstanding anxiety disorder that coincidentally occurs alongside a medical illness, or there could be interplay between the two. There are conditions exacerbated by anxiety, such as the common cold or influenza, and also those that are precipitated by high levels of anxiety, such as angina pectoris or myocardial infarction. Other medical illnesses that commonly accompany an anxiety disorder include cardiovascular illnesses, pulmonary disorders, drug side effects (eg, thyroid hormone replacements, antipsychotics, caffeine, theophylline, selective serotonin-reuptake inhibitors [SSRIs]) or interactions, and hyperthyroidism. Given the complicated clinical picture that results when anxiety and medical disorders coexist, a thorough assessment, including a clinical history, is imperative before treatment begins.

PHARMACOLOGIC MANAGEMENT

Numerous compounds have been used over the years as anxiolytics: alcohol, barbiturates, antihistamines, benzodiazepines, antipsychotic medications, and β-blockers. Although empirical studies of the use of anxiolytics in treating elderly persons are lacking, the efficacy of these medications is inferred from clinical practice with younger patients, and their use is modified by age-appropriate dosing. A brief description of the various classes of compounds currently favored as anxiolytics follows. Table 36.2 summarizes the treatment strategies for anxiety disorders in late life.

Antidepressants

Antidepressants are efficacious in the treatment of panic disorder, obsessive-compulsive disorder, generalized anxiety disorder, and posttraumatic stress disorder in younger patients. Given their relatively favorable side-effect profile, the SSRIs or serotonin–norepinephrine reuptake inhibitors (eg, venlafaxine) should now be considered the drugs of choice for these disorders. Further, SSRIs should also be considered treatments of choice for treating mixed anxiety and depression. Compounds such as venlafaxine should be considered as alternatives for those patients who do

Table 36.2—Treatment Strategies for Anxiety Disorders in Late Life

Disorder	First-Line Treatments	Second-Line Treatments
Panic disorder with or without agoraphobia	SSRIs,* SNRIs,* CBT	Newer antidepressants, benzodiazepines**
Social phobia		
Generalized	SSRIs* or phenelzine[OL] plus CBT	Benzodiazepines**
Specific	β-blockers plus CBT	Buspirone
Simple (specific) phobia	CBT or benzodiazepines**	β-blockers
Obsessive-compulsive disorder	SSRIs* plus CBT	Clomipramine, combination pharmacotherapy
Posttraumatic stress disorder	SSRIs* or SNRIs*	CBT, newer antidepressants
Generalized anxiety disorder	SNRIs,* SSRIs,* CBT	TCAs, benzodiazepines,** newer antidepressants
Anxiety and medical disorders	Identify and treat underlying cause, use SSRIs* or SNRIs* in primary anxiety disorder	Benzodiazepines**
Mixed anxiety depression	SSRIs* or SNRIs*	Buspirone, benzodiazepines,** CBT
Anxiety and agitation in dementia	Atypical antipsychotics[OL] or trazodone[OL]	Benzodiazepines,** anticonvulsants

* Not all SSRIs and SNRIs are approved for anxiety disorders or all types of anxiety disorders. For example, the SSRI escitalopram is not approved for anxiety, nor is the SNRI duloxetine.

** Preferably, benzodiazepines with a short half-life and no active metabolites (eg, lorazepam).

NOTE: CBT = cognitive-behavioral therapy; SNRIs = serotonin–norepinephrine reuptake inhibitors (eg, venlafaxine); SSRIs = selective serotonin-reuptake inhibitors (eg, sertraline); TCAs = tricyclic antidepressants.

not respond to SSRIs or who develop adverse effects. Case reports, open-label trials, and, more recently, controlled trials of serotonergic antidepressants like trazodone and SSRIs have also suggested a modest degree of efficacy in the management of anxiety and agitation in dementia, particularly when patients are not psychotic and comorbid depression is a strong possibility. (See also "Behavioral Problems in Dementia," p 231.)

Benzodiazepines

Over the past several decades benzodiazepines have been the most commonly prescribed anxiolytics for both young and older patients, but their use is now discouraged. When needed because symptoms are severe, benzodiazepines with a short half-life, such as lorazepam and oxazepam, are preferable in treating elderly patients because they are metabolized by direct conjugation, a process relatively unaffected by aging. However, it is preferable to limit the use of even short-acting benzodiazepines to less than 6 months because long-term use is fraught with multiple complications, such as motor incoordination and falls, cognitive impairment, depression, and the potential for abuse and dependence.

[OL] Not approved by the U.S. Food and Drug Administration for this use.

Buspirone, Antihistamines, and Atypical Antipsychotics

Several studies have suggested that buspirone, an anxiolytic medication with some serotonin-agonist properties, is efficacious in the treatment of patients with generalized anxiety disorder, although clinical experience is less positive. Buspirone appears to be a safer choice than benzodiazepines for patients taking several other medications or needing to be treated for longer periods of time. One drawback of buspirone is the amount of time required to see a clinical response (approximately 4 weeks). This suggests that concomitant use of a short-acting benzodiazepine in the initial stage of treatment would be useful for some patients. Buspirone may also be efficacious in reducing symptoms of anxiety and agitation in patients with dementia. Antihistamines such as hydroxyzine and diphenhydramine[OL] are sometimes used to manage mild anxiety, but there are few data that demonstrate efficacy and the anticholinergic properties of these agents can cause serious problems. Finally, atypical antipsychotics, such as risperidone[OL], olanzapine[OL], and quetiapine[OL], are increasingly being used to manage anxiety and agitation associated with dementia, particularly when an underlying psychosis may be present.

PSYCHOLOGIC MANAGEMENT

Although pharmacotherapy is commonly the first-line treatment for late-life anxiety disorders, psychologic treatments are often adequate, either alone or as adjuncts to medication. Techniques generally fall into three categories. Relaxation training can be employed with the use of music, visual imagery, aromatherapy, or instruction in relaxation techniques. Cognitive restructuring helps the patient identify triggers and stimuli that maintain anxiety and helps him or her to slowly gain more control over the effect of such stimuli and develop a range of coping strategies and tools. Finally, exposure, with response prevention, has been shown to be particularly effective with both panic disorder and obsessive-compulsive disorder. Treatment of the elderly person typically includes a combination of these behavioral approaches. Their success depends on the appropriateness of the patient for psychotherapy; the patient's support system, intellectual functioning, and motivation level; the degree of coordination of care with medical professionals; and the nature of the disorder. Consultation with a mental health professional can assist in determining the appropriateness of a referral.

ANNOTATED REFERENCES

■ De Beurs E, Beekman AT, Deeg DJ, et al. Predictors of change in anxiety symptoms of older persons: results from the Longitudinal Aging Study Amsterdam. *Psychol Med.* 2000;30(3):515–527.

This study reviews the clinical course of anxiety over time through comparison of two groups of older adults residing in the community, those suffering from anxiety and those without symptoms. Risks factors were assessed and included vulnerability factors, such as demographics and social support, and stressors, including those life events that occurred during participation in the study. Those who were found to be most likely to become anxious were slightly neurotic females who suffer from a sensory deficit (eg, hearing or eyesight problems) and experienced a stressful life event during the course of the study. These results will aid in targeting at-risk individuals for preventive care.

■ Kogan JN, Edelstein BA, McKee DR. Assessment of anxiety in older adults. *J Anxiety Disord.* 2000; 14(2):109–132.

About 25% of older adults meet criteria for some mental disorder. Of this group, anxiety is the most commonly reported diagnosis. This reality necessitates the understanding of anxiety in the elderly age group, including the prevalence rates for each disorder, clinical presentations, outcomes, and the important role of assessment in each of these factors. This article reviews each of these areas and presents recommendations for assessment and future research.

■ Mostofsky DI, Barlow DH, eds. *The Management of Stress and Anxiety in Medical Disorders.* Needham Heights, MA: Allyn & Bacon; 2000.

This book includes a collection of chapters addressing anxiety associated with various medical conditions. Psychologic components and interventions, including cognitive-behavioral therapy and biofeedback, are reviewed. The various manifestations of anxiety, including insomnia and chronic fatigue syndrome, are discussed in light of current treatment developments. The specific issues associated with geriatric patients' suffering from anxiety, such as polypharmacy and comorbid medical conditions, are included to assist clinicians in identifying these factors early in treatment.

■ Sheikh JI. Anxiety in older adults: assessment and management of three common presentations. *Geriatrics.* 2003;58(5):44–45.

This report discusses the three most common presentations of anxiety in older adults seen in primary care: mixed anxiety-depression, anxiety associated with illness or medications, and anxiety or agitation associated with dementia. Symptom profiles and clinical considerations are given for each condition. Pharmacologic treatment strategies are proposed.

Erin L. Cassidy, PhD
Javaid I. Sheikh, MD

CHAPTER 37—PSYCHOTIC DISORDERS

KEY POINTS

■ Hallucinations are perceptions without stimuli that may occur in any sensory modalities (ie, visual, tactile, auditory, olfactory, gustatory). In late life, multimodal hallucinations are common.

■ Delusions are abnormal beliefs that in late life are often paranoid or persecutory, such as a belief that one's safety is in jeopardy or belongings are being stolen.

■ Psychosis occurring for the first time in late life is often due to dementia or neurologic conditions such as dementia or stroke, as opposed to a primary psychotic disorder, such as schizophrenia.

■ Dementia with Lewy bodies is associated with characteristically vivid visual hallucinations, often consisting of people or animals.

■ When psychotic symptoms arise in the context of depression, the symptoms are often "mood congruent"; examples are delusions that one is penniless or that one is already dead.

Psychotic symptoms are defined as either *hallucinations*, that is, perceptions without stimuli, or *delusions*, that is, fixed, false, idiosyncratic ideas. Hallucinations are abnormal perceptions that can be in any of the five sensory modalities (auditory, visual, tactile, olfactory, gustatory). Delusions are unfounded ideas that can be suspicious (paranoid), grandiose, somatic, self-blaming, or hopeless. This chapter focuses on conditions in which psychotic symptoms are prominent and central to making the diagnosis. It only briefly discusses other disorders, such as dementia, delirium, and the mood disorders, in which psychotic symptoms can occur but whose defining features are in the cognitive or mood realms and which are discussed elsewhere. (See "Dementia," p 221; "Delirium," p 239; "Depression and Other Mood Disorders," p 269.)

Hallucinations and delusions occur in a variety of disorders. The evaluation of a person with hallucinations and delusions (Figure 37.1) should first evaluate for underlying sources such as delirium, dementia, stroke, or Parkinson's disease. An acute onset of altered level of consciousness or inability to sustain attention suggests delirium. Next, a primary mood disorder should be considered. Only after other causes are excluded should the diagnosis of a schizophrenia-like state be made. It should be noted that delirium, most often superimposed on an underlying dementia, is the most common cause of new-onset psychosis in late life.

SCHIZOPHRENIA AND SCHIZOPHRENIA-LIKE SYNDROMES

Schizophrenia is defined as a chronic psychiatric disorder characterized by positive symptoms (eg, hallucinations, delusions, and thought disorder) and negative symptoms (eg, social dilapidation and apathy). Mood disorder and cognitive disorder should be excluded. In men, schizophrenia has a modal onset at age 18; onset after age 45 years is uncommon. In women, on the other hand, modal age of onset is 28, and 20% to 30% of cases begin after age 45. Ten percent to 15% of cases of schizophrenia first come to clinical attention after patients have reached 59 years of age.

In older persons, schizophrenia-like conditions are characterized by onset after age 44, prominent persecu-

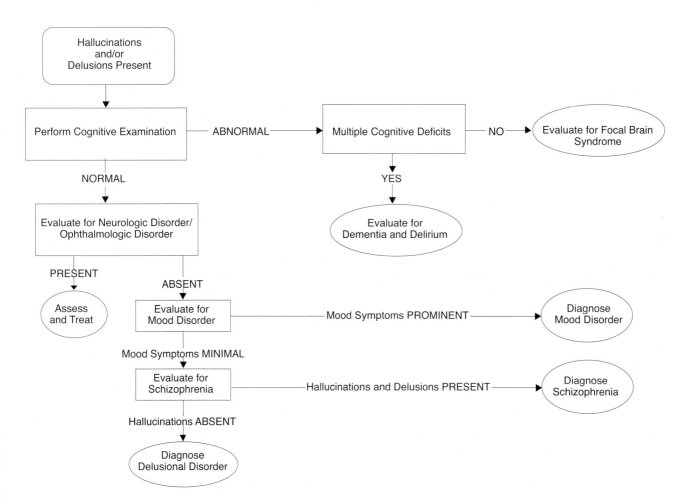

Figure 37.1—Evaluating the patient with hallucinations or delusions, or both.

tory (paranoid) delusions, and multimodal hallucinations. For example, patients commonly complain that items are being stolen or report that they are being persecuted unjustly. Hallucinations often manifest in complaints, for example, that a neighbor is persistently banging on walls or the roof, that someone is pumping gas under the door, or that electrical sensations are being sent through the walls of the person's home and into his or her body. A schizophrenia-like psychosis can be diagnosed only when cognitive disorder, mood disorder, or other explanatory medical conditions such as delirium or focal brain pathology have been excluded (Figure 37.1).

The schizophrenia-like psychoses of late life differ from schizophrenia beginning in early life in two ways. First, thought disorder, a sign described as speech in which a series of thoughts are not connected to one another in a logical fashion, is much less common in elderly patients, comprising only 5% of cases. In early-onset schizophrenia, thought disorder is present in approximately 50% of cases. It is important to note that thought disorder in schizophrenia occurs in the absence of an impaired sensorium (ie, delirium). When illogical speech occurs in late life, a delirium or dementia should be excluded. A second significant difference is the rarity of social deterioration and dilapidation among elderly patients. Thus, personality is often intact in late-onset cases. However, there is a dearth of long-term follow-up studies, so it is unknown whether social deterioration and personality changes occur after many years of symptoms.

Epidemiology and Clinical Characteristics

Late-onset schizophrenia is more common among women. The population-based incidence of late-onset schizophrenia is unknown, but the lifetime prevalence of schizophrenia is 1% among both men and women.

Late-onset schizophrenia-like psychoses affect predominantly women, with the female:male ratio ranging from 5:1 to 10:1. It has been speculated that later onset is due to decreasing natural estrogen levels, but there is little evidence to support this hypothesis. Many persons with late-onset schizophrenia-like psychosis have been able to hold responsible jobs and work efficiently, but premorbid isolation and "schizoid" (socially isolated personality) traits are common. Studies report greater degrees of brain white matter hyperintensities on magnetic resonance imaging scans in late-onset schizophrenia, a finding that suggests that brain vascular disease is a risk factor. However, this finding has not been adequately replicated, and other causes of white matter hyperintensities are plausible.

One condition that may be confused with late-onset schizophrenia is frontotemporal dementia (formerly referred to as Pick's disease), as it may involve features of socially inappropriate and odd behaviors as well as premorbidly odd or "schizoid" personality features. (See "Dementia," p 221.)

Treatment and Management

Nonpharmacologic

Because suspiciousness and paranoid delusions are commonly the most prominent symptoms, the physician's first task in treating late-onset psychosis is often to establish a trusting therapeutic relationship with the patient. On occasion, the suspicious ideas are plausible (eg, the claim that the patient is being financially abused by a relative), but usually the delusions are bizarre and implausible. It is rarely effective to confront the patient with the unreality or implausibility of his or her ideas. The patient is more likely to respond positively if the physician empathizes with the distress that the symptoms cause ("I can see how upset you are by all of this"). If patients ask whether the physician "believes" them, a response such as, "I don't hear anything like that, but I appreciate the fact that you do" is both honest and empathic. The symptoms are usually frightening and distressing to the patients and can lead to unusual behaviors. For example, patients who develop concerns that their food is being poisoned may exhibit unusual eating habits or food avoidance. Furthermore, suspiciousness can isolate the patient from friends and family. Therefore, encouraging patients to maintain important relationships and seeking their permission to discuss the source of symptoms with close family members or friends may help these patients maintain important, supportive relationships.

Pharmacologic

Clinical experience and descriptive case series suggest that antipsychotic drugs are as effective in late-onset schizophrenia as in early-onset cases. Most specialist physicians recommend the newer atypical antipsychotic drugs because they are less likely to cause tardive dyskinesia, a side effect for which older age is a predisposing factor. Doses should be increased at semi-weekly or weekly intervals, as needed. While doses are being titrated, patients should be monitored for the emergence of extrapyramidal side effects (parkinsonian tremor, rigidity, dystonia) and other movement disorders. These should be treated by lowering dosage and switching to an alternative antipsychotic if necessary. Polypharmacy should be avoided by reducing or switching antipsychotic medication rather than adding a medication for extrapyramidal symptoms. The more common side effects with quetiapine are sedation and orthostatic hypotension; with risperidone, extrapyramidal symptoms; and with olanzapine, weight gain and sedation (Table 37.1).

No studies are available to guide the length of treatment. Clinical experience suggests that patients who respond to antipsychotic medications should be continued on the minimal effective dose for at least 6 months. For patients who relapse on treatment or when the dosage is lowered, maintenance over a longer term (at least 1 to 2 years) is recommended. Patients should be monitored for the emergence of tardive dyskinesia, a syndrome characterized by repetitive involuntary movements of the oral and limb musculature. If tardive dyskinesia develops, the dosage of the antipsychotic agent should be lowered, if possible. Depending on the duration of exposure, tardive dyskinesia may worsen or appear when the antipsychotic is discontinued or the dose is lowered, or when switching from one antipsychotic to another. At the time antipsychotic drugs are initiated or as soon as symptoms improve enough so that the patient can understand the risk, he or she should be informed of the risk of tardive dyskinesia and the possibility that it can be irreversible.

PSYCHOTIC SYMPTOMS IN DELIRIUM

Hallucinations, particularly visual hallucinations, can be a symptom of delirium, even when it is mild. The onset of delirium is usually acute, and there is often an identifiable metabolic or infectious cause. The mental status examination reveals multiple cognitive impairments and a diminished level of consciousness. (See "Delirium," p 239.)

PSYCHOTIC SYMPTOMS IN MOOD DISORDER

Delusions can be seen in major depression and in the manic phase of bipolar disorder. These delusions are described as "mood congruent." That is, in patients with depression, the delusional content usually reflects self-deprecation, self-blame, hopelessness, or the conviction of ill health. A patient may complain that she has no blood or that her intestines are not working, for example; another patient may believe that he has caused a terrible wrong and deserves to be punished (a self-blaming delusion). Some patients become convinced that they are dying and that nothing can be done to help them when there is no physiologic evidence to support their concerns. Other common depressive delusions are the conviction that one has no insurance, no clothing, or no money when this is not true (delusion of poverty). Delusions congruent with mania are grandiose. Examples include the person's belief that that he or she is infallible, can do impossible physical or intellectual activities, has skills and abilities that no other human being has, or is a special personage such as Jesus Christ. (See "Depression and Other Mood Disorders," p 269.)

PSYCHOTIC SYMPTOMS IN DEMENTIA

Patients with dementia experience both hallucinations and delusions. These are usually less complex than the delusions seen in schizophrenia or mood disorder. Common delusions in dementia are the belief that one's belongings have been stolen or moved, or the conviction that one is being persecuted. Delusions that one's spouse is unfaithful (delusions of infidelity) are also common. (See "Dementia," p 221.)

Management of psychosis in dementia is particularly challenging, as the use of antipsychotic medication warrants careful consideration of risks and side effects. There has been recent attention to potential side effects of the newer antipsychotic medications in the class of atypical antipsychotics when used in patients with dementia. This group includes aripiprazole, olanzapine, risperidone, clozapine, quetiapine, and ziprasidone. One concern involves the risk of

Table 37.1—Commonly Used Antipsychotic Medications: Dosing and Side Effects

Agent	Starting Daily Dose (*mg*)	Maximum Daily Dose (*mg*)	Side Effects*		
			EPS**	Drowsiness	Weight Gain
Clozapine	12.5	75	1	3	3
Haloperidol	0.5–1	8	3	2	1
Olanzapine	2.5	10	1	2	3
Quetiapine	25	200	1	3	2
Risperidone	0.5–1	4	2	1	2

* Key: 1 = uncommon to 3 = common.

** EPS = extrapyramidal side effects: rigidity, parkinsonian tremor, dystonia, akathisia.

cerebrovascular adverse events (eg, stroke, transient ischemic attack) with risperidone, when such events were observed in clinical trials of risperidone in elderly patients with dementia-related psychosis. It is important to note that these clinical trials included patients with vascular dementia. The mechanism for the risk of cerebrovascular events has not yet been clarified. The observation of increased cerebrovascular events resulted in the addition of a warning to the product information. A class warning regarding atypical antipsychotics has already been applied concerning the risk of hyperglycemia in both younger and older patients with schizophrenia. The U.S. Food and Drug Administration has asked all manufacturers of atypical antipsychotic drugs to include a warning on the increased risk of developing hyperglycemia and diabetes. The mechanism for these adverse effects is unclear, although the fact that weight gain occurs with most of these medications may account for the increased rate of hyperglycemia.

ISOLATED SUSPICIOUSNESS

Suspiciousness can be viewed as a personality trait, that is, an aspect of all human beings that varies among people in its degree of prominence. One epidemiologic study has found that suspiciousness becomes more common in older Americans and affects 4% of those aged 65 and over. It is distinguished from psychotic disorders by the understandable nature of the ideas (for example, excessive worry about safety) and the absence of other psychotic symptoms.

SYNDROMES OF ISOLATED HALLUCINATIONS

Charles Bonnet Syndrome

Between 10% and 13% of patients with significant visual impairment (bilateral acuity worse than 20/60) experience visual hallucinations. These can take the form of shapes such as diamonds or rectangles but more commonly consist of complex hallucinations such as small children, multiple animals, or a vivid scene such as one would see in a movie. This condition, first described more than 200 years ago, goes by the eponym *Charles Bonnet syndrome*. The criteria for this syndrome are as follows:

- visual hallucinations,
- partially or fully intact insight (the patient is aware that the perceptions cannot be real but still reports that they appear absolutely real and vivid),

- visual impairment, and
- lack of evidence of brain disease or other psychiatric disorder.

It has been suggested that this syndrome is a concomitant of the phantom limb syndrome caused by retinal lesions. However, visual hallucinations have also been reported in persons with field defects due to cortical lesions of the visual pathways.

The best treatment of the Charles Bonnet syndrome is information and support. Patients should be told that the hallucinations are a sign of eye disease, not mental illness. An occasional patient has partial insight or loses insight and becomes very distressed by this symptom. When this distress is significant or leads to dangerous behavior, a cautious trial of low doses of an atypical antipsychotic medication is occasionally beneficial.

Organic Hallucinosis

Patients with Parkinson's disease, stroke, and other brain disorders occasionally experience delusions and hallucinations without prominent cognitive impairment or other evidence of psychiatric disorder. Delirium due to a superimposed condition should be excluded. In patients with Parkinson's disease, the symptoms may be secondary to prescribed dopaminergic agent, but some patients experience visual hallucinations prior to the onset of any pharmacotherapy. Education and support should be offered to all patients with these symptoms. If the patients experience significant emotional distress or the symptoms lead to dangerous or upsetting behavior, cautious use of an antipsychotic medication is appropriate. For patients with Parkinson's disease and hallucinations, quetiapine[OL] 12.5 to 75 mg or olanzapine[OL] 2.5 to 5.0 mg daily may be beneficial. Some patients require clozapine[OL] 12.5 to 75.0 mg daily. However, clozapine requires a complete blood cell count once a week for 6 months and then biweekly thereafter because of the risk of granulocytopenia.

Dementia associated with Lewy bodies is increasingly recognized as an important cause of hallucinations in late life. The clinical scenario typically involves cognitive decline accompanied by motor features of parkinsonism. However, prominent visual hallucinations are a key part of the diagnosis. These hallucinations are often vivid and troubling. (See "Dementia," p 221.)

Dementia associated with Lewy bodies presents a challenge similar to that of psychosis in Parkinson's disease because the drugs in the class approved to treat psychosis, the antipsychotics, have been shown to worsen the parkinsonian symptoms. No trial data are available to guide drug choice, but there are case reports of significant improvement through the use of

---

[OL] Not approved by the U.S. Food and Drug Administration for this use.

cholinesterase inhibitors[OL]. If an antipsychotic medication must be used, then the treatment strategies outlined above are appropriate if there is careful attention to the risk of extrapyramidal side effects. Nonpharmacologic treatments include redirection, reassurance, and explanation.

ANNOTATED REFERENCES

■ Howard R, Rabins PV, Castle DJ, eds. *Late Onset Schizophrenia*. Petersfield, UK: Wrightson Biomedical Publishing Ltd.; 1999.

> This is a compilation of presentations at an international consensus conference summarizing current thought on this condition. Chapter topics include epidemiology, clinical presentation, neuroimaging, and treatment. One chapter presents the view that this is not a unique syndrome.

■ Kertesz A, Munoz DG. Frontotemporal dementia. *Med Clin North Am*. 2002;86(3):501–518.

> The clinical features of frontotemporal dementia are described. The under-recognition of this disorder and its pathologic and genetic features are discussed.

■ Marsh L. Neuropsychiatric aspects of Parkinson's disease. *Psychosomatics*. 2000; 41(1):15–23.

> This article nicely reviews the range of psychiatric symptoms seen in association with Parkinson's disease, including hallucinations, delusions, anxiety symptoms, mood symptoms, and obsessive-compulsive phenomena. Treatment is discussed.

■ McKeith IG, Burn DJ, Ballard CG, et al. Dementia with Lewy bodies. *Semin Clin Neuropsychiatry*. 2003;8(1):46–57.

> This review of dementia associated with Lewy bodies addresses the clinical characteristics and criteria for diagnosis as well as the literature on neuropathology and genetic implications.

■ Sachdev P, Brodaty H, Rose N, et al. Schizophrenia with onset after 50 years of age: 2: neurological, neuropsychological and MRI investigation. *Br J Psychiatry*. 1999; 175:416–421.

> This article examines the correlates and risk factors of late-onset schizophrenia in a well-studied sample. It focuses on the question of whether structural brain damage is the primary progenitor of late-onset schizophrenia.

Peter V. Rabins, MD, MPH

CHAPTER 38—PERSONALITY AND SOMATOFORM DISORDERS

KEY POINTS

- Personality disorders persist into late life and pose complex challenges to clinicians across various medical and psychiatric settings.

- Personality disorders may be more difficult to detect in late life because of age-associated changes in symptoms, comorbid psychopathology, and lack of age-adjusted diagnostic instruments.

- The goal of treatment of personality disorders in late life is not to cure the disorder, but to decrease the frequency and intensity of symptoms. To this end, both psychotherapeutic and psychopharmacologic strategies are needed.

- Somatoform disorders represent the presence of physical symptoms without established underlying pathology and with strongly associated psychologic factors. Undifferentiated somatoform disorder and hypochondriasis are likely the most common forms seen in late life.

- Treatment of somatoform disorders must attend to the affected individual's distress and belief in the veracity of his or her symptoms. The prognosis may be guarded, but repeated reassuring clinical visits help to build a therapeutic relationship.

PERSONALITY DISORDERS

Personality disorders are defined in the fourth edition of the *Diagnostic and Statistical Manual of Mental Disorders, Text Revision* (*DSM-IV-TR*) by the presence of chronic and pervasive patterns of inflexible and maladaptive inner experiences and behaviors. These patterns lead to significant disruptions in several spheres of function, including cognitive perception and interpretation, affective expression, interpersonal relations, and impulse control. People with personality disorders are often distinguished by repeated episodes of disruptive or noxious behaviors, and as a result they often receive pejorative labels, depending on their form. Descriptive terms often applied to those with personality disorders include "difficult," "dramatic," and "overbearing," to name just a few. The developmental roots of personality disorders are believed to lie in childhood and adolescence, but their features can present clinically at any age. These features represent the influence of both genetic and environmental factors.

[OL] Not approved by the U.S. Food and Drug Administration for this use.

The *DSM-IV-TR* describes ten personality disorders, grouped into three broad clusters that are based on common phenomenology. Depressive and passive-aggressive personality disorders are two additional categories, but they are considered provisional since they appear to lack the empirical support of the other ten diagnoses. Brief definitions and late-life features of all twelve personality disorders are provided in Table 38.1. Mixed diagnoses and those that do not fit into any existing category are labeled "personality disorder, not otherwise specified" (NOS).

Many older persons with personality disorders can easily become overwhelmed by age-associated losses and stresses, largely because they lack appropriate coping skills and the personal, social, or financial resources to buffer their losses. In particular, admission to a hospital or long-term-care setting poses a unique stress on all persons with personality disorders in late life. The loss of a familiar environment, personal items, privacy, and the control over one's schedule can lead to a sense of disorganization and displacement. Conflict in an institutional setting begins when patients with personality disorders try to cope with the stresses from their new environment by exaggerating their maladaptive behaviors. An obsessive-compulsive person may attempt to maintain a sense of control by demanding rigid adherence to schedules and rules of hygiene. Dependent persons may feel helpless and panicked without enough attention to their needs, and they respond with clinging behaviors and excessive questions or requests for assistance. Paranoid, antisocial, and borderline patients may refuse to cooperate with treatment plans or institutional rules.

Epidemiology

Prevalence rates of late-life personality disorders in the community range from 5% to 10%, which is a slightly lower range than the 10% to 18% prevalence estimates for persons of all ages in the community. Prevalence rates in inpatient settings and with comorbid depression are much higher, ranging from 10% to over 50%, depending on the method of diagnosis. The most common personality disorders in late life are dependent, obsessive-compulsive, paranoid, and NOS. Although most research has demonstrated fewer diagnoses in older age groups, it is unclear whether this represents an actual difference in prevalence or merely reflects the fact that it is more difficult to make a diagnosis in late life. Some researchers have suggested that prevalence rates may be influenced by increased mortality among those with personality traits that are associated with higher rates of reckless, impulsive, and self-injurious behaviors. Other research exploring the neural substrates of emotion has demonstrated an attenuation of emotional reactivity in late life across a

number of physiologic and behavioral parameters. These findings may partially explain the reduction in prevalence of the more impulsive and emotionally reactive personality features, such as those associated with borderline personality disorder.

Diagnostic Challenges

Establishing a diagnosis of personality disorder in the older patient can be especially challenging because it requires a detailed, longitudinal psychiatric and psychosocial history. Elderly patients and their informants are not always able to provide sufficient history, especially when it may span 50 years or more. The history may be distorted by recall bias (the tendency to present more socially desirable traits) or memory impairment. Furthermore, schizotypal and paranoid persons may be reluctant to engage in clinical interviews and share personal history, and antisocial and narcissistic persons who lack insight into their problems may refuse to divulge relevant experiences. Records often do not provide sufficient information to determine prior personality dynamics. Remote diagnoses from previous decades cannot be easily correlated with current ones because the diagnostic criteria for personality disorders have changed significantly in the past 50 years. As a result of all of these limitations, clinicians often are reluctant to make a diagnosis or to make judgments that are based on insufficient information.

A further diagnostic challenge for clinicians is the need to isolate lifelong personality characteristics from a multitude of comorbid problems. Acute and chronic episodes of major depression, psychosis, and other major psychiatric disorders can distort personality features considerably. Even the current diagnostic nomenclature might serve to handicap late-life diagnosis since it is not age adjusted, and many criteria fail to apply in late life. A final barrier to diagnosis may be present if the clinician erroneously considers all older patients to have disruptive personality features as a normal function of age.

Differential Diagnosis

In clinical settings, it is important to remember that not every older person with prominent or troubling personality features has a personality disorder. Those who demonstrate rigid and maladaptive personality traits but without the pervasiveness or severity as represented by *DSM-IV-TR* criteria are better described as suffering from personality dysfunction or an adjustment disorder. An adjustment disorder might best characterize previously healthy and well-adjusted persons who demonstrate acute changes in personality as a result of severe stresses. For example, physical pain

Table 38.1—Features of Personality Disorders

Cluster, Disorder	General Features*	Features Specific to Geriatric Patients
Cluster A: Odd or Eccentric Behaviors		
Paranoid	Pervasive suspiciousness of the motives of others, which often leads to irritability and hostility	Episodes of paranoid psychosis, agitation, and assaultivenes
Schizoid	Disinterest in social relationships, coupled with isolative and sometimes odd behaviors	Poor, strained, or absent relationships with caregivers
Schizotypal	Characteristic appearance, behaviors, and beliefs that are strange, unusual, or inappropriate	Beliefs that may become delusional and that may lead to conflicts with others; relationships with caregivers that may be strained or absent
Cluster B: Dramatic, Emotional, or Erratic Behaviors		
Antisocial	Poor regard for social norms and laws; lack of conscience and empathy for others; frequent reckless and criminal behaviors	Frequent remission of antisocial behaviors with less aggression and impulsivity
Borderline	Impaired control of emotional expression and impulses associated with unstable interpersonal relations, poor self-identity, and self-injurious behaviors	Persistent emotional lability and unstable relationships, but less self-injurious and impulsive behaviors
Histrionic	Excessive emotionality and attention-seeking behaviors, sometimes appearing overly seductive or provocative	Behaviors that may become excessively disinhibited and disorganized, appearing manic
Narcissistic	Pervasive sense of entitlement, grandiosity, and arrogance, coupled with lack of empathy	May present as hostile, rageful, paranoid, or depressed
Cluster C: Anxious or Fearful Behaviors		
Avoidant	Excessive sensitivity to rejection and social scrutiny; social demeanor that may be timid and inhibited	Social contacts that may be extremely limited, providing for inadequate support
Dependent	Excessive dependence on others to help make decisions and provide support	Commonly, comorbid depression; clinical appearance often with demanding or clinging behaviors if dependency needs not met
Obsessive-Compulsive	Pervasive preoccupation with orderliness and cleanliness; a perfectionistic, rigid, and controlling approach that may become more inflexible and indecisive under stress	Obsessive-compulsive traits that may become exaggerated in efforts to maintain control over somatic and environmental changes
Provisional Personality Disorders		
Passive-Aggressive	Pervasive pattern of passive resistance to demands and authority, such as through procrastination; attitudes toward others and responsibilities that are often critical and resentful	No clear changes in late life
Depressive	Outlook on life that is pervasively gloomy and pessimistic; excessively guilt prone with poor self-esteem	Commonly seen with comorbid depression in late life

* Descriptions of the clusters and of the disorders in each cluster are based on the *Diagnostic and Statistical Manual of Mental Disorders*. 4th ed. Text Revision, Washington, DC: American Psychiatric Association; 2000. The provisional disorders are described in the *DSM-IV–TR* appendix.

and disability can lead to dependent or avoidant behaviors that resemble those seen in personality disorders, but without the pervasive pattern and degree of maladaptiveness. There is also considerable overlap between symptoms of major psychiatric disorders and those of personality disorders, and without longitudinal history it can be difficult to distinguish between them. For example, the odd thinking and unusual perceptual experiences seen in psychotic disorders may resemble behaviors seen in schizotypal personality disorder. The emotional lability of bipolar states can mimic behaviors of borderline and histrionic diagnoses, and depressive symptoms from dysthymic and depressive disorders can be almost indistinguishable from depressive personality traits. Diagnosis of a personality disorder becomes more certain when seemingly acute behaviors emerge as enduring and pervasive personality traits. This process depends on the opportunity to observe a person over time and in multiple settings or situations.

Personality disorders as described in *DSM-IV-TR* must also be differentiated from the diagnosis of personality change due to a specific medical condition. When personality change is a direct result of brain damage, it has classically been described within the context of an "organic" personality disorder, although this term is no longer used in *DSM* nomenclature. Most often, personality changes with an "organic" source involve impairments in executive functioning, consisting of poor impulse control, poor planning, and greater vulnerability to irritability or agitation. Along these lines, Alzheimer's disease and other dementias are often associated with personality changes, including apathy, egocentricity, and impulsivity. Frontal lobe injury may result in a disinhibited impulsive syndrome, or conversely, an apathetic, avolitional syndrome may result. Frontotemporal dementia has been associated with distinct personality changes characterized by odd social interactions and compulsive behaviors such as hoarding. (See "Dementia," p 221.) Temporal lobe epilepsy has been associated with personality change, including emotional deepening, verbosity, hypergraphia, hypersexuality, and preoccupation with religious, moral, and cosmic issues.

Long-Term Course

Personality disorders may follow one of four possible courses: they persist unchanged, evolve into a different form or major psychiatric disorder (eg, depression), improve, or remit. Few disorders have actually been studied over time, and rarely into late life. Several studies have suggested that personality disorders may enter a period of relative quiescence in middle age, with fewer and less intense symptoms and increased adaptation. However, this period may precede their reemergence in late life. Other researchers have proposed that personality disorders characterized by emotional and behavioral lability, including antisocial, borderline, histrionic, narcissistic, and dependent, tend to improve over time, although patients remain vulnerable to depression. Personality disorders characterized by an overcontrol of affect and impulses, including paranoid, schizoid, schizotypal, and obsessive-compulsive personality disorders, are thought to either remain stable or to worsen in late life.

Only antisocial and borderline personality disorders have been looked at longitudinally, and both have shown symptom improvement and even remittance into middle and later life for a significant percentage of patients. At the same time, there can be persistent psychopathology that is not recognized within the context of existing antisocial or borderline diagnostic criteria. In other words, longstanding personality dynamics may manifest in new behaviors. For example, those with antisocial personality disorders demonstrate less aggressiveness, violence, and criminal acts as they age, but they still have antisocial tendencies expressed through substance abuse, disregard for safety, and noncompliance with institutional rules. Elderly borderline patients display less impulsivity, self-mutilation, and

risk-taking, but more age-appropriate symptoms, such as the use of multiple medications and nonadherence with treatment.

Treatment

The treatment of personality disorders in late life is complicated and often has limited success. Given the chronic and pervasive nature of personality disorders, the overall goal of treatment in late life is not to cure the disorder, but to decrease the frequency and intensity of disruptive behaviors. The first step should always be to clarify the diagnosis and then to identify recent stressors that may account for the current presentation. The resultant formulation will guide the selection of realistic target symptoms and therapeutic approaches and will allow a treatment team to anticipate future stressors. Treatment of personality disorders in late life uses the same basic approaches as with younger patients, but clinicians must incorporate a much broader understanding of the impact of age-related stressors and comorbid disorders. All forms of psychotherapy have been used to treat personality disorders in older adults, ranging from intensive and long-term insight-oriented approaches to equally intensive but more focused cognitive-behavioral models. In late life, however, there may be more limitations on time and intensity of therapy, and as a result treatment must focus more on short-term, cognitive-behavioral, and pharmacologic approaches. Studies in adults generally find that comorbid personality disorders complicate the treatment of psychiatric illness, but that with consistent treatment, the prognosis is often favorable. The prognosis in late life is more guarded, especially for persons with comorbid major depression. One study of elderly persons with major depression found that those with a concomitant personality disorder were less likely to benefit from psychotherapy.

In outpatient settings, clinicians have limited control over a patient's environment and must therefore rely on one-to-one interventions if the patient is willing to cooperate with treatment. With some patients, it may be necessary to convey a basic formulation of their behaviors, along with suggested approaches, to caregivers and affiliated health care professionals, such as internists, social workers, and visiting nurses. This communication is important when patients are vulnerable to self-harm or likely to cause significant disruptions in other settings when they are not understood and approached in a therapeutic manner. Table 38.2 suggests therapeutic approaches that clinicians can employ with various personality disorders.

Long-term-care settings allow more opportunities for intervention. A staff meeting or case conference often provides the best forum to discuss disruptive persons and to coordinate a consistent treatment plan.

Table 38.2—Therapeutic Strategies for Personality Disorders in Late Life

Cluster A—Paranoid, Schizoid, Schizotypal Personality Disorders

- Always assess for and treat comorbid psychosis.

- Do not force social interactions, but offer support and problem-solving assistance in a professional and consistent manner.

- Do not challenge paranoid ideation; instead, solicit and empathize with emotional responses to the inner turmoil and fear of paranoid states.

Cluster B—Antisocial, Borderline, Histrionic, and Narcissistic Personality Disorders

- Assess for and treat underlying mood lability, depression, anxiety, and substance abuse.

- Adopt a consistent, structured, and predictable approach with strict boundaries to contain disruptive behaviors.

- Adopt a team approach with all involved clinicians to devise a common plan; avoid staff splits between "supporters" and "detractors" of the patient.

- Use behavioral contracts and authority figures when necessary to address recurrent disruptive behaviors.

- Do not personalize belligerent behaviors directed toward staff members; instead, provide opportunities for staff to ventilate frustration and negative thoughts and emotions with professional colleagues.

Cluster C—Avoidant, Dependent, and Obsessive-Compulsive Personality Disorders

- Assess for and treat underlying anxiety, panic, and depression.

- Provide regularly scheduled clinical contacts rather than on an as-needed basis.

- When possible, provide case managers to solicit the needs of avoidant patients and to provide extra reassurance and attention to the needs of dependent and obsessive-compulsive patients.

Depressive and Passive-Aggressive Personality Disorders

- Differentiate between the depressive and negative attitudes and the actual symptoms of major depression. Provide appropriate and adequate antidepressant treatment.

- Avoid becoming too pessimistic or burnt-out with attempts at providing care; shift focus to a supportive and nonjudgmental therapeutic relationship, with minimal expectations as to outcome.

- Encourage individual psychotherapy to identify underlying emotions and to redirect negative attitudes toward more constructive activities.

Disruptive behaviors can sometimes be traced to particular activities or staff interactions, which can be adapted as part of an overall treatment strategy. Sometimes, disengagement from patients will reduce the intensity of disruptive interactions. In other situations, the continuity of staffing and of daily schedules is critical. In all situations, a treatment plan should be well documented and conveyed to the patient, as well as all involved staff and caregivers. All plans must provide appropriate limits to ensure the safety of patients and staff. A written contract, signed by all parties, may be needed with nonadherent persons in order to eliminate ambiguity. Although it is important to involve family members in the treatment plan, clinicians must recognize that patients with personality disorders often have conflictual relationships with them. Attention should also be given to individual staff members who must work with difficult patients. They need opportunities to vent feelings of anxiety and frustration, and to feel acknowledged and supported by administrative and clinical staff.

There have been no studies looking specifically at pharmacologic strategies for personality disorders in late life, so clinicians must instead extrapolate from guidelines used for younger persons. Psychotropic medications can be targeted at a particular personality disorder, specific symptoms or symptom clusters, or comorbid depression, anxiety, or psychosis. The goal is not to cure the disorder, but to reduce the frequency and intensity of targeted symptoms. Antidepressant medication may be helpful for the target symptoms of depression and anxiety found in most personality disorders. Mood stabilizers (eg, lithium carbonate[OL] and divalproex sodium[OL]) and antipsychotic medications have been found to reduce mood lability and impulsivity in borderline patients, and they may be useful with similar symptoms in antisocial personality disorder. Antianxiety agents are commonly used for transient agitation seen in borderline, antisocial, narcissistic, and paranoid disorders, and they may reduce social anxiety and panic in avoidant and dependent patients. Antidepressants are used commonly to treat obsessive-compulsive personality symptoms, although efficacy has not been established for the treatment of these symptoms as opposed to obsessive-compulsive disorder. Antipsychotic agents can treat the transient psychosis, agitation, and impulsivity seen in dramatic

---

[OL] Not approved by the U.S. Food and Drug Administration for this use.

cluster and paranoid disorders, as well as the borderline psychosis and paranoia seen in odd cluster disorders.

For personality disorders, psychotropic medications are best used as adjuncts to psychotherapy. In older persons, multiple medications should be avoided in general, and particularly when there is a history of nonadherence, confusion, or impulsivity. Attention must be given to potential interactions with multiple other medications used to treat medical disorders. It is important to obtain and document informed consent (or consent of family members or guardians) for the use of psychotropics when there is a history of dementia, recent delirium, paranoia, or conflictual doctor-patient relationships.

Finally, clinicians must recognize that in some cases it is best not to prescribe a psychotropic medication. Such cases include older persons with personality disorders and comorbid substance abuse, chronic nonadherence, or a history of or potential for abusive or self-injurious use of medications. Antisocial and borderline persons often demonstrate such behaviors. Dependent patients may insist upon medications as a means of fostering dependency on the clinician, and obsessive-compulsive patients may perpetuate a maladaptive relationship with the clinician through detailed and controlling discussions of medication management. In each example, medication management is corrupted by dysfunctional interpersonal behaviors that lie at the heart of personality disorders.

SOMATOFORM DISORDERS

Somatoform disorders encompass a heterogeneous group of seven diagnoses that have in common the presence of physical symptoms or complaints without objective organic causes, and that are strongly associated with psychologic factors. Clinical characteristics of each diagnosis are summarized in Table 38.3. These disorders are especially relevant to geriatric care because affected older persons are seen in all health care settings, and they tend to overutilize medical services. Somatoform disorders in late life have not been well studied, and existing research has usually focused on select diagnoses, such as hypochondriasis, in limited or biased samples. Research also has looked at somatic symptom reporting rather than at specific diagnoses. Prevalence rates in middle and late life have been found to be less than 1%, except for one study, which found a prevalence rate of more than 36% for somatization disorder in women over 55 years old seen in health care clinics. The presence of these disorders has not been found to be strongly associated with age, although there is weak evidence for a slight increase in hypochondriasis with age. Increased somatic preoccupation and symptoms are, however, associated with

depression in late life, and older age of onset for depression may be most predictive. In addition to depression, increased somatic preoccupation is associated with the presence of the personality trait of neuroticism, in which a person displays a tendency to experience more negative emotions. Somatoform disorders are found more commonly in women and in lower socioeconomic groups. Late onset of a somatoform disorder may suggest associated neurologic illness.

Clinical Characteristics and Causes

It is important to recognize that somatoform disorders do not represent intentional, conscious attempts by older patients to present factitious physical symptoms. Somatoform symptoms are experienced by the affected person as real physical pain and discomfort, usually without insight into associated psychologic factors. Somatoform disorders do not represent delusional thinking as found in psychotic states (although body dysmorphic disorder can be associated with beliefs of delusional quality), and they are different from psychosomatic disorders, which are characterized by actual disease states with presumed psychologic triggers. Rather, somatoform disorders represent a complex interaction between mind and brain in which an affected person is unknowingly expressing psychologic stress or conflict through the body. It is not surprising, then, that depression and anxiety are associated with increased somatic expressions. In late life, somatoform disorders, in particular hypochondriasis, may be a way for a person to express anxiety and attempt to cope with accumulating fears and losses. These may include fears of abandonment by family and caregivers, loss of beauty and strength, financial setbacks, loss of independence, loss of social role (eg, through retirement, loss of spouse, occupational disability), and loneliness. The psychologic distress and anxiety over such losses may be less threatening and more controllable when shifted to somatic complaints or symptoms. In turn, the adoption of a sick role might be reinforced by increased social contacts and support.

The causes of somatoform disorders are usually multifactorial, and often they are rooted in early developmental experiences and personality traits. Psychodynamic approaches suggest that these disorders result from unconscious conflict in which intolerable impulses or affects are expressed through more tolerable somatic symptoms or complaints. One reason for this may be the presence of alexithymia, in which a person is unable to identify and express emotional states, so that the body becomes the available mode of expression.

Although psychodynamic explanations can apply across the life span, these conflicts often begin early

Table 38.3—Clinical Characteristics of Somatoform Disorders*

Somatization Disorder

Multiple physical complaints in excess of what would be expected, given history and examination, prior to the age of 30 and lasting several years; complaints not fully explained by medical work-up; must include four different sites of pain, two gastrointestinal symptoms, one sexual symptom, one pseudoneurologic symptom (not pain).

Undifferentiated Somatoform Disorder

One or more physical complaints, lasting at least 6 months, that cannot be fully explained by appropriate medical work-up and that result in considerable social, occupational, or functional impairment.

Conversion Disorder

One or more motor or sensory deficits that cannot be fully explained by appropriate medical work-up and that appear to be causally related to psychologic factors.

Pain Disorder

Pain is the major focus of clinical presentation, and psychologic factors are believed to be playing a critical role in the onset, severity, exacerbation, and maintenance of the pain.

Hypochondriasis

A preoccupation with fears of having a serious illness, based on misinterpretation of bodily symptoms and resistant to appropriate medical evaluation and reassurance.

Body Dysmorphic Disorder

Preoccupation with an imagined defect in appearance. If there is an actual physical defect, this preoccupation greatly exceeds what would be expected.

Somatoform Disorder, Not Otherwise Specified

The presence of somatoform symptoms that do not meet the criteria for other categories.

* Descriptions of the clusters and of the disorders in each cluster are based on the *Diagnostic and Statistical Manual of Mental Disorders. 4th ed. Text Revision*, Washington, DC: American Psychiatric Association; 2000.

in life, perhaps accounting for the relatively young age of onset for most somatoform disorders. In late life, psychologic conflict that results in significant depression and anxiety are for the most part the same conflicts that can lead to somatization. In addition, the presence of so many comorbid medical problems and the use of multiple medications may provide readily available somatic symptoms around which psychologic conflict can center. In long-term care, older persons are faced with many overwhelming losses, and their own bodies often serve as the last bastion of control. Somatic preoccupation thus serves as a means of coping with stress, even though it is maladaptive and can result in excessive and unnecessary disability.

Treatment

Persons with somatoform disorder do not usually present as such; by their definition they present to clinicians with what appear to be legitimate somatic complaints with an unknown physical cause. It is only after repeated but fruitless work-ups, multiple and persistent complaints and requests, and sometimes angry and inappropriate reactions to treatment that clinicians begin to suspect a somatoform disorder. In

some cases the manner of presentation and symptom complex is more immediately suggestive of a particular somatoform disorder. In any event, it is important for the clinician to remember that from the perspective of the patient, the symptoms and complaints are quite real and disturbing. It is never wise to challenge the patient or to suggest that the symptoms are "all in your mind," even after work-up has made it obvious that psychologic factors are involved. The typical response to such advice is for the patient to seek additional opinions and medical tests, which in turn can perpetuate a cycle of somatization that never addresses the underlying issues.

Instead, the physician should attempt to foster an ongoing, supportive, consistent, and professional relationship with the affected person. Such a relationship will serve to provide reassurance as well as to protect the patient from excessive and unnecessary medical visits and procedures. The physician should focus on responding to individual complaints, perhaps with periodic but regularly scheduled appointments, and to set limits on work-up and treatment in a firm but empathetic manner. This can be difficult to do when patients become demanding and attempt to consume excessive clinic time, but the physician must endeavor to remain professional and not to personalize the situation or to feel that he or she is failing the patient. Overall, the role of the physician is to focus on symptom reduction and rehabilitation, and not to attempt to force the patient to have insight into the potential psychologic nature of his or her symptoms. It would be hazardous to prematurely diagnose a somatoform disorder when there might actually be an underlying medical problem that has eluded diagnosis. For example, disorders such as multiple sclerosis, systemic lupus erythematosus, and acute intermittent porphyria commonly have complex presentations that elude initial diagnostic work-up. Moreover, many somatoform disorders coexist with actual disease states; for example, many persons with pseudoseizures also have an actual seizure disorder. At the same time, it is important for the physician to set limits on what he or she can offer, and to make appropriate referrals to specialists and mental health clinicians.

The mental health clinician will play a more active role in addressing the somatoform disorder. Unfortunately, no particular treatment for any somatoform disorder has been found to have good efficacy, and most disorders tend to be lifelong. As a result, the goal of treatment is not to cure, but to control symptoms. The physician first forms a therapeutic alliance based on empathetic listening and acknowledgment of physical discomfort, without trivializing the somatic complaints. Sometimes an offer to review all available medical records can be a tangible way of conveying one's seriousness to the patient. Underlying anxiety and depression must be identified and treated with psychotherapy and, when necessary, antidepressant or antianxiety medications, or both. Cognitive-behavioral therapy focuses on identifying distorted thought patterns and anxious triggers, and replacing them with more realistic and adaptive strategies. A mental health professional may assist in determining whether cognitive-behavioral therapy may be of benefit. In many cases, however, the supportive nature of regular visits to a primary care provider may be sufficient to meet the needs of persons with somatoform disorders as well as other personality disorders.

ANNOTATED REFERENCES

■ Agronin ME. Somatoform disorders. In: Blazer DG, Steffens DC, Busse EW, eds. *Textbook of Geriatric Psychiatry.* 3rd ed. Washington, DC: American Psychiatric Press; 2004:295–302.

> This chapter provides a comprehensive, up-to-date review of somatoform disorders in late life, including specific features and treatment strategies for each diagnosis. The chapter emphasizes the heterogeneity of both clinical presentation and treatment for these varied disorders, which are placed under a common diagnostic heading.

■ Agronin ME, Maletta G. Personality disorders in late life: understanding and overcoming the gap in research. *Am J Geriatric Psychiatry.* 2000;8(1):4–18.

> This review article provides a comprehensive discussion of diagnostic limitations for personality disorders in late life and of the implications for research. This is a helpful guide to the evolution of diagnostic categories over the successive nosologies in the *Diagnostic and Statistical Manual of Mental Disorders.* The discussion addresses a number of ways in which late-life diagnosis could be improved.

■ Rabinowitz T, Hirdes JP, Desjardins I. Somatoform disorders. In: Agronin ME, Maletta GJ, eds. *Principles and Practice of Geriatric Psychiatry.* Philadelphia: Lippincott Williams & Wilkins; 2006:489–504.

> This unique chapter weaves together a review of somatoform disorders in late life along with illuminating data from the author's own research to underscore many points. Keeping with the focus of the comprehensive textbook in which this chapter appears, there is a particular focus on clinical diagnosis and management.

■ Zweig RA, Agronin ME. Personality disorders. In: Agronin ME, Maletta GJ, eds. *Principles and Practice of Geriatric Psychiatry.* Philadelphia: Lippincott Williams & Wilkins; 2006:449–470.

> This chapter presents a comprehensive review of personality disorders in late life, with a specific focus on clinical diagnosis and management. Both psychotherapeutic and psychopharmacologic approaches are described in detail and supplemented with a practical table.

Marc Edward Agronin, MD

CHAPTER 39—ALCOHOL AND DRUG ABUSE

KEY POINTS

- Alcohol and other substance-abuse problems may remain undetected when screening questions are omitted during routine medical visits.

- Alcohol use may be an unrecognized cause of falls, cognitive decline, and medical problems (eg, anemia, elevated liver function tests, thrombocytopenia).

- It is important to consider a diagnosis of alcohol withdrawal in older persons who develop delirium with hospitalization or facility placement.

- Cognitive impairment from chronic alcoholism in the older adult may improve with sustained abstinence.

The abuse and misuse of alcohol, psychoactive medications, illicit drugs, and nicotine have become significant public health concerns for the growing population of elderly people. This concern is highlighted by the growth in the literature demonstrating that substance abuse and dependence among older people is common. Moreover, elderly adults are particularly vulnerable to the cognitive and physical effects of these substances. Clinicians and researchers therefore may need to change their thinking about the risks of use in this segment of the population. Typically, substance-use problems are thought to occur only in those persons who use substances in high quantities and at regular intervals. Among elderly persons, however, negative health consequences have been demonstrated at consumption levels previously thought of as light to moderate, and certainly not in the amounts usually associated with a diagnosis of substance dependence. A growing number of effective treatments for these problems lead not only to reductions in substance use but also to improvement in general health. Taken together, both the risks and the emergence of new treatments underscore the need to identify problems and provide appropriate treatment for those older adults suffering from the effects of substance misuse.

DEFINITIONS OF SUBSTANCE ABUSE

Establishing valid criteria for determining which older adults would benefit from reducing or eliminating their substance use is the first step in successful intervention. *Substance dependence* has been defined by the medical community as any use that imparts significant disability and warrants treatment. Many older adults are not recognized as having problems that are related to their substance use, partly because the diagnostic criteria are difficult to interpret and to apply consistently to older adults. For instance, many older people drink at home by themselves; thus, they are less likely than younger drinkers to be arrested, to get into arguments, or to have difficulties in employment. Moreover, because many of the diseases caused or affected by substance misuse (eg, hypertension, stroke, and peptic ulcer disease) are common disorders in late life, the clinician may overlook the effects of substance use on the older patient who presents with these disorders. The literature indicates that older problem drinkers are identified less often by clinicians and are less often referred for treatment than are their younger counterparts.

Because of the difficulties in assessing older adults for substance dependence, many of the experts have advocated screening to identify persons who are at risk for problem behaviors or who have at-risk or problem use. *At-risk use* is defined as any use of a substance at a quantity or frequency greater than a recommended level. The level of use is often determined empirically on the basis of association with significant disability. For instance, the recommended upper limit of alcohol consumption for elderly adults has been established as no more than seven standard drinks per week with no more than two episodes of binge drinking (four or more drinks in a day) during a period of 3 months. *Problem substance use* is defined as the consumption of any amount of an abusable substance that results in at least one problem related to this use. For example, the use of benzodiazepines by a patient who has an unsteady gait would be considered problem use.

On the other end of the spectrum, *abstinence* refers to drinking no alcohol in the previous year. Approximately 60% to 70% of older adults are abstinent. If an older patient is abstinent, it is useful to ascertain why alcohol is not used. Some individuals are abstinent because of a previous history of alcohol problems. For this reason, it is particularly important to obtain a history of both current and past use. Some are abstinent because of recent illness; others have lifelong patterns of low-risk use or abstinence. Patients who have a previous history of alcohol problems may require preventive monitoring to determine if any new stresses could exacerbate an old pattern. In addition, a previous history of at-risk drinking or alcohol dependence increases the risk for developing other mental health problems in late life, such as depressive disorders or cognitive problems, and may limit treatment response because of brain damage.

Low-risk or moderate use of alcohol is that which falls within the recommended guidelines for consumption and is not associated with problems. Older adults in this category not only consume amounts that fall within recommended drinking guidelines but are also able to employ reasonable limits on alcohol consumption, that is, they do not drink when driving a motor vehicle or boat, or when using contraindicated medications. It is important to note, however, that a change in physical health or change in prescription medications may elevate even low-risk use to a problem level.

The most practical method for identifying persons who could benefit from intervention is to determine the quantity and frequency of their use of abusable substances. This method has advantages over formal diagnostic interviews because of its brevity, easily interpretable results, and absence of stigmatizing language, such as "addiction," "alcoholism," "alcoholic" or "alcohol dependence." For more on screening, see the section below on identifying substance-use disorders (p 301).

MAGNITUDE OF THE PROBLEM

Drug Use

Little is known about the epidemiology of substance-use disorders among elderly persons other than alcoholism. The general belief is that older drug addicts are only younger addicts grown old and that few older adults initiate drug use in their later years. The Epidemiologic Catchment Area study provides perhaps the only community study of the prevalence of drug abuse and dependence among elderly adults. Using the Diagnostic Interview Schedule to determine prevalence rates for psychiatric diagnoses as defined by the third edition of the *Diagnostic and Statistical Manual of Mental Disorders* (*DSM-III*), the study found the lifetime prevalence rates of drug abuse and dependence to be 0.12% for elderly men and 0.06% for elderly women. The lifetime history of illicit drug use was found to be 2.88% for men and 0.66% for women. No active cases were reported in either gender. In contrast, a more recent study of an elder-specific drug program in a veteran population found that one quarter had either a primary drug problem or concurrent drug and alcohol problems. This study may be a reflection of the growing number of elderly persons who used drugs during a time of expanded drug experimentation in the United States in the 1960s. Recent increases in hepatitis C among patients aged 60 and over may reflect both a history of intravenous drug use as well as increased risk of nosocomial infection with advanced age. Other studies to determine the prevalence and incidence of substance-use disorders involving nicotine, caffeine, benzodiazepines, marijuana, and opiates (in later life) are needed.

Medication Use

Perhaps a unique problem with the elderly age group is the misuse or inappropriate use of prescription and over-the-counter medications. This problem includes the misuse of substances such as sedatives, hypnotics, narcotic and non-narcotic analgesics, diet aids, decongestants, and a wide variety of over-the-counter medications. Community surveys have found that 60% of elderly persons are taking an analgesic, 22% are taking a central nervous system medication, and 11% are taking a benzodiazepine. Many medications used by elderly persons have the potential for inducing tolerance, withdrawal syndromes, and harmful medical consequences, such as cognitive changes, kidney disease, falls, and liver disease. There is a growing body of literature demonstrating a concerning increase in morbidity and mortality associated with the misuse of prescription and nonprescription medications, even though this is not considered as a disorder by *DSM-IV*.

Medication use by all elderly patients needs to be monitored carefully; it is important to avoid prescribing potentially hazardous combinations of drugs, medications with a high risk for adverse effects, and ineffective or unnecessary medications. (See "Pharmacotherapy," p 72.) A practical approach to monitoring psychoactive medications is to reevaluate the older patient's use every 3 to 6 months. Continue on maintenance treatment only those patients with specific target symptoms and a documented response to the treatment. Reevaluate to consider the appropriate diagnosis and further care of patients without a response or partial response. In such cases, consultation with a geriatric mental health professional could be advantageous. (See also "Depression and Other Mood Disorders," p 269; "Anxiety Disorders," p 281; "Psychotic Disorders," p 285; and "Personality and Somatoform Disorders," p 290.)

Alcohol Use

Community-based epidemiologic studies define the extent and nature of alcohol use in the older population by reporting percentages of abstainers, heavy drinkers, and daily drinkers. Abstention from alcohol ranges from 31% to 58%, and daily drinking ranges from 10% to 22% in samples of older patients. "Heavy" drinking, defined as a minimum of 12 to 21 drinks per week, is present in 3% to 9% of the older population; alcohol abuse, as defined clinically, is present in approximately 2% to 4%.

Longitudinally designed community studies give valuable insight regarding the natural course of drinking patterns in elderly age groups. Studies that examined longitudinal alcohol use indicate an incidence of heavy drinking of 0.2% to 4% of older persons per year. It is also important to keep in mind that most of the literature on drinking indicates that although elderly persons are likely to decrease the quantity of alcohol consumed on a given day, the frequency of use or pattern of use changes very little over time.

Cultural and Demographic Factors

Numerous studies have shown that the prevalence of alcohol use and alcohol-related problems among older persons is much higher for men than for women. Among younger adults, however, the ratio of men to women drinkers has changed over the past several decades, with the result that more women present for treatment. These changes are likely to continue to be reflected in the next generation of older women. Similar patterns by gender are seen with illicit drug use, except that benzodiazepines are much more commonly used by older women than by older men.

Conclusions are less clear from the few studies addressing differences among various ethnic groups. Depending on the study, older black Americans and older Hispanic Americans have been found to consume amounts of alcohol similar to or lower than the amounts consumed by older white Americans. The Epidemiologic Catchment Area data demonstrated nonsignificant differences in the 1-year diagnosis of alcohol abuse and dependence among black Americans (2.93% among men, 0.60% among women), white Americans (2.85% among men and 0.47% among women), and Hispanic Americans (6.57% among men and 0.0% among women). More relevant risk factors than race or ethnicity for alcohol consumption among elderly persons are increased leisure time and higher disposable income.

Clinical Settings

Elderly people constitute the majority of admissions to acute-care facilities and are frequent users of outpatient medical services, including primary care. The prevalence rates for alcohol problems among hospital populations are substantially higher than for community dwellers. High prevalence rates for problems related to drinking are also becoming more common in retirement communities. Data from a survey of a Veterans Affairs nursing home has demonstrated that 35% of the patients interviewed had a lifetime diagnosis of alcohol abuse. A significant number of patients seen in outpatient clinics also have been found to have an active alcohol-use disorder. The high prevalence of alcohol-related problems in both hospital and outpatient populations underscores the need for thorough screening of older patients in medical settings.

RISKS AND BENEFITS OF SUBSTANCE USE

Benefits of Alcohol Consumption

Moderate alcohol consumption among otherwise healthy older adults has been promoted as having significant beneficial effects, especially with regard to cardiovascular disease and mortality. The findings from the cardiovascular literature have led to a host of articles in the popular press espousing the benefits of alcohol use.

Alcohol in moderate amounts may promote relaxation and reduce social anxiety. However, even though there are benefits of moderate drinking, the practice of recommending drinking to people who currently do not drink is not advocated. Many older adults do not drink because of past problems with drinking, family problems with drinking, the expense related to drinking, and the adverse effects of intoxication. There is no evidence to support a therapeutic effect of alcohol for heart disease or any other condition in persons who previously did not drink.

Excess Physical Disability

Substance abuse has clear and profound effects on the health and well-being of elderly people in all spheres of life. Older persons are prone to the toxic effects of substances on many different organ systems. The social and economic impact is also tremendous. Substance abuse has adverse effects on self-esteem, coping skills, and interpersonal relationships, which may be compounded by losses that are common in the late stages of life. Elderly adults are particularly prone to these toxic effects because of both the physiologic changes associated with aging and the changes associated with other illnesses common in late life.

Levels of alcohol consumption above seven drinks per week, so called at-risk drinking, have been associated with a number of health problems, including an increased risk of stroke caused by bleeding, impaired driving skills, and an increased rate of injuries, such as falls and fractures. The risk of breast cancer in women who consume three to nine drinks per week has been shown to be increased by approximately 50% over that of women who drink fewer than three drinks per week. Of particular importance to older persons are the potential harmful interactions between alcohol and both prescribed and over-the-counter medications, especially psychoactive medications such as benzodiazepines and antidepressants. Alcohol is also known to interfere with the metabolism of many medications, including digoxin and warfarin.

Older adults who consume more than an average of four drinks per day or whose drinking has led to a diagnosis of alcohol dependence are at greatest risk for excess physical disability and physical illness that are related to the drinking. The most common problems associated with alcohol dependence are alcoholic liver disease, chronic obstructive pulmonary disease, peptic ulcer disease, and psoriasis. Moreover, unexplained multisystem disease should alert the clinician to probe more closely for alcohol use. With smoking, the risks are much clearer, including increased rates of pulmonary disease, especially cancer. Medications such as benzodiazepines are also associated with excess physical disability, with increased rates of falls, and driving-related impairment. Research is beginning to demonstrate that the disability associated with these problems is also reversible with reductions in substance use.

Mental Health Problems

Substance use can be a significant factor in the course and prognosis of nearly all mental health problems of late life. Alcohol, benzodiazepine, opioid, and cigarette use have all been demonstrated to be related etiologically to mood disturbances, but they also complicate the treatment of concurrent mood disorders. Persons with both alcoholism and depression have been shown to have a more complicated clinical course of depression with an increased risk of suicide and more social dysfunction than nondepressed persons with alcoholism. Overall, elderly persons with alcohol abuse or dependence are nearly three times more likely to have a lifetime diagnosis of another mental disorder. Alcoholism has been implicated in mood disorders, suicide, dementia, anxiety disorders, and sleep disturbances.

As might be expected, patients with alcohol-related dementia who become abstinent do not show a progression in cognitive impairment comparable to that of persons with Alzheimer's disease. The complex role of alcoholism in the development of Alzheimer's disease is not fully understood, but certainly alcoholism is known to lead to a syndrome of dementia independently. Interesting new hypotheses implicate glutamatergic toxicity, but overall, the mechanisms are not well understood. The criteria for alcohol-related dementia are as follows:

- clinically evident dementia at least 60 days after last alcohol exposure;
- a history of significant use for at least 5 years, ie, at least 35 drinks per week for men and 28 per week for women;
- the occurrence of this period of significant use within 3 years of the onset of cognitive deficits.

Clinical features supporting the diagnosis include end-organ damage (eg, liver disease), cognitive stabili-

zation or improvement after abstinence, and evidence of cerebellar atrophy in brain imaging. Further research is greatly needed to understand the potential benefits of long-term abstinence in this condition. Similarly, those with comorbid depression and alcohol use are likely to have better depression outcomes if abstinence is achieved. Moderate alcohol use has also been demonstrated to have negative effects on the treatment of late-life depression, further underscoring the need for reducing moderate use in the context of chronic health problems in older adults.

IDENTIFYING SUBSTANCE-USE DISORDERS

Although clinical examination remains the most valuable tool for identifying substance-use problems, screening instruments help increase the sensitivity and efficiency of the diagnosis of various disorders. Several instruments have been developed for identifying alcohol-use disorders, including self-administered questionnaires and laboratory studies. Self-administered questionnaires provide the busy physician with a rapid, sensitive, and inexpensive method of screening for alcohol problems. Two questionnaires—the Michigan Alcoholism Screening Test (MAST) and the CAGE (see Table 39.1)—have been developed with these principles in mind. Both of these instruments have high sensitivity and specificity for identifying alcohol-use disorders in young and middle-aged persons.

Biologic markers of substance use can be useful in managing patients with known substance-use disorders, but they have proved less valuable in detecting illness. These markers include γ-glutamyl transferase, which has a low sensitivity and a moderate specificity for diagnosing an alcohol-use disorder; mean corpuscular volume, which has a low sensitivity but a high specificity; and carbohydrate-deficient transferrin, which has a low sensitivity and low specificity. These markers require further research, but clinically any combination of macrocytic anemia, thrombocytopenia, and elevated γ-glutamyl transferase should flag the need for further

Table 39.1—The CAGE Questionnaire

C	Have you ever tried to **C**ut down on your drinking?
A	Have you ever gotten **A**nnoyed at someone for criticizing your drinking?
G	Do you ever feel **G**uilty about your drinking?
E	Have you ever had an **E**ye-opener to steady your nerves or get rid of a hangover?

A positive answer to one or more questions suggests problem drinking

screening. Urine drug screens are an effective method for screening for or identifying illicit drug use as well as prescription drug use.

TREATMENT

Older persons with a substance-use problem often present with a variety of treatment needs. It is therefore important to have an array of services available for older adults that can be tailored to these individual needs and to have the flexibility to adapt to changing needs over time. The most important aspect to treating an older adult who is misusing a substance is to engage the patient in the intervention. Older adults engaged in treatment have been shown to have very robust improvement, especially in comparison with younger cohorts. The spectrum of interventions for alcohol abuse in older adults range from prevention and education for persons who are abstinent or low-risk drinkers, to minimal advice or brief structured interventions for at-risk or problem drinkers, and formalized alcoholism treatment for drinkers who meet criteria for abuse or dependence. The array of formal treatment options available includes psychotherapy, education, rehabilitative and residential care, and psychopharmacologic agents. An example of the necessity to tailor care is the contrast between the at-risk drinker or benzodiazepine user and the severely dependent patient. It is unlikely that the at-risk user will need the intensity of services required for the severely dependent patient. Indeed, requiring the at-risk drinker to accept a set of rigorous services may be more detrimental than helpful.

Dependency on medications such as benzodiazepines is managed by placing the patient on a 24-hour equivalent of the dosage of the drug on which the patient is dependent, tapering the dosage by 10% every three half-lives, and by providing supportive counseling via groups, psychosocial support, and 12-step programs. Symptoms of withdrawal from narcotics can be controlled when necessary with oral clonidine. Assuring that the patient enters a long-term treatment program increases the likelihood of long-term success. For smoking cessation, it is important to prepare the patient for quitting by discussing management strategies before quitting, setting a quit date, and implementing a monitoring plan for maintaining success.

Detoxification and Stabilization

The assessment of any substance abuser starts with a thorough history, physical, and laboratory examination. Included in the initial assessment is an assessment of the patient's potential to suffer acute withdrawal. Severe withdrawal such as that from alcohol use can be life threatening and warrants careful attention. Patients with severe symptoms of dependency or withdrawal potential and patients with significant medical or psychiatric comorbidity may require inpatient hospitalization for acute stabilization prior to implementing an outpatient management strategy. Detoxification is achieved by placing the patient on the minimum amount of drug that suppresses withdrawal symptoms and then decreasing the dosage by 10% every three half-lives. In general, longer acting formulations of the drug being abused are preferred to shorter acting formulations, but many clinicians find that prescribing the specific drug that a patient was abusing makes the process more acceptable to the patient and minimizes the time needed to determine the initial dose.

For the patient hospitalized for an elective surgery or condition unrelated to the substance problem, it is extremely important to be vigilant for any evidence of withdrawal. Unrecognized alcohol withdrawal can result in serious morbidity and mortality for the elderly patient. Early symptoms include tachycardia, diaphoresis, tremulousness, and hypertension. These symptoms may progress to overt delirium, psychosis, and seizures. Intravenous lorazepam[OL] is most expedient intervention in this scenario, followed by an oral taper.

Outpatient Management

Traditionally, outpatient substance-abuse treatment has been reserved for specialized clinics focused on substance abuse. It is becoming increasingly apparent that this model is inadequate in addressing the broader public health demand, and there is a need to involve a variety of clinicians and clinical settings to deliver substance-abuse treatment. This is particularly important for older adults, who frequently seek medical services but rarely seek specialized addiction services. The traditional addiction clinic is focused on supportive group psychotherapy and encouragement to attend regular self-help group meetings such as Alcoholics Anonymous, Alcoholics Victorious, Rational Recovery, or Narcotics Anonymous. For older adults, peer-specific group activities are considered superior to mixed-age group activities. Outpatient rehabilitation, in addition to focusing on active addiction issues, usually needs to address issues of time management. Abstinence reduces the time spent in maintaining the substance-use disorder. The management of this time, which is often the greater part of a patient's day, is critical to the prognosis of treatment. Clinicians should be wary of focusing on abstinence as the only positive outcome of treatment and should commend patients

---

OL Not approved by the U.S. Food and Drug Administration for this use.

for making progress in cutting down on use as well as stopping. This may be particularly relevant for medications misuse such as benzodiazepines, as it may be more difficult to eliminate the use. For benzodiazepines, remember that the risks of adverse events such as falls are greater with higher doses and medications with a longer half-life such as diazepam or clonazepam. Therefore, using medications with a half-life of 6 to 12 hours reduces the risks for that patient. If benzodiazepines seem to be indicated for an anxiety condition and treatment is initiated for the first time, it is best to avoid the long-acting preparations in favor of shorter-acting agents that do not have active metabolites (eg, lorazepam). However, for patients already receiving long-acting benzodiazepines (eg, 50 mg or more per day of diazepam), there is an increased risk for withdrawal complications, and dose reductions should therefore be made very gradually. If the daily dose is greater than the equivalent of 100 mg of diazepam, then the patient should be hospitalized to initiate withdrawal. Ultimately, a transition to shorter-acting agents is ideal, but this should be initiated very carefully and should involve an equivalent dose initially before any reductions are considered. The use of resources such as day programs and senior centers can be beneficial, especially for cognitively impaired patients. Social services such as financial support are often needed to stabilize the patient in early recovery. Supervised living arrangements, such as halfway houses, group homes, nursing homes, and residing with relatives, should also be considered.

Brief Interventions

Low-intensity, brief interventions have been suggested as cost-effective and practical techniques that can be used as an initial approach to at-risk and problem drinkers in primary care settings. Studies of brief intervention have been conducted in a wide range of health care settings, from hospitals and primary health care locations to mental health clinics. Two trials of brief alcohol intervention with older adults have been reported. Both studies were randomized trials of brief intervention to reduce hazardous drinking by older adults, and both used advice protocols in primary care settings. These studies have shown that older adults can be engaged in brief intervention protocols, that the protocols are acceptable in this population, and that there is a substantial reduction in drinking among the at-risk drinkers receiving the interventions in comparison with a control group.

Pharmacotherapy

The use of medications to support abstinence may be of benefit, but it is not well studied. Small-scale studies

have demonstrated that naltrexone is well tolerated and efficacious in older patients. Studies are currently under way using various antidepressants, including the selective serotonin-reuptake inhibitors. Some of the general principles used in treating younger patients should be applied to older drinkers as well. For example, benzodiazepines are important in the treatment of alcohol detoxification, but they have no clinical place in maintaining long-term abstinence because of their abuse potential and the potential for fostering further alcohol or benzodiazepine abuse. Disulfiram may benefit some well-motivated patients, but cardiac and hepatic disease limits the use of this agent by the older person who abuses alcohol. The use of methadone maintenance has proven efficacy in opioid dependence. Older patients can be initiated and maintained on methadone, following the same principles of use as in younger patients. Comorbid medical and psychiatric disorders must be identified and properly treated, and they may necessitate the need for referral to, or consultation with, a psychiatrist with expertise in these areas. Buprenorphine and buprenorphine with naloxone have been approved for outpatient treatment of opioid dependence. However, given the complexity of the treatment of this condition, systematic training, practice, monitoring, regulation, and evaluation are necessary in a multidisciplinary treatment setting to optimize outcomes. Guidelines for developing treatment programs using buprenorphine are available on the Web site of the Substance Abuse and Mental Health Services Administration (see http:// buprenorphine.samhsa.gov/index.html).

Establishing abstinence from nicotine follows the same principles as that from other addicting substances. Initially, pharmacologic substitution with either nicotine gum or patch is followed by a gradual decrease in dosage. Several trials demonstrated that antidepressant medications improve rates of continued abstinence, but only bupropion has been approved for this purpose by the U.S. Food and Drug Administration. As with other abstinence regimens, psychotherapy plus pharmacotherapy is better than pharmacotherapy alone. See also "Respiratory Diseases and Disorders" (p 326).

ANNOTATED REFERENCES

■ Blow FC, Brower KJ, Schulenberg JE, et al. The Michigan Alcoholism Screening Test–Geriatric Version (MAST-G). *Alcohol Clin Exp Res.* 1992;16:372.

The geriatric version of the MAST (MAST–G), which asks questions relevant to an aging cohort, has been found to be 95% sensitive and 78% specific for identifying older persons with alcohol problems. Other widely used questionnaires include the Alcohol Use Disorders Identification Test (AUDIT) and the Drinking Problems Index. For information about a number of screens for alcohol problems, see http://

www.niaaa.nih.gov/publications/ (accessed October 2005) or the AGS Clinical Practice Committee guidelines (see below).

■ Fleming MF, Manwell LB, Barry KL, et al. Brief physician advice for alcohol problems in older adults: a randomized community-based trial. *J Fam Pract.* 1999;48(5):378–384.

This study demonstrates the efficacy of a brief alcohol intervention among older patients attending primary care. Results from the intervention group were compared with those in usual care in similar primary care practices, and the intervention group showed a 62% greater reduction than the control group by those who were drinking more than 21 drinks per week.

■ Helzer JE, Burnam A, McEvoy LT. Alcohol abuse and dependence. In: Robins LN, Reiger DA, eds. *Psychiatric Disorders in America: The Epidemiologic Catchment Area Study.* New York: The Free Press; 1991.

This chapter reviews the epidemiology of alcohol use, abuse, and dependence from the Epidemiologic Catchment Area (ECA) study. The remainder of the book is also relevant and includes discussion of drug use, abuse, and dependence. The ECA study was a sampling of community residents from five sites representing urban and rural populations. Persons who were sampled were then interviewed with the Diagnostic Interview Schedule for mental health problems. Thus, the results published are broad-based epidemiologic data on all mental health conditions. The alcohol chapter includes analyses of demographic information on age and race.

■ Korper SP, Council CL, eds. *Substance Use by Older Adults: Estimates of Future Impact on the Treatment System* (DHHS Publication No. SMA 03-3763, Analytic Series A-21). Rockville, MD: Substance Abuse and Mental Health Services Administration, Office of Applied Studies; 2002.

This report extensively documents the projected demand for substance abuse treatment services for older Americans over the next three decades. This report highlights the importance of recognizing the relatively greater use of alcohol and illicit substances by the baby-boomer generation than by earlier generations. Electronic access to this report may be obtained via http://www.samhsa.gov (accessed October 2005).

■ Moore AA, and the American Geriatrics Society Clinical Practice Committee. Clinical guidelines for alcohol use disorders in older adults. Updated November 2003. Available at: http://www.americangeriatrics.org./products/positionpapers/alcohol.shtml (accessed October 2005).

The AGS guideline, which updates Substance Abuse Among Older Adults, Treatment Improvement Protocol Series 26 of the Substance Abuse and Mental Health Services Administration, addresses screening recommendations for older adults and age-related physiologic changes that may occur with late-life alcoholism. Medications that may interact adversely with alcohol are outlined, and chronic conditions that may be triggered or worsened by alcohol use are noted. To assist the clinician in early detection, the risk factors for alcoholism in late life are summarized; guidelines for inquiring about alcoholism and specific laboratory values that may be abnormal are also provided. Different risk levels are outlined, and definitions for abuse and dependence are provided. Various interpersonal and pharmacologic intervention strategies are discussed and supplemented by a link to the following resource: http://findtreatment.samhsa.gov (accessed October 2005).

■ Oslin DW, Pettinati HP, Volpicelli JR. Alcoholism treatment adherence: older age predicts better adherence and drinking outcomes. *Am J Geriatr Psychiatry.* 2002:10(6);740–747.

This study, conducted in younger and older adults with alcohol dependence, was a double-blind, randomized controlled trial of naltrexone 100 mg versus placebo. The results of the trial demonstrated that naltrexone is well tolerated by older adults, but more importantly, that older adults are more adherent to treatment and have better treatment outcomes.

David W. Oslin, MD

CHAPTER 40—MENTAL RETARDATION

KEY POINTS

■ Difficulties with behavioral problems and impairment in adaptive skills are a major problem among adults with mental retardation.

■ Poor communication skills often lead to under-recognition of medical problems, which may precipitate behavioral problems.

■ Menopausal symptoms should be considered when women with mental retardation exhibit behavioral changes in later life.

■ Dementia of the Alzheimer's type occurs almost invariably among persons with Down syndrome, but dementia is not a necessary outcome among persons with other types of mental retardation.

Mental retardation continues to be a widely used term to describe the condition of subaverage intellectual function in the presence of deficits in adaptive behavior. Critics have attacked this definition for a variety of reasons. These include reliance on intelligence tests to demonstrate intellectual difficulties, which has been criticized because of difficulties in determining cut-off values for normality, the questionable cultural fairness of the tests, and the questionable relevance of the tests for performance in real-life situations. Similar controversies regarding the imprecision of definition and measurement of adaptive behavior remain unresolved. However, the key concept of a central, biologically based deficit in intellectual function appears to be valid; persons with mental retardation have a condition in which nearly every cognitive process that has been studied is deficient. For mild mental retardation, the same genetic and environmental influences appear to operate that determine individual differences throughout the normal range of variation in general cognitive ability. Importantly, the heritability of general cognitive ability is substantial, probably around 50%; the effects of shared environmental influences in families become negligible after adolescence, and genetic influence increases from infancy to adulthood. Persons with severe degrees of mental retardation are more likely to have structural defects of the brain or metabolic or chromosomal derangements. The challenge for the future is to determine how these biologic abnormalities interact with the aging process.

PREVALENCE

The number of aging persons with mental retardation is increasing, probably because of increased longevity. Life expectancy in mental retardation has increased from 20 years in the 1930s to 60 years in 1980. For those with Down syndrome, life expectancy has increased by about 30 years. The prevalence of mental retardation and developmental disability (cerebral palsy, autism, epilepsy) is generally assumed to be around 1%. Thus, estimates are that in the United States there are 525,000 persons aged 60 and over with these conditions, and the numbers are expected to double by 2030.

PSYCHIATRIC AND MENTAL DISORDERS IN AGING ADULTS WITH MENTAL RETARDATION

The prevalence of psychiatric disorders among adults with mental retardation is about five times that of age-matched control groups. Depending on the exact population studied and the type of diagnoses included, rates range from 10% to 40%.

Dementia

Adults with Down syndrome have an increased risk for the early onset of Alzheimer's disease, with nearly 100% developing the neuropathology by age 40. Although not all develop symptoms in their 40s, approximately 40% aged 50 and over have symptoms of dementia, with 50% developing seizures as a result of

the degenerative changes. Approximately 75% of persons with Down syndrome in their 60s have symptoms of dementia (compared with a prevalence in the general population of 5% at age 65). Symptoms also include loss of adaptive skills and increased maladaptive behavior; the dementia is often associated with depression, indifference, and social inappropriateness. The average age at death for persons with Down syndrome and Alzheimer's disease is approximately 50. One study has demonstrated that in women with Down syndrome, an early age of menopause is associated with earlier dementia symptoms. Menopause may be an important factor among women with mental retardation who experience a behavioral or cognitive change in late life.

The incidence of dementia in persons with mental retardation who do not have Down syndrome is the same as in the general population; however, these persons also have a higher prevalence of the neuropathology of Alzheimer's disease: 54% for ages 50 to 65, 76% for ages 66 to 75, 87% for ages > 75.

Other Major Mental Disorders

For persons with mental retardation, the lifetime prevalence of other major mental illnesses appears to be similar to or slightly higher than that of the general population. In those aged 65 and over, approximately 70% may reach criteria for a psychiatric diagnosis, often with higher rates than for a younger age group. Autistic traits are common, occurring in up to approximately half of adults with learning disability or mental retardation. These traits are more common in those with severe or profound degrees of mental retardation and in younger individuals; they are typically associated with behavioral difficulties.

Adaptive Behavioral Difficulties

Difficulties that adults with mental retardation have with adaptive behavior may be severe, and difficulties may occur with increasing frequency in later life as a consequence of cognitive decline and increasingly impaired mobility. For example, surveys concerning adults with mental retardation have revealed that 25% have no useful speech and 10% have no receptive comprehension. Half do not have basic self-care skills, half have a physical disability, and half have a mobility impairment; 10% are totally dependent. Support services for these people are usually deficient.

Behavioral Disorders

As many as 50% to 60% of adults with mental retardation have a maladaptive behavior (such as withdrawal, self-injury, stereotypy) that is severe or that occurs frequently, and follow-up studies show that these behaviors may persist for years. The proportion decreases with age, except in Down syndrome, in which the proportion is higher and the incidence of behavioral problems increases with the degree of mental retardation. Aggression occurs with similar frequency in all age groups. About half of the persons with behavioral disorders have had an experience in the preceding 12 months that may have precipitated the disorder, such as a change in environment or loss of a familiar companion.

DIAGNOSIS AND TREATMENT

The diagnosis of a mental disorder in the older adult with mental retardation is based on the same principles of history and examination that apply in the general population. However, presentations of mental illness may be different in these patients. Typically, verbal skills are poor, and reports of mood or mental experiences are difficult to obtain. Often, mental disorders present as behavioral changes, for example, social withdrawal, apathy, and vegetative changes occurring in depressed persons, or agitation, sleeplessness, or aggression in those experiencing delusions or hallucinations. It is more difficult for persons with limited coping skills to adjust to changes in living or work situations, and inquiries should be made about whether such changes have occurred.

It is important to identify the cause of the person's mental retardation. Careful physical, laboratory, and neurologic investigation (electroencephalography and neuroimaging) may establish a cause in 40%. Different conditions are associated with different problems (see Table 40.1). Elderly persons with mental retardation who have not been previously evaluated should be referred to a specialist for assessment if asymmetric neurologic signs are present, if there is a history of cognitive or neurologic deterioration, or if behavioral symptoms cannot be reversed. Medical disorders commonly present as psychiatric or behavioral disorders, and they occur in persons with mental retardation twice as commonly as in the average psychiatric population.

Maladaptive behaviors, such as aggression, are common in persons with mental retardation and may not indicate a mental disorder. An impulsive response to a stressor may reflect only suboptimal judgment in a particular situation. An appropriate treatment in such cases would be instructional or behavioral; the preferred behavior programs are ones that reward good behavior. A disorder of impulse control, however, may also produce aggressive responses; diagnosis of such a

Table 40.1—Disorders That Are Associated With Specific Types of Mental Retardation in the Older Adult

Type of Retardation	Associated Disorders
Down syndrome	Hypothyroidism, Alzheimer's disease
Fragile X syndrome	Autistic behaviors, gaze avoidance, attentional difficulty
Frontal lobe damage	Apathy, irritability, distractibility, perseveration, impulsivity
Prader-Willi syndrome	Hyperphagia, obesity, ritualistic behaviors, aggression
Temporal lobe lesions	Gastaut-Geschwind syndrome (an interictal syndrome with hypergraphia, irritability, elation, paranoia) Kluver-Bucy syndrome (hypersexuality, hyperorality, visual agnosia, diminished aggression, anxiety)

disorder requires a pattern of impulsivity that is disproportionate to the degree of intellectual impairment. With an impulse-control disorder, aggression may be preceded by a period of increasing tension and arousal, occur explosively and out of proportion to the stressor, and seem to have a driven, sustained nature. Appropriate treatment would consist of instructional and behavioral methods, but also with pharmacologic interventions to reduce impulsivity (eg, selective serotonin-reuptake inhibitors[OL]) or arousal (eg, β-blockers[OL]). Pharmacologic treatment of aggression is similar to that in the general population and includes the use of mood stabilizers[OL], selective serotonin-reuptake inhibitors[OL], β-blockers[OL], and antipsychotic medications[OL].

The diagnosis of dementia among persons with mental retardation is made according to the same criteria as in the general population. These criteria include the presence of cognitive and adaptive deterioration; demonstration of deficits on examination (preferably with longitudinal follow-up showing progression of deficits); and exclusion of other possible causes of deterioration, such as medical or environmental factors, or other mental disorders, such as depression or delirium. Standardized scales are available that help structure the interview and history and produce a score that indicates the likelihood that dementia is present and its severity. The Washington University Clinical Dementia Rating Scale that is widely used with the general population can also be used in many individuals with mental retardation. Neuroimaging studies may be helpful in establishing the diagnosis and in differentiating Alzheimer's disease from vascular dementia; longitudinal and volumetric studies may help differentiate normal aging from dementia. There are insufficient studies to demonstrate the efficacy of standard treatments (such as donepezil) in persons with mental retardation.

[OL] Not approved by the U.S. Food and Drug Administration for this use.

MEDICAL DISORDERS

Adults with mental retardation have more medical problems than do age-matched persons (approximately five medical conditions per person; those with more severe mental retardation have more problems). Approximately two thirds of those in a community setting have chronic conditions or major physical disability. It is estimated that 50% of these medical conditions go undetected. Prompt detection and treatment is associated with better survival. Visual or hearing impairments are more common in persons with mental retardation; they increase with age and affect approximately 25%.

Persons with Down syndrome and others with mental retardation have similar age-specific mortality until ages 30 to 34, after which there is an exponential increase in mortality with age for those with Down syndrome, probably because of the onset of dementia. Life expectancy decreases with increasing severity of mental retardation, and with other morbidity such as inability to ambulate, lack of feeding skills, and incontinence. Life expectancy for adults with mental retardation is lower than for the general population and is about 65 years. The commonest causes of death are cardiovascular and respiratory disorders, cancer, and dementia (particularly in Down syndrome).

SOCIAL CONDITIONS

At least 80% of adults with mental retardation live at home and are cared for by aging family members; 20% live in residential programs. It is estimated that about 40% of eligible persons may not be served by the formal service system. This situation often leads to a crisis when the parent is no longer able to provide adequate care or is unable to manage a behavioral problem. It is estimated that about half of developmentally disabled adults with a behavior problem need a different living arrangement. Typically, more than half of the families have not made plans for the future care of adult relatives with mental retardation; those in day programs or workshops do not typically have pensions or Social Security benefits to allow retirement. Not surprisingly, the degree of mental retardation, physical health, and functional skills of the aging person correlate with the degree of parental stress and burden, although maternal and family characteristics such as education and income are more correlated with overall life satisfaction and maternal well-being.

ANNOTATED REFERENCES

■ Eastgate G, Lennox NG. Primary health care for adults with intellectual disability. *Aust Fam Physician.* 2003;32(5):330–333.

> This article addresses the clinical challenges in managing adults with intellectual disability. These persons commonly have undiagnosed health problems, and treatment may require a specialized approach to overcome deficits in communication. This article outlines the common physical and psychiatric conditions found in adults with intellectual disability and highlights the need for a structured approach to health care for patients with limited communication skills. An overview of strategies for better assessment and management for older adults with developmental disabilities is provided.

■ Gedye A. *The Dementia Scale for Down Syndrome.* Vancouver, BC, Canada: Gedye Research and Consulting; 1995. (To order, contact A. Gedye, Gedye Research and Consulting, PO Box 39081, Point Grey, Vancouver, BC, Canada V6R 4P1. Phone/Fax: 604-733-1950.)

> This scale assesses the presence or absence of dementia in adults with Down syndrome; it has also been used for the same purpose in mentally retarded persons who do not have Down syndrome. Information is collected from caregivers only. Field testing has demonstrated a concurrent validity coefficient (kappa) of 0.81 and an inter-rater reliability kappa coefficient of 0.91. Diagnosis with the scale was compared with diagnosis by clinicians (see Deb S, Braganza J. Comparison of rating scales for the diagnosis of dementia in adults with Down's syndrome. *J Intellect Disabil Res.*1999;43 [part 50]:400–407), and a sensitivity of 0.85 and specificity of 0.89 for the scale were found.

■ Ryan R, Sunada K. Medical evaluation of persons with mental retardation referred for psychiatric assessment. *Gen Hosp Psychiatry.* 1997;19(4):274–280.

> A total of 1135 people with mental retardation referred for mental health assessment for a behavioral deterioration were medically evaluated by a two-step protocol that involved a screening evaluation plus expanded testing, depending on clinical findings. Medical comorbidity was double that of similar persons without mental retardation, and 75% had one or more medical problems, almost all undiagnosed or undertreated. In 258 patients, treatment of the medical condition caused remission of the psychiatric condition.

■ Sutherland G, Couch MA, Iacono T. Health issues for adults with developmental disability. *Res Dev Disabil.* 2002;23(6):422–445.

> This paper highlights the specific health concerns found in adults with developmental disabilities and reviews the most common untreated conditions that may be recognized with special attention. Other environmental factors that are important in the clinical management of adults with mental retardation are also addressed, including the impact of living arrangements and caregivers on health-promoting activities. The complexity of the interactions among biology, pathology, and behavioral and environmental determinants for the disabled individual are discussed. Greater use of self-reported health studies is suggested, as well as further exploration of effective strategies of health promotion for this population.

Andrew C. Warren, MB, BS, DPhil

DISEASES AND DISORDERS

CHAPTER 41—DERMATOLOGIC DISEASES AND DISORDERS

KEY POINTS

- Seborrheic dermatitis and rosacea are chronic conditions that can be suppressed, but not entirely eliminated.

- Neurodermatitis, or lichen simplex chronicus, occurs most commonly in the age group over 60 years old.

- Stasis dermatitis is most commonly caused by incompetency of venous valves and is best treated by control of venous hypertension.

- Most lower extremity chronic ulcers are caused by venous insufficiency.

- The risk of metastasis from squamous cell carcinoma increases with the size of the lesion, depth of invasion, lack of differentiation, and location of the lesion.

Skin disease increases with aging and sun exposure. Dermatologic care of the older patient requires an awareness of cutaneous changes of aging and the effects of cumulative ultraviolet (UV) radiation exposure, as well as knowledge of the common tumors, inflammatory diseases, and infections seen in older persons.

AGING AND PHOTOAGING

Skin is composed of the epidermis, dermis, basement membrane zone (the area between the epidermis and dermis that serves to hold the two together), and the subcutaneous fat. In normal young skin the epidermis interdigitates with the dermis. Over time these interdigitations are flattened, with decreased contact between the epidermis and dermis. This results in decreased nutrient transfer and increased skin fragility. There is also a change with age in the barrier function because fewer lipids are present in the top layer of the skin, leading to dryness and roughness. The turnover of epidermal cells is slower and may account for the decrease in the rate of wound healing. In aging skin, there is a decrease in the number of immune antigen-presenting cells, such as Langerhans cells, which may have consequences for cutaneous immune surveillance. Changes in the dermis, such as decreased ground substance, correlate with wrinkling and atrophy of the skin in the older person. A decrease in the amount of collagen and elastin is associated with striking changes in fiber orientation, notably a fragmented and more haphazard architecture.

Changes in hair in the older person include graying of hairs that is due to changes in follicular melanocytes, and a decrease in scalp hair density secondary to shortening of anagen (the growth phase of the hair cycle) duration and an increase in the proportion of hairs in telogen (the resting phase).

Photoaging refers to the effects of UV exposure on skin. The depth of penetration of UV light depends on the wavelength, and shorter wavelengths are more biologically active. Ultraviolet B (UVB; 290 to 320 nm) radiation causes most of the acute and chronic damage. Ultraviolet A (UVA; 320 to 400 nm) also plays an important role because it makes up more of the sunlight that reaches the earth's surface and has greater depth of penetration. Mechanisms by which UV light causes changes in the skin probably include DNA injury or decreased DNA repair or both, oxidative damage, lysosomal damage, and altered collagen structure.

Photodamaged skin appears wrinkled, coarse, or rough, and it has mottled pigmentation (due to solar lentigos, seborrheic keratoses, and ephelides or freckles), hypopigmentation, and telangiectasias. Cutaneous malignancies are also more common in photodamaged skin. Prevention of photodamage involves the use of broad-spectrum sunscreens—sunscreens that protect against both UVB and UVA radiation—as well as the avoidance of direct sunlight and use of protective clothing along with hats and sunglasses. Although there are claims that various topical agents decrease photodamage, only topical tretinoin has been shown to increase the thickness of the superficial skin layers, reduce pigmentary changes and roughness, and increase collagen synthesis.

Surgical therapies are used to treat photodamage through controlled partial injury to the skin. These include chemical peeling agents, dermabrasion, and laser resurfacing. All rely on the destruction of surface populations of keratinocytes, followed by repopulation with keratinocytes deep from within the sun-protected follicular structures. Controlled trials to evaluate the effectiveness of these expensive modalities are rare and inconclusive.

SEBORRHEIC DERMATITIS

Seborrheic dermatitis is a common chronic dermatitis that is characterized by symmetric erythema and greasy-looking scales in areas rich in sebaceous glands, such as the hairline (scalp), forehead, nasolabial fold, and the retroauricular and midline chest areas. Dandruff may be an early precursor of this condition. The prevalence of seborrheic dermatitis is higher in persons infected with human immunodeficiency virus (HIV) and those with Parkinson's disease. At all ages, seborrheic dermatitis is more common in males than females.

Although the cause of seborrheic dermatitis is unclear, it is thought that the normal yeast flora (*Malassezia furfur*) play some role in inducing inflammation of the skin, which leads to increased epidermal proliferation and desquamation. The name is misleading, and patients affected with seborrheic dermatitis do not have more seborrhea than the normal population. On the face, it can involve only the eyebrows, glabella, and nasolabial folds, or it can cause a mild blepharitis with red eyelid margins. It should be stressed to patients that seborrheic dermatitis can be suppressed but not cured. It is often treated with medicated shampoos that act against yeast, including selenium sulfide, ketoconazole, and various tar shampoos. Acute forms can also be treated with mild topical corticosteroids such as hydrocortisone 1% to 2%. Once the dermatitis is under control, patients can use the medicated shampoos for maintenance.

ROSACEA

Rosacea (Figure 41.1) is a common condition in fair-skinned persons and affects young to middle-aged as well as elderly persons. The cause of rosacea remains elusive; recurrent facial flushing resulting from a variety of stimuli is a common symptom. The flushing is often induced by sunlight exposure, alcohol, hot beverages, and drugs that cause vasodilatation. Medications such as oral niacin (for hyperlipidemia) and topical steroids can often induce or worsen rosacea. Rosacea has several variants, each of which requires a different approach to treatment. Usually the central convex areas of the face are affected (nose, forehead, cheeks, and chin) with erythema and telangiectasias. More advanced cases show follicular and nonfollicular papules and pustules. Recurrent flushing and edema cause thickening of the skin; in the most severe cases a rhinophyma may develop. Rosacea can also involve the eye, causing irritation and burning that may present as conjunctival injection, blepharitis, episcleritis, chalazion, or hordeolum. Often, rosacea and seborrheic dermatitis coexist.

Figure 41.1—Rosacea. Diffuse erythema and erythematous papules and papulopustules are seen on the cheeks, forehead, and chin. The nose shows thickening of the skin and changes consistent with an early rhinophyma.

The treatment of rosacea is based on the clinical picture. It is important for patients to understand that it is a chronic condition with frequent flares. They should be educated on avoiding skin irritants or strong soaps and cleansers, and instructed to reduce sun exposure and regularly apply sunscreens. Oral antibiotics such as tetracylines (doxycycline, minocycline) and erythromycin are used to treat the moderate to severe papular-pustular rosacea. Topical agents such as azelaic acid cream, erythromycin, clindamycin, and metronidazole can be used for mild rosacea or as maintenance once the oral antibiotics have been tapered. Severe or refractory rosacea can be treated with oral isotretinoin. Lasers, such as the potassium-titanyl-phosphate (KTP) laser, intense pulsed light and the pulsed dye laser, can be used to reduce the redness and improve cosmetic appearance. Rhinophyma occurs less commonly and can be treated with surgical excision or CO_2 laser ablation.

XEROSIS

Dryness of the skin, often a concern for the older patient, is due to the reduction in water content and barrier function of the aging epidermis. It is exacerbated by environmental factors, such as decreased humidity from cold weather or central heating, irritation by hot water, and too frequent washing with harsh soaps and cleansers. Skin findings are often more pronounced on the legs. Depending on the severity of the dryness, xerosis can present as rough, itchy skin or as scales that give the skin a dry, cracked appearance known as *eczema craquelé* (Figure 41.2).

The patient's awareness of exacerbating factors and regular use of tepid showers and emollients immediately after bathing can be quite helpful. Moisturizing agents containing lactic acid or α-hydroxy acids can reduce the roughness and scaliness. When irritation or inflammation is a prominent finding, episodic use of mild topical corticosteroids for a short time provides relief.

NEURODERMATITIS

Neurodermatitis is a nonspecific term that is used to refer to chronic, pruritic conditions of unclear cause. Another term commonly used is *lichen simplex chronicus*. It is most common in adults over the age of 60. The lesions show signs of chronic scratching, such as hyperpigmentation and lichenification (leathery thickness) along with redness and scaling. Scratching these lesions often leads to pleasure and a vicious cycle of skin changes that then induce more pruritus.

Figure 41.2—Eczema craquelé. Dry, erythematous, fissured, and cracked skin is seen on the lower legs of this patient.

OL Not approved by the U.S. Food and Drug Administration for this use.

Treatment consists of potent topical corticosteroids, often under occlusion, emollients, as well as behavior modification. Other causes of pruritus such as irritant or allergic contact dermatitis, drug allergy, or xerosis must be excluded.

STASIS DERMATITIS

Stasis dermatitis can be an early sign of chronic venous insufficiency of the lower extremities. Chronic venous hypertension, caused mostly by incompetency of the venous valves, is the initial trigger for stasis dermatitis. Venous hypertension slows down the flow of blood in the microvasculature, damages the permeability barrier of the small vessels, and allows for the passage of fluid and plasma proteins into the tissue, leading to the edema and extravasation of erythrocytes. These processes lead to decreased oxygen diffusion and metabolic exchange and to activation and attraction of inflammatory cells and mediators to the site. Stasis dermatitis typically occurs in the medial supramalleolar areas. It is often associated with intense pruritus. Initially, pitting edema to the ankle is noted, which is often worse at night. Over time, these events lead to the progressive induration and adherence of the skin and subcutaneous tissues. Venous ulcers can develop spontaneously or secondary to trauma, arising most often in the supramalleolar areas.

The goal of therapy is to control the venous hypertension with the regular use of compression bandages or stockings and exercising the calf muscles to improve venous return. Topical treatment includes the judicious use of corticosteroids and emollients. Sensitization to ingredients in topical medications and emollients, including topical antibiotics, is commonly encountered but frequently overlooked. Patch testing to exclude contact sensitization to these agents should be considered before use.

VENOUS AND ARTERIAL ULCERS

An ulcer is a wound with loss of epidermal and dermal layers, in contrast to an erosion, which is loss of the epidermal layer only. Chronic leg wounds are defined as open wounds that fail to heal within a period of 6 weeks. Venous disease causes 72% of leg ulcers, 22% have a mixed arterial and venous etiology, and only 6% are due to pure arterial disease. (See Table 41.1.)

To achieve healing of arterial ulcers, changes in life style such as increasing exercise, following a diet low in cholesterol, ceasing smoking, losing weight, and achieving better diabetic control should be encouraged. Oral systemic agents that have hematologic effects such as pentoxifylline[OL] or antiplatelet medications such as aspirin[OL] and clopidogrel[OL] can be used,

Table 41.1—The Characteristics of Venous and Arterial Ulcers

	Venous Disease	Arterial Disease
Signs and symptoms	Limb heaviness, aching and swelling that is associated with standing and is worse at end of day	Claudication (pain in leg with walking), poor peripheral pulses, sluggish capillary refill
Risk factors	Age, obesity, history of deep-vein thrombosis or phlebitis	Age > 40, cigarette smoking, diabetes mellitus, hyperlipidemia, hypertension, male gender, sedentary life style
Location of ulcers	Along the course of the long saphenous vein, between the lower medial calf to just below the medial malleolus	Over bony prominences

although their effectiveness has not been proven to decrease the risk of thrombotic events or accelerate the healing of existing ulcers. Occlusive dressings can be used to help the wound heal; the type of dressing used depends on the ulcer type and amount of drainage. Debridement of necrotic and fibrinous debris is key to the healing process and can be achieved by mechanical or chemical methods. Vascular bypass surgery or angioplasty may be necessary to provide revascularization. Other surgical measures such as pinch grafts, split thickness skin grafts, or allografts can be used to cover a wound. Tissue-engineered skin such as Apligraf (composed of an epidermal layer of keratinocytes derived from human neonatal foreskin and a dermal layer containing bovine type I collagen and with cultured human fibroblasts) has been shown to shorten healing time.

PRESSURE ULCERS

See "Pressure Ulcers" (p 259).

INTERTRIGO

Intertrigo (Figure 41.3) is more common in older persons because of the increased skin folds secondary to decreased dermal elasticity; environmental factors such as decreased mobility, moisture, friction, and poor hygiene also contribute. Diabetic and obese patients are more prone to develop intertrigo.

Commonly involved areas, such as the inframammary abdominal folds, groin, and axillae, will appear erythematous, macerated, moist, and mildly malodorous. Often there is secondary candidal or mixed bacterial colonization. Frequent airing, keeping involved areas dry, and using topical antifungal powders and creams, such as 2% miconazole powder or nystatin cream, constitute the treatment. Occasionally, a very mild topical corticosteroid such as 1% to 2% hydrocortisone is needed for a short period to reduce inflammation and irritation. (See also the section, p 315, on candidiasis.)

Figure 41.3—Intertrigo and candidiasis are commonly found in the web space between the 4th and 5th toes. Moist erythema, maceration, and superficial erosion is apparent.

BULLOUS PEMPHIGOID

Most cases of bullous pemphigoid (Figure 41.4) occur in patients in their 60s and 70s. This is a chronic autoimmune blistering disorder characterized by large tense blisters on normal or erythematous skin. The blisters heal without scar formation. They are usually filled with clear fluid but on occasion may be hemorrhagic and can be found anywhere on the body. Mucous membranes are involved in up to a third of patients and show erosions or blisters on the mucosa. In some cases there is intense pruritus, and instead of

Figure 41.4—Bullous pemphigoid. Tense, fluid-filled, and hemorrhagic bullae on an erythematous base were seen on the trunk and extremities. Some of the bullae have ruptured and left a scab with crusting.

blisters, one may find urticarial lesions. Systemic medications such as diuretics, analgesics, antibiotics, and angiotensin-converting enzyme inhibitors can lead to the development of bullous pemphigoid.

The antibodies directed against bullous pemphigoid are antigens in the hemidesmosomes (proteinaceous plaques that help the epidermis adhere to the basement membrane). The cause of antibody formation is still unclear. It is thought that the antibodies bind to the bullous pemphigoid antigen, which then activates the complement cascade. The activated complement components then attract leukocytes and cause degranulation of mast cells, and proteases from these cells cause separation of the epidermis from the basement membrane.

Diagnosis is clinical and confirmed by biopsy and immunofluorescence studies. On histopathology, one sees that the blister occurs below the epidermis. Direct immunofluorescence reveals immunoreactants in a linear pattern at the basement membrane between the epidermis and dermis. The complement component C3 is detected in almost all patients, and immunoglobulin G is found in most patients. One can also measure antibodies to the basement membrane antigens in sera through indirect immunofluorescence; however, the antibody titer does not correlate with disease activity.

Though it may last for months to years, bullous pemphigoid is often a self-limited disease. Treatment depends on severity. When the lesions are localized, they may be treated with topical corticosteroids. More extensive disease can be treated with oral corticosteroids, especially for control of acute flares. Because of the adverse effects of corticosteroids, particularly in older persons, other immunosuppressive, steroid-sparing agents, such as azathioprine or cyclophosphamide, are usually added as steroids are tapered. Combination therapy with tetracylines and niacinamide has been shown to be effective.

PRURITUS

Pruritus, a very common skin complaint, is associated with many cutaneous and systemic conditions. In older persons pruritus at times can be very severe, compromising quality of life. Although xerosis is the most common cause of pruritus in the older patient, it is important to perform a complete history and examination to exclude skin conditions such as scabies, allergic, irritant or atopic dermatitis, or bullous pemphigoid. Systemic diseases such as renal disease, cholestasis or chronic liver disease, thyroid disease, anemia, occult malignancies, or drug side effects must also be considered. Generalized pruritus can also be associated with generalized anxiety disorder, depression, and even psychosis, including delusions of parasitosis.

Treatment depends on the underlying cause; symptomatic relief can often be achieved with topical corticosteroids, emollients, or menthol in calamine preparations. Oral antihistamines should be used with caution in older persons. For severe, refractory cases, UVB phototherapy has been used.

PSORIASIS

Psoriasis (Figure 41.5) affects 2% of the population and has bimodal incidences: one in the mid-20s and the other at about 50 to 60 years of age. There is a genetic predisposition, with multigene mode of inheritance, and environmental factors also play a role in triggering the disease.

The skin findings in psoriasis are rather characteristic: well-demarcated erythematous papules and plaques with overlying silvery scale. Extensor surfaces, areas prone to trauma, scalp, and nails are commonly involved. Various forms of psoriasis exist:

- inverse pattern, where lesions occur in skin folds, such as the neck, axillae, and genital area;

- guttate, where small 1-cm papules appear over the upper trunk and proximal extremities, usually after an infection;

- pustular, which is acute with generalized eruption of 2- to 3-mm sterile pustules and fever;

- palmoplantar; and

- erythrodermic psoriasis, in which the patient has generalized erythema.

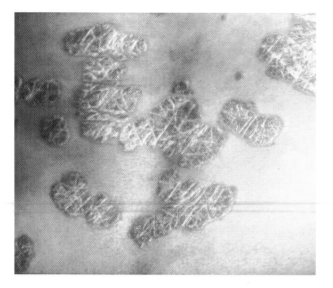

Figure 41.5—Psoriasis. Characteristic well-demarcated beefy red plaques with overlying silvery-white scales are evident on the back of this patient.

Various factors may trigger psoriasis. Physical trauma (known as Koebner's phenomenon), infections, stress, medications (oral corticosteroids, lithium, β-blockers, angiotensin-converting enzyme inhibitors, as well as nonsteroidal anti-inflammatory drugs) have been shown to initiate or exacerbate psoriasis. Five percent to 30% of patients with psoriasis also suffer from psoriatic arthritis, which is characterized by pain, swelling, and stiffness in the small joints. Some patients may also suffer from spondylitis or sacroiliitis.

Several treatment options are available for patients with psoriasis, but each method must be evaluated in terms of risks and benefits for the older patient. Topical treatments such as corticosteroids, vitamin D derivatives (calcipotriene), topical retinoids (tazarotene), salicylic acid, or tar compounds may be sufficient to treat and control mild plaque psoriasis. Some of these treatments may be irritating or messy to apply. Long-term use of topical corticosteroids is limited by the cutaneous atrophy and decreased potency (tachyphylaxis) that occur over time. Patients who do not improve with topical treatments may be candidates for systemic treatment, such as phototherapy or immunosuppressive agents. UV therapy, including PUVA (psoralen with UVA light) and UVB therapies, can be adjunctive treatment along with topical agents; several treatments per week may be required. Patients with longstanding psoriasis who receive phototherapy must be carefully examined for skin cancer. Agents such as cyclosporine and methotrexate are quite effective in treating psoriasis. However, each of these medications has significant side effects that require careful monitoring through laboratory tests and physical examinations. In addition to drug interactions, systemic illnesses such as poor kidney function, hypertension, and lung disease may limit the use of these medications. As the pathophysiology of psoriasis is elucidated, newer and more effective therapies that target specific cytokines and T-lymphocyte surface molecules and that inhibit signaling are showing promise.

ONYCHOMYCOSIS

See "Diseases and Disorders of the Foot" (p 454).

HERPES ZOSTER

More than two thirds of reported cases of herpes zoster (Figure 41.6) occur in persons aged 50 years and older. The incidence of herpes zoster is 20 to 100 times higher in immunosuppressed patients than in other groups, and the severity and likelihood of recurrence is also higher. Patients with herpes zoster are contagious to those who lack immunity, but less so than patients with varicella. Patients with uncomplicated dermatomal zoster spread infection by means of direct contact with their lesions, whereas patients with disseminated zoster may also transmit infection in aerosol and thus need respiratory isolation.

The pathogenesis of zoster is due to the passage of the varicella zoster virus (VZV) from skin and mucosal surfaces into sensory nerves and then into sensory ganglia, where latent infection is established. Although reactivation is associated with several immunosuppressive conditions, such as HIV infection, malignancy, or the use of immunosuppressive drugs or corticosteroids, the most important is the senescence of the cellular immune response to VZV with increasing age. (See Table 44.1, p 333.) These settings lead to reactivation of the virus, with the neuronal necrosis and inflamma-

Figure 41.6—Herpes zoster. This patient had clusters of vesicles and pustules on an erythematous base involving a thoracic dermatome.

tion that account for the severe neuralgia. The infection spreads down the sensory nerve and is released around the sensory nerve endings in the skin, producing the characteristic lesions: a cluster of vesicles on an erythematous base in a dermatomal pattern that is unilateral and does not cross the midline. Patients often complain of symptoms of pain, burning, paresthesias, tenderness, pruritus, or hyperesthesia several days before the rash appears. The vesicles turn into pustules and eventually crust over in 7 to 10 days.

Ten percent to 15% of cases of herpes zoster involve the ophthalmic branch of the trigeminal nerve. Involvement of the nasociliary branch, which presents as vesicles on the tip of the nose (known as Hutchinson's sign), requires careful ophthalmic examination to monitor for complications, such as neurotrophic keratitis and ulceration, scleritis, or uveitis. Involvement of the facial or auditory nerves that presents as herpes zoster of the external ear or tympanic membrane leads to facial palsy with or without tinnitus, vertigo, and deafness. This is known as Ramsay Hunt syndrome. Another complication is secondary bacterial infection. Pain is a chief complaint of patients with zoster; it can precede, be concomitant with, or persist after the rash. Pain that persists or appears after the rash has healed or at 30 days after onset of rash is called *post-herpetic neuralgia*. Age is the most significant risk factor, and post-herpetic neuralgia occurs in 70% of zoster patients aged 70 and older. It is often difficult to treat.

Although the symptoms of herpes zoster can be confused with a variety of conditions causing localized pain (eg, pleurisy, myocardial infarction, renal colic, cholecystitis, and glaucoma), the lesions and their distribution make the diagnosis rather easy. However, it is very difficult, if not impossible in some situations, to differentiate herpes simplex from zoster. In both infections, a Tzanck smear from the base of vesicle (stained with either hematoxylin-eosin, Giemsa, or Papanicolaou) shows multinucleated giant cells and epithelial cells containing intranuclear inclusion bodies. A smear from the base of the vesicle can be sent for direct fluorescent antibody staining. This test can differentiate between herpes simplex virus and the VZV. Definitive diagnosis is made by viral culture; however, isolation of the virus can be difficult.

If the patient's immunity is intact, herpes zoster is usually self-limited. Treatment in all patients should be initiated early, within 72 hours of the onset of rash. Acyclovir is effective, and in patients aged 50 years and older it is dosed at 800 mg five times a day for 7 to 10 days. Valacyclovir or famciclovir are prodrugs of acyclovir that provide greater oral bioavailability and allow less frequent dosing. Early treatment halts progression of disease, increases the rate of clearance of virus from vesicles, decreases the incidence of visceral and cutaneous dissemination, decreases the ocular complications when the eye is involved, and in some cases it may decrease pain and the incidence of post-herpetic neuralgia. Wet compresses and topical antibiotics such as bacitracin or mupirocin can treat secondary bacterial infection.

There is no definitive treatment for post-herpetic neuralgia. Narcotics, nonsteroidal anti-inflammatory drugs, epidural injection of local anesthetics, glucocorticoids, low-dose tricyclic antidepressants, capsaicin, and acupuncture are some of the therapies that are mentioned in literature. Debate over the efficacy of corticosteroids given with antiviral therapy has been fueled by two large randomized controlled trials that reached opposite conclusions. However, risks do not appear to be significantly increased with the use of corticosteroids for zoster, especially when used with antiviral therapy, and the steroids may decrease the acute neuropathic pain and reduce pain medication requirements. Capsaicin, an extract of hot chili peppers that depletes substance P, is the only compound labeled for use in post-herpetic neuralgia. Unfortunately, many patients cannot tolerate the burning associated with this topical medication.

CANDIDIASIS

Factors that contribute to intertrigo also predispose a person to candidiasis. (See the section, p 312, on intertrigo.) Involved areas appear clinically similar to intertrigo, but there may be peripheral satellite pustules. Candida pustules can also occur on the backs of bedridden patients and on other areas prone to moisture and occlusion. Oral thrush may also develop in patients on corticosteroid inhalers, antibiotics, or immunosuppressive medications or with concomitant systemic illnesses, such as diabetes mellitus. To confirm the diagnosis, a KOH preparation of scrapings of the involved site is performed. The presence of spores and pseudohyphae is consistent with candidiasis.

Treatment resembles that of intertrigo: keeping the moist areas dry, improving hygiene, and treating with topical or oral treatment with anticandidal agents such as nystatin or ketoconazole.

SCABIES

Scabies refers to infestation with the human mite *Sarcoptes scabiei*. It is spread by person-to-person contact and is common in institutionalized older persons. Epidemics are described in long-term-care facilities, and eradication can be difficult. The adult female mite becomes fertilized on skin and burrows into the top superficial layer, where she lays eggs. The clinical manifestations occur days to weeks later when the patient develops hypersensitivity reaction to the mite saliva and excretions. Therefore, it is often difficult to pinpoint the initial infested patient, and spreading of mites may have occurred before diagnosis.

Infested patients complain of severe pruritus, especially of the hands, axillae, genitalia, and peri-umbilical region. Clinically one finds erythematous papules and occasionally nodules along with linear burrows (crooked, raised lines). The patient may have scratched to the point of causing bleeding or weeping eczematous lesions. Scabies should be suspected in anyone who complains of pruritus or displays signs of excoriation. Diagnosis is confirmed by performing a scraping on a suspected lesion and finding mite excreta, eggs, or, rarely, the mite itself, under the microscope.

Treatment of scabies is often initiated when there is strong clinical suspicion of infestation. Treatment involves eradicating the mite, decreasing the pruritus, and treating any contacts. Topical permethrin 5% is most commonly used. It is applied from the neck to the toes and rinsed off after 8 to 12 hours. This treatment should be repeated in 1 week to prevent development of resistance. Persons who may have been exposed should also be treated. Topical corticosteroids may help to reduce pruritus, but it is important to reassure patients that the itching may persist for weeks or months. Cleaning the bedding, clothes, and towels (bath, linen) with hot water is sufficient to eradicate the mite from the surroundings.

There have been reports in the literature of treating scabies effectively with an oral dose of an antihelminthic agent called ivermectin (250 to 400 µg per kg) that is repeated in a week. However, there are no long-term studies, and it is not yet approved for this use by the U.S. Food and Drug Administration.

LOUSE INFESTATIONS

Lice can infest the body (pediculosis corporis), scalp (pediculosis capitis), or pubic hair (pediculosis pubis). With pediculosis corporis or capitis, lice are spread from person to person through physical contact or fomites. Pediculosis pubis is usually spread by sexual contact. In all cases, patients complain of pruritus of the involved areas, and there can be secondary infection. In cases of pediculosis corporis, the lice feed on the body but live on clothing, where they lay eggs, often near the seams. In cases of pediculosis capitis, the lice lay eggs on the proximal part of the hair shaft. The eggs (or nits) are visible as white specks cemented to the hair at an oblique angle. Patients with pediculosis pubis also have nits on the pubic hair and commonly have more organisms.

Treatment involves eradicating the lice and larvae, treating close contacts, and treating the secondary infection. Pyrethrin or its derivatives (permethrin) are ovicidal and can be used as single 10-minute topical

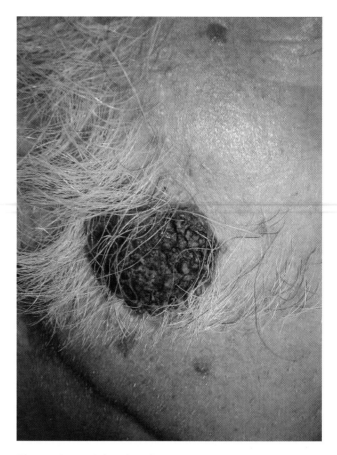

Figure 41.7—Seborrheic keratoses. These lesions present as waxy, warty stuck-on papules in a variety of colors.

treatment for patients and those who have been exposed. Combs, brushes, hats, clothing, bedding, and towels (bath, linen) must be washed with hot water.

BENIGN GROWTHS

Seborrheic Keratoses

Seborrheic keratoses (Figure 41.7) are very common benign growths that present as tan to gray or black waxy or warty papules and plaques. They commonly occur on the trunk and extremities but can be found anywhere on the body. Occasionally some lesions may be darkly pigmented, and differentiation from a melanoma may be difficult without a biopsy. These growths are irksome to patients and can be removed with cryosurgery or shave excision if necessary.

Cherry Angiomas

Cherry angiomas are the most common acquired cutaneous vascular proliferations. They usually appear in persons in their 20s and increase in number over time. Clinically they appear as round to oval, bright red, dome-shaped papules ranging in size from less than 1 mm to several millimeters. Cherry angiomas are benign but can bleed when traumatized. Removal of these lesions can be achieved with excision, electrodessication, or laser ablation.

Actinic Keratoses

Actinic keratoses (also known as *solar keratoses*) are lesions caused by chronic UV radiation (Figure 41.8) that occur in fair-skinned persons. They are considered premalignant growths, precursors of squamous cell carcinoma. It is unclear how many progress to squamous cell carcinoma; reports vary from 0.24% to 20%. They appear as poorly circumscribed, occasionally scaly, erythematous macules and papules on sun-exposed areas, such as the face, ears, and dorsum of hands and arms. Some may have an overlying thick, hard growth known as a *cutaneous horn*. Lesions on the lips are called *actinic cheilitis*.

Actinic keratoses are most often treated to prevent progression to squamous cell carcinoma but also to decrease discomfort. They respond to a variety of treatments, such as cryotherapy with liquid nitrogen, topical agents such as chemical acids, 5-fluorouracil, immunomodulators such as imiquimod[OL], or excision. Although treating the lesions with liquid nitrogen for 10 to 15 seconds is very effective, it can be somewhat uncomfortable and can cause pigmentary changes. When there are several lesions in an area, treatment that the patient can perform at home, such as topical 5-fluorouracil or imiquimod, is helpful because it can also treat subclinical lesions. However, patients must be monitored and warned about the bright erythema and discomfort that can occur with these treatments.

SQUAMOUS CELL CARCINOMA

Squamous cell carcinoma is the second most common form of skin cancer. It affects patients in mid- to late life and occurs most commonly on chronically sun-exposed areas. Squamous cell carcinomas cause local tissue destruction if not treated and have a low risk (but greater risk than basal cell carcinomas) to metastasize. The risk of metastases and recurrence increases with the size of the tumor (greater than 2 cm), poor differentiation, and increased depth of invasion. Squamous cell carcinoma also tends to behave more aggressively when it occurs on sites such as the lip and ear. These tumors present as chronic erythematous papules, plaques, or nodules with scaling, crusting, or ulceration. They also have a propensity to occur in longstanding nonhealing wounds and in burn and radiation scars.

Treatment consists of surgical excision. In cosmetically important areas or with aggressive tumors, Mohs micrographic surgery is performed. In patients who are poor surgical candidates or who have multiple comorbidities, destruction with cryotherapy or local radiation has been used.

BASAL CELL CARCINOMA

Basal cell carcinoma is the most common cancer in the United States. As with other cutaneous malignancies, fair-skinned persons with chronic sun exposure are at risk. It presents in three major clinical patterns:

■ nodular—this is the most common variant and appears as a waxy, translucent papule with overlying telangiectasias;

■ morpheaform—this has a scar-like appearance and can look atrophic;

■ superficial—this appears as an erythematous macule or papule with fine scale or superficial erosion.

Some basal cell carcinomas appear as superficial ulcers with characteristic rolled borders (Figure 41.9).

Figure 41.8—Actinic keratoses are rough, scaly, red-brown macules on sun-exposed skin and are premalignant.

[OL] Not approved by the U.S. Food and Drug Administration for this use.

Others may be pigmented and confused for melanoma, especially in darker skinned individuals.

Treatment of basal cell carcinoma is surgical excision. Some basal cell carcinomas, particularly those located in cosmetically important areas, those that are nodular or morpheaform, and those that are recurrent should be excised by use of Mohs micrographic surgery to ensure adequate excision and tissue sparing. Like squamous cell carcinomas, basal cell carcinomas occurring in poor surgical candidates can also be treated with ablative methods, such as cryosurgery, radiation, and curettage with electrodessication.

MELANOMA

The incidence of melanoma continues to increase, and it affects all adult age groups. The risk factors for melanoma include very fair skin type, family history, dysplastic or numerous nevi, and sunlight exposure, particularly intermittent blistering sunburns in childhood. Melanomas are usually asymptomatic; thus, regular skin examinations and early recognition are key for favorable prognosis.

A new pigmented skin lesion or a change in the color, size, surface, or borders of a preexisting mole should be suspected for melanoma and biopsied. A useful mnemonic is ABCD: **A**symmetry, **B**orders, **C**olor, **D**iameter. There are four clinical types:

- lentigo maligna—the type seen most commonly on atrophic, sun-damaged skin of an elderly patient; this appears as an irregularly shaped tan or brown macule that has been enlarging slowly;

- superficial spreading—this type can occur anywhere and presents often as an irregularly shaped macule, papule, or plaque with great variation in color (Figure 41.10);

- nodular—a papule or nodule, often black or gray, that has been growing rapidly;

- acral lentiginous—this type is found on the palms, soles, or nail beds (Figure 41.11); it is found in all skin types and presents as a dark brown or black patch; its incidence is highest in persons aged 65 or older.

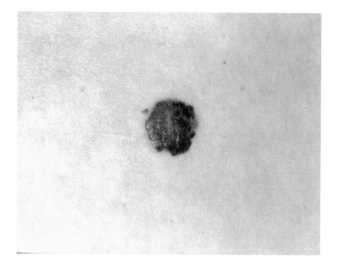

Figure 41.10—Melanoma. This lesion has irregular variegation in pigment (shades of brown and blue-black) as well as irregular borders, suggesting melanoma.

Figure 41.9—Basal cell carcinoma, ulcerated. This is also a pearly, fleshy papule but is ulcerated in the center and has a characteristic rolled border.

Figure 41.11—Acral lentiginous melanoma. This type of melanoma presents as a dark macular growth with irregular borders on volar surfaces of palms and soles (as in this case), and nails.

The treatment of melanoma consists of surgical excision and, depending on depth, may also involve sentinel node mapping and biopsy, lymph node dissection, or adjuvant therapy.

ANNOTATED REFERENCES

■ Chosidow O. Scabies and pediculosis. *Lancet.* 2000; 355(9206):819–826.

This review article describes the epidemiology, causes, clinical manifestations, and treatment of scabies and pediculosis. The author describes the various presentations of scabies in older persons and patients who are immunosuppressed. The topical agents used for treatment are discussed, and management options for pruritus after scabicide therapy are described. The use of ivermectin as an antiscabetic treatment is also discussed.

■ Lebwohl M, Christophers E, Langley R, et al. Alefacept Clinical Study Group. An international, randomized, double-blind, placebo-controlled phase 3 trial of intramuscular alefacept in patients with chronic plaque psoriasis. *Arch Dermatol.* 2003; 139(6):719–727.

This study demonstrated that intramuscular administration of alefacept, a human lymphocyte function–associated antigen 3/immunoglobulin 1 fusion protein, is a well-tolerated and effective therapy for chronic plaque psoriasis.

■ Martin ES, Elewski BE. Cutaneous fungal infections in the elderly. *Clin Geriatr Med.* 2002;18(1):59–75.

This is a comprehensive review of the variety of cutaneous fungal infections that are commonly seen in older persons.

The review includes the evaluation and differential diagnosis of cutaneous fungal infections and an evidence-based guide to therapy in this age group.

■ Schmader K. Herpes zoster in the elderly: issues related to geriatrics. *Clin Infect Dis.* 1999;28(4):736–739.

This article reviews the epidemiology and the clinical and treatment issues regarding herpes zoster in older patients. Covered topics include risk and treatment of post-herpetic neuralgia, age-related decline in immunity to varicella zoster virus, the psychosocial impact of zoster on quality of life, and varicella zoster virus transmission and control in the nursing home.

■ Valencia IC, Falabella A, Kirsner RS, et al. Chronic venous insufficiency and venous leg ulceration. *J Am Acad Dermatol.* 2001;44(3):401–421.

This review discusses current aspects of the epidemiology, pathophysiology, clinical presentation, diagnostic assessment, and current therapeutic options for chronic venous insufficiency and venous ulceration.

■ Yosipovitch G, Tang MB. Practical management of psoriasis in the elderly: epidemiology, clinical aspects, quality of life, patient education and treatment options. *Drugs Aging.* 2002;19(11):847–863.

This article provides an overall review of the different options available to treat psoriasis by focusing on the elderly age group, who often have other medical, social, and economic comorbidities.

Sumaira Z. Aasi, MD

CHAPTER 42—ORAL DISEASES AND DISORDERS

KEY POINTS

■ Since teeth become less sensitive with age, it is not uncommon to observe profound yet asymptomatic untreated dental disease in older persons, which justifies a need for regular dental evaluation every 6 to 12 months.

■ Periodontitis caused by plaque formation within the gingival sulcus may lead to loss of alveolar bone height, decreased support around the tooth, malposition, loosening, and eventual loss of the tooth.

■ Dentures usually aid in speech and restore diminished facial contours, but improved ability to masticate is unpredictable and enhanced oral intake is a less likely outcome.

■ Oral cancer screening is critical to early detection and treatment of asymptomatic early-stage oral cancer, translating into improved outcomes and better survival rates.

The oral cavity is responsible for initiating food intake, producing speech, and protecting the alimentary tract and upper airway. Dysfunction and disease in the mouth can profoundly affect overall health and social functioning and may be particularly important for elderly patients who are frail or nutritionally at risk. Findings prevalent in older patients (eg, decay, missing teeth, periodontal disease, and salivary hypofunction) do not represent normal aging, and patients with such findings should be urged to seek preventive and therapeutic care.

THE AGING OF THE TEETH

Most age-related changes in teeth are subtle (see Table 42.1) but become significant in the presence of envi-

Table 42.1—The Clinical Significance of Selected Age-Related Changes in Oral Tissues

Tissue Affected	Nature of Change	Clinical Significance
Tooth dentin	Increased thickness	Diminished pulp space
	Diminished permeability resulting from sclerosis of dentinal tubules	Diminished sensitivity of dentin; diminished susceptibility to effects of bacterial metabolites; increased tooth brittleness
Dental pulp	Diminished volume	Diminished reparative capacity; diminished sensitivity and alteration in nature of sensitivity
	Shift in proportion of nervous, vascular, and connective tissues	Diminished reparative capacity; diminished sensitivity and alteration in nature of sensitivity
Salivary glands	Fatty replacement of acini	Possibly less physiologic reserve

ronmental factors or disease. For a combination of reasons, the teeth of an older person are typically less sensitive or wholly insensitive to temperature changes and, importantly, to the sensations that commonly herald dental disease in younger adults. It is not uncommon to observe profound yet asymptomatic untreated dental disease in an older person's mouth.

DENTAL DECAY

Dental *caries*, or decay, is a bacterially derived demineralization and cavitation that can attack teeth throughout the life span. *Recurrent caries* refers to decay at the interface between a dental restoration (such as a filling or crown) and the tooth. (See Figure 42.1 for the anatomy of the tooth.) Older persons have more restored teeth (and usually the restorations are older and more extensive) and thus are more likely to have recurrent caries. The teeth of older persons may feature more caries of the root surfaces than are typically observed in younger persons because prior periodontal disease exposes the root surface, thereby predisposing it to demineralization and increased risk for caries. Both recurrent and root caries are generally asymptomatic and may become advanced before discovery, often resulting in destruction of much or all of the tooth.

Advanced caries commonly results in necrosis of the remaining pulp, which usually leads to acute or chronic dental abscess. Even if such infections do not cause pain, they should not be ignored, since severe metastatic infections of dental and oral origin have been reported in virtually every organ system. In particular, α-hemolytic (viridans) streptococci of the oral cavity have long been implicated in close to one third of the cases of bacterial endocarditis reported annually in the United States, and bacteria associated with dental abscesses (eg, *Staphylococcus aureus*) have been cultured from the aspirates of infected hip arthroplasties.

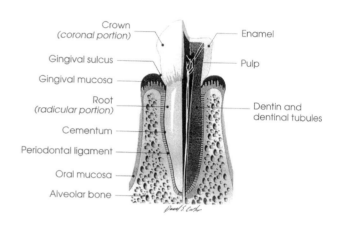

Figure 42.1—Dental and periodontal anatomy.

The risk factors for dental caries are the same at any age, but many of the risk factors increase in prevalence as people age. A primary risk factor is poor oral hygiene, which often occurs in an older person when visual acuity, manual dexterity, or upper extremity flexibility is impaired, or when salivary flow is diminished. Another risk factor is frequent ingestion of sticky foods with a high content of sucrose, such as cake, candy, and cookies. Other risk factors include infrequent dental visits because of financial, access, or educational barriers; the presence of permanent or removable artificial teeth (more common with increasing age); and limited lifetime exposure to fluoride, widely used in the United States only in the past four decades. White elderly Americans display a higher incidence of root caries than either black elderly Americans or Hispanic elderly Americans, but they are more likely to have received dental treatment for the lesions. Recurrent caries are also more common in white elderly Americans because of the greater likelihood that they have received prior dental treatment.

The prevention of caries involves daily oral hygiene with fluoride toothpaste, limitation of sugar intake, and regular dental examinations. The treatment of dental caries includes topical high-potency fluoride for remineralization, removal of demineralized tooth structure ("drilling"), and replacement of removed tooth structure with fillings or crowns. When caries involves the dental pulp, root canal treatment becomes necessary. This in turn usually requires reinforcement of the remaining tooth structure with a crown ("cap").

DISEASES OF THE PERIODONTIUM

The investing tissues of the teeth, termed the *periodontium*, consist of the gingiva, the alveolar bone, and a collagenous sleeve (termed the *periodontal ligament*) located between the tooth root and the surrounding bone. Periodontal disease occurs when microorganic colonies (*plaque*) form on the teeth near the gingiva and between the gingiva and the root surface within the gingival sulcus. The most common form of periodontal disease is gingivitis, in which the inflammatory reaction to plaque is limited to the gingiva. Gingivitis develops more rapidly in healthy older adults than in younger ones, but in both groups the changes—including gingival edema and light bleeding on brushing—are rapidly reversible following removal of plaque. If the inflammatory process extends to the periodontal ligament and alveolar bone, the process is termed *periodontitis*. In periodontitis there is destruction of the hard and soft tissues of the periodontium. In most adults periodontitis is a process marked by long periods of disease quiescence punctuated by bursts of localized destructive inflammation. The prevalence of active periodontitis is 20% to 40% of dentate adults. By their 50s, more than 90% of Americans with teeth show 2 mm or more of lost alveolar bone height, the primary marker of prior periodontal disease activity. In advanced cases of periodontitis, the decreased support around a tooth leads to its malposition, loosening, and eventual loss.

Epidemiologic data support the concept that those who reach advanced age without significant periodontal bone loss will not likely experience a worsening of the disease in senescence. In contrast, other adults who have experienced a more rapid rate of bone loss commonly will have lost teeth in their 40s and 50s. In addition to age, risk factors for periodontitis include smoking and poor oral hygiene. Black and Hispanic Americans have a significantly higher prevalence of advanced periodontitis than do white Americans. Preventing gingivitis and periodontitis is largely a matter of oral hygiene and regular dental examinations and cleanings. Managing periodontal disease involves debriding the roots below the gingiva, which may require surgical access. Topical antibiotics (chlorhexidine, tetracycline) and systemic antibiotics (minocycline, metronidazole) are increasingly used as adjuncts to other periodontal therapy.

Periodontitis has been long reported to be worse in patients with poorly controlled diabetes mellitus. Investigations also support the contention that periodontitis, as an active infection, impairs diabetic control. Periodontal disease may be rapidly destructive in a patient whose immune system is impaired by disease or immunosuppression therapy. Epidemiologic data also correlate osteoporosis and tooth loss due to periodontitis. Periodontal disease and the pathogens responsible for it have been linked epidemiologically and immunologically with peripheral vascular disease, cerebrovascular disease, and pneumonia. Similar correlations have been reported for coronary heart disease, although one report disputes this. There is also epidemiologic association between gram-negative pneumonia, gram-negative periodontal pathogens, salivary hypofunction, and impaired swallowing function.

The prevention and control of periodontal disease revolve around daily oral care: tooth brushing and flossing to remove bacterial plaque on the teeth, particularly within the gingival sulcus. Regular dental evaluation, every 6 to 12 months, is important to ensure that the periodontium is healthy or to provide early intervention if it is not.

TOOTHLESSNESS

Advanced age was once considered synonymous with the need for false teeth, but that stereotype is fading. In the early 1960s more than 70% of adult Americans aged 75 or over were edentulous. By the 1990s fewer than 40% of this group were edentulous, most likely because of a rising tendency for exposure to some level of preventive and restorative dental care in childhood or early adulthood.

Nevertheless, removal of one or more teeth in an older adult may be necessitated by various combinations of physiologic and behavioral factors. The leading cause is inability or unwillingness to access and pay for restorative dental treatment in the face of a symptomatic dental disease, usually stemming from dental caries. A second common cause is loosening of teeth as a consequence of periodontal disease, to the point that mastication becomes painful or ineffective, or both. The third common cause is removal of otherwise healthy teeth that, because of the absence or loss of other teeth for the preceding or other reasons, would hinder the fabrication or function of a dental prosthesis.

Nearly 50% of Americans aged 85 and over have no natural teeth, and there are unique problems associated with the edentulous state. Functionally, the teeth aid in mastication and enunciation. Aesthetically, the teeth support the lips and cheeks and keep the nose and chin at a fixed distance apart. When a person has lost all teeth and there are no prosthetic replacements, the facial appearance is dramatically changed because of the lack of tissue support and diminished vertical height in the lower half of the face. Chewing ability is severely compromised, yet the impact on nutritional intake is difficult to characterize. One longitudinal study employing diet diaries demonstrated a correlation between loss of teeth and increased carbohydrate intake, decreased protein intake, and diminished intake of selected micronutrients.

As a modality of compensation for loss of all of the teeth, removable dentures can aid in speech and restore diminished facial contours, but they are less predictably successful in restoring the ability to masticate. Edentulous persons with dentures are generally capable of eating a wider range of foods than edentulous persons without dentures. Yet dentures restore, on average, only about 15% of the chewing ability of the natural dentition. The range of foods regularly eaten by denture wearers is significantly restricted in comparison with the dietary range of persons with natural teeth. Denture wearers also have to chew more times before they swallow food, and they swallow their food in larger particles. Older patients and their physicians who hope that dentures will restore oral intake in cases of malnutrition or unexplained weight loss are usually disappointed, whereas those who hope for a more socially acceptable appearance, clearer speech, and modest improvement in chewing comfort and range of dietary choices are more likely to be satisfied.

Dentures often are a considerable source of discomfort, dysfunction, and embarrassment for older people. This is because the alveolar processes that originally held the natural teeth continually remodel and diminish in volume once the natural teeth are gone. For most patients, dentures require frequent professional adjustment and periodic replacement. Alveolar ridge resorption is most severe in the oldest patients who have had the longest time without natural teeth; this effect is more pronounced in those with osteoporosis.

For health of the oral mucosa, dentures should be kept clean by removing them and cleaning them after meals, and soaking them in a commercial disinfectant several times each week. Dentures should remain out of the mouth for several hours each day; most people choose to leave their dentures out during sleep. Fractured or broken dentures, as well as denture looseness or soreness, should be brought to a dentist's attention without delay. However, since neither dental services nor dentures are currently covered by Medicare and fewer than 10% of older Americans have private dental insurance, many elderly people continue to use inadequate or even damaging dentures.

SALIVARY FUNCTION IN AGING

Saliva is critical for protecting the tissues of the oral cavity and maintaining their function in speech, mastication, swallowing, and taste perception. Saliva buffers the intraoral pH, contains a wide spectrum of antimicrobial factors, remineralizes and lubricates the oral surfaces, and keeps the taste pores patent. In the absence of disease, the major salivary glands undergo regressive histologic changes with age. Yet data from the Baltimore Longitudinal Study on Aging and the Veterans Affairs Dental Longitudinal Study have demonstrated that with healthy aging, flow from the parotid glands under both resting and stimulated conditions remains essentially unchanged. Both groups of investigators have reported that flow from the submandibular glands undergoes no change with age; other centers have reported a measurable but clinically minor decrease. It has been suggested that the major salivary glands show "organ reserve" in which the capacity of youthful glands exceeds ordinary demands, but that with age-related changes, functional reserves dwindle. By extreme old age, healthy glands function adequately under normal conditions but are more susceptible to factors that impede function, such as dehydration or drug-induced hypofunction.

Complaints of dry mouth are very common among older people. The leading causes are the commonly prescribed drugs that have this adverse effect. Commonly implicated are drugs with anticholinergic effects, including tricyclic antidepressants, opioids, antihistamines, and anti-arrhythmic agents. Separate studies have found that 72% of institutionalized elderly patients received at least one (and some as many as five) potentially xerostomic medications daily and that 55% of more than 4000 rural community-dwelling elderly persons took at least one potentially xerostomic medication daily. Dry mouth may also be due to local disease, such as salivary gland tumors and blocked ducts, or to systemic disease. Sjögren's syndrome affects approximately 3 million Americans—predominantly women—aged 50 or over. Depression has been reported to diminish saliva flow, as have poorly controlled diabetes mellitus and hypothyroidism.

Dry mouth is also an adverse effect of therapeutic irradiation of the head and neck. In the total dose range administered for oral and oropharyngeal squamous cell carcinoma, salivary flow is commonly obliterated as a consequence of short-term direct effects on the glands and long-term fibrosis of their vascular supply. As a result, patients who have undergone radiation of the head may experience rapidly destructive dental caries and painful oral mucositis, which may affect nutritional status.

Treatment of the older person with dry mouth requires attention to both diagnosis and prevention.

Diminished oral secretions increase the risk for serious oral disease. A history of irradiation of the head and neck as well as systemic causes should be excluded. Medications that reduce salivary flow should be decreased, discontinued, or substituted for, if possible. Patients who have had irradiation should be considered for a 3-month course of oral pilocarpine (5 to 10 mg three times a day), which may restore some salivary function. Saliva substitutes and oral lubricants, available without prescription and used as needed, can provide transient relief but have none of the protective properties of saliva. Patients should be counseled on the greatly elevated risk for oral disease and educated on the need to limit sugar in their diet and optimize their daily oral hygiene practices.

ORAL MUCOSAL PROBLEMS

Squamous cell carcinoma accounts for 96% of oral and oropharyngeal malignancies. Of the 28,000 new cases of oral cancer reported in the United States annually, more than 95% occur in people aged 40 or over; age is the primary risk factor identified in epidemiologic analyses. The 5-year survival rate for white Americans is approximately 55% and for black Americans, 34%. Carcinoma of the lip, tongue, and floor of mouth represents more than 65% of all oropharyngeal cases. Lip cancer affects men eight times more frequently than women; most other sites affect men at a ratio slightly below 2:1. Oral cancer is strongly linked with the use of tobacco, particularly cigarettes. Lip cancer has a strong correlation with pipe and cigar smoking. Ethanol is a potent cofactor that enhances the effects of tobacco. Other potential risk factors—dentures, poor oral care, oral viral disease, oral lichen planus, candidosis—have been suggested, but none has shown the unambiguous associations of age, smoking, and alcohol use.

Oral malignancy appears clinically as painless red, white, or mixed red and white areas of the oral mucosa that may be ulcerated or indurated. Red and mixed lesions (termed *erythroplakia*) (Figure 42.2) display cellular atypia in as many as 93% of cases and should be biopsied immediately. White lesions (*leukoplakia*) (Figure 42.3) are malignant or premalignant less than 10% of the time and merit close monitoring; biopsy is indicated if a lesion does not disappear in 14 days or is increasing in size. Clinicians also have less invasive diagnostic tools available for determining whether a white or red lesion in the mouth merits biopsy, such as scraping (exfoliative cytology) and in situ staining. Early identification markedly improves outcome: 5-year survival without nodal involvement in white Americans is 80% and in black Americans is 69%, but survival rates decline with nodal involvement (41% and 30%, respec-

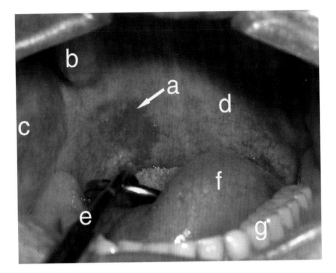

Figure 42.2—Erythroplakia in a 72-year-old man with a history of cigar smoking and alcohol abuse. Lesion confirmed by biopsy to be invasive squamous cell carcinoma, poorly differentiated.

Key: a = erythroplakia; b = right posterior maxillary alveolar ridge; c = inner aspect of right cheek; d = soft palate; e = tongue retractor; f = tongue dorsum; g = mandibular denture.

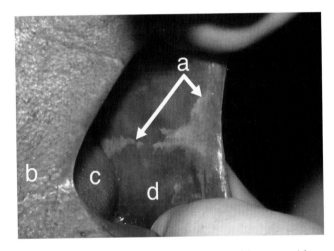

Figure 42.3—Leukoplakia in a 66-year-old man with a history of smoking. Lesion confirmed by biopsy to be carcinoma in situ.

Key: a = leukoplakia; b = right lip commissure; c = tongue; d = inner aspect of left cheek.

tively) and with distant metastases (18% and 12%). A thorough oral cancer screening, which can be completed in less than 2 minutes, consists of a head and neck nodal assessment followed by inspection of the oral cavity using gauze to retract the tongue and tongue blades to enhance visualization of the cheeks, lips, and vestibules. Although oral cancer screening is easy to learn, straightforward to perform, requires minimal instrumentation, and causes no discomfort to the patient, few elderly smokers receive oral evaluations as part of the routine physical examination.

The treatment of localized oral squamous cell carcinoma is generally surgical, although large but localized tumors can be managed with radioactive implants. More extensive disease necessitates surgery followed by beam irradiation. Concern over the deleterious adverse effects of irradiation (described in the preceding section) has led to the development of techniques that seek to limit destruction of healthy tissues surrounding a tumor. Radiation alone has been used to shrink inoperable tumors. Newer protocols combine surgery and chemotherapy with the goal of a cure.

Candidiasis presents as diffuse erythema, cracking at the corners of the mouth, curd-like white patches, or erythema in denture areas; it can result in taste dysfunction, burning, itching, and pain. Older patients are particularly susceptible to candidiasis because of denture use, salivary hypofunction, the prevalence of diabetes mellitus, and the use of antibiotics for pulmonary and urologic diseases. Patients who use inhaled corticosteroids also are at higher risk and should be instructed to rinse out their mouth after using the inhaler. Management of candidiasis involves, first, excluding any immunopathic cause for the disease, followed by administration of topical or systemic antifungal agents and optimal oral and denture hygiene.

Burning mouth syndrome is a chronic oral-facial pain disorder usually without other clinical signs. It typically affects women aged 50 or over, with a particularly high attack rate in Asian Americans and Native Americans. The pain most commonly affects the lips, tongue, and palate. Multiple causes have been suggested, including xerostomia, denture use, candidiasis, nutritional deficiencies, and psychiatric disorders. Treatment is empirical.

CHEMOSENSORY PERCEPTION

Olfactory function declines with age. A decreased ability to identify odors and to rank their intensities affects both elderly men (to the greater extent) and women. Several drugs have been implicated in smell dysfunction, as has Alzheimer's disease, among other disorders common among older persons. Impaired olfaction in older persons has been anecdotally implicated as a risk factor for eating spoiled food or failing to notice gas leaks or domestic fires.

Taste perception changes with aging. The subjective perception of saltiness and sweetness shows blunting with advancing age. This change potentially has

clinical significance, possibly playing a role in a person's tendency to oversalt foods or crave sweets.

Complaints of taste and smell dysfunction are common among older persons. Often the complaint derives from medication use, but other causes are possible (see Table 42.2 and Table 42.3). Some drugs may have no primary effect on taste but cause diminished saliva flow and lead to impaired taste perception. One's sense of "taste" may actually be more accurately termed "flavor"—that is, the full range of sensations that accompany eating, including temperature, texture, sound, and smell in addition to the perception of sweet, salt, sour, and bitter. Flavor perception is prone to impairment in the older person because of changes in olfaction and oral stereognosis, salivary hypofunction, and the presence of dentures, which present physical and thermal barriers. Flavor-enhancement strategies have been shown to have positive effects on both food preference and caloric intake among frail elderly patients.

Table 42.2—Drugs That Interfere With Gustation (Taste) and Olfaction (Smell)

Gustation*		
Acyclovir	Enalapril	Pentoxifylline
Allopurinol	Ethacrynic acid	Phenytoin
Amiloride	Ethambutol	Procainamide
Amitriptyline	Fenoprofen	Prochlorperazine
Amphotericin B	Gemfibrozil	Promethazine
Ampicillin	Hydrochlorothiazide	Propafenone
Baclofen	Imipramine	Propranolol
Buspirone	Labetalol	Ritonavir
Captopril	Levamisole	Saquinavir
Chlorpheniramine	Lomefloxacin	Sulfamethoxazole
Desipramine	Mexiletine	Sulindac
Doxepin	Nabumetone	Terfenadine
Dexamethasone	Nelfinavir	Tetracyclines
Diclofenac	Ofloxacin	Trifluoperazine
Dicyclomine	Nifedipine	Zidovudine
Diltiazem	Pentamidine	

Olfaction**		
Amitriptyline	Enalapril	Pentamidine
Amphetamine	Flunisolide	Pirbuterol
Beclomethasone dipropionate	Flurbiprofen	Propafenone
	Hydromorphone	Tocainide
Cocaine	Levamisole	Zalcitabine
Codeine	Morphine	
Dexamethasone		

* Gustation: source lists more than 250 agents reported to disturb the sense of taste. Agents listed above are limited to those for which taste disturbance was objectively determined through threshold or intensity scaling or both, employing one or more standardized solutions.

** Olfaction: source lists more than 40 agents reported to disturb the olfactory sense. Agents listed above are limited to those for which olfactory disturbance was determined objectively through experiment or clinical trial.

SOURCE: Data from Schiffman SS, Zervakis J. Taste and smell perception in the elderly: effect of medications and disease. *Adv Food Nutr Res.* 2002; 44:247–346.

Table 42.3—Nonpharmacologic Causes of Taste and Smell Dysfunction in Elderly Persons

Gustatory dysfunction
  Oral causes
    Burning mouth syndrome
    Candidiasis
    Laceration
    Malignancy
    Salivary hypofunction
    Therapeutic irradiation of head
    Thermal or chemical burn
  Other causes
    Alzheimer's disease, other neurodegenerative disorders
    Central nervous system tumor
    Endocrinopathies (eg, diabetes mellitus, Cushing's syndrome, adrenocortical insufficiency, hypothyroidism)
    Head trauma
    Nutritional deficiencies (vitamin B_{12}, zinc)
    Psychiatric disorder
    Stroke
Olfactory dysfunction
  Upper aerodigestive and respiratory causes
    Dental infection
    Periodontal disease
    Poor oral hygiene, including poor denture hygiene
    Sinusitis
    Tobacco smoking or use of nasal snuff
    Tumor of airway or sinus
    Upper respiratory infection (bacterial or viral)
  Other causes
    Alzheimer's disease, other neurodegenerative disorders
    Central nervous system tumor
    Exposure to volatile or particulate toxins
    Head trauma
    Nutritional deficiencies (niacin, zinc)
    Psychiatric disorder
    Stroke

ANNOTATED REFERENCES

■ Hujoel PP, Drangsholt M, Spiekerman C, et al. Periodontal disease and coronary heart disease risk. *JAMA.* 2000;284(11):1406–1410.

> Using data from the First National Health and Nutrition Examination Survey Follow-Up Study, the authors examined the relationship between gingival and periodontal health at baseline and the subsequent occurrence of coronary heart disease. A total of 8032 participants with teeth who did not have a history of cardiovascular disease were selected; 1265 had at least one coronary heart disease event, which when correlated with the 1859 participants with periodontitis at baseline, results in a raw hazards ratio (HR) of 2.66 (95% confidence interval [CI], 2.34 to 3.03). Yet the significant correlation dropped beyond statistical significance (HR 1.21, 95% CI, 0.98 to 1.50) with the analysis of confounding variables, such as race, gender, age, education, weight, alcohol intake, smoking, hypertension, diabetes mellitus, hypercholesterolemia, and depression. The authors question the existence of a "moderate to large" causal relationship between periodontal and coronary heart disease, although they acknowledge that a lesser role may be played.

■ Ritchie CS, Joshipura, K, Hung HC, et al. Nutrition as a mediator in the relation between oral and systemic disease:

associations between specific measures of adult oral health and nutrition outcomes. *Crit Rev Oral Biol Med.* 2002;13(3):291–300.

> The authors conducted a MEDLINE search to identify articles relating specific oral indices to nutritional outcomes. A total of 56 articles were reviewed, most of which had significant methodologic shortcomings. The authors were able to conclude, however, that a relationship does exist between tooth loss and diminished oral intake in a manner that may increase the risk of systemic disease. This impact of tooth loss on oral intake seems to be only partly compensated by the introduction of dental prostheses. The negative impact of xerostomia on nutrient intake is suggested by several studies. Compromised dentition may contribute to weight change, although this is strongly dependent on age and demographic considerations. No studies have established links between oral intake and periodontal disease or oral pain. Overall, the number and quality of studies on this topic is inadequate. The authors suggest the need for longitudinal studies on larger populations with sounder consideration of confounding variables.

■ Schiffman SS, Zervakis J. Taste and smell perception in the elderly: effect of medications and disease. *Adv Food Nutr Res.* 2002;44:247–346.

> This is an exhaustive review of the origins of chemosensory disorders and the studies conducted to elucidate them. The authors discuss the latest findings on the physiology, biochemistry, and anatomy of the gustatory and olfactory systems, reviewing what is known of the effects of aging on these senses. Tables recount the subjective and objective findings that associate gustatory and olfactory disorders with medications and disease states. The impacts of cancer and of Alzheimer's disease on taste and smell are also explored. The authors also review studies on flavor-enhancement strategies that demonstrate a salutary effect on not just the subjective preference for food among frail or unwell older patients but also on caloric intake, plasma protein levels, T-lymphocyte counts, salivary flow, and salivary IgA concentration.

■ Sciubba JJ. Oral cancer: the importance of early diagnosis and treatment. *Am J Clin Dermatol.* 2001:2(4):239–251.

> In the United States, mortality of oral and pharyngeal cancers exceeds that of either cutaneous melanoma or cervical cancer. Significant agents involved in the causes of oropharyngeal cancer in Western countries include sunlight exposure, smoking, and alcohol consumption. A wide range of mucosal alterations are termed *leukoplakia*, making the clinical finding of this entity a concerning yet nonspecific predictor of extant disease. An observation of erythroplakia, however, is almost certain to represent dysplasia or invasive carcinoma. Squamous cell carcinoma will develop from antecedent dysplastic oral mucosal lesions if an early diagnosis has not been made and treatment initiated. Early diagnosis (stage I and II lesions) corresponds to a vastly improved 5-year survival rate when compared with later diagnosis (stages III and IV). Early detection of the asymptomatic early-stage oral cancer translates in general terms to satisfactory clinical outcome and cure in most cases.

■ Shay K. Infectious complications of dental and periodontal diseases in the elderly population. *Clin Infect Dis.* 2002;34(9):1215–1223.

> The author reviews the most common oral infectious diseases (caries, gingivitis, and periodontitis) and explores their sys-

temic implications. Untreated dental caries may result in local cellulitis and abscess formation. In addition, metastatic infections originating in the oral cavity have been reported in the brain, lung, pleura, kidneys, heart, and joints. The linkage between oral bacteria and endocarditis has given rise to widespread application of a prophylactic regimen of an antibiotic prior to invasive dental procedures in certain high-risk patients. Periodontitis pathogens have been reported in anaerobic lung infections. Furthermore, the oral cavity (gingiva and mucosa) readily becomes populated by gram-negative rods and other pulmonary pathogens in frail elderly persons residing in health care institutions, contributing to the risk associated with aspiration of oral contents. The author reviews the limited number of investigations that have evaluated oral hygiene interventions as a means for reducing the morbidity and mortality of aspiration pneumonia in frail elderly populations.

Kenneth Shay, DDS, MS

CHAPTER 43—RESPIRATORY DISEASES AND DISORDERS

KEY POINTS

- With age, there is a decline in forced vital capacity, forced expiratory volume in 1 second, and Pao$_2$, while the A-a gradient increases.

- Five percent to 10% of people aged 65 years and over meet criteria for asthma.

- Smoking cessation may slow the decline in lung function at any age.

- Descriptive studies show that older people recover pulmonary physiology at the same rate as their younger cohorts, but in some disease states they may require a longer time to be liberated from the ventilator.

- Most patients with chronic obstructive pulmonary disease derive little or no benefit from routine inhaled corticosteroids, but a brief course of systemic corticosteroids may reduce the duration of an acute exacerbation of the disease.

AGE-RELATED PULMONARY ALTERATIONS

Studies of age-specific alterations in pulmonary function are limited by common and important comorbidities experienced by older persons, including smoking-related diseases, occupational and industrial exposures, and other significant organ dysfunction such as heart failure or deconditioning. These limitations notwithstanding, decrements in various aspects of pulmonary function occur with aging.

Because of alterations in connective tissue, the size of the airways is reduced and the alveolar sacs become shallow. Chest wall compliance is reduced as a consequence of kyphoscoliosis, calcification of the costal cartilage, and arthritic changes in the costovertebral joints. Sarcopenia results in intercostal muscle atrophy and a reduction in diaphragmatic strength by 25%. These processes result in a decline of forced vital capacity and forced expiratory volume in 1 second of 25 to 30 mL per year in nonsmokers and approximately double that (60 to 70 mL per year) in smokers aged 65 years and over. The normal A-a gradient increases with age and can be approximated by the following formula: (Age / 4) + 4. The Pao$_2$ decreases with age and can be approximated by the following equation: Pao$_2$ = 110 − (0.4 × age).

COMMON RESPIRATORY SYMPTOMS AND COMPLAINTS

There is a common misperception that older persons tend to overestimate or exaggerate respiratory symptoms; however, the opposite is more often true. For example, many older persons and their physicians tend to underestimate the importance of dyspnea, which may go undiagnosed until advanced disease is evident. This is partly due to the fact that dyspnea is blamed on deconditioning and age. Older persons will often adjust their activity level to compensate for insidiously shrinking lung function and disabling dyspnea. Such changes in life style often go unnoticed by family, the patient's physician, and even the patient. Pulmonary or cardiac disorders, or both, may underlie such modifications in life style, and testing (eg, pulmonary function tests or chest radiography) may reveal major abnormalities such as asthma, emphysema, or pulmonary fibrosis. Another complicating feature of symptom recognition in older persons is that older persons often have more than one explanation for their problems. A patient may have overlapping symptoms of dyspnea, cough, and wheezing because of a combination of diseases such as asthma or emphysema, obstructive sleep apnea, heart failure, and gastroesophageal reflux.

Dyspnea

Dyspnea becomes prominent in end-stage lung diseases such as chronic obstructive pulmonary disease (COPD) and idiopathic pulmonary fibrosis. Importantly, the level of dyspnea is the best predictor of quality of life, yet it does not correlate with either oxygenation or pulmonary function tests. A thorough history and physical examination can help tailor both testing and empirical treatment choices. For example, in an older person presenting with dyspnea and associated nocturnal cough, one would first consider common diseases such as asthma, emphysema, allergic rhinitis with postnasal drip, and gastroesophageal reflux disease. Minimal testing (eg, pulmonary function tests only) followed by an empiric trial directed toward the most likely cause would be a reasonable approach. In the same patient, the presence of significant weight loss or constitutional symptoms (fever, night sweats) could suggest other diseases, such as malignancy or tuberculosis. At times, the particular language the patient choses to describe the dyspnea can be revealing, such as "heavy" for cardiac dysfunction or deconditioning or "tight" for angina or asthma. The common causes of dyspnea in older persons to consider include COPD, cardiac disease, asthma, interstitial lung disease, and deconditioning.

Chronic Cough

Fortunately, most patients can be reassured that chronic cough, though particularly annoying, usually has a benign cause. By far, the most common causes of chronic cough are postnasal drip, asthma, and gastroesophageal reflux. These three diagnoses account for over 90% of the causes identified in most series, and a reasonable approach to the treatment of chronic cough, then, is empiric treatment for these conditions. Not infrequently, a combination of these conditions may contribute, so treatment for multiple causes may be warranted when single therapies are ineffective. Less common yet important differential diagnostic considerations of cough in older persons would include drug effects (eg, angiotensin-converting enzyme inhibitors), heart failure, laryngeal dysfunction, *Bordetella pertussis* infection, chronic cough after viral upper respiratory tract infection or secondary bacterial infections, recurrent aspiration, or respiratory tract abnormalities such as bronchiectasis or airway tumors.

Wheezing

Though asthma is a common cause of wheezing in all age groups, it is not the most common cause, particularly if the wheezing is not associated with cough or dyspnea. Postnasal drip is another common cause to consider; also, the rates of heart failure rise in the older age groups, and associated pulmonary edema may present as "cardiac asthma." Finally, airway hyper-responsiveness from chronic bronchitis is not uncommon in older patients with a history of wheezing and sputum and tobacco use.

MAJOR PULMONARY DISEASES IN OLDER PERSONS

Asthma

After childhood, there is a second peak in the prevalence of asthma beyond the age of 65; 5% to 10% of older persons meet criteria for obstruction and bronchial hyperreactivity. The rate of death from asthma has increased most significantly in those aged 65 and over, accounting for up to 45% of all asthma deaths. This is likely due to reduced awareness of bronchial constriction on the part of the patient (with delays in seeking medical attention), as well as under-recognition and undertreatment on the part of clinicians. Therapy of asthma in older and younger persons differs in several ways. Paramount to the care of the elderly asthmatic patient is adequate instruction in the proper use of peak expiratory flow monitoring (because of the older person's decreased perception of bronchoconstriction) and in the correct activation of the metered-dose inhaler. Neurologic, muscular, and arthritic diseases in older persons can lead to suboptimal timing and discoordination in the actuation of the inhaler device. The clinician should observe the patient actually using the inhaler. Inhaled corticosteroids (or other controller drugs such as leukotriene receptor antagonists) represent the mainstay of therapy in both older and younger persons. Use the lowest effective dose, and counsel regarding rinsing of the oropharynx to avoid thrush. In older people, theophylline is fraught with adverse effects and drug interactions, and should be considered a third-line drug to be used only as a once-daily medication in the evening for severe asthma or COPD, targeting a serum level of 10 to 12 mg/dL if tolerated. Oral corticosteroids are discussed in the next section on COPD. Although controversy persists as to whether the response to relievers such as β-agonists varies with age, these drugs remain a mainstay as an as-needed reliever medication. The potential for adverse effects of β-agonists—for example, hypokalemia or possible QT prolongation in cardiac patients on digoxin or other medications—warrants adequate controller use by asthmatic patients to minimize their overreliance on the β-agonist. The use of long-acting β-agonists is controversial and should be considered with caution and only in those patients who are reliably able to manage medications. (See Table 43.1 for commonly used medications taken with metered-dose inhalers.)

Table 43.1—Commonly Used Inhaled Medications, With Packaging Colors

Class of Drug	Generic Name	Trade Name	Color (Body/Cap)
β-Agonists	Albuterol	Proventil	Yellow/orange
		Ventolin	Light blue/dark blue
	Formoterol*	Foradil	White/light blue
	Pirbuterol	Maxair	Blue/white
	Salmeterol	Serevent	Teal/light teal
Corticosteroids	Beclomethasone	Beclovent	White/brown
		Vanceril	Pink/dark pink
		QVAR	Mauve/gray
	Budesonide	Pulmicort	White/brown
	Flunisolide	AeroBid	Gray/purple or green
	Fluticasone	Flovent	Orange/light orange
	Triamcinolone	Azmacort	White/white
Combination β-agonist and corticosteroid	Fluticasone propionate and salmeterol	Advair	Purple/light purple
Others	Cromolyn	Intal	White/blue
	Ipratropium	Atrovent	Silver/green
	Tiotropium*	Spiriva	Gray/green
	Nedocromil	Tilade	White/white
	Albuterol-ipratropium	Combivent	Silver/orange

NOTE: Generics may differ.

* Powder for oral inhalation.

Chronic Obstructive Pulmonary Disease

COPD affects approximately 15 million people in the United States and is the fourth most common cause of death after heart disease, cancer, and stroke. The prevalence and mortality rate from COPD is increasing, especially in older persons. Episodes of acute respiratory failure that require mechanical ventilation are associated with mortality rates ranging from 11% to 46%. The National Lung Health Education Program Executive Committee has noted that the morbidity and mortality from COPD accounts for more than $15 billion per year in U.S. medical care expenditures. Hospitalization continues to represent the largest component of cost for COPD patients.

The diagnosis of airflow limitation is challenging in that no single item or combination of items from the history and clinical examination excludes airflow limitation. The finding most strongly associated with a decreased likelihood of airflow limitation is a history of never having smoked cigarettes (especially in patients without a history of wheezing and without wheezing on examination). Wheezing noted on physical examination is the most potent predictor of airflow limitation, and patients with obstructive airflow limitation are 36 times more likely to have wheezing than are patients without this problem. Other findings associated with an increased likelihood of airflow limitation include a barrel-shaped chest, hyperresonance on percussion, and a forced expiratory time of greater than 9 seconds measured during the clinical bedside examination.

Smoking cessation at any age has been shown to slow the decline in lung function, and aggressive cessation efforts are appropriate even in the oldest-old patient. The basic elements of the approach are the "Five As" from the Agency for Health Care Policy and Research:

- **A**sk patients about use of tobacco at every office visit.
- **A**ssess readiness to quit.
- **A**dvise patients to quit.
- **A**ssist patients in the quit attempt with aids such as a local cessation program and pharmacologic agents such as bupropion or nicotine replacement.
- **A**rrange both a quit date and a follow-up visit or contact to discuss the quit attempt.

The chief components of daily drug therapy in emphysema consist of a β-agonist, ipratropium bromide or tiotropium, or both drugs in combination. For more severe disease, the use of long-acting β-agonists such as salmeterol along with a combined albuterol and ipratropium bromide metered-dose inhaler can achieve improved adherence and long-term control by reducing the number of inhalers by one (ie, the patient will have only the long-acting inhaler and the combination short-acting inhaler rather than three inhalers). Inhaled corticosteroids have now been tested in several multicenter randomized controlled trials in COPD with negative results overall; however, there does appears to be a benefit in subgroup analyses of patients with "asthmatic COPD" as defined by spirometry testing with documented bronchodilator responsiveness. A landmark investigation documented that the use of systemic corticosteroids (intravenous followed by oral) reduces the duration and recurrence of acute exacerbations of COPD for up to 6 months. Importantly, there is no benefit to a course of steroids longer than 14 days. For the few patients (5% to 10%) who do benefit or who require prolonged use of corticosteroids, the risks should be considered, discussed, and documented in the patient's chart. These risks include peptic ulcer disease, hypertension, cataracts, diabetes mellitus, osteoporosis, psychosis, seizures, poor wound healing, infections, and aseptic necrosis of the hip. Appropriate preventive measures should also be taken in these circumstances of prolonged use, such as using the lowest possible dose of corticosteroids and using supplemental vitamin D, calcium, and perhaps a bisphosphonate for those at risk for osteoporosis. Other possible beneficial interventions in older emphysema patients include pulmonary rehabilitation via exercise training and respiratory therapy and education. Both major depression and anxiety have been shown to be present in up to 40% of COPD patients, and their treatment must be considered. In fact, unprovoked anxiety attacks often result in patients' seeking help in emergency departments, being admitted to the hospital, and being treated with potentially avoidable courses of oral corticosteroids when the anxiety is not diagnosed and treated.

Obstructive Sleep Apnea

Sleep-related breathing disorders are very common in older persons, and obstructive sleep apnea is the most common type of sleep-related breathing disorder. Obstructive sleep apnea has been associated with cerebrovascular accidents, myocardial infarctions, and a threefold increase in mortality. Most patients with obstructive sleep apnea remain undiagnosed and therefore without treatment of this life-threatening, yet potentially correctable disease. Treatment options include addressing upper-airway obstruction via weight loss, avoidance of alcohol and sedatives, sleeping on one's side or upright, correction of metabolic disorders

such as hypothyroidism, and continuous positive airway pressure (CPAP) via a nasal mask. To increase adherence with the use of CPAP, one might order the treatment with "nasal pillows" to increase comfort and "ramping technique" to give a delayed rise in the applied pressure after the patient has fallen asleep. Treatment issues are generally the same for the young and the old, and the major consideration for the clinician is a high index of suspicion and clinical recognition of this disease.

Idiopathic Pulmonary Fibrosis

There are more than 100 causes of restrictive lung diseases; however, the history, examination, serologic testing, and biopsy often leave the patient with the diagnosis of idiopathic pulmonary fibrosis. This disease is increasing in prevalence with the aging of our population. Rarely is it an inherited disorder. Pulmonary fibrosis is extremely frustrating for all involved because of its relentless progression. The median survival is 3 to 5 years. The presentation is normally one of insidious dyspnea (often unrecognized because of a decrease in the activity level on the part of the patient) and cough. Clubbing is often a prominent finding on physical examination in pulmonary fibrosis, as opposed to emphysema, which rarely causes clubbing (prompting a search for another disease such as occult lung cancer). Oral corticosteroids (0.5 mg/kg/ day) for 3 to 6 months is the initial therapeutic maneuver most commonly taken, yet only 10% to 20% of patients respond and adverse effects are often prominent. Early referral to a subspecialist is warranted if the patient wishes to consider further therapeutic attempts so that steroid-sparing agents such as azathioprine[OL] or enrollment in a randomized controlled trial of newer pharmacologic agents (eg, interleukin-10 or interferon gamma) can be considered.

Pulmonary Thromboembolism

The incidence of pulmonary thromboembolism triples between the ages of 65 and 90 years and has a reported 10% recurrence rate within 1 year. Age above 70 years has been independently associated with missed antemortem diagnosis. Importantly, 10% to 20% of patients with documented pulmonary embolism have an entirely normal blood gas (ie, normal Pao_2 and normal A-a gradient for age). Age-specific risk factors for pulmonary thromboembolism include hypercoagulability due to increases in fibrinogen, activated protein-C resistance due to factor-V Leiden gene mutation, malignancy, stasis (decreased mobility due to

OL Not approved by the U.S. Food and Drug Administration for this use.

Chapter 43: Respiratory Diseases and Disorders **329**

stroke, heart failure, or arthritis), or vessel injury (due to trauma or varicosities). The diagnostic work-up is not different for young and older patients. Anticoagulants are central to therapy and generally guided by the same principles in younger and older patients. Because of lessened cardiopulmonary reserve, it may be even more important to achieve therapeutic levels of heparinization quickly to avoid major adverse hemodynamic or oxygenation defects in older patients. The trend toward increased utilization of outpatient low-molecular-weight heparin preparations, while achieving anticoagulation with warfarin, is supported by large and appropriately designed randomized controlled trials. There should be an overlap of approximately 1 to 3 days between heparinization and adequate warfarin therapy with an INR target of 2 to 3. Warfarin interacts with many drugs that are commonly used in the older age group (for lists of drugs that increase or decrease INR with warfarin, see the section on anticoagulation in the Appendix, p 491). Studies have inconsistently shown that age itself is a risk factor for bleeding risk with use of warfarin. Duration of therapy for at least 6 months has been shown to be superior to 3 months, and the shorter duration should be used only for those patients with either a specific risk factor that is now removed or for those in whom the risk of prolonged anticoagulant therapy clearly outweighs that of completing 6 months of therapy. Indeed, patients with multiple ongoing risk factors for pulmonary thromboembolic disease are to be considered for anticoagulation therapy for up to 2 years or longer. Recurrent pulmonary thromboembolism is usually treated with lifelong anticoagulation.

Pneumonia

See "Infectious Diseases" (p 335).

Lung Cancer

See "Oncology" (p 486).

INTENSIVE CARE OF THE CRITICALLY ILL

There is widespread belief that many patients do not want aggressive care at the end of life. Moreover, eight of ten health care professionals believe that the treatments they offer to patients are often overly burdensome. More consistency in our attempts to obtain patients' preferences for do-not-resuscitate orders might reduce the extent and burden of aggressive medical care for the elderly age group. Clinicians receive little training regarding this topic. Data from the Study to Understand Prognoses and Preferences for Outcomes and Risks of Treatments (SUPPORT) showed that physician error rates in approximating patients' preferences for mechanical ventilation increased from 36% for patients younger than 50 up to 79% for patients older than 80. Furthermore, SUPPORT data also showed that age was a predictor of less aggressive care in the intensive care unit (ICU) even after adjusting for severity of illness, gender, race, and diagnosis.

A report from a cohort of mechanically ventilated patients in a medical ICU, on the other hand, showed that persons older than 75 years spent the same amount of time on the ventilator as did younger patients but had a lower cost of ICU and in-hospital care. These outcomes were not explained by differences in mortality, since both groups had similar survival rates. Accordingly, the decision to use mechanical ventilation should not be based on age alone, and the appropriate use of ventilatory support in the elderly patient requires further prospective evaluation.

When ICU care and mechanical ventilation are chosen to treat an older person with respiratory failure, special issues related to liberation from the ventilator may be important. In contrast to the general medical ICU population, acute lung injury and acute respiratory distress syndrome patients do appear to have a higher mortality with advancing age. Interestingly, three separate studies of more than 1500 patients have shown that older persons recover from their pulmonary physiologic abnormalities such as hypoxemia and ventilatory disturbances at a rate equal to their younger counterparts after acute lung injury. These patients do, however, have a particularly difficult time during the latter stages of ventilatory support and require nearly twice as long to be successfully liberated from the ventilator and discharged from the ICU. Often comorbid conditions contribute to these patients' deaths despite the apparent correction of their acute lung injury-induced physiologic disturbances. Sedative and analgesic medications must be used judiciously, and delirium, heart failure, hypothyroidism, electrolyte disturbances, oropharyngeal dysfunction, and aspiration should be considered in patients with difficulty liberating from the ventilator. For many older people in good physical condition who succumb to an acute illness, cognitive decline is the main threat to their ability to recover their former functional abilities. For those whose physical activities were already limited, cognitive decline may dramatically worsen after an ICU stay and become the major additional threat to quality of life.

Establishing end-of-life care in critically ill patients is treacherous. Numerous studies have documented the tremendous inaccuracy in formulating the prognosis for patients with serious illnesses. At times, in caring for critically ill patients, it may become apparent to the patient, family, and clinician that further intervention would not likely be of substantial benefit, depending on the individual patient's goals, values, and hopes. Thus, a strict definition of *futility* is impossible. The American Medical Association recommends a standardized "fair process" rather than a strict definition of futility. As much as possible, physicians should base futility decisions on factors such as clinical efficacy of treatment, likelihood of mortality, and subsequent quality-of-life considerations rather than on chronologic age alone.

A recent analysis of 6303 ICU-related deaths found that 26% of these deaths occurred in patients receiving full ICU care, including failed cardiopulmonary resuscitation; 24% received full ICU care without cardiopulmonary resuscitation; 14% had life support withheld; and 36% (the single largest group) had life support actively withdrawn. Although there was a wide variation in the practice pattern of different ICUs, the authors concluded that the limitation of life support prior to death is a common practice in teaching ICUs across the country.

In another study of 851 patients receiving mechanical ventilation, 63% were successfully liberated, 17% died while receiving mechanical ventilation, and 20% had mechanical ventilation withdrawn. The top four reasons given for withdrawing the ventilator were 1) physicians' perception that the patient did not want life support, 2) physicians' prediction that ICU survival was lower than 10%, 3) physicians' prediction that future cognitive function would be severely impaired, and 4) the ongoing need for an inotrope or vasopressors. The inability for physicians to accurately prognosticate beyond hours of impending death must again be acknowledged as challenging such decisions and should temper concerns about the application of technology in critically ill older patients.

For preoperative pulmonary evaluation in elderly patients, see "Perioperative Care" (p 102). For other aspects of end-of-life care, see "Palliative Care" (p 133) and "Legal and Ethical Issues" (p 22).

ANNOTATED REFERENCES

■ Chan ED, Welsh CH. Geriatric respiratory medicine. *Chest.* 1998;114(6):1704–1733.

> This review article has an extensive reference list (376) and a thorough discussion of issues related to pulmonary medicine in the aging patient (including pneumonia, tuberculosis, and lung cancer, not covered in this chapter). It would be an excellent resource for geriatric fellows during their training, as well as for practitioners.

■ Cook D, Rocker G, Marshall J, et al. Withdrawal of mechanical ventilation in anticipation of death in the intensive care unit. *N Engl J Med.* 2003;349(12):1123–1132.

> Rather than age or the severity of the illness and organ dysfunction, the strongest determinants of the withdrawal of ventilation in critically ill patients were found to be the physician's perception that the patient preferred not to use life support, the physician's predictions of a low likelihood of survival in the intensive care unit, a high likelihood of poor cognitive function, and the use of an inotrope or vasopressors.

■ Ely EW, Evans GW, Haponik EF. Mechanical ventilation in a cohort of elderly patients admitted to an intensive care unit. *Ann Intern Med.* 1999;131(2):96–104.

> This prospective analysis of 63 patients aged 75 years or older compared with 237 patients younger than 75 years treated with mechanical ventilation demonstrated that older patients remained on the mechanical ventilator a median of 4 days whereas younger patients remained a median of 6 days (P = .14). Older patients recovered from the pulmonary physiologic perspective at least as quickly as did the younger patients. Using multivariate logistic regression analysis to adjust for race, gender, and severity of illness, the researchers found advanced patient age to be predictive of approximately 3 days less on the ventilator, and ICU and hospital costs were lower for the older group. In-hospital mortality in the two groups was not different. These results indicate that the current system of triaging certain elderly patients to the ICU when critically ill appears to be appropriate and that age alone does not portend lesser physiologic recovery of lung function.

■ Lynn J, Ely EW, Zhong Z, et al. Living and dying with chronic obstructive pulmonary disease. *J Am Geriatr Soc.* 2000;48(5 Suppl):S91–S100.

> This report was derived from the 1016 chronic obstructive pulmonary disease (COPD) patients enrolled in the Study to Understand Prognoses and Preferences for Outcomes and Risks of Treatments (SUPPORT) trial, and it is the most in-depth investigation into the dying process of COPD patients to date. One-year survival was 60%; 40% had more than three comorbidities; and 20% of the last 6 months were spent in hospitals. The burden of dyspnea was often under-recognized, and 2 of 3 patients had serious dyspnea throughout their last 6 months of life; 1 in 4 had serious pain. Patients' illnesses had a major impact on over 25% of families. Patients' preferences for do-not-resuscitate orders increased from 40% at 3 to 6 months before death to 80% within 1 month of death; their decisions not to use mechanical ventilation increased from 10% to 30%; and their preferences for resuscitation decreased from 50% to 25%. Patients with advanced COPD often died within a year and had substantial comorbidities and symptoms.

■ Niewoehner DE, Erbland ML, Deupree RH, et al. Effect of systemic glucocorticoids on exacerbations of chronic obstructive pulmonary disease. Department of Veterans Affairs cooperative study group. *N Engl J Med.* 1999;340(25):1941–1947.

> This landmark article represented the first adequately performed, randomized, double-blind, placebo-controlled trial to document that systemic corticosteroids reduce the duration and recurrence rate of acute exacerbations of chronic obstructive pulmonary disease (COPD). From 25 Veterans Affairs

medical centers, 271 patients hospitalized with an acute exacerbation of COPD were enrolled; 80 received an 8-week course of glucocorticoids, 80 received a 2-week course of glucocorticoids, and 111 received placebo. Rates of treatment failure were significantly higher in the placebo group than in the two treatment groups at 30 days and at 90 days. Systemic glucocorticoids were associated with a shorter hospital stay and a higher FEV_1 by about 100 mL within 24 hours of enrollment in the study. The 8-week regimen was not superior to the 2-week regimen, and neither treatment group showed significant benefit beyond 6 months.

E. Wesley Ely, MD, MPH

CHAPTER 44—INFECTIOUS DISEASES

KEY POINTS

- Immune function and host resistance is compromised in elderly persons not only as a consequence of age-related declines in immunity (immune senescence) but more importantly because of comorbid disease.

- Because of the older person's altered febrile response to infection, a redefinition of fever should be considered in the frail older patient (temperature > 2°F over baseline or oral temperature > 99°F).

- The application of minimum criteria for initiating antibiotic therapy for residents of long-term-care facilities is likely to reduce inappropriate antibiotic use without jeopardizing patient safety.

- Careful selection of first-line therapy is warranted in older patients with pneumonia because of the associated high mortality rates and because the causes of pneumonia differ in younger and older patients.

- The response to aggressive, highly active antiretroviral therapy is similar in younger and older adults with human immunodeficiency virus (HIV) infection.

Infection is the major cause of mortality in 40% of those aged 65 years and older, and it contributes to death in many others. Infection is also a significant cause of morbidity in older adults, often exacerbating underlying illness or leading to hospitalization. Four of the top twenty diagnosis-related groups paid by Medicare are infection-related diagnoses (pneumonia, number 2; urinary tract infections, number 14; septicemia, number 15; and other respiratory infections, number 17). Further, because of their increased susceptibility to infection, older adults often herald the arrival of new infections or the return of annual epidemics. Associations of infection and inflammation with age-related chronic diseases suggest that infectious diseases may play an even larger role in the morbidity and mortality of the elderly population than previously realized. This chapter explores the biologic, cultural, and societal factors that influence susceptibility to infection, the presentation of disease, and the management of infections in elderly patients.

PREDISPOSITION TO INFECTION

Fundamental alterations in the immune response occur with aging in large measure because of comorbidities but also because of age-related declines in immunity, a phenomenon known as *immune senescence* (Table 44.1). The main features of immune senescence are depressed T-cell responses and T-cell–macrophage interactions (clinically reflected as delayed-type hypersensitivity responses), but deficits of innate immunity are increasingly being recognized, particularly in frail elderly patients.

Although age itself influences immune function, comorbidities have the greatest impact on innate immune function and nonspecific host-resistance factors; for example, skin integrity and cough or gag reflexes are local defense mechanisms that are often impaired. Perhaps the best example is chronic obstructive pulmonary disease, in which impaired mucociliary clearance and alveolar macrophage dysfunction are likely to be factors that increase the risk of lower respiratory tract infection. Comorbid diseases also indirectly complicate infections in elderly persons. For example, community-acquired pneumonia in otherwise healthy patients under age 50 is typically treated on an outpatient basis and rarely causes mortality; however, in elderly patients with community-acquired pneumonia and multiple comorbid conditions, the greatly increased risk of morbidity and mortality often necessitates hospitalization. Furthermore, cognitive impairment and other barriers to adherence may increase the difficulty of treating elderly patients, increasing complications and costs.

A major influence on immune function in the older person is nutritional status. Global (protein and calorie) undernutrition is present in 30% to 60% of

Table 44.1—Changes in Immune Function Associated With Aging

| | Change With Age | | |
	Direction	Degree	Comment
Innate immunity			
Skin, mucous membranes	decrease	+++	Skin thins and dries with aging
Complement		—	Most changes are due to comorbidity
Polymorphonuclear neutrophils			Most changes are due to comorbidity
Adherence, chemotaxis		—	
Ingestion		—	
Intracellular killing	decrease	+	Most changes are due to comorbidity
Adaptive immunity			
Thymic hormones	decrease	+++	
Lymphocyte subsets			
T cells		+++	Shift from naive to memory subtypes
Natural killer cells	decrease	++	Number increases, but function declines
Lymphocyte functions			
Proliferative responses	decrease	++	
Cytokine production, secretion			
IL-2, IL-2 receptor	decrease	+++	
IL-4, IL-6, IL-10	increase	++	
IFN-γ	increase	+	
PGE$_2$	increase	++	
Delayed-type hypersensitivity	decrease	++	
Autoimmunity	increase	++	Autoantibodies common, but of unclear significance

NOTE: — = no age-related changes; + = mild; ++ = moderate; +++ = marked; IL = interleukin; IFN = interferon; PGE$_2$ = prostaglandin E$_2$.

persons aged 65 years or older on admission to the hospital. In the outpatient arena, 11% of older adults suffer from undernutrition, 90% of which is due to reversible underlying conditions (depression, poorly controlled diabetes mellitus, medication side effects). Delayed wound healing, increased risk of nosocomial infection, extended lengths of hospital stay, and increased mortality are all associated with malnutrition. Even mildly undernourished older adults (those with a serum albumin of 3.0 to 3.5 g/dL) have evidence of immune compromise, poor vaccine responses, and diminished cytokine responses to specific challenges. Nutritional interventions may boost immune function in some older adults, but this remains controversial. Some studies suggest a clinical benefit, particularly in those with subclinical nutritional deficiencies, whereas others do not. Differences in study design, population enrolled, duration of follow-up, and definitions of infection (self-reported versus physician diagnosed) may account for many of these differences. (See "Malnutrition," p 174.)

Institutionalization places elderly persons at greatly increased risk for epidemic disease such as influenza. Widespread antibiotic use also increases their risk for acquiring diseases caused by more resistant organisms. Methicillin-resistant *Staphylococcus aureus,* vancomycin-resistant enterococci, and multiply resistant gram-negative rods are more common causes of infection in institutionalized elderly persons. Resistance is fostered in the nursing home by debilitated hosts, close proximity of residents, and difficulties in implementing infection-control measures in long-term care, as well as high levels of antibiotic use.

DIAGNOSIS AND MANAGEMENT OF INFECTIONS

Presentation

It has long been recognized that older adults may present without typical signs and symptoms, even in the face of very significant infection. Fever, the most readily recognized feature of infection, may be absent in 30% to 50% of frail older adults with serious infections, even pneumonia or endocarditis. The cause of impaired febrile responses in older adults is incompletely understood, but diverse mechanisms of thermoregulation are involved, including blunted thermogenesis by brown adipose tissue.

Because of the altered febrile response to infection, many authors have suggested a redefinition of *fever* in older adults. Given the sensitivity, specificity, and positive and negative predictive values, fever in elderly nursing-home residents can be redefined appropriately as a temperature > 2°F (1.1°C) over baseline (if a baseline is available) or, perhaps more practically, an oral temperature > 99°F (37.2°C) or a rectal temperature > 99.5°F (37.5°C) on repeated measures. This definition of fever has a sensitivity of 82.5% in nursing-home residents, and the specificity remains high at 89.9% (Table 44.2). Although these data were generated in a trial of frail older veteran men in a nursing home, it would seem reasonable to apply the same definitions to frail older adults of either gender in the community. However, the performance characteristics of this definition of fever in otherwise healthy older adults has not been validated.

The absence of fever is only one way that infectious diseases may present atypically in the elderly person. For example, infective endocarditis may be heralded by a nonspecific decline in baseline functional status, such as confusion or falling. Subsequent anorexia and decreased oral intake may follow, and exacerbation of an underlying illness (eg, atrial fibrillation) may become the predominant feature. Cognitive impairment further contributes to the atypical presentation of infections in older adults. Many cognitively impaired older patients are unable to communicate symptoms accurately, and clinicians must be ready to pursue objective assessments such as laboratory and radiologic evaluations at a lower threshold, unless advance directives indicate otherwise.

Antibiotic Management

Drug distribution, metabolism, excretion, and interactions may be altered with age. Aging in the absence of any comorbid disease is associated with a reduction in renal function, and reductions in antibiotic dose may be required in the elderly patient. (See "Pharmacotherapy" p 72.) Furthermore, antibiotic interactions occur with many medications commonly prescribed for elderly persons. Digoxin, warfarin, oral hypoglycemic agents, theophylline, antacids, lipid-lowering agents, antihypertensive medications, and H_2-receptor antagonists all have significant interactions with commonly prescribed antibiotics. Drug concentrations can increase (eg, enhanced digoxin toxicity associated with macrolides, tetracyclines, and trimethoprim) or decrease (eg, reduced absorption of some fluoroquinolones with antacids) with concomitant drug administration. Atrophic gastritis, a common problem in older adults, and H_2 blockers or proton-pump inhibitors can reduce the absorption of some antibiotics, such as ketoconazole or itraconazole. Finally, adherence to prescribed regimens may be limited as a consequence of poor cognitive function, impaired hearing or vision, use of multiple medications, and financial constraints.

The choice and timing of antibiotics may also be important in the treatment of older infected adults. In sepsis, a preponderance of data suggests that initially broad coverage is warranted, since outcomes (mortality, length of stay in intensive care) are improved when the offending organism is covered by the initial antibiotic regimen. In older adults with pneumonia, data suggest that delaying initiation of therapy 4 or more hours after admission to the hospital is associated with an increased risk of mortality. However, these and similar data in other infectious syndromes and the atypical presentation of infection noted above often leads to early initiation of antimicrobials in older adults, particularly in long-term care. However, in long-term care, up to 75% of antibiotic use may be inappropriate. The use of strict, minimum criteria for initiation of antimicrobials in long-term care is most likely to reduce inappropriate antibiotic use without jeopardizing patient safety (Table 44.3).

Table 44.2—Defining Fever in Frail, Older Residents of Long-Term-Care Facilities

Definition	Sensitivity	Specificity	(+) Likelihood Ratio	(−) Likelihood Ratio
T > 101°F (38.3°C)	40.0%	99.7%	133	0.6
T > 100°F (37.7°C)	70.0%	98.3%	41	0.3
T > 99°F (37.2°C)	82.5%	89.9%	8	0.2

NOTE: (+) Likelihood ratio = sensitivity / (1− specificity); (−) Likelihood ratio = (1− sensitivity) / specificity; T = temperature.

SOURCE: Data from Castle SC, Yeh M, Toledo S, et al. Lowering the temperature criterion improves detection of infections in nursing home residents. *Aging Immunol Infect Dis.* 1993;4(2):67–76.

Table 44.3—Suggested Minimum Criteria for Initiation of Antibiotic Therapy in the Long-Term-Care Setting

Condition	Minimum Criteria
Urinary tract infection, without catheter	Fever AND one of the following: new or worsening urgency, frequency, suprapubic pain, gross hematuria, CVA tenderness, incontinence
Urinary tract infection, with catheter	Fever OR one of the following: new CVA tenderness, rigors, or new-onset delirium
Skin and soft-tissue infection	Fever OR one of the following: redness, tenderness, warmth, new or increasing swelling of affected site
Respiratory infection	■ Fever > 102°F (38.9°C) AND one of the following: RR > 25, productive cough ■ Fever > 100°F < 102°F AND one of the following: RR > 25, pulse > 100, rigors, new-onset delirium ■ Afebrile with COPD AND new or increased cough with purulent sputum ■ Afebrile without COPD AND new or increased cough AND either RR > 25 or new-onset delirium
Fever without source of infection	■ At least one of the following: new-onset delirium, rigors ■ If these are not present, evaluate without initiating antibiotics ■ Antibiotics probably should not be instituted as a diagnostic test, but if initiated as such, discontinue in 3–5 days if no improvement and evaluation negative

NOTE: COPD = chronic obstructive pulmonary disease; CVA = costovertebral angle; RR = respiratory rate.

SOURCE: Data from Loeb M, Bentley DW, Bradley S, et al. Development of minimum criteria for the initiation of antibiotics in residents of long-term-care facilities: results of a consensus conference. *Infect Control Hosp Epidemiol.* 2001;22:120–124.

INFECTIOUS SYNDROMES

Bacteremia and Sepsis

Bacteremia is a common cause of hospitalization for older patients. Older patients with bacteremia are less likely than their younger counterparts to have chills or sweating, and fever is commonly absent. Gastrointestinal and genitourinary sources of bacteremia are more common; thus, the causative bacteria are more likely to be gram-negative rods.

Bacteremia carries a poor prognosis in older adults. For example, nosocomial gram-negative bacteremia carries a mortality rate of 5% to 35% for young adults, but in older adults the mortality rate is 37% to 50%. Major contributing factors include coexisting diseases that reduce physiologic reserve and the more common use of invasive devices (eg, intravenous or urinary catheters) that make eradication of organisms difficult.

The management of bacteremia and sepsis in older and younger patients is similar. Rapid administration of appropriate antibiotics aimed at the most likely sources is essential. The use of activated protein C as adjunctive therapy in septic older adults had raised concern about increased bleeding. However, a recent analysis of patients aged 75 and over enrolled in a randomized trial of activated protein C in sepsis demonstrated preservation of the survival benefit in older adults despite a slightly increased risk of serious bleeding.

Pneumonia

Patients aged 65 years and older account for more than 50% of all pneumonia cases, and annual hospital-ization rates for pneumonia range from 12 per 1000 among community-dwelling adults aged 75 and older to 32 per 1000 among nursing-home residents. In fact, the cumulative 2-year risk of pneumonia for long-term-care residents is approximately 30%. Pneumonia mortality in older adults is three to five times that of young adults, but the rate is profoundly influenced by comorbidity. Comorbidity is the strongest independent predictor of mortality in community-acquired pneumonia in older adults, with a relative risk of 4.1 (in the article that determined this relative risk, comorbidity was defined as cancer, collagen vascular disease, or advanced liver disease). Other independent risk factors include age of 85 years and older, debility (decreased motor function), serum creatinine > 1.5 mg/dL, and the presence of hypothermia (< 36.1°F), hypotension (< 90 mm Hg systolic), or tachycardia (> 110 beats per minute) on admission. Long-term follow-up data also suggest that community-acquired pneumonia in older adults indicates a higher risk of subsequent all-cause mortality over the next 12 years as a consequence of both recurrent pneumonia (relative risk 2.1 [1.3 to 3.4]) but also cardiovascular disease (relative risk 1.4 [1.0 to 1.9]).

The causes of pneumonia in younger and elderly adults differ. In elderly patients, *Streptococcus pneumoniae* is still the predominant organism, but gram-negative bacilli (eg, *Haemophilus influenzae, Moraxella catarrhalis, Klebsiella* spp.) are much more common than in younger adults, particularly in patients with chronic obstructive pulmonary disease or who reside in long-term-care facilities. *S. aureus* and respiratory viruses are also common causes of community-acquired pneumonia in nursing-home residents (Figure 44.1).

Pneumonia therapy has changed significantly in the past few years because of the emergence of resistant bacteria, particularly drug-resistant *S. pneumoniae*, leading many practitioners to rely heavily on fluoroquinolones, even for routine community-acquired pneumonia. This practice, however, has led to increased rates of fluoroquinolone resistance in several areas of the world, and some fluoroquinolones can have significant adverse effects, including dizziness and cardiac conduction abnormalities (QT prolongation), that may limit their use in certain older adults. The current Infectious Diseases Society of America treatment guidelines for community-acquired pneumonia suggest the following as first-line therapy in adults over the age of 60 with or without comorbidity: a β-lactam and β-lactamase combination or advanced-generation cephalosporin (ceftriaxone or cefotaxime) with or without a macrolide. Alternatively, one of the newer fluoroquinolones with enhanced activity against *S. pneumoniae* (levofloxacin, sparfloxacin, moxifloxacin, gatifloxacin) may be used. Given the resistance already emerging to fluoroquinolones, it is prudent to use these drugs only in situations with highest risk for drug-resistant *S. pneumoniae* or other resistant organisms. In the outpatient setting, this is limited to residents of long-term-care facilities or patients with marked chronic obstructive pulmonary disease (FEV$_1$ < 30% predicted). In the inpatient setting, the sicker the patient (ie, the closer to needing intensive care), the stronger the justification for use of a fluoroquinolone. This is true because the margin for error is small, fluoroquinolones are currently the most effective therapy for drug-resistant *S. pneumoniae*, they are effective against most gram-negative bacilli, and they can be used to treat atypical organisms such as such as *Legionella* spp. that are more likely in the intensive-care setting.

Nursing-home acquired pneumonia (NHAP) or hospital acquired pneumonia (HAP) in older adults requires more broad initial therapy than community-acquired pneumonia because of the broader spectrum of organisms causing infection (see Figure 44.1). In the nursing-home setting, polymicrobial infection, often due to aspiration, and *S. aureus* are much more common than in the community setting. In the hospital setting, gram-negative bacilli predominate, but *S. aureus* is more common as well and is more likely to affect specific antibiotic choices because of resistance. Outcomes data suggest

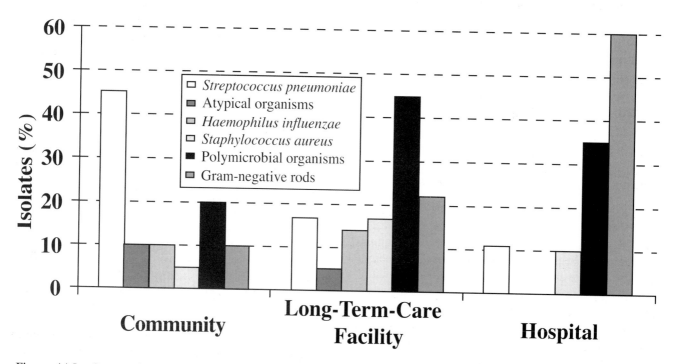

Figure 44.1—Causes of pneumonia by domiciliary setting. A specific cause for pneumonia is isolated only 30% to 50% of the time. Isolates here were pooled from several studies and were microbiologically confirmed. When a specific causative agent is identified, the predominant organisms vary by domiciliary setting, as indicated. Atypical organisms include *Mycoplasma pneumoniae*, *Chlamydia pneumoniae*, viruses, and, rarely, *Legionella* spp.

that response to therapy is greater when the initial antibiotic regimen covers the offending agent. Thus, initial regimens should be broadly inclusive, followed by step-down therapy to more narrow coverage if the causative agent is identified. Importantly, if patients are known to be colonized with methicillin-resistant *S. aureus* (MRSA), initial regimens should include vancomycin or linezolid until MRSA is excluded as the cause. Further, data suggest that patients with clinically improving HAP not caused by nonfermenting gram-negative bacilli (eg, *Pseudomonas*, *Stenotrophomonas*) can be treated with shorter courses of antibiotics, 7 or 8 days, rather than the 2 weeks commonly employed in the past. Shorter courses (8 days versus 15 days) of antibiotics are associated with equivalent efficacy and less antibiotic resistance.

The prevention of pneumonia in older adults is a complex issue, and a multipronged approach is most likely to be effective. Immunization of at-risk persons is far and away the most well-studied measure (see "Prevention," p 69). In addition to vaccines, smoking cessation and aggressive treatment of comorbidities (eg, minimizing aspiration risk in post-stroke patients, limited use of sedative hypnotics) may reduce the risk of infection. Finally, system changes with attention to infection control (isolation, cohorting, skin testing for tuberculosis with purified protein derivative [PPD], and immunization policies) may be particularly effective in the nursing home.

Influenza

Influenza results in approximately 40,000 deaths annually in the United States, and nearly all of these deaths occur in the older adult population. The clinical syndrome of influenza is easily recognized by most clinicians, particularly in the setting of local activity or outbreak settings frequently seen in the nursing home. Annual influenza vaccine is 60% to 80% efficacious in older adults for preventing severe disease, hospitalization, and death. Therefore, annual immunization is recommended for all adults over the age 50, and for anyone of any age who wishes to reduce the risk of serious influenza.

Several drugs are available for treatment and prophylaxis of influenza. M2 inhibitors (amantadine and rimantadine) block the M2 ion channel of influenza and are effective only against influenza A. Amantadine is particularly difficult to use in older adults because of the extensive dose adjustments required for small changes in kidney function and marked adverse effects, particularly central nervous system symptoms. In contrast, neuraminidase inhibitors (zanamivir and oseltamivir) are effective against both influenza A and B; they inhibit the virus by interference with an

essential enzyme, neuraminidase, that cleaves sialic acid to expose host cell receptors for the virus. Oseltamivir, a capsule, is preferred over zanamivir in older adults because zanamivir must be inhaled, and it is difficult for many older adults to properly use the product. Treatment of influenza is effective if initiated in the first 48 hours, but it is most effective if initiated within 24 hours of symptom onset. Amantadine, rimantadine, zanamivir, and oseltamivir also can be used for prevention in outbreak situations (eg, in long-term care) when combined with appropriate vaccination strategies.

Urinary Tract Infection

Urinary tract infection (UTI) is among the most common of clinical illnesses in older adults, with an incidence of 10.9 per 100 person years in men and 14 per 100 person years in women age 65 and older. As in young adults, gram-negative bacilli (eg, *Escherichia coli*, *Enterobacter* spp., *Klebsiella* spp., *Proteus* spp.) are most common, but there is an increase in more resistant isolates, such as *Pseudomonas aeruginosa*, and in gram-positive organisms, including enterococci, coagulase-negative staphylococci, and *Streptococcus agalactiae* (group B strep). In patients with indwelling catheters, the microbes listed still predominate, but it is also common to encounter additional organisms, including enterococci, *S. aureus*, and fungi, particularly *Candida* spp. The organisms colonizing urinary catheters commonly develop biofilms and are difficult to clear with the same urinary catheter in place.

Asymptomatic Bacteruria

Up to 15% of women in the community and 40% of women in nursing homes will have asymptomatic bacteruria; the incidence in men is approximately half that for women. Rates are even higher with the use of condom catheters (87%) or Foley catheters (nearly 100%). Numerous studies have suggested that there is no clinical benefit from the treatment of asymptomatic bacteruria and that treatment is associated with significant adverse effects, expense, and the potential for selection of resistant organisms. Thus, no treatment is recommended. The clinical difficulty faced almost daily by clinicians is deciding what is symptomatic. The presentation of infection can be quite subtle in older adults, and a change in functional status often prompts the collection of a urine specimen even in the absence of fever, dysuria, or other typical clinical features. However, since no controlled trial has ever shown a decreased incidence of urosepsis or mortality with antibiotic treatment of asymptomatic bacteruria, a period of observation rather than a therapeutic trial would seem most prudent when symptoms are not clearly related to bacteruria.

Urinary Tract Infection in Women

In contrast to asymptomatic bacteruria, symptomatic UTI does require therapy. Therapy is based on the location of infection (upper versus lower tract disease) and likely causative agent. Lower tract UTI (cystitis), characterized by dysuria, frequency, and urgency (note: not fever, which generally indicates upper tract disease), is often treated in young women for 1 to 3 days, and recent data suggest 3 days of therapy is sufficient for uncomplicated cystitis in older women. Randomized trials in older women indicate that fluoroquinolones are more efficacious than trimethoprim-sulfamethoxazole (TMP-SMX), likely because of E. coli TMP-SMX resistance rates of 10% to 20% in most areas of the country. Other reasonable choices in some settings include amoxicillin (particularly for enterococcal infection) and first-generation cephalosporins in the patient with multiple antibiotic intolerances. Culture is not required unless first-line therapy fails.

Upper UTI (pyelonephritis), characterized by fever, chills, nausea, and flank pain and commonly accompanied by lower tract symptoms, requires more prolonged therapy, 7 to 21 days. Because of the excellent bioavailability of many antibiotics, particularly the fluoroquinolones, intravenous therapy is not essential if the patient can tolerate oral medications. A study comparing fluoroquinolones with TMP-SMX for upper tract UTI in younger women (aged 18 to 58) suggests that fluoroquinolones are more effective (microbiologic cure rate 99% versus 89% for TMP-SMX; clinical cure rates 96% versus 83%, respectively) because of the presence of TMP-SMX–resistant organisms. This is likely to be true in older adults as well. Intravenous administration of antibiotics remains the standard of care for patients with suspected urosepsis, those with upper tract disease due to relatively resistant bacteria such as enterococci, or those unable to tolerate oral medications. Culture and sensitivity data are more useful in guiding antimicrobial therapy in upper tract UTIs than in lower tract disease and should be obtained in most cases.

Prophylactic antibiotics intended to prevent frequently recurrent UTIs in older women are not recommended because of the high incidence of the development of resistant organisms. Several measures may decrease the frequency of recurrence, including intravaginal or systemic estrogen replacement that changes the vaginal flora, thus reducing the risk of UTI, or perhaps ingestion of at least 300 mL of cranberry juice each day, though data in support of these measures remain preliminary.

Urinary Tract Infection in Men

Prostatic disease (primarily hyperplasia) or functional disability, such as autonomic neuropathy from diabetes mellitus with incomplete bladder emptying, account for the majority of both lower and upper UTIs in elderly men. Thus, short-course therapy for UTIs in elderly men is inappropriate and should be avoided. A minimum of 14 days of therapy should be provided, and if prostatic involvement is suspected (ie, acute or chronic prostatitis), at least 6 weeks of therapy is usually required. The causative organisms and treatment choices are similar to those outlined above for elderly women. Fluoroquinolones and TMP-SMX are most widely used when prostatic involvement is suspected and culture data confirms the organism's susceptibility because, of the available agents, these two penetrate the prostate most adequately. Because treatment for all UTIs in men is generally longer than in women and the prostate is a common reservoir for recurrent UTIs, culture and sensitivity data should guide therapy for virtually all UTIs in men.

Tuberculosis

Worldwide, approximately 1.7 billion persons are infected with *Mycobacterium tuberculosis* (MTB), 16 million in the United States. Adults aged 65 and older account for one fourth of all active tuberculosis cases in the United States. The vast majority of active MTB in older adults occurs in community-dwelling elderly persons, but the rate of infection in long-term-care residents is much higher: skin-test studies show prevalence rates of skin-test reactivity in the range of 30% to 50%. This high prevalence is due to MTB exposure in the early 1900s, when it was estimated that 80% of all persons were infected with MTB by the age of 30. Most active cases of tuberculosis in older adults are, therefore, due to reactivation disease, but primary infection may account for 10% to 20% of cases and is of particular concern in nursing-home outbreaks.

As with most other infections, tuberculosis may not present in classic fashion (cough, sputum, fever, night sweats, weight loss) in the elderly patient. Often fatigue, anorexia, decreased functional status, or low-grade fever are the presenting manifestations. Most tuberculous disease in elderly persons occurs with lung involvement (75%), and pneumonic processes in older adults, particularly those that occur in a postacute manner, should raise a high index of suspicion for MTB. Older adults are more likely than their younger counterparts to have extrapulmonary disease. Other sites include miliary (disseminated) disease, tuberculous meningitis or osteomyelitis, and urogenital disease, but virtually any body structure can be involved, and that organ system can account for the major presenting symptom.

A diagnosis of active disease usually requires isolation of the organism from sputum, urine, or other clinical specimen. Current techniques have improved the speed of diagnosis, particularly for identifying the species of *Mycobacterium* after isolation. This is now typically accomplished within 24 hours of obtaining a positive culture by use of DNA probes. Direct polymerase chain reaction of clinical specimens or other rapid diagnostic techniques are not available or reliable in most local laboratories, but such tests can be obtained in research settings. They are most likely to be helpful for establishing a diagnosis from cerebrospinal or pleural fluid, which yields positive cultures in only 10% to 15% of cases.

The most confusing area of MTB diagnostics for most practitioners is the interpretation of the results of PPD skin tests. In all populations, induration of ≥ 15 mm 48 to 72 hours after placement of a 5-tuberculin-unit PPD indicates a positive test. Induration ≥ 10 mm is considered a positive test in nursing-home residents, recent converters (previous PPD < 5 mm), immigrants from countries with high endemicity of MTB, underserved populations in the United States (homeless persons, black Americans, Hispanic Americans, and Native Americans), and persons with specific risk factors (gastrectomy, > 10% below ideal body weight, chronic kidney failure, diabetes mellitus, or immune suppression, including that caused by corticosteroids or malignancy). In patients infected with human immunodeficiency virus (HIV), those with a history of close contact with persons with active MTB, and those with chest radiographs consistent with MTB, ≥ 5 mm induration is considered a positive PPD test. Anergy panel testing in conjunction with PPD testing is of little value and is not recommended.

Long-term-care facilities should employ a two-step procedure for PPD testing during the initial evaluation of residents. Two-step testing requires retesting of patients with < 10 mm induration within 2 weeks. If the second skin test results in ≥ 10 mm of induration or the increase in the size of the induration from the first to the second skin test is ≥ 6mm, the patient is considered PPD positive.

The treatment of active MTB in the elderly person is similar to that in young adults. Four-drug therapy (usually isoniazid [INH], rifampin, pyrazinamide, and ethambutol or streptomycin) is recommended as initial therapy, with tapering to one of several two- or three-drug regimens once susceptibility testing is available. The most common regimen is INH, rifampin, and pyrazinamide for 2 months, followed by INH and rifampin for an additional 4 months.

Prophylaxis with 9 months of INH for asymptomatic persons with a positive PPD should be provided *regardless of age* in adults who are recent converters (defined in persons > 35 years of age with a PPD that has gone from < 10 mm to ≥ 15 mm within 2 years), or regardless of duration of PPD positivity if one is afflicted with any of the specific risk factors highlighted above. Patients with a positive PPD of unknown duration, particularly those over the age of 35 years, should receive INH prophylaxis with close monitoring for symptoms and signs of peripheral neuropathy (due to INH and preventable by coadministration of pyridoxine) and hepatitis (due to INH, rifampin, or pyrazinamide). Shorter course therapy with 2 months of rifampin and pyrazinamide is effective but has a much higher incidence of hepatotoxicity than INH and thus should be used only in very specific circumstances.

Infective Endocarditis

Since the early part of the 20th century, infective endocarditis (IE) has undergone a transformation, from a disease of young adults primarily due to rheumatic or congenital valve anomalies to one of older adults associated with degenerative valvular disorders and prosthetic valves. Native-valve endocarditis is typically caused by viridans streptococci, *S. aureus*, and occasional infections are due to HACEK organisms (a group of typically nonfermenting gram-negative rods that primarily inhabit the oral cavity and include the genuses *Haemophilus, Actinobacillus, Cardiobacterium, Eikenella,* and *Kingella*). Gastrointestinal and genitourinary organisms, such as enterococci and gram-negative rods, are more common in native-valve IE in older adults, and coagulase-negative staphylococci are a common cause of prosthetic-valve endocarditis, particularly in the first 60 days following placement of a prosthetic valve.

The diagnosis of endocarditis is often difficult in the elderly patient. Fever and leukocytosis are less common in elderly than in younger patients, occurring in only 55% and 25%, respectively, versus 80% and 60%, respectively. Blood culture positivity rates do not vary by age; however, degenerative, calcific valvular lesions and prosthetic valves lower the sensitivity of transthoracic echocardiography (TTE) to 45% in older patients (sensitivity is 75% in younger patients). Transesophageal echocardiography (TEE) improves the diagnostic yield for IE, but the absence of positive findings on TEE never excludes IE. TEE is of particular value in resolving the clinical problem of *S. aureus* bacteremia. Positive findings on TEE support prolonged antibiotic administration (4 to 6 weeks) versus short-course (2-week) therapy. On the other hand, TEE is invasive and expensive. Interestingly, age does not appear to play a major role in mortality risk, with a 2-year survival of 75% for IE in all age groups unless major comorbidities are also present.

Antibiotic treatment of IE is directed at the identified pathogen or the most likely causes, if blood cultures are negative. Therapy is administered intravenously for 2 to 6 weeks. Surgical therapy should be considered for severe valvular dysfunction, recurrent emboli, marked heart failure, myocardial abscess formation, fungal endocarditis, or the failure of appropriate antibiotics to sterilize blood cultures.

Prophylaxis is available for bacterial endocarditis in at-risk patients undergoing dental, upper respiratory tract, gastrointestinal, or genitourinary procedures. Recommendations for endocarditis prophylaxis have been published and are widely available (eg, the American Heart Association, see http://www.amhrt.org).

Prosthetic Device Infections

Permanent implantable prosthetic devices are common in the elderly age group. Prosthetic joints, cardiac pacemakers, artificial heart valves, intraocular lens implants, vascular grafts, penile prostheses, and a variety of other devices are more often placed in older than in younger adults. A discussion of all prosthetic device infections is beyond the scope of this chapter, but several general concepts can be summarized.

Prosthetic device infections are usually separated into early versus late infection because the causative agents differ significantly. Early prosthetic device infection (PDI), most commonly defined as occurring less than 60 days after device implantation, is primarily due to contamination at the time of implantation or events associated with the acute hospitalization (such as occult bacteremias due to intravenous catheters). Thus, coagulase-negative staphylococci predominate, and S. aureus and diphtheroids are common as well; gram-negative bacilli and fungi are relatively rare causes of early PDI. Late PDI is usually caused by organisms that commonly cause transient bacteremia (in the elderly person this is most often skin, respiratory, gastrointestinal, or genitourinary organisms). Staphylococci, including coagulase-negative staphylococci, play a major role in PDIs in both the early and late periods, though their relative importance is greater early. Thus, empiric staphylococcal therapy should be provided in either early or late PDI if a specific causative agent is not identified.

In general, hardware removal is required to clear PDIs. However, early antibiotic intervention, in some instances combined with aggressive surgical drainage, may be successful. Small studies in prosthetic joint infection suggest that initial debridement and culture and a brief course (2 weeks) of intravenous antibiotics followed by combination oral therapy with fluoroquinolones and rifampin for 3 to 6 months may obviate the need for device removal. Until more definitive data are available, it is prudent to restrict this approach to patients with a short duration of symptoms (< 3 weeks), those who are likely to have difficulty tolerating another surgical procedure, or those in whom return to full functional status is not a realistic goal because of comorbidities. In those older adults in whom full functionality is the goal, the best chance for cure is a two-stage procedure in which the device is removed and antibiotics are given for an extended period (6 to 8 weeks), followed by delayed reimplantation. For life-saving devices such as mechanical valves or implantable defibrillators, this is not an option. Infected prosthetic devices are usually surrounded by microbial biofilms, such as microbe-derived glycocalyx. Biofilms reduce antibiotic penetration and greatly increase the bactericidal concentrations of antibiotic without changing the inhibitory concentrations (ie, the amount of drug necessary to inhibit the organism does not change, but it takes tremendously increased concentrations to kill the organism). Furthermore, many conditions associated with infected prostheses are also accompanied by poor blood flow to the area. Thus, it is preferable to use bactericidal antibiotics, often in combination with a second agent that penetrates biofilms and poorly perfused areas (eg, rifampin for staphylococci).

The use of prophylactic antibiotics in situations other than prosthetic heart valves remains a point of contention. Antimicrobial prophylaxis is indicated for dental, gastrointestinal, and genitourinary procedures for patients with prosthetic valves and is probably reasonable for vascular grafts, particularly within the first few months after placement, but no randomized controlled trial has ever clearly shown benefit. The need for prophylaxis for patients with prosthetic joints, intraocular lens implants, cerebrospinal fluid shunts, breast implants, or less common prostheses is even less clear. However, a joint statement by the American Dental Association and American Academy of Orthopaedic Surgeons (AAOS) recommends very limited use of antibiotic prophylaxis in specific patients undergoing dental procedures with a higher bacteremic risk (eg, dental extraction) and who are also at high risk for hematologic seeding (eg, first 2 years after prosthetic joint replacement, immunocompromised or immunosuppressed, or previous prosthetic joint infection). For more information, see the advisory statement posted on the AAOS Web site (http://www.aaos.org/wordhtml/papers/advistmt/1014.htm).

Bone and Joint Infections

Native bone and joint infections in the absence of prostheses occur in older adults. Septic arthritis is more likely to occur in joints with underlying pathology (rheumatoid changes, gout, osteoarthritis), and early arthrocentesis is indicated in any mono- or oligo-articular syndrome to exclude infection. *S. aureus* is the most likely pathogen; only rarely are infections due to gram-negative bacilli and streptococci. Aggressive antibiotic therapy combined with serial arthrocentesis may be as effective as open surgical drainage in uncomplicated septic arthritis, and it preserves better functionality in the joint. Surgical drainage is required for patients failing this more conservative strategy.

Osteomyelitis in older adults can be due to hematogenous seeding from a bacteremia or contiguous spread from an adjacent focus. *S. aureus* is the predominant organism, but gastrointestinal and genitourinary flora are again more common in older adults, which emphasizes the advantage of a specific microbiologic diagnosis to guide therapy. Infections of pressure ulcers and diabetic foot infections are very common, particularly in institutionalized older adults, and they commonly require surgical consultation combined with aggressive antimicrobial therapy aimed at mixed aerobic and anaerobic bacteria.

HIV Infection and AIDS

HIV infection in elderly adults was initially limited to those who had received blood transfusions for surgical procedures. However, increasing numbers of older Americans with HIV have acquired their infection via sexual activity. Older adults constitute approximately 10% of all new diagnoses of acquired immunodeficiency syndrome (AIDS) in the United States, but this group suffers from a lack of HIV awareness among their clinicians. Nonspecific symptoms such as forgetfulness, anorexia, weight loss, and recurrent pneumonia are often dismissed as age-related, and HIV testing can be delayed. Untreated HIV infection in the elderly person tends to pursue a more rapid downhill course, perhaps because of impaired T-cell replacement mechanisms with advanced age and the impact of additional comorbidities. However, if older adults are treated with aggressive highly active antiretroviral therapy (HAART), the response is similar to that seen in young adults. In fact, older adults often are more adherent with complicated HAART regimens than young adults. Treatment regimens and opportunistic infection prophylaxis with the HAART combination are similar to those used in younger persons. Indications that HIV therapies may accelerate atherosclerosis and glucose intolerance suggest that an aggressive approach to cardiovascular prevention in older HIV-infected adults is warranted and may lead to specific recommendations in older adults if associations of metabolic changes with specific HIV therapies become clearer.

HIV prevention is rarely discussed in the geriatric community but is important if the trend of increasing sexual acquisition of HIV in older adults is to be reversed. Most older women do not believe that they are at risk for HIV infection, yet heterosexual activity is the primary mode of infection in this group. The concept of HIV-risky behavior is not pervasive in the geriatric community because HIV was not a problem during their adolescence or young adulthood. Elderly persons must be included in educational programs aimed at ensuring safe sexual practices and increasing awareness of the benefits of testing and effective HIV therapy.

Miscellaneous Infectious Syndromes

Bacterial meningitis is most common at the extremes of life, and older adults account for the majority of meningitis-associated fatalities. *S. pneumoniae* remains the most common cause in older adults, but gram-negative bacilli (20% to 25%), *Listeria* spp. (up to 10%), and tuberculosis are more common than in young adults. Because many *S. pneumoniae* are now resistant to β-lactam antibiotics (up to 30% penicillin resistance and 10% ceftriaxone resistance nationwide), ceftriaxone or cefotaxime *plus* vancomycin are recommended as empiric therapy for bacterial meningitis in older adults until a specific isolate can be tested for antimicrobial susceptibility. Ampicillin is the drug of choice for *Listeria* spp., and more resistant gram-negative rods (eg, *Pseudomonas* spp.) require ceftazidime or an extended-spectrum penicillin with or without intrathecal aminoglycoside therapy.

Neurosyphilis remains one of the most perplexing diagnoses in medicine. It is often raised as a possible underlying process in stroke or dementia in older adults. Syphilis should also be considered in unilateral deafness, gait disturbances, uveitis, and optic neuritis. In reality, there is no gold-standard test to "rule out" neurosyphilis. Neurosyphilis can only be "ruled in" by such tests. However, suspicion is often first raised when a serum rapid plasma reagent or VDRL is positive. A reasonable diagnostic work-up after discovery of such a positive test includes confirmation of nonspecific tests (rapid plasma reagent and VDRL) with a specific test (microhemagglutination–*Treponema pallidum* [MHA-TP], or fluorescent treponemal antibody absorption [FTA-ABS]); if tests are confirmed, lumbar puncture should be performed for cell counts, glucose, protein, and cerebrospinal fluid VDRL. A positive cerebrospinal fluid VDRL is diagnostic of neurosyphilis, but the sensitivity of this test is approximately 75% in most series. Other diagnostic tests are controversial. The ratio of intrathecal to serum-specific treponemal antibody (standardized to the total immunoglobulin G in cerebrospinal fluid and serum) may also be helpful, with ratios of 3.0 or greater indicating likely infection. In the absence of these tests, it must be the judgment of a skilled clinician as to whether minor abnormalities in cerebrospinal fluid (eg, low-level pleocytosis) and the clinical picture support the diagnosis and warrant therapy for neurosyphilis. Optimal treatment of neurosyphilis remains penicillin G, but a study in HIV-infected patients suggests that ceftriaxone may be an acceptable alternative.

Advancing age is the major risk factor for reactivated varicella-zoster virus, herpes zoster or "shingles"; the most disabling complication, post-herpetic neuralgia, is common in elderly persons. (See "Dermatologic Diseases and Disorders," p 314, for diagnosis and treatment.) One study of a zoster vaccine indicates that it can reduce the risk of zoster and post-herpetic neuralgia by > 50%. Recommendations for use of this vaccine in specific age groups are likely to be put forth in the near future.

Facial nerve palsy (Bell's palsy) is common in older adults and associated with at least three infectious causes: herpes simplex virus, varicella zoster virus, and *Borrelia burgdorferi* (which causes Lyme disease). There are no strong data, at present, to suggest benefit of antiviral therapy for facial nerve palsies due to herpes simplex virus, but trials are under way. If facial nerve palsy occurs as part of an episode of varicella zoster virus, treatment is indicated (see "Dermatologic Diseases and Disorders," p 315) If Lyme disease is suspected on a clinical basis, the patient should receive oral amoxicillin, 500 mg four times a day for 14 days; or doxycycline, 100 mg twice a day for 14 days; or intravenous ceftriaxone, 2 g per day for 14 days.

Gastrointestinal infections are common among elderly persons. Diverticulitis, appendicitis, cholecystitis, intra-abdominal abscess, and ischemic bowel can present diagnostic dilemmas in the absence of fever or elevated white blood cell counts. A high index of suspicion is necessary in older adults. Computed tomography or labeled white cell studies are most likely to be of value in establishing the diagnosis of intra-abdominal infection, and ultrasound is an easy, readily available tool to assist in diagnosing cholecystitis, appendicitis, or abscess. Ischemic bowel often requires angiography.

Infectious diarrhea is also common in elderly persons. Older patients with achlorhydria are at particular risk because a lower bacterial inoculum is necessary to cause disease. Decreased intestinal motility associated with specific medications and advanced age may further increase susceptibility to infection. Epidemics occurring in the long-term-care setting are commonly due to *E. coli*, viruses, salmonellae, or *Shigella* spp. Frequent use of antimicrobials in older adults also increases the risk for *Clostridium difficile* colitis. Standard therapies for infectious diarrhea should be used in elderly patients.

FEVER OF UNKNOWN ORIGIN

Fever of unknown origin (FUO) is currently defined as temperature greater than 38.3°C (101°F) that lasts for at least 3 weeks and is undiagnosed after 1 week of medical evaluation. Several studies have examined this syndrome in elderly patients and demonstrated interesting differences between older and younger adults. The cause of FUO can be determined in more than 90% of cases in elderly persons, and one third have treatable infections, such as intra-abdominal abscess, bacterial endocarditis, tuberculosis, perinephric abscess, or occult osteomyelitis, with an incidence of infection similar to that in younger patients. In contrast, collagen vascular diseases are more common causes of FUO in elderly than in younger patients. These are primarily due to giant cell arteritis, polymyalgia rheumatica, and polyarteritis nodosa, but rarely due to Wegener's granulomatosis. In several published series, 28% of all FUOs in elderly persons were due to collagen vascular diseases (Table 44.4). Neoplastic disease accounts for another 20%, but, with rare

Table 44.4—Fever of Unknown Origin in Older Adults

Causes	Approximate % of Cases	
Infections	35	
Intra-abdominal abscess		12
Infective endocarditis		10
Other		7
Tuberculosis		6
Collagen vascular disorders	28	
Giant cell arteritis, polymyalgia rheumatica		19
Polyarteritis nodosa		6
Other		3
Malignancy	19	
Lymphoma		10
Carcinoma		9
Others (pulmonary emboli, drug fever)	9	
No diagnosis	5–10	

SOURCE: Data pooled from multiple studies: Esposito AL, Gleckman RA. Fever of unknown origin in the elderly. *J Am Geriatr Soc.* 1978;26(11):498; Knockaert DC, Vanneste LJ, Bobbaers HJ. Fever of unknown origin in elderly patients. *J Am Geriatr Soc.* 1993;41(11):1187–1192.

exceptions, fever due to cancer is primarily confined to hematologic malignancies (eg, lymphoma and leukemia), and not solid tumors. Drugs are another cause of FUO in elderly persons. Rare causes in this age group include deep-vein thrombosis with or without recurrent pulmonary emboli and hyperthyroidism.

A diagnostic approach to FUO in older adults is presented in Table 44.5.

Table 44.5—Evaluation of Fever of Unknown Origin in Older Adults

1. Confirm fever; conduct thorough history (include travel, MTB exposure, drugs, constitutional symptoms, symptoms of giant cell arteritis) and physical examination. Discontinue nonessential medications.

2. Initial laboratory evaluation: CBC with differential, liver enzymes, ESR, blood cultures × 3, PPD skin testing, TSH, antinuclear antibody, consider antineutrophilic cytoplasmic-antibody or HIV-antibody testing in specific cases.

3. a) Chest or abdomen or pelvic CT scan—if no obvious source; *or*

   b) Temporal artery biopsy—if symptoms or signs consistent with giant cell arteritis or polymyalgia rheumatica and increased ESR; *or*

   c) Site-directed work-up on basis of symptoms or laboratory abnormalities, or both.

4. If 3a is performed and no source is found, then 3b, and vice versa.

5. a) BM biopsy—yield best if hemogram abnormal—send for H&E, special stains, cultures, *or*

   b) Liver biopsy—very poor yield unless abnormal liver enzymes or hepatomegaly.

6. Indium-111 labeled white blood cell or gallium-67 scan—nuclear scans can effectively exclude infectious cause of FUO if negative.

7. Laparoscopy or exploratory laparotomy.

8. Empiric trial—typically reserved for antituberculosis therapy in rapidly declining host or high suspicion for tuberculosis (ie, prior [+] PPD).

NOTE: BM = bone marrow; CBC = complete blood cell count; CT = computed tomography; ESR = erythrocyte sedimentation rate; FUO = fever of unknown origin; HIV = human immunodeficiency virus; H&E = hematoxylin and eosin stain; MTB = *Mycobacterium tuberculosis*; PPD = (tuberculin) purified protein derivative; TSH = thyroid stimulating hormone.

ANNOTATED REFERENCES

- American Thoracic Society and Infectious Diseases Society of America. Guidelines for the management of adults with hospital-acquired, ventilator-associated, and health-care associated pneumonia. *Am J Respir Crit Care Med.* 2005;171(4):388–416.

  This guideline is a joint recommendation of the American Thoracic Society and Infectious Diseases Society of America. It is a very thorough review of the epidemiology, risk factors, diagnostic testing strategies, and treatment regimens for hospital- (HAP) and health-care-associated pneumonia (HCAP). The important findings suggest initial broad antimicrobial therapy with narrowing to pathogen-directed therapy on the basis of culture data whenever available. One major issue often missed when choosing an initial treatment regimen for HAP or HCAP in older adults is the inclusion of specific coverage for methicillin-resistant *Staphylococcus aureus* (MRSA) in persons known to be colonized with MRSA.

- Bentley DW, Bradley S, High K, et al. Practice guideline for evaluation of fever and infection in long-term care facilities. *J Am Geriatr Soc.* 2001;49(2):210–222.

  This comprehensive review of evaluation of fever in residents of long-term-care facilities is an evidence-based compilation of the available literature. The document was approved by the Infectious Diseases Society of America, the American Geriatrics Society, the Gerontological Society of America, and Society for Healthcare Epidemiology of America. It provides guidelines for definition of fever, clinical and laboratory evaluations, criteria for transfer to an acute-care facility, and suggested performance measures for evaluating adequacy of evaluation in long-term-care facilities.

- Ely EW, Angus DC, Williams MD, et al. Drotrecogin alfa (activated) treatment of older patients with severe sepsis. *Clin Inf Dis.* 2003;37(2):187–195.

  This is an analysis of patients with sepsis aged 75 years or older enrolled in the original randomized trials of activated protein C versus placebo. This is an important analysis because of the increased risk of bleeding in older adults, particularly catastrophic intracerebral bleeding. Older adults were found to have a higher incidence of bleeding than young adults, but the survival benefit of active drug versus placebo at 28 days and prior to discharge remained. The relative risk for death within 28 days was 0.68 (95% confidence interval 0.54 to 0.87) and for in-hospital death for patients treated with drotrecogin alfa was 0.70 (95% confidence interval 0.56 to 0.88).

- Loeb MB, Becker M, Eady A, et al. Interventions to prevent aspiration pneumonia in older adults: a systematic review. *J Am Geriatr Soc.* 2003;51(7):1018–1022.

  This evidence-based review comprehensively discusses the available literature on prevention of aspiration in elderly patients. The authors found insufficient data to determine the effectiveness of positioning strategies, modified diets, oral hygiene, or feeding-tube placement for preventing aspiration pneumonia, even though they are widely accepted as effective interventions. Interestingly, only the use of amantadine in nursing-home residents was clearly shown to reduce the risk of aspiration pneumonia and then only in a single trial.

- Lutters M, Vogt N. Antibiotic duration for treating uncomplicated, symptomatic lower urinary tract infections in elderly women. *Cochrane Database Syst Rev.* 2002;(3):CD001535.

  This examined single-dose, short-course (3–6 days) and long-course (7–14 days) therapy for uncomplicated urinary tract infection in older women. It has been widely accepted that 3-day therapy is adequate in young, sexually active adult women, but many practitioners have felt uncomfortable applying these data to older women. The authors conclude that single-dose therapy is less effective, but that there is no difference between short- and long-course therapy. The authors do point out that the quality of the evidence is rather poor and that additional studies would be helpful.

- Oxman MN, Levin MJ, Johnson GR, et al. A vaccine to prevent herpes zoster and postherpetic neuralgia in older adults. *N Engl J Med.* 2005;352(22):2271–2284.

  This landmark study in older adults, age 60 years and over, is the first to demonstrate an intervention that reduced the incidence and severity of zoster. This is a live-virus vaccine, based on the varicella vaccine used in children, but with much higher levels of virus. The vaccine reduces zoster by over 60%, and even if zoster occurs, it is less serious with less pain and post-herpetic neuralgia than the illness seen in unvaccinated patients.

- Perez JL, Moore RD. Greater effect of highly active antiretroviral therapy on survival in people aged ≥ 50 years compared with younger people in an urban observational cohort. *Clin Inf Dis.* 2003;36(2):212–218.

  Untreated human immunodeficiency virus (HIV) infection progresses more rapidly in older adults than in young adults (hazard ratio for death 2.4 for untreated older versus untreated younger adults). Treatment with highly active antiretroviral therapy (HAART) may be difficult in older adults since HAART has been associated with cardiovascular disease, dyslipidemia, osteoporosis, and major health issues in older adults, though a causal relationship has not been established and there are multiple drug-interaction and adherence issues to consider. Data presented in this and other studies suggest that the response and the antiviral and immune-enhancing effects of HAART in adults aged 50 years and older is at least equivalent to that of young adults, and perhaps better. Survival is greatly improved in HAART-treated versus untreated older adults.

- Thompson WW, Shay DK, Weintraub E, et al. Mortality associated with influenza and respiratory syncytial virus in the United States. *JAMA.* 2003;289(2):179–186.

  This report documents the extensive mortality associated with respiratory viral infection in the United States. Although the association is not new, the data in this study suggest that the magnitude of the association has been grossly underestimated. This is due to the fact that only underlying pneumonia and influenza deaths were previously reported. The new data take into account respiratory and circulatory deaths triggered by a respiratory viral illness. Ninety percent of influenza deaths and 78% of respiratory syncytial virus deaths occurred in persons aged 65 or older.

- Zimmerli W, Trampuz A, Ochsner PE. Prosthetic-joint infections. *N Engl J Med.* 2004;351(16):1645–1654.

  This is an outstanding, comprehensive review of prosthetic joint infection management outlining conservative and aggressive strategies, reporting success rates for each strategy that are based on a thorough literature review, and making antibiotic recommendations for specific pathogens. Importantly, conservation of function, not just cure of infection, are endpoints discussed and emphasized by different strategies.

Kevin Paul High, MD, MSc

CHAPTER 45—CARDIOVASCULAR DISEASES AND DISORDERS

KEY POINTS

- Coronary artery disease is the most common cause of death in persons aged 65 years and older. Autopsy studies show that 70% of persons older than 70 have the disease.

- Double-blind, randomized controlled studies have demonstrated that the absolute reduction in cardiovascular mortality and morbidity in elderly persons with dyslipidemia treated with statins is greater than for persons younger than 65 years.

- Heart failure is the most common cause of hospitalization and rehospitalization in persons aged 65 years and older. The prevalence and incidence increase with age.

- Atrial fibrillation is the most common type of arrhythmia in adults and is more common as patients age. Evidence-based recommendations for the management of newly detected atrial fibrillation now exist.

- Older adults with peripheral vascular disease are at increased risk for all-cause mortality, cardiovascular mortality, and mortality from coronary artery disease.

AGE-RELATED CARDIOVASCULAR CHANGES

See Table 45.1.

Table 45.1—Age-Related Changes That Affect Heart Action and Circulation

Structure or Function	Change With Age
Myocytes	Progressive loss of cells; hypertrophy
Left-ventricular stiffness	Increased
Left-ventricular compliance	Decreased
Left-ventricular wall thickness	Increased
Left-ventricular diastolic filling	Decreased, with increased contribution to filling resulting from left atrial systole
Left-ventricular relaxation	Decreased
Maximal heart rate	Progressive decrease
Maximal cardiac output	Progressive decrease
Maximal Vo_2	Progressive decrease
Systemic vascular resistance	Increased
Vasodilator response to exercise	Decreased
Ability to secrete sodium	Decreased

ISCHEMIC HEART DISEASE

Epidemiology

Coronary artery disease (CAD) is the most common cause of death in persons aged 65 years and older. Autopsy studies show that 70% of persons older than 70 years have CAD with $\geq$ 50% atherosclerotic obstruction of one or more coronary arteries. More than 30% of persons aged 65 years and older have clinical manifestations of CAD. In one study the prevalence of CAD among 1802 community-dwelling persons (mean age = 80 years) was 33% for the white Americans, 35% for the black Americans, 35% for the Hispanic Americans, and 38% for the Asian Americans. Eighty percent of deaths from CAD occur in persons aged 65 years and older; 60% of persons hospitalized with acute myocardial infarction (MI) are aged 65 years and older. The prevalence of CAD and the incidence of new coronary events are similar among men and women aged 75 years and older, but they are higher among men who are younger than 75. Eighty-three percent of MIs in women occur after menopause. Women are less likely than men to survive the initial MI.

CAD may be diagnosed in older persons if there is coronary angiographic evidence of significant CAD, a documented MI, a typical history of angina pectoris, or clinical findings of myocardial ischemia. The incidence of sudden cardiac death as the initial manifestation of CAD increases with age.

Risk Factors

It is important to address modifiable risk factors for CAD in older persons. Cessation of cigarette smoking,

treatment of hyperlipidemia, treatment of hypertension, ingestion of a diet low in saturated fat and cholesterol, maintenance of ideal body weight, and regular physical activity will lead to a reduction of CAD and new coronary events. Whether decreasing elevated plasma homocysteine levels by increasing folate supplements will reduce the incidence of new coronary events is not yet known.

If hypertension is present, lower blood pressure to < 140/90 mm Hg. If CAD is present and the serum low-density lipoprotein (LDL) cholesterol is > 125 mg/dL despite use of the American Heart Association (AHA) Step II diet, lipid-lowering drug therapy, preferably statin drug therapy, is recommended. The National Cholesterol Education Program Adult Treatment Panel (ATP) III guidelines have been updated and now recommend that physicians set an LDL goal of less than 70 mg/dL for very high-risk patients, on the basis of studies such as the Heart Protection Study. Very high-risk patients are those with diabetes mellitus and cardiovascular disease, acute coronary syndrome, or multiple severe or poorly controlled risk factors. In high-risk persons, the recommended LDL goal is < 100 mg/dL. High-risk persons are those with cardiovascular disease, diabetes mellitus, or a 10-year risk for CAD of > 20%. If a second lipid-lowering drug is needed in addition to a statin drug to achieve this, preferably the cholesterol absorption inhibitor ezetimibe or a bile acid resin such as colesevelam can be used.

The LDL goals for moderate and low-risk individuals currently remain the same: that is, < 130 mg/dL in older persons with two or more risk factors and a 10-year risk for CAD of 10% to 20%; less than 160 mg/dL for older persons with one or no risk factors.

It may be beneficial to treat hypertriglyceridemia in patients who also have hypercholesterolemia or hypoalphalipoproteinemia, or both. Possible indications for treatment of isolated hypertriglyceridemia include overt CAD, a strong family history of CAD, and multiple coexisting cardiac risk factors. Consider treating with gemfibrozil or nicotinic acid. Persons with CAD and a low serum high-density lipoprotein (HDL) cholesterol in the presence of a normal serum LDL cholesterol should be treated with gemfibrozil. These recommendations may need to be modified in the presence of comorbid conditions.

Presentation

In older persons, myocardial ischemia caused by CAD is more commonly manifested by dyspnea on exertion than by chest pain typical of angina pectoris. The dyspnea is caused by a transient increase in left ventricular (LV) end-diastolic pressure caused by ischemia superimposed on reduced ventricular compliance. Angina pectoris in older persons may cause pain in the back and shoulders or a burning epigastric pain. A substernal location of anginal pain is less commonly observed in older persons. The pain of angina pectoris in older persons may be described as less severe and of shorter duration. Myocardial ischemia may cause clinical heart failure. Acute pulmonary edema in older persons unassociated with acute MI may be a clinical manifestation of unstable angina pectoris resulting from extensive CAD.

In studies of older patients with clinically recognized acute MI, the prevalence of presenting symptoms ranged from 19% to 66% for chest pain, 20% to 59% for dyspnea, 15% to 33% for neurologic symptoms, and 0% to 19% for gastrointestinal symptoms. Other symptoms associated with acute MI in older persons include sudden death, peripheral gangrene, increased claudication, palpitations, kidney failure, weakness, pulmonary embolism, restlessness, and sweating. Older persons with acute MI are more likely than younger persons to die from the MI and to have pulmonary edema, heart failure (HF), LV systolic dysfunction, cardiogenic shock, conduction disturbances requiring insertion of a pacemaker, atrial fibrillation (AF) or atrial flutter, and rupture of the LV free wall, septum, or papillary muscle.

Diagnostic Testing

For terms on interpreting screening and diagnostic tests, see the Appendix, p 502.

Coronary angiography is the gold standard for detecting CAD and determining its severity. Resting electrocardiography (ECG) may be used to diagnose MI or ischemia, whether silent or symptomatic, in older persons. The diagnosis of CAD by treadmill exercise–induced ischemic ST-segment depression ≥ 1.0 mm in older persons has a sensitivity of 84% and a specificity of 70%. The diagnosis of CAD by upright bicycle exercise–induced ischemic ST-segment depression ≥ 1.0 mm in older persons has a sensitivity of 62% and a specificity of 93%. Older persons with the following are more likely to have multivessel CAD and a higher incidence of new coronary events:

- exercise-induced hypotension,
- an inadequate blood-pressure response to exercise,
- marked ischemic ST-segment depression (≥ 2.0 mm),
- ischemic ST-segment depression in both anterior and inferior leads,

- poor exercise duration (< 6 minutes using a standard Bruce treadmill protocol),
- ischemic ST-segment depression occurring within 6 minutes of exercise, and
- persistence of ST-segment depression past 8 minutes in the recovery period.

Older persons with CAD and complex ventricular arrhythmias or silent myocardial ischemia detected by 24-hour ambulatory ECG monitoring have a higher incidence of new coronary events.

Exercise stress testing using thallium perfusion scintigraphy or radionuclide ventriculography may be useful in the diagnosis and prognosis of CAD in older persons, especially for those in whom ST-segment changes cannot be reliably interpreted because of left bundle branch block, LV hypertrophy, or treatment with digitalis. In older persons unable to perform exercise stress testing because of musculoskeletal disorders or pulmonary disease, intravenous dipyridamole-thallium imaging may be used for the diagnosis and prognosis of CAD. The diagnosis of CAD by intravenous dipyridamole-thallium imaging in persons aged 70 years or older has a sensitivity of 86% and a specificity of 75%.

Echocardiography may be useful for detecting regional LV wall motion abnormalities, acute myocardial ischemia, and complications due to acute MI, LV aneurysm, cardiac thrombi, left main CAD, LV hypertrophy, and associated valvular heart disease; it is also useful for evaluating LV systolic and diastolic function and cardiac chamber size in older persons with CAD. Echocardiographic LV hypertrophy and abnormal LV ejection fraction are also associated with an increased incidence of new coronary events in older persons with CAD.

Stress echocardiography using exercise or dobutamine or adenosine is useful in diagnosing CAD and determining the prognosis in older persons. Exercise echocardiography has a sensitivity of 85% and a specificity of 77% in diagnosing CAD in older persons. In persons aged ≥ 70 years, dobutamine stress echocardiography has a sensitivity of 87%, a specificity of 84%, and an accuracy of 86%. In persons aged ≥ 70 years, adenosine stress echocardiography has a sensitivity of 66%, a specificity of 90%, and an accuracy of 73%.

The American College of Cardiology (ACC)/ American Heart Association (AHA) guidelines do not recommend electron-beam computed tomography for diagnosing obstructive CAD because of its low specificity. These guidelines also state that the published data do not answer the question of whether the electron-beam computed tomography score is additive to the Framingham score for defining CAD risk in asymptomatic persons.

Management

The management decisions described below are based on data from randomized controlled trials that included highly variable percentages of older persons. Few trials included older persons with serious comorbidities or frailty.

Stable Angina Pectoris

The physician needs to identify and correct reversible factors that can aggravate angina pectoris and myocardial ischemia, for example: anemia, infection, obesity, hyperthyroidism, uncontrolled hypertension, arrhythmias such as AF with a rapid ventricular rate, and severe valvular aortic stenosis. Smoking should be stopped. Treatment of hypertension and hyperlipidemia can be initiated. An exercise program will improve exercise tolerance. Aspirin 160 to 325 mg daily decreases the incidence of MI, stroke, and vascular death. Patients intolerant to aspirin can be treated with clopidogrel 75 mg daily to reduce the incidence of MI, stroke, and vascular death.

β-Blockers are effective antianginal agents and are the drug of choice to prevent myocardial ischemia. They reduce MI, sudden coronary death, and mortality, and they should be given to all persons with CAD without contraindications to β-blockers.

Nitrates relieve and prevent angina pectoris. Nitroglycerin administered as a sublingual tablet 0.3 to 0.6 mg or as a sublingual spray 0.4 mg is the drug most commonly used to relieve an acute anginal attack. Long-acting nitrates help prevent recurrent episodes of angina. A 12- to 14-hour nitrate-free interval every 24 hours is necessary to avoid nitrate tolerance. If anginal symptoms persist despite treatment with nitrates and β-blockers, a nondihydropyridine calcium channel blocker such as verapamil or diltiazem should be used in persons with normal LV ejection fraction, and amlodipine or felodipine should be used in persons with HF or abnormal LV ejection fraction.

If persons with stable angina have persistent angina interfering with their quality of life despite therapy with nitrates, β-blockers, and calcium channel blockers, consider coronary revascularization by coronary artery bypass graft (CABG) surgery or by percutaneous transluminal coronary angioplasty (PTCA).

Unstable Angina Pectoris and Non-Q-Wave Myocardial Infarction

Persons with unstable angina or non-Q-wave MI are generally admitted to a coronary care unit after treatment has been initiated in the emergency department. Reversible factors are then identified and corrected.

Continuous nasal oxygen should be administered at 1 to 2 liters per minute to persons with cyanosis, respiratory distress, HF, or high risk factors. Aspirin 75 to 325 mg should be given at admission and daily indefinitely. The first dose of aspirin is chewed. A loading dose of 300 mg of clopidogrel should be given at admission and continued in a dosage of 75 mg daily for 9 months. The combination of aspirin plus clopidogrel reduces the incidence of cardiovascular death, nonfatal MI, or stroke by 20% in comparison with aspirin plus placebo. In patients in whom PTCA is performed, the combination of aspirin plus clopidogrel has been shown to reduce the incidence of cardiovascular death, nonfatal MI, or urgent target-vessel revascularization within 30 days of PTCA by 30% in comparison with aspirin plus placebo.

Subcutaneous enoxaparin or dalteparin (low-molecular-weight heparins) can be used instead of unfractionated heparin for the acute phase of management of persons with non-Q-wave MI or unstable angina pectoris. Platelet glycoprotein IIb/IIIa receptor blockade with administration of abciximab is used for 12 to 24 hours in patients in whom PTCA is planned within the next 24 hours. Tirofiban or eptifibatide can be administered to patients with continuing myocardial ischemia, an elevated cardiospecific troponin I or T, or with other high-risk features in whom an invasive management is not planned.

Persons whose anginal symptoms are not fully relieved with three sublingual nitroglycerin tablets should be treated with continuous intravenous nitroglycerin for at least 24 hours. When the person is angina free for 24 hours, he or she can be switched to an oral or transdermal preparation of long-acting nitrates. β-Blockers, unless contraindicated, should be given in the emergency department, intravenously initially and then orally and continued indefinitely. Oral angiotensin-converting enzyme (ACE) inhibitors are another important element in the pharmacologic armamentarium, especially if diabetes mellitus, hypertension, HF, or abnormal LV ejection fraction is present, unless there are contraindications to its use. If the serum LDL cholesterol is ≥ 100 mg/dL 24 to 96 hours after hospitalization, a statin is indicated for long-term use.

Table 45.2 shows the ACC/AHA Class I indications for an early invasive strategy in the treatment of patients with unstable angina pectoris or non-Q-wave MI. Table 45.3 shows the ACC/AHA guidelines for coronary revascularization in the treatment of patients with unstable angina pectoris or non-Q-wave MI.

Acute Myocardial Infarction

Administer aspirin in a dosage of 160 mg to 325 mg daily as soon as acute MI is suspected and continue

Table 45.2—AAC/AHA Class I Indications for Early Invasive Treatment of Patients With Unstable Angina or Non-Q-Wave Myocardial Infarction Without Serious Comorbidity

- Recurrent angina or myocardial ischemia at rest or with low-level activities despite intensive anti-ischemic therapy

- Increased cardiospecific troponin T or I

- New or presumably new ST-segment depression

- Recurrent angina or myocardial ischemia with heart failure symptoms, an S_3 gallop, pulmonary edema, worsening rales, or new or worsening mitral regurgitation murmur

- High-risk findings on noninvasive stress testing

- Abnormal LV systolic function (LV ejection fraction < 40%)

- Hemodynamic instability

- Sustained ventricular tachycardia

- Percutaneous coronary intervention within 6 months

- Prior CABG surgery

NOTE: AAC = American College of Cardiology; AHA = American Heart Association; CABG = coronary artery bypass graft; LV = left ventricular.

SOURCE: Data from Braunwald E, Antman EM, Beasley JW, et al. ACC/AHA 2002 guideline update for the management of patients with unstable angina and non-ST-segment elevation myocardial infarction—summary article: a report of the American College of Cardiology/American Heart Association Task Force on Practice Guidelines (Committee on the Management of Patients With Unstable Angina). *J Am Coll Cardiol.* 2002;40(7):1366–1374.

Table 45.3—ACC/AHA Guidelines for Coronary Revascularization in the Treatment of Patients With Unstable Angina or Non-Q-Wave Myocardial Infarction

- CABG surgery is recommended for patients with left main CAD, three-vessel CAD, or two-vessel CAD with significant proximal left anterior descending CAD and either an LV ejection fraction < 50% or treated diabetes mellitus.

- PTCA or CABG surgery is recommended for patients with one-vessel CAD or two-vessel CAD without significant proximal left anterior descending CAD but with a large area of viable myocardium and high-risk criteria on noninvasive testing.

- PTCA is recommended for patients with multivessel CAD with a suitable coronary anatomy and with normal LV function and without diabetes mellitus.

NOTE: AAC = American College of Cardiology; AHA = American Heart Association; CABG = coronary artery bypass graft; CAD = coronary artery disease; LV = left ventricular; PTCA = percutaneous transluminal coronary angioplasty.

SOURCE: Data from Braunwald E, Antman EM, Beasley JW, et al. ACC/AHA guidelines for the management of patients with unstable angina and non-ST-segment elevation myocardial infarction: a report of the American College of Cardiology/American Heart Association Task Force on Practice Guidelines (Committee on the Management of Patients with Unstable Angina). *J Am Coll Cardiol.* 2000;36(3):970–1062.

indefinitely. The first dose of aspirin should be chewed. Clopidogrel 75 mg daily may be used in persons unable to tolerate aspirin. Intravenous metoprolol or atenolol (the two β-blockers approved by the Food and Drug Administration for intravenous use in acute MI) should be administered at admission to older persons with acute MI without contraindications to

β-blockers. Early intravenous blockade is followed by oral β-blocker therapy continued indefinitely to reduce the incidence of recurrent MI and mortality.

In the absence of contraindications, older persons with ischemic symptoms of at least 30 minutes' duration occurring within 6 to 12 hours of clinical presentation and with at least 1 to 2 mm of ST-segment elevation in two or more ECG leads or the presence of left bundle branch block are potential candidates for reperfusion therapy with either thrombolytic therapy or PTCA. Primary PTCA is the therapy of choice because it is associated with improved survival compared with thrombolytic therapy. There are also data which suggest that thrombolytic therapy increases mortality in patients older than 75 years of age with acute MI.

Intravenous heparin is recommended in persons with acute MI undergoing PTCA or CABG surgery and in persons with acute MI at high risk for systemic embolization, for example, persons with a large or anterior MI, AF, history of pulmonary or systemic embolus, or known LV thrombus. If intravenous heparin is not given, subcutaneous heparin is administered to reduce the incidence of deep-vein thrombosis.

Nitrates may be used for the treatment of chest pain and HF in older persons with acute MI. To reduce mortality, severe HF, or severe LV systolic dysfunction, use ACE inhibitors to treat persons with acute MI who are hemodynamically stable (systolic blood pressure ≥ 100 mm Hg) with HF, a large anterior MI, or an LV ejection fraction ≤ 40%. Calcium channel blockers are not recommended in the treatment of acute MI. Older persons taking calcium channel blockers before the onset of their acute MI should be switched to β-blockers at the time of their acute MI.

Prophylactic use of antiarrhythmic drugs other than β-blockers does not improve clinical outcome in persons with acute MI. The use of lidocaine during MI is limited to the treatment of life-threatening ventricular arrhythmias. Supraventricular tachyarrhythmias may be treated with β-blockers or direct-current cardioversion.

Treatment After Myocardial Infarction

Every attempt to control coronary risk factors must be made after MI. Aspirin 160 to 325 mg daily should be administered indefinitely. Long-term oral anticoagulant therapy is necessary as secondary prevention of MI in persons unable to tolerate daily aspirin or clopidogrel, in persons with persistent AF, and in persons with LV thrombus.

Persons without contraindications to β-blockers should receive them indefinitely after MI. Avoid β-blockers with intrinsic sympathomimetic activity. High-risk subgroups of persons with a history of MI (eg, all older persons and persons with HF, asymptomatic abnormal LV ejection fraction, complex ventricular arrhythmias, peripheral arterial disease, or diabetes mellitus) are most likely to benefit from the use of β-blockers.

ACE inhibitors are recommended for use indefinitely in older persons after MI unless there are specific contraindications to their use. Calcium channel blockers are not to be used after MI unless there is persistent angina pectoris despite the use of β-blockers and nitrates. On the basis of data from the Heart Estrogen-Progestin Replacement study, hormonal therapy is contraindicated in the treatment of postmenopausal women after MI.

β-Blockers are the only antiarrhythmic drugs that reduce mortality after MI. To reduce mortality in older persons with life-threatening ventricular tachycardia or ventricular fibrillation after MI, an automatic implantable cardioverter-defibrillator is indicated.

Risk Stratification After Myocardial Infarction

Clinical factors, including age and coronary risk factors, can be used to classify persons as high or low risk after MI (see Table 45.4). Exercise stress tests using thallium perfusion scintigraphy or radionuclide ventriculography and stress echocardiography using exercise or dobutamine or adenosine are useful for classifying persons as high or low risk after MI.

After MI, older persons with spontaneous episodes of myocardial ischemia or episodes of myocardial ischemia provoked by minimal exertion, before treatment of a mechanical complication of MI (eg, acute mitral valve regurgitation, postinfarction septal deficit, left ventricular free wall rupture, or ventricular aneurysm), or with persistent hemodynamic instability can be referred for coronary angiography and consideration of coronary revascularization.

Coronary Revascularization After Myocardial Infarction

The benefits of revascularization in older persons after MI are prolongation of life and relief of unacceptable symptoms that persist despite optimal medical management.

CABG surgery can improve survival in patients with significant left main CAD; in patients with significant three-vessel CAD, especially if decreased LV ejection fraction and myocardial ischemia are present; in patients with significant two-vessel CAD, proximal left anterior descending CAD, and decreased LV ejection fraction; in diabetic patients with multivessel

Table 45.4—Factors Predicting a High Risk of New Coronary Events in Older Persons With a History of Myocardial Infarction

Findings on Echocardiogram

- Abnormal LV ejection fraction detected by echocardiography or radionuclide ventriculography
- Echocardiographic LV hypertrophy

Findings on ECG

- Abnormal signal-averaged ECG
- Complex ventricular arrhythmias or silent myocardial ischemia detected by a 24-hour ambulatory ECG
- Ischemic ST-segment depression on a resting ECG

Findings on Exercise Tolerance Testing

- Exercise-induced hypotension
- Exercise-induced ischemic ST-segment depression in both anterior and inferior leads
- Exercise-induced marked ischemic ST-segment depression (≥ 2 mm)
- Inadequate blood-pressure response to exercise
- Ischemic ST-segment depression occurring within 6 minutes of exercise
- Persistence of exercise-induced ST-segment depression past 8 minutes in the recovery period
- Poor exercise duration (< 6 minutes using a standard Bruce treadmill protocol)

NOTE: ECG = electrocardiogram; LV = left ventricular.

CAD; and in patients with clinical evidence of HF during ischemic episodes with ischemic but viable myocardium.

PTCA with stenting is preferred in the severely symptomatic patient with significant one-vessel or two-vessel CAD and a normal LV ejection fraction, in patients with multiple medical problems including prior MI, if the patient is at increased risk for developing stroke because of cerebrovascular disease or diffuse aortic disease, if the patient is at increased risk for developing postoperative cognitive dysfunction, and if the patient is frail. See Table 45.3.

DYSLIPIDEMIA

Double-blind, randomized controlled studies have demonstrated that the absolute reduction in cardiovascular mortality and morbidity in older persons with dyslipidemia treated with statins is greater than for persons younger than 65 years of age. In older persons with prior MI and a serum LDL cholesterol of ≥ 125 mg/dL, statins have been demonstrated to reduce new coronary events in persons aged 60 to 100 years and new stroke in persons aged 60 to 90 years. Older persons in whom the serum LDL cholesterol was reduced to < 90 mg/dL had the greatest reduction in new coronary events and in stroke. In the Cardiovascular Health Study, at 7.3-year follow-up of 1250 women and 664 men aged 65 to 80 years with hypercholesterolemia and free of cardiovascular disease, statins were found to significantly reduce all-cause mortality by 44% and cardiovascular events by 56%.

See Table 45.5 and Table 45.6 for treatment indications and drug regimens.

Heart Failure

Epidemiology and Etiology

HF is the most common cause of hospitalization and rehospitalization in persons aged 65 years and older. The prevalence and incidence of HF increase with age. CAD, hypertension, valvular heart disease, and cardiomyopathies are the most common causes of HF in older persons.

Not only do older persons experience an age-related decrease in LV diastolic relaxation and early LV diastolic filling (see Table 45.1), they are more likely to have LV diastolic dysfunction because they have an increased prevalence of hypertension, myocardial ischemia due to CAD, LV hypertrophy due to hypertension, valvular aortic stenosis, hypertrophic cardiomyopathy, and other cardiac disorders. In older persons, the increased stiffness of the LV and prolonged LV relaxation time impair LV early diastolic filling and cause higher LV end-diastolic pressures at rest and during exercise.

In HF associated with LV diastolic dysfunction with normal LV systolic function, the LV ejection fraction is ≥ 50%. The prevalence of a normal LV ejection fraction associated with HF increases with age and is higher in older women than in older men. During exercise, persons with normal LV systolic function but abnormal LV diastolic function are unable to normally increase stroke volume, even in the presence of increased LV filling pressure. Myocardial hypertrophy, ischemia, or fibrosis causes slow or incomplete LV filling at normal left atrial pressures. Left atrial pressure rises to increase LV filling, resulting in pulmonary and systemic venous congestion. The development of AF (the prevalence of which increases with age) may also cause a decrease in cardiac output and the development of pulmonary and systemic venous congestion, because of the loss of left atrial contribution to LV late diastolic filling and reduced diastolic filling time due to a rapid ventricular rate.

In HF associated with LV systolic dysfunction, the LV ejection fraction is < 50%. The amount of myocardial fiber shortening is reduced, the stroke volume is decreased, the LV is dilated, and the patient is symptomatic.

The physician must measure LV ejection fraction in all persons with HF, preferably by echocardiography (because of the additional information provided, eg, the presence and severity of valvular heart disease, LV thrombus), in order to determine appropriate therapy for HF.

Presentation

Increased pulmonary capillary wedge pressure causes pulmonary congestion, resulting in dyspnea. Dyspnea

Table 45.5—Treatment Indications for Dyslipidemia

Risk Category	Conditions	LDL-Cholesterol Goal	Initiate Nonpharmacologic Management	Consider Drug Therapy
Low	0–1 risk factor*	< 160 mg/dL	≥ 160 mg/dL	≥ 190 mg/dL; optional: 160–189 mg/dL
Moderate	2+ risk factors; 10-year CAD risk < 10%†	< 130 mg/dL	≥ 130 mg/dL	≥ 160 mg/dL
Moderately high	2+ risk factors; 10-year CAD risk 10%–20%†	< 130 mg/dL	≥ 130 mg/dL	≥ 130 mg/dL; optional: 100–129 mg/dL
High	CVD‡, DM, or 10-year CAD risk > 20%†	< 100 mg/dL	≥ 100 mg/dL	≥ 100 mg/dL
Very high	DM + CVD‡; acute coronary syndrome; multiple severe or poorly controlled risk factors	< 70 mg/dL	≥ 100 mg/dL	≥ 100 mg/dL; optional: 70–99 mg/dL

NOTE: CAD = coronary artery disease; CVD = cardiovascular disease; DM = diabetes mellitus; HDL = high-density lipoprotein; LDL = low-density lipoprotein.

* Risk factors are cigarette smoking, hypertension, HDL < 40 mg/dL, family history of premature CAD, male age ≥ 45 years, female age ≥ 55 years.

† Calculation of 10-year risk of CAD is available at http://www.nhlbi.nih.gov/guidelines/cholesterol/ (accessed October 2005).

‡ CVD is signified by CAD, angina, peripheral artery disease, transient ischemic attack, stroke, abdominal aortic aneurysm, or 10-year CAD risk > 20%.

SOURCE: Reuben DB, Herr KA, Pacala JT, et al. *Geriatrics At Your Fingertips: 2006*, 8th ed. New York: American Geriatrics Society; 2006:30. Reprinted with permission.

Table 45.6—Drug Regimens for Dyslipidemia

Condition	Drug	Dosage	Formulations
Elevated LDL, normal TG	Statin (HMG-CoA reductase inhibitor*):		
	Atorvastatin	10–80 mg qd	T: 10, 20, 40, 80
	Fluvastatin	20–80 mg qd in PM, max 80 mg	C: 20, 40; T: ER 80
	Lovastatin	10–40 mg qd in PM or bid	T: 10, 20, 40
	Pravastatin	10–40 mg qd	T: 10, 20, 40, 80
	Rosuvastatin	10–40 mg qd	T: 5, 10, 20, 40
	Simvastatin	5–80 mg qd in PM	T: 5, 10, 20, 40, 80
Elevated TG (> 500 mg/dL)	Fenofibrate	54–160 mg qd	T: 54, 160
	Gemfibrozil	300–600 mg po bid	T: 600
	Omega-3-acid ethyl esters	4 g/d in single or divided doses	C: 1 g
Combined elevated LDL, low HDL, elevated TG	Fenofibrate, gemfibrozil, or HMG-CoA if TG < 300 mg/dL	as above	as above
Alternative for any of above	Niacin†	100 mg tid to start; increase to 500–1000 mg tid; ER 150 mg qhs to start, increase to 2000 mg qhs as needed	T: 25, 50, 100, 250, 500, ER 150, 250, 500, 750, 1000; C: TR 125, 250, 400, 500
Elevated LDL or combined with inadequate response to one agent	Lovastatin/niacin combination*†	20 mg/500 mg qhs to start; increase to 40 mg/2000 mg as needed	T: 20/500, 20/750, 20/1000
	Colesevelam	Monotherapy: 1850 mg po bid; combination therapy: 2500–3750 mg/d in single or divided doses	T: 625
	Ezetimibe	10 mg qd	T: 10
	Ezetimibe/simvastatin* combination	1 tab qd	T: 10/10, 10/20, 10/40, 10/80

NOTE: bid = twice a day; C = capsule; d = day; ER = extended release; HDL = high-density lipoprotein; LDL = low-density lipoprotein; max = maximum; po = by mouth; qd = once a day; qhs = each bedtime; T = tablet; TG = triglycerides; tid = three times a day.

*Measure transaminases at baseline and at 3 months, then periodically. Watch for statin-induced myopathy, usually presenting as diffuse, symmetric myalgias. If myopathy is suspected (higher risk at higher statin doses or in combination with fenofibrate, gemfibrozil, or niacin), measure creatinine phosphokinase and transaminases; creatinine phosphokinase levels above 10 times the upper limit of normal indicate serious myopathy or rhabdomyolysis. Even if creatinine phosphokinase and transaminases are normal, myalgias still may be due to statin; if this is the case, myalgias should disappear within 1 week of discontinuing statin.

† Monitor for flushing, pruritus, nausea, gastritis, ulcer. Dosage increases should be spaced 1 month apart. Aspirin 325 mg po 30 minutes before first niacin dose of the day is quite effective in preventing adverse events.

SOURCE: Reuben DB, Herr KA, Pacala JT, et al. *Geriatrics At Your Fingertips: 2006,* 8th ed. New York: American Geriatrics Society; 2006: pp 30–31. Reprinted with permission.

may progress from exertional dyspnea to orthopnea, to paroxysmal nocturnal dyspnea, to dyspnea at rest, and to the development of acute pulmonary edema. Pulmonary congestion may cause coughing and wheezing. Decreased cardiac output may cause weakness, a feeling of heaviness in the limbs, nocturia, oliguria, confusion, insomnia, headache, anxiety, memory impairment, bad dreams or nightmares, and, rarely, psychotic manifestations. Congestive hepatomegaly may cause epigastric or right upper quadrant heaviness or a dull ache, a sense of fullness after eating, anorexia, nausea, and vomiting.

LV failure with transudation of fluid into the alveoli causes moist rales, which are heard over the lung bases posteriorly. Congestion of bronchial mucosa causes rhonchi and wheezes. During acute pulmonary edema, coarse, bubbling rales and wheezes are heard over the lung fields. Signs of pleural effusion may occur with left or right ventricular failure. Systemic venous hypertension causes distention of the jugular veins.

Right ventricular failure may cause an enlarged, tender liver and ascites. Compression of the liver causes the hepatojugular reflux sign. Pressure applied to the middle of the abdomen can cause abdominal jugular reflux sign. A pulsating liver indicates tricuspid regurgitation. Right ventricular failure causes edema that first occurs in the dependent parts of the body. Severe right ventricular failure will cause anasarca.

An LV third heart sound (best heard at the apex) and jugular venous distention are the most sensitive and specific physical findings in HF. Most persons with HF have cardiomegaly. However, HF may develop in persons with acute MI or other conditions before the heart has had a chance to enlarge. Heart murmurs due to valvular heart disease may become faint or absent because of a low cardiac output. Physical examination cannot distinguish between HF associated with abnormal and HF associated with normal LV ejection fraction.

Chest radiographs should be obtained for all persons with suspected HF and will show pulmonary vascular congestion in those with LV failure. When the pulmonary capillary pressure reaches 20 to 25 mm Hg, interstitial pulmonary edema is present. When the pulmonary capillary pressure exceeds 25 mm Hg, alveolar edema and pleural effusion occur.

Older persons, especially women, without HF have higher B-type natriuretic peptide (BNP) levels than younger persons. There is no significant difference in BNP levels between older women with HF and those without HF. BNP levels do not help distinguish older persons with HF with abnormal LV ejection fraction from those with normal LV ejection fraction, although the former group tends to have higher BNP levels. The use of BNP levels in the evaluation of acute HF does not aid in the treatment of older persons.

Management

Precipitating causes of HF, such as excess sodium ingestion, myocardial ischemia, infection, anemia, fever, hypoxia, tachyarrhythmias, bradyarrhythmias, hyperthyroidism, hypothyroidism, and obesity must be identified and treated. Sodium intake should be decreased to 1.6 g (4 g of sodium chloride) daily. Drugs known to precipitate or aggravate HF, such as nonsteroidal anti-inflammatory drugs, calcium channel blockers, and most antiarrhythmic drugs, should be withdrawn.

It is important to identify the underlying causes of HF and treat when possible. Persons with myocardial ischemia due to severely stenotic coronary arteries without contraindications to coronary revascularization who have exercise-limiting angina, frequent episodes of angina occurring at rest, or recurrent episodes of acute pulmonary edema despite optimal medical management can be referred for coronary angiography with CABG surgery or PTCA. Surgical correction of valvular lesions and surgical excision of a dyskinetic LV aneurysm is a potential intervention for some persons with HF.

Anticoagulants should be given if there is prior systemic or pulmonary embolism, AF, or cardiac thrombi detected by echocardiography. Persons with HF who have complete atrioventricular block or severe

bradycardia are candidates for a transvenous pacemaker implanted into the right ventricle.

Persons with HF who are dyspneic at rest or at a low work level may benefit from a formal cardiac rehabilitation program. Disease management strategies, either self-or nurse-directed, have been shown to be effective at reducing rehospitalization rates among older persons with HF. Frequent weighing, careful attention to symptoms, and adjustment of diuretic dosing are components of HF disease management.

Angiotensin-Converting Enzyme Inhibitors

ACE inhibitors improve symptoms, quality of life, and exercise tolerance, and they decrease mortality and hospitalization for HF in persons with HF associated with abnormal LV ejection fraction. A review of 32 randomized trials of ACE inhibitors in persons with HF and abnormal LV ejection fraction revealed that ACE inhibitors have been found to significantly reduce total mortality by 23% and mortality or hospitalization for HF by 35%. ACE inhibitors should be administered to all persons with HF and abnormal LV ejection fraction unless there are specific contraindications to their use.

ACE inhibitors also improve symptoms, exercise tolerance, and LV systolic and diastolic function in persons with HF and normal LV ejection fraction. ACE inhibitors are indicated for persons with HF and normal LV ejection fraction if HF persists despite diuretic and β-blocker therapy. One study reported that persons with HF and normal LV ejection fraction treated with ACE inhibitors for 6 months had a 63% significant reduction in mortality if the LV ejection fraction was 40% to 49% and a 39% insignificant reduction in mortality if the LV ejection fraction was ≥ 50%. In this study, ACE inhibitors significantly improved quality-of-life scores in patients with LV ejection fractions of 40% to 49% and ≥ 50%.

Asymptomatic hypotension with a systolic blood pressure between 80 and 90 mm Hg and a serum creatinine level that increases but is < 2.5 mg/dL are side effects of ACE inhibitors that should not necessarily cause cessation of this drug, but require the physician to decrease the dose of diuretic if the jugular venous pressure is normal and to consider reducing the dose of ACE inhibitor. Contraindications to the use of ACE inhibitors are symptomatic hypotension, progressive azotemia, angioneurotic edema, hyperkalemia, intolerable cough, and rash.

Angiotensin II Type 1 Receptor Antagonists

Studies have found that older patients with HF and abnormal LV ejection fraction treated with losartan have fewer adverse effects, such as cough, rash, or altered taste sensation, than do patients treated with captopril. In the second Evaluation of Losartan in the Elderly study, patients with HF and abnormal LV ejection fraction treated with losartan or with captopril were found to have a similar mortality and hospitalization for HF. This study found a significant reduction in mortality in persons receiving captopril who were also receiving β-blockers. Older persons with HF should be treated with an angiotensin II type 1 receptor antagonist if they are unable to tolerate ACE inhibitors because of cough, rash, altered taste sensation, or angioneurotic edema. Treatment with a β-blocker plus an ACE inhibitor plus an angiotensin II type 1 receptor blocker is not recommended because the Valsartan Heart Failure Trial showed that administration of these three drugs together significantly increases mortality.

β-Blockers

Chronic administration of β-blockers after MI reduces mortality, sudden cardiac death, and recurrent MI, especially in older persons. These benefits are more marked in persons with a history of HF. One study showed that after 6 to 12 months of therapy, carvedilol caused a 65% significant reduction in mortality in patients with HF and abnormal LV ejection fraction treated with diuretics, ACE inhibitors, and digoxin. At 1-year follow-up of those with New York Heart Association class II, III, or IV HF and abnormal LV ejection fraction who were treated with diuretics, ACE inhibitors, and optional digoxin, metoprolol CR/XL was shown to cause a 34% significant reduction in mortality. Older persons with HF and abnormal LV ejection fraction should be treated with diuretics, ACE inhibitors, and β-blockers.

β-Blockers are beneficial in the treatment of HF associated with normal LV ejection fraction by:

- reducing the ventricular rate to < 90 beats per minute, thereby increasing LV diastolic filling time and causing an increase in LV end-diastolic volume;
- decreasing myocardial ischemia;
- reducing elevated blood pressure;
- decreasing LV mass; and
- improving LV relaxation.

The increase in ventricular rate that occurs with exercise can also be prevented with modest doses of β-blockers, especially in older persons.

β-Blockers have also been demonstrated at 32-month follow-up of elderly patients with New York Association class II or III HF and a normal LV ejection fraction treated with diuretics and ACE inhibitors to significantly reduce mortality by 35%.

β-Blockers along with loop diuretics should be used to treat older persons with HF and normal LV ejection fraction.

Diuretics

Diuretics are used in the treatment of HF associated with abnormal or normal LV ejection fraction. Mild HF may be treated with a thiazide diuretic. However, the thiazide diuretic is ineffective if the glomerular filtration rate is < 30 mL per minute. Older persons with moderate or severe HF should be treated with a loop diuretic such as furosemide. Persons with severe HF or concomitant renal insufficiency may need metolazone in addition to the loop diuretic. The minimum effective dose of diuretic should be given. Older persons with HF associated with abnormal LV ejection fraction tolerate higher doses of diuretics than do older persons with normal LV ejection fraction. Older persons with HF and normal LV ejection fraction need high LV filling pressures to maintain an adequate stroke volume and cardiac output, and they cannot tolerate intravascular depletion.

Aldosterone Antagonists

One study showed that among persons with severe HF and abnormal LV ejection fraction who were treated with diuretics, ACE inhibitors, and digoxin, those randomized to spironolactone 25 mg daily had a 30% significant decrease in mortality and a 35% significant reduction in hospitalization for HF at 2-year follow-up. However, only 10% of patients were treated with β-blockers. In the Eplerenone Post-Acute Myocardial Infarction Heart Failure Efficacy and Survival Study, 86% of patients were treated with ACE inhibitors or angiotensin II type 1 receptor blockers and 75% with β-blockers. In comparison with placebo, eplerenone significantly reduced mortality by 15%. The ACC/AHA guidelines recommend (with a Class IIa indication) the use of an aldosterone antagonist in patients with systolic HF and class IV symptoms despite diuretics, ACE inhibitors, β-blockers, and digoxin, preserved kidney function, and normal serum potassium.

Digoxin

Digoxin may be used in the treatment of older persons with HF and supraventricular tachyarrhythmias such as AF. In the Digitalis Investigator Group trial, digoxin in comparison with placebo was found to significantly increase mortality by 23% in women with HF and an abnormal LV ejection fraction. In this study, in men with HF and an abnormal LV ejection fraction, digoxin was found to significantly reduce mortality by 6% if the serum digoxin level was 0.5 to 0.8 ng/mL, insignificantly increase mortality by 3% if the serum digoxin level was 0.9 to 1.1 ng/mL, and significantly increase mortality by 12% if the serum digoxin level was ≥ 1.2 ng/mL. On the basis of these data, digoxin can be administered to men with HF and an abnormal LV ejection fraction if they have persistent HF despite diuretics, ACE inhibitors, and β-blockers. However, the serum digoxin level must be maintained between 0.5 to 0.8 ng/mL.

Digoxin should not be used for treating persons with HF in sinus rhythm associated with a normal LV ejection fraction. By increasing contractility through an increased intracellular calcium concentration, digoxin may increase LV stiffness in these persons, increasing LV filling pressure and aggravating HF with normal LV ejection fraction. In the Digitalis Investigator Group trial, digoxin was found to insignificantly increase all-cause hospitalization by 4% in patients with HF and a normal LV ejection fraction.

Isorbide Dinitrate Plus Hydralazine

The combination of oral isosorbide dinitrate and hydralazine may be beneficial in the treatment of HF and abnormal or normal LV ejection fraction. Isosorbide dinitrate plus hydralazine is indicated if:

- HF with abnormal ejection fraction persists despite treatment with diuretics, ACE inhibitors, β-blockers, and digoxin, or
- HF with normal LV ejection fraction persists despite treatment with diuretics, β-blockers, and ACE inhibitors.

The ACC/AHA guidelines recommend with a Class IIa indication the use of isosorbide dinitrate plus hydralazine in patients with HF who cannot be given an ACE inhibitor or angiotensin II type 1 receptor blocker because of hypotension or renal insufficiency.

Calcium Channel Blockers

Calcium channel blockers such as nifedipine, diltiazem, and verapamil exacerbate HF in patients with HF and abnormal LV ejection fraction. Studies show that diltiazem significantly increases mortality in patients with pulmonary congestion and abnormal LV ejection fraction after MI and that the vasoselective calcium channel blockers amlodipine and felodipine do not significantly affect survival in patients with HF and abnormal LV ejection fraction. In these studies, a significantly higher incidence of pulmonary edema and peripheral edema was observed in patients treated with amlodipine than in those treated with placebo, and a significantly higher incidence of peripheral edema was observed in patients treated with felodipine than in those treated with placebo. Therefore, calcium channel blockers are not indicated in older persons with HF and abnormal LV ejection fraction. However, calcium channel blockers may be given to persons with HF and normal LV ejection fraction if they have persistent HF despite the use of diuretics and are unable to tolerate β-blockers, ACE inhibitors, and isosorbide dinitrate plus hydralazine. Felodipine is the only calcium channel blocker labeled for the treatment of heart failure by the Food and Drug Administration.

Self-Management

The number-one cause of recidivism in HF patients is volume and sodium retention. Patients must be instructed to adhere to a low-sodium diet. They need to weigh themselves daily and call the primary care clinician immediately if they gain more than 2 pounds in 1 day. Over-the-counter drugs to avoid that can exacerbate sodium and fluid retention include sodium-based antacids, high-dose aspirin, nonsteroidal anti-inflammatory drugs, ginseng (germanium), ginkgo, echinacea, and decongestants. Black licorice has the same effect.

VALVULAR HEART DISEASE

Valvular Aortic Stenosis

Valvular aortic stenosis (AS) in older persons is usually due to stiffening, scarring, and calcification of the valve leaflets.

Angina pectoris, syncope or near syncope, and HF are the three classic manifestations of severe AS. Doppler echocardiography is used to diagnose AS and determine the severity.

Older persons with AS have an increased incidence of new coronary events; those with symptomatic severe AS have a poor prognosis. However, those with asymptomatic severe AS are at low risk for death and can be followed until symptoms develop.

The American Heart Association guidelines for the use of prophylactic antibiotics to prevent bacterial endocarditis are available at http://www.amhrt.org. Older persons with HF, exertional syncope, or angina associated with moderate or severe AS can be considered for aortic valve replacement. Persons with asymptomatic AS should report the development of symptoms possibly related to AS immediately to their physicians. Use nitrates with caution in persons with AS and angina to prevent orthostatic hypotension and syncope; vasodilators should be avoided. Prescribe diuretics cautiously in persons with AS and HF to prevent a decrease in cardiac output and hypotension.

If LV systolic dysfunction in persons with severe AS is associated with critical narrowing of the aortic valve rather than with myocardial fibrosis, it often improves after successful aortic valve replacement. Balloon aortic valvuloplasty is a potential intervention for older persons with symptomatic severe AS who are not candidates for aortic valve surgery and possibly for persons with severe LV dysfunction as a bridge to subsequent aortic valve surgery.

Aortic Regurgitation

Acute aortic regurgitation (AR) in older persons may be due to infective endocarditis, rheumatic fever, aortic dissection, trauma following prosthetic valve surgery, or rupture of the sinus of Valsalva. It causes sudden severe HF. Chronic AR in older persons may be caused by aortic valve leaflet disease (secondary to any cause of AS, infective endocarditis, rheumatic fever, congenital heart disease, rheumatoid arthritis, ankylosing spondylitis, following prosthetic valve surgery, or myxomatous degeneration of the valve) or by aortic root disease.

The prevalence of AR increases with age; in one study it was found to be 31% among 554 older men and 28% among 1243 older women. The AR murmur is typically a high-pitched blowing diastolic murmur that begins immediately after the aortic second sound. The diastolic murmur is best heard along the left sternal border in the third and fourth intercostal spaces when AR is due to valvular disease and is best heard along the right sternal border when AR is due to dilatation of the ascending aorta. The severity of AR correlates with the duration of the diastolic murmur, not with the intensity of the murmur. Doppler echocardiography is used to diagnose the presence and severity of AR.

Persons with acute AR develop symptoms as a consequence of the sudden onset of HF. Persons with acute AR should have immediate aortic valve replacement because death may occur within hours to days. Persons with chronic AR may be asymptomatic for many years. The prognosis of older persons with HF and severe AR is poor.

Prophylactic antibiotics should be used to prevent bacterial endocarditis in older persons with chronic AR, according to American Heart Association guidelines (available at http://www.amhrt.org). Older persons with asymptomatic chronic severe AR should be treated with ACE inhibitors to reduce the LV volume overload. Echocardiographic evaluation of LV end-systolic dimension should be performed yearly if the measurement is < 50 mm, but every 3 to 6 months if the measurement is 50 to 54 mm. Aortic valve replacement should be considered if the LV end-systolic dimension exceeds 55 mm, even in the absence of cardiac symptoms. Aortic valve replacement should also be considered when the LV ejection fraction approaches 50% before the decompensated state.

Mitral Regurgitation

One study found mitral regurgitation (MR) to be present in 32% of 554 older men and in 33% of 1243 older women. The most common cause of MR in older persons is mitral annular calcium deposition. Other disorders causing MR in older persons include CAD, mitral valve prolapse, and rheumatic heart disease. Symptoms associated with severe MR are primarily those of HF, especially dyspnea. The heart murmur associated with MR is heard as an apical holosystolic murmur, late systolic murmur, or early systolic murmur beginning with the first heart sound but ending in mid-systole. The presence of an LV third heart sound suggests that the MR is severe. Doppler echocardiography is used to diagnose the presence and monitor the severity of MR.

In MR, the LV ejection fraction should be > 55% to 60% and the LV end-systolic dimension < 45 mm. Mitral valve surgery should be considered in older persons with New York Heart Association class III or IV symptoms caused by MR or in older persons with severe MR and an LV ejection fraction < 50% or an LV end-systolic dimension above 45 to 50 mm.

Mitral Stenosis

The most common cause of mitral stenosis (MS) in older persons is mitral annular calcium. The prevalence of MS in older adults is low. Older persons with MS have a low-pitched mid-diastolic murmur heard at the point of maximum apical impulse with or without presystolic accentuation. Doppler echocardiography is used to diagnose the presence and severity of MS.

Long-term oral warfarin therapy to reduce thromboembolic events must be considered for all older persons with MS, especially those with AF. Mitral valvular surgery or valvuloplasty may be indicated if the person has recurrent embolization on anticoagulants. A β-blocker will slow the ventricular rate if AF is present. Diuretics will control congestive symptoms.

In the absence of clot, MR, and severe subvalvular involvement, the therapy of choice for symptomatic MS is balloon valvuloplasty. However, many older persons with symptomatic MS have poor valve morphology for valvuloplasty (heavy calcification) and require mitral valve replacement. Older persons with MS and a critical valve area of 1.0 cm^2 need interventional therapy. Mitral valve replacement is usually necessary since stenotic mitral valves in older persons are

ARRHYTHMIAS

Ventricular Arrhythmias

The presence of three or more consecutive ventricular premature complexes on an ECG is diagnosed as ventricular tachycardia (VT). VT is considered sustained if it lasts $\geq$ 30 seconds and nonsustained if its lasts < 30 seconds. Complex ventricular arrhythmias (VAs) include VT or paired, multiform, or frequent ($\geq$ 30 per hour on a 24-hour ambulatory ECG or $\geq$ 6 per minute on a 1-minute rhythm strip of an ECG) ventricular premature complexes. Researchers using a 24-hour ambulatory ECG to detect VAs in older persons found a prevalence of 10% for nonsustained VT (N = 554) and a rate of 55% for complex VAs (N = 843).

Nonsustained VT and complex VA are not associated with an increased incidence of new coronary events in older persons with no clinical evidence of heart disease, and asymptomatic persons should not be treated with antiarrhythmic drugs. Simple VA (ie, VAs that are not paired, multiform, or frequent) in older persons with heart disease should also not be treated with antiarrhythmic drugs. Nonsustained VT and complex VA are associated with an increased incidence of new coronary events in older persons with heart disease, especially in those with abnormal LV ejection fraction, LV hypertrophy, or silent myocardial ischemia.

Available data show that older persons with nonsustained VT or complex VA and heart disease should be treated with β-blockers if there are no contraindications. They should not be treated with any of the class I antiarrhythmic drugs (ie, encainide, flecainide, lorcainide, moricizine, propafenone, quinidine, procainamide, disopyramide, mexiletine, phenytoin, or tocainide), calcium channel blockers, d-sotalol, or d,l-sotalol. Amiodarone was found to not reduce mortality in persons with VT or complex VA associated with prior MI or HF, and it had a high incidence of toxicity.

Analysis of data from the Cardiac Arrhythmia Suppression Trial showed that β-blockers are an independent factor for decreasing arrhythmic death or cardiac arrest by 40%, for reducing all-cause mortality by 33%, and for decreasing occurrence of new or worsened HF by 32%. However, the automatic implantable cardioverter-defibrillator (AICD) is the most effective treatment for reducing mortality in older persons with life-threatening VT or ventricular fibrillation.

The Multicenter Automatic Defibrillator Implantation Trial II randomized 1232 patients, mean age 64 years, with a prior MI and a LV ejection fraction of $\leq$ 30% to an AICD or to conventional medical therapy. Compared with conventional medical therapy, the AICD was found to significantly reduce all-cause mortality by 31%. Table 45.7 lists the ACC/AHA indications for an AICD.

Atrial Fibrillation

AF is the most common type of arrhythmia in adults. It is more common as patients age; the prevalence is 1% among those younger than 60 years and increases to more than 8% in those older than 80 years. Data, when adjusted for age, indicate that more men are affected than women. Cardiac conditions associated with the development of AF are hypertension, rheumatic mitral valve disease, CAD, and HF. Noncardiac causes include hyperthyroidism, hypoxic pulmonary conditions, surgery, and alcohol intoxication. Patients with AF may have symptoms of hemodynamic compromise, such as irregular palpitations and lightheadedness, or more vague symptoms, such as malaise, but they may be asymptomatic. Patients with AF are at increased risk for thromboembolic disease.

The Joint Panel of the American Academy of Family Physicians and the American College of Physi-

---

Table 45.7—ACC/AHA Indications for an Automatic Implantable Cardioverter-Defibrillator

- Cardiac arrest due to VF or VT not due to a transient or reversible cause*

- Spontaneous sustained VT in association with structural heart disease*

- Syncope of undetermined origin with clinically relevant, hemodynamically significant sustained VT or VF induced at electrophysiologic study when drug therapy is ineffective, not tolerated, or not preferred*

- Nonsustained VT in patients with coronary disease, prior MI, LV dysfunction, and inducible VF or sustained VT at electrophysiologic study not suppressible by a class I antiarrhythmic drug*

- Spontaneous sustained VT in patients without structural heart disease not amenable to other therapy*

- An LV ejection fraction $\leq$ 30% at least 1 month post-MI and 3 months post–coronary artery surgery**

NOTE: AAC = American College of Cardiology; AHA = American Heart Association; LV = left ventricular; MI = myocardial infarction; VF = ventricular fibrillation; VT = ventricular tachycardia.

* Class I indication.

** Class IIa indication.

SOURCE: Data from Gregoratos G, Abrams J, Epstein AE, et al. ACC/AHA/NASPE 2002 guideline update for implantation of cardiac pacemakers and antiarrhythmia devices: summary article: a report of the American College of Cardiology/American Heart Association Task Force on Practice Guidelines (ACC/AHA/NASPE Committee to Update the 1998 Pacemaker Guidelines). *Circulation.* 2002;106(16):2145–2161.

---

cians, in collaboration with the Johns Hopkins Evidence-based Practice Center, systematically reviewed the available evidence on the management of newly detected AF and developed recommendations for adult patients with first-detected AF. The recommendations do not apply to patients already taking antiarrhythmic drugs or patients with valvular disease. They graded the recommendations using the Guyatt Approach to Grading Recommendations. (For explanation and details, see *Ann Intern Med.* 2003;139[12]:1009–1017.)

The recommendations are as follows:

- Rate control with chronic anticoagulation is the recommended strategy for the majority of patients with atrial fibrillation. Rhythm control has not been shown to be superior to rate control (with chronic anticoagulation) in reducing morbidity and mortality and may be inferior in some patient subgroups to rate control. Rhythm control is appropriate when based on other special considerations, such as patient symptoms, exercise tolerance, and patient preference. Grade: 2A

- Patients with atrial fibrillation should receive chronic anticoagulation with adjusted-dose warfarin, unless they are at low risk of stroke or have a specific contraindication to the use of warfarin (thrombocytopenia, recent trauma or surgery, alcoholism). Grade 1A

- For patients with atrial fibrillation, the following drugs are recommended for their demonstrated efficacy in rate control during exercise and while at rest: atenolol, metoprolol, diltiazem, and verapamil (drugs listed alphabetically by class). Digoxin is effective only for rate control at rest and therefore should only be used as a second-line agent for rate control in atrial fibrillation. Grade: 1B

- For those patients who elect to undergo acute cardioversion to achieve sinus rhythm in atrial fibrillation, both direct-current cardioversion (Grade: 1C+) and pharmacologic conversion (Grade: 2A) are appropriate options.

- Both transesophageal echocardiography with short-term prior anticoagulation followed by early acute cardioversion (in the absence of intracardiac thrombus) with postcardioversion anticoagulation versus delayed cardioversion with pre-and postanticoagulation are appropriate management strategies for those patients who elect to undergo cardioversion. Grade: 2A

- Most patients converted to sinus rhythm from atrial fibrillation should not be placed on rhythm maintenance therapy since the risks

outweigh the benefits. In a selected group of patients whose quality of life is compromised by atrial fibrillation, the recommended pharmacologic agents for rhythm maintenance are amiodarone, disopyramide, propafenone, and sotalol (drugs listed in alphabetical order). The choice of agent predominantly depends on specific risk of side effects determined on the basis of patient characteristics. Grade: 2A

For more information on anticoagulation, see the Appendix (p 491).

The management of AF includes treatment of the underlying disease (such as pneumonia, hyperthyroidism, or pulmonary embolus) when possible and treatment of precipitating factors. Immediate direct-current cardioversion should be performed in persons with paroxysmal AF with a very rapid ventricular rate associated with acute MI, chest pain caused by myocardial ischemia, hypotension, severe HF, or syncope. Intravenous β-blockers, verapamil, or diltiazem may be used to slow immediately a very rapid ventricular rate associated with AF.

Amiodarone may be used in persons with symptomatic life-threatening AF refractory to other drug therapy. Radiofrequency catheter modification of atrioventricular conduction or complete atrioventricular block produced by radiofrequency catheter ablation followed by permanent pacemaker implantation can be performed in persons with symptomatic AF in whom a rapid ventricular rate cannot be slowed by drug therapy.

Paroxysmal AF associated with the tachycardia-bradycardia syndrome is indication for treatment with a permanent pacemaker, in combination with drugs used to slow a rapid ventricular rate in AF. A permanent pacemaker should also be considered in persons with AF who develop cerebral symptoms such as dizziness or syncope associated with ventricular pauses > 3 seconds that are not drug induced, as documented by a 24-hour ambulatory ECG.

BRADYARRHYTHMIAS

Numerous drugs can cause bradyarrhythmias and conduction disturbances. Hyperkalemia, hypokalemia, hypothyroidism, and hypoxia can also depress cardiac impulse formation and conduction. Drugs and endocrine and metabolic disorders causing reversible cardiac impulse formation and conduction abnormalities must be considered before a decision to implant a permanent pacemaker can be made.

A 12-lead ECG with a 1-minute strip may diagnose bradyarrhythmias caused by a sick sinus syndrome, atrioventricular block, right and left bundle branch block, bifascicular block, and trifascicular block.

ECG manifestations of sick sinus syndrome include severe sinus bradycardia, sinus pause or arrest, sinus exit block, sinus node reentrant rhythm, AF or atrial flutter with a slow ventricular rate not drug induced, failure of restoration of sinus rhythm after cardioversion for tachyarrhythmias, a pause longer than 3 seconds after carotid sinus massage, and a tachycardia-bradycardia syndrome. The tachycardia-bradycardia syndrome is characterized by paroxysmal AF, atrial flutter, or supraventricular tachycardia followed by periods of sinus bradycardia, sinus arrest, or sinoatrial block.

Dyspnea, weakness, fatigue, falls, angina pectoris, HF, episodic pulmonary edema, dizziness, faintness, slurred speech, personality changes, paresis, and convulsions in older persons may be caused by bradyarrhythmias. Death may result from prolonged ventricular asystole. Older adults with symptoms that may be due to bradyarrhythmias should have a 12-lead ECG with a 1-minute rhythm strip. Since ECG abnormalities may be intermittent, a 24-hour ambulatory ECG may need to be performed.

In some older persons without clinical evidence of heart disease and recurrent episodes of unexplained syncope, a patient-activated memory loop event recorder may be used to capture the ECG tracings preceding and during syncope. Those with unexplained syncope and heart disease should undergo an electrophysiologic study.

Table 45.8 shows ACC/AHA class I indications for permanent pacemaker implantation in patients with bradyarrhythmias. Telephone telemetry can be used to evaluate the pacemaker battery and determine that the pacemaker functions appropriately. However, reprogramming the pacemaker cannot be performed over the telephone and is best performed in an office where expertise and equipment are available.

Single-chamber pacemakers should be checked by telephone telemetry twice in the first month after implantation, every 3 months from month 2 to 48 after implantation, every 2 months from month 49 to 72 after implantation, and monthly thereafter. Dual chamber pacemakers should be checked by telemetry twice in the first month after implantation, monthly from month 2 to 6 after implantation, every 2 months from month 7 to 36 after implantation, and monthly thereafter.

PERIPHERAL ARTERIAL DISEASE

Aneurysms and Dissections

Aneurysms and dissections are primarily disorders of older persons. Aneurysms most commonly occur in the abdominal aorta, thoracic aorta, popliteal arteries, and

Table 45.8—ACC/AHA Class I Indications for Permanent Pacemaker Implantation in Patients With Bradyarrhythmias

- Third-degree and advanced second-degree AV block associated with:
  - —bradycardia with symptoms
  - —necessity for drugs that result in symptomatic bradycardia
  - —documented period of asystole ≥ 3 seconds or any escape rate < 40 beats per minute in awake, symptom-free patient
  - —after catheter ablation of the AV junction
  - —postoperative AV block not expected to resolve
  - —neuromuscular diseases with AV block
- Chronic bifascicular and trifascicular block with:
  - —intermittent third-degree AV block
  - —type II second-degree AV block
  - —alternating bundle branch block
- AV block after acute myocardial infarction with:
  - —persistent second-degree AV block in the His-Purkinje system with bilateral bundle branch block or third-degree AV block within or below the His-Purkinje system
  - —transient advanced (second- or third-degree) infranodal AV block and associated bundle branch block
  - —persistent and symptomatic second- or third-degree AV block
- Sinus node dysfunction with documented symptomatic bradycardia or with symptomatic chronotropic incompetence

NOTE: AAC = American College of Cardiology; AHA = American Heart Association; AV = atrioventricular.

SOURCE: Data from Gregoratos G, Abrams J, Epstein AE, et al. ACC/AHA/NASPE 2002 guideline update for implantation of cardiac pacemakers and antiarrhythmia devices: summary article: a report of the American College of Cardiology/American Heart Association Task Force on Practice Guidelines (ACC/AHA/NASPE Committee to Update the 1998 Pacemaker Guidelines). *Circulation*. 2002;106(16):2145–2161.

iliac arteries, and they are usually atherosclerotic. Symptomatic aneurysms are medical emergencies that require immediate surgery. Asymptomatic aneurysms should be followed for rate of growth. Older persons with an abdominal aortic aneurysm > 5 cm are potential candidates for surgical repair. Elective surgical repair of a descending thoracic aortic aneurysm or a thoracoabdominal aortic aneurysm in older persons should be considered if the aneurysm is ≥ 5 cm in maximal diameter. All older persons considered for elective surgical repair must be evaluated for coexistent CAD. The treatment of abdominal aortic aneurysms with endovascular stent-graft prostheses has been demonstrated to be efficacious as an alternative to major open abdominal surgery. Endovascular techniques are especially useful in the elderly patient with multiple comorbidities.

The pain associated with thoracic aortic dissection is severe and often tearing. Stroke, paraplegia, syncope, pulse loss with or without ischemic pain, and HF resulting from severe AR secondary to the dissection may occur. Diagnosis is best made by transesophageal echocardiography, magnetic resonance imaging, or computed tomography. Surgical intervention is the treatment of choice for acute proximal dissection and for complicated acute distal dissection (ie, complicated by rupture, expansion, saccular aneurysm formation, vital organ or limb ischemia, or continued pain). Endostenting, a new procedure for treating aneurysm, is under investigation. Medical treatment with afterload reduction and β-blockers is the treatment of choice for uncomplicated distal dissection, for stable, isolated arch dissection, and for uncomplicated dissection presenting 2 weeks or later after onset.

Occlusive Peripheral Vascular Disease

The prevalence of occlusive peripheral vascular disease (PVD) increases with age. Significant independent risk factors for symptomatic PVD in older men and women are age, cigarette smoking, hypertension, diabetes mellitus, and serum LDL cholesterol and serum HDL cholesterol (inverse association). Persons with diabetes mellitus commonly have more distal and diffuse atherosclerosis.

Atherosclerotic vascular disorders, especially CAD, may coexist with PVD. If CAD is present, the prevalence of severe CAD is higher in elderly persons with PVD than in elderly persons without PVD. Elderly persons with PVD are at increased risk for all-cause mortality, cardiovascular mortality, and mortality from CAD.

Atherosclerotic vascular disease affecting the lower extremities may cause asymptomatic arterial insufficiency or symptomatic disease presenting as intermittent claudication or pain at rest, ulceration, and gangrene. Since the superficial femoral and popliteal vessels are most commonly affected by the atherosclerotic process, the pain of intermittent claudication is most often localized to the calf. Atherosclerotic narrowing of the distal aorta and its bifurcation to the two iliac arteries may cause pain in the buttocks or thighs, as well as the legs. Persons with rest pain are at increased risk for developing ulcers and infection.

Only one half of older persons with documented PVD are symptomatic. Older persons with PVD may not walk far or fast enough to induce muscle ischemic symptoms because of comorbidities such as arthritis or pulmonary disease, may have atypical symptoms unrecognized as intermittent claudication, or may have sufficient collateral arterial channels to tolerate their arterial obstruction.

The diagnosis of PVD is usually made by a thorough history and physical examination. Persons with asymptomatic arterial insufficiency are identified by a low ankle-brachial index (ABI), which is determined by dividing the systolic blood pressure measured at the ankle by that obtained in the brachial artery. Lower extremity arterial disease is defined as an ABI < 0.9. An ABI of < 0.90 is 95% sensitive and 99% specific for the diagnosis of PVD. The lower the ABI, the more severe the restriction of arterial blood flow and the more serious the ischemia. An ABI < 0.4 is indicative of severe disease that would require intervention to promote wound healing. With ABIs below 0.25 to 0.40, rest pain and tissue loss are often found. Patients with calcified arteries from diabetes mellitus or kidney failure occasionally have relatively noncompressible arteries leading to falsely elevated ABI values in the normal range.

Doppler flow velocity measurements may be useful in grading the severity of vascular obstructions, predicting the healing of ischemic ulcers, and studying diabetic patients with noncompressible arteries. Ultrasonic duplex scanning with color provides detailed information about the arterial system and should be performed when the person is scheduled for balloon angioplasty or direct arterial surgery; it is also useful in follow-up studies of these persons.

Medical therapy of PVD includes cessation of cigarette smoking and treatment of other risk factors. Exercise therapy is the most effective medical treatment for intermittent claudication. In the Scandinavian Simvastatin Survival Study, simvastatin, in comparison with placebo, was found to reduce the risk of new or worsening intermittent claudication by 38%. Statins have been demonstrated to reduce the incidence of new coronary events in older persons with PVD and a serum LDL cholesterol ≥ 125 mg/dL with and without CAD. Compared with placebo, simvastatin has also been shown to significantly increase the treadmill exercise time until the onset of intermittent claudication by 24% at 6 months and by 42% at 1 year after treatment in older persons with PVD, a serum LDL cholesterol ≥ 125 mg/dL, and a mean ABI of 0.63.

Aspirin therapy will delay the progression of PVD and will reduce the incidence of stroke, MI, or vascular death. The Clopidogrel versus Aspirin in Patients at Risk for Ischaemic Events trial compared aspirin 325 mg daily with clopidogrel 75 mg daily; clopidogrel was found to significantly reduce the annual incidence rate of stroke, MI, or vascular death by 24% in patients with significant PVD. Therefore, clopidogrel 75 mg daily is preferable to aspirin in the treatment of PVD. Vasodilators should be avoided. The use of pentoxifylline has generally been disappointing. Cilostazol has been demonstrated in numerous studies to increase exercise capacity in persons with intermittent claudication and has been shown to be superior to pentoxifylline. However, cilostazol is a phosphodiesterase inhibitor and is contraindicated if HF is present.

Persons with PVD must wear properly fitted shoes. Careless nail clipping or injury from walking barefoot must be avoided. Feet should be washed daily and the skin kept moist with topical emollients to prevent cracks and fissures, which may have portals for bacterial infection. Fungal infection of the feet must be treated. Socks should be wool or other thick fabrics, and padding or shoe inserts may be used to prevent pressure ulcers. When a wound of the foot develops, specialized foot gear, including casts, boots, and ankle foot orthoses, are helpful in unweighting the affected area.

Indications for percutaneous transluminal angioplasty with intravascular stenting or lower extremity bypass surgery include:

- incapacitating claudication interfering with work or quality of life;
- limb salvage in persons with life-threatening ischemia, as indicated by one or more of the following: pain at rest, nonhealing ulcer, infection, or gangrene;
- vasculogenic impotence.

VENOUS DISORDERS

Chronic deep venous insufficiency usually results from prior deep-vein thrombosis (DVT). Symptoms of chronic deep venous insufficiency include edema of the lower extremities, with resolution following nighttime recumbency. Chronic edema with pigmentation of the leg may develop. Compression treatment is the mainstay of therapy. Venous insufficiency predisposes patients to stasis ulcer formation. Venous ulcers occur in the lower aspect of the tibial region, typically above the medial malleolus. Treatment of venous stasis ulcers include different methods of ulcer debridement using gels, proteolytic enzymes, and mechanical debridement. Venous ulcers that fail these therapies may be treated with surgical intervention. Adjunctive procedures include skin grafting of the ulcers using autogenous or tissue-engineered skin with or without venous surgery.

Persons with chronic deep venous insufficiency are at increased risk for developing DVT, a potentially life-threatening disorder. The gold standard diagnostic test for DVT of the lower extremity is ascending phlebography. Other diagnostic tests include impedance plethysmography and venous Doppler duplex ultrasonography.

See also the Appendix (p 491) for more on anticoagulation.

Superficial venous insufficiency with development of varicose veins may be caused by primary valvular degeneration of veins or by chronic deep venous insufficiency. The most common symptom is aching leg pain, most often exacerbated by standing. Ulcers rarely occur unless deep venous insufficiency is present. Stasis dermatitis may also occur. Superficial phlebitis develops in severe cases as a result of localized clotting of the vessels. Treatment consists of limb elevation, elastic supportive stockings, and exercise to increase muscle tone. Anticoagulation is not indicated in the absence of deep venous disease.

ANNOTATED REFERENCES

- Aronow WS. Hypercholesterolemia: the evidence supports use of statins. *Geriatrics.* 2003;58(8):18–20,26–28,31–32.
  This review examines the available evidence supporting the use of statins to treat older men and women with coronary artery disease. Evidence demonstrates that their use reduces all-cause mortality, cardiovascular mortality, coronary events, coronary and noncoronary revascularization, stroke, intermittent claudication, and heart failure.

- Aronow WS. Epidemiology, pathophysiology, prognosis, and treatment of systolic and diastolic heart failure in elderly patients. *Heart Disease.* 2003;5(4):279–294.
  Older patients with systolic heart failure should be treated with angiotensin-converting enzyme (ACE) inhibitors or—for patients who cannot be given ACE inhibitors because of cough, rash, altered taste sensation, or angioneurotic edema—angiotensin receptor blockers (ARBs) and with β-blockers. Add digoxin in men and maintain the serum digoxin level between 0.5 and 0.8 ng/mL. If symptoms persist, add an aldosterone antagonist and isosorbide dinitrate plus hydralazine. Avoid calcium channel blockers. Treat patients with diastolic heart failure with cautious use of diuretics and with β-blockers. If symptoms persist, add an ACE inhibitor or ARB. If symptoms persist, add isosorbide dinitrate plus hydralazine. If symptoms persist, add a calcium channel blocker. Avoid digoxin.

- Aronow WS. Management of peripheral arterial disease of the lower extremities in elderly patients. *J Gerontol A Biol Sci Med Sci.* 2004;59(2):M172–M177.
  Elderly persons with peripheral arterial disease (PAD) are at increased risk for all-cause mortality, cardiovascular mortality, and mortality from coronary artery disease (CAD). Modifiable risk factors should be treated. Aspirin or clopidogrel should be given to all patients with PAD. Statins reduce coronary events and improve exercise performance. Patients with PAD should be treated with angiotensin-converting enzyme inhibitors and also with β-blockers if CAD is present. Cilostazol should be given to patients with intermittent claudication unless heart failure is present. Exercise rehabilitation programs should be used in patients with intermittent claudication. Indications for lower extremity angioplasty, preferably with stenting, or bypass surgery and for amputation are discussed.

- Braunwald E, Antman EM, Beasley JW, et al. ACC/AHA 2002 guideline update for the management of patients with unstable angina and non-ST-segment elevation myocardial infarction—summary article: a report of the American College of Cardiology/American Heart Association Task Force on Practice Guidelines (Committee on the

Management of Patients With Unstable Angina). *J Am Coll Cardiol.* 2002;40(7):1366–1374.

This article presents ACC/AHA guidelines in 2002. Antiplatelet therapy with aspirin plus clopidogrel, platelet glycoprotein IIb/IIIa antagonists, anticoagulation therapy, lipid-lowering therapy, and an early invasive versus an early conservative strategy are discussed.

■ Gregoratos G, Abrams J, Epstein AE, et al. ACC/AHA/NASPE 2002 guideline update for implantation of cardiac pacemakers and antiarrhythmia devices: summary article: a report of the American College of Cardiology/American Heart Association Task Force on Practice Guidelines (ACC/AHA/NASPE Committee to Update the 1998 Pacemaker Guidelines). *Circulation.* 2002;106(16):2145–2161.

This article discusses the 2002 guidelines for implantation of an automatic implantable cardioverter-defibrillator. It also discusses the 2002 guidelines for permanent pacemaker implantation.

■ Grundy SM, Cleeman JI, Merz CN, et al. Implications of recent clinical trials for the National Cholesterol Education Program Adult Treatment Panel III Guidelines. *Circulation.* 2004;110(2):227–239.

The Adult Treatment Panel III (ATP III) of the National Cholesterol Education Program issued an evidence-based set of guidelines on cholesterol management in 2001. Since the publication of ATP III, five major clinical trials of statin therapy with clinical end points have been published. These trials addressed issues that were not examined in previous clinical trials of cholesterol-lowering therapy. This document reviews the results of these more recent trials and assesses their implications for cholesterol management.

■ Hunt SA, Baker DW, Chin MH, et al. ACC/AHA guidelines for the evaluation and management of chronic heart failure in the adult: executive summary: a report of the American College of Cardiology/American Heart Association Task Force on Practice Guidelines (Committee to Revise the 1995 Guidelines for the Evaluation and Management of Heart Failure). Developed in collaboration with the International Society for Heart and Lung Transplantation. Endorsed by the Heart Failure Society of America. *J Am Coll Cardiol* 2001;38(7):2101–2113.

The guidelines for the treatment of systolic heart failure include treatment of hypertension and dyslipidemia, cessation of smoking, and stopping drugs such as nonsteroidal anti-inflammatory drugs, calcium channel blockers, and most antiarrhythmic drugs. Class I indications for drug therapy include use of diuretics in patients with fluid retention, angiotensin-converting enzyme inhibitors and β-blockers in patients without contraindications, and digoxin for the treatment of symptoms of heart failure unless contraindicated.

Wilbert S. Aronow, MD

CHAPTER 46—HYPERTENSION

KEY POINTS

■ Treating hypertension is beneficial in older adults, as it leads to reductions in heart attack, stroke, heart failure, and overall mortality.

■ Thiazide-type diuretics are more effective in preventing cardiovascular disease than other agents and are the preferred first-line therapy in most older adults.

■ α-Receptor antagonist agents may increase morbidity and should not be used for first-line therapy. β-Blockers should not be used as first-line therapy in most older adults. Both α-receptor antagonists and β-blockers may be useful in specific patients, depending on comorbid conditions.

■ Caution is needed in treating older adults with antihypertensives. Monitoring for falls, orthostatic hypertension, and other adverse drug events is essential. "Start low and go slow."

EPIDEMIOLOGY AND PHYSIOLOGY

Blood pressure, particularly systolic pressure, increases with increasing age. The risk associated with hypertension does not decline with age, and the criteria that define hypertension, outlined in the Seventh Report of the Joint National Committee on Prevention, Detection, Evaluation, and Treatment of High Blood Pressure (JNC 7; see references at end of chapter and Table 46.1), are not age adjusted. Epidemiologic studies, including the National Health and Nutrition Examination surveys, suggest that the prevalence of hypertension in persons aged 65 years and older is between 50% and 70%; the prevalence is highest among older black Americans. In contrast to younger hypertensive populations, among whom men predominate, in the older hypertensive population the prevalence rate is higher for women, particularly for those above the age of 75 years. Over the past 50 years the use of antihypertensive medications has increased, and the prevalence rates of elevated blood pressure, left ventricular hypertrophy, and cardiovascular and stroke

Table 46.1—Classification of Blood-Pressure Levels

Category	Systolic (mm Hg)		Diastolic (mm Hg)
Normal	< 120	and	< 80
Prehypertension	120–139	or	80–89
Hypertension			
Stage 1	140–159	or	90–99
Stage 2	≥ 160	or	≥ 100

NOTE: Diagnoses should be based on the average of two or more readings taken at each of two or more visits after an initial screening.

SOURCE: Data from *JNC 7 Express: the seventh report of the Joint National Committee on Prevention, Detection, Evaluation, and Treatment of High Blood Pressure*. Bethesda, MD: National High Blood Pressure Education Program, National Heart, Lung, and Blood Institute, National Institutes of Health, US Department of Health and Human Services; May 2003:3 (Table 1).

mortality have all declined. However, these trends have been delayed among the older population, and blood pressure remains poorly controlled in many older patients despite treatment for hypertension.

Many of the physiologic changes that occur with aging contribute to the increase in blood pressure, but life-style factors such as obesity and physical inactivity and the presence of comorbid diseases are also important contributors. Several physiologic changes combine to increase peripheral vascular resistance, the physiologic hallmark of hypertension in older persons. Several mechanisms contribute to the age-associated increase in arterial vascular stiffness. Arterial stiffness, or reduced vascular compliance, provides the best explanation for the relatively greater increase in systolic pressure and the increase in pulse pressure (the difference between systolic and diastolic pressure) observed with aging. Decreased sensitivity of the baroreflex, perhaps related to decreased arterial distensibility, contributes to an increase in blood-pressure variability and sympathetic nervous system activity. The dynamic regulation of vascular tone is affected by impairments in vasodilator systems (eg, production of nitric oxide by vascular endothelial cells and vasodilatation mediated by β-adrenergic receptors) and heightened vasoconstriction mediated by α-adrenergic receptors. Alterations in kidney function as well as in neurohumoral systems that are involved in sodium balance combine to increase the proportion of older hypertensive persons whose blood pressure increases with increased sodium intake. Approximately two thirds of older hypertensive persons have sodium-sensitive hypertension.

The regulation of blood-pressure homeostasis may be impaired in older hypertensive persons, making older people with elevated systolic blood pressure more likely to develop both orthostatic and postprandial hypotension. Maintaining normal blood pressure and cerebrovascular and coronary perfusion in the face of hypotensive stimuli related to postural challenge, meals, or medications requires the integrated coordina-

tion of multiple compensatory mechanisms. The age-associated decline in baroreflex sensitivity and alterations in sympathetic nervous system function impair the dynamic regulation of blood pressure. Because of the blunted sensitivity of the baroreflex, a greater reduction in blood pressure occurs before the increase in heart rate and other compensatory mechanisms are activated. Other pathophysiologic changes that impair blood-pressure regulation include arterial and cardiac stiffness and a decrease in early diastolic filling.

CLINICAL EVALUATION

Accurate measurement of blood pressure is the most critical aspect of the diagnosis of hypertension in the older patient. Because variability in blood pressure increases with age, the diagnosis of hypertension should be made by using the average of several blood-pressure readings taken on each of three visits. Ambulatory blood-pressure monitoring may be necessary for patients with extreme blood-pressure variability or possible "white-coat" hypertension. Clinicians should be aware of an auscultatory gap, which can lead to underestimation of the true systolic blood pressure and can indicate arterial stiffness. Determining the systolic blood pressure by palpation avoids this problem.

Once a diagnosis of hypertension has been made, the remainder of the clinical evaluation centers on excluding secondary forms of hypertension (using an approach similar to that used in younger patient populations), identifying target organ damage, and determining cardiovascular risk factors and the presence of comorbid conditions. Although most older patients have essential hypertension, secondary forms of hypertension should be suspected in the presence of malignant hypertension, a sudden increase in diastolic blood pressure, worsening level of control, or poorly controlled blood pressure on a regimen of three antihypertensive medications. Renovascular disease is the most common secondary form of hypertension among older patients. Treatment decisions should take into account cardiovascular disease, target-organ damage (eg, left ventricular hypertrophy), diabetes mellitus, and other comorbid diseases. Finally, the patient's smoking history, dietary intake of sodium and fat, alcohol intake, and the level of usual physical activity should be determined to allow the clinician to individualize advice about life-style modifications to help control blood pressure as well as reduce overall cardiovascular disease risk factors.

TREATMENT

The overwhelming consensus derived from the results of several randomized placebo-controlled clinical trials is that treatment of hypertension in older persons is safe and effective. Meta-analyses of more than forty randomized clinical trials of antihypertensive therapy have provided compelling evidence that treatment is effective in reducing cardiovascular (eg, chronic heart failure) and cerebrovascular (eg, stroke) morbidity and mortality. A meta-analysis of outcome trials in systolic hypertension among older patients demonstrated that treatment was associated with significant reductions in overall mortality, cardiovascular events, and stroke. The treatment effect was largest in men, in those aged 70 years and over, and in those who had greater pulse pressures. Of note, few participants in randomized controlled trials of hypertension treatment were over 80 years old and almost none were over 85 years. As the treatment effect is delayed about 5 years, consideration needs to be given to initiating or continuing antihypertensive medication in very elderly persons.

As with other chronic conditions in older patients, it is important to balance the recognized beneficial effects of antihypertensive therapy with the potential impact on the patient's functional status and quality of life (eg, with the development of orthostatic hypotension). A treatment approach using modalities least likely to produce adverse effects and targeting a reduction in systolic blood pressure to 135 to 140 mm Hg and diastolic blood pressure to 85 to 90 mm Hg should be developed. For individuals with type 2 diabetes, a systolic blood pressure goal of less than 130 mm Hg is recommended. For persons with markedly elevated systolic blood pressure, an intermediate target, such as 160 mm Hg, may be an appropriate initial goal in the absence of target-organ damage. The focus of treatment should be on the systolic blood pressure and pulse pressure, since among older hypertensive persons, they are stronger predictors than the diastolic blood pressure of adverse outcomes. The systolic blood pressure alone correctly classifies the blood-pressure stage of more than 99% of older hypertensive patients. In addition, analysis of data from the Systolic Hypertension in the Elderly Program study demonstrates a significant relationship between pulse pressure and the risk for stroke and overall mortality that is independent of the level of mean arterial pressure.

Life-Style Modification

Nonpharmacologic therapy may be effective for older persons with stage 1 hypertension (140 to 159 mm Hg systolic or 90 to 99 mm Hg diastolic blood pressure) and is an important adjunct to drug treatment because of synergistic effects with antihypertensive drugs and the benefits realized through the reduction in other cardiovascular risk factors (see Table 46.2). Life-style modifications that

Table 46.2—Nonpharmacologic Therapy for Stage 1 Hypertension

- Weight reduction
- Aerobic and strength-training exercise programs
- Smoking cessation
- Moderation of alcohol intake
- Dietary changes to decrease sodium, saturated fat, and cholesterol while maintaining adequate intake of potassium, magnesium, and calcium

target the typical characteristics of the older hypertensive person—overweight, sedentary, and salt-sensitive—are likely to be effective. The randomized Trial of Nonpharmacologic Interventions in Elderly study, which evaluated the effects of dietary sodium restriction and weight loss in elderly patients, demonstrated that relatively modest reductions in dietary sodium intake (40 mmol per day) and in body weight (4 kg) are accompanied by a 30% decrease in the need to reinitiate pharmacologic treatment. A meta-analysis of randomized trials assessing the effects of dietary sodium restriction demonstrated a significant reduction in systolic (a mean decrease of 3.7 mm Hg for each decrease of 100 mmol per day in sodium intake) but not in diastolic blood pressure. This differential reduction in systolic pressure is particularly well suited for the older hypertensive patient. Persons with stage 1 hypertension who do not have diabetes mellitus should complete a 6-month trial of nonpharmacologic therapy before adding an antihypertensive medication if the target blood pressure is not achieved. (See also "Physical Activity," p 56; "Malnutrition," p 174.)

Pharmacologic Treatment

The general approach to pharmacologic management of the older hypertensive patient is presented in the JNC 7. General principles regarding drug selection are reviewed here and summarized in Table 46.3. Drug selection may be affected by whether the patient has simple hypertension or hypertension complicated by any of several comorbid conditions (eg, diabetes mellitus, coronary artery disease or history of myocardial infarction, heart failure, prostatism) that may influence the choice of drug. Racial and ethnic background likely has an effect on an individual's response to antihypertensive drug therapy; the blood-pressure reduction resulting from monotherapy with angiotensin-converting enzyme (ACE) inhibitors or angiotensin receptor blockers is somewhat attenuated among blacks. Given the available evidence to date, for those with simple, uncomplicated hypertension, the initial antihypertensive drug choice is a low-dose thiazide-type diuretic. A majority of patients will not

- Begin with a nonpharmacologic approach (see Table 46.2).

- Use a low-dose diuretic as the first choice for initial pharmacologic therapy.

- Base alternative drug selection or combination therapies on individual patient characteristics.

- When initiating drug therapy, begin at half of the usual dose, increase dose slowly, and continue nonpharmacologic therapies.

- Focus treatment goal on systolic blood-pressure reduction to 135 to 140 mm Hg.

- Avoid excessive reduction in diastolic blood pressure (below 70 mm Hg).

- Do not use aggressive therapy whenever adverse effects (eg, postural hypotension) cannot be avoided.

reach their systolic blood pressure goal on a single drug; JNC 7 recommends considering starting patients on two drugs if the initial blood pressure is more than 20 mm Hg above the target level. In this circumstance, partly in light of the results from the Second Australian National Blood Pressure Study, adding an ACE inhibitor to a low-dose thiazide-type diuretic is a combination that is reasonable to consider. Beyond these general recommendations for initial therapy, there is no universally accepted approach to choosing alternative agents or combination therapies; these decisions should be made on an individual basis that considers the advantages and disadvantages of the drug together with the patient's comorbidities. Finally, centrally acting agents (eg, clonidine, methyldopa) and those more likely to produce orthostatic hypotension should be avoided in most older patients.

Diuretics

Therapy with low-dose thiazide-type diuretics (eg, hydrochlorothiazide ≤ 25 mg daily, or the equivalent) has demonstrated significant benefits in mortality, stroke, and coronary events in randomized clinical trials in older hypertensive patients. The two thiazide-type diuretics in common usage—the benzothiadiazine hydrochlorothiazide and the benzene sulfonamide chlorthalidone—differ markedly in their chemical structure, potency, and pharmacokinetics. The effectiveness of both drugs has been demonstrated in clinical trials, although many recent trials, such as the Antihypertensive and Lipid-Lowering Treatment to Prevent Heart Attack Trial (ALLHAT), have used chlorthalidone. Although the direct comparability of these two diuretics has not been rigorously examined, the available evidence suggests that their blood-pressure lowering and other effects are comparable. These beneficial effects, combined with their relative safety, favorable adverse-effect profile (their adverse

metabolic effects—hypokalemia, hyperuricemia, and glucose intolerance—are attenuated at lower doses), once-daily dosing, and low cost have led to the recommendation that diuretics are preferred for initial therapy. Another advantage is that diuretic therapy leads to a disproportionate reduction in systolic relative to diastolic blood pressure, and it is better than other agents at achieving a reduction in systolic blood pressure. Thiazide diuretics are also well suited for use in combination therapies because of synergistic effects with other antihypertensive drug classes. The importance of maintaining a normal potassium level during therapy with thiazide-type diuretics deserves emphasis. Adequate potassium replacement during diuretic-based treatment has been shown to prevent the risk of arrhythmias as well as decrease the impairment in glucose tolerance.

Angiotensin-Converting Enzyme Inhibitors

ACE inhibitors have been demonstrated to be effective in lowering blood pressure in older hypertensive patients. Given the results from the Second Australian National Blood Pressure randomized controlled trial, there is support for using ACE inhibitors as initial monotherapy for simple hypertension in older hypertensive patients, especially in men. Drugs in this class are generally well tolerated (with the exception of cough during ACE inhibitor therapy), and they do not adversely affect the central nervous system or metabolic profile. There are compelling benefits from using ACE inhibitors in those patients with coexisting diabetes mellitus (particularly when there is microalbuminuria), as well as in those with left ventricular systolic dysfunction.

Angiotensin-Receptor Blockers

There have been no randomized controlled trials that have compared outcomes from treatment with angiotensin receptor blockers (ARBs) with diuretics among older hypertensive patients. The recently completed ALLHAT study did not include an ARB arm. Results from a network meta-analysis suggest that diuretic therapy is superior to ARBs for most outcomes. In the absence of data from randomized controlled trials to support their benefit with respect to cardiovascular events and mortality, therapy with an ARB generally should not be considered as initial monotherapy for simple hypertension. ARB therapy may be considered in patients with underlying diabetes, heart failure, or chronic kidney disease, especially if they are not able to tolerate ACE inhibitor therapy.

Calcium Channel Antagonists

Therapy with calcium channel antagonists (CCAs), in particular, long-acting agents in the dihydropyridine (nifedipine-like) class, has been shown in the Systolic Hypertension in Europe and China trials to lead to significant reduction in stroke risk in older hypertensive patients. The pathophysiologic (reduction in peripheral vascular resistance) and adverse-effect (absence of central or metabolic effects) profiles of the CCA class are other factors that support their use in this patient population. Although these agents are not recommended as first-step therapy, they may be considered as second-line drugs, generally in combination with a thiazide-type diuretic. Because of age-related changes in their pharmacokinetics, lower doses of CCAs should be used. Short-acting CCAs should not be used to treat hypertension.

β-Receptor Antagonists

β-Receptor antagonists are recommended in the JNC 7 report as another option for second-line drug therapy. β-Receptor antagonists should not be considered as first-line monotherapy for simple hypertension in older patients. Analysis of evidence from randomized controlled trials has questioned the efficacy of β-blockers in older hypertensive persons. Results from these studies suggest that therapy with a β-receptor antagonist is less effective than therapy with low-dose thiazide diuretics with respect to blood-pressure reduction and in the prevention of cardiovascular events, stroke, and death. In addition, β-blockers are more likely to be discontinued because of adverse effects. Because of their effectiveness in the management of symptomatic coronary artery disease, in secondary prevention following myocardial infarction, and in certain heart failure settings, β-receptor antagonists should be considered for older patients whose hypertension is complicated by these comorbid conditions.

α-Receptor Antagonists

Although the reduction in peripheral vascular resistance that occurs with therapy using an α-receptor antagonist is particularly appropriate for the pathophysiologic profile of geriatric hypertension, and although these agents are effective in blood-pressure reduction, the development of postural hypotension has limited the widespread use of this class of antihypertensive for treating elderly patients. The treatment arm that included persons randomized to therapy with the α-receptor antagonist doxazosin in the ALLHAT study was stopped early because of a higher rate of cardiovascular end points, including a twofold greater likelihood of being hospitalized for heart failure. α-Receptor antagonist therapy, usually in combination with another drug, might be considered for treating older hypertensive men with prostatism since these drugs have been shown to be efficacious in improving obstructive urinary symptoms.

The J-Curve Hypothesis

Although it is clear that an increase in blood pressure above normal (> 130/85 mm Hg) is positively and linearly associated with morbidity and mortality, concerns have been expressed that reduction of blood pressure below a given threshold level may be linked to adverse outcomes. Some studies have shown an increase in mortality with blood-pressure reduction below a certain threshold, creating a J-shaped curve of mortality. The significance of these concerns remains controversial. Many of the studies that have suggested a J-curve relationship have been confounded by comorbid illnesses among those with the lowest blood pressures. However, the results from several longitudinal studies have identified an increased risk for stroke and overall mortality in persons in the lowest systolic and, particularly, diastolic blood-pressure levels. Until additional prospective data are available to provide guidance in this therapeutic dilemma, it is prudent to use caution in lowering blood pressure in older persons with hypertension much below 140/90 mm Hg. Excessive reductions in blood pressure (eg, diastolic levels below 70 mm Hg) and treatment-induced postural hypotension should be avoided.

Follow-Up Visits

The frequency of follow-up visits should reflect the patient's degree of blood-pressure elevation at presentation, with closer follow-up indicated for those with more severe hypertension (ie, a systolic blood pressure greater than 180 mm Hg). With the exception of hypertensive emergencies (discussed below), attempts to reduce the patient's blood pressure to target levels too rapidly are unnecessary and likely deleterious. For most patients, an interval of 1 to 2 months is appropriate between visits to determine the need for dose adjustment.

Given the age-related changes in systems that regulate blood pressure and impaired blood-pressure homeostasis, overtreatment of hypertension may result in situational (postural or postprandial) hypotension. At all follow-up visits, it is imperative to determine the supine and standing blood pressure (Table 46.4). It is good practice to adjust antihypertensive drug doses to achieve the target (seated) blood pressure only after determining whether postural hypotension is present.

The patient's adherence to the current antihypertensive medication regimen should be assessed before an increased dosage is recommended or an alternative medication is considered. For some patients, additional information derived from blood-pressure measurements taken at home or another nonclinical setting may be important; home blood-pressure monitoring may also aid in promoting a

Table 46.4—Hypertension Management: Follow-Up Visits

- Assess adherence to therapy.
- Monitor for adverse effects, especially postural hypotension.
- Measure supine and upright blood pressure.
- Encourage self-monitoring of blood pressure.
- Reinforce life-style modifications (eg, diet, exercise).
- Adjust dose cautiously.
- Evaluate for refractory hypertension.

patient's adherence to therapy. Patient education regarding the significant benefits to be gained from adequate blood-pressure control is of particular importance, since hypertension is usually asymptomatic. The interdisciplinary geriatric team is well suited to promote this approach (eg, nurses to provide feedback on the degree of blood-pressure control, dietitians to review dietary information and adherence, pharmacists to promote adherence to the medical regimen, and social workers to review and, where possible, alleviate the financial burden associated with the cost of medical therapy). This evaluation should include a careful review of the patient's other medications to identify those (eg, nonsteroidal anti-inflammatory drugs and corticosteroids) that may worsen blood-pressure control.

When a patient's blood pressure has not been successfully reduced to the target level, cautiously increasing the dose, adding another agent (particularly a thiazide diuretic, if the patient is not already receiving this drug), or switching to another class of medication should be considered. Patients also should be counseled to continue their life-style modifications. It may take many months to achieve the target blood-pressure goal. When this goal is not attained despite adherence to a three-drug regimen, an evaluation for refractory hypertension (especially renovascular disease) should be considered. Once a patient has achieved appropriate stable blood-pressure control for more than a year, step-down treatment may be considered; a cautious downward dosage adjustment may be attempted, with close blood-pressure monitoring. Patients who have been successful at achieving weight loss or other nonpharmacologic interventions are most likely to be successfully weaned from antihypertensive medications.

SPECIAL CONSIDERATIONS

Hypertensive Emergencies and Urgencies

Elevated blood pressure per se in the absence of signs or symptoms of target-organ damage does not consti-tute a hypertensive emergency or urgency. Rapidly and too aggressively reducing blood pressure in a patient with incidentally discovered elevated blood pressure is potentially harmful and may produce complications, such as coronary or cerebral hypoperfusion syndromes.

Examples of true hypertensive emergencies in older patients include hypertensive encephalopathy, acute heart failure with pulmonary edema, dissecting aortic aneurysm, and unstable angina. These situations present with symptoms and signs of vascular compromise of the affected organs. The management of these emergencies requires an acute hospital setting, with the parenteral administration of an antihypertensive agent and continuous blood-pressure monitoring to achieve an immediate reduction in blood pressure, although not initially to a normal target level. Blood pressure should not be lowered emergently more than 25% within the first 2 hours, with a goal of achieving 160/100 mm Hg gradually over the first 6 hours of therapy.

Hypertensive urgencies, situations in which blood pressure should be lowered within 24 hours to prevent the risk of target-organ damage, are more common than true emergencies. The majority may be managed with oral administration of antihypertensive medications to achieve a gradual blood-pressure reduction.

Hypertension in the Long-Term-Care Setting

Approximately one third to two thirds of residents in long-term-care facilities have hypertension. Special considerations are warranted in the care of residents with respect to making the correct diagnosis and defining the goals of therapy and its effects on quality of life. Blood-pressure measurements in long-term-care settings may not be accurate. Inaccuracies result from measurement errors and from the temporal variability in blood pressure, particularly in relation to meals. Blood pressure appears to be highest in the morning before breakfast. Postprandial hypotension is common among long-term-care residents, affecting about one third of this population. The presence of postprandial hypotension has been associated with otherwise unexplained syncope, and it has been found to be a significant independent risk factor for falls, syncope, stroke, and overall mortality.

There are several factors to consider in the management of hypertension in this setting. First, the advanced average age of persons in long-term care raises controversy surrounding the question whether the benefits of antihypertensive therapy extend to the very old (ie, those aged 80 years and older). If the beneficial effects of treatment are less evident, the potential adverse effects and risks of therapy should be weighed more heavily in defining the goals of therapy.

Even an intervention as seemingly innocuous as a sodium-restricted diet needs to be evaluated in the context of the high prevalence of protein-energy malnutrition among nursing-home residents. Second, the average resident in long-term care takes seven medications, and most have three or more comorbid conditions. The addition of an antihypertensive medication increases the possibility of an adverse drug event in this frail, at-risk group. Third, several studies have identified the use of antihypertensive medications, particularly vasodilators, as a risk factor for falls in this high-risk population, who experience an average of two falls each year. It is therefore important to assess both postural and postprandial blood pressure in this population. Randomized controlled trials that could provide clear risk-benefit evidence to support an approach to antihypertensive management in the long-term-care population have not yet been conducted. The available data suggest that diuretic therapy is effective in controlling systolic blood-pressure elevations and that blood-pressure reduction with diuretics lowers the prevalence of postural hypotension.

ANNOTATED REFERENCES

■ Chobanian AV, Bakris GL, Black HR, et al. The Seventh Report of the Joint National Committee on Prevention, Detection, Evaluation, and Treatment of High Blood Pressure; The JNC 7 Report. *JAMA*. 2003;289(19):2560–2572. Available at http://www.nhlbi.nih.gov/guidelines/hypertension (accessed October 2005).

A concise treatment algorithm applicable to older hypertensive patients is presented in this update of the comprehensive recommendations of the National High Blood Pressure Education Program. A classification of prehypertension—systolic blood pressure 120 to 139 mm Hg—was added to emphasize the importance of early initiation of life-style modifications in the prevention of cardiovascular disease. The report emphasizes the implications of the aging of our population by pointing out that 90% of people who are normotensive at the age of 50 years will develop hypertension in their lifetime (see Vasan et al., discussed below, for more information on this topic). The primary treatment goal is to reduce systolic blood pressure to less than 140 mm Hg since systolic blood pressure confers greater risk than diastolic, and since the diastolic blood pressure will likely also achieve a level of less than 90 mm Hg as the systolic level is reduced. With respect to drug treatment, thiazide-type diuretics remain the preferred initial drug choice for most patients. This report emphasizes that for most patients, more than one antihypertensive drug is often needed to achieve the goal blood pressure, and that for stage 2 hypertension (systolic blood pressure greater than 160 mm Hg), two drugs—one of which is a thiazide-type diuretic—should be started at the outset of therapy. Beyond this, an individualized approach to therapy based on the patient's risk factors and comorbidities is emphasized.

■ Domanski MJ, Davis BR, Pfeffer MA, et al. Isolated systolic hypertension: prognostic information provided by pulse pressure. *Hypertension*. 1999;34(3):375–380.

This study analyzed baseline blood-pressure readings obtained in persons enrolled in the Systolic Hypertension in the Elderly Program (*JAMA* 1991;265(24):3255–3264) and determined the independent relationships among systolic, diastolic, and mean blood pressure and the pulse pressure and the outcomes of stroke and death. In this population, higher pulse pressure was due to a combination of higher systolic and lower diastolic blood pressure. Using a Cox proportional hazards model that adjusted for the significant univariate predictors, including mean arterial blood pressure, the authors identified pulse pressure as an independent significant predictor of both stroke and overall mortality. An increase of 10 mm Hg in pulse pressure was found to be associated with an 11% increase in the risk of stroke and a 16% increase in mortality. These findings supplement the observation from other studies that identified the importance of systolic blood pressure as the more significant prognostic indicator than diastolic blood pressure. Since pulse pressure provides a surrogate indicator of arterial stiffness, these findings suggest that decreased arterial compliance and the resultant increase in both systolic and pulse pressure is of major pathophysiologic significance in older persons with hypertension.

■ Psaty BM, Lumley T, Furberg CD, et al. Health outcomes associated with various antihypertensive therapies used as first-line agents: a network meta-analysis. *JAMA*. 2003;289(19):2534–2544.

This study reports results of a network meta-analysis of 42 randomized controlled trials (including the Antihypertensive and Lipid-Lowering Treatment to Prevent Heart Attack Trial [ALLHAT] and the Second Australian National Blood Pressure study [ANBP2]) to address the relative benefits of seven treatments (including placebo) with respect to cardiovascular outcomes and mortality. In this analysis, therapy with low-dose diuretics was found to be effective in comparison with placebo for all outcomes. In addition, diuretic therapy was better for all outcomes in comparison with β-blockers, angiotensin-converting enzyme inhibitors, calcium channel blockers, α-blockers, and angiotensin-receptor blockers. Although this analysis did not report findings specific to older hypertensive patients, many of the randomized controlled trials were conducted primarily in older patient populations such that these results should apply to geriatric hypertension. These findings underscore the recommendation that low-dose thiazide-type diuretics be used as the first-step antihypertensive for older patients with hypertension.

■ The ALLHAT Collaborative Research Group. Major outcomes in high-risk hypertensive patients randomized to angiotensin-converting enzyme inhibitor or calcium channel blocker vs. diuretic. *JAMA*. 2002;288(23):2981–2997.

This study was designed to determine the optimal initial antihypertensive drug for persons aged 55 years and older at risk for cardiovascular disease on the basis of age and one or more additional cardiovascular risk factors. The mean age of the 33,357 subjects was 67 years; about one third were black and one fifth Hispanic, and one third had diabetes mellitus. Subjects were randomized in double-blind manner to receive chlorthalidone, amlodipine, or lisinopril. (The α-blocker doxazosin arm was prematurely closed because of an excess of hospitalizations for heart failure in those subjects in comparison with the chlorthalidone group.) The chlorthalidone-treated group achieved a greater reduction in blood pressure than the other two groups. The primary outcome (fatal coronary heart disease or nonfatal myocardial infarction) did not differ between groups. The chlorthalidone group had lower rates of many secondary outcomes (lower heart failure rates than in the amlodipine group, and lower rates of cardiovascular disease, stroke, and heart failure than in the lisinopril group). These findings were similar for analyses conducted in subjects older than 65 years of age. The results from this trial reinforce the recommendation that thiazide-type diuretics be used as the first step in antihypertensive therapy.

■ Vasan RS, Beiser A, Seshadri S, et al. Residual lifetime risk for developing hypertension in middle-aged women and men. *JAMA*. 2002;287(8):1003–1010.

This study examined the risk of developing hypertension using Framingham study data from individuals who were normotensive at the time they entered the study when they were between 55 and 65 years of age. In this cohort, the residual lifetime risk of developing hypertension (defined as a blood pressure in excess of 140/90 mm Hg or the initiation of antihypertensive therapy) was 90%. These findings underscore the enormously high prevalence of hypertension among older persons. More than half (range 52% to 72%) of the residual lifetime risk for developing hypertension in these subjects who were between 55 and 65 years of age at study entry occurred within the first 10 years of follow-up. These results suggest that major public health initiatives should be directed toward the primary prevention of hypertension in this high-risk population.

■ Wing LM, Reid CM, Ryan P, et al. A comparison of outcomes with angiotensin-converting–enzyme inhibitors and diuretics for hypertension in the elderly. *N Engl J Med*. 2003;348(7):583–592.

The Second Australian National Blood Pressure study (ANBP2) was conducted in 6083 subjects aged 65 to 84 years who were randomized in an open-label design to treatment with either an angiotensin-converting–enzyme (ACE) inhibitor or a thiazide-type diuretic. In addition to being older (mean age 72 years), other differences in the subject population in comparison with the ALLHAT population were that 95% were white, and their blood pressure at entry was much higher (mean 167/91 mm Hg). The two treatment groups achieved comparable reductions in blood pressure. The group treated with ACE inhibitors had a lower incidence of primary end points of all cardiovascular events or all-cause death and myocardial infarction. These differences were evident only in men, in whom the event rate was twice as high as in women. There was no difference in the incidence of cerebrovascular events or stroke between the two treatment groups, except that the rate for fatal stroke was higher in the ACE inhibitor group. These findings demonstrate that, depending on the outcome being examined, ACE inhibitor therapy may offer benefits relative to thiazide-type diuretics, but that the treatment difference may apply only to men.

Mark A. Supiano, MD

CHAPTER 47—ENDOCRINE AND METABOLIC DISORDERS

KEY POINTS

■ Older adults with severe hypothyroidism should undergo testing to exclude concomitant adrenal insufficiency before receiving thyroid hormone replacement.

■ Vitamin-D deficiency not only contributes to osteoporosis but has been associated with muscle weakness and falls.

■ Malignant causes of hypercalcemia include squamous cell cancers, breast cancer, lymphoma, and myeloma.

■ There is little evidence of long-term benefit from supplementation with growth hormone, testosterone, or estrogen in older adults.

Impaired homeostatic regulation, a hallmark of aging, occurs in many endocrine systems but may become manifest only during stress. For example, fasting blood glucose levels change little with normal aging, increasing 1 to 2 mg per dL per decade of life. In contrast, glucose levels after a glucose challenge increase much more in healthy older persons than in young adults. In some cases, a loss of function in one aspect of endocrine function may result in a compensatory

change in endocrine regulation and associated alterations in catabolism that maintain homeostasis. For example, the reduction in testicular testosterone production that occurs in many older men may be partially compensated for by an increase in pituitary luteinizing hormone secretion and a decrease in testosterone metabolism. In other instances, compensatory changes or alterations in hormone catabolism do not fully offset age-related impairment in endocrine functions, as illustrated by the age-related decline in basal serum aldosterone levels. In this case, a decline in aldosterone clearance fails to offset the decrease in aldosterone secretion.

As with diseases in other organ systems, endocrine disorders in older adults often present with nonspecific, muted, or atypical symptoms and signs. Some of these presentations are well-defined syndromes that are seen almost exclusively in older adults, such as apathetic thyrotoxicosis or hyperosmolar nonketotic state in patients with diabetes mellitus. However, more commonly, endocrine disorders present with subtle, nonspecific symptoms, such as cognitive impairment, or an absence of any complaints. Indeed, the diagnosis of endocrinopathies such as hyperparathyroidism, diabetes mellitus, hypothyroidism, and hyperthyroidism in older adults is commonly established as a result of abnormalities found on routine laboratory screening.

Laboratory evaluation of older adults for endocrine disorders may be complicated by coexisting medical illnesses and medications. For example, the presence of serious acute nonthyroidal illness may lead to the mistaken impression of a thyroid disorder because of the reduction in free thyroxine (T_4) levels and sometimes increased or decreased thyrotropin (TSH) levels in sick but euthyroid older patients. Furthermore, ranges of normal laboratory values for endocrine testing are commonly established in younger adults, and even age-adjusted norms for laboratory tests may be confounded by the inclusion of older adults who are ill. Therefore, normal ranges for healthy older people are not available for most laboratory tests.

THYROID DISORDERS

With aging, a reduction in T_4 secretion is balanced by a decrease in T_4 clearance, resulting in unchanged circulating T_4 levels. Triiodothyronine (T_3) levels are unchanged until extreme old age, when they decrease slightly. However, T_3 levels are commonly reduced in the setting of nonthyroidal illness because of decreased T_4-to-T_3 conversion. TSH levels are unchanged or minimally changed in healthy older people.

Nonspecific, atypical, or asymptomatic presentations of thyroid disease are common in older adults. In the outpatient setting, laboratory testing in the stable outpatient is the most reliable way to identify hypothyroidism or hyperthyroidism in older adults who are not acutely ill. Given a 1.4% prevalence of thyroid disease in ambulatory women aged 50 and over, some clinicians recommend routine screening with a highly sensitive TSH test, although treatment may not affect outcomes. In addition, the prevalence of hypothyroidism or hyperthyroidism is sufficiently high to warrant TSH testing in all older adults with a recent decline in clinical, cognitive, or functional status, or upon admission to the nursing home. However, the results of thyroid function testing may be confusing in euthyroid patients with significant concurrent illnesses, as discussed below.

Hypothyroidism

Most prevalence estimates of hypothyroidism in older adults range from 0.5% to 5% for overt disease, and from 5% to 10% for subclinical hypothyroidism, depending on the population studied. As in younger people, most cases of hypothyroidism in older people are due to chronic autoimmune thyroiditis.

Symptoms of hypothyroidism are often atypical in older adults. Some clinical features of hypothyroidism (eg, dry skin, decreased skin turgor, slowed mentation, weakness, constipation, anemia, hyponatremia, arthritis, paresthesias, gait disturbances, elevated myocardial band of creatine phosphokinase) may misleadingly suggest other diseases. Furthermore, these symptoms usually have an insidious onset and a slow rate of progression. As a result, the diagnosis of hypothyroidism is recognized on clinical examination in only 10% to 20% of cases in older adults, and laboratory screening is necessary to detect most cases of hypothyroidism in this population. In addition, older patients with mild hypothyroidism who develop serious nonthyroidal illness may rapidly become severely hypothyroid, and older adults are more susceptible to myxedema coma in this setting. Demented older people with hypothyroidism rarely recover normal cognitive function with thyroid replacement, but cognition, functional status, and mood may improve with treatment of the hypothyroidism.

Subclinical hypothyroidism, with elevated serum TSH and normal free T_4 levels, occurs in up to 15% of people aged 65 and over, and is more common in women. Subclinical hypothyroidism is associated with impaired left ventricular diastolic and systolic function, and is an important risk factor for atherosclerosis and myocardial infarction in older women. An approach to the management of subclinical hypothyroidism is outlined in Figure 47.1. The presence of elevated thyroid peroxidase antibody titers portends the eventual development of thyroid failure and overt hypothyroidism, and it is appropriate to initiate T_4 replacement therapy in these patients. In addition, T_4 replacement is indicated in older adults with progressively increasing TSH levels or a TSH level persistently above 10 mIU/L.

By itself, an increased TSH level is usually due to primary hypothyroidism, but TSH levels may be transiently elevated during recovery from acute illnesses. Therefore, the diagnosis of hypothyroidism should be confirmed with the combination of an elevated TSH level and a decreased free T_4 or free T_4 index, or by the demonstration of a persistently increased TSH level, or both. Other potentially confusing scenarios in the diagnosis of hypothyroidism include the *low T_4 syndrome*, seen in euthyroid patients with severe nonthyroidal illnesses and presenting with a decreased free T_4 index without an increase in TSH levels. Free T_4 levels are usually normal in the low T_4 syndrome, with elevated levels of reverse T_3. Thyroid hormone supplementation has not been shown to be beneficial in these patients. A normal (or low) TSH together with a low free T_4 level may also suggest *secondary hypothyroidism*, which is differentiated from the low T_4 syndrome by the presence of hypopituitarism (deficiencies in other pituitary hormones) and decreased reverse T_3 levels. Rarely, older people with primary

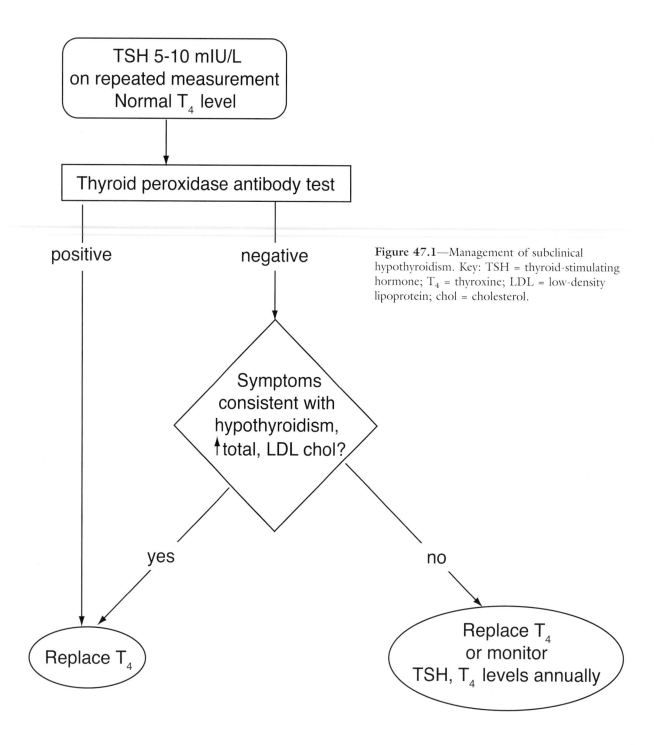

Figure 47.1—Management of subclinical hypothyroidism. Key: TSH = thyroid-stimulating hormone; T_4 = thyroxine; LDL = low-density lipoprotein; chol = cholesterol.

Flowchart text:

TSH 5-10 mIU/L on repeated measurement Normal T_4 level

Thyroid peroxidase antibody test

positive

negative

Symptoms consistent with hypothyroidism, ↑total, LDL chol?

yes

no

Replace T_4

Replace T_4 or monitor TSH, T_4 levels annually

---

hypothyroidism may also present with inappropriately normal TSH levels resulting from suppression of TSH by fasting, acute illnesses, and medications such as dopamine, phenytoin, or glucocorticoids.

T_4 replacement is usually initiated at a low dosage (eg, 25 μg per day) in older adults, increasing the dose every few weeks until TSH levels normalize. However, in patients with cardiac disease, it is prudent to begin replacement therapy at even lower dosages (eg, 12.5 μg per day). In these patients, thyroid replacement

should not be withheld for fear of exacerbating cardiac disease; instead, the goal is to reduce or eliminate symptoms of hypothyroidism without causing intolerable exacerbation of cardiac symptoms, such as angina. Older adults who are severely hypothyroid at presentation should receive larger initial T_4 replacement doses of 50 to 100 μg, or as high as 400 μg intravenously for those with myxedema stupor or coma, even if there is preexisting heart disease. Such patients should also receive testing to exclude concomitant adrenal insufficiency as well as stress doses of glucocorticoids before receiving T_4 to avoid precipitating an adrenal crisis with T_4 replacement.

Thyroid hormone requirements decrease with aging because of a reduction in clearance rate, and T_4 replacement doses are as much as a third lower in older than in younger adults. The average T_4 replacement dosage in older adults is approximately 110 µg per day. Overreplacement of thyroid hormone should be avoided, because osteopenia related to increased bone turnover and exacerbation of heart disease may occur. With correction of the hypothyroid state, the clearance rate of medications such as anticonvulsants, digoxin, and opiate analgesic agents may be affected, necessitating dosage adjustments. T_4 supplementation may have beneficial effects on some parameters of cognitive and cardiac function in some older adults with subclinical hypothyroidism, although randomized trials of such treatment have yielded mixed results. Finally, elevations in total and low-density lipoprotein cholesterol levels in hypothyroid patients may resolve with restoration of the euthyroid state, even in those with subclinical hypothyroidism, suggesting that T_4 replacement may reduce the risk of atherosclerotic vascular disease in older adults with good long-term survival prospects.

Hyperthyroidism

Hyperthyroidism develops in 0.5% to 2.3% of older people, and 15% to 25% of all cases of thyrotoxicosis occur in adults aged 60 and over. In the United States, most cases in older adults are due to Graves' disease, but toxic multinodular goiter and autonomously functioning adenomas are more common in older than in young adults, especially in populations with low iodine intake.

Hyperthyroidism often presents with vague, atypical, or nonspecific symptoms in frail older patients. Many findings that are common in younger adults (eg, tremor, heat intolerance, tachycardia, ophthalmopathy, increased perspiration, goiter, brisk reflexes) are less common or absent in older persons, whereas other manifestations, such as atrial fibrillation, heart failure, constipation, anorexia, muscle atrophy, and weakness, are more common in older adults. Older persons may present with *apathetic thyrotoxicosis*, a well-known clinical presentation of hyperthyroidism that is rarely seen in younger persons, in which the usual hyperkinetic presentation is replaced by depression, inactivity, lethargy, or withdrawn behavior, often in association with symptoms such as weight loss, muscle weakness, or cardiac symptoms. A low TSH level is associated with a threefold higher risk of developing atrial fibrillation within 10 years, and hyperthyroidism is present in 13% to 30% of older people with atrial fibrillation. Hyperthyroidism is a cause of secondary osteoporosis and should be considered in the evaluation of patients presenting with decreased bone mass.

A highly sensitive TSH test is adequate as an initial test for hyperthyroidism in relatively healthy older patients, but the diagnosis should be confirmed with a free T_4 test. Figure 47.2 illustrates the approach to diagnosing the cause of a low TSH level. Most asymptomatic older adults with low serum TSH levels are clinically euthyroid and have normal T_4 and T_3 levels, with normal TSH on repeat testing 4 to 6 weeks later. T_3 *thyrotoxicosis*, with elevated T_3 but normal T_4 levels, occurs in a minority of hyperthyroid patients, but it is more common with aging, especially in patients with toxic adenomas or toxic multinodular goiter. However, in contrast to young adults, many older persons with hyperthyroidism do not have increased T_4 or T_3 levels, probably because of decreased conversion of T_4 to T_3 associated with aging and nonthyroidal illness. Diagnostic confusion may occasionally occur in euthyroid patients with conditions or medications causing elevated T_4 levels (*high T_4 syndrome*). The high T_4 syndrome may occur with drugs or illnesses that decrease T_4-to-T_3 conversion (high-dose glucocorticoids or β-blocking agents, acute fasting) or that increase circulating levels of thyroid-binding globulin (estrogens, clofibrate, hepatitis).

Subclinical hyperthyroidism is present in less than 2% of older people and is associated with adverse cardiovascular events such as atrial fibrillation, increased left ventricular mass, and impaired ventricular relaxation; osteoporosis; neuropsychiatric problems including dementia; and excess cardiovascular and all-cause mortality. Accordingly, treatment for this condition may be justifiable, but there is a lack of data from randomized controlled trials to support this approach.

Thyroid scanning and measurement of radioactive iodine uptake may be useful in confirming hyperthyroidism and defining the cause (Figure 47.2). Radioactive iodine therapy is the treatment of choice for most older people with hyperthyroidism. Higher or repeated doses are often necessary for patients with toxic multinodular goiter. Antithyroid drugs such as methimazole or propylthiouracil are given before radioactive iodine, to control symptoms and to avoid a worsening of thyrotoxicosis due to transient release of thyroid hormone after radioactive iodine. β-Blocking agents are helpful to manage symptoms such as tachycardia, tremor, and anxiety, but patients should be monitored for changes in cardiopulmonary function. Following radioactive iodine therapy, patients should be followed with serial TSH levels for the eventual development of hypothyroidism, or persistent or recur-

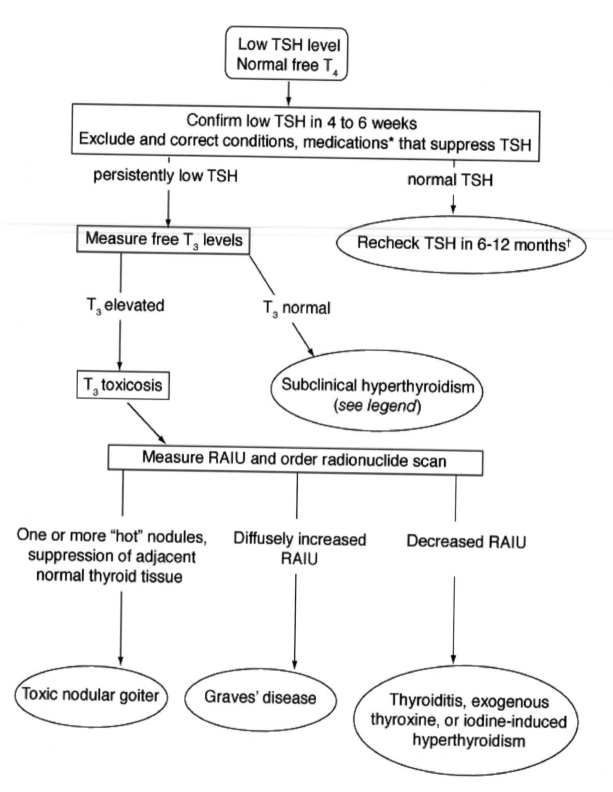

Figure 47.2.—Diagnostic algorithm for a low TSH level.

Key: TSH = thyroid-stimulating hormone; T_4 = thyroxine; T_3 = triiodothyronine; RAIU = radioactive iodine uptake.

* Glucocorticoids, dopamine agonists, and phenytoin.

† If TSH is again normal, discontinue monitoring.

NOTE: The management of subclinical hyperthyroidism is controversial. If subclinical hyperthyroidism is diagnosed, the patient should be assessed for clinical findings consistent with thyrotoxicosis, such as atrial fibrillation, osteoporosis, and neuropsychiatric symptoms. If these findings are present, the clinician may wish to consider further evaluation as suggested for T_3 toxicosis. Otherwise, it is reasonable to recheck TSH, free T_4, and free T_3 and monitor clinically for manifestations of thyrotoxicosis every 6 months.

rent hyperthyroidism. With resolution of hyperthyroidism, the clearance rate of other drugs may decrease, necessitating dosage adjustments to avoid excessive drug levels.

Nodular Thyroid Disease and Thyroid Cancer

The incidence of multinodular goiter increases with aging, and approximately 90% of women aged 70 years and over, and 60% of men aged 80 years and over have thyroid nodules. Most of these are nonpalpable. Multinodular goiters often have autonomously functioning areas, so that administration of exogenous thyroid hormone to suppress these goiters may cause iatrogenic hyperthyroidism. Older persons with multinodular goiter may develop iodine-induced thyrotoxicosis after receiving radiocontrast or amiodarone.

Solitary thyroid nodules are more likely to be malignant in people over 60 years of age, especially men. The incidence of differentiated thyroid cancers is similar in older and younger adults, whereas anaplastic thyroid carcinomas occur almost exclusively in older adults. However, even well-differentiated papillary and follicular carcinomas are more aggressive and are associated with increased mortality in older persons. Accordingly, a new solitary nodule or an enlargement of an existing nodule warrants a careful evaluation, including a fine-needle aspiration. An approach to the management of a solitary thyroid nodule is outlined in Figure 47.3. Levothyroxine suppressive therapy is indicated to reduce the risk of cancer recurrence and mortality for some patients with thyroid cancer (eg, those at highest risk), but adverse effects on the heart and osteoporosis may occur with long-term thyroid suppression. β-Blocking agents and bone antiresorptive agents may be useful to minimize these untoward effects.

DISORDERS OF PARATHYROID AND CALCIUM METABOLISM

Important changes occur with aging in several systems that regulate calcium homeostasis, ultimately leading to a reduction in bone mass and in some cases osteoporosis in older people (Table 47.1). The net effect of these changes is to increase circulating levels of parathyroid hormone (PTH), which increases 30% between 30 and 80 years of age. Serum calcium levels remain normal as a result of the increase in PTH, but the balance between bone resorption and bone formation is altered in favor of resorption, resulting in a decrease in bone mass and an increased risk of osteoporosis with aging.

Vitamin-D Deficiency

Dietary calcium intake is inadequate in most older people. However, as a consequence of factors mentioned in Table 47.1, older people are less able than younger adults to compensate by increasing their intestinal absorption of ingested calcium. In addition, vitamin-D deficiency is common in older adults, especially in hospitalized patients, nursing-home residents, and homebound community-dwelling people. Increased bone turnover and bone loss, especially of cortical bone, is a major consequence of secondary hyperparathyroidism in vitamin D-deficient older adults. Furthermore, vitamin-D deficiency is associated with muscle weakness and may contribute to fall risk in some patients.

Adequate dietary calcium and vitamin-D supplementation may reverse age-related hyperparathyroidism, increase bone mineral density, and reduce falls and osteoporotic fracture rates, although the effectiveness of vitamin D alone in preventing osteoporotic fractures is unclear. For many older people, an elemental calcium intake of at least 1000 to 1500 mg per day is desirable, together with at least 400 IU of vitamin D per day. High-dose supplementation may cause vitamin-D intoxication with hypercalcemia, hypercalciuria, impairment of kidney function, and bone loss. A few patients who are unable to take daily oral supplements may benefit from 100,000 IU of oral or parenteral vitamin D every 6 months with minimal risk of hypercalcemia. (See also the section on prevention and treatment of osteoporosis in "Osteoporosis and Osteomalacia," p 214.)

Hypercalcemia

Primary hyperparathyroidism and malignancy are the most common causes of hypercalcemia in older adults. The annual incidence of primary hyperparathyroidism is approximately 1 per 1000, and the disease is threefold more prevalent in women than in men. Most patients with primary hyperparathyroidism are asymptomatic, and the diagnosis is made after an incidental finding of hypercalcemia. When the disease is symptomatic, older persons are more likely than younger adults to present with neuropsychiatric symptoms such as depression and cognitive impairment, neuromuscular symptoms such as proximal muscle weakness, or osteoporosis. Typical laboratory findings in primary hyperparathyroidism and other common causes of hypercalcemia are described in Table 47.2. The diagnosis of primary hyperparathyroidism is confirmed with an elevated or high normal PTH level by the use of an assay for intact PTH, in the presence of hypercalcemia.

Surgery is the treatment of choice for primary hyperparathyroidism with total serum calcium levels

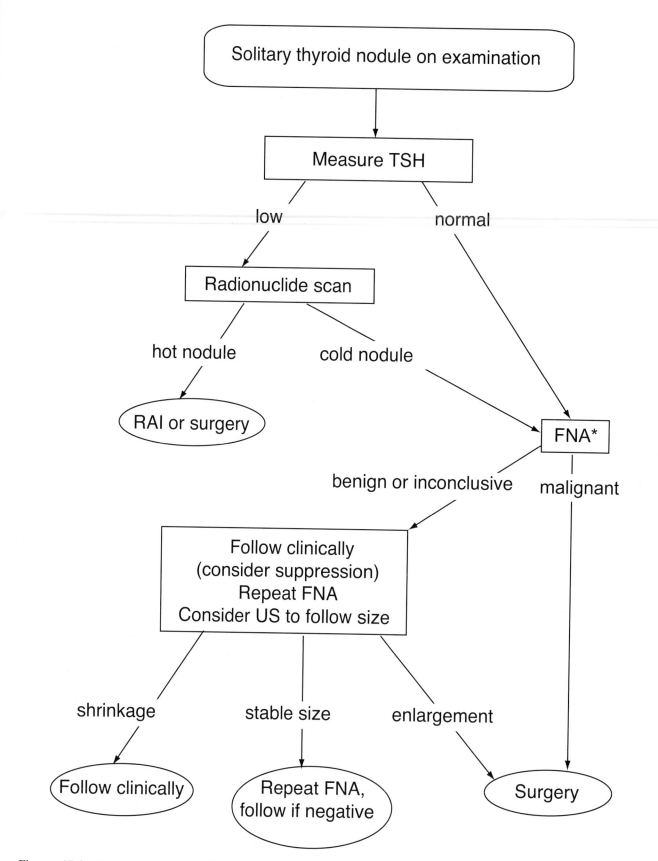

Figure 47.3—Management of a solitary thyroid nodule. This evaluation should be performed in consultation with an endocrinologist.

Key: TSH = thyroid-stimulating hormone; RAI = radioactive iodine; FNA = fine needle aspiration biopsy; US = ultrasound.
* Repeat FNA if inadequate specimen.

Table 47.1—Age-Related Alterations in Calcium Homeostasis

Factors leading to decreased 1,25(OH)$_2$D levels

  Decreased renal 1α-hydroxylase activity, leading to decreased renal parathyroid hormone responsiveness

  Decreased vitamin-D synthesis by the skin

  Decreased sunlight exposure (housebound and institutionalized elderly persons)

Factors leading to decreased intestinal absorption of dietary calcium

  Inadequate dietary calcium and vitamin-D intake

  Decreased intestinal responsiveness to 1,25(OH)$_2$D

  Decreased gastric acid secretion

  Lactase deficiency (avoidance of dairy products)

Factors leading to age-related increase in serum parathyroid hormone levels

  Slight decrease in serum calcium levels

  Decreased renal clearance of parathyroid hormone

  Decreased 1,25(OH)$_2$D levels

NOTE: 1,25(OH)$_2$D = 1,25 dihydroxyvitamin D.

more than 1 mg/dL above the normal range, 24-hour urine calcium levels above 400 mg, creatinine clearance reduced by more than 30% in comparison with normal persons of the same age, markedly decreased bone density (T score below −2.5 at any site on bone densitometry), or nephrolithiasis. Patients with serum calcium levels less than 1 mg/dL above the normal range who are asymptomatic and managed conservatively should avoid thiazide diuretics, dehydration, and immobilization. Baseline assessment in these patients should include blood pressure, serum calcium and creatinine, creatinine clearance, 24-hour urine calcium, abdominal radiography, and bone densitometry. Follow-up assessments should include blood pressure and serum calcium every 6 months, and serum creatinine and bone densitometry can be considered periodically. In addition, these patients should be followed clinically for the development of nephrolithiasis, minimal trauma fractures, and neuropsychiatric or neuromuscular symptoms. Medical management op-

tions for hyperparathyroidism also include β-blocking agents, oral phosphate in patients with low serum phosphate levels and good kidney function, and possibly bisphosphonates or raloxifene.

In hospitalized patients, the most common cause of hypercalcemia is a malignancy that produces PTH-related peptide, with hypercalcemia resulting primarily from increased net bone resorption. The presence of an underlying cancer is usually evident on examination and routine diagnostic testing. Squamous cell cancers of the lung or head and neck are common causes of hypercalcemia due to PTH-related peptide production. Other common malignancies associated with hypercalcemia include breast cancer, lymphoma, and myeloma, although the mechanism of the hypercalcemia is different for many of these cancers. Acute treatment for hypercalcemia includes volume replacement with intravenous saline, followed by diuresis with a loop diuretic when rehydration is complete. A parenteral bisphosphonate such as pamidronate should be given, along with treatment of the underlying malignancy, if possible. In addition to their usefulness in the treatment of hypercalcemia, bisphosphonates may decrease bone pain and the risk of pathologic fractures in patients with osteolytic bone metastases from a variety of cancers.

Paget's Disease of Bone

Paget's disease is characterized by localized areas of increased bone remodeling, resulting in a change in bone architecture and an increased tendency to deformity and fracture. Its prevalence increases with aging, affecting 2% to 5% of people aged 50 years and over. Paget's disease is usually asymptomatic and is often diagnosed as an incidental finding on radiographs or during evaluation for an unexplained elevation in serum alkaline phosphatase. The most commonly affected sites are the pelvis, spine, femur, tibia, and skull. When Paget's disease is symptomatic, pain is the most common presenting symptom, either localized to the affected bones or resulting from secondary osteoarthritic changes, often in the hips, knees, and

Table 47.2—Typical Laboratory Results in the Differential Diagnosis of Hypercalcemia

Laboratory Test	Primary Hyperparathyroidism	Humoral Hypercalcemia of Malignancy	Local Osteolytic Hypercalcemia
Serum calcium	↑	↑ or ↑↑	↑ or ↑↑
Serum phosphate	↓ or low-normal	↓	↑
Urine calcium	↑	↑	↑
Parathyroid hormone	↑	↓↓	↓↓
Parathyroid hormone-related peptide	0	↑	0

NOTE: The diagnosis of malignancy-related hypercalcemia is normally straightforward, and extensive diagnostic testing is rarely required. ↑ = increased; ↓ = decreased; ↑↑ = markedly increased; ↓↓ = markedly decreased; 0 = undetectable.

vertebrae. When bone deformities occur, the long bones of the lower extremities are usually affected, often with a bowing of the involved extremity. Skull involvement may result in compression of the eighth cranial nerve and sensorineural hearing loss. The most devastating complication of Paget's disease is malignant transformation of the affected bone, especially osteosarcoma. Treatment is not usually necessary for asymptomatic disease, unless there is concern for hearing loss from skull involvement, nerve root or spinal cord compression from vertebral involvement, or hip fracture from femoral neck involvement. Bisphosphonates suppress the accelerated bone turnover and bone remodeling that is characteristic of this disease, and they are the treatment of choice. During treatment, patients should be monitored clinically for changes in bone pain, joint function, and neurologic status, and with biochemical indices of bone formation (eg, serum osteocalcin or bone-specific alkaline phosphatase) or resorption (eg, urinary N-telopeptide), or both.

HORMONAL REGULATION OF WATER AND ELECTROLYTE BALANCE

Unlike young adults, older persons are predisposed to both volume depletion and free water excess. This impairment in regulation of volume status and osmolality is multifactorial, reflecting decreased total body water content as well as alterations in antidiuretic hormone (ADH) secretion, osmoreceptor and baroreceptor systems, urine-concentrating capability, renal hormone responsiveness, and thirst sensation. ADH secretion tends to be excessive in older people, with normal to elevated basal ADH levels, increased ADH responses to osmoreceptor stimuli such as hypertonic saline infusion, and decreased ethanol-induced inhibition of ADH secretion. This state of relative ADH excess with aging, together with the common occurrence of renal insufficiency, heart failure, hypothyroidism, and diuretic use, predisposes older adults to hyponatremia by impairing free water clearance. (Medications causing syndrome of inappropriate antidiuretic hormone or SIADH include the selective serotonin-reuptake inhibitors, sulfonylureas, carbamazepine, oxcarbazepine, and tricyclic antidepressants.)

Under other circumstances, older people are at increased risk of volume depletion. With aging, basal aldosterone secretion declines disproportionately to the decrease in clearance, with a net reduction in circulating aldosterone levels of about 30% by the age of 80 years. At the same time, atrial natriuretic hormone secretion (and renal responsiveness to this hormone)

increases with aging. Atrial natriuretic hormone inhibits aldosterone production and causes natriuresis and diuresis through its effects on the kidneys. Taken together, these changes predispose older people to volume depletion by decreasing the ability of the kidneys to conserve sodium under conditions of fluid deprivation. Baroreceptor ADH responses to hypotension and hypovolemia are decreased in older people, placing them at additional risk of dehydration. Moreover, renal responsiveness to ADH is decreased with aging, resulting in a decreased ability of the kidneys to maximally concentrate urine. Finally, even healthy older adults have decreased thirst sensation and may not be aware that they are becoming dehydrated. Demented and immobile older people are at the highest risk for severe dehydration.

In addition to predisposing to volume depletion, age-related hyporeninemic hypoaldosteronism also increases the risk of hyperkalemia, especially in patients with diabetes mellitus or renal insufficiency. The addition of angiotensin-converting enzyme inhibitors, nonsteroidal anti-inflammatory drugs, β-blocking agents, and diuretics with aldosterone-antagonist properties may lead to potentially lethal hyperkalemia in some of these patients.

DISORDERS OF THE ADRENAL CORTEX

Basal serum cortisol levels do not change with aging, because decreased cortisol secretion is balanced by a decrease in clearance. Adrenocorticotropic hormone (ACTH) stimulation of cortisol production is unchanged, and cortisol and ACTH responses to stress and secretagogues are unimpaired with aging. Clinically, acute cortisol responses to stress may be higher and more prolonged in older than in younger adults. Accordingly, unless it is emergent, adrenal function testing should be deferred at least 48 hours after major stressors, such as surgery or trauma. In older patients with a normal ACTH stimulation test in whom adrenal insufficiency is suspected, endocrinology consultation is recommended to assist with further testing.

Hypoadrenocorticoidism

Chronic glucocorticoid therapy is also the most common cause of adrenal failure in older adults, because of chronic suppression of adrenal function. Recovery of adrenal axis function is variable and may take several months to occur. Autoimmune-mediated adrenal failure is less common in older than in younger adults, but tuberculosis, adrenal metastases, and adrenal hemorrhage in anticoagulated patients are more common causes of adrenal insufficiency in older persons. Older patients with chronic adrenal insufficiency may present with nonspecific symptoms such as anorexia, weight loss, or impaired functional status, and hyperkalemia may not be present initially. Accordingly, a high index of suspicion is required to make the diagnosis. When adrenocortical insufficiency is suspected, the ACTH stimulation test should be performed and therapy initiated, although the best test to exclude secondary adrenal insufficiency (decreased pituitary ACTH secretion) is controversial. In older people who are stopping chronic glucocorticoid therapy, the replacement regimen should be tapered gradually, and stress dose coverage should be given for major surgery and other acute physiologic stresses until adrenocortical function has normalized.

Hyperadrenocorticoidism

Exogenous glucocorticoids are the most common cause of Cushing's syndrome in older adults, often causing adverse effects, including psychiatric and cognitive symptoms, osteoporosis, myopathy, and glucose intolerance. For patients beginning long-term glucocorticoid therapy, baseline and follow-up bone densitometry measurements are indicated, and calcium, vitamin D, and antiresorptive treatments such as bisphosphonates should be initiated as appropriate. Management of subclinical glucocorticoid hypersecretion is discussed in the following section.

Adrenal Neoplasms

In autopsy studies, the prevalence of clinically inapparent adrenal masses (*adrenal incidentalomas*) ranges from less than 1% of people younger than 30 years of age to 7% of persons older than 70 years of age. Most adrenal incidentalomas are benign adrenocortical adenomas, although pheochromocytomas and adrenocortical carcinomas also occur.

The goals of assessment are to determine whether the tumor is functional (hormone-secreting) (Table 47.3), and whether it is benign or malignant. Screening for *subclinical glucocorticoid hypersecretion* is controversial. Many adrenocortical adenomas have a degree of functional autonomy, and some patients may

develop hypertension, insulin resistance, and other metabolic derangements. However, it is unclear whether subclinical glucocorticoid hypersecretion is associated with long-term morbidity, or whether adrenalectomy or medical management of metabolic derangements improves outcomes. Moreover, screening all older adults with adrenal incidentalomas for glucocorticoid hypersecretion would yield a high proportion of false-positive results. Accordingly, it may be prudent to limit testing to patients with a symptom complex suggesting Cushing's syndrome and patients scheduled for major surgery who are at risk for postoperative adrenal crisis.

The assessment of malignancy risk in adrenal incidentaloma patients is based on lesion size, its imaging characteristics, and its rate of growth. The prevalence of adrenal cortical carcinoma in these patients increases from 2% of lesions smaller than 4 cm to 25% of lesions larger than 6 cm. Surgical excision is generally recommended for adrenal masses larger than 6 cm, and for imaging findings including rapid growth rate that suggest the mass is not an adenoma. However, the individual's treatment preferences and clinical condition must be taken into account before recommending treatment.

Adrenal Androgens

In contrast to cortisol, circulating levels of the principal adrenal androgen, dehydroepiandrosterone (DHEA), decline progressively with aging and in octogenarians are only 10% to 20% of young adult levels. Low DHEA levels are associated with poor health, whereas DHEA levels are positively correlated with some measures of longevity and functional status. Given these associations, there has been interest in the potential therapeutic effects of DHEA administration in older adults.

Most studies involving physiologic to mildly supraphysiologic DHEA supplementation in middle-aged and older persons have not found beneficial effects on body composition, although bone mineral density was found to increase modestly in postmenopausal women after 1 year of DHEA. DHEA

Table 47.3—Screening Tests for Hormone Hypersecretion in Patients With Adrenal Incidentalomas

Diagnosis	Test	Indications
Functional adrenocortical adenoma	24-hour urine free cortisol 1 mg overnight dexamethasone suppression test	Cushing's syndrome manifestations Before major surgery
Pheochromocytoma	24-hour urine metanephrines and catecholamines Plasma metanephrines	Patients with incidentaloma
Primary aldosteronism	Serum potassium Ratio of morning plasma aldosterone concentration to plasma renin activity	Hypertension

improved mood and subjective well-being in patients with primary adrenal insufficiency and mid-life dysthymia, but improvements in mood and well-being were not consistently observed in healthy middle-aged and older persons. DHEA decreased circulating high-density lipoprotein cholesterol levels in older women, suggesting potential long-term atherogenic effects. Furthermore, DHEA is metabolized to estrogens and to androgens, including testosterone and dihydrotestosterone, and its effects on the risk of breast cancer in women and prostate cancer in men are unknown. Finally, higher doses of DHEA may cause androgenization in some women and gynecomastia in men. Thus, the safety and efficacy of DHEA supplementation in older adults have not been established, and its use is inappropriate outside of clinical studies.

TESTOSTERONE

Despite former controversy, there is now general agreement that total and free testosterone levels and testosterone secretion are lower in healthy older men than in younger men. Many healthy older men exhibit moderate primary testicular failure, with decreased sperm production, testosterone levels, and testosterone secretory responses to gonadotropin administration. In addition, many of these men have inappropriately normal (ie, not increased) gonadotropin levels in the presence of low testosterone levels, suggesting secondary (hypothalamic or pituitary) testicular failure. Overt testicular failure is common in chronically ill and debilitated older men, manifested by total testosterone levels well below the normal range and symptoms suggesting androgen deficiency, including decreased libido and potency, gynecomastia, and hot flushes. Testosterone replacement therapy is generally warranted in these patients, as in hypogonadal young men. However, it is more common to encounter older men with low-normal or mildly decreased serum testosterone levels and nonspecific manifestations, such as decreased libido, weakness, decreased muscle mass, osteopenia, and memory loss. In most cases, these manifestations have multiple causes, but it has been hypothesized that declining testosterone levels with aging contribute to their development, and that testosterone supplementation may help to prevent or treat these disorders.

Men with suspected hypogonadism should be evaluated with a serum free or bioavailable (non–sex hormone–binding globulin-bound) testosterone level, either measured by equilibrium dialysis or calculated from measurements of total testosterone and sex hormone–binding globulin. Concentrations of sex hormone–binding globulin, the main circulating binding protein for testosterone, increase with age. Therefore, the age-related decline in serum free or bioavailable testosterone is greater than that of total testosterone, and total testosterone measurements do not accurately reflect the decrease in biologically active testosterone with aging. Direct radioimmunoassays using "analog" kits for free testosterone are widely used but are not recommended because they may underestimate androgen deficiency in older men and overestimate androgen deficiency in men with low sex hormone–binding globulin (eg, moderately obese men). Luteinizing hormone and follicle-stimulating hormone levels should be obtained. In addition, a review (and if possible, discontinuation) of medications that may suppress gonadotropins (eg, glucocorticoids and central nervous system–active drugs) and a prolactin level are indicated if gonadotropins are low-normal or low in the presence of low testosterone levels. High prolactin levels inhibit gonadotropin secretion and could be due to either a pituitary adenoma or hypothalamic disorder. Further studies may be warranted in such patients, including magnetic resonance imaging of the pituitary fossa and assessment of other pituitary functions (eg, cortisol response to ACTH and T_4). Baseline bone densitometry measurements should be obtained in men with decreased testosterone levels to exclude osteoporosis.

Data from controlled studies of testosterone supplementation of up to 3 years' duration in older men with low-normal or mildly decreased serum testosterone levels are summarized in Table 47.4. However, it is unknown whether these potential benefits and risks are clinically important, or whether the benefits outweigh the risks. Bearing these uncertainties in mind, a trial of testosterone supplementation may be appropriate in older men with serum total testosterone levels below 3.0 ng/mL and clinical features suggesting hypogonadism (eg, osteoporosis, muscle wasting or weakness, mild anemia of unclear cause, loss of libido), although the U.S. Food and Drug Administration has not labeled the use of testosterone for this indication. Notably, bisphosphonates have clearly demonstrated efficacy in treating older men with osteoporosis. Androgen replacement therapy is inappropriate in asymptomatic older men with low-normal total testosterone levels who do not have clinical manifestations consistent with androgen deficiency. Men should be monitored closely for adverse androgenic effects of treatment, including erythrocytosis and potential exacerbation of prostatic disease. However, there is no direct evidence that testosterone therapy increases the risk of prostate cancer or symptomatic benign prostatic hyperplasia. (See also "Disorders of Sexual Function," p 415.)

Table 47.4—Potential Short-Term Benefits and Risks of Testosterone Supplementation in Older Men With Low-Normal or Mildly Decreased Testosterone Levels

Study End Point	Effect of Testosterone
Lean body mass	Increased
Fat mass	Decreased
Bone mineral density	Variable
Strength	Variable Improved strength and performance of some functional tasks in some studies
Sexual function	Variable Activation in sexual behavior and increased libido (most consistent findings)
Mood	Variable Mood, subjective well-being improved (in some studies)
Cognitive	Some cognitive domains improved Worsened effect of practice on verbal fluency
Lipid profile	Decreased total, LDL cholesterol HDL cholesterol unchanged
Coronary heart disease	In men with established disease, improved ECG evidence of exercise-induced coronary ischemia (in most studies) Variable effect on angina pectoris
Prostate	PSA increased slightly in many patients No effect on voiding symptoms, prostate examination
Hematocrit	Increased 2.5% to 5% versus baseline Erythrocytosis developed in 6% to 25% of subjects
Long-term clinical outcomes	Unknown

NOTE: This table summarizes results of placebo-controlled studies. LDL = low-density lipoprotein; HDL = high-density lipoprotein; ECG = electrocardiographic; PSA = prostate-specific antigen.

ESTROGEN REPLACEMENT THERAPY

Many of the symptoms and signs of hormone deficiency mimic those classically associated with aging. The fact that many hormones also decline with aging has led to an enthusiasm for attempting to reverse unwanted changes associated with aging by the use of hormonal replacement. Based on very compelling epidemiologic data, replacement of estrogen, with or without progesterone, was once standard care for postmenopausal women, but this practice has fallen out of favor in the past several years given new data from randomized clinical trials. Estrogen replacement therapy (ERT) now is largely limited to treatment of menopausal symptoms (See the section on treatment of menopausal symptoms in "Gynecologic Diseases and Disorders," p 411).

Three meta-analyses of observational studies have demonstrated an association of ERT use in women with a reduction in heart disease by half. Current use of estrogen is the factor most strongly associated with reducing risk, and prolonged use is the second most important factor. Preliminary studies suggest that the effects are similar when progesterone is added. However, a few long-term prospective studies are now available, and further studies are being completed to determine if the cardiovascular benefit of ERT is present, as suggested by epidemiologic studies. A randomized controlled trial of estrogen with progesterone replacement in women with established coronary disease did not find that estrogen improves cardiac outcome. In fact, the estrogen treatment group demonstrated increased mortality in the first year on therapy, with improved survival in years 2 through 5, leading to no net benefit. Another trial of women with coronary artery disease found no benefit from estrogen for angiographic changes of atherosclerosis.

The Women's Health Initiative (WHI) is a set of clinical trails to test primary prevention of coronary artery disease with estrogen and estrogen-progesterone combinations. In the WHI, the estrogen-progesterone arm was discontinued early because of the increased risk of coronary disease, breast cancer, stroke, and deep-vein thrombosis in this group. Aspirin and lipid-lowering agents were not found to have an effect on the outcomes. The estrogen-alone arm of the study was discontinued early (February 2004 rather than March 2005) because the hormone increased the risk of stroke and did not reduce the risk of coronary heart disease.

Some observational studies also suggested that estrogen may have a role in preventing dementia. Studies of estrogen in women with mild dementia demonstrate improved memory, orientation, and calculation skills, but these studies are small and limited by selection bias. A placebo-controlled trial of estrogen replacement given for 1 year to 120 women with early to moderate Alzheimer's dementia found no improvement in affective or cognitive outcomes. In the WHI, more women in the estrogen-progesterone arm of the trial had clinically important declines in their Mini–Mental State Examination scores. Similarly, in the estrogen-alone arm of the cognitive substudy, 76 women taking estrogen developed mild cognitive impairment, compared with 58 women receiving placebo (hazard ration [HR], 1.34; 95% confidence interval [CI], 0.95 to 1.89), and when this was combined with the estrogen-plus-progestin trial, the HR was 1.25 (95% CI, 0.97 to 1.60), not clear evidence of harm. Conjugated equine estrogen (CEE) alone did not protect against dementia, as 47 participants were diagnosed with probable dementia, 28 assigned to CEE, and 19 to placebo (HR, 1.49; 95% CI, 0.83 to 2.66). When the estrogen-alone trial was combined with the estrogen-plus-progestin trial, per the original WHI mental status protocol, the overall HR for probable dementia was 1/76 (95% CI, 1.19 to 2.60; P = .005).

The risks of breast cancer, endometrial cancer, and deep-vein thrombosis associated with the use of estrogen have been well established. Meta-analyses suggest that women who used estrogen for 5 years or less have no increased risk of breast cancer, but that treatment for 15 years or more is associated with a 30% increased risk. Information about estrogen-progesterone combinations, with various derivatives and dosing schedules, are incomplete; it is therefore not possible to conclude that any particular formulation may lessen these risks compared to other formulations. Unopposed estrogen increases the risk for endometrial cancer by 2% to 8%, and the risk increases with increasing duration of use. Risk may be decreased with lower doses than in standard use. Progesterone reduces or negates the risk of endometrial cancer associated with estrogen. Finally, data demonstrate a two- to fourfold increase in risk of thromboembolic disease with the use of estrogen. (See also the section on estrogen replacement therapy for osteoporosis prevention in "Osteoporosis and Osteomalacia," p 217.)

GROWTH HORMONE

Growth hormone secretion declines with aging, and by 70 to 80 years of age, about half of adults have no significant growth hormone secretion over 24 hours. A corresponding decline occurs in levels of insulin-like growth factor 1, which mediates most of the effects of growth hormone; it falls to levels comparable to those in growth hormone–deficient children in 40% of adults aged 70 to 80 years.

Adults with growth hormone deficiency due to hypothalamic-pituitary disease exhibit decreased muscle strength, lean body mass, and bone density; increased abdominal obesity; unfavorable lipid profiles; and an increased risk of cardiovascular disease. All improve with growth hormone replacement. Older adults without hypothalamic-pituitary disease have many of the same conditions, which leads to the hypothesis that growth hormone supplementation may have a beneficial effect on these clinically important age-related disorders.

Randomized controlled trials of growth hormone supplementation in older adults have reported increased lean body mass and bone density and decreased fat mass. However, growth hormone was not found to augment improvements in muscle strength achieved with exercise alone, and no improvements in functional status were demonstrated. Furthermore, significant adverse effects were common, including carpal tunnel syndrome, arthralgias, edema, and gynecomastia. The long-term efficacy and safety of growth hormone administration in older people are unknown. Short-term growth hormone supplementation may improve nitrogen balance in older persons with severe illness and catabolic states. However, growth hormone is very expensive, and at present it is not recommended for clinical use in older people who do not have established hypothalamic-pituitary disease.

MELATONIN

Melatonin, a hormone secreted by the pineal gland, is thought to be involved in the regulation of circadian and seasonal biorhythms. Melatonin secretion is inhibited by exposure to light, resulting in a marked circadian variation in circulating melatonin levels, and its sedative effects suggest a role in sleep induction. Most studies show that plasma melatonin levels decline throughout life after early childhood, but the physiologic significance of this decline in melatonin secretion is unclear. Numerous claims have been made in the lay press regarding the "anti-aging" benefits of melatonin supplementation for various conditions, including insomnia, immune deficiency, cancer, and the aging process itself. Although melatonin may have sleep-inducing properties in older people with insomnia, the long-term risks and benefits of melatonin supplementation have not been established for insomnia or any other indication.

ANNOTATED REFERENCES

■ Bilezikian JP, Potts JT Jr, Fuleihan Gel-H, et al. Summary statement from a workshop on asymptomatic primary hyperparathyroidism: a perspective for the 21st century. *J Clin Endocrinol Metab.* 2002;87(12):5353–5361.

> This statement summarizes the proceedings of a consensus conference on asymptomatic primary hyperparathyroidism held at the National Institutes of Health in April 2002. Covered topics included the epidemiology of primary hyperparathyroidism, pathophysiology, clinical presentations, differential diagnosis, bone mass measurements, fracture incidence, natural history, new surgical and localization procedures, and new approaches to specific medical management of primary hyperparathyroidism. Revised recommendations for surgical intervention in asymptomatic hyperparathyroidism and monitoring recommendations for patients who are followed without surgery are presented.

■ Grady D, Wenger NK, Herrington D, et al. Postmenopausal hormone therapy increases risk for venous thromboembolic disease. *Ann Intern Med.* 2000;132(9):689–696.

> This analysis of venous thromboembolic events from 2763 women with known coronary artery disease receiving estrogen with progesterone or placebo for 4 years revealed that women receiving the estrogen and progesterone combination were more likely to experience a thrombotic event (34 events versus 13 events in the placebo group; relative hazard 2.7). There was no trend for decreasing relative hazard over time for deep-vein thrombosis (in contrast to the suggestion that any thrombotic event from estrogen would occur in the first few months following the initiation of therapy), but there was decreasing trend for pulmonary emboli after the first 2 years. Baseline characteristics that predicted venous thrombosis in multiple regression analysis were advanced age and assignment to hormone therapy. During the study, risk for thrombosis increased among women with a lower extremity fracture or cancer, and increased in the first 90 days following inpatient surgery or nonsurgical hospitalization and following myocardial infarction. Risk was substantially diminished in women using aspirin or statins. These findings are consistent with observational studies that suggest that estrogen therapy increases the risk of thrombotic events approximately two- to fourfold.

■ Gruenewald DA, Matsumoto AM. Aging of the endocrine system. In: Hazzard WR, Blass JP, Halter JB, et al., eds. *Principles of Geriatric Medicine and Gerontology.* 5th ed. New York: McGraw-Hill; 2004:819–835.

> Clinical management issues and the physiology of aging are reviewed in this chapter on endocrine and metabolic disorders in older adults. Principles of geriatric endocrinology are covered, followed by age-related changes in neurotransmitter and neuropeptide regulation of endocrine systems. Hormonal changes in Alzheimer's disease are briefly discussed. The remainder of the chapter delves into age-related disorders of the anterior and posterior pituitary, the hypothalamic-pituitary-adrenal axis, the sympathoadrenal system, the renin-angiotensin-aldosterone system, the growth hormone axis, and the hypothalamic-pituitary-testicular axis. The reader is referred to other chapters in the textbook for information on estrogen and androgen replacement therapy and for the management of thyroid disease and disorders of calcium and lipid regulation.

■ Gruenewald DA, Matsumoto AM. Testosterone supplementation therapy for older men: potential benefits and risks. *J Am Geriatr Soc.* 2003;51(1):101–115.

> This is a qualitative systematic review of controlled trials of testosterone therapy in older men with low-normal to moderately decreased baseline testosterone levels.

■ Grumbach MM, Biller BM, Braunstein GD, et al. Management of the clinically inapparent adrenal mass ("incidentaloma"). *Ann Intern Med.* 2003;138(5):424–429.

> This is a summary report from a National Institutes of Health consensus conference held February 2002. The panel developed recommendations for the biochemical evaluation of all patients with adrenal incidentaloma and criteria for surgical intervention. A summary of 10 "take-home points" is presented.

■ Rossouw JE, Anderson GL, Prentice RL, et al. Writing Group for the Women's Health Initiative Investigators. Risks and benefits of estrogen plus progestin in healthy postmenopausal women: principal results from the Women's Health Initiative randomized controlled trial. *JAMA.* 2002;288(3):321–333.

> The estrogen plus progestin component of the Women's Health Initiative (WHI) reports its major findings following the early discontinuation of the trial in May 2002. The WHI is a randomized controlled primary prevention trial (planned duration, 8.5 years) in which 16,608 postmenopausal women aged 50 to 79 years with an intact uterus at baseline were recruited by 40 U.S. clinical centers from 1993 to 1998. The primary outcome was coronary heart disease (CHD), that is, nonfatal myocardial infarction and CHD death, and invasive breast cancer was the primary adverse outcome. The data and safety monitoring board recommended stopping the trial of estrogen plus progestin versus placebo because the test statistic for invasive breast cancer exceeded the stopping boundary for this adverse effect and the global index statistic supported risks exceeding benefits. The hazard ratios for the major clinical outcomes are summarized in the article. Overall, all-cause mortality was not affected during the trial, and the risk-benefit profile found was not believed to be consistent with the requirements for a viable intervention for primary prevention of chronic diseases.

David A. Gruenewald, MD

Alvin M. Matsumoto, MD

Anne M. Kenny, MD

(estrogen replacement therapy section)

CHAPTER 48—DIABETES MELLITUS

KEY POINTS

- Diabetes mellitus, one of the most common chronic ailments in older adults, results in decreased life expectancy, excess complications and comorbidities, and a higher risk of geriatric conditions (polypharmacy, urinary incontinence, falls, cognitive impairment, depression, chronic pain), functional impairment, and disability.

- Both diabetes and impaired glucose tolerance are important to identify and address by changes in life style.

- Because of the great heterogeneity in the older population, treatment goals for older diabetic patients must be carefully individualized.

- Though the target blood pressure is debated, attempts to lower blood pressure, as tolerated, are important for older hypertensive diabetic patients.

- Diabetes self-management is an important part of diabetes care, and annual self-management training is a covered benefit under Medicare Part B.

Diabetes mellitus is a group of metabolic diseases characterized by hyperglycemia due to abnormalities in insulin secretion, insulin action, or both. It is one of the most common chronic diseases affecting older persons. Estimates of the prevalence among persons aged 65 years and over range between 15% and 20%. Because the general population is aging and rates of obesity are increasing among middle-aged adults, people aged 65 and older will constitute the majority of diabetic persons in the United States and in other developed countries in the coming decades. In the United States, people aged 65 and older now account for more than 40% of all people with diabetes.

The age-adjusted prevalence of diabetes mellitus is higher among black Americans and Hispanic Americans than white Americans. Further, black Americans have been found to suffer from complications of diabetes at disproportionately higher rates than white Americans. Research is only starting to decipher the effects of race on diabetes development and outcomes.

Because diabetes may be asymptomatic for many years, it is estimated that up to one third of older adults with diabetes mellitus are unaware of their condition. Despite the early asymptomatic period, diabetes mellitus is a serious condition associated with significant morbidity and a shortened survival. Older persons with diabetes can expect a 10-year reduction in life expectancy and a mortality rate nearly twice that of persons without this disease. In addition, older adults disproportionately experience the clinical complications and comorbidities associated with diabetes. These complications include atherosclerosis, neuropathies, loss of vision, and renal insufficiency. The rates of myocardial infarction, stroke, and kidney failure are increased approximately twofold, and the risk of blindness is increased approximately 40% in older persons with diabetes. Most patients aged 65 and older who require dialysis have diabetes.

Recent research is accumulating about important clinical consequences of diabetes that are common in older adults and have serious consequences to health status and quality of life. When diabetes is poorly controlled in older patients, hyperglycemia alone can be the cause of insidious decline characterized by fatigue, weight loss, muscle weakness, and decline in function. Older adults with diabetes are at higher risk than those without diabetes for geriatric syndromes, including incontinence, falls, frailty, cognitive impairment, and depressive symptoms. They also have a higher prevalence of functional impairment and disability than older adults without diabetes. Mobility disability is about 2 to 3 times more likely, and disability in activities of daily living is about 1.5 times more likely, in older adults with diabetes than in those without.

PATHOPHYSIOLOGY OF DIABETES IN OLDER ADULTS

The American Diabetes Association classifies diabetes mellitus affecting older adults into three types. Type 1 is the result of an absolute deficiency in insulin secretion due to autoimmune destruction of the β cells of the pancreas. Type 2 is most commonly due to tissue resistance to insulin action and relative insulin deficiency. A third category is reserved for other specific types of diabetes: injuries to the exocrine pancreas; endocrinopathies characterized by excesses of hormones, such as growth hormone, cortisol, glucagon, and epinephrine, which antagonize insulin action; drug- or chemical-induced diabetes; and infections leading to the destruction of the β cells of the pancreas.

In about 90% of cases, older adults with diabetes have the type 2 form of the disease. Most older adults with type 2 diabetes have had years of glucose intolerance, insulin resistance, and the metabolic syndrome. This "pre-diabetes" syndrome is also associated with increased risk for atherosclerotic disease, as well as development of type 2 diabetes.

The prevalence of both type 2 diabetes and glucose intolerance increases with age. The reasons for the increased prevalence of glucose intolerance and type 2 diabetes among older persons are not fully known; there appears to be an interaction among several factors, including genetics, life style, and aging influences. Obesity and decreased physical activity, common among older persons, contribute to impairments in insulin action. Glucose intolerance has also been shown to be related to aged-associated decline in pancreatic β-cell function and to reductions with aging of the insulin-signaling mechanisms that limit the mobilization of glucose transporters needed for insulin-mediated glucose uptake and metabolism in muscle and fat. Changes in body composition that occur with aging, such as increased visceral fat leading to insulin resistance, may also contribute to alterations in carbohydrate metabolism in aging. Decreased levels of physical activity that may occur in some older adults may exacerbate age-related changes in body composition and increased carbohydrate intolerance. An altered inflammatory environment with aging may also contribute to the higher rates of diabetes in older adults.

In addition to intrinsic physiologic mechanisms, external factors may contribute to glucose intolerance and type 2 diabetes. Some medications commonly used by older adults—diuretics, estrogen, sympathomimetics, glucocorticoids, niacin, and olanzapine—alter carbohydrate metabolism and increase glucose levels. Intercurrent illnesses, such as infections, myocardial infarction, and stroke, as well as other physiologic stresses can lead to worsened hyperglycemia. The heterogeneity in the severity of hyperglycemia among older patients with type 2 diabetes is related to the varying contributions of each of these factors in each individual.

The pathophysiology of the complications of diabetes is similar in younger and older persons. Prolonged hyperglycemia leads to glycosylation of proteins; the accumulation of these abnormal proteins can cause tissue damage. Also, metabolic products of the aldose-reductase system, such as sorbitol, accumulate in the presence of hyperglycemia. These products can impair cellular energy metabolism and contribute to cell injury and death.

Physiologic changes that occur with diabetes and its complications may interact with physiologic changes associated with aging to further decrease physiologic reserve. Type 2 diabetes and obesity are associated with inflammatory dysregulation, which may also be associated with aging and lead to clinical sequelae such as sarcopenia. Aging is associated with decreased physiologic reserve in multiple organ systems (renal, cardiovascular, central nervous system), which may interact with end-organ damage due to diabetes, resulting in increased vulnerability to physiologic stressors.

DIAGNOSIS AND EVALUATION

The current American Diabetes Association diagnostic criteria for diabetes mellitus do not include any adjustments that are based on age. Three ways to establish the diagnosis of diabetes mellitus are possible, and each must be confirmed, on a subsequent day, by any one of the three methods:

- Symptoms of polyuria, polydipsia, and unexplained weight loss plus a casual plasma glucose concentration of ≥ 200 mg/dL (11.1 mmol/L). *Casual* is defined as any time of day without regard to time since last meal.
- A plasma glucose concentration after an 8-hour fast of ≥ 126 mg/dL (7.0 mmol/L).
- A plasma glucose concentration of ≥ 200 mg/dL (11.1 mmol/L) measured 2 hours after ingestion of 75 g of glucose in 300 mL of water administered after an overnight fast.

In clinical practice, the presence of two fasting glucose levels of ≥ 126 mg/dL is the most common method of diagnosis. Older adults with fasting blood glucoses from 110 to 125 mg/dL are defined as having impaired fasting glucose (IFG), a condition associated with increased risk for diabetes development. Some older adults have isolated postchallenge hyperglycemia (IPH) but do not have high fasting blood glucoses; many of these people would be diagnosed as type 2 diabetes by oral glucose tolerance testing criteria. IPH does appear to confer increased risk for atherosclerotic complications, but not as much as diagnosed type 2 diabetes.

Several recent diabetes prevention trials demonstrated that in people with glucose intolerance, progression to type 2 diabetes can be prevented by medications and life-style changes. Life-style changes were found to be slightly more efficacious in older than in younger adults and superior to medications in the older group. These results demonstrate the importance of preventive measures and life-style changes in older adults who are at risk for developing type 2 diabetes.

MANAGEMENT

Clinical Evaluation

Older patients with diabetes require a comprehensive evaluation, which in the primary care setting may be done over several patient visits. For patients with significant functional impairments and comorbidities, including those with psychosocial problems and caregiver requirements, a formal, comprehensive geriatric assessment may be needed. Regardless of how the comprehensive evaluation of an older adult with diabetes mellitus is handled, four issues deserve special attention.

First, the history and physical examination must include evaluation of risk factors for atherosclerotic disease and the presence of all comorbid diseases. Diabetes is a well-established risk factor for atherosclerotic cardiovascular disease, so other risk factors such as smoking, family history, hypertension, and hyperlipidemia should also be explored. Diabetes is also associated with multiple vascular complications that may be subclinical or clinical. The presence of coronary artery disease, peripheral vascular disease, neuropathy, foot problems, and medical eye disease must be determined. In many cases, subspecialty consultation (as for retinopathy) and laboratory testing will be indicated. In addition, older adults with diabetes are also likely to have prevalent chronic diseases that are not necessarily associated with their diabetes, such as osteoarthritis.

Second, a thorough drug history is important. As previously stated, certain medications can contribute to hyperglycemia. More often, older patients may be on multiple medications for multiple comorbidities and may experience adverse drug effects or trouble with medication management or finances.

Third, an assessment of functional status is important in order to help determine whether the patient is able to independently manage his or her diabetes, or whether caregiver input is also needed. Functional assessment will also assist the clinician and the patient in setting diabetes management targets.

Fourth, older patients should be screened for the use of multiple medications, depression, cognitive impairment, urinary incontinence, injurious falls, and pain. Multiple observational studies have shown that these geriatric conditions are more common in older people with diabetes than without. Finally, assess each patient's needs for diabetes education and self-management support, and whether to involve a caregiver.

General Principles of Diabetes Management

The clinician develops goals for diabetes management and individualized clinical targets with each older adult with diabetes, involving the caregiver when appropriate. The goals of diabetes management in older adults include

- control of hyperglycemia and its symptoms,
- evaluation and treatment of associated risks for atherosclerotic and microvascular disease,
- evaluation and treatment of diabetes complications,

- support for diabetes self-management and education, and
- maintenance or improvement of general health status.

Although these goals are similar for older and younger people with diabetes, the management of older patients is complicated by the medical and functional heterogeneity of this group. In fact, this heterogeneity is a key consideration for clinicians in developing individualized diabetes management interventions and clinical targets for older diabetes patients. Some may have developed diabetes in middle age and have developed multiple related comorbidities. Functional heterogeneity is found among older diabetics. Some may be recently diagnosed but may have had undiagnosed diabetes for years and have complications at diagnosis. Others may have just converted from impaired glucose tolerance to diabetes and may have few complications or comorbidities, may be disabled and frail, with advanced cognitive impairment, multiple comorbidities and complications, or significant limitations in functioning. Still others may be healthy and active with minimal comorbidities and excellent function. Many older diabetes patients are in between, with mild or early functional limitations, several related comorbidities, and multiple risks for worsening morbidity.

Another consideration in treating older diabetic patients is life expectancy and the time needed for clinical benefit from a specific intervention. Clinical trials have demonstrated that approximately 8 years are needed before the benefits of glycemic control are reflected in a reduction in microvascular complications such as diabetic retinopathy or kidney disease, but that only 2 to 3 years are required to see benefits from better control of blood pressure and lipids. It is important to remember that the median remaining life expectancy for a 70-year-old woman is 14 years, which is plenty of time for the development of diabetes complications. Therefore, for a person in her or his early 70s who is newly diagnosed or highly functional, diabetes management is no different from that of younger people. However, management must be designed to fit the clinical status of older adults who are significantly functionally impaired or have multiple comorbidities. In all cases, patient preferences and quality of life must be considered.

Solid evidence supports the effectiveness of several components of diabetes care, including control of lipids and blood pressure, control of hyperglycemia, aspirin use, smoking cessation, appropriate eye and foot care, prevention of nephropathy, and diabetes education and self-management support for medication adherence, blood-glucose self-management, appropriate nutrition, weight loss if indicated, and increased physical activity. However, very few of the data supporting these interventions were obtained from research studies of older people. It is likely that many management guidelines can be generalized to many older adults with diabetes, particularly those who are healthy and functional. These older adults should have the same opportunity as younger adults for intensive diabetes management, reduction of the risks associated with diabetes, and treatment of comorbid conditions that can lead to worse disease and poorer health status in the future. However, intensive diabetes management of all diabetes-associated conditions may not be feasible for some older patients, and clinicians may have to prioritize the reduction of some risks over others. For some older patients, particularly those with severe comorbidities and disabilities, aggressive management is not likely to provide benefit and may even result in harm, such as hypoglycemia with aggressive glycemic control or hypotension with aggressive blood-pressure control.

Therefore, it is important to establish individual diabetes management goals and clinical targets with patients, to re-evaluate the clinical, functional and social status of the patient if these goals and targets are not being met, and to determine if caregiver support or specialty input is needed (Table 48.1).

The California Healthcare Foundation and the American Geriatrics Society collaborated to develop guidelines for improving the care of the older person with diabetes mellitus (see the annotated references at the end of the chapter). Many of the specific management interventions outlined below are adapted from this guideline.

Prevention and Management of Atherosclerotic Complications

Older adults with diabetes are at high risk for atherosclerosis and its complications. In fact, virtually all older adults with diabetes have been shown to have either clinical or preclinical atherosclerotic disease. Therefore, interventions that reduce the risk of atherosclerotic diseases are extremely important (Table 48.2). Smoking cessation counseling and pharmacologic intervention should be offered to any older diabetic person who smokes. Daily aspirin therapy should be offered to older adults with diabetes if there is not a contraindication to aspirin. Available evidence suggests that doses from 81 to 325 mg per day are appropriate.

There is strong evidence from a number of randomized controlled trials that the management of hypertension in older adults reduces cardiovascular events and mortality; some of these studies included substantial numbers of older people with diabetes. The best target blood pressure for older diabetic patients is

Table 48.1—Key Elements of Care for Older Persons with Diabetes Mellitus

■ Individualized care and education

■ Prevention and management of cardiovascular risk factors

■ Glycemic control; prevention and management of microvascular complications

■ Screening for and treatment of geriatric syndromes

Table 48.2—Preventing and Managing Cardiovascular Risk Factors in Older Diabetic Patients

Counsel the patient regarding:

■ Maintenance of appropriate weight

■ Increasing physical activity

■ Discontinuing smoking

■ Limiting fat and carbohydrate intake

Consider drug therapy to:

■ Treat hypertension

■ Prevent myocardial infarction (ie, aspirin)

■ Treat dyslipidemia

not clear, but in the majority of patients the target blood pressure should be 140/80. Observational studies suggest that lowering blood pressure to less than 130/80 may provide increased benefit. Because some older adults may not be able to tolerate aggressive blood-pressure lowering, hypertension should be treated gradually to avoid complications. Patient preference and medication side effects should be considered. (See also "Hypertension," p 361.)

Evidence for medication choice in older patients with diabetes suggests that most classes chosen (diuretics, angiotensin-converting enzyme inhibitors, β-blockers, and calcium channel blockers) have comparable effectiveness in reducing cardiovascular disease and mortality. Evidence suggests that angiotensin-converting enzyme inhibitors and angiotensin II receptor blockers have cardiovascular and renal benefit for persons with diabetes.

Evidence supports the use of lipid-lowering therapy and therapy to increase high-density lipoprotein (HDL) in older adults with diabetes; randomized controlled trials and meta-analysis have confirmed the benefit of the statin drugs. The use of fibrates in the setting of low HDL may also be of benefit. Therefore, lipid abnormalities should be corrected in the older adult with diabetes, as long as this is reasonable after considering the individual's overall health status. Evidence suggests that target low-density lipoprotein (LDL) level is 100 mg/dL. Dietary modification can be tried for 6 months if the LDL level is 100 to 129 mg/dL. If the LDL level is 130 mg/dL or over, pharmacologic therapy is needed in addition to life-style modifications in diet and activity level. Older persons are always at risk for adverse drug effects, so when an older person with diabetes is prescribed a statin or niacin, or when the dose is increased, an alanine aminotransferase levels should be measured within 12 weeks of the dose initiation or change. Also, some people may develop muscle inflammation with the statins, so symptoms of muscle pain and weakness in the presence of statin therapy must be evaluated. If a fibrate has been started or increased, liver enzymes should be evaluated annually.

Prevention and Management of Microvascular Complications

Microvascular complications of diabetes are major problems among older adults with diabetes and may be important contributors to disability. Diabetic retinopathy may result in decreased vision in older people with diabetes. It is important to remember that other medical eye diseases, such as glaucoma and cataracts, are also very common in older diabetic persons. Any older person with new-onset diabetes should have a screening dilated-eye examination by an eye-care specialist. If there is evidence of retinopathy, other medical eye disease, eye symptoms, or high risk (poorly controlled hyperglycemia or blood pressure), a dilated-eye examination should be done every year. If there is no eye disease or high risk, eye examinations can be performed every other year.

Serious foot problems and amputations are more common among older people with diabetes, so these patients should have a careful foot examination at least annually. The foot examination should be done more frequently if there is evidence of any problems. To screen for kidney disease, a test for the presence of microalbuminuria should be performed at diagnosis and annually if no abnormalities are detected. (See also "Kidney Diseases and Disorders," the section on kidney disease and the vascular system, p 404.) Finally, given an elevated mortality among diabetic patients who develop pneumonia, pneumococcal vaccination is strongly recommended.

Management of Hyperglycemia

There are many options for drug therapy in older persons with type 2 diabetes and no clearly preferred algorithm. Regimens can consist of any of the classes of drugs shown in Table 48.3 and Table 48.4, used alone or in combination. It is important to adjust the regimen over the course of the illness as goals change, the disease progresses, or complications develop. Sulfonylurea preparations have a long record of safety and effectiveness. Hypoglycemia is a serious adverse effect, and these drugs must be used cautiously in patients with significant renal and hepatic insufficiency, since the liver is the primary site of metabolism and they are excreted by the kidneys. α-Glucosidase inhibitors impair the breakdown of carbohydrates in the gut and limit absorption. The residual carbohydrates in the intestinal lumen are responsible for diarrhea in about 25% of patients who use this drug. The biguanide preparations also have gastrointestinal side effects and can cause lactic acidosis in patients with renal insufficiency. Metformin is contraindicated for older men with a serum creatinine level of 1.5 mg/dL or higher, or older women with a serum creatinine level of 1.4 mg/dL or higher. If an older patient receives metformin, the serum creatinine should be measured at least annually and with any increase in dose. For those aged 80 or older or those suspected to have reduced muscle mass, a timed urine collection for creatinine clearance should be obtained. The thiazolidinediones are generally well tolerated, but there is a risk of idiosyncratic hepatic toxicity. Finally, insulin can be used effectively in patients with type 2 diabetes. It is often possible to achieve good glycemic control with one or two injections a day of an intermediate-acting insulin preparation. The greatest risk of insulin therapy is hypoglycemia, and some evidence suggests that frail older adults are at higher risk for serious hypoglycemia than are healthier, more functional older adults. The management plan for an older adult with diabetes who has severe or frequent hypoglycemia should be evaluated. The patient may require referral to subspecialty diabetes care, or more frequent contact with the health care team. Psychosocial reasons for hypoglycemia must be investigated and treated, such as an inability to understand self-management that is due to cognitive problems, inadequate diabetes knowledge, difficulty in implementing therapy that is due to disability, or lack of caregiver support.

EDUCATION AND SELF-MANAGEMENT SUPPORT

It is important that the patient understands the mechanisms of the metabolic derangements and their management and becomes fully involved in diabetes self-management, that is, monitoring and treating the disease and its complications. Therefore, diabetes education about diabetes and particularly diabetes self-management is a key part of effective care. Often, this can be accomplished in the primary care setting. However, for patients who are clinically complex, referral to a diabetes educator for one-on-one counseling or group classes, a comprehensive diabetes disease management program, or specialty physician care may

Table 48.3—Non-insulin Agents for Treating Diabetes Mellitus

Drug	Dosage	Formulations	Comments (Metabolism)
Oral Agents			
2nd-Generation Sulfonylureas			Increase insulin secretion; lower HbA_{1c} by 1.0%–2.0%
Glimepiride (Amaryl)	4–8 mg once, begin 1–2 mg	T: 1, 2, 4	Numerous drug interactions, long-acting (L, K)
Glipizide (generic or Glucotrol)	2.5–40 mg once or divided	T: 5, 10	Short-acting (L, K)
(Glucotrol XL)	5–20 mg once	T: ER 2.5, 5, 10	Long-acting (L, K)
Glyburide (generic or Diaβeta, Micronase)	1.25–20 mg once or divided	T: 1.25, 2.5, 5	Long-acting, risk of hypoglycemia (L, K)
Micronized glyburide (Glynase)	1.5–12 mg once	T: 1.5, 3, 4.5, 6	(L, K)
α-Glucosidase Inhibitors			Delay glucose absorption; lower HbA_{1c} by 0.5%–1.0%
Acarbose (Precose)	50–100 mg tid, just before meals; start with 25 mg	T: 25, 50, 100	GI adverse effects common, avoid if Cr > 2 mg/dL, monitor liver enzymes (gut, K)
Miglitol (Glyset)	25–100 mg tid, with 1st bite of meal; start with 25 mg qd	T: 25, 50, 100	Same as acarbose but no need to monitor liver enzymes (L, K)
Biguanides			Decrease hepatic glucose production; lower HbA_{1c} by 1.0%–2.0%
Metformin (Glucophage)	500–2550 mg divided	T: 500, 850, 1000	Avoid in patients > 80 yr, Cr > 1.5 in men, Cr > 1.4 in women, HF, COPD, elevated liver enzymes; hold before contrast radiologic studies; may cause weight loss (K)
(Glucophage XR)	1500–2000 mg qd	T: ER 500	Same as above
Meglitinides			Increase insulin secretion; lower HbA_{1c} by 1.0%–2.0%
Nateglinide (Starlix)	60–120 mg tid	T: 60, 120	Give 30 min before meals
Repaglinide (Prandin)	0.5 mg bid–qid if HbA_{1c} < 8% or previously untreated	T: 0.5, 1, 2	Give 30 min before meals; adjust dose at wkly intervals; potential for drug interactions, caution in hepatic, renal insufficiency (L)
	1–2 mg bid–qid if HbA_{1c} ≥ 8% or previously treated		
Thiazolidinediones			Insulin resistance reducers; lower HbA_{1c} by 0.5%–1.0%; risk of HF; avoid if NYHA Class III or IV cardiac status; D/C if any decline in cardiac status
Pioglitazone (Actos)	15 or 30 mg qd; max 45 mg/d as monotherapy, 30 mg/d in combination therapy	T: 15, 30, 45	Check liver enzymes at start, q 2 mo during 1st yr, then periodically; avoid if clinical evidence of liver disease or if serum ALT levels > 2.5 upper limit of normal (L, K)
Rosiglitazone (Avandia)	4 mg qd–bid	T: 2, 4, 8	Check liver enzymes at start, q 2 mo during 1st yr, then periodically; avoid if clinical evidence of liver disease or if serum ALT levels > 2.5 upper limit of normal (L, K)

(table continued on next page)

Table 48.3—Non-insulin Agents for Treating Diabetes Mellitus (continued)

Drug	Dosage	Formulations	Comments (Metabolism)
Combinations			
Glipizide and metformin (METAGLIP)	2.5/250 once; 20/2000 in 2 divided doses	T: 2.5/250, 2.5/500, 5/500	Avoid in patients > 80 yr, Cr > 1.5 in men, Cr > 1.4 in women; see individual drugs (L, K)
Glyburide and metformin (Glucovance)	1.25/250 mg initially if previously untreated; 2.5/500 mg or 5/500 mg bid with meals; max 20/2000/d	T: 1.25/250, 2.5/500, 5/500	Starting dose should not exceed the total daily dose of either drug; see also individual drugs
Rosiglitazone and metformin (Avandamet)	4/1000–8/2000 in 2 divided doses	T: 1/500, 2/500, 4/500, 2/1000, 4/1000	Avoid in patients > 80 yr, Cr > 1.5 in men, Cr > 1.4 in women; see individual drugs (L, K)
Injectable Agents			
Exenatide *(Byetta)*	5–10 µg SC bid	1.2-, 2.4-mL prefilled syringes	Incretin mimetic; lowers HbA1c by 0.4%–0.9%; nausea and hypoglycemia common; less weight gain than insulin; avoid if CrCl < 30 mL/min (K)
Pramlintide (Symlin)*	60 µg SC immediately before meals	0.6 mg/mL in 5-mL vial	Amylin analogue; lowers HbA_{1c} by 0.4%–0.7%; nausea and hypoglycemia common; reduce pre-meal dose of short-acting insulin by 50% (K)

NOTE: ALT = alanine aminotransferase; bid = twice a day; Cr = creatinine; CrCl = creatinine clearance; d = day; D/C = discontinue; ER = extended release; GI = gastrointestinal; HF = heart failure; K = renal elimination; L = hepatic elimination; max = maximum; min = minute(s); qd = each day; qid = four times a day; SC = subcutaneously; T = tablet; tid = three times a day; wkly = weekly; yr = year(s).

*Although patients up to 78 years were enrolled in the pramlintide clinical trials, the manufacturer states that no consistent age-related differences in pramlintide activity were identified. Hypoglycemia can be severe; hence, pramlintide should be prescribed only for patients who are able to recognize and respond to the signs and symptoms of hypoglycemia and for whom close monitoring and supervision are available.

SOURCE: Reuben DB, Herr KA, Pacala JT, et al. *Geriatrics At Your Fingertips: 2006,* 8th ed. New York: American Geriatrics Society; 2006:Table 35. Reprinted with permission.

improve control. It is important to note that annual diabetes self-management training is a covered benefit under Medicare Part B. Diabetes mellitus education programs may be particularly important in older adults with diabetes who are members of minority groups, particularly black Americans or Hispanic Americans, in whom diabetes is more prevalent than in white Americans. It is critically important to recognize when caregiver involvement in diabetes self-management activities is required. The caregiver must be highly involved and educated about diabetes and its self-management when the patient is cognitively impaired, is significantly disabled or frail, or has limited proficiency in English.

Diabetes self-management and support must cover several important areas. It is important that the older patient, and caregiver if appropriate, be educated about hypo- and hyperglycemia, including precipitating factors, prevention, symptoms, monitoring, treatment, and when to notify the physician. Although hypoglycemia is unusual in older adults when they are treated with sulfonylurea or insulin, older adults with diabetes are still at higher risk than middle-aged diabetics. When appropriate, the patients and caregiver should be taught blood-glucose self-monitoring, and their technique should be reassessed and reinforced periodically.

Diet and physical activity remain important components of the initial and ongoing management of patients with diabetes. Specific dietary recommendations must be tailored for each individual and includes assessment of cholesterol intake and weight management. Physical activity programs should also be individualized. The patient should be assessed regularly for level of physical activity and informed about the benefits of exercise and available resources for becoming more active.

An older adult with diabetes who is prescribed a new medication (and any caregiver) should receive education about the purpose of the drug, how to take it, the common side effects, and important adverse reactions, with reassessment and reinforcement periodically as needed. Finally, every older adult with diabetes and any caregiver should receive education about risk factors for foot ulcers and amputation. Physical ability to provide foot care should be evaluated, with periodic reassessment and reinforcement.

Table 48.4—Insulin Preparations

Preparations	Onset	Peak	Duration
Insulin lispro (Humalog)	15 min	0.5–1.5 h	6–8 h
Insulin (eg, Humulin, Novolin)*			
Regular	0.5–1 h	2–3 h	8–12 h
NPH	1–1.5 h	4–12 h	24 h
Insulin aspart (NovoLog)	30 min	1–3 h	3–5 h
Long-acting (Ultralente)	4–8 h	16–18 h	> 36 h
Insulin Glargine (Lantus)**	1–2 h	—	24 h
Insulin, zinc (Lente)	1–2.5 h	8–12 h	18–24 h
Isophane insulin & regular insulin inj. (Novolin 70/30)	30 min	2–12 h	24 h

NOTE: h = hour(s); inj = injectable; min = minute(s); NPH = neutral protamine Hagedorn (insulin).

* Also available as mixtures of NPH and regular in 50 : 50 proportions.

** To convert from NPH dosing, give same number of units once a day. For patients taking NPH twice a day, decrease the total daily units by 20% and titrate on basis of response. Starting dose in insulin-naive patients is 10 U once daily at bedtime.

SOURCE: Reuben DB, Herr KA, Pacala JT, et al. *Geriatrics At Your Fingertips: 2006,* 8th ed. New York: American Geriatrics Society; 2006:Table 36. Reprinted with permission.

ANNOTATED REFERENCES

■ American Diabetes Association: Clinical Practice Recommendations 2005. *Diabetes Care.* 2004;28(Suppl 1):S1–S79.

This supplement is published annually and provides a concise summary of the American Diabetes Association's diabetes mellitus care standards and guidelines. Topics include an expert committee report on diagnosis and classification of the disease, and position statements regarding screening, standards of medical care, nutrition, exercise, drug therapy, and managing the complications of diabetes.

■ Brown AF, Mangione CM, Saliba D, et al.; California Health Care Foundation/American Geriatrics Society Panel on Improving Care for Elders with Diabetes. Guidelines for improving the care of the older person with diabetes mellitus. *J Am Geriatr Soc.* 2003;51(5 Suppl Guidelines):S265–S280.

The American Geriatrics Society joined the California Health Care Foundation to support development of a diabetes management guideline specifically targeted to older adults. An expert panel that included geriatricians, primary care physicians, diabetologists, diabetes educators, and researchers reviewed evidence for diabetes management interventions, particularly as these interventions related to older adults. Not only does it recommend evidence-based management of diabetes in older people, but it gives well-considered rationales for all recommendations and has an extensive bibliography of randomized clinical trials and high-quality observational studies that form the basis for the current recommended management of diabetes. It breaks new ground by emphasizing the need for prevention and management of atherosclerotic and microvascular risks and complications in older adults with diabetes, highlighting the clinical diversity of older people with diabetes, recommending individualized therapy targets, and advocating the consideration of geriatric syndromes in older diabetic patients.

■ DeFronzo RA. Pharmacologic therapy for type 2 diabetes mellitus. *Ann Intern Med.* 1999;131(4):281–303.

This is a comprehensive review of the many different drug regimens used in the management of patients with type 2 diabetes. There is an overview of the pathophysiology of the disease and its complications, followed by details of pharmacologic therapy. For each class of medication, there is a review of the mechanism of action, efficacy, side effects, dosing schedule, safety, and costs. Combination therapies with multiple oral agents and with insulin and oral agents are also reviewed.

■ Halter JB. Diabetes mellitus. In: Hazzard WR, Blass JP, Halter JB, et al., eds. *Principles of Geriatric Medicine and Gerontology.* 5th ed. New York: McGraw-Hill Professional; 2003:949–965.

Clinical management issues and the pathophysiology of the disease are reviewed in this chapter on diabetes mellitus in older adults. There is particular emphasis on the interactions of diabetes with aging and the consequences of aging to altered metabolism in older adults.

Caroline S. Blaum, MD, MS

CHAPTER 49—GASTROINTESTINAL DISEASES AND DISORDERS

KEY POINTS

- Though physiologic changes of aging may affect gastrointestinal function, most gastrointestinal symptoms and signs are due to pathologic conditions.

- Drugs used to treat many of the illnesses affecting older persons can cause gastrointestinal symptoms and disorders.

- Colon cancer is a common and often preventable cause of death.

The structure and function of the gastrointestinal tract are affected both by physiologic changes of aging and by the effects of accumulating disorders involving many body systems. In association with advancing age, there can be changes in connective tissue that limit the elasticity of the gut and alterations in the nerves and muscles that impair motility. Accumulating disorders and diseases are often associated with increased use of medications by older persons, many of which have direct effects on intestinal mucosa and motility. Some disease states, like atherosclerosis and diabetes mellitus, can adversely influence gastrointestinal function and lead to symptoms and complications. Gastrointestinal problems may quickly compromise the older person's ability to maintain adequate nutrition and lead to fatigue and weight loss.

ESOPHAGUS

Dysphagia

Dysphagia implies either the inability to initiate a swallow or a sensation that solids or liquids do not pass easily from the mouth into the stomach; it is a common problem among older adults. Dysphagia in a patient with dyspepsia requires immediate evaluation and therapy. Patients with oropharyngeal dysphagia complain of foods getting stuck shortly after they swallow, inability to initiate a swallow, impaired ability to transfer food from the mouth to the esophagus, nasal regurgitation, and coughing. Cerebrovascular accidents, Parkinson's disease and other neuromuscular disorders, Zenker's diverticulum, oropharyngeal tumors, and prominent cervical osteophytes are the most common causes of oropharyngeal dysphagia in elderly persons. In particular, hesitancy in swallowing and defects in swallowing related to tremor of the tongue occur in patients with Parkinson's disease. In contrast, patients with esophageal dysphagia usually point to the sternum when asked to localize the site. Dysphagia for both solids and liquids from the onset usually implies a motility disorder of the esophagus. In contrast, dysphagia for solids which progresses later to involve liquids suggests mechanical obstruction. Progressive dysphagia results from either cancer or peptic stricture, whereas intermittent dysphagia is most often related to a lower esophageal ring or esophageal dysmotility, such as achalasia or diffuse esophageal spasm. It is particularly important to obtain a detailed review of medications, because anticholinergics, antihistamines, and certain antihypertensive agents can reduce salivary flow. Slurred speech may indicate weakness or incoordination of muscles involved in articulation and swallowing. Dysarthria and nasal regurgitation of food suggest weakness of the soft palate or pharyngeal constrictors. Food regurgitation, halitosis, a sensation of fullness in the neck, or a history of pneumonia accompanying dysphagia may be the result of a pharyngoesophageal (or Zenker's) diverticulum, which may be associated with a poorly relaxing or hypertensive upper esophageal sphincter. Painful swallowing (odynophagia) typically results from infection or malignancy.

Endoscopy is the best first test to evaluate dysphagia; it allows biopsies and therapeutic interventions, such as dilation. However, lower esophageal rings or extrinsic esophageal compression can be overlooked during endoscopy. In such cases, radiologic evaluation with a 13-mm barium tablet or a solid bolus with barium, such as a marshmallow or bread, may identify the level and nature of obstruction. If results of these tests are normal, an esophageal motility study should be performed. For patients with oropharyngeal dysphagia, videofluoroscopy allows detailed analysis of swallowing mechanics, identifies whether aspiration is present, and evaluates the effects of different barium consistencies. Naso-pharyngo-laryngoscopy is a bedside procedure that evaluates the oropharynx, vallecula, and piriform sinuses, as well as the larynx and perilaryngeal regions, for pooled secretions or retained food; its utility is uncertain.

The treatment of dysphagia depends on its underlying cause. Esophageal cancer requires resection, chemotherapy, or radiation therapy. For patients who are poor surgical candidates, palliative endoscopic techniques, such as endoscopic mucosal resection for early esophageal cancer, photodynamic therapy for high-grade dysplasia in Barrett's esophagus, and stent placement in obstructing esophageal cancer, may be considered. Following stroke or head or neck surgery, or in degenerative neurologic diseases, swallowing rehabilitation and dietary modifications to facilitate oral intake are required. In some cases, feeding with a cup, straw, or spoon may improve swallowing. Endoscopic dilation is performed in patients with esophageal webs or strictures. Cricopharyngeal myotomy may benefit patients who have inadequate pharyngeal contraction, pharyngoesophageal diverticulum, or lack coordination between the pharynx and the upper esophageal sphincter. Endoscopic incision of the septum between the pharyngoesophageal (Zenker's) diverticulum and the esophagus with a flexible endoscope and needle-knife may also be performed. Botulinum toxin[OL] injection to the cricopharyngeus muscle is an alternative to surgery for patients with cricopharyngeal achalasia. (See also "Eating and Feeding Problems," p 181.)

Gastroesophageal Reflux Disease

Gastroesophageal reflux disease (GERD) is defined as chronic symptoms or mucosal damage produced by the abnormal reflux of gastric contents into the esophagus. Highly specific symptoms for GERD include heartburn, regurgitation, or both, which occur often after meals and are aggravated by recumbency and relieved by antacids. Among persons aged 65 and over, symptoms of heartburn or acid regurgitation occur at least weekly in 20% of the population and at least monthly in 59%, rates similar to those observed in younger adults.

In more than 80% of patients, GERD is caused by transient inappropriate lower esophageal sphincter relaxations that lead to acid reflux into the esophagus. Some patients may have reduced lower esophageal sphincter tone, which permits reflux when intra-abdominal pressure rises. Sliding hiatal hernia occurs in about 30% of patients aged 50 years or over and may contribute to acid reflux and regurgitation. Poor esophageal peristalsis leads to delayed clearance of the refluxate and increased acid exposure time. In patients receiving anticholinergic drugs, reduced salivary secretion decreases the buffering capacity of the esophagus against refluxed acid and may aggravate mucosal injury.

Patients with uncomplicated heartburn or regurgitation should be treated empirically with acid-suppressing drugs. If such therapy is unsuccessful, or if there are symptoms suggesting complicated disease, an upper endoscopy should be performed. Individuals, particularly white men, who have longstanding symptoms or who require continuous therapy for reflux need endoscopic screening for Barrett's esophagus. The frequency and severity of reflux symptoms are poorly predictive of the presence of Barrett's esophagus, particularly in patients aged 65 or over.

The presence of anemia, dysphagia, gastrointestinal bleeding, recurrent vomiting, and weight loss suggests complicated GERD. Patients with these signs and symptoms should be considered for endoscopy. This is the procedure of choice to evaluate mucosal integrity and confirm the diagnosis of dysplasia or cancer in cases of Barrett's esophagus. However, many patients with reflux symptoms do not have esophagitis. In such cases, 24-hour ambulatory esophageal pH testing helps to confirm the diagnosis. This noninvasive test is also useful for patients with noncardiac chest pain or reflux-associated pulmonary and upper respiratory symptoms or to monitor the esophageal acid exposure in patients with refractory symptoms. Esophageal manometry is used to document the presence of effective esophageal peristalsis in patients in whom antireflux surgery is being considered and to exclude underlying esophageal motility disorder, such as achalasia, as the cause of the patients' symptoms.

Proton-pump inhibitors are the treatment of choice for patients with GERD, but they are expensive. One of them, omeprazole, is now available over the counter. The use of these drugs heals esophagitis in 85% of cases and eradicates heartburn and regurgitation in 80%. In comparison, H_2 antagonists ameliorate symptoms and heal esophagitis in only 60% of cases. For the dysphagic elderly patient, various formulations of proton-pump inhibitors, such as orally disintegrating tablets, are available. Regardless, therapy should be maintained for at least 8 weeks. After acute medical therapy alleviates symptoms, the patient should be given a trial off medication. Endoscopy, esophageal motility, and ambulatory 24-hour pH monitoring should be performed if the most potent medical therapy still results in a poor response.

Recurrence of symptoms is common after therapy is stopped, and lifelong therapy is commonly needed. Intermittent therapy with an H_2 antagonist or proton-pump inhibitor may be successful in some patients with mild to moderate symptoms without severe esophagitis. Depending upon the initial therapy rendered, the medical regimen is adjusted in a step-up or step-down fashion to the most cost-effective regimen. The need for maintenance medical therapy is determined by the rapidity of recurrence. Among patients whose symptoms recur less than 3 months after stopping therapy, their disease may best be managed with continuous drug therapy. Patients whose symptoms recur 3 months or more after stopping treatment may be adequately managed with intermittent use of drugs. The induction of hypergastrinemia and gastric carcinoid tumors in rats treated with omeprazole has raised safety concerns about the long-term safety of proton-pump inhibitors. However, although patients treated with omeprazole for up to 5 years have shown gastritis and gastric atrophy, no neoplastic changes have been seen. Since gastric acidity normally protects against ingested pathogens, another concern with gastric acid inhibition is an increased risk of enteric infections. In a similar fashion,

[OL] Not approved by the U.S. Food and Drug Administration for this use.

acid-suppressive therapy also allows pathogen colonization of the upper gastrointestinal tract with an increased risk of community-acquired pneumonia.

Older patients with large hiatal hernia, with persistent regurgitation despite proton-pump inhibitor therapy, or who do not wish to take proton-pump inhibitors over the long term, should be considered for antireflux surgery. This can be performed laparoscopically, with success rates of more than 90%. Endoscopic anti-reflux procedures may also be used to treat reflux symptoms in selected patients who are not controlled by anti-secretory drugs.

Drug-Induced Esophageal Injury

Decreased esophageal peristaltic clearance, which is common among older persons, may be associated with pill retention. Esophageal injury may then occur as a result of prolonged contact of the caustic contents of the medication with the esophageal mucosa. The site of injury is commonly at the level of the aortic arch, of an enlarged left atrium, or of the esophagogastric junction. Because salivation and swallowing are markedly reduced during sleep, pill intake immediately before lying down and without adequate fluid bolus favors pill retention and injury. Taking medications with at least 8 fluid ounces of water helps dissolve tablets or capsules and may also reduce the risk of injury or gastrointestinal complaints. Patients with medication-induced esophageal injury present with sudden odynophagia to a degree that even swallowing saliva is difficult. A classic example is the elderly patient in a nursing home given a number of medications with a small amount of water while recumbent before sleep.

Tetracyclines, particularly doxycycline, are the most common antibiotics that induce esophagitis. Aspirin and all of the nonsteroidal anti-inflammatory drugs (NSAIDs) can also damage the esophagus. Other offenders include potassium chloride, quinidine, iron, and alendronate, an agent increasingly used for the treatment of osteoporosis in older adults. Because of this, alendronate should be used cautiously in patients with esophageal dysfunction and taken with at least 8 ounces of water to minimize the risk of the tablet's getting stuck in the esophagus and causing damage. In addition, patients should stand or sit upright for at least 30 minutes and should not eat during this interval. Etidronate, another bisphosphonate used to treat postmenopausal osteoporosis and Paget's disease, has not been associated with esophageal injury.

Upper endoscopy, the most sensitive diagnostic tool, may reveal a discrete ulcer of variable size with normal surrounding mucosa. These lesions typically heal spontaneously within a few days, and it is unclear

whether therapy is needed. Suspension of sucralfate^{OL} provides a protective coat on the esophageal mucosa and promotes healing. (Sucralfate is approved only for treating duodenal ulcers, so its use for treating stomach or esophageal ulcers would be off label.) Strictures may be noted in users of NSAIDs. Endoscopic dilation may be needed if a stricture is found. If possible, discontinue potentially caustic oral medications or substitute with a liquid preparation.

Esophageal Cancer: Endoscopic Palliation

Esophageal cancer is commonly diagnosed at an advanced, incurable stage in older patients who are not candidates for tumor resection. These patients are plagued by symptoms of esophageal obstruction or fistula formation, dysphagia, aspiration, and weight loss. In such instances, endoscopic palliation can be achieved with either laser therapy or a single stent placement. Laser therapy with neodymium-yttrium-aluminum-garnet (Nd:YAG) laser fulgurates the malignant obstructing tissue and restores luminal patency in more than 90% of cases, with a 5% risk of perforation. Relief may last for up to several months; treatments may be repeated. Photodynamic therapy uses a photosensitizing agent in combination with endoscopic laser exposure. It is more effective than Nd:YAG laser for palliation and has fewer complications, but it may cause skin photosensitivity.

Stenting with self-expanding metal stents is preferable therapy for patients with a malignant stricture or an esophago-bronchial fistula, as it relieves dysphagia and aspiration in up to 95% of patients and has a low complication rate. The disadvantages of stents include their high cost, tumor ingrowth, and stent migration.

STOMACH

Dyspepsia

Dyspepsia implies chronic or recurrent pain or discomfort in the upper abdomen. The major causes of dyspepsia are gastric or duodenal ulcer, gastroesophageal reflux, and gastric cancer. Because symptom pattern is inadequate for accurate diagnosis, endoscopy is the test of choice. Endoscopy is normal in up to 60% of patients, who are then classified as having functional dyspepsia. It is unclear whether *Helicobacter pylori* gastritis causes symptoms of dyspepsia.

Because the incidence of gastric cancer increases with age, upper endoscopy should be considered in

---

^{OL} Not approved by the U.S. Food and Drug Administration for this use.

older patients presenting with new onset of dyspepsia. Treatment is then targeted at the underlying diagnosis. For patients with ulcer and documented *H. pylori* infection, a trial of anti-*H. pylori* therapy should heal the ulcer and abolish the ulcer diathesis. For the majority of patients with functional (or nonulcer) dyspepsia, reassurance and a course of antisecretory therapy using either H_2-receptor antagonists or proton-pump inhibitors is recommended.

Treatment of *H. pylori* may lead to or possibly exacerbate reflux esophagitis. One possibility is that ammonia production by *H. pylori* buffers acid. Alternatively, reversal of *H. pylori*–induced gastritis (and associated hypochlorhydria) may increase gastric acid secretion and precipitate previously asymptomatic reflux. Despite this association, eradication of *H. pylori* should not be avoided solely to prevent the development or exacerbation of reflux esophagitis.

NSAID-Induced Gastric Complications

The risk of ulcers and their complications is three times greater in NSAID users than in nonusers. For those aged 60 or over, the relative risk increases even more, to fivefold. Older patients, particularly women, are two to four times more likely than younger patients to be hospitalized with peptic ulcer disease. The presence of *H. pylori* infection may have a synergistic effect on NSAID-induced ulcer disease. Elderly patients with NSAID-induced ulcers tend to present with anemia, bleeding, or perforation without the warning symptoms of dyspepsia or abdominal pain. In addition, elderly NSAID users commonly require emergency surgery for serious complications and have higher rebleeding rates, greater transfusion requirements, longer hospital stays, and higher mortality rates than do younger patients. When NSAIDs are used in older patients, the concomitant use of misoprostol or a proton-pump inhibitor may reduce the risk of gastric bleeding. Risk factors for upper gastrointestinal complications of NSAIDs use are shown in Table 49.1. COX-2 inhibitor therapy with celecoxib may be substituted for selected patients at risk for gastric complications from conventional NSAIDs, but a careful evaluation of underlying cardiovascular risk and risk-to-benefit assessment is mandatory.

Peptic Ulcer Disease

In the United States, *H. pylori* infection is responsible for about 80% of duodenal ulcers and approximately 60% of gastric ulcers. The majority of older patients with ulcers complain of dyspepsia, although bleeding, anemia, and acute abdominal pain may also occur. Typically, the diagnosis of peptic ulcer is made by

Table 49.1—Risk Factors for Upper Gastrointestinal Adverse Events in Patients Treated With Nonsteroidal Anti-Inflammatory Drugs

Age 65 years and older

Comorbid medical conditions

Use of oral glucocorticoids

History of peptic ulcer disease

History of upper gastrointestinal bleeding

Use of anticoagulants

SOURCE: Data from American College of Rheumatology Subcommittee on Osteoarthritis Guidelines: recommendations for the medical management of osteoarthritis of the hip and knee, 2000 update. *Arthritis Rheum.* 2000;(43):1905–1915.

upper gastrointestinal radiography or endoscopy. Endoscopy is more sensitive and specific than double-contrast barium study (92% versus 54% and 100% versus 91%, respectively). It is important to differentiate benign gastric ulcers from gastric cancer by obtaining multiple endoscopic biopsies.

The goal in evaluating an older patient with upper gastrointestinal symptoms is to quickly establish a definitive diagnosis, avoiding costly and risky diagnostic procedures. Drugs that may cause dyspepsia, especially NSAIDs, should be eliminated when possible. If early satiety, weight loss, occult gastrointestinal bleeding, or otherwise unexplained anemia is present, an endoscopy should be performed to exclude malignancy.

Among patients with dyspepsia who test positive for *H. pylori*, antibiotic therapy may be beneficial for up to 30% of those with underlying peptic ulcer, but those with nonulcer (functional) dyspepsia will have a variable response. *H. pylori* testing should not be performed in asymptomatic people.

Biliary Disease

Gallstones primarily form in the gallbladder and may obstruct the cystic or common bile duct, causing biliary pain, cholecystitis, and cholangitis. When stones obstruct the ampulla, pancreatitis may occur. Biliary pain is acute, severe upper abdominal pain, usually in the epigastrium or right upper quadrant, and it may last for more than 1 hour. The pain may radiate to the back or scapula and is often associated with restlessness, nausea, or vomiting. Episodes are typically separated by several weeks. Postprandial epigastric fullness, fatty food intolerance, and regurgitation are nonspecific symptoms and are not related to gallstones. If biliary disease is suspected in older patients, ultrasonography should be the initial imaging modality. Computed abdominal tomography scanning may be used if common bile duct stones or ductal obstruction are suspected. Magnetic resonance cholangiography (MRC) and endoscopic ultrasonography are two new, very accurate imaging modalities to detect common bile duct pathology, including gallstones. However, for patients with obstructive jaundice, cholangitis, or suspected biliary pancreatitis where the probability of common bile duct stones is high, therapeutic endoscopic retrograde cholangiopancreatography (ERCP) is preferred.

Isolated alkaline phosphatase elevation without jaundice may be a presenting manifestation of biliary obstruction in older patients and should always be evaluated. If cholelithiasis is detected in patients with biliary pain, laparoscopic cholecystectomy is the procedure of choice. However, this procedure is not indicated in patients with gallstones without biliary pain or complications. The incidental finding of gallstones in a patient with dyspepsia may lead to an unnecessary cholecystectomy and a poor long-term outcome. In the rare older patient who is unable to undergo surgery, treatment with ursodeoxycholic acid or lithotripsy, or both, may be attempted. In patients with common bile duct obstruction due to gallstones, endoscopic sphincterotomy and bile ductal drainage is adequate in preventing recurrent cholangitis, and the gallbladder may be left *in situ*. In any older patient with gallstones, the possibility of gallbladder cancer should be entertained. In older patients presenting with biliary pain who have had a cholecystectomy, a retained common bile duct stone should be suspected and evaluated by ERCP, MRC, or endoscopic ultrasonography. In patients with abnormal liver function tests, right upper quadrant pain, and an increased common bile duct diameter, biliary manometry should also be considered. If sphincter of Oddi dysfunction is confirmed, endoscopic sphincterotomy should be performed. For patients with malignant jaundice, treatments are mostly palliative, with either surgery or percutaneous or endoscopic stenting. Such drainage improves quality of life, decreases pruritus, and improves the nutritional state of the patient, but it does not improve survival.

COLON

Constipation

Chronic constipation affects about 30% of adults aged 65 years or older, more commonly women. Although it commonly occurs as a side effect of drugs, it may be a manifestation of metabolic or neurologic disease. Regardless, colonic obstruction must always be excluded. Constipation has been defined as a stool frequency of less than three per week. However, some individuals may complain of straining at defecation or a sense of incomplete defecation despite a daily bowel evacuation. A more objective diagnosis of constipation is based upon colonic transit times.

Patients with irritable bowel syndrome often complain of constipation, which alternates with periods of diarrhea or normal bowel evacuation. Such patients have normal colonic transit times. Lumbosacral spinal disease may lead to colonic hypomotility and dilatation, decreased rectal tone and sensation, and impaired defecation. Older patients with Parkinson's disease may have constipation worsened by physical inactivity or medication use. In middle-aged and older women, the pelvic floor muscles that contribute to the external sphincter of the rectum may acquire laxity that contributes to problems with fecal incontinence.

Most patients with prolonged colonic transit have colonic inertia, defined as the delayed passage of radiopaque markers through the proximal colon. Outlet delay is a form of idiopathic constipation in which markers move normally through the colon but stagnate in the rectum. This is typically seen in older female patients with fecal impaction and megarectum, and in women with pelvic floor dyssynergia who demonstrate abnormal responses of the pelvic floor muscles during defecation. Older patients with megacolon or megarectum have chronic fecal retention, increased rectal compliance and elasticity, and blunted rectal sensation, all leading to fecal impaction and soiling.

Defecography is a technique in which thick barium simulating stool is introduced into the rectum and evacuation is monitored by fluoroscopy while the patient sits on a commode. Assessment of the anorectal structure and function is then made at rest and during barium expulsion. Anorectal manometry evaluates rectal sensation and compliance, reflex relaxation of the internal anal sphincter, and the competence of the anal sphincters.

For most patients with constipation and normal colonic transit time, fluids, dietary fiber, and bulk laxatives, such as psyllium seed or calcium polycarbophil, are effective in increasing the frequency and softening the consistency of stool with a minimum of adverse effects. Patients who respond poorly or who do not tolerate fiber may require laxatives. Chronic use of stimulant laxatives such as bisacodyl and senna may lead to hypokalemia, protein-losing enteropathy, and impairment of bowel motility. Stool softeners such as docusate sodium have few side effects but are less effective than laxatives. Constipation among patients with dementia is common, especially if psychotropic medications are being used. Because the patient cannot be relied upon to describe symptoms, a proactive approach is needed.

Management of slow-transit constipation requires daily osmotic laxatives, such as sorbitol, lactulose, or a polyethylene glycol solution. Tegaserod, a 5-HT^4 agonist, is also effective. Severe intractable colonic inertia with megacolon may require subtotal colectomy and ileorectostomy. Pelvic floor dysfunction requires biofeedback, relaxation exercises, and the use of suppositories.

Patients with fecal impaction should first have their colon evacuated with enemas or polyethylene glycol electrolyte solution until cleansing is complete. Recurrence of fecal impaction is then prevented with a fiber-restricted diet together with cleansing enemas twice weekly or daily oral intake of 12 to 16 fluid ounces of polyethylene glycol solution.

Fecal Incontinence

Fecal incontinence, defined as the recurrent uncontrolled passage of fecal material for at least 1 month, is a disturbing disability because it affects quality of life and may lead to social isolation. Fecal incontinence may be minor, with inadvertent passage of flatus or soiling of underwear with liquid stool, or it may be major, with involuntary leakage of feces. Fecal incontinence affects 2% to 7% of adults, mostly older persons in poor general health.

Fecal continence depends on many factors, such as physical and mental function, stool consistency, colonic transit, rectal compliance, internal and external anal sphincter function, as well as anorectal sensation and reflexes. Normal defecation is a complex sequential process that starts with the entry of stool into the rectum that leads to reflex relaxation of the internal anal sphincter. If defecation is desired, the anorectal angle is voluntarily straightened, and abdominal pressure is increased by straining. This results in descent of the pelvic floor, contraction of the rectum, and inhibition of the external anal sphincter, which causes evacuation of the rectal contents.

Decreased anal sphincter tone can result from trauma (eg, anal surgery) or neurologic disorders (eg, spinal cord injury or a secondary effect of diabetes mellitus). Vaginal delivery associated with anal sphincter tears or trauma to the pudendal nerve may result in fecal incontinence immediately or after many years. Decreased rectal compliance resulting from ulcerative or radiation proctitis leads to increased fecal frequency and urgency. Impaction is a common cause of fecal incontinence in elderly persons because it inhibits the internal anal sphincter tone, permitting leakage of liquid stool. Idiopathic fecal incontinence caused by denervation of the pelvic floor musculature occurs most commonly in middle-aged and elderly women.

The history and physical examination often provide clues to the cause of fecal incontinence. A flexible sigmoidoscopy may be considered in order to exclude inflammation or tumor. The next step is anorectal manometry, which measures resting anal sphincter tone, the squeeze pressure, the rectoanal inhibitory reflex, rectal sensation, and rectal compliance. Abnor-

malities of the anal sphincters, the rectal wall, and the puborectalis muscle can be further evaluated by the use of endorectal ultrasound. Typically, a defect in the internal anal sphincter is associated with low resting sphincter pressure, whereas defects in the external sphincter are associated with lower anal squeeze pressure.

Medical therapy is aimed at reducing stool frequency and improving stool consistency. The former is achieved with antidiarrheal drugs, such as loperamide; the latter, by supplementing the diet with a bulking agent, such as methylcellulose. Older patients with incontinence related to cognitive impairment or physical debility may benefit from a regular defecation program. Biofeedback therapy is a painless noninvasive method of retraining the pelvic floor and the abdominal wall musculature and is recommended for patients with fecal incontinence associated with structurally intact sphincter. Surgery may involve sphincter repair or implantation of an artificial sphincter. Colostomy may be needed for patients with intractable symptoms in whom other treatments have failed. A synthetic sphincter device, consisting of an inflatable cuff that maintains continence, is a valve that allows the cuff to deflate for defecation. Radiofrequency energy delivery to the anal sphincters (Secca procedure) may also improve continence in selected patients.

Diverticular Disease

The prevalence of diverticular disease is age dependent, increasing to 30% by age 60 and to 65% by age 85. Although most patients remain asymptomatic, 20% develop diverticulitis, and 10% may develop diverticular bleeding. Therefore, the mere presence of diverticulosis does not require specific therapy. A diet high in fiber appears to be associated with a reduced risk of the development of diverticular disease and may reduce the risk of subsequent complications.

Uncomplicated diverticulosis is often an incidental finding on screening sigmoidoscopy, colonoscopy, or barium enema. Some patients may complain of nonspecific abdominal cramping, bloating, flatulence, and irregular bowel habits. Diverticular bleeding is usually painless and self-limited, and it rarely coexists with acute diverticulitis. Diverticulitis usually presents with left lower quadrant pain, although nausea, vomiting, constipation, diarrhea, and dysuria or frequency may occur. The physical examination usually reveals left lower quadrant tenderness, a tender mass, and abdominal distention. Generalized tenderness suggests perforation and peritonitis. Low-grade fever and leukocytosis are common, but their absence in older patients does not exclude the diagnosis. Urinalysis may reveal sterile pyuria induced by adjacent colonic inflammation; the presence of mixed colonic flora on urine culture suggests a colovesical fistula. Other complications that can occur include perforation, obstruction, and abscess formation.

Computed tomographic (CT) scanning is the optimal imaging method in acute diverticulitis. CT features of acute diverticulitis include increased density of soft tissue within pericolic fat and colonic diverticula, bowel wall thickening, soft-tissue masses (phlegmon), and pericolic fluid collections (abscess formation). CT can also identify peritonitis, obstruction, and fistula to the bladder, vagina, and abdominal wall. However, in approximately 10% of patients, diverticulitis cannot be distinguished from colon cancer, since both may show focal thickening of the bowel wall. In such cases, upon resolution of the acute inflammation, a colonoscopy is indicated. In older persons, CT-guided percutaneous drainage of localized abscesses may obviate emergent surgery and permit single-stage elective surgical resection.

The majority of patients (85%) with simple diverticulitis respond to medical therapy. In contrast, all patients with complicated diverticulitis require surgery. Indications for emergency surgery are free perforation with peritonitis, obstruction, clinical deterioration or failure to improve with conservative management, and an abscess that cannot be drained percutaneously. Indications for elective surgical intervention are recurrent or intractable symptoms, persistent mass, obstruction, and fistula or abscess formation.

Mild diverticulitis with left lower quadrant pain, low-grade fever, and minimal physical findings is often treated on an outpatient basis, with clear liquids and oral antibiotics, such as ciprofloxacin 500 mg twice a day or metronidazole 500 mg three times a day, or both. Hospitalization is needed only if the patient fails to improve. Once the episode resolves, solid food is reintroduced and the colon is evaluated, preferably by colonoscopy. For patients with moderate to severe symptoms, treatment with bowel rest, fluids, and intravenous antibiotics is initiated, with the aim to avoid urgent surgery. Antibiotics should be active against gram-negative rods and anaerobes. Possible regimens include cefoxitin, piperacillin-tazobactam, or gentamicin plus clindamycin. If there is no improvement, the diagnosis is incorrect or an abscess, peritonitis, fistula, or obstruction is present. Older immunosuppressed patients with multiple underlying medical conditions may present with minimal symptoms or signs even with frank peritonitis, and the diagnosis is commonly delayed. In such cases, early surgical intervention should be considered. Diffuse peritonitis requires fluid resuscitation, broad-spectrum antibiotics, and emergency laparotomy. Colonic resective surgery removes the septic focus, corrects the obstruction or fistula formation, and restores bowel continuity. In most elective cases, resection and primary anastomosis are possible, if the disease is well localized or has significantly resolved.

After successful medical therapy of the first episode of diverticulitis, one third of patients will remain asymptomatic, another third will have episodic abdominal cramps (painful diverticulosis), and the remaining will proceed to a second attack of diverticulitis. Therefore, elective surgery is not necessary for all patients with diverticulitis who respond to medical therapy. If surgery is performed, progression of diverticulosis in the remaining colon occurs in only 15%, and the need for further surgery is reduced to less than 10%.

Irritable Bowel Syndrome

Irritable bowel syndrome (IBS) is a functional gastrointestinal disorder with remissions and exacerbations, characterized by abdominal pain (A), bloating (B), and either constipation (C) or diarrhea (D), or both. IBS results from altered bowel motility, visceral hypersensitivity, and enhanced perception by the brain of many visceral stimuli. A common mediator for all these abnormalities is serotonin, and serotonin-receptor agonists and antagonists are used in the management of IBS. Although psychosocial factors are commonly involved in IBS, they are not known to have a causative role.

Since the clinical symptoms characteristic of irritable bowel syndrome are not specific, it is important to be mindful of features that are not consistent with IBS. These include weight loss, first onset of symptoms after age 50, nocturnal diarrhea, family history of cancer or inflammatory bowel disease, rectal bleeding or obstruction, and laboratory abnormalities, such as anemia, leukocytosis, abnormal chemistries, positive fecal cultures, or the presence of parasites in the stool. In the older patient the diagnosis should be made only after other conditions (ie, ischemia, diverticulosis, colon cancer, or inflammatory bowel disease) have been carefully excluded. An appropriate work-up of an older person with symptoms consistent with IBS should include a colonoscopy to exclude structural abnormalities of the colon. A CT scan of the abdomen and a small bowel series may also be useful. If the history, physical examination, and laboratory or imaging studies are negative, the diagnosis of IBS can then be made and subcategorized as IBS with constipation (IBS-C) or diarrhea (IBS-D) or IBS with alternating constipation and diarrhea.

Depending on the IBS subtype, treatment includes reassurance, antispasmodics, antidiarrheals, fiber supplements, and serotonin-receptor agents (alosetron and tegaserod). Although quite effective, the latter drugs may precipitate intestinal ischemia and should be used with caution, particularly in the elderly patient. Try to establish a definitive diagnosis of IBS, avoid repetitive investigations, and clarify that although IBS is not life threatening, it can certainly negatively impact quality of life. As part of chronic disease management, it is also important that clinicians listen actively to patients' symptoms, validate their feelings, provide empathy, set realistic shared goals, negotiate treatment strategies instead of issuing directives, help patients take responsibility for treatment decisions, establish limits on the duration and frequency of visits and phone calls, and maintain a continuing relationship.

Occult Gastrointestinal Bleeding

Older patients are commonly noted to have a positive stool test for occult blood or are diagnosed with unexplained iron-deficiency anemia. Although colorectal cancer is a leading concern in such patients, many other causes, such as esophagitis, peptic ulcers, esophageal and gastric malignancies, intestinal or colonic angiodysplasia, benign colon polyps, inflammatory bowel disease, or hemorrhoids may be the cause. A positive fecal occult blood test should not be attributed to esophageal varices or colonic diverticula, because it is rare for such lesions to bleed in an occult fashion. The presence of fecal occult blood should not be attributed to aspirin or warfarin use or alcohol ingestion.

Detection of occult blood in the stool has a low sensitivity and a high rate of false-positive results, leading to more invasive and expensive tests. Despite these limitations, annual screening is currently recommended and has been associated with up to a 33% reduction in mortality from colorectal cancer. Because of the high prevalence of colorectal cancer and adenomatous polyps in older adults with a positive fecal occult blood test, colonoscopy is performed and, if negative, is followed by an upper endoscopy. If symptoms of upper gastrointestinal disease are present, there is a high likelihood for a positive endoscopy. However, in older patients at risk for colon cancer, the presence of a proximal lesion should not preclude evaluation of the colon. Patients with normal upper and lower tract may require evaluation for a small bowel source. The most common cause for bleeding from the small bowel is angiodysplasia, followed by tumors or ulcers that are commonly caused by NSAIDs. Unrecognized gluten-sensitive enteropathy can result in iron-deficiency anemia, since iron is absorbed in the proximal small bowel.

In one prospective study that evaluated patients with iron-deficiency anemia with colonoscopy, endoscopy, and, if these tests were negative, radiographic examination of the small intestine, a source of bleeding was identified in 62%. A lesion was seen on colonoscopy in 25%, on upper endoscopy in 36%, and on both in 1% of patients. Peptic ulcer disease was the primary abnormality in the upper gastrointestinal tract, but cancer was detected on colonoscopy in 11% of patients. Even after endoscopic examination of both the upper and lower parts of the gastrointestinal tract, the source of bleeding remains unidentified in approximately 10% of older patients presenting with iron-deficiency anemia and occult gastrointestinal bleeding. In such cases, video capsule endoscopy has a high diagnostic yield and is simple and noninvasive.

Colonic Angiodysplasia

The terms angiodysplasia, arteriovenous malformation, and vascular ectasia have been used interchangeably. Angiodysplasias occur most often in the cecum and ascending colon, where they may cause bleeding, particularly in patients aged 60 or over. However, angiodysplasias occur throughout the gastrointestinal tract and may be multiple or coexist in several different regions of the gastrointestinal tract. They may be asymptomatic or cause occult or clinically overt gastrointestinal bleeding.

Angiodysplasias are dilated, thin-walled vessels in the mucosa and submucosa that are lined by endothelium or by smooth muscle. Although they are mostly tortuous veins, arteriovenous communications or enlarged arteries may be present, leading to brisk bleeding. The pathogenesis of angiodysplasias is not well understood. They may result from local ischemia associated with cardiac, vascular, or pulmonary disease. Researchers have detected increased expression of angiogenic factors, basic fibroblast growth factor and vascular endothelial growth factor, in segments of colon with angiodysplasia.

Angiodysplasias are usually diagnosed during colonoscopy, appearing as 5- to 10-mm cherry-red, ectatic blood vessels radiating from a central vascular core. Angiodysplasias can also be diagnosed by angiography. If they are serendipitously detected during routine endoscopy or colonoscopy, angiodysplasias should not be treated. However, an actively bleeding angiodysplasia should be treated. Whether angiodysplasias were the cause of bleeding in patients who have stopped bleeding and, in particular, in patients who are found to have both angiodysplasias and diverticula is a more difficult problem. In such cases, bleeding from angiodysplasias is almost always from the cecum or ascending colon.

Many endoscopic ablation techniques have been used in the treatment of angiodysplasias. Although acute bleeding can be successfully controlled with these approaches, rebleeding is common. Angiography may localize the site of active bleeding and allows embolization or infusion of vasopressin. Surgical resection is definitive for lesions that have been clearly identified as the source of bleeding. However, recurrent bleeding may occur from other proximal or distal lesions in more than 30% of cases. Hormonal therapy with estrogen (with or without progesterone) has also been used in women, but its benefit should be weighed against the potential risks of thromboembolic disease, estrogen-dependent tumors, or uterine bleeding.

Colonic Ischemia

Ischemic colitis is typically encountered in patients aged 65 years and older who have atherosclerosis or atrial fibrillation or who have had surgical bypass or vascular grafting procedures. The main symptoms at presentation are abdominal pain and lower gastrointestinal bleeding. Colonoscopy reveals segmental edema, hemorrhages, gray-black pseudomembrane formation, and focal ulcers, mostly in the region of the splenic flexure and typically sparing the rectum. Treatment is mostly supportive, but even with treatment colonic strictures may ensue. The development of peritoneal signs calls for surgical intervention with colonic resection of the involved segment.

Clostridium difficile Infection and Pseudomembranous Colitis

C. *difficile* infection is becoming increasingly recognized among hospitalized patients and as the source of epidemics in hospitals and long-term-care facilities for elderly persons. The infection is often precipitated by the use of antibiotics, such as cephalosporins, penicillins, or clindamycin. Clinically it presents with watery diarrhea, crampy abdominal pain, fever, abdominal tenderness and distention, and an elevated white blood cell count. Serious complications, such as ileus with dehydration and electrolyte abnormalities, toxic megacolon, perforation, and death, may occur. C. *difficile* infection should be considered when acute abdominal distention occurs in older hospitalized adults without diarrhea but with associated severe leukocytosis; it carries high mortality. C. *difficile* infection can be recognized endoscopically by the appearance of diffuse or segmental pseudomembranes coating an edematous mucosa, but the diagnosis is often made by the detection of C. *difficile* cytotoxins in the stool either by cytotoxin tissue culture assay, latex agglutination, or enzyme-linked immunoassays. Metronidazole 250 mg orally every 6 hours is effective in 85% of cases, and it may be given intravenously in severe cases of ileus or megacolon. Vancomycin (125 mg every 6

hours) is also highly effective but only if given orally. Antibiotic treatment for C. *difficile* colitis should be for 10 to 14 days to reduce the risk of relapse. Relapses may occur in up to 20% of cases and require repeat treatment with metronidazole, vancomycin, or a combination of vancomycin and rifampin. In order to prevent the disease in predisposed individuals and to avoid relapses, restitution of the colonic flora with lactobacilli or *Saccharomyces boulardii* has been used.

Acute Colonic Pseudo-Obstruction

Acute colonic pseudo-obstruction is manifested by acute massive dilation of the colon without evidence of mechanical obstruction. In the older adult, it is often related to neurologic disease, such as Parkinson's or cerebrovascular disease, trauma, recent orthopedic surgery, or use of narcotics. Infections, particularly C. *difficile*, and colonic ischemia need to be excluded. Urgent colonoscopy not only can assist with the diagnosis but allows placement of a decompression colonic tube. Parenteral fluids and supportive measures, discontinuation of narcotics, and the use of neostigmine intravenously often lead to rapid resolution.

Colonic Polyps and Colon Cancer

Polyps are usually asymptomatic, but they may bleed or predispose the patient to cancer. Colonic polyps are usually classified as neoplastic (adenomas) or non-neoplastic (hyperplastic). Approximately 40% of the U.S. population aged 50 or over have one or more adenomas. Detection and removal of adenomas significantly decreases the morbidity and mortality associated with colorectal cancer. Old age and male gender are major risk factors. First-degree relatives of patients with adenomas are also at increased risk for colorectal cancer and should undergo screening. Adenomas are most often detected by colon cancer screening tests, primarily sigmoidoscopy. Because adenomas do not typically bleed, the fecal occult blood test is an insensitive screening method. Older age, villous histology, and size are independent risk factors for malignancy within an adenoma. The risk of colon cancer also increases with the number of high-risk adenomas that are present.

Colorectal cancer is the third leading cause of cancer in the United States and the second leading cause of cancer death. The risk of colorectal cancer increases dramatically with age, with more than 90% of cases occurring in people over age 50. Women are more likely than men to harbor right-sided colonic adenomas. The risk of colorectal cancer in patients with rectal bleeding is age related and may reach to 25% in patients aged 80 and over. Up to 40% of colorectal cancer arises proximal to the splenic flexure, and less than 10% is within the reach of the digital rectal examination. Since it is impossible to identify the source of bleeding by clinical criteria, a colonoscopy should be performed in all cases of hematochezia, occult gastrointestinal bleeding, iron-deficiency anemia, or even melena after a negative upper endoscopy. Other symptoms, such as abdominal pain, altered bowel habits, or pencil-thin stools are less predictive of colorectal cancer but do require thorough investigation, starting with a colonoscopy. Typically, right-sided cancers present with iron-deficiency anemia and occult gastrointestinal bleeding, whereas left-sided cancers lead to obstructive symptoms, changes in bowel habits, and overt hematochezia.

Colonoscopy with endoscopic polypectomy is the ideal examination for the detection and removal of adenomatous polyps. Large adenomas that cannot be safely or completely resected endoscopically should generally be removed by segmental colectomy. If a polyp is detected by barium enema, colonoscopy is recommended to establish the histology, remove the polyp, and search for other lesions. If a single polyp is detected by sigmoidoscopy, it should be biopsied. If the polyp is hyperplastic, colonoscopy is not required. If the polyp is adenomatous, full colonoscopy is warranted.

A 3-year interval for surveillance colonoscopy is safe and cost-effective for most patients with adenomas. If only a small tubular adenoma is found, the interval may be extended to 5 years; in contrast, after removal of a large villous adenoma, a 1-year follow-up is recommended. After a negative screening or surveillance colonoscopy, an examination interval of 5 years appears to be safe. Patients with colorectal cancer should also have regular colonoscopic surveillance for adenomas starting 1 year after surgery, since these patients have adenoma or cancer recurrence rates of 25% to 30% at 3 years. Because the greatest impact of colorectal cancer on life expectancy occurs between the ages of 70 and 80 years and the protective effect of colonoscopy on colorectal cancer mortality is approximately 10 years, the optimal and most cost-effective age for one-time colonoscopic screening is 60 to 65 years of age.

Colonoscopic screening for cancer and subsequent surveillance lose their cost-effectiveness after the age of 80 years. Screening for colorectal cancer should also cease when the risk of screening outweighs any potential benefits, in patients with less than 10 years' estimated survival, or when tests are unlikely to prolong patient survival. In patients with known history of polyps, discontinuation of surveillance should be considered in those aged over 75 years in whom a follow-up examination is normal or shows only small tubular adenomas.

ANNOTATED REFERENCES

■ American Gastroenterological Association medical position statement: evaluation of dyspepsia. *Gastroenterology.* 1998;114(3):579–581.

>   This is an exhaustive review of the approach to the patient with dyspepsia. It summarizes the causes, clinical evaluation, and the use of endoscopy or imaging studies and discusses the pros and cons of empirical versus specific drug therapy.

■ De Lillo AR, Rose S. Functional bowel disorders in the geriatric patient: constipation, fecal impaction, and fecal incontinence. *Am J Gastroenterol.* 2000; 95(4):901–905.

>   The authors review the causes and pathophysiology of constipation, fecal impaction, and fecal incontinence and emphasize the aspects of the history and physical examination as well as the pertinent physiologic, radiologic, and endoscopic studies needed for the evaluation of these common problems. The review also provides recommendations for therapy that is based on underlying pathogenetic mechanisms.

■ Fireman Z, Friedman S. Diagnostic yield of capsule endoscopy in obscure gastrointestinal bleeding. *Digestion.* 2004;70(3):201–206.

>   In this cohort study, 293 patients with obscure gastrointestinal bleeding were identified in a company-sponsored clinical study database with data from more than 50 clinical studies. Capsule endoscopy detected definitive findings in 213 of the patients (72%), proving its high diagnostic yield.

■ Gostout CJ. Gastrointestinal bleeding in the elderly patient. *Am J Gastroenterol.* 2000; 95(3):590–595.

>   This review of the evaluation and resuscitation of the elderly patient with gastrointestinal bleeding focuses on the use of endoscopy, diet, and medications for evaluation and treatment, and on issues of informed consent, hospitalization, and discharge planning.

■ Miller KM, Waye JD. Approach to colon polyps in the elderly. *Am J Gastroenterol.* 2000;95(5):1147–1151.

>   This article reviews the magnitude of the problem of colon polyps and colon cancer in the older population and the principles of surveillance of patients with adenomatous polyps.

■ Richter JE. Gastroesophageal reflux disease in the older patient: presentation, treatment and complications. *Am J Gastroenterol.* 2000;95(2):368–373.

>   This is an authoritative and evidence-based review of the epidemiology, pathogenesis, and clinical presentations of gastroesophageal reflux disease. It provides an update on the evaluation of patients with the disease and on the use of

physiologic, radiologic, and endoscopic tests. It also summarizes the medical and surgical therapy.

- Schoenfeld P, Cash B, Flood A, et al. Colonoscopic screening of average-risk women for colorectal neoplasia. *N Engl J Med.* 2005;352(20):2061–2068.

    The authors sought to determine the prevalence and location of large adenomas by offering colonoscopy instead of flexible sigmoidoscopy to consecutive asymptomatic women referred for colon-cancer screening. Only 35.2 % of women with large adenomas would have had their lesions identified if they had undergone flexible sigmoidoscopy alone, as compared with 66.3% of a cohort of men from another Veterans Affairs trial of similar design.

- Tendler DA. Acute intestinal ischemia and infarction. *Semin Gastrointest Dis.* 2003; 14(2):66–76.

    Acute intestinal ischemia is a gastrointestinal emergency resulting from a sudden decrease in intestinal blood flow; it carries a high mortality unless early angiography and surgical intervention are performed. Acute colonic ischemia is often a reversible condition with lower mortality rate. This article reviews the pathophysiology, clinical features, diagnostic, and therapeutic options applicable to patients with acute intestinal ischemia.

George Triadafilopoulos, MD

CHAPTER 50—KIDNEY DISEASES AND DISORDERS

KEY POINTS

- The older kidney is capable of maintaining homeostasis of body fluids and electrolytes under most circumstances.

- Therapies directed at controlling blood pressure and minimizing proteinuria are key in patients with chronic kidney disease.

- Adjusting medication doses appropriately and avoiding nephrotoxic medications are important aspects of the management of patients with chronic kidney disease.

- Early referral to a nephrologist is useful for optimal planning for kidney replacement therapy.

Kidney function declines after age 40 years at a mean rate of approximately 1% per year, accelerating some in the later years. This observation was first reported in cross-sectional studies and confirmed in a population of normal aging persons followed over time. However, although two thirds of individuals followed for up to 20 years in the Baltimore Longitudinal Study developed a decline in glomerular filtration rate (GFR) with aging, one third had no decline, indicating that a decline in kidney function with age is not inevitable.

Although there is loss of glomerular mass with aging, the loss of tubular mass is proportional, so that glomerular-tubular balance is usually maintained. Despite significant anatomic and functional changes, the older kidney is capable of maintaining homeostasis of body fluids and electrolytes under most circumstances. However, under environmental and disease-related stresses, such as volume changes or alterations in acid-base status, the older kidney is slower to respond to correct the abnormality.

FLUID AND ELECTROLYTE DISTURBANCES

Hyponatremia and Hypernatremia

Surveys of older adults in both acute and long-term-care facilities show a high prevalence of hyponatremia (serum sodium concentration < 132 mmol/L). By definition, these persons have an excess of water relative to solute. Clinically, older adults with hyponatremia can be separated into those with decreased extracellular fluid (ECF) volume (eg, gastrointestinal losses, adrenal and renal salt-losing conditions), increased ECF volume (eg, heart failure), or normal ECF volume (eg, syndrome of inappropriate antidiuretic hormone, or SIADH). The last is the most common. Regardless of cause, nonosmotic (baroreceptor) stimulation of arginine vasopressin (AVP) release is a major factor in the development of hyponatremia. Older persons appear to have an increased osmoreceptor sensitivity, as evidenced by the greater increase in serum AVP in response to any given increase in serum osmolality. Postoperative and diuretic-induced hyponatremia are much more common in older than in younger persons.

Hyponatremia does not usually produce symptoms until the serum sodium concentration falls below 125 mmol/L. At about this level, central nervous symptoms begin to appear, including somnolence, cognitive impairment, seizures, and ultimately coma, secondary to brain edema. Although therapy is not different for older adults, it is important to proceed slowly and to monitor regularly the older patient's response to avoid the development of cardiovascular or neurologic symptoms, or both.

Hypertonic dehydration (serum sodium > 148 mmol/L) is common in older adults, especially among acutely hospitalized and nursing-home patients. It also is largely avoidable. A number of factors may contribute to this condition. Body water is decreased as a proportion of total body weight because of the relative increase in fat content of normal older adults. Although AVP release from the posterior pituitary is normal (or even supernormal) in response to hypertonicity in older adults, the ability to concentrate the urine in response to AVP is decreased. Probably most important is the blunted or even absent thirst response to hypertonicity seen in normal older adults. This thirst response is even more impaired in patients with cerebral disease, such as stroke. In hot weather and in the absence of air conditioning, it is therefore important to make certain that older adults know to increase their consumption of fluids. An inability to obtain water because of functional or cognitive barriers may further limit the older person's ability to adequately replenish lost body fluids. It is helpful to instruct older adults to drink a specific amount of water each day. For institutionalized older adults, particularly those with decreased mobility or impaired cognition, placing a specific amount of fluid within easy reach and assuring that it is gone by the end of the day is helpful. In addition, on very hot days, it may be wise to hold or decrease the dose of diuretics in some patients. Symptoms of hypernatremia (obtundation, lethargy, coma) are predominantly neurologic, presumably because of shrinkage of the brain cells. As intravascular volume is preserved at the expense of cell water, changes in blood pressure, pulse rate, and skin turgor may not be evident early on.

Hypokalemia and Hyperkalemia

There is a long list of potential causes of hypokalemia in older adults. A low serum potassium measurement usually represents total body potassium depletion. This may be secondary to gastrointestinal losses, as occurs with vomiting, diarrhea, nasogastric suction, or fistula drainage. Vomiting produces a metabolic alkalosis that shifts potassium into cells and increases urinary potassium losses. Another commonly overlooked cause of hypokalemia is excessive use of purgatives and enemas.

Total body depletion of potassium may also occur secondary to renal losses. In older adults this is commonly secondary to diuretic usage and may be completely avoided with supplemental potassium. Although the liquid form of potassium supplement has an unpleasant taste, it is generally absorbed better than potassium tablets and is not associated with the same risk of gastric ulceration. Potassium wasting may also result from excessive adrenal hormone production or a primary underlying kidney disease. Primary and secondary aldosteronism (the latter from renal artery stenosis or volume contraction resulting from diuretic usage in patients with heart, liver, or kidney disease) may be a contributing factor. Hypomagnesemia-induced hypokalemia with ongoing renal potassium wasting is also seen with diuretic usage.

Potassium deficiency affects the cardiovascular system, neurologic system, muscles, and kidneys. The major side effects affecting the cardiovascular system are hypokalemia-induced ventricular arrhythmias. Muscle symptoms include weakness, easy fatigability, cramping, myalgias, and muscle tenderness secondary to rhabdomyolysis. Effects on the kidneys result in polyuria and development of a metabolic alkalosis with paradoxical aciduria (low urine pH).

Since an alkalosis (chloride depletion) usually accompanies hypokalemia and is responsible for a shift of potassium intracellularly, replacement therapy should be with potassium chloride. The exception is the patient with renal tubular acidosis, in which case the alkaline salts of potassium should be given. Azotemia and age are the two significant risk factors for life-threatening hyperkalemia in potassium-supplemented patients. The latter may be related to the lower levels of aldosterone seen in the elderly patient under any given set of conditions (low-salt versus high-salt diet, supine versus upright posture).

Most episodes of hyperkalemia are seen in patients with chronic kidney disease (CKD). However, significant hyperkalemia is uncommon until the azotemia becomes life threatening or another factor contributes, such as an increased endogenous or ingested potassium load, severe acidosis, administration of a diuretic to block sodium potassium exchange (triamterene, spironolactone), a deficiency of endogenous aldosterone or mineralocorticoid, or, importantly, administration of drugs, such as nonsteroidal anti-inflammatory drugs (NSAIDs) or angiotensin-converting enzyme (ACE) inhibitors. Older persons with an interstitial nephritis, especially diabetic patients, develop a failure of the renin-aldosterone system with a hyperkalemia and mild metabolic acidosis, often referred to as *type IV renal tubular acidosis*.

CLINICAL PRESENTATIONS OF KIDNEY DISEASES

In general, the presentation of kidney disease in older and younger adults is not significantly different. It is important to recognize a decline in kidney function to permit early diagnosis of treatable causes of renal insufficiency. If no treatment is available, then interventions to retard disease progression should be started whenever possible. As detailed below, national guidelines have been developed to guide pre–end-stage renal disease (ESRD) care. Equally important, the impact of kidney function on other aspects of a person's health care needs to be considered. For example, medications that are excreted by the kidney may need a dose adjustment to prevent toxic drug levels. In addition, some medications may adversely affect kidney function or complicate kidney disease. In patients with CKD there may be alterations in feelings of well-being and changes in functional status that must be addressed.

The medical history and physical examination may be very helpful in determining the cause of renal insufficiency. The clinical symptoms and signs are variable but often are related to the underlying disease. Nephrotic syndrome may present with edema and hypertension. Kidney stones may present with flank pain, hematuria, nausea, and vomiting. These same symptoms are also seen with acute renal artery embolization. Renal artery stenosis may be silent or present with multiple episodes of pulmonary edema. The symptoms commonly reported as a direct result of CKD (eg, fatigue, nausea, cognitive difficulties) are generally not experienced until the creatinine clearance (CrCl) is less than 20 mL/min. However, complications of CKD, including anemia, metabolic acidosis, and alterations in calcium-phosphate metabolism, may develop as the GFR falls below 60 mL/min.

The first hint of kidney disease may be seen on a screening urinalysis with asymptomatic abnormalities (hematuria, proteinuria, pyuria, casts). It may also present with an asymptomatic elevated serum urea nitrogen or serum creatinine concentration. It is important to remember that muscle mass decreases with age. Therefore, a normal serum creatinine may represent a decline in kidney function. For example, a serum creatinine of 1.0 mg/dL in an 80-year-old person weighing 65 kg corresponds to an estimated CrCl of 54 mL/min. It also is helpful to look for changes in serum creatinine over time. A change in serum creatinine from a steady-state level of 0.7 mg/dL to 1.4 mg/dL indicates that the kidney function has decreased by 50% and signals the need for further evaluation.

In summary, the finding in an older adult of hematuria, proteinuria, abnormal urinary sediment, or a decreased CrCl indicates the need to more fully evaluate kidney function. Although it is not clear that age alone is a risk factor for CKD, the comorbidity associated with the aging process, including vascular disease, diabetes mellitus, and cardiac disease, places older adults at increased risk for a renal insult.

Hematuria

Whether macroscopic or microscopic (> 3 to 5 red blood cells per high-power field), hematuria in older adults deserves evaluation. A microscopic examination of the urine may suggest the source of the hematuria.

Dysmorphic red blood cells (normal biconcave shape is distorted) or red cell casts in freshly voided urine suggest a glomerular source. Associated proteinuria or an elevated serum creatinine concentration also suggest kidney parenchymal disease. Biconcave red blood cells suggest a disease of the collecting system. It is also important to consider systemic coagulation defects. In addition to a microscopic urine evaluation, the work-up of isolated hematuria should include a urine culture, imaging (kidney ultrasound or intravenous pyelography) to exclude a renal parenchymal mass, and, if these are nondiagnostic, a urologic consultation for cystoscopy. In addition, a platelet count, prothrombin time, and partial thromboplastin time should be obtained to exclude a coagulopathy. In approximately 80% of older adults, the source of hematuria is the bladder, prostate, or urethra. Malignancies, most often bladder but also hypernephroma and prostate, account for one third of the cases of hematuria. Less than 10% of the hematuria is glomerular in origin (in the absence of proteinuria). It is important to remember that hematuria in patients on warfarin is not normal and suggests underlying pathology. Hematuria with proteinuria in a patient with diabetic nephropathy also needs evaluation to exclude underlying malignancy. Where hematuria is noted on dipstick examination of the urine and no red blood cells are seen on the microscopic examination, the clinician needs to consider the presence of myoglobin.

Proteinuria

Normal protein excretion in older and younger adults does not differ significantly. Significant proteinuria is defined as greater than 150 mg per 24 hours. The urine dipstick is a good screening method for the detection of proteinuria, but it detects only albumin; light chains, which would be present in a patient with multiple myeloma, and low-molecular-weight protein (tubular protein) need to be detected by the use of a sulfa salicylic acid test. This test may be easily performed in the outpatient clinical setting.

When urinary proteins are primarily albumin and higher-molecular-weight proteins, the pathology is likely glomerular. Three grams of protein in a 24-hour urine sample is used to distinguish nephrotic from non-nephrotic proteinuria. The evaluation of proteinuria should begin with a careful examination of fresh urinary sediment (cells, casts), as this can provide helpful clues as to the mechanism of the proteinuria.

The urine dipstick method for detection of proteinuria is relatively insensitive, requiring urinary albumin concentrations of nearly 30 mg/dL. This means that a person with a urine output of 1 liter per day must be excreting nearly 300 mg of albumin per day before proteinuria can be detected. Microalbuminuria, defined as a urinary albumin excretion of more than 30 mg per day (less than that detectable with the dipstick method), is an early indicator of progressing renal injury. This has become important because antihypertensive therapy, specifically ACE inhibitors, are being used to lower glomerular capillary pressures. This therapy reduces the proteinuria, which itself may be nephrotoxic, and retards the further development of renal damage, not only in diabetic but in nondiabetic kidney disease. Quantification of the severity of microalbuminuria does not require a 24-hour urine sample, as accurate enough estimates can be obtained with a timed early morning sample or simultaneous measurement of urinary creatinine concentration, or both.

Chronic Kidney Disease

The most useful measure of kidney function is an estimate of the GFR, as reductions in other functions (eg, tubular functions, concentrating ability, acid excretion) tend to parallel decline in GFR. The CrCl is the most reproducible measure of GFR available for clinical decision making. In older persons creatinine production falls at nearly the same rate as the renal clearance of creatinine and, as noted previously, a normal serum creatinine may actually reflect a decline in kidney function. This pattern of change is important to recognize when the older patient is using drugs cleared primarily by the kidney. The relationship between serum creatinine and GFR has prompted a number of investigators to suggest that one could properly correct for the confounding variables, so they have developed formulas to estimate CrCl as a measure of GFR. The most widely used formula is that of Cockcroft and Gault:

$$CrCl = \frac{(140 - age) \times weight}{72 \times serum\ creatinine}$$

Weight in kg; serum creatinine in mg/100 mL; 85% less in women.

This formula was developed and validated on highly selected samples of older adults that did not include many very old individuals. Only moderate correlations have subsequently been found between calculated and actual CrCls, especially in older populations.

Currently, no available method of estimating GFR from easily obtainable variables, such as age, sex, weight, and serum creatinine, is very accurate, and no method will be available until we have an easy method for estimating muscle mass. In older adults, the lower limit of a normal GFR is not well defined. Neverthe-

less, in clinical practice, the use of an estimated GFR from the Cockcroft and Gault formula will provide a prompt and reasonable guide for clinical decision making in most situations. Finally, it is important to recognize that certain commonly prescribed drugs (trimethoprim-sulfamethoxazole, cimetidine, and cefoxitin) compete with creatinine for tubular secretion, causing an increase in serum creatinine concentration without changing GFR. (See also the section on elimination in "Pharmacotherapy," p 73.)

IMAGING TECHNIQUES AND KIDNEY BIOPSY

A variety of imaging techniques are available to evaluate the genitourinary system. Ultrasonography is noninvasive and safe, and it can provide many diagnostic clues, showing kidney size, hydronephrosis of the collecting system, and solid and cystic parenchymal renal masses. An intravenous pyelogram shows more detail of the collecting system, including sites of obstruction and other pathology, such as papillary necrosis. However, it is best to avoid intravenous contrast in older adults with diabetes mellitus, CKD, hypertension, and, most notably, multiple myeloma, given the increased risk for contrast media–induced acute renal failure (ARF), especially if the person is dehydrated. If intravenous contrast absolutely must be used, the patient should be well hydrated before the procedure and for at least 24 hours after the procedure. Although the studies are controversial, most clinical centers now use N-acetylcysteine prior to procedures with contrast dye in high-risk patients. Computed tomography scans, magnetic resonance imaging, isotopic renography, and angiography are additional techniques available to further evaluate selected kidney disorders.

For patients with suspected primary glomerular disease or unexplained kidney failure, a kidney biopsy may be indicated after all other available means for establishing a diagnosis have been exhausted. Kidney biopsy should not be withheld because of age alone. At least half of all primary glomerular lesions responsible for the nephrotic syndrome are potentially treatable (eg, membranous glomerulopathy, minimal-change disease, vasculitis), and trials of immunosuppressive or corticosteroid therapies, or both, are warranted. On the other hand, when a lesion unresponsive to these agents is diagnosed, such as primary amyloidosis, it is important not to subject older adults to the potentially serious side effects of these medications. One study looked at more than 200 kidney biopsy samples in adults aged 60 and over with ARF to evaluate whether the biopsy was useful in predicting organ and patient survival. The authors found that in more than 90% of the biopsies, a diagnosis was made for ARF; in many of these cases, a treatment was available; and in 30% of the cases, the diagnosis on biopsy did not match the clinical diagnosis. In summary, when a cause for ARF is unclear on the basis of clinical and laboratory evaluation, a kidney biopsy is warranted. The exception would be the older adult who is unable to tolerate the indicated treatment for ARF because of comorbidity. It is important to work with the nephrologist and make certain that the patient is clinically stable for the procedure. This includes optimum blood-pressure control and holding medications that might increase the risk of bleeding, for example, aspirin.

DISEASES OF THE KIDNEY AND VASCULAR SYSTEM

A retrospective analysis examining the reason for kidney biopsy in 1368 older adults showed that the three most common reasons for referral were nephrotic syndrome (31%), acute renal insufficiency (26%), and chronic renal insufficiency (25%).

The incidence of nephrotic syndrome is at least as common in older adults as it is in younger persons. The most common cause in older adults is membranous nephropathy (35%), followed by minimal-change disease (16%) and primary amyloidosis (12%). The incidence rates for membranous nephropathy, crescentic glomerulonephritis (GN), and amyloidosis are higher in older adults, those for proliferative GN and immunoglobulin A nephropathy are lower, and the incidence rate for minimal-change disease is comparable to that for young adults but much lower than the rate seen in children. Diabetic nephropathy is probably the most common cause of nephrotic syndrome in older adults. The diagnosis is usually made on the basis of a long (15- to 20-year) history of diabetes mellitus and the finding of diabetic retinopathy, and a biopsy is not necessary. Glomerulopathies resulting from systemic disease are more common in older adults because of the increased incidence of underlying diseases, such as amyloidosis (dysproteinemias), collagen vascular diseases (vasculitis), and neoplastic disease.

Membranous nephropathy (MN) is the most common form of primary kidney disease in older adults and is twice as common in older than in younger persons. In a cohort of 155 patients over age 60 years followed for 20 years, older patients were found more likely to be hypertensive, have worse kidney function, and experience more thrombotic complications than younger patients. Possible causes of MN include medications (eg, NSAIDs, penicillamine), malignancies, and hepatitis B infection. One review reported that 11% of patients with MN had an underlying malignancy. In most patients the malignancy is clinically evident when the diagnosis of MN is made, and probably only 1% to 2% of patients have an occult malignancy. Screening older adults with MN for malignancy should probably include a complete history and physical examination, chest radiograph, fecal occult blood tests, and colonoscopy. It does appear that older patients are more susceptible to the extra-renal complications of the nephrotic syndrome and its treatment, most notably, cardiovascular, thrombotic, and infectious events. As the primary care physician is likely the first person called when acute symptoms develop, it is essential he or she be aware of these potential complications.

Minimal-change nephropathy presents similarly in young and old patients, but older persons are more likely to have nonselective proteinuria, microscopic hematuria, hypertension, and renal insufficiency.

Most older adults with diabetic nephropathy have type 2 (non-insulin-dependent) diabetes. Control of blood pressure is important in slowing the rate of deterioration of kidney function. The use of ACE inhibitors or angiotensin-II receptor blockers, even in normotensive diabetic patients, promotes efferent arteriolar vasodilatation and decreases glomerular capillary pressure, which also slows the rate of deterioration of kidney function. Current recommendations are that in most patients with hypertension and CKD, an ACE inhibitor or an angiotensin-II receptor blocker in combination with an ACE inhibitor should be used.

After diabetes, the next most common group of systemic diseases associated with kidney disease in older adults is the dysglobulinemias. These include amyloidosis, multiple myeloma, fibrillary GN, essential mixed cryoglobulinemia, and macroglobulinemia.

Acute Renal Insufficiency or Failure

ARF is at least as common in older as in younger adults. Controversy remains as to whether the prognosis is poorer in older adults, but there are no reasons to deny treatment for ARF, using any of the available techniques, on the basis of age. In older adults, azotemia and other consequences of ARF may induce acute behavioral changes that are usually reversible, and treatment should not be stopped on the assumption that the patient's mental status is irreversible. The primary physician is in a unique position to impact acute renal insufficiency, both in terms of prevention and early detection. With a comprehensive medical history, physical examination, laboratory values, and urinalysis, it is usually possible to determine whether the cause of acute renal insufficiency is pre-renal, intra-renal, or post-renal. In general, a normal urinalysis suggests the cause is either pre-renal or post-renal.

There are two clinical situations to consider. The first is the development of acute renal insufficiency in the hospitalized or institutionalized patient being treated for a non-nephrologic illness. In this setting, intravascular volume depletion and acute tubular necrosis (ATN) are the major contributors—both of which may often be avoided with appropriate measures. The diagnosis is usually made on the basis of the history, physical examination, and laboratory data, so that a kidney biopsy is not necessary. ARF has been reported in up to 8% of acutely hospitalized older adults aged 60 years and older. Although the studies vary, in general, ATN accounts for approximately 40% to 50% of the cases of ARF, and intravascular volume depletion for most of the remaining cases.

The second clinical situation to consider is whether acute renal insufficiency results from a primary kidney disease or is secondary to a systemic disease, such as diabetes mellitus, hypertensive or atherosclerotic vascular disease, or collagen vascular disease. Post-renal obstruction should always be excluded, as it is usually amenable to treatment.

Pre-Renal Acute Renal Insufficiency

Pre-renal ARF occurs when poor perfusion is causing the failure of kidney function. This type of ARF is of special importance in older adults. With acute hypotension, the decrease in kidney perfusion stimulates sympathetic activity and release of vasoconstrictor substances that further reduce GFR, contributing to ARF. Once the hemodynamic disturbances are corrected, the patient usually, but not always, recovers from the ARF. Loss of fluids (intravascular volume depletion), internal redistribution, decreased cardiac output, sepsis, and certain drugs (diuretics, ACE inhibitors) are responsible for the vast majority of cases of pre-renal ARF. In several series, intravascular volume depletion alone was found to account for more than half of the cases of pre-renal ARF in older adults. The slow response to sodium retention, the decreased urinary concentrating ability, and, most importantly, the impairment of thirst regulation, all characteristics of the older patient, contribute to this high incidence.

The use of drugs that alter intrarenal hemodynamics is a growing cause of pre-renal ARF in older adults. The rapid development of pre-renal ARF in a patient recently started on an ACE inhibitor should make the physician think about bilateral renal arterial stenosis. However, in one series, two thirds of the ACE inhibitor–related cases of ARF were found to have occurred in persons without renal arterial stenosis. Other factors that alter intrarenal hemodynamics include cardiac failure, concomitant use of NSAIDs (which inhibit prostaglandin production, an important regulator of kidney blood flow and GFR), diabetes mellitus, and volume depletion from any cause. (See the section on kidney diseases associated with NSAID use, p 407.)

It is important to distinguish between pre-renal ARF and ATN, which can develop in the more severe cases. In patients who are oliguric, a urinary osmolality > 500 mOsm/kg, a urinary sodium concentration of < 20 mEq/L, a urine-to-plasma creatinine ratio > 40, or a fractional excretion of sodium < 1% suggests pre-renal ARF. Generally, with pre-renal ARF the ratio of blood urea nitrogen to serum creatinine is > 20. These urinary indices are not always reliable in differentiating pre-renal ARF from other forms of ARF. Probably the most reliable indicator of the pre-renal state is the response to treatment with volume (salt and water) repletion, but, again, older patients may have a delayed response to volume expansion.

Acute Tubular Necrosis

ATN can be either ischemic or nephrotoxic in origin. The causes of ischemic ATN are basically the same as those described in the preceding section as causes of pre-renal ARF, only more severe. In addition, surgical interventions, most notably cardiac surgery and repair of aortic aneurysms, as well as sepsis, account for most of the remaining cases in older adults. Hypotension during and after surgery, postoperative fluid loss, and arrhythmias may be important contributors. Measures to decrease the risk of ATN in the postoperative patient include careful attention to nutritional issues, avoidance of hypotension, prevention and treatment of postoperative infection, appropriate medication dosing, and hydration. (See also "Perioperative Care," p 103.)

Most of the antibiotics effective in treating serious infections have been associated with nephrotoxic ATN. Age is a well-known risk factor for the development of aminoglycoside nephrotoxicity. Preexisting kidney disease and volume depletion may contribute to medication accumulation, leading to ATN. When it is necessary to use an aminoglycoside antibiotic in an older person, monitoring blood levels is essential.

Older adults also are at increased risk of developing radiocontrast-induced ARF. Although the non-ionic contrast dye has been reported in the literature to be less toxic to the kidneys, in practice, the risk of an acute renal insult is likely not significantly reduced. As mentioned earlier, it is best to avoid the use of intravenous contrast dye in any person with preexisting impairment of kidney function, multiple myeloma, vascular disease, intravascular volume depletion, or diabetes. Hydration before and after procedures employing use of contrast agents has been reported to be effective in reducing the incidence and severity of ARF in high-risk patients.

Clearly, when ARF develops, it needs to be dealt with promptly—but perhaps one of the most important roles of the clinician is preventing hospital-acquired ARF. With daily attention to changes in fluid intake, urine production, weight, and orthostatic blood-pressure measurements, the development of intravascular volume contraction in many older adults may be identified before significant symptoms develop. Another common cause of intravascular volume depletion is the order for "nothing by mouth" written in anticipation of a procedure, or the order for enemas written as a bowel preparation. When a procedure is delayed and maintenance intravenous fluids are not given, symptomatic intravascular volume depletion may develop in the frail older adult, with all the associated risks, including falls. (See also "Perioperative Care," p 99.)

Although the older kidney is able to defend against changes in volume, the response to correction is delayed. Avoiding the simultaneous use of multiple medications that may interact also is of benefit. For example, in the treatment of heart failure, the combination of a diuretic and an ACE inhibitor together with an NSAID is a recipe for the potential development of renal insufficiency unless the patient is carefully monitored. When an older hospitalized patient is being treated by several physicians, it may be prudent to write orders for "no NSAIDs" when appropriate.

Other Intrarenal Causes of Acute Renal Failure

In one review of 259 kidney biopsies done for ARF on adults aged 60 and older (remembering that when the cause of ARF has been established by the history, physical examination, and laboratory data, a kidney biopsy is not done), the following diagnoses were made: pauci-immune crescentic GN (with or without arteritis) in 31% of the biopsy samples, acute interstitial nephritis (AIN) 19%, ATN with nephrotic syndrome 8%, atheroemboli 7%, ATN alone 7%, light chain cast nephropathy 6%, postinfectious GN 5.5%, antiglomerular membrane antibody nephritis 4%, and immunoglobulin A nephropathy or Henoch-Schönlein syndrome 4%.

Acute GN in older adults often presents with circulatory congestion that suggests heart failure, in contrast to the hypertension and edema seen in younger patients. This observation, together with low urinary sodium concentrations and high ratios of blood urea nitrogen to serum creatinine that suggests pre-renal ARF, results in the misdiagnosis of acute GN as heart failure.

Acute or subacute GN may be an immunologic consequence of a systemic disease, for example, lupus erythematosus, vasculitis, Wegener's granulomatosis, mixed cryoglobulinemia, or a primary kidney disease of unknown cause, for example, crescentic GN with or without glomerular immune deposits. Other forms of proliferative GN include mesangioproliferative GN (including immunoglobulin A nephropathy), focal prolif-

erative GN, crescentic GN (including antiglomerular basement membrane disease), and vasculitis. It is important to remember that acute postinfectious GN remains a common entity.

AIN is caused by a variety of agents and probably has no special implications for older adults except for the higher prevalence of NSAID-induced AIN, discussed below, and the fact that older adults tend to be on multiple medications.

Renal vascular causes of ARF are discussed below. Rhabdomyolysis with ARF is seen in the setting of acute immobilization, infectious diseases, stroke, hyperosmolar states, hyponatremia, and hypernatremia, and after falls associated with muscle trauma.

Obstructive Nephropathy

Urinary obstruction is one of the most common causes of ARF in older adults. It is an important diagnosis to make because it is usually reversible. Prostatic hypertrophy or carcinoma is the most common cause, but one should also consider retroperitoneal or pelvic neoplasia, such as lymphoma and carcinoma of the bladder, cervix, uterus, ovaries, or rectum. Another cause of post-renal obstruction may be a blocked indwelling Foley catheter.

Laboratory findings with obstructive ARF tend to be nonspecific, with high urinary sodiums and decreased osmolalities and a nondiagnostic urinalysis. The ratio of blood urea nitrogen to serum creatinine is usually increased. Ultrasonography is safe and readily available, and it has become the initial evaluation of choice in most settings. In most cases, but not all, the diagnosis of obstruction can be made on the basis of a dilated collecting system or large distended bladder.

Renal Vascular Disease

Nearly half of both normotensive and hypertensive person aged 60 and over with evidence of atherosclerotic aortoiliac or peripheral vascular disease, or both, show some obstruction (> 50% narrowing) of the renal artery. In most of these patients, the obstruction goes unrecognized and is not clinically important. However, in some individuals, severe hypertension or progressive kidney disease, or both, may develop. Correction of stenosis may reverse these consequences. Therefore, any patient with suspected severe renal artery stenosis should have a diagnostic work-up. If a significant stenosis is found, the patient should be referred for evaluation for either percutaneous transluminal renal angioplasty or surgical revascularization of the renal artery. Clues suggesting hemodynamically significant renal artery stenosis include the new onset of severe hypertension, significant worsening of preexistent hypertension, failure to control hypertension on previously effective medications, repeated episodes of pulmonary edema, and renal insufficiency in the absence of urinary abnormalities or other known cause. The last may be most dramatic in patients started on ACE inhibitors. A vascular bruit may be heard in the mid-abdomen or flank.

Occlusive arterial disease can cause either acute or chronic kidney failure with or without changes in the urinalysis and urinary sediment. Renal arterial embolization or thrombosis may occur in patients with acute myocardial infarction, chronic atrial fibrillation, and subacute bacterial endocarditis. Symptoms vary from a slowly progressive, clinically silent event to severe acute flank pain and tenderness, hematuria, hypertension, fever, nausea, and vomiting. Serum lactic dehydrogenase concentrations increase dramatically after 1 to 2 days and remain elevated for a week or more.

Renal cholesterol embolization may occur after vascular manipulation (ie, aortic surgery or angiography) or in association with anticoagulation or thrombolytics. Although less common, cholesterol emboli may also occur spontaneously. The usual course is a progressive kidney disease and worsening hypertension, but it can be acute with a vasculitic picture, including oliguria or anuria, fever, eosinophilia, eosinophiluria, hypocomplementemia, and embolization to other organs, including the extremities (digital infarctions). Hints to this diagnosis include livedo reticularis and cholesterol emboli on a dilated funduscopic examination (which should be performed on every patient when this diagnosis is suspected). The urinalysis is usually unremarkable, although hematuria and mild proteinuria may be seen. If the diagnosis remains unclear or other diagnoses exist as valid possibilities (radiocontrast nephropathy, endocarditis with left-sided emboli, vasculitis, thrombotic emboli), a definitive diagnosis may be made on visualization of cholesterol crystals on a biopsy of the skin or kidney.

Kidney Diseases Associated With NSAID Use

NSAIDs are widely consumed by older adults because of their effectiveness in relieving pain in a variety of common chronic musculoskeletal disorders. Older persons are more predisposed than younger adults to the adverse effects of NSAIDs on the kidneys because of the age-associated decline in kidney function, the increased prevalence of such comorbid conditions as heart failure, hypertension, cirrhosis, and CKD, and the high use of concomitant drugs that affect kidney function (eg, diuretics, antihypertensives). It should be possible to use these drugs safely in older adults and maintain a low risk-to-benefit ratio, as those who are at risk for NSAID-induced kidney disease can be identified and monitored.

As mentioned above, NSAIDs may alter intrarenal hemodynamics and decrease GFR. NSAIDs may induce a variety of acute and chronic renal lesions. AIN can follow the use of nearly all NSAIDs. The typical clinical picture includes the nephrotic syndrome with acute renal insufficiency in a patient who has been on NSAIDs for months. An increase in eosinophils in blood or urine, or both, with NSAID-induced AIN is not nearly as common as in AIN due to penicillin and other agents. The kidney abnormalities usually improve after discontinuation of the medication, with or without corticosteroid therapy, but chronic renal insufficiency and even ESRD may occur. The AIN results primarily from a delayed hypersensitivity response to NSAIDs, and the nephrotic syndrome results from changes in glomerular permeability mediated by prostaglandins and other hormones. Less commonly, nephrotic syndrome may occur without AIN; rarely, an immune complex glomerulopathy is observed. Patients taking NSAIDs for months or years may develop papillary necrosis, chronic interstitial nephritis, and even ESRD. Case-control studies show that patients at increased risk are older men with chronic heart disease and kidney hypoperfusion. Impaired medullary circulation and direct toxicity due to a drug metabolite appear to play a critical role in inducing interstitial fibrosis, which can be facilitated by a sustained production of some growth factors and cytokines. The newer COX-2 inhibitors may also be injurious to the kidneys.

Chronic Kidney Failure

An examination of kidney biopsy results in older adults with chronic kidney failure showed that the most common histologic findings are hypertensive nephrosclerosis, focal segmental glomerulosclerosis, interstitial nephritis, and amyloidosis. Again, in persons with chronic kidney failure where a cause is clear from the history and physical examination (eg, diabetes mellitus), no biopsy would be necessary.

There are several points to be made with regard to chronic renal insufficiency in the older adult. First, although chronic elevation of serum creatinine represents a loss of kidney function that likely will not be recovered, defining the underlying pathology may help to prevent further decline in function. Second, the degree of kidney failure may be much greater than indicated by the serum creatinine, so that cognitive difficulties may develop at lower-than-expected serum creatinine levels. Third, although this area needs considerable research, some data suggest that erythropoietin serum levels do not change with age. Data also suggest that anemia secondary to erythropoietin deficiency may occur with more mild cases of renal insufficiency than previously thought. Preventing a further decline in kidney function or the development of "acute or chronic" kidney failure is critical. This requires careful attention to medication dosing, measurement of serum blood levels of medications when available, and avoidance of medications known to accumulate in renal insufficiency, including magnesium-containing compounds and meperidine. In addition, the older adult with renal insufficiency is even less able than the healthy older adult to defend against physiologic stress, including a free water load, salt challenge, or acidosis; this should be taken into consideration during acute illness. Lastly, as detailed below, early referral to a nephrologist and pre-ESRD care is very important.

Early Referral to a Nephrologist and Pre-ESRD Care

Early referral of older adults with evidence of kidney disease to a nephrologist is important. In general, when the serum creatinine is greater than or equal to 1.5 mg/dL, patients should be referred for a nephrology consultation. There is currently a national effort to improve pre-ESRD care. National guidelines have been established by the Kidney Disease Outcomes Quality Initiative (KDOQI). The goal of the nephrology consultation is to determine the type of kidney disease, to define any associated comorbid conditions, and to assess the severity of renal dysfunction and any associated risk factors. A plan should be developed to address specific therapies for CKD and associated complications, maximize GFR, treat comorbid conditions, prevent cardiac disease, and, when indicated, begin planning for replacement therapy. In addition, data suggest that beginning dialysis early in older adults may improve clinical outcomes and patient survival; early referral contributes to this positive outcome.

With regard to blood-pressure control, in patients with CKD the goal blood pressure is less than 130/80 mm Hg. High blood pressure is both a cause and consequence of CKD. Poorly controlled blood pressure may accelerate a decline in kidney function and exacerbate underlying cardiovascular disease. Whenever tolerated, an ACE inhibitor or angiotensin receptor blocker (ARB) should be used together with a diuretic. Attention to life-style change, including weight control, smoking, and an adherence to a low-salt diet, is also very important.

Anemia (normocytic, normochromic) is associated with CKD and is usually secondary to either decreased production of erythropoietin (EPO) or possibly inhibitors of erythropoiesis. However, before this diagnosis is made other common causes of anemia need to be excluded. All patients should have peripheral blood smear, screening for fecal occult blood, serum B_{12}, and iron studies. If folate deficiency is suspected, a red blood cell folate should be measured. After other causes for anemia are excluded, a patient may be considered for EPO therapy. The goal hematocrit/hemoglobin is 33–36/11–12 to reduce the risk of heart disease, cognitive dysfunction, higher hospitalization rates, and increased mortality.

Individuals with CKD (GFR less than 60 mL/min) are at risk for alterations in calcium-phosphate metabolism that place them at risk for underling bone disease. The histologic types of bone disease vary in different clinical setting. There are several therapies available that need to be individualized, again, depending on bone histology and clinical setting. All patients should have a serum phosphate, calcium, and parathyroid hormone measurement done before referral to a nephrologist.

Individuals with CKD are also at risk for metabolic acidosis and loss of bone mineral. The national guidelines include recommendations that the serum CO_2 be greater than 22 mEq/L to protect bone loss.

It is important for older adults with a GFR less than 60mL/min to have a consultation with an expert in nutrition. The U.S. Multicenter Modification of Diet in Renal Disease Study has shown a benefit of a low-protein diet (0.7 g/kg of body weight) to those with a CrCl < 55 mL/min/L in slowing the progression of chronic kidney failure. However, the benefits must be weighed against the nutritional consequences, as this study showed there were also small declines in various indices of nutritional status (protein-calorie malnutrition). It is important for the clinical team, including a nephrologist and dietitian, to determine what is best given each patient's individual nutritional needs. Again, these goals in pre-ESRD care are developed by a team effort between the patient's primary care physician and a consulting nephrologist.

Dialysis and Transplantation

A 1999 report from the U.S. Renal Data System indicates that in 1997 more than half of all patients on chronic dialysis were aged 65 years or older. Diabetes mellitus, hypertension, GN, and obstructive nephropathy are the most common causes of ESRD in this group. The increased number of older adults started on dialysis has occurred for two reasons. First, there is increased referral and acceptance of older adults, especially those with serious comorbid conditions. Second, the increased survival rates of other competing diseases, such as coronary artery disease or diabetes, increase the chances that a person will survive to develop ESRD.

The results of studies looking at life satisfaction and functional status in older adults on dialysis have varied. One prospective cohort study found that life satisfaction of older adults on dialysis and those in the control group did not differ significantly at 3 years. For some older adults living alone or in isolation, time spent on dialysis was a time to interact both with their "neighbors" on dialysis and with nursing staff; in a sense, this becomes their social life. It is also clear that rehabilitation (occupational and physical therapy) is important in slowing the loss of function in the dialysis patient. The choice of hemodialysis or peritoneal dialysis (chronic ambulatory peritoneal dialysis) depends on the patient's wishes and overall condition, the physician's expertise, and available resources. Neither method offers any advantage in survival rates when patients with similar risk factors are compared.

An alternative therapy for ESRD in older adults is kidney transplantation. The results have improved because of better patient selection, improved perioperative care, and the use of safer, more effective immunosuppression. Despite improved survival, kidney transplantation in persons aged 65 years and over remains uncommon and controversial, largely because of a reluctance to allocate a scarce resource (the donor kidney) to an older adult with a limited life expectancy. As older adults have a senescent immune system, they may require less aggressive immunotherapy.

One report comparing older adults with a kidney transplant with those on dialysis (matched by age, underlying diagnosis leading to ESRD, and number of comorbid conditions) showed that after adjusting for known prognostic factors, the transplant patients had a much better (twofold) survival probability than did the patients on dialysis. The 5-year survival rates were 81% and 51% for transplant and dialysis patients, respectively. In addition, a study comparing graft survival in patients aged 18 to 59 with that in patients 60 years and older found that in the absence of risk factors (pretransplant history of nonskin cancer, vascular disease, or being an active smoker), the survival rates were similar. These findings will have important implications in the future for the management of ESRD patients aged 60 years and older.

ANNOTATED REFERENCES

■ Brown WW, ed. Aging and the kidney. *Adv Renal Replacement Ther*. 2000;7(1):1–92.

> The entire issue is dedicated to the aging kidney. It includes articles on a broad range of issues, including the biology of renal aging, hypertension, diabetes mellitus, kidney replacement therapy, and ethical issues in aging and renal disease, as well as information on healthy aging and disease prevention.

■ Johnson DW, Herzig K, Purdie D, et al. A comparison of the effects of dialysis and renal transplantation on the survival of older uremic patients. *Transplantation*. 2000;69(5):794–799.

> The purpose of this clinical study was to evaluate survival for transplant versus dialysis in persons aged 60 years and older in Australia. Sixty-seven patients were randomized to kidney transplant and 107 to dialysis. The two groups were matched for age, gender, body mass index, cause of renal disease, comorbidity, and dialysis duration. The authors conclude that kidney transplantation confers a significant survival advantage over dialysis in patients who are rigorously screened for kidney transplantation.

■ Levey AS, Coresh J, Balk E, et al. National Kidney Foundation practice guidelines for chronic kidney disease: evaluation, classification and stratification. *Ann Intern Med*. 2003;139(2):137–147.

> This paper reviews the current criteria for classification of chronic kidney disease and summarizes current recommendations on early diagnosis of kidney disease in older adults.

■ Loos C, Briancon S, Frimat L, et al. Effect of end-stage renal disease on the quality of life of older adults. *J Am Geriatr Soc*. 2003;51(2):229–233.

> This is a controlled cross-sectional study to assess the quality of life of older adults on dialysis. The authors conclude that in in older patients with a planned initiation for dialysis, the impact of end-stage renal disease on quality of life is no different from the impact of other diseases but that in patients with unplanned dialysis, the quality of life is impaired.

■ Luckey AE, Parsa CJ. Fluid and electrolytes the elderly. *Arch Surg*. 2003;138(10):1055–1060.

> This is a comprehensive review of the common electrolytes abnormalities experienced by older adults.

■ Wolfson M. Nutrition in elderly dialysis patients. *Semin Dial*. 2002;15(2):113–115.

> This article discusses the special challenges posed by the aging process, including concurrent illness, mobility, and cognitive dysfunction, that may impact nutrition in the growing number of older patients on dialysis.

Catherine Lee Kelleher, MD
Robert Dean Lindeman, MD

CHAPTER 51—GYNECOLOGIC DISEASES AND DISORDERS

KEY POINTS

- Many older women do not spontaneously discuss gynecologic problems, yet many of these problems are treatable.

- Symptomatic urogenital atrophy is common in postmenopausal women and is readily reversed with the administration of local estrogen.

- Half of all cases of invasive cancer of the vulva occur in women over the age of 70 years.

- Pessaries may improve comfort and bladder function in some older women with pelvic organ prolapse.

Most older women do not seek regular gynecologic care. This may be in part because they are reticent about discussing personal gynecologic problems. Important and treatable disorders consequently go undiagnosed until they become severely disabling. For example, although urinary incontinence affects 16 million adults in the United States, the average time between onset and reporting to a physician is 8.5 years; gynecologic problems such as genital prolapse and atrophic vaginitis often exacerbate urinary incontinence. Full gynecologic examination should be a routine part of a complete history and physical examination for all older women who are amenable to screening.

HISTORY AND PHYSICAL EXAMINATION

The latest American College of Obstetrics and Gynecology recommendations for primary care of women aged 65 and older include inquiring about not only routine gynecologic issues but also about involuntary loss of urine or feces, sexual behavior patterns and potential exposure to sexually transmitted diseases, and use of alternative medical treatments.

Nongynecologic medical problems that can have significant gynecologic effects should be noted in the history. For example, breast cancer therapy typically leads to severe urogenital atrophy, obesity can result in hyperestrogenic states due to peripheral conversion of androgens to estrogen, and osteoporotic lordosis causes increased intra-abdominal pressure and resultant predisposition to genital prolapse. Previous obstetrical events may cause pelvic floor neuromuscular damage and eventual development of urinary incontinence and genital prolapse.

If a woman is on hormone replacement, the regimen should be reviewed annually to assure adherence, need for continued therapy, and absence of abnormal side effects. If the uterus is present, estrogen must be combined with a progestin in order to prevent the development of endometrial hyperplasia (see the section on hormone replacement therapy in "Endocrine and Metabolic Disorders," p 379). The history should also include inquiry about abdominal distention (sign of ovarian cancer) and abnormal vaginal discharge or bleeding (signs of endometrial, cervical, or vaginal cancer).

The pelvic examination also presents an opportunity to discuss sexual function with the patient. Although the lack of available, sexually capable men may limit an elderly woman's sexual activities, many older women are interested in maintaining sexual relationships. Issues related to sexual activity such as atrophy-related dyspareunia, postcoital bleeding, and sexually transmitted diseases should be addressed. Many women require reassurance that enjoyable sexual activity is possible and normal at their age. Also, women who maintain regular sexual activity are less likely to have significant vaginal atrophy.

Most ambulatory elderly women can assume the lithotomy position. Because the vaginal introitus may be small and stenotic, smaller speculums may be needed. The dorsal position, in stirrups for a pelvic examination, requires flexion and external rotation of the hips. Patients with osteoarthritis who find the lithotomy position uncomfortable or impossible to assume will need to use an alternative position. The left lateral decubitus position is one alternative. The patient lies on her left side, with knees flexed. The upper hip (right) is flexed to a greater degree and the right leg is elevated, exposing the perineum. An adequate speculum and bimanual examination can usually be done in this position. To examine a bedbound patient, position an inverted bedpan under the sacrum to elevate the pelvis. Water-based lubricants facilitate the examination and can be used if a Pap smear will be performed.

In performing the pelvic examination of an older woman, the examiner should:

- examine the vulva for abnormal pigmentation, erythema, or raised lesions;

- look for signs of urogenital atrophy, including urethral caruncle, vaginal dryness, pale vaginal mucosa, loss of rugae, and reduced vaginal caliber and depth;

- have the patient perform Valsalva's maneuver to evaluate for pelvic organ prolapse and urinary incontinence;

- carefully palpate for pelvic masses or ovarian enlargement on bimanual examination;
- perform a Pap smear if indicated (see the section on cervical cancer in "Prevention," p 67).

The presence of significant vaginal mucosal atrophic changes may lead to inadequate or abnormal Pap smear interpretation. In this situation, the Pap smear should be repeated after 2 to 3 months of local estrogen therapy. Bimanual examinations and perineal inspection performed annually may detect vulvar, vaginal, or ovarian pathology. A rectal examination could also be performed at the same time in order to identify masses, detect occult bleeding, and evaluate the anal sphincter.

Ovaries become smaller with aging, and any palpable adnexal tissue should prompt consideration of malignancy. Although uterine fibroids are common, any increase in uterus size should be investigated. An ovarian or uterine mass could be evaluated by abdominal or pelvic ultrasound (using a vaginal probe) to determine location and character. Sonography, however, cannot definitively establish the nature (benign or malignant) of the mass, so further evaluation with laparoscopy ultimately depends on clinical judgment.

TREATMENT OF MENOPAUSAL SYMPTOMS

Estrogen is labeled by the U.S. Food and Drug Administration (FDA) for the treatment of menopausal symptoms and urogenital dryness and for the prevention of osteoporosis, but estrogen replacement therapy (ERT) has historically been used by clinicians for other reasons as well. The common short- and long-term uses, common prescribing practices, and risks of ERT are reviewed herein.

Menopause on average occurs at age 51 in the United States. With a life expectancy of 78 years, the average woman is postmenopausal one third of her life. Despite some controversy about the risks and benefits of ERT, many women and their physicians choose to treat or prevent the sequelae of estrogen deficiency in menopause, although the popularity of this therapy is waning in response to findings of the Women's Health Initiative (WHI) trial.

Vasomotor symptoms or hot flushes are the most common symptom of the climacteric, occurring in up to 80% of perimenopausal women. Symptoms persist beyond 5 years in 25% of women and are lifelong in a small minority. Although the cause of the vasomotor response remains unknown, vasomotor symptoms are usually relieved within the first cycle of estrogen

treatment. Low-dose therapy can be initiated and estrogen doses titrated until symptoms improve. When estrogen is contraindicated or not acceptable, selective serotonin-reuptake inhibitors or progestins are considered the second most effective therapies. Clonidine[OL], methyldopa[OL], or herbal remedies such as yams and black cohosh have also been tried with little evidence to support their use.

See also the section on hormone replacement therapy in "Endocrine and Metabolic Disorders" (p 379) and the section on ERT and osteoporosis prevention in "Osteoporosis and Osteomalacia" (p 217).

TREATMENT OF UROGENITAL SYMPTOMS

Estrogen deficiency causes atrophy of both the vaginal and urethral mucosa. Both have a high density of estrogen receptors. Although randomized trials are few and have yielded variable results, a Cochrane Database Review suggests that estrogen may improve urge incontinence more than placebo.

See also "Disorders of Sexual Function" (p 415) and "Urinary Incontinence" (p 184).

UROGENITAL ATROPHY

The lower genital tract is exquisitely sensitive to estrogen. Urogenital atrophy occurs in all postmenopausal women. Proliferation and maturation of the vaginal epithelium depends on adequate estrogen stimulation. With reduction of estrogen production, genital blood flow decreases, leading to further decline in delivery of estrogen to those tissues. This reduction in microvascularity leads to vaginal dryness, mucosal pallor, decreased rugation, mucosal thinning, inflammation with discharge, and, ultimately, decreased vaginal caliber and depth. With progressive atrophy, the vaginal Pap smear–maturation index shows atrophic changes with a decrease in mucosal superficial cells and an increase in intermediate and basal cells. Many women experience dyspareunia, burning, and even vaginal bleeding in some cases (Figure 51.1).

These changes are readily reversed with the administration of local estrogen. The intravaginal use of estrogen cream, one half an applicator (1 to 2 g) as infrequently as two nights per week, allows topical estrogen therapy with minimal (if any) absorption, endometrial proliferation, or other systemic effects. The available prescription estrogen creams appear to be therapeutically equivalent. The estrogen ring may be used for 3 months per ring, and vaginal tablets are available for use twice a week. Estrogen cream is also an excellent lubricant for use during intercourse or for pessary insertion. (See also "Disorders of Sexual Function," p 415.)

[OL] Not approved by the U.S. Food and Drug Administration for this use.

Figure 51.1—Severe vulvovaginal atrophy, including labial fusion secondary to lichen sclerosus.

VULVOVAGINAL INFECTION AND INFLAMMATION

Postmenopausal women are susceptible to a broad range of vulvovaginal infections. Candidal infection, common in diabetic and obese patients who are plagued with moisture and irritation, can be treated with oral, intravaginal, and topical antifungal agents. Patients should be questioned about their ability to insert a vaginal applicator before beginning therapy. Topical corticosteroids can be used to hasten relief of symptoms. Combination therapy may be necessary, as older women commonly present with more chronic, untreated candidal infections that spread from the vulva to the inguinal areas. Other vaginal infections common in reproductive age women such as trichomonas and *Gardnerella* vaginosis are less common in elderly women, likely because of the higher vaginal pH. A wet preparation revealing sheets of inflammatory cells without bacterial forms may represent advanced atrophy rather than an infectious cause. Local estrogen cream in the case of a symptomatic woman with atrophic vaginitis is effective.

DISORDERS OF THE VULVA

With aging, the skin of the vulva loses elasticity, and the underlying fat and connective tissues undergo degeneration, with loss of collagen and thinning of the epithelial layer. Consequently, postmenopausal women not on estrogen are predisposed to a variety of dermatologic disorders and symptoms. The assessment of vulvar complaints must include direct examination. Any pigmented lesion or lesions that do not respond to topical corticosteroid or estrogen treatment *must* be promptly biopsied.

Vulvar skin irritation occurs from a variety of agents and causes burning, itching, and edema. Hy-gienic products used for urinary or fecal incontinence may lead to chemical dermatitis, as does urine itself. Treatment of incontinence is important to solving this problem. Vulvar burning or pain is rarely due to estrogen deficiency, and this complaint should be investigated rather than treated with ever-increasing doses of estrogen. Vulvar excoriation can result from scratching of an inflamed vulva. Local corticosteroids such as hydrocortisone 1% ointment applied daily, sitz baths, or use of a bidet can help alleviate vulvar irritation. Any chronically irritated area should be biopsied to exclude a malignancy.

Vulvar dystrophy is a somewhat outdated term used to describe both benign and malignant vulvar squamous changes. The preferred terminology set out by the International Society for the Study of Vulvovaginal Disease outlines three classes of non-neoplastic vulvar lesions. These are lichen sclerosus, squamous cell hyperplasia, and other dermatoses. A separate classification is used for biopsy-proven dysplastic lesions. These vulvar intraepithelial neoplasias (VIN) are graded on the basis of the level of atypia (dysplasia).

Nonneoplastic Vulvar Lesions

Lichen sclerosus causes over one third of all vulvar dystrophies and may extend beyond the vulva to the perirectal areas. It is rarely precancerous. There is epithelial thinning with edema and fibrosis of the dermis. It can progress to shrinkage and adherence of the labia minora with reduction in introital caliber. Lesions are typically shiny, white or pink, and parchment-like. Lesions may be asymptomatic or may cause itching, vaginal soreness, and dyspareunia. Diagnosis is confirmed on biopsy of the involved vulvar areas. Recommended treatment involves daily application of a rather potent topical corticosteroid, clobetasol propionate 0.05%. Treatment should be continued for at least 3 months. Testosterone had been the mainstay of therapy but has been shown to be significantly less effective than clobetasol. Further measures include wearing cotton underwear and avoiding irritant soaps. Topical emollient agents including lanolin can be helpful, but petroleum jelly should be avoided.

Squamous hyperplasia appears as thickened, hyperplastic, elevated white keratinized lesions that can be difficult to distinguish clinically from VIN or condylomata. However, it is benign. Biopsy should precede treatment. Topical mid-potency corticosteroids such as triamcinolone 0.1% twice daily for a few weeks (or longer with thick lesions) resolves the lesions; intermittent therapy may be necessary.

Other vulvar lesions include lichen simplex chronicus, which presents with vulvar pruritus, and lichen planus, which presents as erosive, ulcerative lesions that can result in significant vulvar scarring. Mid-potency corticosteroids applied topically or intravaginally are recommended. In lichen planus involving the vagina, local estrogen cream should also be used.

Vulvar Neoplasia

All suspicious, unusual, or symptomatic vulvar lesions should be biopsied. VIN lesions are not usually precancerous. VIN is most often seen in postmenopausal women, but the incidence of VIN does not increase with age. Over half of cases are asymptomatic. When symptoms are present, the most common is pruritus. The clinical appearance is the same as squamous hyperplasia or may be simply pigmentation. Lesions are often multifocal.

Invasive cancer of the vulva is an age-related malignancy; half of all cases occur after age 70. The vast majority are squamous cell carcinomas. Malignant melanoma, sarcoma, basal cell, carcinoma, and adenocarcinoma account for under 20% of cases. Treatment involves surgery (radical vulvectomy), occasionally accompanied by radiation.

DISORDERS OF PELVIC FLOOR SUPPORT

Child bearing and activities that increase intra-abdominal pressure cause progressive weakening of the connective tissue and muscular supports of the genital organs and can lead to genital prolapse. Conditions such as constipation, chronic coughing, and heavy lifting commonly increase intra-abdominal pressure. Common symptoms of prolapse include pelvic pressure, lower back pain, urinary or fecal incontinence, difficulty with rectal emptying, or a palpable mass. Traditional classification of vaginal prolapse differentiated protrusion of the posterior vaginal wall (enterocele or rectocele), descent of the anterior vaginal wall (cystocele), and prolapse of the vaginal apex. These conditions are demonstrated by having the patient bear down or cough while in the dorsal lithotomy position, but the full extent of prolapse is better appreciated with a standing Valsalva's maneuver. Vaginal prolapse represents a pelvic organ hernia through the vaginal hiatus.

The 1995 American College of Obstetrics and Gynecology classification of pelvic organ prolapse is outlined in Table 51.1. The International Continence Society and the American Urogynecologic Association adopted a new, rather complex prolapse classification system that is based on measurement of the distance between vaginal anatomic sites and the hymeneal ring. The purpose of this classification, which is used by specialty societies, is to more objectively and reproducibly describe a patient's degree of prolapse.

Mild prolapse (1st or 2nd degree; see Table 51.1) can be retarded with adequate estrogenization and Kegel's exercises to strengthen the pelvic floor musculature (see the Appendix, p 500, for exercise instructions for the patient). Genital prolapse does not always lead to bladder dysfunction and should not be assumed to be the cause of incontinence (see "Urinary Incontinence," p 184). Correcting the prolapse will in some cases cause or exacerbate incontinence. On the other hand, large cystoceles or rectoceles may produce urinary retention, and reduction of the cystocele may restore normal bladder function.

Pessaries

Pessaries are commonly employed in an effort to delay or avoid surgery. Their use in older women may be indicated to provide comfort and restore bladder function when comorbid illness makes surgery undesirable. Such women may elect long-term pessary use under medical supervision. Available pessaries are made from rubber, plastic, or silicone. A variety of shapes and sizes are available: doughnuts, rings, cubes, inflatable balls, and foldable models. Pessary care requirements often influence the selection of a device and the amount of follow-up required.

The choice of pessary is influenced by the degree of prolapse, presence of incontinence, type of accompanying tissue relaxation, and ease of care. Patients with prolapse and no incontinence require only space-occupying types. Those with stress incontinence benefit from a foldable type, which restores bladder neck support. Ring pessaries are easier to insert and remove and may be preferred by older women.

Pessary selection often proceeds by trial and error; the optimal pessary fits snugly but comfortably and allows voiding and defecating without difficulty. After pessary selection and insertion, clinical follow-up within a few days is essential to ascertain satisfactory usage. After initial fitting and recheck, pessaries should be removed and cleaned, and the vaginal walls inspected. Pessary care requirements often influence the selection

Table 51.1—Classification of Pelvic Organ Prolapse

Class	Description
1st degree	Extension to the mid-vagina
2nd degree	Approaching the hymenal ring
3rd degree	At the hymenal ring
4th degree	Beyond the hymenal ring

SOURCE: Data from American College of Obstetricians and Gynecologists. *Pelvic Organ Prolapse.* Washington, DC: American College of Obstetricians and Gynecologists. Technical Bulletin No. 214; 1995.

of a device and the amount of follow-up required for individual patients. If an older woman's mobility or manual dexterity permit, she should be advised to remove the pessary twice a week, wash it with soap and water, and reinsert it with a water-soluble lubricant; she should use 1 g vaginal estrogen cream twice a week as well. Patients who cannot provide this level of self-care should be assisted at periodic office visits or by a visiting nurse. All patients with pessaries should be instructed to report any unusual discharge, bleeding, or discomfort, and any changes in bladder or bowel function, and all should have a pelvic examination once or twice a year. If discomfort is present or the device becomes uncomfortable, a different size or type should be tried. Pessaries do not work as well with marked vaginal outlet relaxation. If a pessary is left in place for long periods without monitoring, fibrous tissue may form around the pessary, and removal under anesthesia may be necessary.

Surgery for Prolapse

Surgical treatment of vaginal prolapse can be classified as either reconstructive or obliterative. Reconstructive procedures are designed to restore normal anatomy, whereas obliterative procedures result in closure of the vaginal canal. Vaginal reconstructive procedures include sacrospinous fixation (for apical prolapse), anterior repairs (for a cystocele), and posterior repairs (for a rectocele). These can safely be done under regional anesthesia, which minimizes anesthetic risks. Abdominal reconstructive procedures include sacrocolpopexy (for apical prolapse) and paravaginal repairs (for a cystocele). They typically require general anesthesia. Urinary incontinence procedures can be done either vaginally or abdominally at the time of the prolapse surgery. (See also "Urinary Incontinence," p 184.)

Obliterative procedures are restricted to elderly women who are not, and will not be, sexually active. In a LeFort colpocleisis, the anterior and posterior vaginal walls are sutured together, obliterating the vaginal canal. The simplicity and safety are very attractive for the oldest-old women, as the procedure can be done under local anesthesia in the outpatient setting. Anti-incontinence procedures can be done at the same time, as well. Limitation of physical activities and intra-abdominal pressure increase for 6 to 12 weeks postoperatively, the performance of pelvic floor exercises, and use of vaginal estrogen cream are key in optimizing the success rate of surgical therapy. The impact on quality of life of prolapse surgery for the patient can be quite remarkable, as a large, exteriorized prolapse can markedly limit a woman's ability to perform physical and social activities.

Age, in itself, is not a contraindication to surgery for genital prolapse. When a proven protocol for perioperative care, including preoperative medical clearance, regional anesthesia, infection prophylaxis, and deep-vein thrombosis prophylaxis, is followed, vaginal surgery offers a safe alternative to pessary use for elderly women with symptomatic genital prolapse. (See also "Perioperative Care," p 99.)

POSTMENOPAUSAL VAGINAL BLEEDING

Postmenopausal bleeding (defined as bleeding after 1 year of amenorrhea) occurs in a significant number of older women. The challenge is not only to exclude gynecologic malignancies but also to alleviate the symptoms and eliminate the cause of benign conditions. Causes of bleeding can be grouped according to anatomic areas and endocrine dysfunction (Table 51.2). Not all complaints of postmenopausal bleeding are related to the reproductive organs but may be confused by the patients as originating from these areas. Proper evaluation involves complete physical examination and directed diagnostic studies. Endometrial hyperplasia and cancer can be evaluated with endometrial biopsy or by measuring the endometrial thickness on vaginal probe ultrasound. Though neither ultrasound nor biopsy is 100% specific, an endometrial thickness of less than 5 mm on

Table 51.2—Causes of Postmenopausal Vaginal Bleeding

Cervical
  Carcinoma
  Cervicitis
  Polyp

Endocrinologic
  Exogenous hormones
  Perimenopausal ovarian function

Ovarian
  Functioning ovarian tumor

Uterine
  Endometrial atrophy
  Hyperplasia
  Neoplasia
  Polyp
  Submucosal leiomyoma

Vaginal
  Atrophy
  Inflammation
  Tumor
  Ulceration

Vulvar
  Carcinoma
  Laceration or ulceration
  Urethral caruncle

Other
  Coagulation disorder
  Rectal lesion
  Urinary tract infection

ultrasound essentially excludes hyperplasia and malignancy. Dilation and curettage is reserved for cases where tissue cannot otherwise be adequately sampled or when bleeding persists. The use of direct visualization (hysteroscopy) during the procedure is the most accurate method for tissue sampling. New techniques for destruction of the endometrial lining (ablation) by heat, cold, or excision may be helpful in women whose bleeding is proven to be due to nonmalignant conditions.

Exogenous hormone replacement is a common cause of postmenopausal bleeding. Women on continuous combined estrogen-progesterone replacement who continue to have bleeding after 1 year must be evaluated. Some specialists recommend biopsy if bleeding persists beyond 6 months. Women on cyclic hormone therapy who bleed at an unexpected time during the cycle should also be evaluated. (See also the section on hormone replacement therapy in "Endocrine and Metabolic Disorders," p 379.)

CLIMACTERIC SYNDROMES

See the section on estrogen replacement therapy in "Endocrine and Metabolic Disorders" (p 379).

ANNOTATED REFERENCES

■ Adams E, Thomson A, Maher C, et al. Mechanical devices for pelvic organ prolapse in women. *Cochrane Database Syst Rev.* 2004(2):CD004010.

  This review is the most up-to-date information regarding the state of evidence involved in treating pelvic organ prolapse with devices. The authors found that the evidence is sparse and the data are insufficient to recommend particular devices for particular indications.

■ American College of Obstetricians and Gynecologists. *Vulvar Non-neoplastic Epithelial Disorders.* ACOG Educational Bulletin No. 241. Washington, DC: American College of Obstetricians and Gynecologists; 1997.

  Vulvar disorders typically found in elderly women are classified and described, and treatment options are discussed. No illustrations are provided. Because of the variable physical appearance of vulvar changes, a biopsy is recommended for any suspicious or changing lesion. Strong corticosteroid ointments are commonly required for treatment of lichen sclerosus.

■ Bash KL. Review of vaginal pessaries. *Obstet Gynecol Surv.* 2000;55(7):455–460.

  This is a practical, useful review for practitioners. All of the major pessary types and their usage are described, with helpful illustrations.

■ Neimark M, Davila GW, Kopka SL. Le Fort colpocleisis: a feasible treatment option for pelvic organ prolapse in the elderly woman. *J Pelv Surg.* 2003;9(2):83–89.

  As the population ages, it is increasingly important to evaluate treatment options for disorders prevalent among elderly women, such as pelvic organ prolapse. Bowel and bladder function and overall quality of life were investigated in elderly women who received a Le Fort colpocleisis. The results showed that Le Fort colpocleisis is a viable treatment option for severe vaginal prolapse in the elderly patient. Low postoperative quality-of-life impact scores, despite irritative bladder symptoms and constipation, demonstrate the beneficial outcome of colpocleisis in elderly women with advanced genital prolapse who are not sexually active.

■ Tabor A, Watt HC, Wald NJ. Endometrial thickness as a test for endometrial cancer in women with postmenopausal vaginal bleeding. *Obstet Gynecol.* 2002;99:663–670.

  A literature review was performed to assess the value of endometrial thickness measurement as a test for endometrial cancer in postmenopausal women with vaginal bleeding. The authors conclude that with a 4% false-negative rate and a 50% false-positive rate, endometrial thickness measurement in postmenopausal women with vaginal bleeding should not replace invasive diagnostic testing (ie, dilatation and curettage).

G. Willy Davila, MD

CHAPTER 52—DISORDERS OF SEXUAL FUNCTION

KEY POINTS

■ Normal age-associated changes in sexuality lead to declines in sexual function; however, sexual dysfunction should not be viewed as part of healthy aging.

■ Physiologic changes in sexual response occur in both men and women. It is important to distinguish between normal age-associated changes and pathologic conditions that may be related to medications or medical disorders.

■ Many older women have sexual dysfunction but may not report it to their primary care practitioners unless asked.

■ Multiple options are available for the treatment of erectile dysfunction.

■ Sexuality is an important part of quality of life for older adults; treatment of sexual dysfunction in older adults may lead to improvements in quality of life.

Our understanding of sexual function and dysfunction in older men has increased significantly in recent years. However, there is less scientific information on the sexuality of older women, possibly because of the difficulty of measuring the female sexual response and the exclusion of older adults from research. For example, the National Health and Social Life Survey, a study of adult sexual behavior, sampled adults only up to age 59.

FEMALE SEXUALITY

Age-Associated Changes

Many factors play an important role in the sexual response of older women, including changes that occur with menopause, cultural expectations, relationship problems, previous sexual experiences, chronic illnesses, and depression. American women live about 29 years after menopause and outlive their spouses an average of 8 years. Although the frequency of intercourse decreases with aging, sexuality remains important for older women. One study found that among Swedish women aged 61 years, 59% were sexually active, but 43% experienced vaginal dryness and 10%, vaginal burning. In a study of British women aged 55 to 85, only 24% were found to be sexually active; 62% did not have a sexual partner. Lack of sexual activity among women with partners was found to be due to lack of the woman's interest in intercourse (43%), lack of the man's interest (24%), or the man's illness or erectile dysfunction (29%).

The female sexual response cycle changes with aging. During the excitement phase, the clitoris may require longer direct stimulation, and genital engorgement is decreased. Vaginal lubrication is reduced, although with increased foreplay and gentle stimulation lubrication is usually adequate for intercourse. During the plateau phase, there is less expansion and vasocongestion of the vagina. During orgasm, fewer and weaker contractions occur, although older women can still achieve multiple orgasms. Occasionally during orgasm, the older woman experiences spastic and painful contractions of the uterine musculature. During the resolution phase, vasocongestion is lost more rapidly. Most of these changes are thought to be due to a decline in serum estrogen concentration after menopause, but a vasculogenic component may contribute to postmenopausal sexual dysfunction.

Female Sexual Dysfunction

For the most part, menopause is accompanied by decreased sexual function, with decreased sexual inter-

est, responsiveness, and coital frequency. In addition, there is an increase in urogenital symptoms, often not discussed with the physician. For example, a study of older British women found that 16% reported urinary urgency, dysuria, or frequency, 9% urinary incontinence, 11% vaginal itching, 8% vaginal dryness, and 2% painful intercourse. Among the women affected by vaginal dryness or painful intercourse, 33% did not seek professional advice and 36% resorted to over-the-counter medication (ie, lubricating jelly).

Dyspareunia, defined as pain with intercourse, can be due to organic or psychologic factors, or a combination of the two. For example, a woman may experience an episode of dyspareunia because of postmenopausal vaginal atrophy. With each subsequent sexual encounter she anticipates pain, causing inadequate arousal with decreased lubrication. Because of this cycle, the woman continues to experience dyspareunia, even after the vaginal atrophy has been treated. The most common organic cause of dyspareunia is atrophic vaginitis due to estrogen deficiency. Other causes include localized vaginal infections, cystitis, Bartholin cyst, retroverted uterus, pelvic tumors, excessive penile thrusting, or improper angle of penile entry.

Estrogen replacement can improve vaginal lubrication and sense of well-being, but it has little effect on libido. Libido is thought to be dependent on testosterone (even in women), rather than estrogen. The ovaries and adrenals are the main sources of androgens in women. Many investigators believe that there is a "female androgen deficiency syndrome," with impaired sexual function, loss of energy, depression, and serum total testosterone concentrations in the lower end of normal for women (< 15 ng/dL), but there is no clear-cut definition. The effects of female androgen deficiency were originally identified in women treated for advanced breast cancer with oophorectomy and adrenalectomy. When deprived of androgens, these women reported loss of libido. In a double blind, randomized controlled trial, surgically menopausal women on estrogen replacement were randomized to placebo or testosterone patches that deliver 150 or 300 μg of testosterone daily. After 12 weeks, only the women randomized to the higher dose reported improvements in frequency of sexual activity, pleasure, orgasm, sexual fantasies, masturbation, and positive well-being. This dose increased mean serum free testosterone into the upper normal range for healthy younger women. In naturally postmenopausal women, some, but not all, studies have shown that the addition of testosterone[OL] to estrogen replacement therapy improves sexual function. (Testosterone has not been approved by the U.S. Food and Drug

---

[OL] Not approved by the U.S. Food and Drug Administration for this use.

Administration [FDA] for the treatment of sexual dysfunction in women.)

Older women commonly have multiple medical ailments, some of which affect sexuality. However, there are limited scientific studies of the effect of chronic diseases and medications on the sexuality of older women. Women with diabetes mellitus report decreased libido and lubrication, and longer time to reach orgasm. Rheumatic diseases affect sexuality via functional disability. After mastectomy for breast cancer, 20% to 40% of women experience sexual dysfunction, possibly because of disruption of body image, marital and family problems, spousal reaction, adjuvant therapy, or the psychologic impact of a breast cancer diagnosis. Several drugs can adversely affect sexual function, including antihistamines, antihypertensives, antidepressants, antipsychotics, antiestrogens, central nervous system stimulants, narcotics, alcohol, and anticholinergic drugs.

Psychosocial factors have an important role in sexual dysfunction. Women commonly marry men older than themselves and live longer than men. Consequently, heterosexual older women are likely to spend the last years of their lives alone. Even when a partner is available, he might have erectile dysfunction. Finally, lack of privacy may be a problem when the older couple lives with their children or in a nursing home.

Evaluation and Treatment

The history is the most important part of the evaluation of sexual function, and careful questioning can detect problems that the woman might not otherwise volunteer. First, it is important to attempt to provide a comfortable atmosphere. Clinicians should ask about dyspareunia, lack of vaginal lubrication, and previous negative experiences, like rape, child abuse, or domestic violence. Medications should be carefully reviewed. A woman with dyspareunia should undergo a pelvic examination to exclude organic causes.

Dyspareunia due to atrophic vaginitis and decreased lubrication responds well to topical or systemic estrogen therapy. However, it is important to explain to the patient that complete restoration of vaginal tissue function may take up to 2 years. A vaginal estradiol ring delivers low-dose estrogen locally with lower systemic absorption and risks of systemic side effect than do vaginal estrogen creams. The ring is inserted into the upper third of the vaginal vault and replaced every 3 months. If the patient is not a candidate for or does not want to use estrogen, water-soluble vaginal lubricants (eg, Replens, Astroglide, K-Y jelly) are beneficial. Importantly, local stimulation through regular intercourse helps maintain a healthy vaginal mucosa. Longer foreplay allows more time for vaginal lubrication, just as older men often need longer and more direct stimulation to achieve an adequate erection.

Decreased libido may respond to testosterone, but no androgen preparation is approved by the FDA for female sexual desire disorders. Testosterone for women is available only in combination with estrogens and is FDA approved for moderate to severe vasomotor symptoms that are not improved with estrogens alone. Therapy is usually initiated with oral esterified estrogen 0.625 mg and methyltestosterone 1.25 mg. If symptoms do not improve, the dose can be doubled to esterified estrogen 1.25 mg and methyltestosterone 2.5 mg. Pharmacokinetic studies identifying appropriate replacement doses are lacking. The masculinizing side effects of testosterone, such as increased facial hair, are infrequent, dose dependent, and, for the most part, reversible upon discontinuation. Hepatic toxicity has been noted only in female-to-male transsexuals receiving very high doses of oral methyltestosterone. Oral

Table 52.1—Treatment Options for Sexual Dysfunction in Older Women

Symptom	Possible Cause	Therapy
Decreased desire	Postmenopausal status	Estrogen ± testosterone[OL]
	Chronic illness	Treatment of underlying illness
	Depression	Antidepressant medication
	Relationship problems	Marital therapy
	Drugs	Review of drugs ingested
Decreased lubrication	Postmenopausal status	Longer foreplay, regular intercourse, lubricants, estrogen
	Anticholinergic drugs	Review of medications, including over-the-counter drugs
Delayed or absent orgasm	Postmenopausal status	Estrogen ± testosterone[OL]
	Psychological problems	Sex therapy, antidepressant medication[OL]
Pain with intercourse	Organic cause	Treatment of underlying physical condition
	Vaginal dryness, atrophy	Longer foreplay, regular intercourse, lubricants, estrogen
	Vaginismus (involuntary vaginal contractions)	Sex therapy

[OL] Not approved by the U.S. Food and Drug Administration for this use.

methyltestosterone should not be used in women with liver disease and uncontrolled hyperlipidemia, as it may decrease high-density lipoproteins. In a 9-week study of postmenopausal women, esterified estrogens (1.25 mg a day) were found to decrease low-density lipoproteins and increase high-density lipoproteins, while the same dose of estrogens plus oral methyltestosterone (2.5 mg a day) decreased high-density lipoproteins. Lipid profile and liver function should be checked at baseline and every 6 months during therapy. Further studies of the best dosage, delivery system, long-term efficacy, and safety of testosterone are needed.

Randomized trials of sildenafil for female sexual dysfunction yielded conflicting results. The manufacturer has therefore decided not to apply for a license to use sildenafil in women.

Finally, the older woman should receive education about male sexual aging in addition to female sexual aging. Otherwise, she might mistakenly attribute her partner's diminished erection and need for more genital stimulation to her own inability to arouse her partner. Other psychologic issues, including depression, history of sexual abuse, and relationship problems, should be addressed and treated with antidepressants, psychotherapy, and marital therapy, as necessary. Table 52.1 summarizes treatments for female sexual dysfunction.

MALE SEXUALITY

Age-Associated Changes

As men age, their sexuality changes. The frequency of sexual intercourse and the prevalence of engaging in any sexual activity decrease. Young men report having intercourse three to four times per week, whereas only 7% of men aged 60 to 69 years and 2% of those aged 70 years and older report the same frequency. Fifty percent to 80% of men 60 to 70 years old engage in any sexual activity, a prevalence rate that declines to 15% to 25% among those aged 80 years and older. However, sexual interest often persists despite decreased activity. The man's level of sexual activity, interest, and enjoyment in younger years often determines his sexual behavior with aging. Factors contributing to a man's decreased sexual activity include poor health, social issues, partner availability, decreased libido, and erectile dysfunction.

Aging is associated not only with changes in sexual behavior but also with changes in the stages of sexual response. During the excitement phase, there is a delay in erection, decreased tensing of the scrotal sac, and loss of testicular elevation. The duration of the plateau stage is prolonged, and pre-ejaculatory secretion is decreased. Orgasm is diminished in duration and

intensity, with decreased quantity and force of seminal emission. During the resolution phase, there is rapid detumescence and testicular descent. The refractory period between erections is also prolonged. However, erectile dysfunction is not a part of healthy aging.

Erectile Dysfunction

Erectile dysfunction is the inability to achieve or maintain an erection adequate for sexual intercourse. The prevalence of erectile dysfunction increases with age; by age 70 years, 67% of men have erectile dysfunction. This high prevalence is important; in a study comparing affected and unaffected men, men with sexual dysfunction reported impaired quality of life. The causes of sexual dysfunction in men are summarized in Table 52.2.

The most common cause of erectile dysfunction in older men is vascular disease. Risk for vascular erectile dysfunction increases with traditional vascular risk factors such as diabetes mellitus, hypertension, hyperlipidemia, and smoking. In fact, erectile dysfunction is a predictor of future major atherosclerotic vascular disease (ie, myocardial infarction and stroke).

Obstruction from atherosclerotic arterial occlusive disease likely impedes the intracavernosal blood flow and pressure needed to achieve a rigid erection. In addition, atherosclerotic disease may cause ischemia of trabecular smooth muscle and result in fibrotic changes leading to failure of venous closure mechanisms. Venous leakage leading to vascular erectile dysfunction may also result from Peyronie's disease, arteriovenous fistula, or trauma-induced communication between the glans and the corpora. In anxious men who have excessive adrenergic-constrictor tone and in men with injured parasympathetic dilator nerves, erectile dysfunction can occur from insufficient relaxation of trabecular smooth muscle.

The second most common cause of erectile dysfunction in older men is neurologic disease. Disorders that affect the parasympathetic sacral spinal cord or the peripheral efferent autonomic fibers to the penis impair penile smooth muscle relaxation and prevent the vasodilation necessary for erection. In patients with spinal cord injury, the extent of erectile dysfunction largely depends on the completeness and the level of the spinal injury; those who have complete lesions or injury to the sacral spinal cord are more likely to have loss of erectile function. Common health problems such as diabetes mellitus, stroke, and Parkinson's disease can cause autonomic dysfunction that results in erectile failure. Finally, surgical procedures such as radical prostatectomy, cystoprostatectomy, and proctocolectomy commonly disrupt the autonomic nerve supply to the penis, resulting in postoperative erectile dysfunction.

Table 52.2—Causes of Sexual Dysfunction in Older Men

Causes (in order of prevalence)	Characteristics
Vascular disease	Gradual onset Vascular risk factors: diabetes mellitus, hypertension, hyperlipidemia, tobacco use
Neurologic disease, eg, spinal cord injury, autonomic dysfunction, surgical procedures	Gradual onset Neurologic risk factors: diabetes mellitus, history of pelvic injury, surgery, or irradiation, spinal injury or surgery, Parkinson's disease, multiple sclerosis, or alcoholism Loss of bulbocavernosus reflex
Medications, eg, anticholinergics, antihypertensives, cimetidine, antidepressants	Sudden onset Lack of sleep-associated erections or lack of erections with masturbation Temporal association with a new medication
Psychogenic, eg, relationship conflicts, performance anxiety, childhood sexual abuse, fear of sexually transmitted diseases, "widower's syndrome"	Sudden onset Sleep-associated erections or erections with masturbation are preserved
Hypogonadism	Gradual onset Decreased libido more than erectile dysfunction Small testes, gynecomastia Low serum testosterone concentration
Endocrine, eg, hypothyroidism, hyperthyroidism, hyperprolactinemia	Rare, < 5% of cases of erectile dysfunction

Numerous commonly used medications have been associated with erectile dysfunction for which the mechanism, for the most part, is unknown. Those medications with anticholinergic effects, such as antidepressants, antipsychotics, and antihistamines, may cause erectile dysfunction by blocking parasympathetic-mediated penile artery vasodilatation and trabecular smooth muscle relaxation. Almost all antihypertensive agents have been associated with erectile dysfunction; of these, β-blockers, clonidine, and thiazide diuretics have higher incidence rates. One mechanism may be the lowering of blood pressure below the critical threshold needed to maintain sufficient blood flow for penile erection, especially in those men who already have penile arterial disease. Over-the-counter medications such as cimetidine and ranitidine may also cause erectile dysfunction. Cimetidine, an H_2-receptor antagonist, acts as an antiandrogen and increases prolactin secretion and thus has been associated with loss of libido and erectile failure. Ranitidine can also increase prolactin secretion, although less commonly than does cimetidine.

The prevalence of psychogenic erectile dysfunction correlates inversely with age. Psychogenic erectile dysfunction may occur via increased sympathetic stimuli to the sacral cord, inhibiting the parasympathetic dilator nerves and thus inhibiting erection. Common causes of psychogenic erectile dysfunction include relationship conflicts, performance anxiety, childhood sexual abuse, and fear of sexually transmitted diseases. Older men may have "widower's syndrome," in which the man involved in a new relationship feels guilt as a defense against subconscious unfaithfulness to his deceased spouse.

The role of androgens in erection is unclear. Hypogonadal men show smaller and slower developing erections in response to fantasy, which is improved with androgen replacement. However, even men with castrate levels of testosterone can attain erections in response to direct penile stimulation. It may be that erection to certain types of sexual stimuli (ie, direct penile stimulation) are androgen independent, whereas response to fantasy may be androgen sensitive. Overall, testosterone appears to play a minor role in erectile function and a larger role in libido. In addition, hypogonadal patients respond better to phosphodiesterase inhibitors after testosterone replacement therapy.

Hyperthyroidism, hypothyroidism, and hyperprolactinemia have been associated with erectile dysfunction. However, less than 5% of erectile dysfunction is caused by endocrine abnormalities. Thus, endocrine evaluation of men with erectile dysfunction but intact libido is of limited value.

Evaluation of Erectile Dysfunction

The initial step in evaluation is to obtain a sexual, medical, and psychosocial history. Sexual history should clarify whether the problem consists of inadequate erections, decrease in libido, or orgasmic failure. The onset and duration of erectile dysfunction, the presence or absence of sleep-associated erections, and associated decline in libido may lead the clinician to the likely cause.

Sudden onset suggests psychogenic or drug-induced erectile dysfunction. A psychogenic cause is likely if there is sudden onset but sleep-associated erections or if erections with masturbation or another partner are intact. However, if the sudden onset is accompanied by lack of sleep-associated erections and lack of erection with masturbation, temporal association with new medication should be sought. A gradual onset of erectile dysfunction associated with loss of libido suggests hypogonadism.

Medical history is directed at discerning those factors likely to be contributing to erectile dysfunction. Vascular risk factors include diabetes mellitus, hypertension, coronary artery disease, peripheral arterial disease, hyperlipidemia, and smoking. Neurogenic risk factors include diabetes mellitus, history of pelvic injury or surgery, spinal injury or surgery, Parkinson's disease, multiple sclerosis, and alcoholism. An extensive medication review, including over-the-counter medications, is also essential. Finally, the psychosocial history should assess the patient's relationship with the sexual partner, the partner's health and attitude toward sex, economic or social stresses, living situation, alcohol use, and affective disorders.

On physical examination, signs of vascular or neurologic diseases must be sought. Peripheral pulses should be palpated. Signs of autonomic neuropathy and loss of the bulbocavernosus reflex suggest neurologic dysfunction. The genital examination includes palpating the penis for Peyronie's plaques and assessing for testicular atrophy. A femoral bruit and diminished (or absent) pedal pulses suggests arterial insufficiency. An absent bulbocavernosus reflex in a patient with diabetes mellitus suggests penile neuropathy. A loss of secondary sexual characteristics, small testes, and gynecomastia suggest hypogonadism.

Appropriate laboratory evaluation are those that target relevant comorbid conditions such as diabetes mellitus and vascular disease or that evaluate neurologic disorders if suggested by the physical examination. Consider the measurement of total testosterone in the setting of other symptoms of androgen deficiency. (See "Endocrine and Metabolic Disorders," p 378.)

An office-based diagnostic tool that can help direct the treatment of erectile dysfunction is intracavernous injection of a vasoactive drug, such as papaverine or alprostadil (formerly prostaglandin E_1, or PGE_1). An initial test dose of 15 to 30 mg of papaverine is used if the history and examination suggest a neurogenic cause. A 30-gauge needle and 1-cc syringe are typically used for the injection. Hold the glans of the penis with one hand and clean the injection site with an alcohol swab. Then, holding the needle parallel to the floor, insert the needle into the side of the penis to avoid the urethra. Inject the vasoactive agent over 30 to 60 seconds. After withdrawing the needle, apply pressure to the injection site for 1 minute to prevent bruising. An erectile response will occur within 15 minutes and may last up to 40 minutes. A poor response suggests arteriogenic or venogenic erectile dysfunction, inadequate dose of vasoactive agent, or anxiety with excessive adrenergic tone. A second trial injection at the next office visit with a higher dose (30 to 60 mg papaverine) or alprostadil (5 to 20 μg) may be used.

An at-home therapeutic trial of a phosphodiesterase inhibitor (sildenafil or vardenafil) is easier than the in-office diagnostic penile injection of a vasodilator. The initial dose should be low (sildenafil 25 to 50 mg or vardenafil 5 to 10 mg) in men suspected of having neurogenic erectile dysfunction. A poor response suggests vasculogenic erectile dysfunction. Further therapeutic trial with sildenafil 100 mg or vardenafil 20 mg may prove to be effective. An at-home therapeutic trial using tadalafil (5 to 10 mg) can be considered, but the long half-life complicates matters if an adverse reaction occurs with the first dose.

More extensive diagnostic tools are available but not commonly used. Nocturnal penile tumescence testing is of little value, except to confirm a psychogenic cause. The penile brachial pressure index may be helpful in assessing arteriogenic erectile dysfunction. This index measures the loss of systolic pressure between the arm and the penis. When measured before and after exercise, it can be used to assess for a pelvic steal syndrome, which is the loss of erection associated with initiation of active pelvic thrusting, presumably due to the transfer of blood flow from the penis to the pelvic musculature. More invasive and expensive tests such as Doppler ultrasound to assess penile arterial function, dynamic infusion cavernosometry to assess venous leakage syndrome, and penile arteriography are generally reserved for research or penile vascular surgery candidates.

Treatment of Erectile Dysfunction

Multiple effective therapeutic options are now available for the treatment of erectile dysfunction. Treatment should be individualized and based on cause, personal preference, partner issues, cost, and practicality of the therapeutic modality (Table 52.3).

Oral therapy for erectile dysfunction consists of sildenafil, vardenafil, or tadalafil. Sildenafil is a type-5 phosphodiesterase inhibitor that potentiates the penile response to sexual stimulation. It is effective in improving the rigidity and duration of erection. It is taken 1 hour before sexual activity and has no effect until sexual stimulation occurs. Because absorption is attenuated when sildenafil is ingested with a fatty meal, patients need to be educated about this issue.

Table 52.3—Treatment Options for Erectile Dysfunction

Treatment	Administration	Applicable Conditions	Onset	Duration of Action	Dosage	Selected Side Effects
Sildenafil*	Oral	N, A?, V?	60 min	4 hours	25–100 mg	Headache, flushing, rhinitis, dyspepsia, transient color blindness; contraindicated with nitrate use; precaution with α-blockers
Vardenafil*	Oral	N, A?, V?	45 min	4 hours	5–20 mg	Headache, flushing, rhinitis, dyspepsia; contraindicated with nitrate use and precaution with α-blockers
Tadalafil*	Oral	N, A?,V?	45–60 min	24–36 hours	5–20 mg	Headache, dyspepsia, flushing, rhinitis; contraindicated with nitrate use and precaution with α-blockers (except tamsulosin)
Vacuum device	External	P, N, V, A?	< 5 min	30 min	—	Petechiae, bruising, painful ejaculation
Papaverine[OL]	Intracavernosal	N, A?, V?	10 min	30–60 min	15–60 mg	Prolonged erection, fibrosis, ecchymosis
Alprostadil	Intracavernosal	N, A?, V?	10 min	40–60 min	5–20 µg	Prolonged erection, pain, fibrosis
Phentolamine[OL]	Intracavernosal	N, A?, V?	10 min	30–60 min	0.5–1 mg	Prolonged erection, fibrosis, headache, facial flushing
MUSE	Intraurethral	N, A?, V?	10–15 min	60–80 min	250–1000 µg	Penile pain or burning, hypotension
Penile prosthesis	Surgical	N, A, V		replacement in 5–10 years		Infection, erosion, mechanical failure
Sex therapy	Counseling	P	weeks	years	weekly	Anxiety

NOTE: A = arteriogenic; min = minutes; MUSE = medicated urethral system for erection; N = neurogenic; P = psychogenic; V = venogenic; ? = possibly.

On July 8, 2005 the U.S. Food and Drug Administration issued a statement approving label changes for all three PDE5 inhibitors that reflect a small number of cases of nonarteritic ischemic optic neuropathy (NAION) that were reported postmarketing. It is not possible at this time to determine causality of PDE5 inhibitors and NAION since other factors are associated with NAION, such as underlying anatomic or vascular risk factors, including but not necessarily limited to: low cup-to-disc ratio ("crowded disc"), age over 50, diabetes mellitus, hypertension, coronary artery disease, hyperlipidemia, and smoking. It is not possible to determine whether these events are related directly to the use of PDE5 inhibitors, to the patient's underlying vascular risk factors or anatomical defects, to a combination of these factors, or to other factors. Men who experience visual changes or loss of vision in one or both eyes are advised to stop the medication and contact their doctor or health care provider immediately.

Vardenafil is a more potent and specific phosphodiesterase inhibitor. A lower effective dose and better side-effect profile (no effect on color vision) make vardenafil a reasonable option. Tadalafil is a longer acting phosphodiesterase inhibitor with a similar side-effect profile. All three of these agents are contraindicated for concomitant use with nitrate drugs, since the combination can produce profound and fatal hypotension. Choosing between the three currently available phosphodiesterase inhibitors should likely be based on price. There are also labeling differences with the α-blockers that need to be taken into consideration.

Vacuum tumescence devices are an effective and accepted treatment. The apparatus consists of a plastic cylinder with an open end into which the penis is inserted. A vacuum device attached to the cylinder creates negative pressure within the cylinder, and blood flows into the penis to produce penile rigidity. A penile constriction ring placed at the base of the penis then traps the blood in the corpora cavernosa to maintain an erection for about 30 minutes. The vacuum device is effective for psychogenic, neurogenic, and venogenic erectile dysfunction, but it requires manual dexterity. Local pain, swelling, bruising, coolness of penile tip, and painful ejaculation are potential side effects. It is important to remove the constriction ring after 30 minutes.

Intracavernous injection of vasoactive drugs such as papaverine, phentolamine, and alprostadil are effective in producing erections adequate for sexual activity. Alprostadil, which is the only agent approved by the FDA for intracavernous injection, produces erections that last 40 to 60 minutes. Phentolamine[OL] is mainly used in combination therapy with papaverine[OL] or alprostadil, or both. Potential side effects are bruising, ecchymoses or hematoma, local pain, fibrosis from repeated injections, and priapism. Alprostadil appears to cause less scarring and priapism than papaverine. If an erection lasts longer than 4 hours, detumescence is necessary by aspiration of blood from the corpora cavernosa or injection of phenylephrine, since there is the potential for intracavernous hypoxia and fibrosis of trabecular smooth muscle, which may prevent future

[OL] Not approved by the U.S. Food and Drug Administration for this use.

erections. In general, intracavernosal therapy should probably be reserved for patients who fail oral therapy with a phosphodiesterase inhibitor. Alprostadil can also be administered intraurethrally using MUSE (medicated urethral system for erection). This system contains a small pellet of alprostadil that is placed within the urethra and is rapidly absorbed through the urethral mucosa to produce an erection within 10 to 15 minutes. Possible side effects are penile pain, urethral burning, and a throbbing sensation in the perineum.

Testosterone supplementation increases libido and may improve erectile dysfunction in men with true hypogonadism. It is available as an intramuscular injection (testosterone enanthate or cypionate) or topical transdermal patch and gel. Possible side effects associated with testosterone include polycythemia, increase in prostate size, gynecomastia, and fluid retention. It is important to perform a digital rectal examination to assess the prostate and obtain a baseline prostate-specific antigen level prior to initiation of therapy. If there is a rise in prostate-specific antigen or hematocrit with testosterone therapy, it usually occurs within 6 months. Therefore, it is advisable to check these levels at 3-month intervals during the first year of therapy, then every 12 months thereafter.

Surgical implantation of a penile prosthesis is another therapeutic option. Mechanical failure, infection, device erosion, and fibrosis are possible complications. However, since the availability of alprostadil and, more recently, phosphodiesterase inhibitors, surgical implantation of a penile prosthesis is rarely used (ie, men with severe arterial occlusive disease). Penile revascularization surgery has limited success.

Psychogenic erectile dysfunction should be referred for further evaluation and treatment.

ANNOTATED REFERENCES

- Bodie J, Lewis J, Schow D, et al. Laboratory evaluations of erectile dysfunction: an evidence based approach. *J Urol.* 2003;169(6):2262–2264.

  There is considerable conflict regarding the most cost-effective approach to the evaluation of erectile dysfunction. For example, in the absence of low libido, some would advocate no assessment other than a trial of sildenafil. On the other hand, some clinicians obtain numerous laboratory tests, most of which have normal results. This evidence-based review suggests that most patients should be evaluated with a complete blood cell count, electrolytes, and hemoglobin A_{1c}, cholesterol, and testosterone levels.

- Matthias RE, Lubben JE, Atchison KA, et al. Sexual activity and satisfaction among very old adults: results from a community-dwelling Medicare population survey. *Gerontologist.* 1997;37(1):6–14.

  This survey investigated the relationship of sexual activity, sexual satisfaction, and psychosocial factors among 1216 well-educated, relatively affluent people with a mean age of 77. About one third reported sexual activity in the past month, and current level of sexual activity was satisfactory in 67%. The men were more likely to be sexually active, with younger age and higher educational level predicting greater activity. For the women, being married was the strongest predictor of sexual activity. Regardless of gender, the main predictors for sexual satisfaction were being sexually active and having positive mental health scores.

- Mulligan T, Reddy S, Gulur PV, et al. Disorders of male sexual function. *Clin Geriatr Med.* 2003;19(3):473–481.

  Sexuality remains an important issue in the older population. Sexual desire in men continues in spite of a decreased ability to achieve an erection. Many studies suggest that erectile dysfunction in the older man is caused primarily by age-associated chronic disease rather than by normal healthy aging. Therefore, preventive measures that are aimed at the underlying diseases should be sought. Nevertheless, effective treatment options are now available to successfully regain sexual function and thereby improve quality of life.

- Padero MC, Bhasin S, Friedman TC. Androgen supplementation in older women: too much hype, not enough data. *J Am Geriatr Soc.* 2002; 50(6):1131–1140.

  This review critically examines the literature on androgen supplementation in older women. Androgen supplementation may improve some aspects of cognitive function, sexual function, muscle mass, strength, and sense of well-being in older women. Measurement of free testosterone in women is not widely used because of methodologic difficulty; therefore, androgen deficiency in women is hard to define. More studies are needed to determine whether physiologic testosterone replacement in older women can improve important outcomes like physical function, muscle mass and performance, fracture risk, and cognitive and sexual function.

- Rajpurkar A, Dhabuwala CB. Comparison of satisfaction rate and erectile function in patients treated with sildenafil, intracavernous prostaglandin E_1, and penile implant surgery for erectile dysfunction in urology practice. *J Urol.* 2003;170(1):159–163.

  This study investigated patient satisfaction after 1.5 years of treatment for erectile dysfunction using any of the three commonly used approaches. Surprisingly, patients who had undergone penile implant surgery were more satisfied than patients who were using either sildenafil or intracavernous prostaglandin E_1. Prior to treatment, almost all patients opt for oral rather than surgical therapy. Nevertheless, this study suggests that we should not neglect implant surgery as a viable option.

- Seftel AD. Erectile dysfunction in the elderly: epidemiology, etiology and approaches to treatment. *J Urol.* 2003; 169(6):1999–2007.

  Erectile dysfunction is very common in older men. This paper reviews the normal age-associated physiologic changes, as well as the prevalence, pathophysiology, and treatment of erectile dysfunction in older men. It provides a good review of recently released treatments (ie, phosphodiesterase inhibitors), as well as a discussion of potential future approaches (ie, gene therapy).

Angela Gentili, MD
Thomas Mulligan, MD

CHAPTER 53—PROSTATE DISEASE

KEY POINTS

- A number of treatment options exist for benign prostatic hyperplasia (BPH), including watchful waiting, drug therapies, minimally invasive procedures, and more extensive operations. The choice is influenced by the extent of symptoms, the presence of complications from outflow obstruction, and the preferences of the patient.

- The use of 5α-reductase inhibitors for BPH is especially indicated when the prostate gland is large.

- Recommendations regarding screening for prostate cancer using PSA differ among experts, and patients should be educated about the risks and benefits of this screening strategy so that they can make a well-informed decision.

- Several treatment options exist for men with localized prostate cancer, including watchful waiting, resection of the gland and seminal vesicles, and radiation therapy. How the patient balances the potential benefits and burdens of the various options will influence the choice of therapy.

- For patients with chronic prostatitis, efforts should be made to identify the causative organism, and even with a prolonged course of appropriate antibiotics, a cure can be expected in fewer than half the patients.

With advancing age, the prevalence of prostate diseases increases dramatically. The three most common conditions are benign prostatic hyperplasia (BPH), prostate cancer, and prostatitis. Self-reported prostate disease affects about 3 million Americans. BPH develops in over half the men aged 65 years and older and affects the overwhelming majority of men after age 85 years. Prostate cancer is the second leading cause of cancer death in men, and many men have asymptomatic or low-grade tumors that cause few or no health problems. The prevalence of prostatitis is similar to that of ischemic heart disease or diabetes mellitus. The three common prostatic conditions are reviewed herein, with special attention to diagnosis and management.

BENIGN PROSTATIC HYPERPLASIA

Epidemiology

BPH is a noncancerous enlargement of the epithelial and fibromuscular components of the prostate gland. The epithelial component normally makes up 20% to 30% of prostate volume and contributes to the seminal fluid. The fibromuscular component comprises 70% to 80% of the prostate and is responsible for expressing prostatic fluid during ejaculation. Age and long-term androgen stimulation induce BPH development. Microscopic appearance of BPH may occur as early as age 30, is present in 50% of men by age 60, and is present in 90% of men by age 85. In half of these cases, microscopic BPH develops into palpable macroscopic BPH. Of those with macroscopic BPH, only half develop into clinically significant disease brought to medical attention. BPH is one of the most common conditions in aging men; in the United States annually it accounts for more than 1.7 million office visits and 250,000 surgical procedures.

Prostatism, or Lower Urinary Tract Symptoms

The symptoms of BPH are nonspecific; other diseases can result in identical symptoms. The pathophysiology of BPH symptoms is not completely understood, but presumably it involves the periurethral zone of the prostate gland, which results in obstructed urine flow and compensatory responses of the urinary bladder, such as hypertrophy and decreased capacity. The urethral obstruction has both mechanical (obstructing mass) and dynamic (smooth muscle contractions) components. The resulting lower urinary tract symptoms are divided into irritative (frequency, urgency, nocturia) and obstructive (hesitancy, intermittency, weak stream, incomplete emptying) manifestations. The American Urological Association developed a quantitative symptom index for severity assessment and treatment response monitoring, which was adopted by the World Health Organization and is known as the International Prostate Symptom Score (IPSS). Although tracking symptom severity is useful in the longitudinal management of patients, symptom severity has not been found to correlate with prostate size, urine flow rates, or postvoid residual volume. BPH primarily affects quality of life, although complications such as recurrent urinary tract infection, bladder stones, urinary retention, chronic renal insufficiency, and hematuria can develop.

Diagnosis

Differential diagnosis of lower urinary tract symptoms includes endocrine disorders (especially diabetes mellitus), neurologic disorders, urinary tract infections, sexually transmitted diseases, kidney or bladder stones, and medications (especially drugs with anticholinergic and diuretic effects). Digital rectal examination (DRE) may be unremarkable or reveal an enlarged, smooth, rubbery, symmetrical gland. Urinalysis is routinely performed to evaluate for urinary tract infection, hematuria, and glycosuria. A baseline serum creatinine assesses kidney function and the possibility of obstructive uropathy or intrinsic renal disease, or both. Additional optional tests include postvoid residual urine volume, urine flow rates, and pressure flow studies. These tests may be considered when the diagnosis is uncertain or an invasive treatment is being planned.

Treatment Approaches

BPH therapy is patient dependent and driven by the impact of symptoms on the patient's quality of life (see Table 53.1). All patients should be educated regarding life-style modification: fluid adjustments (avoid caffeine) and avoidance of medications (especially anticholinergics) that aggravate symptoms. Patients with mild to moderate symptoms may be satisfied with life-style modification only. Both medical and surgical treatments are also available, with medication the usual first approach. Indications for surgical treatment include patient preference, dissatisfaction with medication, and refractory urinary retention, as well as renal dysfunction, bladder stones, recurrent urinary tract infections, or hematuria if these are clearly due to prostatic obstruction.

Medical Treatment

The two main pharmacologic approaches are α-adrenergic antagonists and 5α-reductase inhibitors.

α-Adrenergic antagonists, or α-blockers, are directed at the dynamic component of urethral obstruction. Smooth muscle of the prostate and bladder neck has a resting tone mediated by α-adrenergic innervation. α-Blockers relax the smooth muscle in the hyperplastic prostate tissue, prostate capsule, and bladder neck, thus decreasing resistance to urinary flow. Of the two major α-adrenergic receptors, α_1 receptors predominate in the prostate, and the α_{1a} subtype comprises 70% of these receptors. α-Blockade development for BPH therapy has progressed from selective α_1 agents (prazosin[OL], alfuzosin) to long-acting selective α_1 agents (terazosin, doxazosin) and now to long-acting α_{1a} subtype selective agents (tamsulosin). The most common adverse effects of α_1 agents are dizziness, mild asthenia (fatigue or weakness), and headaches. Postural hypotension occurs infrequently and can be minimized by careful dose titration.

The enzyme 5α-reductase is required for the conversion of testosterone to the more active dihydrotestosterone. Finasteride is an inhibitor of this enzyme and reduces tissue levels of dihydrotestosterone, thus reducing prostate gland size. Improvements in symptom scores and urine flow rates may not be evident for up to 6 months. Finasteride is most effective in men with larger prostates (> 40 g,

Table 53.1—Management Options for Benign Prostatic Hyperplasia

Category	Interventions	Rationale	Comments
Life-style modification	Reduce nighttime fluids to manage nocturia Eliminate bladder irritants (eg, caffeine, alcohol, nicotine)	Factors outside the urinary tract contribute to urinary symptoms	Often sufficient management for mild symptoms Complements management for moderate to severe symptoms
Pharmacologic management	α-Adrenergic antagonists Selective α_1: prazosin[OL], alfuzosin Long-acting selective α_1: terazosin, doxazosin Long-acting selective α_{1A} subtype selective: tamsulosin	Relaxation of the smooth muscle in hyperplastic prostate tissue, prostate capsule, and bladder neck decreases resistance to urinary flow	Adverse effects: dizziness, mild asthenia, headaches, postural hypotension (reduced with careful dose titration, not present with tamsulosin), abnormal ejaculation, rhinitis
	5α-Reductase inhibitors: finasteride, dutasteride	Reduced tissue levels of dihydrotestosterone result in prostate gland size reduction	Most effective for men with larger prostates (> 40 g) Results may not be evident for up to 6 months
Surgery	Transurethral resection of the prostate Transurethral incision of the prostate Open prostatectomy Transurethral vaporization of the prostate Stent placement	Removal or expansion of peri-urethral prostate tissue reduces obstruction to urinary flow	Indicated for BPH-induced recurrent UTI, recurrent or persistent gross hematuria, bladder stones, renal insufficiency

NOTE: BPH = benign prostatic hyperplasia; UTI = urinary tract infection.

[OL] Not approved by the U.S. Food and Drug Administration for this use.

about the size of a plum). Because finasteride reduces serum prostate-specific antigen (PSA) levels an average 50%, baseline serum PSA determination is advocated for men in whom prostate cancer surveillance is planned. Subsequently, after a 6-month trial if continued finasteride therapy is desired, a PSA level on treatment is obtained and then measured annually for cancer surveillance.

When used together over years, the combination of α-adrenergic antagonists with 5α-reductase inhibitors has been shown to be safe and to reduce clinical progression of BPH better than either agent alone. In particular, a lower risk of urinary retention, urinary incontinence, renal insufficiency, and recurrent bladder infections is associated with combination therapy. Also, consistent results from a number of trials demonstrate that the herbal preparation *Serenoa repens,* or saw palmetto, improves urinary symptoms and flow measures in men with BPH. The improvements are similar to those associated with treatment with finasteride, and there are fewer reported adverse effects with *S. repens.* (See also "Complementary and Alternative Medicine," p 80.)

Surgical Treatment

Surgical management includes transurethral resection of the prostate, transurethral incision of the prostate, open prostatectomy, transurethral vaporization of the prostate, and device insertion such as stent placement. Surgical approaches offer the best chance for symptom improvement but also have the highest rates of complications. The benefits of surgical treatments are generally considered equivalent, but complication rates differ. Transurethral resection of the prostate is the standard of care to which other BPH treatments are compared and has an 80% likelihood of successful outcome in properly selected patients. Usually performed under spinal anesthesia, a transurethral resection of the prostate involves the passage of an endoscope through the urethra to remove surgically the inner portion of the prostate. Long-term complications may include retrograde ejaculation, urethral stricture, bladder neck contracture, incontinence, and impotence. Transurethral incision of the prostate is an endoscopic procedure via the urethra to make one to two cuts in the prostate and prostate capsule, relieving urethral constriction. Limited to small prostate glands (< 30 g), transurethral incision of the prostate offers lower rates of retrograde ejaculation, bleeding, and contractures. Open prostatectomy involves removal of the inner portion of the prostate through a retropubic or suprapubic incision. It is best used for patients with larger prostates or with complicating conditions such as bladder stones or urethral strictures. Open prostatectomy is associated with incisional morbidity, longer

hospitalization, and greater risk of impotence. Transurethral vaporization of the prostate uses a high-energy electrode inserted via the urethra to vaporize the prostate. This approach has little bleeding but creates more prolonged irritative voiding. Prostatic stents are used to maintain expansion of the prostatic urethra and are employed for temporary and permanent uses.

PROSTATE CANCER

Incidence and Epidemiology

Cancer of the prostate is the most common noncutaneous cancer and the second leading cause of cancer deaths among men in the United States. It was estimated that in 2005, 232,090 men would be diagnosed and 30,350 men would die from prostate cancer. The incidence increases with age and is rare in men younger than 40 years. In autopsy studies where the entire prostate is examined, incidental histologic evidence of cancer of the prostate is found in 30% of men over 50 and 80% of men over 80. The incidence of disease varies according to race, with American blacks having the highest risk in the world. Among black men cancer of the prostate occurs at an earlier age, has a higher mortality rate, and tends to be at a more advanced stage of disease at diagnosis. Family history is a contributing factor. Men with one first-degree relative affected have more than a twofold increased risk, and with two first-degree relatives affected, more than an eightfold increased risk. Androgens are necessary for prostate cancer pathogenesis; the disease does not occur in men castrated before puberty. Diets high in total fat consumption are associated with increased risk. The association between cancer of the prostate and early onset of sexual activity, sexually transmitted disease, or vasectomy is inconclusive.

Symptoms

Cancer usually arises in the peripheral zone of the prostate. The majority of patients, especially those with early-stage, potentially curable disease, are asymptomatic. Cancer of the prostate spreads by three routes: direct extension, the lymphatics, and the blood stream. Direct invasion of the urethra and bladder can lead to irritative voiding symptoms, urinary incontinence, and hematuria. Extension of disease to adjacent nerves may cause impotence and pelvic pain. Nodal metastasis may cause extrinsic ureteral obstruction. Leg edema may develop from lymphatic obstruction. Hematogenous metastasis to bone may cause severe local pain, normochromic normocytic anemia, pathologic fractures, and spinal cord compression. Less commonly, hematogenous metastasis involves viscera—namely, the lung, liver, and adrenal glands.

Screening Controversy

The benefit of early detection and the best approach to treatment of prostate cancer are controversial. At the heart of the screening debate is the fact that no direct evidence exists to show that early detection decreases prostate cancer mortality rates. There is a large reservoir of cancer of the prostate that does not need to be diagnosed because the majority of men with prostate cancer die with the disease, not from it. The well-recognized burden of progressive cancer of the prostate is the impetus for early detection and management. The American Urological Association and the American Cancer Society advocate annual screening, recommending the PSA test and DRE beginning at age 50 for men with at least a 10-year life expectancy and earlier (age 40) for men at high risk (black men, first-degree relative affected). Groups that use explicit criteria to develop evidence-based practice guidelines (U.S. Preventive Services Task Force, American College of Physicians, and Canadian Task Force on the Periodic Health Examination) have recommended against routine PSA screening for cancer of the prostate. Guidelines are in agreement that the controversy surrounding screening should be discussed with patients in order to achieve individualized, informed courses of action. The effectiveness of PSA screening is particularly questionable in elderly men.

Screening and Diagnostic Tests

DRE of the prostate allows palpation of the posterior surfaces of the lateral lobes, where cancer most often begins. Cancer characteristically is hard, nodular, and irregular. DRE enhances screening efforts by detecting some cancers with a normal PSA level. DRE is inherently inaccurate because parts of the prostate gland cannot be reached. About half of the cancers thought to be "confined" to the prostate on the basis of DRE are found during surgery to have already spread. DRE produces many false-positive results; about one third of positive DRE tests are shown to be cancer by biopsy. Local extension of cancer of the prostate into the seminal vesicles can often be detected by DRE. Despite its limitations, DRE remains important for screening and staging.

The serum PSA test is not specific for cancer of the prostate. PSA elevations occur in benign conditions of the prostate, namely, hypertrophy and prostatitis, and in transient response to conditions such as ejaculation and prostatic massage. The sensitivity of the PSA test is also imperfect. Declines in PSA values have been associated with acute hospitalization and use of medications such as finasteride and saw palmetto. Normal PSA levels are found in 30% to 40% of men with cancer confined to the prostate (false-negative tests). The reported positive predictive value of PSA in

screening studies is 28% to 35%: about one third of men with elevated PSA levels have cancer of the prostate demonstrated by fine-needle biopsy.

Several approaches to improve the accuracy of PSA testing have been developed. PSA density is derived from the PSA concentration divided by the volume of the gland (measured by ultrasound). Cancer of the prostate produces higher PSA levels per unit volume than BPH and should therefore yield a higher PSA density. The PSA rate of change or velocity is more specific for cancer of the prostate than a single PSA measurement. Using a PSA velocity value of ≥ 0.75 ng/mL/year achieves 90% specificity, whereas using a single PSA level > 4 ng/mL achieves 60% specificity. This high specificity for PSA velocity is realized even in normal-range serum PSA levels (< 4 ng/mL). Another approach involves age-adjusted PSA reference ranges because PSA values increase with age. Finally, one can measure the ratio of free to complexed PSA, recognizing that PSA bound to α_1-antichymotrypsin accounts for a larger proportion of total PSA with cancer of the prostate than with BPH.

Abnormal DRE or PSA tests lead to transrectal ultrasound–guided biopsy of the prostate for pathologic diagnosis. Cancer may appear as a hypoechoic density, but ultrasound is not specific enough to be used as a screening tool. Spring-loaded core needle biopsies are routinely taken from the base, middle, and apex of each lobe (six samples total). Biopsies may also be taken from specific palpable nodules.

Grading

The Gleason grading system is the most commonly used system that is based on the histologic appearance of prostate cancer. The Gleason grade ranges from 1, or well differentiated, to 5, or poorly differentiated. The Gleason score is the sum of the most common Gleason grade observed plus the next most common Gleason grade seen. The Gleason score ranges from 2 to 10. Gleason scores are sometimes grouped as 2–4, well differentiated; 5–7, moderately differentiated; 8–10, poorly differentiated. Well-differentiated tumors have a favorable prognosis; poorly differentiated tumors, an unfavorable prognosis. Most clinically detected tumors are moderately differentiated.

Staging

Staging of cancer of the prostate is necessary for planning disease management. Two classification systems are used: the tumor, regional node, metastasis (TNM) system and the Jewett-Whitmore (ABCD) system (Table 53.2). Usually detected by transurethral resection of the prostate, incidentally discovered cancers are staged according to the amount of tissue involved (T1 or A). Stage T1c reflects the growing number of tumors detected because of an elevated PSA level. Tumors detectable by DRE and confined to the prostate (T2 or B) are subdivided on the basis of the amount of tumor that is palpable. The degree of extension and invasion of surrounding structures stage tumors that extend beyond the prostatic capsule (T3 to T4 or C). Advanced disease (M1 or D) has metastasized.

The initial staging evaluation includes PSA level, DRE findings, and transrectal ultrasonography results. Bone scans may be performed on patients with PSA values greater than 10 ng/mL or complaints of bone pain. For patients electing active treatment, surgical assessment of lymph node involvement (pelvic lymphadenectomy) is performed by itself or in conjunction with prostate surgery or implantation of radioactive seeds. Computed tomography (CT) scans are often employed for active treatment planning.

In the past, CT scans, magnetic resonance imaging scans, pedal lymphangiography, and pelvic lymph node dissection were routinely employed in various combinations to evaluate the extent of cancer of the prostate. These tests should be eliminated in the initial staging evaluation of prostate cancer patients because they have been associated with unacceptably high false-negative and false-positive results. A subset of patients appears to benefit from CT scans combined with fine-needle aspiration. Patients who have a PSA > 25 ng/mL, a Gleason score > 6, and a palpable abnormality on DRE are currently recommended to undergo a CT scan with fine-needle aspiration if a lymph node larger than 6 mm is present. Many of these patients will be diagnosed with nodal metastasis and thus spared the need for bilateral pelvic lymph-node dissection and its associated morbidity.

The serum PSA level should be used to eliminate the staging radionuclide bone scan. In the asymptomatic, newly diagnosed, previously untreated prostate cancer patient, a PSA concentration ≤ 10 ng/mL has been associated with rare (0% to 0.8%) findings of skeletal metastases. Adopting recommendations to eliminate the staging radionuclide bone scan in this population will substantially reduce testing, because 50% to 60% of men with newly diagnosed cancer of the prostate have a serum PSA concentration in this range.

Management of Localized Disease

Localized cancer lends itself to cure, but the prevalence of men dying with cancer of the prostate (often asymptomatic) but not from the disease questions the necessity of treatment. No trials have shown that treatment prolongs life when treatment is compared with watchful waiting. Thus, three approaches to

Table 53.2—Staging Systems for Prostate Cancer

TNM Stage	Jewett-Whitmore Stage	Description
T1	A1, A2	Tumor is an incidental finding
T2	B1, B2	Tumor is palpable, confined to prostate
T3	C1, C2	Tumor extends beyond the prostate capsule, may involve seminal vesicles
T4	C2	Tumor invades adjacent structures (eg, bladder neck, rectum, pelvic wall)
N	D1	Lymph node metastasis present
M	D2	Distant metastasis present

NOTE: TNM = tumor, regional node, metastasis.

SOURCE: For further details, see AUA Prostate Cancer Clinical Guidelines Panel. *Report on the Management of Clinically Localized Prostate Cancer.* Baltimore, MD: American Urological Association; 1995.

localized prostate cancer are routinely advocated: watchful waiting, radical prostatectomy, and radiation therapy (see Table 53.3).

Watchful waiting (also called *expectant* or *conservative management; surveillance*) is the approach offered most commonly to men with less than a 10-year life expectancy, who have significant medical comorbidities, or whose tumor is small and well to moderately differentiated. Conservative management studies have shown that 10-year disease-specific survival is 89% to 96% for Gleason score 2–5 tumors, 70% to 82% for Gleason score 6 tumors, 30% to 58% for Gleason score 7 tumors, and 13% to 40% for Gleason score 8–10 tumors. Because most men with cancer of the prostate are asymptomatic, watchful waiting attempts to spare men the burden of unnecessary treatment. However, awaiting symptoms in men with prostate cancer before initiating treatment means sacrificing the opportunity for cure. Patients are offered palliation if and when symptoms develop.

Radical prostatectomy involves the surgical removal of the entire prostate gland and the seminal vesicles. It can be performed through a perineal (incision near the rectum) or retropubic (lower abdominal incision) approach. The perineal approach allows an easier vesicourethral anastomosis and less bleeding, whereas the retropubic approach allows access to the pelvic lymph nodes and spares the neurovascular supply to the corpora cavernosa (with improved potency). The major morbidities of this treatment are urinary incontinence and erectile dysfunction. Surgery is thought to have the highest incidence of post-treatment sexual dysfunction. A population-based study of 1291 men undergoing radical prostatectomy for clinically localized prostate cancer found that 18 months later, 59.9% reported erections not firm enough for sexual intercourse and 8.4% were incontinent. Patients following

Table 53.3—Management Approaches for Localized Prostate Cancer

Management	Description	Comments
Watchful waiting	Prostate cancer is not treated until symptoms develop	Offered to men with less than a 10-year life expectancy; significant medical comorbidities; small, well-differentiated tumors; or unwillingness to bear treatment burdens Awaiting symptoms sacrifices opportunity for cure
Radical prostatectomy	Surgical removal of the entire prostate gland and seminal vesicles	Offered to men with an absence of surgical contraindications Adverse effects realized immediately
External beam radiation therapy	Standard regimen delivers 6000 to 7000 rads of pelvic radiation over a 7-week period	Radiation reaches tissues outside the prostate including pelvic lymph nodes Adverse effects develop over time
Brachytherapy	Radioactive seeds (eg, iridium, palladium) are implanted into the prostate gland using computed tomography scan guidance	Most adverse effects realized immediately

radical prostatectomy are more likely to experience stress incontinence, with symptoms ranging from occasional leakage to no urinary control. Bladder neck contractures also occur, resulting in obstructive voiding symptoms and urinary retention. Both sexual dysfunction and urinary symptoms have a negative impact on quality of life. The relationship between these morbidities and sense of bother is not direct; for example, those with the most leakage may have little bother while those with minimal leakage may report substantial bother. The goal of surgery is cure. Biochemical progression (PSA $\geq$ 0.4 ng/mL) has been reported in 40% of men 10 years after radical prostatectomy for localized disease. Actuarial metastasis-free survival at 15 years is 82%. Thus, this treatment can be offered to men with locally confined disease, with greater than a 10-year life expectancy, and without contraindications to operative therapy.

Radiation therapy is provided through external beam radiation or through implantation of radioactive sources (known as *brachytherapy*). The standard regimen of external beam radiation delivers a total of 6000 to 7000 rads over a 7-week period. Pelvic lymph nodes can be radiated as well. Proctitis and urethritis are common acute side effects. Chronic complications include erectile dysfunction, urinary incontinence, and chronic proctitis. The incidence of urinary stress incontinence after radiation therapy is significantly less than with surgery, but the presence of irritative voiding dysfunction is greater. Bowel dysfunction, uncommon after surgery, affects more than half of patients after radiation. Bowel symptoms include diarrhea, rectal urgency, and fecal soiling. The majority of patients classify these bowel symptoms as minor with little to no effect on quality of life. Local control and cancer survival rates are comparable to those of radical prostatectomy. Conformal radiation therapy is a mode of high-precision external-beam radiation that uses high-resolution CT scan data and advanced computer technology to conform the radiation dose to the three-dimensional configuration of the tumor. This new technology shows promise in reducing complications and adverse effects.

Brachytherapy involves retropubic or perineal implantation of radioactive seeds, usually iridium or palladium. Improvements in three-dimensional imaging of the prostate through CT scan or ultrasound guidance have allowed more uniform distribution of seeds throughout the prostate and overcome many of the past limitations of brachytherapy. Potency is better preserved with seed implants. Urinary symptoms include frequency, dysuria, and urge incontinence. Bowel symptoms include rectal urgency and rectal bleeding. The morbidity of seed implants appears to improve over time following the initial seed placement. Currently no evidence suggests that brachytherapy is more effective than external beam radiation or prostatectomy.

Management of Locally Advanced Prostate Cancer

Locally advanced prostate cancer extends beyond the capsule or invades the seminal vesicle, without evidence of distant or nodal metastasis. Radiation therapy is the recommended treatment, and adjuvant androgen deprivation provides additional benefit toward increased survival and freedom from metastases. However, controversy exists as to when androgen deprivation should be initiated. Patients may have a prolonged asymptomatic cancer period, while significant negative quality-of-life changes from long-term androgen deprivation occur, including loss of stamina, increased fatigue, hot flashes, diminished muscle mass, and premature osteoporosis. Patients should therefore be given the choice of early versus delayed androgen deprivation.

Management of Advanced Disease

Advanced disease is treated with androgen ablation and symptom-specific approaches, such as focal radiation therapy to painful bone metastasis. Androgen ablation aims to eliminate prostate cancer growth stimulation and includes orchiectomy or luteinizing hormone-releasing hormone (LHRH) agonists with antiandrogens. Orchiectomy and LHRH agonists are equally effective at reducing androgens to castration levels. Orchiectomy is the oldest, safest, least expensive approach but is rejected by nearly half of U.S. men. LHRH agonists such as leuprolide and goserelin produce castration levels about a month after an initial increase in serum testosterone levels. Antiandrogens (eg, flutamide) are often given before initiation of LHRH agonists to blunt the effects of the initial testosterone increase. Antiandrogens inhibit the binding of androgen to its receptor. After castration a small amount of adrenal androgen exists and may allow continued stimulation of prostate cancer growth. Antiandrogens may be combined with chemical or surgical castration, a practice called *complete androgen ablation*. Survival rates for antiandrogens alone are inferior to those for chemical or surgical castration alone; complete androgen ablation offers slight improvement in survival over that offered by castration only.

Radiation therapy is useful for relieving the pain of isolated bone metastasis and reducing the risk of fracture of bones with significant destruction. Diffuse bone metastases require alternative approaches. Bone-seeking radiopharmaceuticals such as strontium can be beneficial for pain control. Androgen deprivation decreases bone pain in two thirds of symptomatic patients.

PROSTATITIS

Etiology

Prostatitis is an inflammatory condition of the prostate that may represent acute bacterial, chronic bacterial, or nonbacterial causes. The most common sources of acute or chronic infection are ascending urethral infection or reflux of infected urine into the prostatic ducts, or both. Direct extension or lymphatic spread from the rectum or hematogenous spread also occurs. Acute prostatitis is an infectious process that is more common in young men. Pathogens in men 35 years and younger often include *Neisseria gonorrhea* and *Chlamydia trachomatis*. In older men acute prostatitis is associated with indwelling urethral catheter use, and coliforms are the suspected bacterial cause. More than 80% of patients with prostatitis have no identifiable infectious agent.

Diagnosis

Acute bacterial prostatitis is characterized by fever, chills, dysuria, and a tense or boggy, extremely tender prostate. Because bacteremia may result from manipulation of the inflamed gland, minimal rectal examination is indicated. Gram's stain and culture of the urine can identify the causative agent.

Chronic bacterial prostatitis presents classically as recurrent bacteriuria caused by the same organism, although most patients will not have this presentation. Patients have varying degrees of obstructive or irritative voiding symptoms and perineal pain. The prostate often feels normal. First-void or midstream urine is compared with expressed prostatic secretion or urine collected postmassage. The expressed sample should reveal leukocytosis and the causative agent. Sterile expressant with leukocytosis suggests nonbacterial prostatitis.

Treatment

Acute bacterial prostatitis is treated with antibiotics and may require hospitalization. The severe inflammation allows antibiotics to penetrate the prostate, and prompt response to empiric therapy is expected. CT or magnetic resonance imaging should be considered to evaluate for an abscess if recovery is delayed. Antibiotic selection should be based initially on urine Gram's stain results, with subsequent consideration of sensitivity profiles. Fluoroquinolones are highly effective in most cases.

Antibiotics are less effective for chronic bacterial prostatitis because of the poor penetration of the prostate by most of these drugs. Prolonged therapy of 6 to 16 weeks offers a cure rate of 30% to 40%. Continuous low-dose antibiotic suppression therapy can be offered for those with frequent symptomatic relapse. Total prostatectomy offers cure but at a high risk-to-benefit ratio. Transurethral resection of the prostate is safer but cures only one third of patients.

Nonbacterial prostatitis is treated symptomatically. A small percentage of cases may involve occult infections, and empiric antibiotic therapy is often used. Efforts to reduce pain and discomfort include anti-inflammatory agents, sitz baths, fluid adjustments (avoid caffeine), anticholinergic agents, and α-adrenergic antagonists.

ANNOTATED REFERENCES

■ AUA Practice Guidelines Committee. AUA guideline on management of benign prostatic hyperplasia (2003). Chapter 1: Diagnosis and treatment recommendations. *J Urol*. 2003;170(2 Pt 1):530–547.

This article provides a review of the diagnostic and therapeutic approaches to benign prostatic hyperplasia with a section on emerging therapies. The American Urological Association panel of experts noted that the Agency for Health Care Policy and Research 1994 guideline is still valid with five minor adjustments.

■ Harris R, Lohr KN. Screening for prostate cancer: an update of the evidence for the U.S. Preventive Services Task Force. *Ann Intern Med.* 2002;137(11):917–929.

This article reports the U.S. Preventive Services Task Force updated review of the evidence of benefits and harms of screening and earlier treatment for prostate cancer patients. The task force concluded that the data are insufficient to recommend for or against routine screening for prostate cancer.

■ Penson DF, Litwin MS. The physical burden of prostate cancer. *Urol Clin North Am.* 2003;30(2):305–313.

This article provides a comprehensive description of the physical burden of prostate cancer and its treatments, covering both metastatic and localized disease. This information may be useful for patients and their physicians as they discuss treatment alternatives.

■ Schaeffer AJ, Datta NS, Fowler JE, et al. Advances in the diagnosis and treatment of prostatitis: overview summary statement. *Urology.* 2000; 60(Suppl 6):1–4.

This is the lead article of an entire supplement on chronic prostatitis. The authors review the diagnostic criteria and then review recommendations for the initial assessment of patients presenting with symptoms of chronic prostatitis. There is a helpful overview of treatment options along with references to other articles in the supplement that provide additional details.

Lisa J. Granville, MD

CHAPTER 54—MUSCULOSKELETAL DISEASES AND DISORDERS

KEY POINTS

■ Most musculoskeletal complaints in older adults are not caused by true arthritis but rather by disorders resulting from derangement of tendons, bursae, muscles, connective tissue, and nerves. Symptoms typically involve a region of the body rather than discrete joints.

■ Among those aged 65 and older, osteoarthritis is the most prevalent articular disease.

■ Most blood testing in rheumatologic conditions can, at best, only help confirm the clinical impression or provide prognostic data. Studies show that laboratory testing tends to be overused.

■ Well-designed studies have now shown the value of exercise in the management of rheumatoid arthritis, osteoarthritis, polymyositis, and systemic lupus erythematosus. Exercise preserves function, reduces symptoms, and reduces sick days. Prescribed exercise must now be considered an essential part of the treatment of all the rheumatologic disorders.

Musculoskeletal complaints are among the most common reasons that older adults seek medical attention. About 1 in 4 of all patients seen by primary care physicians presents with a musculoskeletal condition. Osteoarthritis (OA), whether based on radiographic findings, clinical symptoms, or self-report, is overwhelmingly prevalent in older persons. Depending upon the source of data and which joint is involved, OA is present in anywhere from 50% to 90% of older

adults. In 1996, diseases of the musculoskeletal system and connective tissue accounted for about 7% of all Medicare spending.

DIAGNOSING MUSCULOSKELETAL DISEASE IN OLDER ADULTS

The rheumatologic disorders can be broadly classified as those that present with predominantly musculoskeletal symptoms and those that present with symptoms suggesting a systemic illness. True joint disease (arthritis) is characterized by symptoms and physical examination findings localized to the joints. A patient's history of joint swelling is strong evidence from the outset that true joint involvement is present. History of pain in a joint with motion or weight bearing is suggestive of arthritis. Further questioning about patterns of joint involvement, the presence of morning stiffness, stiffness after periods of inactivity, the effect of activity, and the effect on sleep can greatly narrow diagnostic possibilities.

Musculoskeletal symptoms that seem to be located in a joint are instead often due to a variety of disorders of periarticular tissues, muscles, nerves, and metabolism. These soft-tissue disorders include chronic postural strain, acute muscular and ligamentous strain, bursitis, and fibromyalgia plus conditions not directly related to joints, such as endocrinopathies and neuropathies. Pain complaints in soft-tissue disorders often involve anatomic regions, such as the shoulder girdle or a whole extremity, and rarely include a history of joint swelling; the patient commonly cannot clearly indicate which joint is involved.

When symptoms of pain and fatigue are generalized and not specifically referable to joints or classic bursal areas, differentiating between inflammatory and noninflammatory conditions is paramount. In the inflammatory disorders that may present with generalized aching and pain, there are usually historical and physical findings that lead to the correct diagnosis. The presence of rash, fever, stomatitis, dysphagia, Raynaud's phenomenon, or true muscle weakness suggests one of the autoimmune rheumatologic disorders. The absence of such symptoms make generalized conditions such as fibromyalgia or regional conditions such as chronic postural strain or myofascial pain more likely.

Laboratory Testing

Laboratory testing plays a small role in the diagnosis of rheumatologic diseases in older adults because of the lack of tests that are specific, the high background incidence of OA, and increased seroreactivity in later life, especially in women. Tests for erythrocyte sedimentation rate (ESR) and rheumatoid factor are neither sensitive nor specific. The antinuclear antibody test has such a high sensitivity in systemic lupus erythematosus (SLE) that a negative test essentially excludes it; however, a positive antinuclear antibody is of very low specificity. A few blood tests are specific. For example, either high titers of anti–double-stranded DNA antibodies or the presence of the anti-Sm antibody is specific for SLE, but unfortunately neither is sensitive. Most blood testing in rheumatologic conditions can, at best, only help confirm the clinical impression or provide prognostic data. Studies show that laboratory testing tends to be overused.

The Role of Exercise in Treatment

Clinicians who treat older adults have long understood the value of exercise. Exercise helps preserve muscle and bone mass, reverses the increased fat-to-muscle ratio associated with aging, and preserves physical function. In contrast, classic teaching in rheumatoid arthritis (RA) as recent as the mid-1980s was that exercise should be avoided and even that total bed rest was a mainstay treatment for severe flares. Conventional wisdom also held that weight bearing in OA would accelerate joint degeneration and that exercise in polymyositis would aggravate muscle inflammation. Increasingly, well-designed studies have disproved these beliefs and have now shown the value of exercise in the management of RA, OA, polymyositis, and SLE. Rather than worsening these disorders, exercise preserves function, reduces symptoms, and reduces sick days. Prescribed exercise must now be considered an essential part of the treatment of all the rheumatologic disorders.

SOFT-TISSUE RHEUMATISM

The variety and number of conditions that present with musculoskeletal symptoms is impressive. This section describes the general approach to a patient with a regional musculoskeletal complaint and then discusses a selection of clinically common soft-tissue disorders.

Evaluating Reports of Pain

Most musculoskeletal complaints in older adults are not caused by true arthritis but rather by disorders resulting from derangement of tendons, bursae, muscles, connective tissue, and nerves. Symptoms typically involve a region of the body rather than discrete joints. It makes sense to evaluate a new musculoskeletal complaint as likely soft-tissue rheumatism. The physical examination can begin with observation of the patient performing active range of motion of the affected region. Interpreting abnormal range of motion requires an understanding of the anatomy of the relevant muscles, tendons, bones, and nerves.

The shoulder, for example, is not a simple ball-in-socket joint, but an extremely mobile system of three bones (scapula, clavicle, and humerus) that is attached to the rest of the skeleton only at the sternoclavicular joint. The rest of the shoulder girdle floats and slides over the body and is controlled by a complex set of muscles and associated innervation. To analyze a painful shoulder, instruct the patient to abduct the shoulder from 0 degrees at the side through 90 degrees to 180 degrees, with hand above the head. Test shoulder internal and external rotation by having the patient put the backs of the hands on the sacrum and then the palms on the occiput. Depending on the result of these active range-of-motion tests, the examiner can further pinpoint the likely site of pathology by selectively moving the shoulder components for the patient. Passive motion is most informative when active motion has been demonstrated to be painful or limited. The glenohumeral joint can be isolated while the patient completely relaxes the shoulder; the examiner holds one hand over the upper scapula to prevent scapular motion and simultaneously slowly abducts, extends, flexes, and rotates the shoulder joint. True shoulder (glenohumeral) joint disease would be indicated should isolated passive joint motion be painful. In the case that active motion proved to be painless, then the examiner can first palpate key periarticular structures and then engage the patient with a series of selective resisted active movements that stress particular anatomic elements of the shoulder apparatus. Figure 54.1 shows an algorithm for analyzing the complaint of shoulder pain. A similar method can be applied to other regions of the musculoskeletal system.

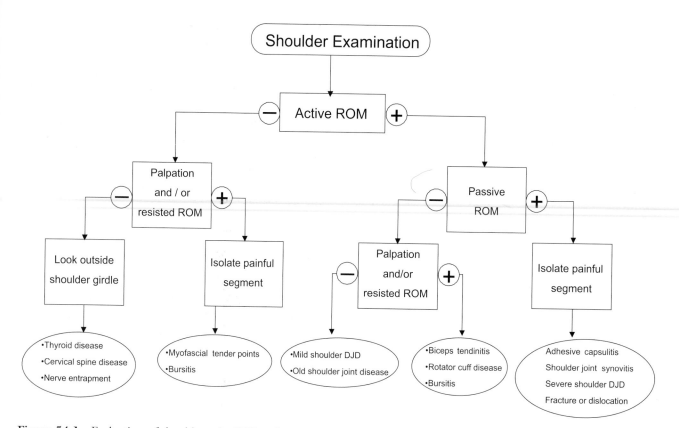

Figure 54.1—Evaluation of shoulder pain. DJD = degenerative joint disease; ROM = range of motion; + = limitation or pain; − = no limitation or pain.

Myofascial Trigger Points

When examination does not reveal arthritis, tendinitis, bursitis, or nerve impingement as the cause of regional pain, careful palpation may locate indurated, and sometimes crepitant, trigger points. Myofascial trigger points are distinct from the symmetrical multiple tender points of fibromyalgia in that palpation of trigger points reproduces the pain syndrome. Trigger points are most common over the upper back at upper or medial edges of a scapula. Similar trigger points can sometimes be discovered over the anterior chest, lower back, sacral, and iliac areas. The cause is poorly understood. Anesthetic injection into a trigger point can confirm the diagnosis. Treatment includes repeated ice application to the trigger points or injection with anesthetic or glucocorticoid, or both.

Fibromyalgia

Fibromyalgia is a generalized pain syndrome that occurs at nearly all ages; prevalence rates of 2% to 10% are similar around the world, independently of nationality or ethnicity and cultural factors. Although there is no pathophysiologic explanation of the condition, the uniform worldwide incidence is persuasive that the condition is real. It was originally termed *fibrositis* in

the early 20th century; more recent usage favors the term *fibromyalgia*, as there is no demonstrable inflammation in symptomatic tissues. A conceptual breakthrough was made nearly 30 years ago with seminal publications by Smythe and Moldofsky that demonstrated characteristic changes in sleep polysomnography in individuals who were defined by the classic "fibrositis" tender points (see Figure 54.2). Furthermore, it was found that electroencephalographic (EEG) changes and classic tender points could be induced by experimental disruption of deep sleep in normal volunteers. Researchers also learned that the EEG changes could be normalized and tender points could be resolved by aerobic exercise and by medications that tend to deepen deep sleep. Over the next 15 years, a multitude of symptoms were associated with fibromyalgia that tended to overlap with those of patients with irritable bowel syndrome and chronic fatigue syndrome. Some experts incorporated these symptoms as secondary criteria for diagnosis.

In 1990 the American College of Rheumatology (ACR) issued criteria for fibromyalgia diagnosis that were about 88% sensitive and 81% specific (see the caption for Figure 54.2). The criteria allow for the coexistence of fibromyalgia with other musculoskeletal disorders. With this approach, fibromyalgia is not

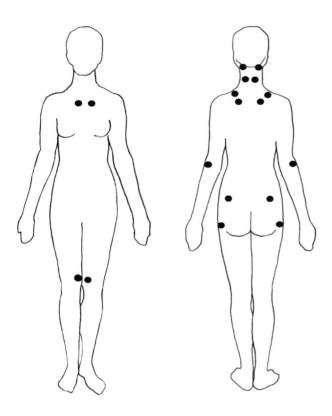

Figure 54.2—Fibromyalgia tender point sites.

For a diagnosis of fibromyalgia, both of the following must be present: (1) a history of widespread pain for at least 3 months; (2) pain in 11 of 18 tender points on digital palpation. For a tender point to be considered positive, the patient must state that the palpation was "painful"; "tender" is not considered synonymous with "painful."

SOURCE: Diagnostic criteria are from Wolfe F, Smythe HA, Yunus MB, et al. The American College of Rheumatology 1990 criteria for the classification of fibromyalgia: report of the multicenter criteria committee. *Arthritis Rheum.* 1990;33:160–172.

simply a diagnosis of exclusion. No laboratory studies can help confirm the diagnosis. Despite the skepticism of many observers who believed fibromyalgia to be an artificial construct, research in the past decade has helped to develop an understanding of fibromyalgia as a condition of altered pain processing by the central nervous system. This research has paralleled advances in understanding the neurologic basis of pain itself. These advances have not yet led to new treatment, but there is ground for optimism.

The average age of fibromyalgia patients is around 45 years, and the majority are female. The condition seems to be a primary and persistent disorder that afflicts adults well into their 80s. Research indicates that the distress experienced by fibromyalgia patients diminishes with advancing age, suggesting that management in older adults may be less challenging. Mainstays of treatment have changed little in recent years. Reassurance that the condition is not life threatening and can be improved is indicated. Aerobic

exercise is recommended, partly because of the original findings of Smythe and Moldofsky but also because of the deconditioning and muscle weakness seen in fibromyalgia. Analgesics give benefit; the role of narcotics is not yet well defined. Tramadol has been investigated and found to give benefit without serious adverse effects. Tricyclic antidepressants have long been used with benefit, but other antidepressants of different classes are also effective. Also, the muscle relaxant cyclobenzaprine and the benzodiazepine alprazolam[OL] have given benefit. Some patients find benefit from rotating medications every 6 months if tolerance seems to emerge. (See also "Persistent Pain," p 140.)

Biceps Tendinitis

Pain in the anterior shoulder with associated exquisite tenderness over the proximal biceps tendon and exacerbation with supination of the forearm (with elbow flexed to 90 degrees) against resistance (Yergason sign) is diagnostic of biceps tendinitis. Also, anterior flexion of the shoulder against resistance is likely to exacerbate the pain in biceps tendinitis. The condition is usually associated with repetitive motions but can be associated with bony impingement problems in the shoulder apparatus. Biceps tendinitis responds well to tendon sheath infiltration with glucocorticoid with or without anesthetic. Steroid iontophoresis can also be effective. Stretching and range-of-motion exercises are indicated during and following healing.

Rotator Cuff Disease

The shoulder rotator cuff is formed superiorly by a common tendinous insertion on the humeral greater tuberosity of the supraspinatus, infraspinatus, and teres minor muscles and inferiorly by the insertion of the subscapularis muscle on the lesser humeral tuberosity. Vascular supply to the upper portions of the rotator cuff is somewhat limited and easily compromised by impingement. Several bursae are associated with the rotator cuff and contribute to symptoms in rotator cuff problems. Rotator cuff disorders tend not to be as acute in older as in younger adults. A history of a recent acute event is not likely to be elicited, but a past episode of a fall with direct blow to the shoulder or falling with the arm outstretched may be recalled. Rotator cuff derangement can involve partial tear or degeneration or complete degenerative destruction. Although trauma is commonly an important factor, tissue ischemia from impingement and changes in bony relationships with advanced shoulder joint degeneration are more likely to be dominant factors in older patients. With complete loss of the rotator cuff,

---

[OL] Not approved by the U.S. Food and Drug Administration for this use.

initiation of active abduction of the hanging arm is severely impaired. With partial tear or degeneration, only pain and giving way with the shoulder abducted to 90 degrees may be present. Management of rotator cuff degeneration should include identification of aggravating factors that can be avoided, especially sleeping with the arm outstretched. Initiation of tailored physical therapy to maintain shoulder range of motion is essential. Injection of a mixture of anesthetic and glucocorticoid into related bursal areas can be helpful in relieving pain and allowing progressive physical therapy to be successful. Surgery is an intervention of last resort in the treatment of rotator cuff disorders in older adults.

Lower Cervical Nerve Impingement

Intermittent pain in the shoulder, deltoid, and upper arm area in the absence of shoulder joint or associated musculotendinous structures should raise suspicion of cervical nerve impingement. The C5 level is most commonly involved. A cervical compression test (Spurling maneuver) can help identify cervical nerve impingement. In this maneuver the seated person tilts and turns the head slightly to the affected side. Steady vertical downward pressure on the top of the head is exerted by the examiner for 10 to 15 seconds. Reproduction of the symptoms on the affected side is a positive test. With more advanced impingement, sensory changes over the upper arm can be demonstrated on examination. Further evaluation would include cervical spine plain radiographs, including oblique views to optimally show the neuroforamina and detect bony impingement. Cervical disk disease can occur and might best be discovered with magnetic resonance imaging. Electrodiagnostic testing may also help sort out more obscure cases. Cervical traction twice daily at home, use of a cervical pillow, and avoidance of aggravating activities are the mainstays of conservative treatment. When muscle spasm is associated with cervical impingement, hot or cold applications plus injection of any identified trigger points can aid in the control of symptoms during recovery. Rarely, surgical intervention is needed for cervical nerve impingement.

Adhesive Capsulitis

Adhesive capsulitis (frozen shoulder syndrome) is an acute process of obscure cause that involves inflammation of the shoulder joint capsule. The condition can follow other shoulder disorders or injury. ESR may acutely increase. Unilateral shoulder involvement can help differentiate this condition from polymyalgia rheumatica. Shoulder pain and tenderness plus severely restricted active and passive range of motion are present. Early intervention with aggressive range-of-motion exercises combined with intra-articular glucocorticoids are important to preserve shoulder motion and reduce inflammation. Although not essential, shoulder arthrography with glucocorticoid and anesthetic injection at the time of arthrogram should be both diagnostic and therapeutic. In addition to intra-articular injection, percutaneous glucocorticoid injections anteriorly, posteriorly, and laterally into the glenohumeral joint capsule and shoulder bursal areas can also be effective. Adhesive capsulitis usually follows a course of several months that includes three phases: freezing, frozen, and thawing. With timely treatment, the outcome should be good, but physical therapy needs to extend well beyond the thawing phase.

Olecranon Bursitis

Enlargement of the olecranon bursa with marked distension due to effusion with or without inflammation and surrounding cellulitis is common regardless of age. In younger adults occupational factors are often present, supporting the notion that olecranon bursitis can have an origin based in repetitive trauma. Olecranon bursitis is also commonly associated with RA and gout, with or without nodules in the former case and tophi in the latter. Infection of the bursa is also common, usually with staphylococci. Evaluation of an inflamed olecranon begins with sterile aspiration of fluid for cultures and cell count. The presence of surrounding cellulitis could be due to infection or acute gout; diagnostic aspiration of the bursa through affected skin mandates initiation of an antibiotic and continuation until culture results are in hand. Antibiotic selection should provide *Staphylococcus aureus* coverage, with modification that is based on culture results. Repeated aspiration during treatment may help recovery from infection. The course of recovery can be prolonged, with frequent relapses. The bursa often spontaneously drains, and complete healing of the cutaneous fistula may require many months. Olecranon bursitis associated with RA or gout is managed in accordance with the underlying disease once infection is excluded. Noninfectious olecranon bursitis suspected to be of traumatic origin should be treated with padding and avoidance of further trauma; aspiration and injection of the bursa could be considered. Close follow-up is indicated because olecranon bursae are so prone to spontaneous infection.

Carpal Tunnel Syndrome

Entrapment of the median nerve where it passes through the carpal tunnel of the wrist is one of the most common nerve-entrapment syndromes in older adults. Symptoms of median nerve compression can occur with wrist synovitis due to RA, gout, or pseudogout. Hypothyroidism and diabetes mellitus are predisposing factors. Amyloidosis is an infrequent but well-known cause of carpal tunnel syndrome. The most common cause, however, is repetitive trauma. Carpal tunnel syndrome presents with nocturnal hand pain, tingling, and numbness involving the median nerve distribution in the hand. Pain during the day, even with radiation proximally to the shoulder, is occasionally seen and can confound diagnosis. In addition to the sensory deficits almost always present, atrophy of the thenar eminence can develop in longstanding median nerve compression. Evaluation should include inquiry into factors in the patient's daily activities that could exacerbate carpal tunnel disease. Untreated or unrecognized hypothyroidism and diabetes should be tested for. A cock-up wrist splint, especially at night, can lessen symptoms. Some clinicians recommend isometric flexion exercises of metacarpal phalangeal joints and the affected wrist joint in which the tense flexor tendons act like a bowstring to stretch the transverse ligament overlying the carpal tunnel. Injection of glucocorticoids into the carpal tunnel, taking care not to inject the median nerve, can be of benefit and is highly recommended by some clinicians. Injection of the wrist joint when carpal tunnel syndrome is related to active wrist synovitis due to RA, gout, or pseudogout is usually quite effective. Surgical release of the transverse ligament can relieve symptoms when conservative measures fail.

Trochanteric Bursitis

Several bursae surround the hip joint and femoral trochanteric areas. Two bursa are of particular interest in soft-tissue rheumatism. The first is the bursa that directly overlies the greater femoral trochanter, and the second is deep to the gluteus maximus and posterior and slightly superior to the trochanter. Presenting symptoms of trochanteric bursitis include hip pain that is localized over the lateral proximal thigh. Pain on the affected side during sleep is usually present. The cause of trochanteric bursitis is not well understood. Significant predisposing factors may include local trauma, strain, and obesity. Treatment in elderly persons should include physical therapy, evaluation of transferring techniques to minimize excessive gluteal muscle stress, stretching exercises, and the use of a pillow positioned posterolaterally behind the involved side to discourage inadvertent resting on the affected bursa during sleep. Infiltration of the trochanteric areas with glucocorticoids is very helpful.

Anserine Bursitis

There are several bursae associated with the knee. In elderly persons the two most important are both associated with knee joint arthritis: the gastrocnemius and semimembranosus bursae in the popliteal fossa (see next section) and the anserine bursa anteromedially distal to the knee. The anserine bursa is located in relation to the insertion of the medial collateral ligament on the proximal tibia. Anserine bursitis presents with the complaint of knee pain that may bother the patient especially at night. Palpation over the area of the bursa should reveal marked local tenderness. Swelling, induration, or effusion may exist in association with anserine bursitis. Knee OA may be symptomatic as well. Cold applications may be of benefit. A pillow placed between the knees at night can lessen both nocturnal pain and recurrence in susceptible individuals. Injection of the bursa with a mixture of glucocorticoid and anesthetic is effective and can provide prompt relief.

Popliteal Cyst

A popliteal cyst (Baker cyst) may develop at any age. A symptomatic cyst can present with knee pain with pressure in the posterior knee; occasionally, a popliteal cyst can present with acute rupture. A popliteal cyst develops as an extension of the knee joint synovial space posteriorly into the gastrocnemius and semimembranosus bursae. Knee arthritis is almost always a precursor. Knee effusions in arthritis result in high resting intra-articular pressure that increases many-fold with knee flexion or with weight bearing. High knee synovial pressure tends to force fluid into one of the popliteal bursa. The communication between joint and bursa also tends to behave like a ball valve, with one-way movement of fluid from knee to bursa. This process leads to progressive popliteal cyst formation and enlargement, with eventual emergence of pain behind the knee. In addition to pain, the cyst can become a space-occupying lesion and can impede deep venous return from the lower leg.

Inspection for the presence of a popliteal cyst should be part of the routine knee examination in patients with known OA or who present with knee pain. Often a popliteal cyst is not distinctly palpable. Inspection of both popliteal fossae with the patient standing may reveal asymmetric fullness on one side. Hyperextension of the ankle while the knee is fully extended can accentuate the bulge of a popliteal cyst. Ultrasound examination of the popliteal fossa easily demonstrates the presence of a cyst. Though highly accurate, magnetic resonance imaging of the knee is rarely necessary to evaluate for a popliteal cyst.

A popliteal cyst can rupture spontaneously or with exertion. The result can be dramatic, with acute pain, swelling, warmth, and erythema of the lower leg that mimics all the signs of deep-vein thrombosis. In a few days bruising can surface in the lower leg and form a bruise below the lateral malleolus on the affected side (crescent sign). Occasionally, true deep-vein thrombosis can develop following acute popliteal cyst rupture. Venography or serial venous Doppler studies, or both, may be required to correctly interpret the course of popliteal cyst rupture. Glucocorticoid injection into the knee may be of benefit with acute cyst rupture, as presumably the same mechanisms that direct fluid from the knee to the popliteal cyst will carry the injected steroid into the area of the ruptured cyst. Similarly, knee arthrocentesis followed by glucocorticoid instillation for a symptomatic, but intact, popliteal cyst may reduce synovial fluid production and intra-articular pressure and give a few months' improvement in popliteal symptoms. In the case of associated knee OA, a series of knee hyalin injections (see the next section) could ameliorate the factors driving popliteal cyst formation. Correction of the underlying knee disease that has led to development of the popliteal cyst is required to control cyst recurrence. Aspiration of the cyst itself, taking care to avoid the popliteal neurovascular bundle, with injection of glucocorticoid directly into the cyst is recommended by some clinicians.

JOINT DISEASE

Osteoarthritis

OA, whether based on radiographic findings, clinical symptoms, or self-report, is overwhelmingly prevalent in older persons. Depending upon the source of data and which joint is involved, OA is present in anywhere from 50% to 90% of older adults. OA is the major cause of knee, hip, and joint pain, as well as back pain in older adults. Knee pain alone, according to data from NHANES III (the third National Health and Nutrition Examination Survey) affects more than 20% of adults aged 60 or over, with an incidence approaching 30% for those aged 80 and over. Sequential NHANES data suggests that the rising incidence of knee pain can be attributed to the worsening obesity and decreasing physical activity of Americans in recent decades.

OA is a degenerative disease of cartilage that correlates strongly with aging, yet pathologic changes in osteoarthritic cartilage are quite distinct from changes seen in normal aging cartilage. OA is also a heterogenous group of related joint disorders that have a variety of causes; these may be inborn, associated with metabolic disease, or due to joint malformation, joint trauma, or damage from other joint diseases. Distinct patterns of joint involvement are used to classify OA, ranging from isolated finger interphalangeal joint bony enlargement, to severe deterioration of weight-bearing joints, to isolated spinal involvement, and to generalized axial and peripheral

joint degeneration. Primary OA appears to be genetically determined, with dominant expression in woman and recessive expression in men, and it tends to avoid wrists, elbows, shoulders, and ankles. Involvement of these joints with OA is suggestive of the presence of another disease or factor contributing to joint degeneration.

Underlying pathology in OA does not feature inflammation, though hypertrophy of synovium and accumulation of joint effusions is typical. Progressive changes in cartilage include poor chondrocyte function and death, altered cartilage composition with poor mechanical properties, cartilage surface fibrillation, and eventual gross cartilage destruction. Associated boney proliferation at the cartilage-bone interface leads to palpable and radiographically distinct osteophytes around affected joints.

Pain and reduced joint motion are the hallmarks of OA, with attendant ligamental instability and muscle atrophy. OA in weight-bearing joints is associated with gait abnormalities, and it increases the risk for falling and injury, contributing substantially to OA morbidity, especially in the oldest and most frail patients. Disability can be profound. The ACR diagnostic criteria for OA of the knee and hip are summarized in Table 54.1.

The management of OA usually begins with efforts to control pain. Rarely do analgesics alone accomplish pain control. By the time of physician evaluation for symptomatic OA, function has likely worsened because of muscle atrophy and joint motion limitation. These collateral changes put an affected joint at biomechanical disadvantage that both increases pain and predisposes the joint to ever more rapid deterioration. Early efforts to strengthen atrophied muscles related to the diseased joint and improve joint motion are critical. Analgesics play a role in allowing physical therapy to be used effectively in the long-term management of OA. Early referral to a physical therapist for evaluation and

Table 54.1—Diagnostic Criteria for Osteoarthritis

Knee Pain	Hip Pain
plus at least one of the following:	*plus at least two of the following:*
▪ Age > 50 years	▪ ESR < 20 mm/hour
▪ Stiffness < 30 minutes	▪ Femoral or acetabular osteophytes
▪ Crepitus	▪ Joint-space narrowing
▪ Osteophytes on radiography:	▪ Osteophytes on radiography:
91% sensitive	89% sensitive
86% specific	91% specific

NOTE: ESR = erythrocyte sedimentation rate (Westergren).
SOURCES: Data from Altman R, Asch E, Bloch D, et al. The American College of Rheumatology criteria for the classification and reporting of osteoarthritis of the knee. *Arthritis Rheum.* 1986;29:1039–1049, and Altman R, Alarcon G, Appelrouth D, et al. The American College of Rheumatology criteria for the classification and reporting of osteoarthritis of the hip. *Arthritis Rheum.* 1991;34:505–514.

to define a set of exercises the patient can do daily at home is usually indicated. With OA of the weight-bearing joints, especially the knees, early remobilization and an ongoing walking exercise program may result in progressive functional improvement and reduction in pain rather than the often feared inevitable deterioration of the affected joints. Weight reduction can help reduce pain and improve function, especially if the lumbar spine or weight-bearing joints are involved. Joint injection with corticosteroids, joint injections with hyaluronic acid derivatives, and joint lavage can be of temporary benefit with low risk for toxicity. If there is a high interest in avoiding knee arthroplasty, a cartilage-preserving lateral tibial wedge osteotomy can be considered, provided there is isolated medial compartment knee osteoarthritis and the lateral knee compartment is intact. If conservative management proves to be inadequate with knee or hip disease, total arthroplasty is an excellent ultimate solution.

Recommendations about which analgesics to use for OA have changed over the past decade. Research shows that acetaminophen is often as effective as any of the nonsteroidal anti-inflammatory drugs (NSAIDs). Considerable gastrointestinal and renal toxicity can be associated with NSAID use in older adults. The ACR recommends that acetaminophen be the first analgesic chosen in treating OA. Similar recommendations have been issued by the American Geriatrics Society. Clinical studies over the past 2 years suggest an emerging consensus that NSAIDs may be slightly more effective in treating OA of the knee, especially when analgesia is still required after 3 to 6 months of treatment.

Controversy continues regarding possible kidney and liver damage from acetaminophen. There is no disagreement about the severe hepatic toxicity of acetaminophen overdose; however, hepatotoxicity is not seen when dosing guidelines are followed. Of course, with cognitively impaired elderly patients, there is always the possibility of inadvertent or accidental overdose of any prescribed medication. The possibility that chronic acetaminophen use contributes to renal insufficiency continues to intrigue investigators. Possibly because phenacetin was banned by the Food and Drug Administration more than 20 years ago because of the high risk of nephropathy, suspicions about acetaminophen (the active metabolite of phenacetin) persist. Nearly all studies of the renal effects of acetaminophen use have been retrospective and are impaired by numerous methodologic problems. The preponderance of data suggests that the risk of nephropathy from acetaminophen is quite low when it is used in modest doses by those without preexisting kidney disease. Acetaminophen, given under physician supervision, is still the analgesic of choice for patients with existing renal insufficiency, according to the National Kidney Foundation recommendations.

If acetaminophen is initially ineffective, nonacetylated salicylates such as salsalate or magnesium choline salicylate, which have lower gastrointestinal toxicity than most older NSAIDs, can be given. The selective COX-2 inhibitors are more expensive. COX-2 inhibitors have the same risk of unwanted renal effects as the other NSAIDs. They may also be associated with increased risk of myocardial infarction. The COX-2 inhibitors are further discussed in the section on RA (see p 440).

Hyaluronic acid is a major constituent of synovial fluid and is a major contributor to synovial fluid viscosity and a contributor to cartilage elasticity. Hyaluronic acid and hyaluronan polymers were approved for intra-articular injection for OA of the knee in 1997. This viscosupplementation therapy is given in a series of weekly knee joint injections, five for hyaluronic acid and three for hyaluronan polymers. The benefits of these preparations typically last for 6 months, which is substantially longer than for corticosteroid injection.

Glucosamine and chondroitin sulfate are components of glucosaminoglycan molecules that are important in maintaining mechanical properties of connective tissue and cartilage. When given orally, these compounds are absorbed and incorporated into cartilage. Both have been studied separately as treatments for OA, with evidence of benefit. In OA of the knee, the effectiveness of glucosamine is equivalent to that of ibuprofen, with less gastrointestinal toxicity. The therapeutic benefit of chondroitin sulfate does not become apparent for several weeks after it is started, and improvement lasts for several weeks after it is stopped. Long-term studies will be needed before chondroitin sulfate can be considered a disease-modifying drug for OA. Glucosamine and chondroitin sulfate are available in combination as nutriceuticals. Though both compounds are nontoxic, the dosage and bioavailability of these nutriceuticals are not established; therefore, the benefit seen in therapeutic trials cannot be predicted with these over-the-counter preparations.

Gout

Gout is perhaps the oldest recognized form of arthritis; it was unmistakably described in Hippocrates, and Sydenham's clinical description of his own experience of gout in the late 17th century can hardly be improved upon today. Through the 19th century, the classification of arthritis had rheumatic fever as a distinct form of arthritis, and other forms of joint disease were considered to be subtypes of gout. Hence, terms like *rheumatoid gout* were used for the disease now called *rheumatoid arthritis*. These views prevailed until about 150 years ago when the relationship of classic gout with high levels of uric acid in blood was recognized. Proof of intra-articular monosodium urate crystals as the specific cause of acute gout was not established until the early 1960s.

Gout often presents as acute monarthritis, usually of the first metatarsal phalangeal joint, mid-foot, or ankle. With subsequent attacks, the knee, elbow, or wrist can be involved. Later in the course of untreated disease, attacks tend to be less intense and to last longer, and they may feature simultaneous involvement of more than one joint. Late in untreated disease, chronic low-grade inflammation in multiple joints appears and tophi (gross subcutaneous urate deposits on extensor surfaces) develop. In this late phase of untreated gout, the condition can be mistaken for nodular RA, with the tophi being mistaken for rheumatoid nodules. This can be a sad error, as gout and RA do not occur together, and the two conditions are treated differently. Thus, a strong case is made for microscopic evaluation of samples of joint fluid in the initial evaluation of chronic polyarticular, as well as acute monarticular, arthritis.

With rare exceptions, the clinical emergence of gout is preceded by a period of asymptomatic hyperuricemia. However, hyperuricemia is not uniformly present at the time of an acute gout attack, nor does the presence of hyperuricemia confirm a diagnosis of gout. Acute attacks can be precipitated by trauma, acute nonarticular illness requiring hospitalization, dehydration (acute gout is particularly common postoperatively), or medications that can perturb serum uric acid levels.

A diagnosis of gout is most directly and unequivocally established by observing the presence of strongly negatively birefringent needle-shaped crystals in a sample of joint fluid. Needle-shaped urate crystals can often be seen by ordinary or dark field microscopy of joint fluid, but confirmation of negative birefringence requires the use of a polarizing microscope equipped with a compensator plate. Many laboratories and most rheumatologists have access to such a microscope. This type of microscope is essential in diagnosing pseudogout, described in the next section.

The treatment of gout is biphasic. The acute episode is best managed with a short course of an NSAID. The choice of the NSAID is not critical, as the risk of gastrointestinal toxicity is less likely to emerge during the 10 to 21 days needed for an acute attack to respond. Drugs such as allopurinol or probenecid, which can acutely lower uric acid levels, should not be used in the management of acute gout, as premature lowering of uric acid level will paradoxically intensify and prolong an acute gout attack.

Once the acute attack is resolved, attention can be turned to correcting the underlying problem of urate deposition. Urate accumulation in body tissues can be due to uric acid overproduction in the body, reduced renal elimination, or a combination of both. Ninety percent of chronic hyperuricemia is a consequence of reduced renal excretion that is due to renal disease or drugs, especially diuretics. Uric acid overproduction in older adults is seen in disorders with increased tissue turnover, such as lymphoproliferative disease, chronic hemolytic anemia, and psoriasis, as well as rare genetic enzymatic defects.

Drugs, for example probenecid, that promote renal uric acid excretion can correct hyperuricemia in young adults who have normal kidney function. In older adults, reduced kidney function renders uricosuric drugs less effective. The most effective treatment for uric acid reduction is allopurinol, which acts by blocking the formation of uric acid. Allopurinol dose can be adjusted upward from a starting dosage of 100 mg daily, increasing the daily dose by 100 mg at 2- to 4-week intervals until serum uric acid levels are 5 or below. Because of the high likelihood of decreased kidney function with aging, somewhat lower allopurinol doses may be adequate in older patients to depress uric acid to the desired therapeutic level.

During treatment to lower uric acid levels, the risk of recurrent acute gout attacks is raised. Prophylaxis against acute attacks is advisable for 3 to 6 months while treatment to lower uric acid is introduced and optimized. Although NSAIDs could be used for prophylaxis, the risk of gastrointestinal toxicity with chronic use must be considered. Colchicine can be effective for prophylaxis in older adults at a reduced dosage of 0.6 mg daily. This low dose is well tolerated and does not have an associated risk of gastrointestinal ulceration. Colchicine should be avoided in individuals with hepatic disease or advanced renal insufficiency and is contraindicated if both hepatic and renal diseases are present.

Chondrocalcinosis

Radiographically evident deposition of calcium pyrophosphate dihydrate (CPPD) crystals in articular tissue is markedly related to aging and can be seen in up to 50% of adults aged 90 and over. CPPD crystals can be found in synovial fluid and are associated with several clinical syndromes. CPPD crystals can cause attacks of acute monarthritis, most commonly the knee, wrist, and shoulder, termed *pseudogout* because of the resemblance to acute (urate) gout. CPPD deposition can occur simultaneously in multiple joints and be responsible for chronic polyarticular synovitis reminiscent of RA. Radiographic chondrocalcinosis with or without CPPD crystals in the synovial fluid can also be present in joints with OA without any evidence of inflammation. The coexistence of CPPD crystals and OA is not surprising, as both conditions are common in older adults; however, controversy persists regarding the relationship of the two disorders. Differentiation of CPPD deposition arthropathy from urate gout and RA is important, as the treatment approaches are different.

Acute pseudogout attacks can be treated with a limited course of oral colchicine[OL] or an NSAID in a manner similar to the treatment for acute urate gout. Similarly, intra-articular corticosteroids will halt an attack in patients for whom an NSAID is contraindicated. Parenteral corticosteroids have been shown to be effective for acute pseudogout when NSAIDs and intra-articular corticosteroid injections are both contraindicated. Given once with possible repeat in 1 to 2 days, triamcinolone acetonide 60 mg IM, betamethasone 7 mg IM, or methylprednisolone 125 mg IV have all proven to be safe and effective. Although a single intravenous dose of colchicine of 1 to 2 mg is long acting and can be effective in treating acute pseudogout, the risk of tissue necrosis with accidental extravasation and of bone-marrow suppression in older adults with renal or hepatic impairment suggests this should be considered very carefully in individual cases. Recurrent attacks of pseudogout can be prevented by the use of prophylactic oral colchicine. Any combination of oral and IV colchicine is absolutely contraindicated.

INFLAMMATORY DISORDERS

Polymyalgia Rheumatica

Polymyalgia rheumatica (PMR) is a distinct syndrome that occurs in older adults, as early as age 50 but predominantly after age 60. The onset tends to be insidious, with corresponding delays in diagnosis. The classic symptom of PMR is remarkable proximal limb girdle stiffness and aching pain upon arising in the morning. ESR is so often markedly elevated that a high ESR is one of the essential diagnostic criteria. The syndrome may be accompanied by fatigue, low-grade fever, weight loss, and variable expression of synovitis of proximal joints of the upper, more than lower, extremities. Studies of PMR in recent years have confirmed the presence of synovitis identical to that seen in RA, with synovial thickening, effusions, and lymphocytic synovial infiltration. PMR can progress to chronic polyarthritis that fulfills criteria for RA. Of more immediate clinical importance is the common coexistence of PMR with giant cell arteritis (GCA), a more serious, potentially life-threatening disease. This relationship is discussed in the next section. Even with uncomplicated PMR, treatment with corticosteroids is associated with significant iatrogenic long-term morbidity, including diabetes mellitus, osteoporotic frac-

ture, muscle atrophy, hypertension, glaucoma, and acceleration of cataracts and skin atrophy.

The cause of PMR is unknown. Studies for infectious agents responsible for triggering the syndrome have been inconclusive. Type II HLA gene associations have been found, but associations differ from those for RA.

The standard treatment of PMR is oral prednisone beginning at 15 mg daily. Dramatic improvement is so much to be expected that some have proposed that low-dose corticosteroid responsiveness confirms the diagnosis of PMR. ESR normalization corresponds to initial symptomatic improvement. Prednisone dose can be tapered over succeeding months on the basis of control of symptoms. PMR often runs a course of 2 to 3 years, and many patients are able to discontinue prednisone by then. Unfortunately, mean time to the first adverse event on corticosteroid therapy for PMR is about 1.6 years. Occasional patients with PMR respond to NSAIDs. Though long-term prednisone has significant toxicity, prednisone may be safer in older adults than NSAIDs, provided the prednisone dose can be minimized and parallel efforts are made to protect bone mass. In a randomized trial of methylprednisolone acetate, a dosage of 120 mg IM every 3 to 4 weeks has been found to control PMR with fewer fractures, less weight gain, and lower cumulative dose than a daily oral prednisone regimen.

Giant Cell Arteritis

Giant cell arteritis (GCA) is the most common form of vasculitis to affect older adults. This form of vasculitis predominantly affects proximal branches of the aorta. Therefore, inflammatory and ischemic manifestations are mostly seen in the head and upper extremities. Occasionally, gross inflammation with tender, nodular swelling and erythema of the temporal arteries can be seen. In the absence of gross findings, symptoms of temporal headache, jaw and tongue claudication, and sudden vision loss may be seen. Diagnosis can be confirmed by biopsy of a temporal artery, thus the often-used synonym *temporal arteritis*. ACR criteria for the diagnosis of GCA are available on the ACR Web site (http://www.rheumatology.org/publications/classification). The recognition of GCA is often preceded by several months of a nonspecific systemic illness that includes weight loss, fever, and muscle aching that is indistinguishable from PMR. GCA can also present with sudden blindness with no prior systemic illness or with upper-extremity limb claudication. Other manifestations can include stroke, ischemic necrosis of tongue or scalp, or, rarely, myocardial infarction. Aortic aneurysm, predominantly thoracic, is a late manifestation of GCA even when previously appropriately treated. The incidence of aneurysm in

---

[OL] Not approved by the U.S. Food and Drug Administration for this use.

GCA is about 10%, with thoracic and abdominal aneurysm discovery 5.9 and 2.5 years, respectively, after GCA diagnosis.

The cause of GCA is unknown. Infectious agents have long been suspected, but none has yet been confirmed as causative. Recent studies of biopsy material revealed the presence of parvovirus B19 DNA. In another study, serum IgM antibodies (implying recent infection or reinfection) against type I parainfluenza virus correlated very well with biopsy-positive GCA.

The diagnosis of GCA may require a high index of suspicion combined with the finding of an otherwise unexplained elevated ESR above 40 mm/hour. Combined elevation of ESR and C-reactive protein is more specific (97%) than elevated ESR alone for biopsy-positive GCA. Because of the risk of sudden blindness, most clinicians would start high-dose oral prednisone as soon as the possibility of GCA is seriously considered, and then proceed to biopsy. Administration of prednisone does not change arterial histology for weeks. Diagnosis can sometimes even be established or reestablished after a few years of prednisone treatment. Arterial involvement is patchy, and diagnostic histologic changes can be missed by biopsy. This oversight can be minimized by biopsy of the symptomatic side and by obtaining a several centimeters length of artery. Multiple longitudinal sections as well as cross-sections of artery should be examined by a pathologist. Still, on occasion biopsies are negative in cases where suspicion remains high. Biopsy of the opposite side is recommended by some; however, in a study of bilateral temporal artery biopsy in 150 patients suspected of GCA, results from the two sides were found to agree in 97% of the cases.

Since 25% of cases of GCA are associated with PMR, there is a longstanding controversy as to which patients with PMR should undergo temporal artery biopsy. There are no clear data to guide decision making in this situation. One reasonable criterion would be to obtain temporal artery biopsies in cases of PMR in which there are symptoms or physical findings suggestive of arteritis (ie, temporal headache; visual changes; tongue, jaw, or limb claudication; neck or chest pain; or neurologic changes suggestive of central nervous system ischemia). The temporal artery can also be involved with other forms of systemic vasculitis. Vasculitides other than GCA should be considered whenever the temporal artery biopsy shows necrotizing vasculitis but an absence of giant cells.

The treatment of GCA requires high-dose prednisone initially. No other treatment has been so clearly proven to be effective. Clinicians differ on the definition of high dose, with some recommending starting dosages as high as 120 mg daily. There are no data that show dosages above 40 mg daily to be more effective. Older adults are highly susceptible to

corticosteroid toxicity, and toxicity increases markedly with total dose. The use of higher doses should be individualized and considered when there is resistance to initial treatment or disease is unusually severe. Response is confirmed when ESR falls rapidly over the first month of therapy. Tapering of the steroid should begin at the rate of 10% to 20% of the total dose per month as soon as the ESR is normalized. Published studies of methotrexate as a steroid-sparing agent have not consistently proven methotrexate to be effective.

Rheumatoid Arthritis

Late-onset RA appears to be clinically different from the same disease with onset earlier in life. The condition in the older adult is more likely to be of rapid onset, involve fewer and more proximal joints, and to be rheumatoid-factor negative. Nodules are less likely and joint destruction may be less severe. Overall prognosis may be better than with earlier onset, seropositive, nodular, erosive disease. Nevertheless, RA is a chronic disease that persists indefinitely, with high risk for progressive joint damage and functional impairment, and more recent reviews confirm that late-onset RA is still a serious disease. Criteria to aid in the diagnosis of RA are listed in Table 54.2.

Treatment is almost always indicated, and therapeutic options have increased since 1998 with the introduction of a variety of entirely new drugs for the management of RA. In more severe cases, consultation with a rheumatologist is indicated.

NSAIDs are often recommended as first-line medications for symptom control in RA. The older nonselective NSAIDs, such as ibuprofen, naproxen, diclofenac, and several others, nonspecifically inhibit both cyclooxygenase isoenzymes. Celecoxib was approved in late 1998 as the first of a new class of NSAIDs, the selective cyclooxygenase-2 enzyme (COX-2) inhibitors. Rofecoxib was approved in mid-1999 for OA and pain and more recently for RA. Valdecoxib was the third COX-2 inhibitor to become

Table 54.2—Criteria for Diagnosing Rheumatoid Arthritis

The presence of at least four of the following signs and symptoms:

- Morning stiffness for at least 6 weeks
- Arthritis of three or more joint areas for at least 6 weeks
- Arthritis of the hand joints for at least 6 weeks
- Symmetric arthritis for at least 6 weeks
- Subcutaneous rheumatoid nodules
- Elevated serum rheumatoid factor
- Radiographic changes that include erosions or unequivocal bony calcification in periarticular bone

SOURCE: Data from Arnett FC, Edworthy SM, Bloch DA, et al. The American Rheumatism Association 1987 revised criteria for the classification of rheumatoid arthritis. *Arthritis Rheum.* 1988;31:315–324.

available for RA and was approved for marketing in late 2001.

The hope for the selective COX-2 inhibitors was that they would be substantially free of antiplatelet effects, gastric toxicity, and renal toxicity. Clinical studies have confirmed that the incidence of serious gastric toxicity was about half that of nonselective COX NSAIDs. However, if COX-2 inhibitors are used concomitantly with mini-dose aspirin, the risk of gastric toxicity becomes similar to that of older NSAIDs. Renal toxicity, unfortunately, has proved to be as serious with the COX-2 inhibitors as with older NSAIDs.

In 2004 reports emerged that there was an increased risk of myocardial infarction during the first 6 weeks after starting rofecoxib. Subsequent studies of rofecoxib for prevention of adenomatous polyps confirmed an increased risk of stroke and myocardial infarction with long-term use of rofecoxib versus placebo. These reports led to the withdrawal of rofecoxib from the market in late 2004. Valdecoxib was voluntarily withdrawn from the market by the manufacturer in early 2005. Celecoxib is still marketed. The mechanism of increased cardiovascular adverse effects from COX-2 inhibitors is uncertain. The lack of inhibition of platelet function could be a partial explanation, as older NSAIDs at least reversibly inhibit platelet aggregation.

Certainly, NSAIDs can no longer be considered first-line therapy for arthritis or other chronic, painful conditions. Alternatives to old NSAIDs and selective COX-2 inhibitors might include the relatively selective COX-2 inhibitors: nabumetone, etodolac, and meloxicam. Nabumetone and etodolac were introduced prior to celecoxib, and meloxicam was introduced in 2004. These three agents have generally lower serious gastric adverse effects than older NSAIDs and have less renal toxicity than either older NSAIDs or the selective COX-2 inhibitors. At this time, they are not known to cause an increased risk of stroke and myocardial infarction with long-term use. Therapy with a low-dose corticosteroid such as prednisone may be a preferable option, provided doses can be limited to 5 mg daily and precautions are taken to preserve bone density. The nonacetylated salicylate, salsalate, has minimal gastric mucosal toxicity yet has preserved anti-inflammatory activity.

RA is recognized as a lifelong systemic disease associated with progressive joint and extra-articular organ involvement that leads to functional decline and shortened longevity. Mere symptomatic treatment is no longer considered appropriate. Disease-modifying drugs should be considered for treating all cases of RA. Longitudinal studies have confirmed the preservation of function when disease-modifying drugs are instituted early and maintained over the long term.

Parenteral gold, penicillamine, azathioprine, and cyclophosphamide use has markedly declined in the past decade because of the availability of safer effective drugs. Methotrexate has been approved for use in RA for more than a decade and has become established as the disease-modifying agent of choice. When given daily, methotrexate can cause hepatic injury, with cirrhosis and end-stage liver failure. Low-dose, weekly, oral pulse therapy dramatically reduces the risk of hepatic toxicity, provided ethanol intake is completely avoided. Methotrexate can be used in combination with other immunosuppressive agents to yield proven additive or synergistic benefit. Since 1991, more than 100 cases of lymphoproliferative disease have been reported in patients with RA who are under treatment with methotrexate. Usually, the lesion is extranodal non-Hodgkin's lymphoma, and remission is often seen when methotrexate is stopped. At least one population-defined study did not find excess cancer in RA patients treated with methotrexate in comparison with RA patients who never received methotrexate.

Randomized controlled studies have now confirmed that minocycline 100 mg twice daily is effective in treating RA with minimal toxicity. Minocycline[OL] would be a good choice for mild disease or when there is a need to start therapy even when the initial phase of diagnostic uncertainty has not passed. Similarly, hydroxychloroquine is well tolerated and does not require blood-test monitoring for toxicity. When dosages are limited to 5 mg/kg/day, the risk of retinal toxicity is very low. Weekly oral methotrexate is well tolerated by the older adult and can be added if hydroxychloroquine alone is ineffective. Sulfasalazine (only the enteric coated tablets are approved for RA) is more effective than hydroxychloroquine but requires divided daily dosing, has a high incidence of gastrointestinal intolerance, and cannot be given in the presence of sulfa allergy.

Cyclosporine is approved for use in severe RA alone or in combination with methotrexate. Toxicity remains a concern, and the role of cyclosporine in treating RA is still evolving.

Leflunomide, approved in 1998, is the first disease-modifying antirheumatic drug introduced for over a decade and is the first such drug approved both for symptomatic improvement of RA and to prevent radiographic progression in joint damage. It has relatively fast onset of action (about 4 weeks) in comparison with older disease-modifying drugs.

Etanercept was approved in late 1998 for use in treating RA that had failed at least one other disease-modifying agent. Etanercept is a tumor necrosis factor receptor blocker produced by recombinant DNA techniques. It is given in twice-weekly subcutaneous

OL. Not approved by the U.S. Food and Drug Administration for this use.

injections and is expensive. Clinical benefit is seen within 1 to 12 weeks, and it must be given indefinitely to maintain benefit. The major risk of etanercept is the development of serious granulomatous infections (see discussion below under infliximab). Headache is a common, less severe adverse effect.

Infliximab was approved in late 1999 in combination with methotrexate for treatment of RA. Infliximab is a monoclonal antibody that prevents interaction of tumor necrosis factor alpha with its receptor. Infliximab must be given by intravenous infusion. Clinical trials show marked initial response to a single infusion, but continued response to bimonthly infusions requires concomitant administration of oral methotrexate.

Both etanercept (0.07%) and infliximab (0.24%) are associated with an increased incidence of granulomatous infections with organisms such as tuberculosis, atypical mycobacterium, yeast, listeria, and nocardia. Other adverse effects associated with infliximab include systemic postinfusion reactions of fever, chills, headache, chest pain, and dyspnea. Antibody formation is common but reduced by the concurrent use of methotrexate.

Adalimumab was approved in 2002. It is similar to infliximab except that this therapeutic antibody is entirely human. Adalimumab is given by subcutaneous injection every other week and does not require concomitant methotrexate therapy. Serious infections similar to those seen with infliximab have been reported, but data about relative incidence are not available.

Anakinra was introduced in 2001 as a recombinant form of the human interleukin-1 receptor antagonist IL-1Ra. Anakinra is administered as daily subcutaneous injections. Infections during anakinra therapy are mostly bacterial respiratory tract infections with no opportunistic infections.

Systemic Lupus Erythematosus

Though thought of as a disease in younger women with a higher prevalence among black women, SLE can present in later life. SLE is a multisystem disorder that can have a wide variety of presentations and predominant organ system involvement at any age. SLE is diagnosed with high specificity when any four or more of eleven criteria are documented singly or together at any time during the patient's life (for a detailed description of the ACR criteria, see http://rheumatology.org/publications/classification).

Criteria include malar rash, photosensitivity, stomatitis, nonerosive arthritis, serositis (pleurisy or pericarditis), seizure, nephropathy (urinary casts or heavy proteinuria), cytopenias (leukopenia, hemolytic anemia, or thrombocytopenia), positive antinuclear antibody, and any one of other immunologic abnormalities (anti-double stranded DNA, anti-SM, or false positive test for syphilis). Fever, Raynaud's phenomenon, alopecia, migraine, antiphospholipid syndrome, and Sjögren's syndrome are also often seen in SLE.

It is not surprising that patterns of organ involvement in SLE are different in older adults. Numerous studies suggest that late-onset SLE affects women and men more equally (3:1 in older adults versus 10:1 in young adults); relatively more white than black older adults are affected. Late-onset SLE is less likely to present with rash, arthritis, Raynaud's phenomenon, nephropathy, and the involvement of the central nervous system and more likely to present with serositis, Sjögren's syndrome, and positive rheumatoid factor. In older adults, SLE onset may be more insidious, involve fewer organ systems, and have fewer relapses. As nephropathy and central nervous system involvement are related to mortality in younger women, late-onset lupus has been sometimes thought of as a milder disease. Despite the impression of milder disease in older adults, immunosuppressive and cytotoxic medications are required as often in managing late-onset SLE.

Hormonal factors may be partly responsible for the differences between early- and late-onset SLE. Estrogens are suspected of being an aggravating factor in young women. Studies of the administration of postmenopausal estrogen for 2 years or more in women is associated with a fivefold increase in SLE risk. The increased risk is somewhat lower if estrogen is combined with a progestational agent. In a population-based study, SLE in women was found to be associated with a doubled overall incidence of cancer.

The treatment of SLE in older adults is similar to the treatment given in early-onset disease. Corticosteroids are less well tolerated by the older adult and should be reserved as much as possible for organ- or life-threatening SLE flares. Hydroxychloroquine has been shown to be of benefit in SLE skin involvement and to reduce the overall number of disease relapses in younger adults. Hydroxychloroquine is well tolerated and has few serious adverse effects in dosages of 5 mg/kg/day or less. Dapsone, azathioprine, and weekly oral methotrexate are used by some clinicians as alternatives to corticosteroids or as corticosteroid-sparing agents. Monthly intravenous pulse cyclophosphamide is reserved for severe or life-threatening disease.

Sjögren's Syndrome and Sjögren's Disease

Sjögren's syndrome with xerostomia and keratoconjunctivitis sicca has been long recognized as occasionally complicating RA. The incidence of Sjögren's syndrome in other connective-tissue diseases is also increased. Dry eye and dry mouth symptoms without confirmation of Sjögren's syndrome occur in up to 40% of older adults who do not have a connective-tissue disease, and these symptoms are undoubtedly contributed to by many of the medications often prescribed to older adults. The treatment of sicca symptoms and uncomplicated Sjögren's syndrome is targeted to the symptoms and includes artificial tears and artificial saliva and ophthalmologic and dental preventive care. Pilocarpine 5 mg three times a day can help stimulate saliva flow.

Sjögren's disease (SD) is a systemic, multiorgan chronic disease that features lymphocytic infiltration of exocrine glands throughout the body, including lacrimal, salivary, respiratory tree, intestinal tract, pancreatic, hepatic, renal, and vaginal glands. In addition, cutaneous vasculitis and central nervous system involvement are often seen. The involvement of salivary and lacrimal glands is responsible for the sicca symptoms seen in Sjögren's syndrome that is associated with other connective-tissue diseases. The peak onset of SD is in mid-life to early late life.

There is no single diagnostic test for SD. Unexplained interstitial lung disease, renal impairment, hepatic dysfunction, esophageal dysfunction, malabsorption, or central nervous system disease resembling multiple sclerosis should raise the suspicion of SD. Antinuclear, anti-SSA, and anti-SSB antibodies are usually present. Rheumatoid factor and a variety of autoantibodies against gastric parietal cells, mitochondria, smooth muscle, and thyroid are often seen. An ophthalmologic examination can confirm the presence of keratoconjunctivitis, and biopsy of a lip or lacrimal gland can confirm the presence of characteristic lymphocytic infiltration. Biopsy of a rash can verify the presence of cutaneous vasculitis.

Symptomatic and preventive treatment is indicated for sicca symptoms, as described above. Trial therapy with hydroxychloroquine may help stabilize disease activity, as in SLE. Dapsone may be effective for cutaneous vasculitis. Corticosteroids and other cytotoxic drugs should be reserved for organ- or life-threatening disease.

Polymyositis and Dermatomyositis

Polymyositis (PM) is a heterogeneous group of inflammatory diseases of striated muscle that are not unique to older adults; however, late-onset PM is evaluated and treated somewhat differently in older adults. The onset of PM is often insidious. The cardinal symptom is muscle weakness, most marked in proximal muscle groups. Muscle tenderness is usually not prominent. Exercise tolerance is reduced, and an inability to perform simple tasks such as reaching above the head or ascending stairs may be present. Other system

involvement is common in PM and reminiscent of other connective-tissue diseases, including rash, arthritis, esophageal dysmotility, and Raynaud's phenomenon. Cardiac involvement is not rare and usually presents with dysrhythmias. Rash may involve the eyelids (heliotrope) or the nose and malar areas, or be more generalized. Rash with dorsal thickening over the interphalangeal joints (Gottron's papules) are distinctly different from the dorsal phalangeal rash of systemic lupus that spares the interphalangeal joints. When rash is present, PM is referred to as dermatomyositis (DM).

In contrast to childhood PM, adult-onset PM affects women more often than men, and blacks more often than whites. Also, esophageal involvement and respiratory failure complicated with bacterial pneumonia are more likely in older PM patients. Up to 50% of cases of late-onset PM, and especially DM, are associated with underlying malignancy. No one cancer type seems most strongly associated: Colon, lung, breast, prostate, uterus, and ovary are all well represented with PM and DM. Ovarian cancer is the most commonly associated gynecologic cancer underlying PM and DM. Mortality in adult PM and DM is usually associated with esophageal disease, respiratory failure with bacterial pneumonia, and malignancy.

Serum levels of muscle enzymes are usually markedly elevated in PM. Electromyography will reveal changes consistent with myositis, provided affected muscle is tested. Paraspinal muscle involvement is typical and should be included in the muscles tested. The diagnosis is confirmed with muscle biopsy that reveals inflammatory cellular infiltrates. The diagnosis of PM or DM in older adults entails a search for underlying malignancy. Minimum evaluation would include chest radiography and colon examination. In women, a pelvic examination and imaging plus mammography is included; in men, a prostate examination and prostate-specific antigen testing.

An important histologic and clinical subtype of PM is inclusion-body myositis. Rimmed vacuoles and an accumulation of amyloid in muscle fibers are seen on muscle biopsy. Inclusion-body myositis predominantly affects men and is more likely to involve distal muscle groups including the volar forearm flexor and ankle dorsi flexor muscles. The onset and progression is slower than in PM. Inclusion-body myositis is also thought to be relatively resistant to anti-inflammatory therapy.

Remission of PM and DM after treatment of an underlying malignancy is seen. Therapy should also generally be directed at the inflammatory process itself. Corticosteroids are almost always the first drug of choice. Prednisone at 1 mg/kg/day is a typical starting dosage. Some clinicians advocate three daily intravenous doses of methylprednisolone 1000 mg initially for severe disease. In the absence of prospective data, this high-dose regimen should be individualized. Prednisone can be tapered after an initial phase of improvement of muscle strength and normalization of muscle enzyme levels. Rates of tapering of 10% to 20% of the total dose per month are typical. Methotrexate, given parenterally, in a weekly pulse regimen can be combined with corticosteroids. Somewhat higher methotrexate doses than those used in treating RA are given by some clinicians, up to 50 mg weekly. Methotrexate may also have a steroid-sparing effect in long-term therapy. Weekly oral methotrexate is effective in managing refractory skin manifestations of DM. Azathioprine may also have a steroid-sparing effect, but it is not as well accepted in the treatment of PM. Supervised exercise over 6-week and 6-month study periods has proven to be beneficial in PM, improving function without aggravating the underlying disease.

ANNOTATED REFERENCES

■ Agudelo CA, Wise CM. Crystal-associated arthritis in the elderly. *Rheum Dis Clin North Am.* 2000;26(3):527–546.

This is an accessible review of gout, calcium pyrophosphate deposition arthropathy, and basic calcium phosphate deposition (hydroxyapatite) arthropathy. Each of these disorders has a variety of clinical manifestations, and each requires a different approach for managing acute presentation and chronic symptoms.

■ American Geriatrics Society Panel on Exercise and Osteoarthritis. Exercise prescription for older adults with osteoarthritis pain: consensus practice recommendations. *J Am Geriatr Soc.* 2001;49(6):808–823.

This is a thorough review of osteoarthritis management that emphasizes nonpharmacologic approaches. It also represents American Geriatrics Society practice guidelines for osteoarthritis. The entire article can be accessed at the society Web site (http://www.americangeriatrics.org).

■ Evans JM, Hunder GG. Polymyalgia rheumatica and giant cell arteritis. *Rheum Dis Clin North Am.* 2000;26(3):493–515.

Much clinical lore and mystique surround polymyalgia rheumatica and giant cell arteritis and their interrelationship. This review provides a concise summary of what is scientifically known about these conditions and their management. Much of this body of knowledge derives from the extensive population-based experience of the Mayo Clinic.

■ Lawrence RC, Helmick CG, Arnett FC, et al. Estimates of the prevalence of arthritis and selected musculoskeletal disorders in the United States. *Arthritis Rheum.* 1998; 41(5):778–799.

As arthritis is the leading cause of disability in adults aged 65 years old or older, this report is important. Arthritis prevalence is 45% (9.9% with activity limitation) in adults aged 65 to 74, 55% (13.1% with limitation) aged 75 to 84, and 57.1% (18.5% with limitation) aged 85 and over. Prevalence data for the full spectrum of rheumatologic disorders are provided in this review.

■ Mishra N, Kammer GM. Clinical expression of autoimmune diseases in older adults. *Clin Geriatr Med.* 1998;14(3):515–542.

This review includes discussion of late-onset systemic lupus erythematosus, Sjögren?s syndrome or disease, and the inflammatory myopathies. It covers the epidemiology, pathology, evaluation, and treatment of each of the three disorders. Extensive references are included.

■ Rexrode KM, Buring JE, Glynn RJ, et al. Analgesic use and renal function in men. *JAMA.* 2001;286(3):315–321.

This report is a large prospective study of chronic analgesic use by more than 11,000 males; analgesics included both acetaminophen and nonsteroidal anti-inflammatory drugs. The authors conclude that their "findings provide assurance to clinicians and patients that moderate analgesic use is unlikely to contribute to increased risk of renal dysfunction among individuals without a history of renal impairment."

■ Sewell KL. Rheumatoid arthritis in older adults. *Clin Geriatr Med.* 1998;14(3):475–494.

Despite the impression that late-onset rheumatoid arthritis is a milder disease, it still must be considered a lifelong multisystem disease with serious morbidity and increased mortality. Disease-modifying drugs are required as often in late-onset rheumatoid arthritis as in early-onset disease, and older adults are more vulnerable to the toxicity of these agents. This article is a comprehensive review of late-onset rheumatoid arthritis; however, it predates release of the newest agents: leflunomide, etanercept, infliximab, anakinra, and adalimumab.

■ Solomon DH, Schneeweiss S, Glynn RJ, et al. Relationship between selective cyclooxygenase-2 inhibitors and acute myocardial infarction in older adults. *Circulation.* 2004;109(17):2068–2073.

For several years, a series of reports raised increasing concerns about thromboembolic adverse effects of cyclooxygenase-2 (COX-2) inhibitors. The authors analyzed large databases of Medicare beneficiaries who were enrolled in comprehensive medication benefits programs. The COX-2 inhibitor rofecoxib was found to be associated with an increased risk of acute myocardial infarction in comparison with celecoxib, another COX-2 inhibitor, or with nonselective nonsteroidal anti-inflammatory medications. This will be an important area of scrutiny because of the high rates of cardiovascular and musculoskeletal disease in elderly patients and resulting widespread use of nonsteroidal anti-inflammatory medications in this age group.

John W. Rachow, PhD, MD

CHAPTER 55—BACK AND NECK PAIN

KEY POINTS

- Back problems are the third most common reason for physician visits by older persons, and degenerative conditions of the spine are the most common cause of these problems.

- Pain that is insidious in onset, progressive in its course, and nonpositional, that is associated with night pain and systemic symptoms or signs, and that persists for more than 1 month should raise concerns about tumor or infection. Nonsystemic causes of pain are characterized by intermittent, often positional pain that is worse at onset and usually improves with time.

- The physical examination of the back, hips, and legs is essential in the assessment of an older patient with back pain. Plain radiographs remain the most useful starting point in a back pain work-up of an older patient.

- Management requires a therapeutic approach that addresses the structural problems most likely to be causing the pain.

- Neck pain is most often due to mechanical disease of the cervical spine and is best diagnosed on physical examination.

Back problems are the third most common reason for physician visits by older persons, and degenerative conditions of the spine are the most common cause of these problems. Less common conditions that can cause back pain, such as tumors, infections, and visceral lesions, occur more often in older than in younger patients and may require emergent treatment. Anatomic abnormalities are commonly found in diagnostic imaging tests of an older person's lumbar spine but may be unrelated to the patient's complaints.

The causes, natural history, and prognosis of back pain in older and younger persons are different. For example, although herniation of the nucleus pulposus of the lumbar disk is a common cause of back pain in younger adults, this herniation is unlikely to occur above the age of 60 because of changes in the water content of the nucleus pulposus. Although the natural history of mechanical lower back pain in younger people has been well outlined in the literature, it has not been well defined in older people. Mechanical instability of the lumbar spine, osteoporotic fractures, lumbar spinal stenosis, and systemic causes of pain are more common in the older age group.

A systematic approach to the diagnosis of lower back pain in older patients requires knowledge of the typical presentation of common back conditions of elderly persons, an understanding of the anatomy of the lumbar spine, the identification of physical findings associated with common abnormalities, and the judicious use of diagnostic imaging studies. (See Table 55.1.)

SYSTEMIC CAUSES OF BACK PAIN

Back pain due to systemic causes merits immediate attention and intervention. The pattern of pain with these conditions can be distinctive. Tumors or infections of the spine usually have an insidious onset of

Table 55.1—Conditions Causing Back Pain in Older Persons

Condition	History	Examination	Laboratory Tests, Imaging
Tumor	Persistent, progressive pain at rest; systemic symptoms	No focal abnormalities	Anemia, elevated ESR, abnormal bone scan or MRI
Infection	Persistent pain, fever; at-risk patient (eg, indwelling catheter)	Tender spine	Elevated ESR, WBC; positive bone scan or MRI
Unstable lumbar spine	Recurring episodes of pain on change of position	Pain going from flexed to extended position	One disc space narrowed and sclerotic spondylolisthesis
Lumbar spinal stenosis	Pain on standing and walking relieved by sitting and lying	Immobile spine; L4, L5, S1 weakness	MRI or CT scan showing stenosis
Sciatica	Pain in the posterior aspect of leg; may be incomplete	Often positive straight leg raise; L4, L5, S1 weakness	Variable diagnostic imaging findings
Vertebral compression fracture	Sudden onset of severe pain; resolves in 4–6 weeks	Pain on any movement of spine; no neurologic deficits	Vertebral end-plate collapse; compression fracture seen on plain film
Osteoporotic sacral fracture	Sudden lower back, buttock, or hip pain	Sacral tenderness	H-shaped uptake on bone scan

NOTE: CT = computed tomography; ESR = erythrocyte sedimentation rare; MRI = magnetic resonance imaging; WBC = white blood cell count.

pain that becomes more and more persistent with time. This pain is usually nonpositional and associated with systemic systems and signs; it often persists through the night. The likelihood of cancer as a cause of back pain increases in patients aged 50 and older, those with a previous history of cancer, and those with pain that persists for longer than 1 month.

Fever, discrete local vertebral tenderness, upper lumbar or thoracic pain, and nonpositional pain may indicate vertebral infection. Approximately 10% of patients with endocarditis have back pain. Infection may produce back pain in patients at risk for endovascular infections, such as those on hemodialysis, with chronic indwelling venous access catheters, with a history of recent or chronic urinary tract infections, or with a history of intravenous drug abuse.

A number of visceral problems, from abdominal aortic aneurysms to intra-abdominal infections or tumor, can present with back pain. Referred pain from these conditions should be suggested by the historical pattern of the pain, the absence of positional changes, and a normal physical examination of the lumbosacral spine.

NONSYSTEMIC CAUSES OF BACK PAIN

Lumbar Spinal Stenosis

Lumbar spinal stenosis results from a narrowing of either the central or lateral aspect of the lumbar spine canal. This narrowing may be due to facet joint osteophytes, encroachment of the annulus fibrosus of the lumbar disc, or hypertrophy of the ligamentum flavum. Diagnostic imaging tests often demonstrate spinal stenosis in patients without back pain or with other causes of pain; the clinician must recognize the characteristic historical and physical features of this condition.

Flexion of the lumbar spine causes an increase in spinal canal volume and decrease in nerve root bulk. Extension of the lumbar spine produces a decreased volume of the spinal canal with an increased nerve root bulk. As a result of these anatomical changes, positions that flex the spine, such as sitting, bending forward, walking uphill, and lying in a flexed position, all relieve symptoms. Extension of the lumbar canal, which occurs with prolonged standing, walking, and walking downhill, exacerbates symptoms.

Lumbar spinal stenosis produces pain either in the back or in the legs, made worse by standing or walking. Pain in the calf when walking can often mimic the claudication of arterial insufficiency and is referred to as *pseudoclaudication*. Continued walking after this point may produce combinations of paresthesia, numb-

ness, and weakness in one or both legs. Walking uphill is easier than walking downhill, and walking with an assistive device, such as a shopping cart, which allows some flexion of the lumbar spine, is usually better tolerated. These symptoms are usually progressive and consistent, not intermittent. There is often subtle weakness in the muscles innervated by the L4, L5, and S1 nerve roots. (See Table 55.2 and the assessment section, below.)

Sciatica

Sciatica describes a lancinating pain, usually felt from the buttock down the posterior aspect of the leg to the foot; it may occur only in isolated regions of the distribution of the sciatic nerve. In older persons there are two common patterns of sciatica. Sciatic pain that comes on only with standing and walking and that limits the person's ability to walk at a relatively constant distance is usually a result of lumbar spinal stenosis. Other older patients may develop the relatively sudden onset of sciatic pain, present at rest and exacerbated by sudden maneuvers, such as getting out of a bed or chair. This abrupt and persistent pain, not necessarily related to the erect position, usually resolves spontaneously in several weeks. The diagnosis of sciatica can be confirmed by the demonstration of muscle weakness of the L4, L5, and S1 innervated muscles of the foot, ankle, and hip. (See Table 55.2 and the assessment section, below.)

Unstable Lumbar Spine

Lumbar degenerative disc disease may produce an unstable lumbar spine. Patients with this condition often have episodes of severe pain in the back or in the distribution of the sciatic nerve. This pain usually comes on suddenly, often following abrupt movements. It usually lasts only minutes to hours, but recurs frequently. This pain also comes on with significant flexion or extension of the lumbar spine. On physical examination, the patient often has guarded movements of the lumbar spine and pain when moving from the flexed to the extended position. Diffuse disk space narrowing and vertebral osteophytosis are common in older persons and not related to back pain. When there are significant disk and bone changes at one disk and facet joint level that are out of proportion to the other disk spaces, instability of the lumbar spine may be the cause of the patient's back pain.

Osteoporotic Vertebral Compression Fracture

Vertebral compression fractures are a common cause of back pain in older persons. Many of these fractures, however, are found incidentally and are asymptomatic.

Table 55.2—Innervation of Lower Extremities

Function	Muscle	Peripheral Nerve	Nerve Root
Great toe dorsiflexion	Extensor hallucis longus	Deep peroneal	L5
Ankle dorsiflexion	Tibialis anterior	Deep peroneal	L4, L5
Ankle eversion	Peroneus longus, brevis	Superficial peroneal	L5, S1
Ankle plantar flexion	Gastrocnemius, soleus	Tibial	S1, S2
Knee extension	Quadriceps	Femoral	L3, L4
Hip flexion	Iliopsoas	Femoral	L2, L3
Hip adduction	Adductor magnus, brevis, longus	Obturator	L3, L4
Hip abduction	Gluteus medius	Superior gluteal	L4, L5
Hip extension	Gluteus maximus	Inferior gluteal	L5, S1

The pain from an acute vertebral fracture usually lasts from 2 weeks to 2 months. The onset of pain is abrupt and pain is intense; it is felt deep at the site of the fracture. There is often marked tenderness over the involved vertebra. The pain is usually worse on standing and walking, and relieved with lying down. Although the pain commonly radiates to the flank, abdomen, and legs, neurologic sequelae should not occur in patients with spontaneous osteopenic fractures. Symptomatic fractures most often affect the lower thoracic and lumbar vertebrae.

The acute pain resolves slowly. One study found that analgesic use decreased by 16% by day 5 and 33% by day 14. Patients often have trouble walking for 2 weeks and have approximately 1 month of restricted activity.

The impact of these fractures, and osteoporosis in general, on chronic back pain and the function of older persons is unclear. Some studies have found that multiple fractures are associated with more disability, frailty, and back pain; others have not demonstrated a correlation between osteoporosis and chronic back pain.

Osteoporotic Sacral Fractures

Lower back pain in elderly women may be due to osteoporotic sacral fractures. This pain often occurs spontaneously, usually involving the lower back. Pain can also be felt in the buttock or hip area. Sacral tenderness on physical examination is found in a majority of patients. There is a high incidence of associated additional osteoporotic fractures.

Plain radiographs are usually negative. Technetium bone scans show a characteristic H-shaped uptake over the sacrum. A computed tomography (CT) scan shows displacement of the anterior border of the sacrum. These fractures have an excellent prognosis for recovery, with no neurologic deficits. The pain usually resolves in 4 to 6 weeks.

ASSESSMENT OF BACK PAIN

See Table 55.3.

History

Pain that is insidious in onset, progressive in its course, and nonpositional, that is associated with night pain and systemic symptoms or signs, and that persists for more than 1 month should raise concerns about tumor or infection. Nonsystemic causes of pain are characterized by intermittent, often positional pain that is worse at onset and that usually improves with time.

Diseases of the hip often produce pain in the back and leg in a distribution that resembles that of back disease. Back disease is more apt to cause pain when a patient goes from the supine to the sitting position or when bending or stooping. Hip disease can cause pain after prolonged sitting and when moving from a sitting to a standing position.

Physical Examination

The physical examination of the back, hips, and legs is essential in the assessment of an older patient with back pain. (See Table 55.4.) The finding of subtle but asymmetric weakness of the hip, ankle, and feet muscles innervated by the lumbar and sacral nerves can help elucidate the cause of back and lower extremity pain.

A thorough back examination begins with the patient in the upright position. The back should be moved through all four planes of movement of the lumbar spine, side flexion to the right, side flexion to the left, forward flexion, and extension. Asymmetric limitation of the range of motion of the lumbar spine, or reproduction of the patient's pain with these maneuvers, often indicates mechanical disease of the lumbar spine. The pain of lumbar spinal stenosis is often produced by spinal extension.

The remainder of the examination is performed with the patient in the supine position. A straight leg raise test can be informative if positive, but a negative test does not exclude any condition. Each patient with a back complaint should have a complete examination of the hips, as hip disease often mimics back disease. The passive range of motion of the hip should be

Table 55.3—Assessment of Lower Back Pain in Older Persons

Symptoms	Conditions
Acute pain	Vertebral compression fracture
	Disk displacement
	Osteoporotic sacral fracture
	Visceral pain (eg, aortic aneurysm)
Positional pain	Increased with standing and walking and relieved with sitting—lumbar spinal stenosis
	Brought on by bending, lifting, or unguarded movements—unstable lumbar spine
Persistent pain (gradually increasing, nonpositional)	Tumor
	Infection

Table 55.4—Physical Examination of Older Persons With Lower Back Pain

Sign	Condition
Paravertebral muscle spasm	Mechanical disease
Asymmetric range of motion of the lumbar spine	Mechanical disk disease
	Unstable lumbar spine
Spinal tenderness	Vertebral compression fracture
	Infection
Weakness of the L4–L5 and L5–S1 muscles	Mechanical disk disease
	Lumbar spinal stenosis
Normal examination of lumbar spine	Osteoporotic sacral fracture
	Hip disease
	Tumor
	Referred visceral pain

assessed. The examiner should be able to abduct the hip to 40 degrees before the pelvis starts to tilt. The hip should flex beyond 110 degrees, externally rotate 50 to 60 degrees, and internally rotate 15 to 20 degrees.

The manual examination of the muscles of the lower extremities can be helpful. This examination should distinguish between weakness due to a nerve root problem and weakness due to a peripheral neuropathy. (See Table 55.2). Great toe extension, ankle dorsiflexion, and ankle eversion weakness with no involvement of the hip abductors and hip extensors suggests a peripheral neuropathy rather than lumbar spine disease. A patient with lumbar spine disease is more likely to have weakness of lumbar and sacral innervated hip, as well as of ankle and foot, muscles.

A patient should be closely observed both rising from a chair and walking. Unless the patient has significant sciatica, back disease should not cause a limp. A significant limp suggests hip disease as a cause of the patient's pain.

Laboratory Tests and Imaging

Plain radiographs remain the most useful starting point in a back pain work-up of an older patient. Although these films are not recommended in the initial evalua-

tion of back pain in younger patients, they are appropriate for patients aged 70 and over. This single test can demonstrate degenerative disk and joint disease, vertebral compression fractures, deformities such as spondylolisthesis and scoliosis, systemic disorders such as osteoporosis and Paget's disease, and, in some cases, infectious processes and neoplasms. A complete blood cell count with erythrocyte sedimentation rate is perhaps the most useful screening laboratory test for an underlying systemic disease.

A technetium bone scan is useful in evaluating a suspected infection or neoplasm. CT and magnetic resonance imaging (MRI) have largely replaced myelography in assessing the neural canal. CT imaging is, in many cases, slightly superior in demonstrating the bony architecture of the spine, whereas the MRI is more sensitive to morphology of soft tissue, including disk, ligamentum flavum, neoplasm, and infection. Either CT or MRI studies are necessary to document spinal stenosis should surgical treatment be contemplated.

The utility of diagnostic imaging studies is tempered by the high false-positive rates of these studies in older persons. A diagnostic imaging study simply identifies an anatomic abnormality; it does not demonstrate that this abnormality is the cause of the patient's pain. One study found that 57% of persons aged 60 and older, with no history of lower back pain or sciatica, had abnormal lumbar spine MRIs. Of these persons, 36% had a herniated nucleus pulposus and 21% had lumbar spinal stenosis. Another study found that only 36% of asymptomatic persons had normal disks at all levels; the prevalence of disk abnormalities did increase in older persons. Other studies have shown similarly high rates of abnormal findings in asymptomatic persons. These studies reinforce the need to correlate carefully the patient's history and physical examination with the findings on diagnostic imaging studies.

MANAGEMENT OF BACK PAIN

Management of back pain is hampered by the common difficulty of making a definitive diagnosis. Patients can do well, however, with a therapeutic approach that addresses the structural problems most likely to be causing their pain.

Treatment of an unstable lumbar spine is symptomatic. Nonopioid analgesics are often helpful in the early stages. As soon as the acute symptoms subside, a gentle, progressive exercise program should be initiated that is designed to strengthen and improve the efficiency of the spinal and abdominal musculature. An aquatic program offers the dual benefits of rapid rehabilitation with a low incidence of reinjury. Walking in chest-high water against resistance and performing the flutter kick are two simple aquatic exercises.

Chronic mechanical pain is based on excessive vertebral motion that is more pronounced and repetitive. The pain is usually associated with advanced degenerative disc and facet joint disease. Management is aimed at eliminating or reducing motion. This can be done internally by strengthening the paraspinous and abdominal muscles, thus providing an internal "brace" for the lumbar spine. It must be stressed that this exercise should be a lifetime commitment. Lumbar sacral corsets and braces provide an external method of immobilizing the lumbar spine. The third option, a structural alteration to limit motion, is accomplished by surgical fusion.

Analgesia is the most important goal of treatment of vertebral compression fractures, while trying to avoid the complications of the bed rest required by the patient's pain. Braces and corsets are rarely required, as the natural history of the acute pain is relatively brief. Corsets may offer symptomatic relief if the pain is persistent. Spinal extension exercises also may be helpful. Calcitonin[OL] can act as an analgesic and may shorten the period of acute pain.

Vertebroplasty is the percutaneous injection of bone cement into a collapsed vertebra. Although there

[OL] Not approved by the U.S. Food and Drug Administration for this use.

are encouraging reports of this procedure in patients with substantial vertebral compression lesions, the long-term efficacy of these procedures has not been established in randomized controlled trials. In view of the good short-term natural history of pain following fractures, most clinicians suggest vertebroplasty only for patients with persistent pain despite conservative management with rest, analgesics, and calcitonin.

Because of the mechanical encroachment on lumbar nerve roots which causes lumbar spinal stenosis, conservative therapy is limited. Uncontrolled European studies advocate marked immobilization of the lumbar spine. Epidural corticosteroid injections have been used extensively for the sciatica associated with lumbar spinal stenosis, but a review of controlled trials of this therapy failed to demonstrate efficacy of injection over controls.

Lumbar spinal stenosis is the most common indication for spinal surgery in older adults. Long-term benefit from laminectomy, or laminectomy combined with fusion, is about 50% to 70%, regardless of whether the stenosis is central or lateral. In a prospective study of surgery for spinal stenosis, the ideal candidates for surgery were found to be those patients with severe narrowing of the spinal canal, minimal associated back pain, no coexisting conditions that affect walking, and symptom duration of less than 4 years.

NECK PAIN

Causes

Although neck pain can be due to inflammatory and systemic conditions, it is most often due to mechanical disease of the cervical spine. Inflammatory conditions, such as polymyalgia rheumatica and rheumatoid arthritis, are characterized by morning stiffness, systemic complaints such as fatigue, fever, and weight loss, and muscle and joint complaints elsewhere in the body. Most importantly, these patients do not have the characteristic physical findings of patients with mechanical disease of the cervical spine.

Mechanical disease of the cervical spine can cause neck and occiput pain, scapula and trapezius pain, radicular pain down the arm, as well as spastic paraparesis due to cervical spinal stenosis.

A number of injection studies have demonstrated the referral pain pattern of cervical spine disease. C2–C3 disease is felt in the occiput; C3–C4 and C4–C5 problems are referred into the posterior and lateral aspects of the neck. C5–C6 lesions are referred into the trapezius and upper cervical region; C6–C7 disease is felt in the retroscapular region, often felt as far down as the mid- to lower thoracic region. This referral process produces not only pain in these regions but also local muscle spasm and tenderness, often mistaken for "trigger points."

Irritation of a cervical nerve root produces lancinating pain and numbness in the neck and upper scapular region, radiating into the arm in a dermatomal distribution. Characteristic muscle weakness of the upper extremity muscles (see below) confirms the specific nerve root involved.

Narrowing of the cervical canal (cervical spondylosis or cervical spinal stenosis) can produce a syndrome of lower extremity clumsiness and weakness, spasticity of the legs, bladder spasticity, and upper motor neuron signs of the lower extremities (clonus, hyperreflexia, and Babinski's signs). Although progressive signs and symptoms call for an aggressive diagnostic and therapeutic approach, the natural history of this problem can be quite stable, and surgical intervention is not always necessary.

Assessment

Mechanical disease of the cervical spine is best diagnosed on physical examination. There are four planes of movement of the cervical spine: rotation to the right, rotation to the left, flexion, and extension. Mechanical disease of the cervical spine is demonstrated if there is asymmetric limitation of the range of motion of the cervical spine in some but not all of these movements, and if there is weakness of the upper extremity muscles innervated by the cervical nerve root. The shoulder abductor and elbow flexor muscles are innervated by C5 and C6 nerve roots, the wrist extensor and thumb opponens muscles by C6 and C7, and the elbow extensor and finger abductors muscles by C7 and C8. Weakness of the C7- and C8-innervated muscles is most common with cervical disk disease, because the C7–T1 interspace is the most common site of cervical spine lesions. Patients with mechanical disease of the cervical spine often awake in the morning with this discomfort, have difficulty with full rotation of the cervical spine, and have difficulty with such activities as backing an automobile out of a driveway.

Diagnostic Imaging

The role of diagnostic imaging tests in the diagnosis and management of neck pain is unclear. Among persons older than 55 years, 80% have signs of degenerative cervical disk disease on cervical spine radiography. These films, therefore, are often unhelpful in the assessment of neck pain. Although MRIs of the cervical spine more completely define anatomical abnormalities in this region, these abnormalities are quite common in older persons. Anatomical abnormalities call for interventions only if they are consistent with the historical and physical features of the patient's condition.

Management

There is much controversy about the therapy of mechanical disease of the cervical spine. Studies of manipulation, cervical traction, cervical collars, local physical modalities, acupuncture, and injection therapies have not shown consistent efficacy for any of these modalities. Two studies from the Netherlands and Finland have shown promising results for manual therapy and active neck muscle training in the treatment of neck pain. These studies were both done, however, on younger patients. Because many patients notice that their neck pain is worse in the morning, a trial of several weeks of a soft cervical collar to be worn at nighttime is worthwhile before proceeding with more aggressive interventions.

ANNOTATED REFERENCES

- Atlas SJ, Deyo RA. Evaluating and managing acute low back pain in the primary care setting. *J Gen Intern Med.* 2001;16(2):120–131.

  Although the authors talk primarily about younger patients, this is a good overview of the assessment and management of back pain.

- Cherkin DC, Sherman KJ, Deyo RA, et al. A review of the evidence for the effectiveness, safety, and cost of acupuncture, massage therapy, and spinal manipulation for back pain. *Ann Intern Med.* 2003;138(11):898–906.

  This article challenges the evidence for any benefit of spinal manipulation or acupuncture in the management of lower back pain.

- Hoving JL, Koes BW, deVet HC, et al. Manual therapy, physical therapy, or continued care by a general practitioner for patients with neck pain. *Ann Intern Med.* 2002;136(10):713–759.

  This study demonstrated that manual therapy is a favorable therapy option for patients with neck pain. Most of these patients, however, were under the age of 70 years.

- Jarvik JG, Hollingworth W, Martin B, et al. Rapid magnetic resonance imaging vs. radiographs for patients with low back pain. *JAMA.* 2003;289(21):2810–2818.

  Rapid MRIs were found to offer little benefit over plain spinal radiographs in the outcome of primary care patients with lower back pain.

- Koes BW, Scholten RJ, Mens JM, et al. Efficacy of epidural steroid injections for low-back pain and sciatica: a systematic review of randomized clinical trials. *Pain.* 1995;63(3):279–288.

This review points out that the efficacy of epidural corticosteroid injections has not yet been established.

■ Rao R. Neck pain, cervical radiculopathy, and cervical myelopathy: pathophysiology, natural history, and clinical evaluation. *J Bone Joint Surg Am.* 2002;84-A(10):1872–1881.

This is an excellent review of the anatomy of the cervical spine and referral patterns of cervical spine pain.

■ Ylinen J, Takala EP, Nykanen M, et al. Active neck muscle training in the treatment of chronic neck pain in women. *JAMA.* 2003;289(19):2509–2516.

This study showed that a strength and endurance training program is an effective method of decreasing pain and disability in women with chronic nonspecific neck pain. These patients, however, were between the ages of 25 and 53 years.

Leo M. Cooney, Jr., MD

CHAPTER 56—DISEASES AND DISORDERS OF THE FOOT

KEY POINTS

- Foot problems, both orthopedic problems and skin and nail changes, are common and have important functional consequences for older persons.

- Many orthopedic foot problems can be adequately addressed with orthotics and proper shoes.

- Skin problems may require debridement and topical medications in addition to orthotics and proper footwear.

- Systemic illnesses can be associated with serious foot problems, for which regular podiatric care is advised.

Foot problems lead to some of the most distressing symptoms and disabling conditions affecting older patients. Foot and related problems and their sequelae may be local, or they may be associated with systemic conditions. The ability to remain pain free and ambulatory is a key element in successful aging.

Feet are fairly rigid structures that carry heavy physical workloads, both static and dynamic. The foot, though shaped like a rectangle, bears static forces in a triangular pattern. Flat and hard surfaces force the foot to absorb shock; over the lifespan, the foot is subjected to both prolonged and repetitive micro- and macrotrauma. When the foot is unable to adapt to stress, inflammatory changes in bone and soft tissue are produced that may manifest in one or more of many mechanical disorders, including synovitis, fasciitis, and arthritis. In addition, vascular, neurologic, dermatologic, rheumatologic, and endocrinologic diseases increase the older person's risk of serious foot problems.

ORTHOPEDIC DISORDERS OF THE FOOT

For the older person, disease or decreased activity, or both, may cause osteopenia, progressive loss of muscle mass, and atrophy of tissue, and these may affect the structure and function of the foot. Manifestations of degenerative processes affecting older persons that are specific to the foot include plantar fasciitis, atrophy of the plantar fat pad, and hammertoe (digiti flexus) formation (see Table 56.1 for definitions and descriptions of several foot disorders and deformities). When these and other conditions cause foot pain, the older person's mobility and ambulatory status may be further limited, and as the ambulatory status of the person changes, foot problems may worsen.

Common orthopedic foot disorders in the elderly person are the consequences of severe or repeated trauma, inflammation, metabolic change, strain, obesity, osteoarthritis, rheumatoid arthritis, gout, and osteoporosis. Manifestations of these processes in the foot include stress fractures, tendonitis, residual deformities (including rotational digital deformities), joint swelling, anterior imbalance, bursitis, neuritis, and neuromas. Because even minor trauma can result in a fracture, a stress fracture should be suspected when foot pain is severe, prolonged, and not otherwise explained.

Disorders of the Mid- and Forefoot

Deformities such as flat feet (pes planus), high arched feet (pes cavus), bunions (hallus valgus), and hammertoes create pain and reduce the older person's ability to walk. *Hammertoe* is a general term applied to several types of contracture deformities of the toes. It is usually seen in the lesser toes, but a hallux (great toe) hammertoe may develop in the presence of coexistent neurologic abnormalities. The classic hammertoe is dorsiflexion at the metatarsophalangeal joint and plantar contraction of the proximal interphalangeal joint. Mallet toes and claw toes are different variations. A cock-up toe occurs when the contracture provides no contact between the toe and plane of support.

Rotational deformities and overlapping toes (see Figure 56.1) due to hallux valgus and arthritis are also referred to clinically as hammertoes. These deformities

Table 56.1—A Glossary of Foot Disorders

Disorder	Definition or Description
Calcaneal spur	A calcification of the attachment of the plantar fascia, usually at the medial plantar tuberosity of the calcaneus. The spur projects anteriorly and is the consequence of chronic repetitive trauma or stress resulting from biomechanical and pathomechanical change. When ligamentous calcification occurs, inflammation and associated pain at the attachment are the result. This may be referred to as *heel pain syndrome* and may be related to plantar fasciitis.
Cystic erosion	Areas of radiolucency usually noted with arthritic changes, such as rheumatoid arthritis, and usually occurring in the metatarsal heads with associated joint changes.
Digiti flexus	May be fixed or flexible flexion at the metatarsal phalangeal joints; ie, hammertoe.
Digiti quinti varus	Refers to a valgus displacement or splaying of the fifth metatarsal, with a resulting varus or inward deviation of the fifth toe.
Entrapment syndrome	Occurs when a nerve is compressed by ligamentous or other soft-tissue inflammation, resulting in pain and possibly numbness and neuropathic symptoms. The most common sites are the posterior tibial nerve and the intermetatarsal nerves, plantarly.
Haglund's deformity	A hyperostosis of the posterior and superior portion of the calcaneus, which expands the shape of the calcaneus, which can in turn place pressure on the attachment of the Achilles tendon. The presence of the deformity also can produce a pressure area for the counter of the shoe. It is easily demonstrated on a lateral radiograph of the foot and is clinically significant, with pain associated with tendonitis or bursitis, usually resulting from an incompatibility of foot to shoe last.
Hallux abducto valgus	An alternative clinical diagnosis for hallux valgus, or bunion. There is a varus splaying of the first metatarsal with a valgus and rotational deformity of the phalanges of the great toe.
Hallux limitus and rigidus	A degenerative joint change involving the first metatarsal phalangeal joint, resulting from dorsal spurs, with a marked limitation or absence of any range of motion. The difference between hallux limitus and rigidus is based on the radiographic interpretation and difference in function.
Hallux valgus	Deviation of the tip of the great toe, or main axis of the toe, toward the outer or lateral side of the foot; ie, *bunion.*
Metatarsal prolapse	Marked prominence of the metatarsal head, usually associated with atrophy or posterior displacement, or both, of the anterior plantar fat pad, pes cavus, or digital contractures, which force the metatarsal heads in a plantar projection.
Metatarsalgia	Pain in the forefoot near the heads of the metatarsals.
Morton's syndrome	A congenital shortening of the first metatarsal shaft, which creates an abnormal metatarsal arc. Excessive weight is placed on the second metatarsal head during gait and stance. The dynamics and pathomechanics of the foot are modified and provide one of the causes of hallux valgus, abducto valgus, and rotational deformity of the hallux.
Periostitis	Inflammation of the periosteum.
Pes cavus	Represents a higher than normal arch and is commonly associated with neurologic change. In the older patient, excessive pressure is usually placed on the metatarsal heads. With atrophy of the plantar fat pad and displacement, pressure is increased, which can serve as a predisposing cause for pain and ulceration.
Pes planus	A flattening of the medial longitudinal arch, where the calcaneal pitch on a radiograph is usually below 15 degrees; ie, *flat feet.*
Pes valgo planus	Represents the same clinical picture as pes planus, with an addition of pronation, demonstrated by a lateral deviation of the Achilles tendon and an outward and rotational deformity of the foot, which presents a compensatory deformity due to complex biomechanical imbalance.
Plantar fasciitis	An inflammation and pain involving repetitive microtrauma to the plantar fascia, particularly at its posterior calcaneal attachment; associated with biomechanical and pathomechanical changes in the function of the foot. It is related to calcaneal spurs, ligamentous calcification, and tissue atrophy.
Tailor's bunion	An enlargement of the fifth metatarsal phalangeal joint, usually with a lateral deviation of the fifth metatarsal shaft and head and a medial and rotational deformity of the fifth toe. It is usually associated with a splaying of the fifth metatarsal and can present with bursitis, capsulitis, and degenerative joint change.
Tenosynovitis	Inflammation of a tendon and enveloping sheath.

Figure 56.1—Hallux abducto valgus, hammertoe, subluxated second toe, xerosis onychodystrophy, onychodysplasia.

are related to atrophy of interossei muscles of the foot and contractures of the long extensor tendons. The deformities can be classed as flexible, semi-rigid, or rigid, depending on the motion demonstrated and the ability to reduce the deformity. The toes may also become rotated, and with arthritic changes, they may become dislocated and subluxed (as in rheumatoid arthritis). These deformities increase the formation of corns, especially in the presence of ill-fitting footwear or incompatible shoe lasts (the *last* is the model over which shoes are made). In older patients the heads and bases of the phalanges are commonly enlarged, and degenerative changes can often be demonstrated at the tufted end of the distal phalanx.

The management of all deformities should be directed toward relief of pain and improvement of the ability to walk. The choice of management strategies depends on the causes and symptoms. When deformity is noted, shoe modification is important and should include a high toe box (a deep and rounded covering over the toe area). Silicone molds can be used to maintain a more normal position of the toes, acting as a digital brace. Where hyperkeratosis is noted, debridement should be completed to reduce the possibility of ulceration. Padding with materials such as lamb's wool, silicone, or foam can help reduce pressure. For most older patients, nonoperative treatment strategies are

effective in controlling the pain associated with the deformity. Surgical revision remains an option when these measures are not successful.

Metatarsalgia refers to pain in the anterior metatarsal area. It can be functional in nature or associated with metatarsophalangeal abnormalities. It can be associated with anterior fat pad atrophy or displacement, retrograde pressure from hammertoe deformities on the metatarsal heads, and other pathomechanical changes. It may also be due to degenerative changes, deformities that increase the angle at which the foot makes contact with the plane of support. It may be associated with obesity, a consequence of the increase in weight bearing and imbalance. Incompatibility of foot to shoe last and ill-fitting footwear are additional possible causes.

Management depends on the cause and includes padding, orthotics such as a metatarsal pad, shoe modifications, physical therapy, local corticosteroid injection, digital molds to help transfer an anteriorly displaced fat pad, and analgesics if the problem is related to degenerative joint changes. A metatarsal bar is a transverse bar used to transfer weight over the metatarsal heads and is usually placed on the plantar surface or sole of the shoe. It may be placed between the insole and outsole.

Heel and Arch Pain

Plantar fasciitis is a common syndrome that causes pain in the sole of the foot. This heel pain is usually due to a strain of the plantar fascial attachment, which inserts on the medial plantar tuberosity of the calcaneus. A calcaneal spur may develop as a result of chronic stress on the attachment. Conservative management is usually effective for the older patient. Oral analgesics, injectable corticosteroids, pressure reduction (heel cups and night splints), and physical medicine are the initial forms of therapy. Orthotics can reduce pressure on the heel by changing biomechanics during the gait cycle and transferring weight elsewhere.

Heel pain may also be caused by the rubbing of the shoe on the back of the heel. This may result in inflammation known as posterior Achilles bursitis. This can occur between the calcaneus and the Achilles tendon or between the tendon and skin. Constant pressure can result in bursal formation. Haglund's deformity or disease, which is an osseous enlargement of the posterior–superior segment of the calcaneus, complicates this condition and its management. Nonoperative management is usually effective.

DISORDERS OF THE SKIN AND NAILS

With aging, the skin, ligaments, muscles, neurovascular structures, and bones undergo changes. The skin is one of the first structures to demonstrate change with aging. Trophic changes, such as a loss of hair below the knee and on the dorsum of the foot and toes, are common. The skin may become atrophic and resemble parchment. It also loses the normal lubricants and becomes xerotic. Brownish pigmentations are often related to the deposition of hemosiderin. A combination of physiologic changes in the skin coupled with continuing repetitive trauma, pressure, and atrophy of soft tissue prompts hyperkeratosis to form as a normal protective function. When the hyperkeratosis becomes excessive, it tends to act as a foreign body, increasing pressure and creating local ischemia, which can lead to tissue breakdown. Localized pressure can create subkeratotic hemorrhage, and the resultant hematoma becomes the predisposing factor for the development of ulcerations.

Hyperkeratosis

Common foot complaints of elderly persons concern the many forms of hyperkeratotic lesions, such as tyloma (calluses) and heloma (corns). The biomechanical and pathomechanical factors that create these problems are associated with compressive, tensile, and shearing stresses. Soft-tissue loss associated with aging and atrophy of the plantar fat pad increases pain and limits ambulation. Contractures, gait changes, deformities, the incompatibility of foot type to the shoe last, and arthritis are additional factors that need consideration. A multiplicity of conditions, including skin tone and elasticity, result in the development of keratotic lesions in elderly persons.

Management should be directed toward the functional and activity needs of the patient. Treatment includes debridement, padding, weight dispersion and diffusion, emollients, shoe modifications and last changes, orthoses, and surgical revision. Keratotic lesions can become primary irritants and can produce local avascularity that can precipitate ulceration. Pressure ulcers in the foot usually begin with subkeratotic hemorrhage. Once debrided and managed properly, they usually heal, but they may recur unless adequate measures are instituted to reduce pressure to the local areas of ulceration. Despite all measures, the problem may persist because of residual deformity and systemic diseases, such as diabetes mellitus. (See also "Pressure Ulcers," p 259.)

Xerosis

Excessive dryness, or xerosis, is associated with a lack of hydration and lubrication and is a related keratin dysfunction. Fissures develop as a result of dryness and associated stress on the heel. Management aims to prevent infection and further complications. A 10%, 20%, or 40% urea cream or solution or 12% ammonium lactate may be helpful as a mild and safe keratolytic. A heel sleeve or pad made with mineral oil or a heel cup can help to minimize trauma to the heel, thus reducing the potential for complications.

Nail Problems

Disorders of the toenails are common in older persons. Toenails undergo changes much more than do fingernails as a consequence of trauma, the environment of the shoe or sock, and the forces associated with ambulation. The toenails undergo degeneration and trophic changes (onychopathy) with thickening or longitudinal ridging (onychorrhexis) that is the consequence of repeated microtrauma, disease, and nutritional impairment. Nail malformation (onychodystrophy and onychodysplasia), subungual hematoma, discoloration, loosening or separation of the nail from the nail bed (onycholysis), nail thickening (onychauxis and onychogryphosis) (see Figure 56.2 and Figure 56.3), and subungual keratosis are all prevalent among older adults. Deformities of the toenails may become more pronounced and may be complicated by xerotic changes in the periungual nail folds as onychophosis (hyperkeratosis) and tinea unguium (onychomycosis) with periungual infection.

Fungal infections account for 20% of all nail disease and are almost exclusively found in adults. Onychomycosis (Figure 56.4) can be caused not only

Figure 56.2—Onychauxis, subungual diabetic ulcer, xerosis, with arterial insufficiency and onychomycosis.

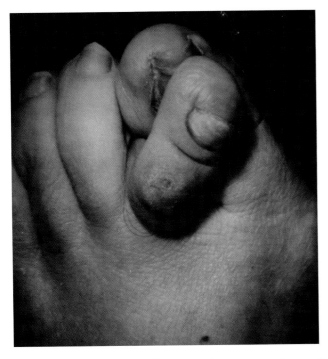

Figure 56.3—Onychogryphosis, onychomycosis, subungual debris, and tinea pedis.

Figure 56.4—Onychomycosis. Nails infected by fungi are often yellow, thickened, and friable, with yellow-brown debris under the nail plate.

by dermatophytes (fungi that infect keratinized tissues), but also by certain yeasts and nondermatophytic molds. The most common dermatophytes causing onychomycosis are *Trichophyton rubrum*, *Trichophyton mentagrophytes* var. *interdigitale*, and *Epidermophyton floccosum*. *Candida albicans* can infect the nails in chronic mucocutaneous candidiasis; however, other candida species (such as *C. parapsilosis*) can infect the nails of otherwise healthy persons. Nondermatophytic onychomycosis usually occurs in previously diseased nails or aged nails. It can often be difficult to determine whether a positive nondermatophytic nail culture is truly infection or contamination. In most cases of onychomycosis, there is preceding or concomitant tinea pedis.

Onychomycosis can be divided into four clinical subtypes: distal subungual onychomycosis, proximal subungual onychomycosis, white superficial onychomycosis, and candidal onychomycosis. Distal subungual onychomycosis is most common, and proximal subungual onychomycosis is least common. On clinical examination, infected nails have whitish or brownish-yellow discoloration. In response to the infection, hyperproliferation of the nail bed occurs, leading to subungual hyperkeratosis (yellow-brown debris under the nail bed). Diagnosis can be confirmed by potassium hydroxide (KOH) preparation or fungal culture of the nail plate or subungual debris.

A decision to treat is usually made because of the cosmetic concern of a yellow friable nail, other comorbidities (particularly diabetes mellitus, where the break in the epidermal barrier due to the fungal infection can serve as a route for bacterial infections), and occasionally because of pain. Topical agents have not been effective. A topical nail lacquer, ciclopirox (which is applied daily for 1 year) has been made available to treat onychomycosis, but in clinical studies it was found that less than 12% of patients achieved clear or almost clear toenails with its use. Griseofulvin is a systemic medication administered orally, but poor absorption, side effects, and drug interactions have limited adherence and efficacy. Regimens with newer agents, such as oral terbinafine, fluconazole, and itraconazole, have fewer side effects and drug interactions. Fluconazole can be used to treat candidal infections. It is well tolerated and has an excellent safety profile. When prescribing itraconazole, it is imperative to review all other medications the patient is taking; itraconazole interacts with warfarin, digoxin, and many other drugs through the cytochrome P-450 liver enzyme system. Terbinafine is the only orally active fungicidal agent that can be administered orally. It has fewer drug interactions but may interact with tricyclic antidepressants. Regardless, treatment can take 3 to 4 months, and the rate of relapse of onychomycosis is high.

Ingrown toenails are relatively common in elderly persons and are usually the consequence of deformity, disease, or onychopathy (onychodysplasia, or involution) and improper self-care. When the nail penetrates the skin, an abscess may result. If an ingrown nail is not managed early, periungual granulation tissue may form and complicate treatment. Onychia, inflammation of the soft tissue adjacent to the nail plate, is usually precipitated by local trauma or pressure but may be a complication of systemic disease or an early sign of infection. Mild erythema, swelling, and pain are the most prevalent findings. Management includes removing all pressure, applying tepid saline compresses, and using antibiotics if needed. Lamb's wool, tube foam, or shoe modification may reduce pressure. Paronychia, inflammation of the nail matrix plus the deeper and surrounding structures, may develop with infection and abscess of the posterior nail wall. It is a serious problem because of the potential for bone involvement as a result of the close association of the nail with the distal phalanx. Management includes surgical debridement and antibiotic treatment, if needed.

Elderly patients may also develop subungual hemorrhage from direct or constant trauma of the shoes, coagulopathies, or bed covers. Bleeding under the nail may result in an ulcer or loss of the toenail (onycholysis) if it is substantial.

Subungual heloma (also known as a corn or clavus) is usually associated with a subungual exostosis, spur, or hypertrophy of the tufted end of the distal phalanx. Initial management includes debridement and protection of the toe involved, as well as the use of a shoe with a high toe box (deep and rounded). Surgical excision of the osseous deformity may be required if the condition cannot be successfully treated in a conservative manner.

SYSTEMIC DISEASES AND THE FOOT

Diabetes Mellitus

Diabetes is the most important disease affecting foot health in older persons. (See also "Diabetes Mellitus," p 382.) It has been estimated that 50% to 75% of all amputations in diabetic patients could be prevented by periodic assessment, early intervention, and foot health education. The ocular complications of diabetes may affect the ability of the older person to see ingrown toenails, corns, and ulcers. The slower wound healing also contributes to the foot problems common to patients with diabetes.

These problems include neuropathy, vascular insufficiency,, dermopathy, atrophy of the muscles and soft tissues, and deformity. Neuropathy, especially sensory impairment, is a precursor to ulcers. Insensitivity, paresthesias, decreased vibratory sense, and loss of protective sensation are among the most important neuropathic changes.

Arterial insufficiency causes pallor, a loss or decrease in the posterior tibial and dorsalis pedis pulse, dependent rubor, and decreased capillary filling time in the toes. Severe vascular disease may result in rest pain that typically occurs at night. A loss of the plantar metatarsal fat pad is associated with vascular insufficiency and predisposes the patient to ulcerations at the site of bony prominences or deformities of the foot.

Prevention and early recognition are key in managing foot ulcers. Clinicians should examine the feet of diabetic patients at each visit and instruct patients and caregivers in the importance of daily foot inspections. Preventive strategies include optimizing glycemic control, and monitoring and treating peripheral neuropathy, arterial disease, limited joint mobility, bony deformities, hyperkeratosis, and onychodystrophy. Using the Semmes-Weinstein monofilament, assessing vibratory sensation, and monitoring reflex changes all help the clinician to assess the risk for and help prevent foot ulcers in patients with diabetes. Reducing excessive pressure, shock, and shear by accommodating, stabilizing, and supporting deformities by weight diffusion and dispersion is also important in ulcer prevention.

When prevention fails and an ulcer develops, the history should focus on duration, inciting event or trauma, prior ulcerations, wound care, and pressure off-loading procedures. The examination can include an assessment of the location and depth, the presence of infection, ischemic or neuropathic changes, edema, and the presence of a Charcot joint. Imaging is essential to exclude osteomyelitis and may include plain radiography, computed tomography, technetium bone scans, indium scans, and magnetic resonance imaging. Noninvasive vascular studies include Doppler and transcutaneous oxygen tension. Consultation with a vascular specialist may be needed when vascular insufficiency is severe or the wounds are nonhealing.

The general principles of management include debridement, pressure relief, off-loading, avoidance or limitation of weight bearing, proper wound management, management of infection with early antibiotics, management of ischemia, medical management of comorbidities, and hospitalization and surgical management when necessary. Weight bearing can be modified by the use of crutches, wheelchairs, and bed rest, as well as contact casts, walkers, boots, braces, total contact orthosis, modified surgical shoes and boots, and appropriate dressings. A wide variety of dressings and topical agents are available; selection is guided by nature of the ulcer and its complications. Topical agents include saline, antiseptics, topical antibiotics, enzymes, growth factors, and dermal skin substitutes. Empiric antibiotic therapy should be instituted early, especially if infection may become limb threatening. With osteomyelitis or limb-threatening infection, hospitalization is usually indicated. The choice of antibiotic is based on the clinical symptoms, culture and sensitivity, and the presence of deep infection, bone exposure, or sepsis, as well as whether soft tissue or bone is infected.

Peripheral Vascular Disease

Older adults with peripheral vascular disease demonstrate many of the same signs and symptoms as those with diabetes mellitus. (See "Cardiovascular Diseases and Disorders," p 359.) In contrast to neuropathic ulcers, vascular ulcers are extremely painful.

Arthritis

Osteoarthritis is common in older adults. It occurs in weight-bearing joints and causes pain, swelling, stiffness, limitation of movement, and deformity. It may be worsened by chronic trauma, strain, or obesity. Gouty arthritis results early in intense pain and erythema and later in joint damage.

Rheumatoid arthritis affects the hands and feet equally and results in muscle wasting and marked deformity. The metatarsophalangeal joints become dislocated or subluxed; there is increased protrusion of the metatarsal heads, and walking becomes painful. If conservative treatment with orthotics and special shoes does not relieve the pain, surgery may help to allow less painful ambulation. (See "Musculoskeletal Diseases and Disorders," p 440.)

SPECIAL SHOES AND ORTHOTICS

Foot pain and stress can be relieved through weight diffusion and weight dispersion. Weight diffusion is accomplished with an increase in the thickness of an orthosis or sole of a shoe that is placed between the foot and the plane of support, such as the floor. Weight dispersion is accomplished by diverting pressure away from painful areas of the foot by making specific adjustments to an orthosis or insole or by some form of internal or external shoe modification. Examples include balance padding, metatarsal padding, and external shoe wedges or bars. The primary treatment goals of both approaches are to relieve pain, restore maximum function, and maintain restored function once it is achieved.

Special footwear and orthotics aim to reduce shock and shear, transfer weight from painful areas, correct or support flexible deformities, accommodate fixed deformities, and control or limit joint motion. Shoes with depth or extra-depth lasts are usually suggested to accomplish these objectives. A *depth shoe* is a shoe that usually has a filler or insole that extends from heel to toe and that provides at least 3/16″ of additional depth in the shoe and a high toe box, so that an orthotic or customized insole can be placed in the shoe and prevent the top of the foot from being compressed against the underside of the toe box. An extra-depth shoe provides 1/4″ of additional depth, and a super-depth shoe provides an additional 1/2″ of depth

for total-contact orthoses or inserts. Custom shoes are recommended for patients with severe deformity, amputation, or other foot problems for which special lasts are required.

Shoe modifications that are often useful for older patients include mild calcaneal wedges to limit motion and alter gait, metatarsal bars to transfer weight, Thomas heels to increase calcaneal support, long shoe counters to increase mid-foot support and control foot direction, heel flares to add stability, shank fillers or wedges to produce a total weight-bearing surface, steel plates to restrict motion, and rocker bars to prevent flexion and extension. Additional internal modifications include longitudinal arch pads, wedges, bars, lifts, and tongue or bite pads. Orthoses are available in rigid, semi-rigid, and flexible varieties; they are made from an array of materials, of which plastic, leather, and laminates are the most useful.

Medicare provides for what are termed *therapeutic shoes* (depth, super-depth, or custom) and *multidensity inserts*. To be eligible, patients must have a history of diabetes mellitus or other disease affecting foot health, evidence of a comprehensive management plan for the disease process that specifies that therapeutic shoes are needed, and documentation that he or she has one or more of the following conditions: peripheral neuropathy with evidence of callus formation, a history of pre-ulcerative calluses, a history of a previous ulceration, a foot deformity, previous amputation of all or part of the foot, or poor circulation. Appropriate footwear is effective in the prevention of serious foot complications.

THE ROLE OF THE PRIMARY CLINICIAN IN FOOT CARE

Foot impairment, including diseases and disorders of the foot that are common in elderly patients, may affect the general health and functioning of older patients. Periodic comprehensive podogeriatric assessment is recommended for older patients. Practitioners should be aware of local conditions and the complications of systemic diseases, such as diabetes mellitus, peripheral arterial disease, arthritic changes, neurologic disorders, and mental health symptoms that manifest as foot symptoms and signs. Primary practitioners should recognize common foot problems and should refer patients for podiatric care and management in a timely and appropriate manner. The quality of life for older persons can be significantly improved by early detection and comprehensive management of foot problems.

ANNOTATED REFERENCES

■ Bowker JH, Pfeifer MA. *Levin and O'Neal's The Diabetic Foot*. 6th ed. St. Louis, MO: Mosby; 2001.

This is a text dedicated to the management of the diabetic foot. It covers diabetes mellitus, epidemiology of foot ulcers, neuropathic problems of the lower extremity, atherosclerosis and thrombosis in diabetes mellitus, hemorheology, biomechanics, cutaneous aspects of diabetes mellitus, nutrition, pathogenesis and general management, diabetic foot problems, classification and staging, diabetic foot ulcer care including assessment and management, total contact casting, alternative weight distribution, imaging, noninvasive vascular testing, radiologic intervention in peripheral vascular disease, wound healing, hyperbaric oxygen, footwear and orthotics, Charcot foot, infection, surgical pathology, medical management, vascular surgery, plastic surgical reconstruction, amputation, rehabilitation, education, self-management, psychosocial and psychological aspects of care, and medicolegal aspects of care.

- Helfand AE, ed. Clinical podogeriatrics: assessment, education, and prevention. *Clin Podiatr Med Surg.* 2003;20(3).

  This focuses on the assessment of geriatric foot problems. Included are segments dealing with an overview of geriatrics, nursing and long-term-care considerations, foot pain in later life and its psychosocial correlates, podiatric assessment protocols, onychial disorders, hyperkeratotic lesions, skin disorders, arthritis and related diseases, foot deformities, biomechanical and pathomechanical changes, orthotic considerations, peripheral vascular considerations, neurologic evaluation, diabetic foot assessment in the older patient, geriatric primary podiatric medicine, geriatric footwear, and surgical considerations in treating the geriatric patient.

- Helfand AE. Foot problems in older patients—a focused podogeriatrics assessment study in ambulatory care. *J Am Podiatr Med Assoc.* 2004;94(3):294–304.

  The Assessment Protocol Form can be duplicated without permission inasmuch as the study was funded by the Pennsyl-

vania Department of Health. In addition, the protocol is also on Temple University's Institute of Aging Web site (available at http://www.temple.edu/aging/courses.htm) and the University of Pennsylvania's School of Nursing Web site (available at http://www.nursing.upenn.edu/centers/hcgne/gero_tips/tls_assessment.htm) (both accessed November 2005).

- Lorimer D, French G, O'Donnell M, et al. *Neale's Common Foot Disorders, Diagnosis and Management.* 6th ed. New York: Churchill Livingstone; 2002.

  This general text covers the structure and functions of the foot, examination and diagnosis in clinical management, radiologic assessment, pediatrics, adult foot disorders, podiatric management of the elderly patient, dermatologic conditions, nail disorders, diabetic and high-risk patients, patient education, sports medicine and injuries, clinical therapeutics, orthoses, injectable silicone, physical therapy, infection control, local anesthesia, nail surgery, digital surgery, genetic disorders, circulatory disorders, metabolic diseases, rheumatic diseases, neurologic disorders, leprosy, and tropical diseases.

- Veves A, Giurini JM, LoGerfo FW. *The Diabetic Foot: Medical and Surgical Management.* Totowa, NJ: Humana Press; 2002.

  This is a text dedicated to the management of the diabetic foot. It covers principles of care, epidemiology, physiology and pathophysiology, polyneuropathy, microvascular changes, clinical features, foot-pressure abnormalities, biomechanics, examination and identification of the at-risk foot, radiographic changes, microbiology and treatment of diabetic foot infections, Charcot changes, chronic wound care, local care, amputations and rehabilitation, surgical reconstruction, growth factors and skin equivalents, vascular surgery, angioplasty, footwear, and prevention of foot problems.

Arthur E. Helfand, DPM

CHAPTER 57—NEUROLOGIC DISEASES AND DISORDERS

KEY POINTS

- Cerebrovascular disease is the leading cause of disability and death among older persons.

- Control of systolic hypertension is the most important factor in preventing stroke.

- Common causes of late-life seizure include vascular disease, new mass lesions, and alcohol or medication withdrawal.

- Parkinson's disease may be recognized by an insidious onset of asymmetrical tremor or muscular rigidity.

The number of disorders that affect the nervous system increases rapidly with advancing age. Subtle neurologic abnormalities often are detected on examination. In one study of nearly 500 older adults the following signs were found which could not be attributed directly to any specific medical or a neurologic disease: diminished arm swing (present in 29% of those examined), diminished toe vibration sense (21%), hyperreflexia in arms (10%), unequal nasolabial folds (9%), absent pupillary response (9%), Babinski's sign (7%), diminished toe position sense (7%), and reduction in arm strength (5%). False findings imply that the diagnosis of neurologic disease may be more difficult in the setting of these "normal" signs. Still, a large percentage of elderly persons will have neurologic disease that cause a variety of impairments. The goal of the clinician is to determine the significance of these abnormalities and to make an accurate diagnosis and implement appropriate treatment.

CEREBROVASCULAR DISEASES

Stroke is a leading cause of disability and death among older persons. The incidence of stroke increases with advancing age, approximately doubling with each decade. The incidence of stroke for men is 2.1 per 1000 at ages 55 to 64 years, 4.5 per 1000 at ages 65 to 74 years, and 9.3 per 1000 at ages 75 to 84 years. The incidence of stroke for women is 25% to 30% lower than that for men in comparable age groups, but it surpasses that of men in the age group 85 years and older.

Throughout the latter half of the 20th century the incidence of stroke declined in the United States, Canada, and Western Europe. This drop may be attributable to better control of modifiable risk factors, including hypertension, heart disease, diabetes mellitus, cigarette smoking, elevated blood lipids, and alcohol use. Hypertension is the most prevalent risk factor for stroke, and its treatment results in a substantial reduction in the risk of stroke. Treatment of isolated systolic hypertension in elderly persons reduces the risk of stroke by nearly 40%. (See "Hypertension," p 361.) Heart disease is also an important risk factor for stroke, including atherosclerotic coronary heart disease, left ventricular hypertrophy, valvular heart disease, valve replacement, and valvular and nonvalvular atrial fibrillation. (See "Cardiovascular Diseases and Disorders," p 344.) Several studies have confirmed a two- to fourfold increased risk of stroke in patients with diabetes mellitus. Studies suggest that tight control of blood-sugar levels might reduce the risk of stroke in patients with diabetes mellitus, although the evidence for reduction of other vascular complications (eg, retinopathy, nephropathy) is somewhat more compelling. (See "Diabetes Mellitus," p 382.) Cigarette smoking independently increases the risk of stroke as much as threefold, according to the Framingham Study. The incidence of stroke declines significantly even after 2 years of cessation of smoking, and after 5 years the level of risk returns to that of nonsmokers. Elevated blood lipids and alcohol use are other important risk factors for stroke. (See "Alcohol and Drug Abuse," p 298.)

Besides being the most common acute, serious neurologic disease, stroke also is a leading cause of death. The fatality rate within 1 month of an acute stroke is 20% to 30% across all age groups; mortality is highest among older persons. Survival in part depends on the location and severity of the stroke. The most important predictor is the severity of neurologic signs. The severity of the neurologic deficits following stroke can be quantified by use of an instrument such as the NIH Stroke Scale (see http://www.vh.org/adult/provider/neurology/Stroke/Scaleind.html or http://www.strokecenter.org/trials/scales/nihss.pdf). In general, a score of less than 5 in this scale, which ranges from 0 to 42, is associated with a very good prognosis. Persons with a score greater than 20 have a very poor prognosis and a high likelihood of major complications.

Neurologic causes of death include the brain injury itself or resultant brain edema. Common medical causes of death are myocardial infarction, arrhythmia, heart failure, aspiration pneumonia, and pulmonary embolism. Age in itself does not influence the gross neurologic aspects of stroke, but older age is associated with lesser recovery in activities of daily living. Older stroke patients can benefit from formal rehabilitation.

Internal Carotid Artery Disease

A lesion at the origin of the internal carotid artery, most commonly secondary to atherosclerosis, can lead to transient monocular blindness (amaurosis fugax) or a cerebral hemispheric deficit (eg, focal motor, sensory, or cognitive symptoms or signs) because both the retina and cerebral hemispheres derive their blood supply from the internal carotid artery. Hemispheric deficits include hemiparesis or hemisensory loss, homonomous hemianopia or aphasia, or apraxia. The initial evaluation of patients with these symptoms or signs usually includes a neuroimaging study (computed tomography or magnetic resonance imaging) and noninvasive imaging of the carotid arteries (B-mode ultrasonography and Doppler ultrasonography or magnetic resonance angiography). Data from the North American Symptomatic Carotid Endarterectomy Trial (NASCET) indicate that the optimal treatment for symptomatic carotid stenosis of greater than 70% is carotid endarterectomy, provided the patient has few comorbidities and the institution performs a high number of endarterectomies. The operation can be performed with reasonable safety in elderly persons provided medical comorbidity is relatively low. The optimal treatment for symptomatic carotid stenosis of less than 70% or of asymptomatic carotid stenosis is still not clear; treatment options include carotid endarterectomy or medical management. Medical management should seek to optimize blood pressure, lipid status, and antiplatelet agents.

Aspirin is the mainstay of antiplatelet therapy for atherosclerotic stroke prevention. Studies on the use of aspirin in stroke prevention suggest that higher dosages than 325 mg of aspirin per day do not add therapeutic benefit, but the minimum necessary dosage has not been fully investigated. Many physicians routinely prescribe 81 to 325 mg per day, although even the lower dosage may cause gastrointestinal irritation and blood loss. Patients who fail aspirin monotherapy are usually advanced to other platelet-inhibiting medications. These may include sustained-release dipyridamole combined with aspirin. Clopidogrel 75 mg once daily is an alternative for patients who cannot tolerate aspirin.

The only clear role for warfarin is primary or secondary stroke prevention in the setting of cardioembolic disease. Specific indications include atrial fibrillation, severe valvular disease, and known intracardiac clot secondary to myocardial infarction.

Vertebrobasilar Arterial Diseases

Syndromes associated with vascular lesions in the posterior circulation (vertebral and basilar arteries) result in cranial nerve impairment or dysfunction of the descending motor or ascending sensory tracks within the brain stem. Because of the large number of pathways passing through the brain stem, vertebrobasilar occlusion results in myriad signs, including abnormal eye movements; Horner's syndrome; unilateral or bilateral or crossed motor and sensory abnormalities in the face, arm, or leg; ataxia; dysarthria; dysphagia; and even stupor or coma. Because the thalamus and inferior portions of the cerebral hemispheres also are supplied by the vertebrobasilar system, behavioral and visual symptoms also can occur. Treatment of posterior circulation cerebrovascular disease is medical, as no surgical approach to improving the posterior circulation has been shown to improve outcomes. Although many clinicians prefer warfarin anticoagulation over antiplatelet agents for patients with vertebrobasilar disease, no formal studies have confirmed better clinical outcomes with warfarin. A large trial (Warfarin-Aspirin Recurrent Stroke Study) found aspirin and warfarin to be equally efficacious (unless the cause is cardioembolic, in which case warfarin is superior).

Lacunar Disease

Lacunar disease secondary to occlusion of small penetrating vessels is presumably the consequence of lipohyalinosis (lipid deposition and hyalinization) or local atherosclerosis. Lacunar strokes may result in several well-defined syndromes, including pure motor hemiplegia, pure hemisensory stroke, ataxic hemiparesis, and dysarthria–clumsy hand syndrome. Risk factors include hypertension and diabetes mellitus. The most effective means of managing lacunar disease is aggressive treatment of these risk factors. Although aspirin also is prescribed for stroke prevention in patients who have suffered lacunar strokes, it has not been shown to prevent lacunar strokes specifically. Lacunar strokes may occur independently or concurrently with large-vessel cerebrovascular disease.

Intracerebral Hemorrhage

Intracerebral hemorrhage accounts for 15% to 20% of all strokes. Approximately 80% occur between the ages of 40 and 70. A racial distribution suggests that black Americans and Asian Americans may be at slightly higher risk than white Americans.

The most common risk factor for intracerebral hemorrhage is hypertension, which is present in 75% to 80% of the cases. Excessive use of alcohol is also associated with a higher incidence. Common locations for hypertensive bleeds are the putamen, thalamus, cerebellar hemisphere, pons, and cerebrum. In elderly patients a common cause of cerebral lobar hemorrhage is cerebral amyloid angiopathy, which usually occurs without systemic amyloidosis. In these cases intracranial bleeds tend to be recurrent. Hemorrhage also can complicate the use of antiplatelet agents and anticoagulants. Other secondary causes of intracerebral hemorrhage should not be overlooked. These include trauma, arteriovenous malformations, and aneurysms. Acute treatment is supportive, with interim control of severe hypertension and discontinuation or antiplatelets. Large lobar or intraventricular hemorrhages may be considered for neurosurgical drainage.

Treatment Following Ischemic Stroke

The current protocol for care of the elderly stroke patient includes optimizing hydration status; controlling blood pressure while avoiding acute hypotension; preventing deep-vein thrombosis; detecting and treating coronary ischemia, heart failure, and cardiac arrhythmias; and initiating long-term treatment with antiplatelet agents or oral anticoagulation to prevent recurrent stroke, depending upon the presumed cause. Dehydration on presentation is common, but rehydration must be gradual to reduce the risk of cerebral edema. In patients with clinically evident cerebrovascular disease immediately after the occurrence of an ischemic cerebral infarction, it is appropriate to withhold treatment of hypertension (unless blood pressure is very high, eg, higher than 220/110 mm Hg) until the situation stabilizes. Even when treatment has been withheld temporarily, the eventual goal is to reduce blood pressure gradually while avoiding orthostatic hypotension. The target systolic blood pressure should be 10 to 20 points higher than the patient's baseline pressure; if the baseline is unknown, systolic pressure should not be lowered beyond 160 mm Hg. Patients with acute ischemic stroke who are treated with fibrinolytic agents require careful blood-pressure monitoring, especially over the first 24 hours after treatment is started. Elevated blood pressure should gradually be brought down to the upper end of the normal range. Patients with a history of ischemic heart disease or arrhythmia and patients with large strokes should be monitored by electrocardiography for 48 hours. For large cardioembolic strokes (eg, involving most of the middle cerebral artery territory or involving both middle and anterior cerebral artery territories), one generally waits 48 hours before beginning anticoagulation. Earlier anticoagulation does not improve outcome. Early initiation of aspirin[OL] therapy has a low risk of bleeding side effects and might improve outcome, modestly.

The only therapy approved by the U.S. Food and Drug Administration for ischemic stroke is recombinant tissue–plasminogen (rt-PA) activator (its generic name is alteplase). Infusion of this medication within 3 hours of stroke onset approximately doubles the chances of a favorable outcome at 3 months. The benefits of this treatment, however, must be weighed against the increased the risk of intracranial hemorrhage, which can be fatal or can result in worsened neurologic status. Most hemorrhagic events occur among patients with severe strokes, and outcomes among persons with severe strokes are very poor without treatment. Use of this medication requires careful assessment by a physician experienced in the treatment of stroke. Tissue-plasminogen activator should be considered when patients present within 3 hours of onset of neurologic deficit and computed tomography confirms the absence of intracranial hemorrhage. Major contraindications include infarction of greater than one third of a hemisphere, major surgery within 2 weeks, previous intracranial hemorrhage, sustained systolic blood pressure above 185 or diastolic above 110, symptoms of subarachnoid hemorrhage, recent urinary or gastrointestinal tract bleeding, coagulopathy, thrombocytopenia, or INR above 1.7. The NIH Stroke Scale is helpful for stratifying ischemic stroke patients according to risk and benefit for rt-PA. Scores below 5 generally have a favorable outcome regardless of treatment. Scores higher than 20 have a substantially increased hemorrhagic complication rate. Even though older patients might have a higher rate of bleeding complications than persons younger than 65, the risk is not sufficiently high to preclude treatment. (See also the section on stroke rehabilitation in "Rehabilitation," p 113.)

SUBDURAL HEMATOMA

A collection of blood between the dura and the arachnoid is referred to as a *subdural hematoma*. It is usually due to head trauma, although the trauma may be mild, particularly in older adults. In approximately 15% of cases, the hematomas are bilateral.

[OL] Not approved by the U.S. Food and Drug Administration for this use.

Perhaps most relevant in the elderly patient is the chronic subdural hematoma. The incidence of chronic subdural hematoma increases with age, from 0.13 per 100,000 for those in their 20s to 7.4 per 100,000 for those in their 70s. In 50% of chronic subdural hematomas, there is no history of head injury, although other risk factors include clotting disorders, shunting procedures (eg, ventriculo-peritoneal shunting for normal-pressure hydrocephalus may separate the blood vessels from the dura, resulting in tears), and seizures.

The symptoms of chronic subdural hematoma are headache, slight or severe impairment in cognition, and hemiparesis. Some patients may have seizures. Focal neurologic signs (weakness, sensory loss, and change in sensation) may be present. Neuroimaging studies reveal an extra-axial collection of blood.

The treatment of the hematoma varies depending on whether it is symptomatic or an incidental finding on a neuroimaging study. If symptomatic and the patient's condition is worsening, then removal of the clot may be attempted. If asymptomatic or if the patient's condition is improving, then clinical monitoring is appropriate, as the hematoma may shrink and disappear without surgery.

HEADACHES

There is evidence to suggest that the prevalence of headaches diminishes with age. One study demonstrated that although 74% of men and 92% of women between the ages of 21 and 34 years have headaches, these proportions drop to 22% and 55% after the age of 75 years. Headache is one of the most common medical complaints in young persons, and yet one study suggests that it is the 10th most common symptom in older women and the 14th most common symptom in older men. Headache incidence also declines with age; only 2% of all sufferers of an initial migraine are over the age of 50 years.

Persistent headaches are more likely to represent systemic or intracranial lesions (ie, nonbenign conditions) in older adults than in younger adults. One study demonstrated that among younger patients, 10% of headaches represent systemic or intracranial lesions; in older adults, this proportion was found to be 34%. These nonbenign conditions include intracranial masses (eg, primary or secondary tumors, subdural hematomas), cervical spondylosis, chronic obstructive pulmonary disease, carbon monoxide poisoning, and giant cell arteritis. In addition, many commonly used medications can cause headaches that are dull, diffuse, and nondescript, including vasodilators (eg, nitrates), hypotensives (eg, reserpine, atenolol, and methyldopa), antiparkinsonian agents, and stimulants.

One secondary cause of headache specific to older adults is giant cell (temporal) arteritis. This disease does not appear to occur below the age of 50 and peaks in incidence between the ages of 70 and 80. Women are affected twice as often as men. Pain may be centered at temporal or occipital arteries. Palpation of the scalp arteries may reveal focal tenderness and nodularity. Complaints of visual changes, low-grade fever, polymyalgia, and constitutional symptoms further suggest the diagnosis. Twenty percent of patients suffer visual loss that is generally irreversible. Peripheral markers of inflammation are typically elevated; however, nearly 10% of patients have a normal erythrocyte sedimentation rate. Elevated C-reactive protein may be more sensitive. Patients with the proper presentation should be promptly evaluated by temporal artery biopsy. Prednisone 40 to 60 mg daily day relieves symptoms within a few days. The dose is gradually tapered with close serologic monitoring.

As in younger persons, the common primary headache disorders may be classified into migraines (with or without aura) and tension-type headaches. Migraines are often unilateral, pulsating headaches of moderate or severe intensity associated with nausea, vomiting, or photophobia. Auras, when they occur, usually precede the headache and are manifested by transient neurologic symptoms that are localizable to the cerebral cortex or brain stem. Visual phenomena are among the most common types of auras. In contrast to migraines, tension-type headaches are often more diffuse, have a pressing or a tight quality, and are not associated with nausea or vomiting.

Headaches in older adults, however, may present in atypical ways. With migraines in particular, auras tend to disappear with age, and in some individuals the reverse occurs (headaches disappear while auras remain). The occurrence of an isolated visual or sensory aura in the absence of a headache can be diagnostically challenging in the sense that these symptoms may be signs of transient ischemic attacks as well.

The treatment of headaches may be categorized as either abortive (ie, treating an attack that has already begun) or preventive. Apart from various over-the-counter preparations, abortive therapies include ergotamines or triptans (eg, sumatriptan), which act by central serotonergic mechanisms. These medications are mild vasoconstrictors and contraindicated in the setting of uncontrolled hypertension, stroke, and coronary artery disease. Generally, safety data in geriatric populations is lacking. Preventive therapies include β-blockers (propranolol, atenolol[OL]), valproic acid, topiramate, tricyclic antidepressants, and calcium channel blockers. The choice of an agent should be guided

by an effort to avoid adverse effects and drug interactions.

Older adults may not tolerate headache medications as well as younger patients do; moreover, in some older patients a medication may be contraindicated by comorbidities or existing drug regimens. For example, β-blockers and tricyclic antidepressants, which are often used as preventive therapy, may be associated with lethargy or sedation.

MOVEMENT DISORDERS

A movement disorder may be defined simply as abnormal involuntary movements. These movements are not the result of weakness or sensory deficits; they are the result of dysfunction of the basal ganglia or the extrapyramidal motor system. Movement disorders may be classified as hyperkinesias (excessive movement) or hypokinesias (paucity of movement). A particular movement disorder (eg, Parkinson's disease) may be characterized by several types of involuntary movements (eg, tremor, bradykinesia). Several movement disorders are especially common among older persons.

Parkinson's Disease

Parkinson's disease is a progressive neurodegenerative disease in which cell death in the substantia nigra and consequent reduction in brain dopamine levels results in a constellation of signs, including tremor at rest, bradykinesia, rigidity, and postural instability. The pathologic hallmark of the disease is the Lewy body, an intracellular inclusion body found in the substantia nigra.

The incidence increases dramatically with age, and the incidence among people in their 70s and 80s in the United States is approximately 200 cases per 100,000 (0.2%). The incidence among those in their 70s and 80s in other countries (Iceland, India, Scotland, Australia) has been estimated to be even higher, approaching 1000 to 2000 per 100,000 (1% to 2%). The disease most commonly appears between the ages of 50 and 79 years. In a small proportion of cases, the disease clusters within families and has a genetic basis. In a small number of these families, the disease has been linked to a region on the long arm of chromosome 4 that encodes the neuronal protein α-synuclein. In addition, environmental toxins (eg, manganese and pesticides) have been associated with some forms of the disease.

The disease begins insidiously and asymmetrically. The clinical manifestations include tremor, usually in one hand or sometimes in both, classically involving the fingers in a pill-rolling motion. The tremor (usually 3 to 5 Hz) is present at rest and usually decreases with

---

active, purposeful movement. Muscular rigidity is usually readily evident on passive movement of a limb. Passive movement may demonstrate a smooth resistance or superimposed ratchet-like jerks (cogwheel phenomenon). The term *bradykinesia* is often used to describe either a slowness in initiating movement (ie, a paucity of spontaneous movements) or movements themselves that are slow, and the term *freezing* is used to describe sudden interruption of movement. Other clinical features of Parkinson's disease may include the following:

- tachykinesia: the tendency for movements to become smaller and faster;

- tachyphemia: the tendency to speak more and more rapidly until all of the words run together into a mumble;

- micrographia: the tendency to make loops that become smaller and tighter when drawing loops across a page, to exhibit handwriting that is very small;

- festinating gait: to take steps that inadvertently quicken and become smaller, and

- impaired finger tapping: in which the amplitude lessens and the movements become more rapid until the fingers seem stuck together.

Postural abnormalities are evident in the standing and sitting positions, and an erect posture is not readily assumed or maintained. The head tends to fall forward on the trunk. The tendency to fall forward (propulsion) or backward (retropulsion) results from the loss of postural reflexes. Bradykinesia prevents the patient from stopping the fall, either by taking a step or moving the arms. The face can become mask-like, with lack of expression and diminished eye blinking.

Mood abnormalities, usually depression or anxiety, are common, as are cognitive impairment and dementia. These may place severe restrictions on the medications that might be used to relieve the tremor, bradykinesia, and rigidity.

One of the diagnostic challenges may be distinguishing mild early parkinsonism from the changes that often accompany normal aging (slowing down, loss of balance, stiffness, difficulty walking, stooped posture). However, the bradykinesia and rigidity of Parkinson's disease are usually asymmetric at onset, with one side slightly affected and the other remaining normal. In addition, tremor at rest is not a feature of normal aging, and although elderly persons may complain of stiffness, true extrapyramidal rigidity is otherwise uncommon.

The diagnosis is made clinically. Neuroimaging should be considered in atypical presentations such as the abrupt onset of tremor, focal weakness, sensory disturbances, or reflex abnormalities not attributed to muscle tone asymmetry.

Treatment programs must be individualized. This caution applies especially to elderly patients, who have reduced tolerance for dopaminergic and anticholinergic agents, the mainstays of parkinsonism therapy. Nonpharmacologic therapy includes a regular exercise program. Many elderly patients benefit from a course of physical therapy aimed at restoring their confidence in walking and maintaining balance, as well as teaching them simple tricks to help them manage unpredictable and disabling freezing episodes, and, when needed, selecting a cane or walker of the appropriate size and weight. A home visit by an occupational therapist may help to plan the appropriate placement of wall rails, grab bars, and other such assistive devices that reduce the possibility of falling.

Treatment of the motor manifestations of parkinsonism is important, but many elderly patients also complain of difficulty with constipation and insomnia. Constipation is particularly bothersome to elderly patients taking levodopa, which tends to exacerbate the constipation associated with reduced levels of physical activity. Treatment includes a diet rich in fruit and fiber, prune and other juices, frequent consumption of liquids, and use of osmotic laxatives. Elderly Parkinson's disease patients with insomnia should also be given individualized treatment. Some patients wake up at night because of a low dopamine state, which results in feelings of stiffness and malaise that are severe enough to awaken the patient. Higher bedtime doses of levodopa or even sustained-release forms of levodopa are appropriate. Patients may also experience insomnia because they are sleeping too much during the day, which may be a side effect of levodopa therapy. In these cases, it may be important to reduce the dosage of levodopa and correct the reversed sleep-wake cycle. Because urinary urgency may be a feature of Parkinson's disease, this may be the cause of the frequent night-time awakenings.

The major factor influencing the treatment of elderly patients with Parkinson's disease is their propensity to develop confusion and psychosis on antiparkinsonian medications. In general, the therapeutic regimen should be kept simple. Rather than prescribing small doses of multiple medications, prescribe higher doses of one or two medications; toxic side effects are less likely to occur. Levodopa provides the most improvement in the motor manifestations of Parkinson's disease relative to its toxic side effects on the central nervous system, whereas those with anticholinergic properties (agents such as trihexyphenidyl and amantadine) provide the least benefit. The dopamine agonists (bromocriptine, ropinirole, pramipexole) fall in between. Although psychosis may be treated effectively with clozapine, olanzapine, or quetiapine, which have fewer extrapyramidal side effects than other antipsychotic agents, confusion and disorientation may be treated more simply by lowering the doses of antiparkinsonian medications. In this setting, anticholinergic medications should be the first to be discontinued, followed by selegiline, dopamine agonists, and, finally, levodopa.

The most effective step in treating patients with Parkinson's disease is to accomplish dopamine replacement by using levodopa combined with carbidopa. Levodopa is converted to dopamine in both the central nervous system and the periphery. To reduce peripheral conversion, levodopa is combined with carbidopa (a peripheral decarboxylate inhibitor), which does not cross the blood-brain barrier. Treatment usually begins with a half tablet of the 25:100 combination (ie, 25 mg carbidopa to 100 mg levodopa) once or twice a day. Every 1 to 2 weeks, the dose can be increased by one half to one tablet, to reach a dose of one full tablet three times a day, if needed and if side effects are tolerable. If disabling bradykinesia, rigidity, postural instability, or tremor are still present, the dose can be gradually increased further, with cautious observation of side effects. Older adults, particularly if cognitively impaired, rarely tolerate more than 1000 mg per day of levodopa. Common adverse effects include nausea, abdominal cramping, orthostatic hypotension, and confusion. A controlled-release form (25:100 and 50:200) generally requires a slightly higher total daily dose. By approximately 5 years of levodopa therapy, half of patients will develop dyskinesias from the drug. Because of this, less effective dopamine agonists should be considered for initial therapy when the patient's life span is projected to be significantly more than 5 years such that dyskinesias will likely develop.

For patients with milder disease and no signs of dementia, dopamine agonists may be used initially as monotherapy. A cautious induction period with each is required, as nausea, orthostatic hypotension, and confusion are common side effects. Bromocriptine is begun with 1.25 mg per day and gradually increased by 1.25-mg increments every 2 to 5 days, to a total daily dose of 10 to 30 mg. Other newer dopamine agonists include ropinirole (given in starting dosages of 0.25 mg per day and increased as needed to dosages of 3 mg per day) and pramipexole (given in starting dosages of 0.125 mg per day and increased as needed to dosages of 4.5 mg per day). All dopamine agonists, and to a lesser extent levodopa, have been associated with sudden sleep attacks in which patients may fall asleep abruptly while driving. Patients should be warned of this rare but potentially serious adverse effect of therapy. As Parkinson's disease progresses, patients eventually require a switch from dopamine agonists to levodopa. Later in the disease when the

response to levodopa becomes variable, dopamine agonists may be reintroduced to manage periods of off-time.

Selegiline in dosages of 5 mg twice a day (8 AM and noon) may be used in an early stage to slow disease progression. The drug inhibits oxidative metabolism of dopamine. Trials indicate that selegiline can delay the need for additional antiparkinsonian agents. However, whether selegiline slows the disease progression or just suppresses symptoms is controversial. The drug is generally well tolerated, although some patients may experience side effects, including nausea, insomnia, confusion, anxiety, and feeling "revved up." Although chemically related to other monoamine oxidase inhibitors, selegiline does not require dietary restrictions.

Amantadine, a drug particularly useful for treating tremor, is generally prescribed at 100 mg two to three times daily. Amantadine's mild anticholinergic effects appear to play a role in its antiparkinsonian effects. It also promotes dopamine release in the corpus striatum. Elderly patients can develop cognitive side effects, including hallucinations.

Surgical options are increasingly being utilized for Parkinson's disease patients who have symptoms uncontrollable by medical therapies. Depending on a patient's most troubling symptoms, brain stimulators or stereotactic lesioning may be considered. Subthalamic nucleus stimulation is achieved by attaching an embedded pacemaker-like generator to a wire with the tip located deep to the thalamus. High-frequency stimulation results in improvement in tremor, akinesia, rigidity, and gait. Several sites have been identified which, when lesioned, can help certain symptoms of Parkinson's disease. Lesioning of the pallidum is often successful in the treatment of contralateral dyskinesias. Lesioning of the ventral intermediate nucleus of the thalamus has been successful in the treatment of contralateral tremor. Generally, the morbidity of these procedures is low among patients in otherwise fair to good health who do not have dementia.

Multiple System Atrophy

A histopathologic understanding of three parkinsonisms—olivopontocerebellar atrophy, Shy-Drager syndrome, and striatonigral degeneration—has permitted these overlapping syndromes to be carried under the rubric multiple system atrophy (MSA). Sometimes called a *Parkinson's plus disease*, MSA is characterized by parkinsonism (rigidity, tremor, bradykinesia, and postural instability) plus autonomic symptoms, cerebellar signs, and sometimes myoclonus. Other features that may accompany MSA are upper motor signs, severe dysarthria, stridor, dystonia, and an amyotrophic lateral sclerosis (ALS)–like picture. The diagnosis is clinical and can initially be indistinguishable from idiopathic Parkinson's disease. The mean age of onset for MSA is 55. It has a slight male preponderance and is progressive to death in approximately 7 years.

Autonomic symptoms are often the first to allow MSA to be differentiated from Parkinson's disease. Patients complain of dizziness, lightheadedness, or syncope on standing, and of postexertional weakness, gait unsteadiness, and dimming of vision. Impaired temperature control, reduced sweating, sphincter disturbance with urinary or fecal incontinence, diarrhea, constipation, impotence, iridic atrophy, impaired eye movements, Horner's syndrome, and anisocoria may also occur.

Orthostatic hypotension is often the most disabling symptom. Nonpharmacologic treatment of the autonomic dysfunction includes eating small meals, getting up slowly, and avoiding excessive straining at stool. Compressive clothing and elastic stockings, increased salt and fluid intake, and sleeping in a reverse Trendelenburg position may ameliorate some of the orthostatic symptoms. Drugs that are sometimes useful in treating the orthostatic hypotension include midodrine and fludrocortisone[OL]. Use of these medications occasionally results in supine hypertension, which requires close blood-pressure monitoring. Levodopa may initially help the rigidity, bradykinesia, and postural instability. Unfortunately, dopamine replacement often worsens the orthostatic hypotension.

Progressive Supranuclear Palsy

Progressive supranuclear palsy accounts for approximately 4% of cases of parkinsonism. It is marked by supranuclear gaze palsy, square wave jerks (defined below), and cognitive impairment. Onset usually occurs during the late 50s or early 60s. The pathogenesis is unknown. The disease usually progresses rapidly, with marked incapacity occurring within 3 to 5 years and death within 10 years, generally as a result of intercurrent infection or other complications of immobility.

This disease derives its name from progressive impairments of voluntary gaze. The majority of patients develop eye movement restrictions at approximately year 4 of the disease course. Patients are unable to voluntarily look downward or upward (upward gaze is less severely involved). Limitation of voluntary gaze is termed *supranuclear*. Because the vestibular nuclei are still able to direct eye movements, when the examiner abruptly tips the head, the eyes can be driven to look downward or upward. In addition to gaze palsy, patients with progressive supranuclear palsy often

exhibit macro-square wave jerks. During fixation, small brief saccadic-appearing eye movements occur every few seconds. These eye movements are involuntary and give the appearance of scanning eye movements around a small target.

As the disease progresses out of the early stages, it differentiates from the appearance of idiopathic Parkinson's disease. Resting tremor is usually mild, and the rigidity is more pronounced at the neck and trunk. Axial rigidity is often striking, giving patients a hyperextended neck with contracted facial muscles bearing an expression of sustained surprise. Gait is disturbed early in the course, with frequent falls in the majority of patients. Cognition is often affected, with personality changes, impaired judgment, and sometimes inappropriate laughing and crying. Unlike MSA, other than urinary incontinence, autonomic dysfunction is atypical.

No fully effective treatment is available. Treatment with levodopa may be partially effective at reducing the rigidity, although the dramatic response to levodopa that is experienced by patients with Parkinson's disease is usually lacking. Generally, any improvement is transient.

Chorea

Chorea is a flowing, continuous, random movement that flits from one part of the body to another. A variety of conditions are associated with chorea in the elderly patient. The pathologic basis for chorea is dysfunction of the striatum.

Choreiform movements that sometimes occur as an isolated symptom in persons 60 years and older are then called *senile chorea*. Involuntary complex movements of the face, mouth, and tongue may occur alone or with unilateral or bilateral limb movements. Neither mental disturbance nor family history of Huntington's chorea is associated with senile chorea. Pathologic findings often include degeneration of the putamen or caudate nucleus, or both.

Chorea may be treated with dopamine-receptor blocking medications (eg, haloperidol[OL]), but a potential adverse effect is tardive dyskinesia. Agents that block the release of dopamine presynaptically (eg, reserpine[OL]) are another option, as they are not associated with tardive dyskinesias; however, reserpine can be associated with depression and orthostatic hypotension. Metyrosine[OL] is an agent that inhibits the enzyme tyrosine hydroxylase, which catalyzes the conversion of tyrosine to dihydroxyphenylalanine (DOPA). Therefore, metyrosine blocks the formation of dopamine and can be effective in treating chorea. Though not associated with tardive phenomena, the medication may cause some somnolence. All of these medications can produce parkinsonism as a side effect,

OL Not approved by the U.S. Food and Drug Administration for this use.

Chapter 57: Neurologic Diseases and Disorders **465**

which is usually dose dependent and reversible when the medication is discontinued.

Drug-Induced Movement Disorders

A variety of different types of involuntary movements may arise as a result of the use of medications. It is important to distinguish acute drug effects, chronic but reversible drug effects, and chronic and irreversible drug effects. One acute drug effect that may happen with antipsychotic medications is an acute dystonic reaction resulting in oral, lingual, or nuchal dystonia. If it is severe enough, treatment with intravenous diphenhydramine or lorazepam may be required, although this approach in older adults should be exercised with caution, given the propensity for this agent to produce somnolence or confusion. Fortunately, acute dystonia occurs less frequently in older than in younger adults. Chronic reversible drug effects (effects that resolve upon discontinuation of the causative medication) include action tremor (eg, lithium, theophylline, valproic acid), parkinsonism (antipsychotic, antiemetic medications), chorea (estrogen, antiepileptic medications), or dystonia (dopamine replacement therapy in Parkinson's disease). Chronic irreversible drug effects or tardive phenomena often begin after the medication (usually an antipsychotic medication) has been in use for weeks to months. Movements may include orobuccal dyskinesias, dystonia, akathisia (sensation of needing to move), myoclonus, and tics. Advanced age and duration of treatment with antipsychotic medications are the only well-established risk factors for developing tardive movement disorders. Once the diagnosis of a tardive phenomenon is established, the clinician should attempt to reduce the dosage of medication or discontinue it. Treatment for tardive dyskinesia or tardive dystonia includes anticholinergic agents (trihexyphenidyl), baclofen[OL], reserpine[OL], or clozapine[OL], each of which must be used with caution in older adults. In cases of severe tardive dystonia in which there is neck jerking or sustained eye closure, intramuscular injections of botulinum toxin[OL] may reduce the frequency and severity of movements.

Essential Tremor

Essential tremor is the most common form of abnormal tremor. The tremor is an action tremor, which is present when the limbs are in active use (eg, while writing or while holding a cup). The tremor most commonly involves the arms, although the head and voice are also commonly involved. Other areas of the body may include the chin, tongue, and legs. The tremor is often slightly worse in one arm than in the other. One of the striking features of the tremor is that it has a varying amplitude so that during some moments the tremor is mild or even absent and during others it is severe. The tremor disappears when the arms are relaxed, that is, when the person is sitting with hands in the lap or when standing or walking with arms held at the sides. Functionally, the tremor may interfere with many daily activities, such as eating, writing, or fastening buttons. Stress or anxiety can exacerbate the tremor. The frequency of the tremor is in the 4- to 12-Hz range; because age is inversely related to the frequency of the tremor, older persons have slower tremor, which is often in the 4- to 8-Hz range.

The prevalence of the disorder increases with advancing age, with as many as 1% to 5% of persons aged 60 years and older affected. The age of onset seems to have a bimodal distribution, with peaks in the teens and 20s and in the 50s through the 70s. The prevalence rates among men and women are similar, although head tremor may be more common among women.

Between 17% and 100% of affected persons report having an affected relative, which suggests that there is a familial form of the tremor. In some families, many individuals are affected over several generations. Familial forms of the tremor have been linked to regions on chromosomes 2p and 3q. There are no apparent clinical differences between the familial and sporadic forms of essential tremor. The cause of the sporadic form of the illness is not known; age is the only known risk factor for essential tremor.

It may be difficult to distinguish essential tremor from several other conditions. Physiologic tremor, which is present in all people, varies in amplitude, and it may be more noticeable in some individuals. It may also be enhanced by anxiety, stimulants, hypoglycemia, medications, or certain illnesses (eg, hyperthyroidism). The tremor is often faster than that of essential tremor (8 to 12 Hz) and the amplitude lower. Although patients with Parkinson's disease most typically have a tremor at rest, they may also have an action tremor. In addition, if essential tremor is severe enough, it may even be present at rest. However, other features of Parkinson's disease (bradykinesia and rigidity) should not be present in persons with essential tremor.

The main indications for treatment of essential tremor are embarrassment and disability. The latter may manifest itself either as difficulty performing certain tasks (eg, eating and writing), modification in the way the task is performed (eg, only drinking with a straw out of closed cups), and even avoidance of certain tasks. Initial therapy includes β-blocking agents (eg, propranolol, atenolol[OL]), primidone[OL],

---

[OL] Not approved by the U.S. Food and Drug Administration for this use.

phenobarbital[OL], diazepam[OL], and newer agents, including gabapentin[OL] and clozapine[OL]. The response to these agents is variable (ie, some patients experience moderate improvement, whereas others experience none), and the tremor is rarely reduced to asymptomatic levels. Some patients with severe, medically refractory tremor may undergo deep brain (thalamic) stimulator surgery in which the ventral intermediate (VIM) nucleus of the thalamus is stimulated at high frequency with an implanted electrode. The treatment has been shown to be effective in controlling tremor.

EPILEPSY

A seizure is a paroxysmal excessive or hypersynchronous cerebral neuronal discharge, or both, that results in a transient change in motor function, sensation, or mental state. Recurrent seizures are the defining feature of epilepsy. Depending on whether the seizure discharges involve only a portion of the cortex or the entire cortex, seizures are broadly classified as partial or generalized. Partial seizures are subdivided on the basis of whether or not the seizure is associated with impairment of consciousness. Simple partial seizures do not impair consciousness and most often are associated with focal rhythmic motor twitching. Complex partial seizures are associated with alteration of consciousness and commonly amnesia for the event. Automatisms and other motor manifestations may occur with complex partial seizures. Generalized seizures in older adults are almost invariably convulsive ("grand mal").

New-onset seizures occur in a bimodal pattern with respect to age, with an initial peak in incidence within the first year of life and a second peak after the age of 60 years. Disease-specific causes of epilepsy are more common in older adults, and one-half or more of older adult patients with new-onset epilepsy have an underlying cause. Common causes include vascular disease, space-occupying lesions, brain trauma, alcohol withdrawal, and neurodegenerative diseases. Related to this is the observation that the incidence of partial seizures increases in older adults, whereas the incidence of generalized tonic-clonic seizures remains constant with respect to age. Beyond the age of 65, approximately one half of new-onset cases of epilepsy have a complex partial pattern. This pattern may be explained by the greater incidence of underlying focal lesions in older age groups.

Because of this propensity for new-onset cases of epilepsy to be harbingers of focal lesions, the work-up of older adults to exclude an underlying treatable cause is particularly important. The neurologic history and examination should aim to clinically characterize the seizure and localize its source, as well as elicit other signs of a focal lesion or a metabolic disturbance (eg, uremia, hepatic failure). Blood studies (blood urea nitrogen; serum levels of sodium, glucose, magnesium, calcium; and liver function tests), magnetic resonance imaging, and electroencephalography play important roles.

The treatment of epilepsy in older adults is particularly challenging. The prevalence of adverse drug-disease and drug-drug interactions increases with age. One example of a drug-disease interaction is that between anticonvulsants such as divalproex sodium and hepatic disease, given the tendency of divalproex and other anticonvulsants such as carbamazepine to exacerbate preexisting liver dysfunction, particularly in the older patient. In terms of drug-drug interactions, cimetidine and propranolol increase the serum concentrations of phenytoin and carbamazepine, respectively. Age-related changes in renal and hepatic function may alter drug metabolism significantly, so that older adults must often be placed on lower doses of antiepileptic drugs (AEDs). A sizable fraction of many AEDs is bound to plasma proteins. Since aging causes a reduced synthesis of albumin, it may be important to monitor free (unbound) levels of AEDs (eg, phenytoin). Older persons may be particularly sensitive to medication side effects. For example, AEDs may intensify an underlying dementia or exacerbate mild cognitive decline. Management questions invariably arise when treating older adults with AEDs. Even an experienced neurologist may seek the assistance of a clinical pharmacist to resolve issues of drug interactions, dosages, and side effects. Finally, there are a variety of reasons why older adults may have difficulty with adherence. It is particularly important in treating older adults to involve caregivers so that the goals of the treatment, side effects, and monitoring of progress may be understood.

There are a variety of AEDs, and most must be started slowly and the dose increased gradually (see Table 57.1). Reduction in seizure frequency and severity and the onset of side effects are the parameters that should be followed, not the blood level. If monotherapy has not adequately controlled the seizures and the dose has been maximized, then monotherapy with another agent should be tried before resorting to add-on therapy. Epilepsy surgery has become an increasingly common choice of patients whose seizures have proven refractory to pharmacologic management. The utility of surgery in elderly patients is not known. Discontinuing AEDs should be considered if the patient has not had a seizure for several years, particularly if the original seizure activity was a single or poorly characterized event.

[OL] Not approved by the U.S. Food and Drug Administration for this use.

Table 57.1—Antiepileptic Therapy in Older Adults

Drug	Dosage (*mg*)	Target Blood Level (μg/mL)	Comments (Metabolism, Excretion)
Carbamazepine	200–600 bid	4–12	Many drug interactions; mood stabilizer; occasional hyponatremia; thrombocytopenia, SIADH, leukopenia; sustained-release form available (L, K)
Gabapentin	300–600 tid	n.a.	Used as adjunct to other agents; adjust dose on basis of creatinine clearance (K)
Lamotrigine	100–300 bid	2–4	When used with valproic acid, begin at 25 mg qod, titrate to 25–100 mg bid (L, K)
Levetiracetam	500–1500 bid	n.a.	Adjust dose on basis of creatinine clearance (K)
Oxcarbazepine	300–1200 bid	n.a.	Many drug interactions; can cause hyponatremia, leukopenia (L)
Phenobarbital	30–60 bid–tid	20–40	Many drug interactions; not recommended for de novo use in older adults (L)
Phenytoin	200–300 qd	5–20*	Many drug interactions; exhibits nonlinear pharmacokinetics (L)
Tiagabine	2–12 bid–tid	n.a.	Adverse-event profile in older adults less well described (L)
Topiramate	25–100 qd–bid	n.a.	May affect cognitive functioning at high doses (L, K)
Valproic acid	250–750 tid	50–100	Can cause weight gain; several drug interactions; mood stabilizer; follow LFTs and platelets (L)
Zonisamide	100–400 qd	n.a.	Anorexia; contraindicated in patients with sulfonamide allergy

NOTE: bid = twice a day; K = metabolized via kidneys; L = metabolized via liver; LFTs = liver functions tests; n.a. = not available; qod = every other day; SIADH = syndrome of inappropriate secretion of antidiuretic hormones; tid = three times a day.

* Phenytoin is extensively bound to plasma albumin. In cases of hypoalbuminemia or marked renal insufficiency, calculate adjusted phenytoin concentration (C):

$$C_{adjusted} = \frac{C_{observed}\ (\mu g/mL)}{0.2 \times albumin\ (g/dL) + 0.1.}$$

If creatinine clearance < 10 mL/min, use:

$$C_{adjusted} = \frac{C_{observed}\ (\mu g/mL)}{0.1 \times albumin\ (g/dL) + 0.1.}$$

Obtaining a free phenytoin level is an alternate method for monitoring phenytoin in cases of hypoalbuminemia or marked renal insufficiency.
SOURCE: Adapted from Reuben DB, Herr K, Pacala JT, et al. *Geriatrics At Your Fingertips: 2006*. 8th ed. New York: American Geriatrics Society; 2006:141–142. Adapted with permission.

MOTOR NEURON DISEASE

Amyotrophic lateral sclerosis (ALS) is a neurodegenerative condition involving both upper and lower motor neuron cell bodies; it is characterized clinically by a progressive weakness and wasting of skeletal muscles, often in combination with bulbar palsy and respiratory failure. The incidence increases with age but reaches a plateau in the 60s. To date, age remains the single most clearly identifiable risk factor for this progressive and fatal disorder.

Patients commonly present with gait disturbance, falls, foot drop, weakness in grip, dysphagia, or dysarthria. On neurologic examination, patients may have a combination of upper motor neuron signs (hyperreflexia, clonus, extensor plantar responses) and lower motor neuron signs (weakness, atrophy fasciculations). Although cranial nerves may be involved, with weakness of the face tongue and pallet, the extraocular movements are usually spared. The electromyogram demonstrates findings consistent with diffuse denervation (diffuse fibrillation potentials, positive sharp waves) and poor recruitment of motor units. The differential diagnosis includes lesions at the level of the foramen magnum or the high cervical cord and vitamin-B_{12} deficiency. The prognosis is poor, with the average survival on the order of 2 to 3 years. The presence of bulbar signs carries a poorer prognosis.

Although most new cases of ALS occur in older adults, the incidence and prevalence of this disorder relative to other more common neurologic disorders is low. Therefore, gait disturbance and focal motor weakness may be attributed to the more common cerebrovascular diseases or to cervical radiculomyelopathy rather than to ALS. Older adults are also more likely to have coexisting neuropathology, adding to the challenge of and delay in diagnosing ALS. One study showed that those over the age of 65 years were diagnosed after 19 months, in comparison with those who were less than 65 years of age, who were diagnosed after 3 months.

The treatment is mostly supportive. Riluzole, which has demonstrated modest effects upon survival or time to tracheostomy, is now in widespread use. The action of riluzole is thought to protect against glutamate toxicity, which may be involved in the pathogenesis of ALS.

MYELOPATHY

In older persons, myelopathy or spinal cord dysfunction is most often the result of compression of the spinal cord. Most commonly affected is the cervical region. Intrinsic spinal cord lesions are often the result of spinal cord tumors or vascular events (infarcts or hemorrhages). Extrinsic compressive lesions are more prevalent; common causes among older patients are cervical spondylosis (with resultant osteophyte formation and degenerative disc disease), disc prolapse or herniation, rheumatoid arthritis resulting in vertebral body subluxation, or spinal metastases. Nearly 80% of patients aged 70 years or older have radiographic evidence of osteophyte formation with significant narrowing of the spinal canal; the majority of these cases are asymptomatic. Spinal stenosis is a congenitally, abnormally narrow spinal canal. When disc protrusion occurs in a patient with spinal stenosis, it further compromises the capacity of a spinal canal that is already limited. Narrowing of the cervical canal may lead to neck stiffness and pain; radicular pain, sensory loss, or weakness in the arm; and weakness and upper motor neuron signs (hyperreflexia, spasticity, Babinski's sign) in the lower extremities. Narrowing of the lumbar canal may lead to lower back pain, to radicular pain, sensory loss, or weakness in the legs, and to upper motor neuron signs in the legs. Other symptoms of spinal cord compression include gait disturbance, falls, or complaints of "numb, clumsy hands." On examination, the patient may exhibit spastic paraparesis (symmetric or asymmetric), sensory loss at a particular cord level, or problems with micturition.

Magnetic resonance imaging is the key diagnostic step. If the patient cannot tolerate this procedure because of the presence of metallic objects, a pacemaker, or severe claustrophobia, then spinal computed tomography with intrathecal contrast should be performed.

Conservative management, particularly if neck pain is an associated feature, includes activity modification, neck immobilization with a cervical collar, massage, heat treatment, physical therapy, and medications (muscle relaxants and pain medications, including nonsteroidal anti-inflammatory agents). Decompressive surgery is recommended for persistent pain or a progressive neurologic deficit. Older patients are more prone to have multiple levels of involvement, and some studies have suggested that their prognosis after surgery is poorer than that of younger patients.

RADICULOPATHY

Radiculopathy results from compression of a spinal root as it exits the spinal cord. Among older adults,

this may be the result of herniated discs or osteophyte formation. Symptomatic nerve root compression may result in complaints of pain radiating down the neck, back, arm, or leg, and on neurologic examination, this may be accompanied by motor and sensory deficits as well as diminution of reflexes in the distribution of a particular spinal root or roots. (See also "Back and Neck Pain," p 445.)

PERIPHERAL NEUROPATHY

The prevalence of peripheral neuropathy in older adults has been estimated to be as high as 20%, and some degree of subclinical decrement in peripheral nerve function on electromyography is probably universal in healthy older adults. Peripheral neuropathy may be particularly devastating in older adults because of gait impairment due to sensory and motor deficits and thus a propensity to fall. In developed countries, diabetic neuropathy is the most common form of neuropathy; up to 60% of patients who have diabetes mellitus and who are over the age of 60 years have a peripheral neuropathy. Several types of neuropathy are associated with diabetes mellitus, including a distal symmetric neuropathy, asymmetric neuropathies that may involve cranial nerves, roots, or plexus, and mononeuropathy multiplex. Other common causes of peripheral neuropathy in older adults are medications (eg, amiodarone, colchicine, phenytoin, lithium, vincristine, isoniazid), alcohol abuse, and nutritional deficiencies (eg, of vitamins B_6 and B_{12} as well as of thiamine, folate, and niacin), renal disease (ie, uremia), monoclonal gammopathy (eg, multiple myeloma), and neoplasm (eg, infiltration of peripheral nerves by malignant cells, paraneoplastic syndromes associated with oat cell carcinoma of the lung, breast cancer, ovarian cancer, renal cell carcinoma, and prostate cancer).

The treatment of the neuropathy depends on the cause, ranging from withdrawal of the causative agent (alcohol, medications) to nutritional supplementation (nutritional deficiency), or treatment of the primary cancer (neoplastic neuropathy). There is some evidence that optimizing glucose control may lessen the severity of diabetic neuropathy. Treatment of neuropathic pain includes the use of tricyclic antidepressants, anticonvulsant medications (eg, carbamazepine[OL], gabapentin[OL]—both are off-label uses except for specific neuropathies), and selective serotonin-reuptake inhibitors. Topical agents include capsaicin cream and local anesthetic medications. Another alternative may include the antidepressant duloxetine. Duloxetine is a serotonin-norepinephrine reuptake inhibitor (SNRI) in the same class as the antidepressant venlafaxine. It has

---

[OL] Not approved by the U.S. Food and Drug Administration for this use.

recently been approved by the U.S. Food and Drug Administration for the management of neuropathic pain.

MYOPATHY

Myopathies are characterized by proximal muscle weakness, wasting, and diminished or absent reflexes, and they may be accompanied by elevations in serum enzymes (creatinine kinase) and a myopathic pattern on electromyogram and on muscle biopsy (ie, fiber degeneration follows a random pattern). Older adults may attribute mild or moderate muscle weakness to aging and therefore may not immediately consult a physician. Proximal muscle weakness, which results in difficulty rising from a chair, difficulty in climbing stairs, or difficulty washing the hair, is particularly likely to be attributed to aging or arthritis.

The most common myopathies in older adults are polymyositis, endocrine myopathies, toxic myopathies, and myopathies associated with carcinoma. Polymyositis is a disorder of skeletal muscle of diverse causes characterized by an infiltration of the muscles with lymphocytes. Muscle biopsy usually shows signs of degeneration, regeneration, and infiltration by lymphocytes. Treatment with prednisone should be used with caution in older adults because of its propensity to produce psychosis. In thyrotoxic myopathy, weakness and wasting are greatest in the pelvic girdle muscles and to some extent in the muscles of the shoulder region. Reflexes may be normal, and the diagnosis is made by the distribution of muscle weakness in a patient with thyrotoxicosis. Improvement of the myopathy follows treatment of the underlying endocrine disorder. Hypothyroidism may also cause a myopathy that improves with thyroid replacement therapy. Myopathy may occasionally be the result of a remote effect of a cancer (ie, a paraneoplastic disorder), with complaints of weakness often preceding the establishment of a diagnosis of cancer. Several drugs cause myopathy, including corticosteroids, lipid-lowering agents, procainamide, and diuretics that produce hypokalemia.

RESTLESS LEGS SYNDROME

See "Sleep Problems" (p 252).

ANNOTATED REFERENCES

■ Edmeads J. Headaches in older people: how are they different in this age group? *Postgrad Med.* 1997;101(5):91–100.

> Although there is a decline in the prevalence of headaches with age, headaches are still a common condition in older adults. There are a number of special considerations in the diagnosis and management of older adults with headaches, including recognition of atypical ways that migraines may present, treatment with special regard for a reduced tolerance to medications, and diagnosing underlying systemic illness. The author discusses the more common causes of headaches in older adults, including migraine and tension headache, as well as those caused by diseases (eg, chronic obstructive pulmonary disease, intracranial mass lesions).

■ Olanow CW, Watts RL, Koller WC. An algorithm (decision tree) for the management of Parkinson's disease (2001): treatment guidelines. *Neurology.* 2001; 56(11 Supp 5):S1–S87.

> The short monographs in this series address the diagnosis and the nonpharmacologic, pharmacologic, and surgical therapies of Parkinson's disease. Particularly helpful are decision trees that address therapeutic options across the spectrum of disease severity and trees to assist the clinician in avoiding various therapeutic failures and combating medication side effects.

■ Pancioli AM, Broderick J, Kothari R, et al. Public perception of stroke warning signs and knowledge of potential risk factors. *JAMA.* 2000;279(16):1288–1292.

> Using random digit dialing, the authors interviewed 1880 persons to determine respondents' knowledge of stroke warning signs and risk factors. Over 1000 of the respondents were aged 65 years and older. Only 57% of the respondents correctly knew at least one of the established stroke warning signs, and 68% correctly listed at least one established stroke risk factor. Older patients, especially those 75 years or older, were less likely to correctly identify stroke warning signs or risk factors. The study implies that the education of adults, especially those who are elderly, regarding stroke warning signs and risk factors would improve stroke prevention and the timely management of acute strokes.

Coleman O. Martin, MD
Harold P. Adams, Jr., MD

CHAPTER 58—HEMATOLOGIC DISEASES AND DISORDERS

KEY POINTS

- The reserve capacity of hematopoiesis diminishes with advancing age.
- The possibility of a multifactorial cause should be considered when a patient with anemia of chronic disease has a hemoglobin below 10 g/dL.
- Concentrations of coagulation enzymes increase with age and lead to increased hypercoagulability.
- Polycythemia vera, essential thrombocythemia, and idiopathic myelofibrosis occur primarily in older persons and have a slow rate of spontaneous transformation to leukemia.

Hematopoiesis is regulated by a complex series of interactions between hematopoietic cells, their stromal microenvironment, and diffusible regulatory molecules that affect cellular proliferation. The orderly development of the hematopoietic system in vivo and the maintenance of homeostasis require that a strict balance be maintained between self-renewal, differentiation, maturation, and cell loss. Within the hematopoietic system, populations of terminally differentiated cells are continually entering the peripheral blood, to be replaced by cells from a transit or amplification compartment. Evaluation of the effect of age on hematopoiesis at the organ or cellular level demonstrates evidence of a diminished reserve capacity. Abnormalities in function, not evidenced in the basal state, become apparent in the stimulus-driven state. In addition to being lower, the aged response tends to be more variable. Given a comparable stress, hematologic abnormalities are likely to occur earlier and to be of greater severity in elderly than in younger persons. Thus, the rate of return of the hemoglobin to normal following phlebotomy is blunted, and the ability to mount a granulocyte response to infection is reduced. Numerous animal studies have shown a reduced ability of the aged hematopoietic system to respond to stimulation. Studies in humans have not been as conclusive. (See also "Biology," p 8.)

Although, there is no significant change in basal blood cell counts with aging, there does tend to be a modest increase in the prevalence of anemia. This is particularly noted in men 75 years and older, who in cross-sectional studies have significantly lower values than their younger counterparts (65 or younger). This large effect has not been noted in longitudinal studies. The mechanism for the difference is unclear but is thought to reflect the presence of comorbid illness or reduced erythropoietin (EPO) drive, or both, as a result of declines in androgen concentrations. There does not appear to be an impaired ability of older persons to increase their hematocrit in response to exogenous EPO or increase their granulocyte count following the administration of granulocyte colony-stimulating factor. There is also little evidence to suggest that leukocyte counts are consistently lower in older persons with bacterial infections or in response to a surgical insult. Thus, the severity of neutropenia following chemotherapy in older cancer patients is greater in those who are underweight and malnourished than in those who are not. Age appears to reduce the hematopoietic reserve capacity. This, however, is of clinical relevance only in the presence of other comorbidities (occult or latent) that also adversely effect functioning. In several observational studies, protein energy malnutrition has been reported as being in part responsible for age-related anemia. Thus, the evidence is that aging and illness combined lead to significant abnormalities.

Aging does not appear to affect the circulating concentrations of EPO and colony-stimulating factors; the increase in response to anemia or infection in older people is equal to that noted in their younger counterparts. However, in response to stress, the blunted hematopoietic response seen with age has been attributed to an impaired ability to release growth factors. This might explain the age-related reduced neutrophil response to infection seen in animal studies and may contribute to increased infection-induced morbidity with aging. The production of certain growth factors, particularly interleukin-6, appears to increase with aging. (See Table 44.1, p 333.) This has led to the notion that aging is accompanied by dysregulation of growth factor production, with overproduction of some and underproduction of other cytokines. An important question is whether aging affects the ability of the hematopoietic system to respond to injected growth factors such as EPO and granulocyte colony-stimulating factor. Current information suggests that in the absence of comorbidity, the response is unaffected by age.

ANEMIA

Clearly, the most common age-related hematologic abnormality, anemia, occurs in both older men and women. Studies have shown a high prevalence of anemia in hospitalized older persons, patients attending geriatric clinics, and institutionalized older persons. However, if stringent criteria are employed for the selection of apparently normal subjects, the prevalence drops. An analysis of the second National Health and Nutrition Education Survey demonstrated a significant reduction in hemoglobin levels with advancing age in apparently healthy men and a minimal although significant decrease in older women. There are few reports on the incidence of new cases of anemia in the elderly population. In the general population, the annual incidence of anemia is estimated to be 1% to 2%. Compared with this, the incidence of anemia in a well-defined population of elderly (> 65 years of age) whites attending the Mayo Clinic was reported to be four- to sixfold higher. Anemia was diagnosed in accordance with World Health Organization criteria, if the hemoglobin concentration was < 13 g/dL in men and < 12 g/dL in women. In this study, in every age group over 65 years, the incidence of anemia in men was higher than that in women. It has been suggested that reduced sensitivity to EPO occurs because of declines in testosterone concentrations. In several studies, the prevalence rate before age 80 is reported as being 8% to 10% in women and 12% to 14% in men. In the over-80-year cohort, the prevalence of anemia is 12% to 16% in women and 18% to 22% in men. At the time of diagnosis, > 50% of the patients had mild anemia (hemoglobin > 11.0 g/dL for women, and > 12.0 g/dL for men), and only 2% had a hemoglobin concentration lower than 10 g/dL. In over 80% of patients, the anemia was normocytic, with the cause either being multifactorial or anemia of chronic disease. Significantly, despite an exhaustive work-up, in 16% of the elderly persons the cause of the anemia remained uncertain. Whether this subset of patients represents the true anemia of aging remains unclear.

Presentation of Anemia

The presence of multiple pathologies in older persons often makes the evaluation of anemia difficult. In hospitalized patients, multiple disorders can contributed to the anemia. A classic example is a patient with active rheumatoid disease who has lost blood from aspirin ingestion. Similarly, protein-energy malnutrition or blood loss will markedly aggravate the anemia associated with neoplasia. Iron deficiency and vitamin-B_{12} deficiency may coexist, presenting confusing red blood cell indices. The possibility of a multifactorial causation—including blood loss, malnutrition, folate deficiency, or hemolysis—should always be considered when the anemia of chronic disease or inflammation is associated with a hemoglobin below 10 g/dL. In this circumstance, laboratory investigations commonly give equivocal results; hence, a bone marrow examination may be required. Clinical judgment is critically important in deciding how aggressive the work-up for anemia ought to be.

Work-up of Anemia

For practical purposes, we recommend 12 g/dL as a lower limit of normal for hemoglobin for both elderly men and elderly women. Attempting to define the cause of anemia when the hemoglobin concentration is between 12 and 14 g/dL rarely yields a cause. Even at a level of 12 g/dL, a decision as to how aggressively evaluate a patient with borderline low hematocrit must rest on clinical judgment. The complex nature of the problems that present in older persons, together with the high risk of simultaneous multiple pathologies, makes this decision much more critical. On the other hand, once a decision has been made to investigate low hemoglobin in an older person, the principles involved in assessment and evaluation are very similar to those that would be used in patients of any age.

The causes of the various anemias seen in elderly persons are summarized in Table 58.1. The initial approach to the patient with anemia must include a complete history and physical examination, as well as a complete blood cell count to allow evaluation of the production rate of red blood cells. Microcytosis (mean corpuscular volume [MCV] < 84) indicates an impairment of hemoglobin synthesis, and macrocytosis (MCV > 100) may be caused by reticulocytosis or more

Table 58.1—Physiologic Classification of Anemia

Hypoproliferative	Ineffective	Hemolytic

■ Iron-deficient erythropoiesis
  Iron deficiency
  Chronic disease
■ Erythropoietin lack
  Renal
  Endocrine
■ Stem-cell dysfunction
■ Aplastic anemia
	■ Macrocytic
	  Vitamin B_{12}
	  Folate
	  Myelodysplastic syndrome (refractory anemia)
	■ Microcytic
	  Thalassemia
	  Sideroblastic
	■ Normocytic
	  Myelodysplastic syndrome
		■ Immunologic
		  Idiopathic
		  Secondary
		■ Intrinsic
		  Metabolic
		  Abnormal hemoglobin
		■ Extrinsic
		  Mechanical

SOURCE: Data from Chatta GS, Lipschitz DA. Aging and hematopoiesis. In: Hazzard WR, Blass JP, Ettinger WH Jr., et al., eds. *Principles of Geriatric Medicine and Gerontology.* 5th ed. New York: McGraw-Hill Health Professions Division; 2003:763–770.

commonly by an abnormality in nuclear maturation. Red cell production is estimated from the reticulocyte production index. Hemolytic anemia usually has a reticulocyte index greater than 3, whereas a failure of production is indicated by a reticulocyte index of less than 2. Decreased production is caused by the hypoproliferative anemias or by ineffective erythropoiesis. An elevated lactate dehydrogenase (LDH) level and indirect hyperbilirubinemia result from the increased destruction of red cell precursors in the marrow and may be used to distinguish ineffective erythropoiesis from hypoproliferative anemia. A rational approach to the laboratory work-up of anemia is illustrated in Figure 58.1. A significantly elevated reticulocyte count, indirect hyperbilirubinemia, and an elevated LDH level are diagnostic of hemolytic anemia. A low reticulocyte count, elevated indirect bilirubin, and an elevated LDH level suggest ineffective erythropoiesis. In older persons with ineffective erythropoiesis, macrocytosis strongly suggests vitamin-B_{12} or folate deficiency, and microcytosis should suggest sideroblastic anemia.

The Hypoproliferative Anemias

Iron is the only nutrient that limits the rate of erythropoiesis. Thus, inadequate iron supply for erythropoiesis, the commonest cause of anemia in older persons, results in a hypoproliferative anemia. This is diagnosed by the presence of a decreased serum iron and a reduced transferrin saturation (serum iron divided by the total iron binding capacity, or TIBC, expressed as a percentage). Absolute iron deficiency (blood loss) is the commonest cause of iron-deficient erythropoiesis in younger persons. In the elderly person, the cause is more likely to be the "anemia of chronic disease" or anemia associated with inflammation. Iron-deficient erythropoiesis in these disorders results from a defective ability of the reticuloendothelial system to reutilize iron derived from senescent red cells. Thus, tissue iron stores are normal or increased, resulting in a serum ferritin concentration above 50 ng/mL and a reduction in the TIBC. This contrasts with a low serum ferritin and high TIBC, which reflect absent iron stores in blood-loss anemia. Blood-loss anemia, the anemia of inflammation and chronic disease, and the anemia associated with protein-energy malnutrition are the most prevalent anemias in elderly populations. Nutritional iron deficiency is very rare in the elderly age group, despite the prominence of other nutritional problems. When unexplained iron deficiency does occur, it is almost exclusively due to blood loss from the gastrointestinal tract. Angiodysplasia of the large bowel and diverticular disease are common causes but should be considered only once a neoplasm has been excluded. Rarely, iron deficiency can result from malabsorption or urinary losses of iron, which occur in the face of intravascular hemolysis.

The pathophysiology of the anemia of chronic disease is complex and is due to an inability of macrophages to release iron from the breakdown of senescent red cells. As a consequence, the serum iron falls and, as with blood-loss anemia, there is inadequate iron supply for erythropoiesis. In contrast to blood-loss anemia, in which iron stores are absent, in the anemia of chronic disease iron stores are normal or increased. Laboratory features include a mild anemia, a low serum iron, low transferrin saturation, and normal to increased iron stores (ferritin > 100 ng/mL). The term *anemia of chronic disease* is often used to explain an anemia associated with some other major disease process. Examples include cancer, collagen vascular disorders, rheumatoid arthritis, and inflammatory bowel disease. Occasionally, the anemia may be the initial manifestation of an occult disease. It is critical that this condition be distinguished from iron-deficiency (blood-loss) anemia, to avoid unnecessary gastrointestinal tests to identify a cause for blood loss and to prevent the inappropriate prescription of oral iron therapy.

Decreased EPO production accounts for the anemia of end-stage renal disease. EPO has been in clinical use since 1985 for patients with end-stage renal disease. In some instances, the anemia of cancer and chronic diseases is associated with inappropriately low EPO levels. Many cancer patients have anemia independently of any myelosuppressive therapy. The anemia is characterized by an inability to use iron stores and an inadequate EPO response. In addition, a component of the erythroid suppression is mediated by cytokines like interleukin-1, tumor necrosis factor alpha, and transforming growth factor beta. The precise incidence of cancer-related anemia is not known. However, a number of studies have documented a decrease in transfusion frequency, following treatment with EPO. Depending on symptoms, erythroid support is recommended for hemoglobin levels below 11 g/dL. EPO treatment should be instituted after excluding hemolysis and iron deficiency. Typically, the starting dose of EPO ranges from 20,000 to 40,000 units subcutaneously every week. If required, the dosage can be escalated to 60,000 units per week. Conversely, some patients require treatment only every 2 to 3 weeks. Hemoglobin levels should be monitored weekly, to avoid the vascular sequelae of an iatrogenic polycythemia. A target hemoglobin of 12 to 13 gm/dL is usually safe. Most patients respond within 4 to 6 weeks. Iron should be added to the regimen if ferritin levels fall below 50 ng/mL. If there is no reticulocyte response after 4 to 6 weeks of EPO treatment, therapy should be discontinued. Although it

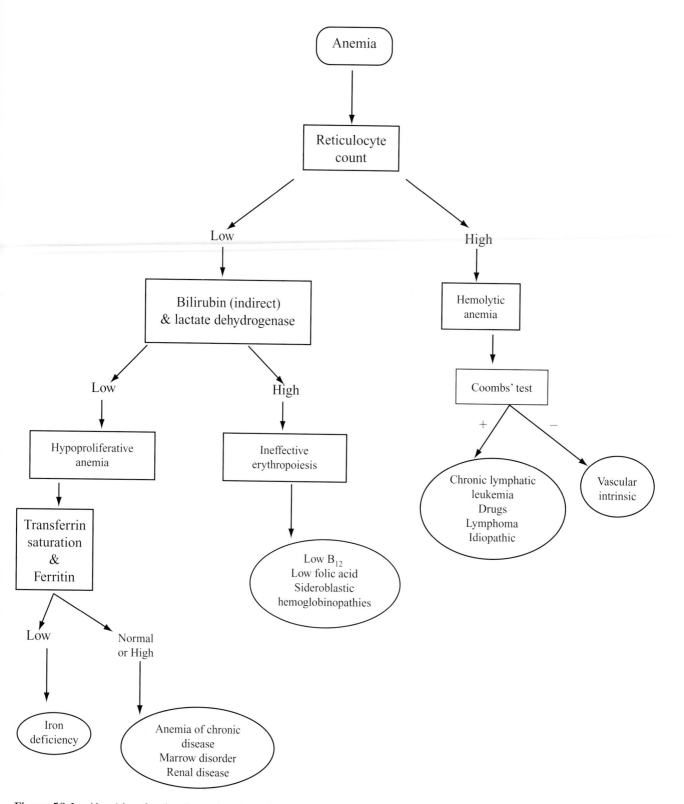

Figure 58.1—Algorithm for the diagnosis of anemia.

is difficult to prospectively identify responders, it has been reported that patients with endogenous EPO levels of < 200 mU/mL are most likely to respond to treatment with EPO.

Marrow failure due to interference with the proliferation of hematopoietic cells occurs in elderly persons. The disorder is generally associated with suppression of all marrow elements and is suggested by the presence of peripheral pancytopenia. Common causes include drugs, immune damage to the stem-cell population, intrinsic marrow lesions, and marrow replacement by malignant cells or fibrous tissue. The latter is usually associated with a myelophthisic blood picture (nucleated red cells, giant platelets, and metamyelocytes on smear) as a reflection of the disruption of marrow stromal architecture. The presence of pancytopenia and the absence of iron-deficient erythropoiesis is an indication for bone marrow aspiration and biopsy. Occasionally isolated suppression of erythropoiesis occurs, which is referred to as *pure red cell aplasia*. This disorder may be drug-related or may be caused by benign or malignant abnormalities of lymphocytes, including thymoma. These patients present with isolated anemia, an elevated serum iron, and absent erythroid precursors on bone marrow examination.

Ineffective Erythropoiesis

Macrocytic anemias in the elderly person result from vitamin-B_{12} and folate deficiency. The prevalence of pernicious anemia increases with advancing age. The disorder results from malabsorption of vitamin B_{12} as a consequence of the action of antibodies against gastric parietal cells and intrinsic factor. Atrophic gastritis and decreased secretion of intrinsic factor occur, resulting in failure of vitamin-B_{12} absorption. Pernicious anemia occurs most commonly in persons over the age of 60 and is more common in women. Although cobalamin deficiency is common with aging, anemia secondary to this is rare (see the section on vitamin B_{12}, folate and homosysteine, p 476). The presence of pancytopenia, macrocytosis, hypersegmented neutrophils in the peripheral smear, a decreased reticulocyte index, an increased LDH level, and indirect hypobilirubinemia suggests a diagnosis of megaloblastic anemia. The bone marrow classically shows giant metamyelocytes, hypersegmented neutrophils, and enlarged erythroid precursors with more hemoglobin than would be expected from the immaturity of their nuclei (nuclear cytoplasmic dissociation). Chronic pancreatitis and diseases of the distal ileum (blind loop syndrome) may also cause vitamin-B_{12} deficiency. The Schilling test is able to distinguish a deficiency of intrinsic factor (malabsorption corrected by ingested vitamin B_{12} and intrinsic factor) from an abnormality in the ability of the ileum to absorb the vitamin B_{12}–intrinsic factor complex (absorption still impaired with intrinsic factor plus vitamin B_{12}). Folate deficiency of sufficient severity to cause anemia in the elderly person is rare. Alcohol and various other drugs are also known to interfere with folate absorption and metabolism. Vulnerability to deficiency is significantly greater when folate requirements are increased as a result of inflammation, neoplastic disease, or hemolytic anemia.

The major causes of ineffective erythropoiesis and microcytosis are thalassemia and the sideroblastic anemias. Although thalassemia is generally diagnosed at an earlier age, there are reports of its initial detection in older people. Mild anemia, a disproportionately low MCV, and the absence of iron deficiency usually points to a diagnosis of thalassemia trait, a condition of little or no clinical consequence. Iron supplements have no role in the treatment of thalassemia trait; on the contrary, they can be detrimental. Acquired sideroblastic anemia is primarily a disease of elderly persons. It is a heterogenous group of disorders characterized by the presence of iron deposits in the mitochondria of normoblasts. The disorder is a consequence of impaired heme synthesis. It usually reflects an intrinsic marrow lesion (idiopathic) but may be secondary to inflammation, neoplasia, or drug ingestion. The common finding is the presence of a dimorphic red cell population, in part markedly hypochromic and in part well filled with hemoglobin. The diagnosis is made by the demonstration of ringed sideroblasts in the bone marrow as well as the presence of maturation abnormalities of myeloid and erythroid precursors. A fraction of elderly patients with sideroblastic anemia show some response to pharmacologic doses of pyridoxine (200 mg three times daily). This dosage should be given to all patients until it becomes apparent that a rise in hemoglobin concentration will not occur. For patients who are unresponsive to pyridoxine, the anemia must be treated symptomatically.

The myelodysplastic syndromes (MDS) are a group of stem-cell disorders characterized by disordered hematopoiesis that occur primarily in the elderly age group. Refractory anemia and refractory anemia with ringed sideroblasts account for 25% to 30% of the MDS syndromes. Refractory anemia commonly presents as a macrocytic anemia with marrow erythroid hyperplasia and relatively normal myeloid and megakaryocytic lineages. Cytogenetic abnormalities are relatively common in MDS, and one of particular interest in elderly patients is deletion of the long arm of chromosome 5 (5q−). The median age at presentation is 66 years, and the 5q− syndrome is characterized by macrocytic anemia, modest leukopenia, normal or increased platelet counts, marrow erythroid hypoplasia or hyperplasia, and female preponderance. Treatment of MDS in the elderly person tends to be supportive. The 5q− syndrome has a relatively good prognosis with a low propensity for transformation to an acute leukemia. Di Guglielmo's syndrome is another stem-cell disorder that is more common in older people; patients present with anemia that is characterized by megaloblastic erythroid precursors, dysplastic myeloid cells, and hyperplasia in the marrow. The disease usually evolves into an erythroleukemia, with an associated pancytopenia and the presence of nucleated red cells, and immature myeloid and megakaryocytic precursors in the circulation. Treatment is usually supportive.

Hemolytic Anemias

The causes of hemolytic anemia in elderly persons are somewhat different than in younger persons. Although most patients with congenital disorders will have been previously identified, an occasional older patient with congenital hemolytic anemia may present for the first time with symptoms related to cholelithiasis. Autoimmune hemolytic anemia is the commonest cause in the elderly age group: the diagnosis is made by the presence of a positive Coombs' test. In younger persons, a cause of the autoimmune hemolysis is only rarely identified. In the elderly person, on the other hand, the anemia is more likely to be associated with a lymphoproliferative disorder (non-Hodgkin's lymphoma or chronic lymphocytic leukemia), collagen vascular disease, or drug ingestion. Corticosteroids and splenectomy are usually effective in patients with red cell antibodies of the immunoglobulin G (IgG) type. Patients with red cell antibodies of the IgM variety are more likely to be refractory to such treatment. A disorder of some importance in older adults is microangiopathic hemolytic anemia, secondary to either disseminated intravascular coagulation (DIC) or occurring as a manifestation of the syndrome of thrombotic thrombocytopenic purpura (TTP). DIC is usually associated with severe infections or disseminated neoplasm and presents not only with hemolysis but also a consumptive coagulopathy. The presence of red cell fragmentation, thrombocytopenia, a prolonged prothrombin time and prolonged partial thromboplastin time, and hemosiderinuria suggests this diagnosis. Treatment of DIC entails treating the underlying disorder, as well as blood product support (including fresh frozen plasma and cryoprecipitate as needed). TTP is characterized by the pentad of fever, intravascular hemolysis, thrombocytopenia, neurologic symptoms, and renal dysfunction. In contrast to DIC, in TTP both the prothrombin time and partial thromboplastin time are normal. Early diagnosis is imperative, as TTP responds very well to treatment with plasmapheresis.

VITAMIN B₁₂, FOLATE, AND HOMOCYSTEINE

Older persons are more likely than younger persons to have lower levels of vitamin B_{12} and folate. In epidemiologic studies, approximately 10% of apparently healthy persons aged 70 and over were found to have vitamin-B_{12} levels that are deficient, and 5% to 10% were found to have low folate values. These low values may be clinically important. Methylmalonic acid levels are increased in the urine and serum, marrow deoxyuridine suppression is abnormal, and excretion of formiminoglutamic acid is increased. These tests tend to indicate functional abnormalities as a direct consequence of low vitamin B_{12} or folate. Pernicious anemia is rarely caused by vitamin-B_{12} deficiency. Atrophic gastritis leading to vitamin-B_{12} malabsorption is the likely cause in the majority of cases. This can also contribute to low folate levels in older persons. However, alcohol abuse, drug interactions with folate absorption, and inadequate dietary intake are the most common causes of low folate levels. Low vitamin-B_{12} and folate levels are not necessarily accompanied by macrocytosis or evidence of megaloblastic anemia. There is some evidence to suggest that low vitamin-B_{12} levels may contribute to cognitive decline in older persons. There is no question that severe vitamin B_{12}-deficiency can result in cognitive loss and significant neurologic deficits. In the older population with low vitamin-B_{12} levels, there is little evidence at the current time to indicate an important relationship between the vitamin and dementia. Nevertheless, aggressive replacement must always be undertaken when a demented patient presents with low levels of vitamin B_{12} or folate.

Low levels of vitamin B_{12} or folate are accompanied by increased levels of homocysteine. In recent years a great deal of attention has focused on the role of raised homocysteine levels in coronary artery disease risk. A relationship may exist between coronary artery disease and low vitamin B_{12} and elevated homocysteine in older persons. Levels of homocysteine can be reduced by prescribing 400 μg of folate acid once or twice daily. It is clear that deficiencies of vitamin B_{12} and folate are common in older persons and that the reductions have clinical relevance. Empiric prescription of vitamin B_{12} or folate for older persons with ischemic heart disease may be reasonable. Even in patients with atrophic gastritis, oral vitamin B_{12} is generally adequate; 10% will be absorbed by mass action alone and not require the presence of intrinsic factor. Thus, a daily dose of 1 mg vitamin B_{12} will replete a person with levels in the low-to-normal range. Parenteral replacement should be used in severe deficiencies with vitamin B_{12}, that is, levels below 100 pg/mL. It has been suggested that in elderly patients with low normal (< 350 pg/mL) B_{12} level, methylmalonic acid (MMA) levels be checked to exclude metabolically active B_{12} deficiency. Kidney failure can artificially raise the serum MMA level. Those patients with low-normal B_{12} levels and macrocytosis (with or without anemia) or neurologic changes should be considered for vitamin replacement, particularly if the MMA level is elevated.

PLATELETS AND COAGULATION

Platelet counts do not change with aging, but the concentrations of a large number of coagulation enzymes have been shown to increase with age. These include factors VII, VIII, and fibrinogen. In centenarians, highly significant increases in the concentrations of these factors are noted, as are levels of factors IX, X, and thrombin-antithrombin complexes. Fibrin formation is also increased, as evidenced by higher concentrations of fibrinopeptide A. In addition, elevated levels of D-dimers suggest increased hyperfibrinolysis. These facts suggest that aging may be accompanied by increased hypercoagulability. Hyperhomocysteinemia, secondary to low B_{12} levels, is also more common in the elderly age group and may be an additional factor associated with hypercoagulability. However, the very high level of clotting factors and evidence of hypercoagulability in remarkably healthy centenarians have also led to the suggestion that elevated coagulation factors may not be markers of increased risks of thrombosis.

Bleeding diatheses are not uncommon in older persons. Unexplained bruises, repeated nosebleeds, gastrointestinal losses, or excessive blood loss during surgery or following dental extraction are common presentations. In these patients, screening platelet counts and coagulation studies should be obtained. Tests of platelet aggregation are useful in detecting disorders of platelet function. Thrombocytopenia is a common cause of bleeding problems in older persons. A level less than 150,000 mL is considered significant, but bleeding usually occurs at much lower levels. Common causes include decreased production of platelets in the bone marrow, sequestration in enlarged spleens, and increased peripheral destruction. Decreased production of platelets occurs in the leukemias, marrow aplasia, or most commonly in older persons in association with drugs that suppress platelet production. The major cause of increased peripheral destruction is immune thrombocytopenia. A lymphoma, collagen vascular disease, or a drug-induced cause is common in older persons with autoimmune thrombocytopenia. Treatment of thrombocytopenia depends upon the cause. For decreased production, platelet transfusion should be considered if there is significant blood loss, irrespective of the platelet count. Generally, bleeding occurs when the count drops to 20,000 per μL or less. Since the immune thrombocytopenia is usually secondary in older persons, the initial approach is to identify and treat the primary cause. If no cause is found, a trial of corticosteroids is warranted. Isolated thrombocytopenia in the elderly person should prompt a work-up to exclude MDS, particularly when the low platelet count is thought to be secondary to inadequate production. DIC and TTP are also important causes of thrombocytopenia in the elderly age group, which ought to be recognized and treated appropriately.

Platelet function disorders (thrombopathy), although uncommon, can cause significant bleeding in older persons on aspirin therapy. Aspirin irreversibly acetylates cyclooxygenase, affecting arachidonic acid metabolism. The net effect is significant loss of platelet function. In the rare circumstance, spontaneous bleeding may occur or may be precipitated by injury or surgery. Platelet transfusions may be needed. Hereditary von Willebrand's disease may present initially in older persons. The disease is caused by a reduction in concentration of von Willebrand's factor (vWF) that is accompanied by reductions in factor-VIII concentrations. vWF is essential for normal platelet function, so bleeding occurs because of a platelet function defect. Acquired von Willebrand's disease, although rare, is a disease of older persons. It is commonly associated with monoclonal gammopathies, lymphomas, or myeloma. Monoclonal factor VIII does not contain the vWF factor, and viral contamination may occur with cryoprecipitates (which used to be the treatment of choice for von Willebrand's disease). When treatment is necessary, desmopressin acetate may be used. This synthetic analogue of arginine vasopressin stimulates endothelial cells to release stored vWF. Treatment is often successful, but adverse effects are common. In this circumstance, factor VIII concentrates that have high doses of vWF should be used.

Bleeding can also occur because of clotting factor deficiencies, which in the elderly person are usually acquired and caused by the presence of circulating clotting factor inhibitors. The most common is an acquired inhibitor to factor VIII. The onset is often sudden, titers to anti-factor VIII antibodies can be very high, and presentation is with bleeding into joints and muscle, similar to that in hemophilia A. Treatment involves factor replacement; depending on the severity, prednisone or cyclophosphamide may also be needed. Deficiency of the vitamin K–dependent clotting factors tends to occur in older persons with major illnesses. Disorders of the hepatobiliary tree, antibiotics that neutralize bowel bacteria (a major source of the vitamin), malabsorption, and severe malnutrition are the causes. Even if the patient was not prescribed warfarin, inappropriate use must be considered. The deficits are readily treated with vitamin K. (See the anticoagulation information in the Appendix, p 491). Liver disease must always be considered in patients who present with excessive bleeding. The prothrombin time is prolonged even in mild to moderate liver disease. The partial thromboplastin time remains normal until liver disease becomes severe. With the exception of factor VIII (which is produced by endothelial cells), liver disease causes reductions in all clotting factors. Liver disease is also associated with DIC. Fibrin degradation products are not cleared as well, and platelet function may be affected. The treatment of a bleeding diathesis in liver disease is fresh frozen plasma. A bleeding disorder will be thought of only if it is appropriately included in a differential diagnosis. This particularly applies to chronic blood loss from the gastrointestinal system. In those in whom endoscopic evaluation does not identify a cause, careful evaluation of platelets, including platelet functions and coagulation, should always be considered.

CHRONIC MYELOPROLIFERATIVE DISORDERS

The Philadelphia chromosome–negative chronic myeloproliferative disorders—polycythemia vera (PV), essential thrombocythemia (ET), idiopathic myelofibrosis (IMF)—have overlapping clinical features but exhibit different natural histories and different therapeutic requirements. All three disorders occur primarily in the elderly age group and are characterized by the involvement of a multipotent hematopoietic progenitor cell, marrow hypercellularity, overproduction of one or more marrow lineages, thrombotic and hemorrhagic diatheses, exuberant extramedullary hematopoiesis, and a slow rate of spontaneous transformation to acute leukemia. Thus PV, ET, and IMF have a long natural history, distinguishing them from chronic myeloid leukemia, the Philadelphia chromosome–positive myeloproliferative disorder, which progresses and transforms much more rapidly. The main cause of morbidity and mortality in PV and ET is thrombosis, which occurs more commonly in older patients or in those with previous vascular complications. Severe bleeding is rare and limited to patients with a very high platelet count or to those taking antiplatelet drugs. Cytotoxic therapy is effective in preventing thrombosis but increases the risk of leukemic transformation. Since there is no curative therapy for PV and ET, the goals of therapy are to minimize thrombotic risk and prevent progression to marrow fibrosis or acute leukemia, or both.

Several different treatment strategies for PV have been tested in randomized clinical trials. In the PV Study Group (PVSG-01) trial, 431 patients were randomized to one of the following: phlebotomy alone, 32P plus phlebotomy, or chlorambucil plus phlebotomy. The median survival in the three arms was 13.9 years, 11.8 years, and 8.9 years, respectively. In the phlebotomy-only arm, thrombotic deaths were higher, particularly in the first 2 to 3 years. In the other two arms, there was a higher incidence of leukemic transformation. The risk of thrombotic events is highest in patients aged 60 years or older and those with a prior history of thrombosis. The PVSG currently recommends:

- phlebotomy in all patients to keep the hematocrit below 0.45;

- myelosuppressive agents like 32P or busulfan in patients at high risk of thrombosis (> 60 years of age) and in those with excessive phlebotomy requirements;

- anagrelide, an antiplatelet agent for symptomatic thrombocytosis.

Finally, given the results of the European Collaboration on Low-dose Aspirin in Polycythemia Vera trial, in all patients with PV an antithrombotic strategy with low-dose aspirin is recommended. In this trial, 531 patients with PV with a hematocrit in the 0.46 range were randomized to no aspirin or low-dose aspirin. In the aspirin arm there was a 59% reduction in cardiovascular mortality, with a nonsignificant risk of increased bleeding.

The incidence of thrombotic and hemorrhagic complications in ET was recently analyzed in 1850 patients from 21 retrospective cohort studies. Rates of thrombosis and hemorrhage ranged from 7% to 17% and 8% to 14%. Age over 60 years, a prior thrombotic event, and a long duration of thrombocytosis are the major risk factors for thrombotic events. A very high platelet count ($1500 \times 10^9/L$) is a risk factor for bleeding. Consensus-based practice guidelines for ET include, first, observation in asymptomatic low-risk patients with platelet counts below $1500 \times 10^9/L$, and second, hydroxyurea plus aspirin in high-risk patients, which has been shown to be superior in a recent randomized clinical trial. Anagrelide, a new antiplatelet agent, is very effective at reducing high platelet counts. However, its efficacy as compared with hydroxyurea in reducing thrombotic events remains to be proven in a randomized controlled trial.

ET, like PV, has a long natural history with a low incidence of leukemic transformation. On the other hand, IMF progresses much more rapidly, with median survival in the 3.5- to 5.5-year range. Neoangiogenesis is a hallmark of IMF and is characterized by increased microvessel density in the marrow. It is also the basis of thalidomide-based trials in IMF, preliminary results from which look promising.

ANNOTATED REFERENCES

■ Ania BJ, Suman VJ, Fairbanks VF, et al. Incidence of anemia in older people: an epidemiologic study in a well defined population. *J Am Geriatr Soc*. 1997;45(7):825–831.

These investigators followed an inception cohort of older persons in Olmstead County, Minnesota, to determine the incidence of anemia. They conclude that anemia is significantly more common than it is suspected clinically and that the incidence rises with advancing age and is more common in men than in women. About half the cases were due to blood loss. The association of anemia with reduced survival was believed to be related to comorbid conditions rather than the low blood cell count.

■ Balducci L. Epidemiology of anemia in the elderly: information on diagnostic evaluation. *J Am Geriatr Soc*. 2003;51(3 Suppl):S2–S9.

This article, in a special edition of the journal devoted to anemia in elderly patients, offers a comprehensive review of the evaluation and treatment of the anemias. The suggested diagnostic algorithm places emphasis on red cell indices in the evaluation of patients whose reticulocyte count is low. There is a useful discussion of anemia of unknown cause, which may represent as many as a third of the cases of anemia among older persons in the ambulatory care setting.

■ Carmel R. Anemia and aging: an overview of clinical, diagnostic and biological issues. *Blood Reviews*. 2001;15(1):9–18.

This is an excellent overview of the causes and work-up of anemia in the elderly patient. It is particularly good at highlighting the controversies and recommending thoughtful solutions.

■ Chatta GS, Lipschitz DA. Aging and hematopoiesis. In: Hazzard WR, Blass JP, Ettinger WH Jr., et al., eds. *Principles of Geriatric Medicine and Gerontology*. 5th ed. New York: McGraw-Hill Health Professions Division; 2003:763–770.

This chapter provides a comprehensive review of age-related changes in hematopoiesis. The importance of external variables contributing to anemia is emphasized. Changes in growth factors and cell maturation in the lymphoid, myeloid, and erythroid lines are specified.

■ Clark R, Grimley Evans J, Schneede J, et al. Vitamin B_{12} and folate deficiency in later life. *Age Ageing*. 2004;33(1):34–41.

In this population-based cross-sectional analysis in Britain, the prevalence of deficiencies in vitamin B_{12} and folate was measured. As many as 5% of patients aged 65 to 74 have low levels of B_{12}, and the prevalence rises to 10% of patients aged 75 and older. Similar findings are reported for folate deficiency, but combined deficiencies are very uncommon.

Gurkamal S. Chatta, MD
David A. Lipschitz, MD, PhD

CHAPTER 59—ONCOLOGY

KEY POINTS

- Older patients and black Americans of all ages are more likely to develop cancer and present with more advanced disease.

- Epidemiologic data have not supported the long-held clinical dogma that cancers in older people are less aggressive or slower growing.

- There has been no demonstrated age-associated resistance to chemotherapy; further, acute toxicities (nausea, vomiting, and hair loss) are less prominent in older patients.

- Surgery, radiation, chemotherapy, and biologic therapy are safe and effective treatment modalities for older cancer patients when appropriate precautions are taken on the basis of the patient's comorbidities, vital organ functions, and medications.

Prevalence studies indicate that cancer is primarily a burden for geriatric populations. In fact, the median age for cancer in the United States is 70 years. Though cancer has long been recognized as a disease of older people, emphasis on geriatric issues and cancer is a recent development.

Three questions have arisen that form the underpinnings of this new emphasis:

- Why are tumors more common in elderly persons?

- Is there a difference in tumor aggressiveness with advancing age?

- Should treatment be different for the older patient?

Experimental data and clinical experience have indicated that tumors are not resistant to treatment by virtue of age alone. However, age is associated with slight reductions in certain organ functions, and these deficiencies in physiologic reserve might be magnified by comorbid conditions. Cancer treatments, especially chemotherapy, may therefore be associated with an increase in adverse events, and treatment should be tailored to the individual, taking into consideration potential increased toxicities and balancing this with expectations of survival in the context of comorbidities.

A review of the National Cancer Institute's Surveillance, Epidemiology and End Results (SEER) data revealed that more than 50% of all cancers are diagnosed in patients aged 65 years and older, and this older patient population incurs more than 60% of all cancer deaths. The data also reveal important trends. Whereas between 1968 and 1985 cancer mortality decreased 23% in patients younger than 55 years (primarily reflecting advances in the therapy of acute leukemias, Hodgkin's disease, non-Hodgkin's lymphomas, and testicular cancers), cancer mortality for those aged 55 years and older increased by 17%. Thus, in the older age groups we are faced with an increasingly prevalent disease for which modern therapies have not improved overall survival. We have much to learn about providing optimal management of cancer in elderly persons, but an emphasis on disease prevention and screening remains a logical priority.

CANCER BIOLOGY AND AGING

Explaining the Increased Prevalence of Cancer With Age

There are at least three reasons for the increased prevalence of cancer with age. First, cancers, particularly those that occur after menopause, are thought to develop over a long period, perhaps decades. This is best exemplified by the current understanding of colon cancer, which has been shown to develop because of an accumulation of several damaging genetic events occurring in a stochastic manner over time. Thus, if mutations are acquired at a constant rate, older people are more likely to have lived long enough to develop the 8 to 10 genetic lesions it takes to develop a malignancy. In contrast, lymphomas are just as likely to occur in young as old people. Lymphocytes normally undergo gene rearrangements and mutations to generate antigen receptors, and these processes appear to be particularly vulnerable to errors that may lead to lymphoma at any age.

A second reason for the greater prevalence of cancer with advancing age is that DNA repair mechanisms are thought to decline with age. As a consequence, cells may accumulate damage. Normally, a dividing cell pauses in G1 (the gap following mitosis [M] and before DNA replication [S]) and in G2 (the gap following S and before M) to take inventory and repair any damage before proceeding to the next phase. These are the G1 and G2 checkpoints. Older cells may fail to detect or repair damage and fail to

control DNA replication accurately. This leads to aneuploidy and to uncontrolled proliferation. In younger people, these aberrations may trigger the death of the cell; in older people, the errors may be tolerated and fail to signal cell death. Cells without functioning checkpoints are vulnerable to loss of growth control.

A third contribution to increased cancer incidence in older people may be a decline in the function of the immune system, particularly in cellular immunity. A number of findings suggest that the immune system can recognize and control certain cancers. A decline in immune function may lead to the emergence of a cancer in an older person that was controlled when that person was younger.

The Different Characteristics of Cancer With Age

There has been a long-held but incompletely documented clinical dogma that cancers in older people are less aggressive or slower growing. However, epidemiologic data from tumor registries or large clinical trials have not supported this notion. Such data may be confounded by geriatric problems that shorten survival independently of the cancer (eg, comorbidity, multiple medications, physician or family bias regarding diagnosis and treatment in elderly persons, and age-associated life stresses). These factors may counter any primary influence that aging might have on tumor aggressiveness. However, there is experimental support for the contention that there is reduced tumor aggressiveness with age. Data obtained from laboratory animals with a wide range of tumors under highly controlled circumstances demonstrate slower tumor growth, fewer experimental metastases, and longer survival in old mice. Tumor growth involves several levels of interaction between the tumor and the host. It may be that tumor angiogenesis is impaired in older people, thereby controlling the rate of tumor growth. The clinical importance of this is limited, inasmuch as it is difficult to know in any given patient whether the course of the disease will be characterized by an indolent or aggressive pattern of growth.

Breast cancer is the most notable clinical example of age-associated decline in tumor aggressiveness. Older patients are more likely to have more favorable histologic types, higher levels of estrogen and progesterone receptor expression, lower growth fraction, and less frequent metastases. In a published series on breast cancer patients with primary tumors of 1 cm (diameter) or less, the single most important predictor of metastasis to axillary nodes has consistently been found to be patient age: patients under the age of 50 years have the highest likelihood of spread, whereas those over the age of 70 years have the lowest likelihood of spread. Stage for stage, older patients seem to have longer survival than younger patients.

By contrast, Hodgkin's disease seems to be a more aggressive disease in older patients. The most likely reason for the age-associated differences in prognosis is that Hodgkin's disease is a different disease in patients aged 45 years and over than in younger patients. Incidence data demonstrate two distinct peak incidence rates, one at age 32 years and one at age 84 years. The frequency of particular histologic subtypes of Hodgkin's disease is different in younger and older patients; nodular sclerosis is the most common subtype in younger patients, mixed cellularity is the most common in older patients. In all reported treatment series, older age is an independent prognostic factor. Additional study is necessary to document age-associated differences in tumor cell biology.

Acute leukemia, like Hodgkin's disease, appears to be a different disease in older people; the MDR1 drug resistance pump is more commonly expressed, patients respond less well to treatment, and survival is shorter than in younger patients. However, for most cancer types, the molecular biology and clinical behavior of the tumor is similar across the age span.

Ethnic Differences in Cancer Incidence and Mortality

As the demographics of the U.S. population changes, additional information is needed on incidence and natural history differences in cancers occurring in different ethnic and racial groups. The U.S. Census Bureau estimates that by 2050, Hispanic Americans will account for nearly 25% of the population and black Americans, Asian Americans, and Native Americans will combine to total another 25%. Overall, black Americans have the highest cancer incidence and mortality rates. Cancer incidence among black Americans is 10% higher than among white Americans, 50% to 60% higher than among Hispanic Americans and Asian Americans, and more than twice as high as among Native Americans. The cancer death rate for black Americans is about 30% higher than for white Americans and more than twice as high as for Hispanic Americans, Asian Americans, and Native Americans. For the period from 1992 to 1998, 5-year survival for all cancers was 64% for white Americans and 53% for black Americans.

The factors contributing to the ethnic differences are not defined. However, certain data suggest that when the quality of the health care delivered to white and black Americans is similar, disease outcomes in the two groups are comparable. Specific incidence, diagnosis, and survival data for common cancers in different ethnic groups are provided in Table 59.1 and Table 59.2.

PRINCIPLES OF CANCER MANAGEMENT

Current forms of cancer treatment include surgery, radiation, cytotoxic chemotherapy, hormone manipulation, and biologic therapy. Age alone does not pre-

Table 59.1—Ethnic and Racial Differences in Cancer Incidence, United States, 1996–2000 *(per 100,000 population)*

Site	White Americans		Black Americans		Hispanic Americans		Asian Americans	
	Male	Female	Male	Female	Male	Female	Male	Female
All	555.9	431.8	696.8	406.3	419.3	312.2	392.0	306.9
Breast	—	140.8	—	121.7	—	89.8	—	97.2
Colon	64.1	46.2	72.4	56.2	49.8	32.9	57.2	38.8
Lung	79.4	51.9	120.4	54.8	46.1	24.4	62.1	28.4
Prostate	164.3	—	272.1	—	137.2	—	100.0	—

SOURCE: Data from: Ward E, Jemal A, Cokkinides V, et al. Cancer disparities by race/ethnicity and socioeconomic status. *CA Cancer J Clin.* 2004;54(2):78–93.

Table 59.2—Racial Differences in Cancer Diagnosis and Survival

Site	Advanced Disease at Diagnosis (%)		5-Year Survival (%)	
	White Americans	Black Americans	White Americans	Black Americans
Breast	33	43	88	74
Colon	19	24	63	53
Lung	38	40	15	12
Head and neck	55	73	60	36
Bladder	21	35	83	64
Endometrial	22	39	86	60

SOURCE: Data from: Jemal A, Tiwari RC, Murray T, et al. Cancer statistics, 2004. *CA Cancer J Clin.* 2004;54(1):8–29.

clude any of these approaches, but because of normal changes with age in certain organs and also age-associated conditions (comorbidities), special considerations are warranted.

Randomized clinical trials are the most reliable instrument to study medical intervention, and treatment decisions are best founded on the results of such work. However, despite efforts from the cooperative oncology groups, patients entered onto trials are by and large younger and presumably healthier than the typical geriatric patient with the same disorder. Furthermore, common end points of these trials are length of survival (for therapeutic interventions) or disease-specific deaths (for prevention studies), and these end points are not always the most appropriate outcomes for older patients (because of their inherently limited life expectancies on the basis of age alone).

Clinical researchers are making a start at addressing issues of geriatric oncology. New, more geriatrics-oriented trials focus more on symptom reduction and quality-of-life outcomes than on life expectancy. Surveys have indicated that older patients, when fully informed, most often choose life-extending treatments, even at the risk of toxicity. It is the physician and the patient's family that are most focused on quality-of-life issues. Furthermore, for the most part, tumors are not more resistant to treatment in older patients. It is also commonly appreciated that acute toxicities (nausea, vomiting, hair loss) are less prominent in older patients. Thus, although quality of life remains a primary treatment consideration, efforts at extending life should not be denied older patients on the basis of their age alone.

Cancer Screening

Screening is designed to detect disease in asymptomatic individuals with the hope that early-stage disease is more readily curable. Thus, to be useful, screening needs to identify mainly people who actually have disease, and the disease needs to have been shown to be more readily cured when found in asymptomatic people than in symptomatic people. Screening for colon cancer, cervical cancer, and probably breast cancer has been shown to save lives. Controlled prospective randomized trials are the only method of documenting the value of screening, and the study populations must be followed for many years to document the cancer cause-specific survival advantage to the screened group.

A screening test is evaluated on the basis of its capacity to distinguish people with authentic disease from those without disease. (For the terms used to assess screening tests, see the Appendix, p 502.) Screening is of greatest value when the disease being sought is common in the population being screened and the test being used is highly specific. The use of weakly specific tests in populations with low disease prevalence does not save lives. In some instances, more harm is done through morbidities and mortality associated with the diagnostic evaluation of positive screening tests than the good associated with early detection of cancer.

Screening is subject to three main types of bias: lead time, length, and selection biases. These biases can make a test appear to be effective when it actually is not. Lead time bias occurs when the underlying disease is not able to be affected by treatment. It results in earlier diagnosis but does not alter the time of death. Thus, the person spends more time as a patient, but the course of the disease is basically unaltered.

Length bias occurs when a test identifies clinically slowly progressive or nonprogressive disease that would never have become a symptomatic problem for the patient. Screening for prostate cancer is affected by length bias. Elevated prostate-specific antigen levels can detect cancers that will never cause the patient's death. This leads to overdiagnosis, the detection of "disease" that is of no consequence, also called *pseudodisease*.

Selection bias is based on the observation that people willing to be screened for cancer may not reflect the population as a whole. Volunteers may be more health conscious or have other personal habits that favorably influence prognosis. Thus, their outcome from screening may be better than what would be seen in a random population.

In addition to these biases, two additional issues are barriers to screening older persons for cancers. First, most of the large cancer clinical studies that have documented the efficacy of screening have systematically omitted the study of older people. Thus, it is not clear whether the benefits of a particular screening test initiated at age 50 extends to people at age 70 or 75. For prostate cancer, it is believed that screening is not indicated for someone with less than 10 years' life expectancy. For men without other comorbidities, this rule would suggest that men older than age 80 should not be screened. Data are not available in other cancers.

A second issue that complicates screening older persons is adherence to the screening schedule. Barriers to screening include a person's lack of information about the nature and value of screening and limited availability of economic and social support. The primary care physician has a central role in promoting screening. Published investigations have revealed that physician recommendation is the most important factor influencing cancer-screening adherence.

Several methods of improving adherence have been investigated. These include personal invitation letters, a plastic pocket-sized card as a reminder of screening deadlines, and personal visits with members of volunteer organizations who escort the person through the screening process. Adherence may be improved by streamlining the process, avoiding redundancies, prolonging the time interval between screening sessions, and coupling screening sessions with other office visits. An increase in the percentage of women aged 65 and older undergoing mammography may indicate the success of these approaches. (See also "Prevention," p 69.)

Chemotherapy

Aging may be associated with changes in key pharmacologic parameters of antineoplastic agents and in the susceptibility to end-organ toxicity (see Table 59.3).

The most consistent pharmacokinetic change of aging is a progressive delay in the elimination of renally excretable drugs because of a reduction in glomerular filtration rate. The more prolonged half-life of these agents may account in part for more severe toxicity. In a study of women aged 65 and older with metastatic breast cancer, doses of methotrexate and cyclophosphamide were modified according to the creatinine clearance. As a consequence, the myelotoxicity was markedly reduced without compromise of the therapeutic effect.

Owing to differences in their pharmacokinetics and pharmacodynamics, certain drugs may be particularly suitable for treating aged patients. Oral etoposide provides valuable palliation for small cell cancer of the lung and large cell lymphoma, with minimal risk of complications. Fludarabine, which is very active in lymphoproliferative neoplasms, induces apoptosis of cancer cells, a process that may be altered in malignancies occurring in older persons. Vinorelbine and gemcitabine are two newer agents that are active against lung and breast cancer and are well tolerated and effective in older patients.

Hormonal Therapy

Hormonal treatment is effective in cancers of the breast, the prostate, and the endometrium. Tamoxifen, a selective estrogen receptor modulator, has antagonistic and partial agonistic effects. It is a useful therapy in adjuvant treatment of breast cancer and also has estrogen-like positive effects on cardiovascular risk factors and bone disease. Other more selective drugs in this category, such as raloxifene, are in clinical testing. Although inactive as single agent, tamoxifen is syner-

Table 59.3—Chemotherapy Issues in Geriatric Oncology

Issue	Comments
General	Comorbidities and multiple medications add complexity
Pharmacokinetic changes	A progressive delay with age in the elimination of renally excreted drugs, due to a reduction in glomerular filtration rate, may account in part for more severe toxicity
Pharmacodynamic changes	Possible enhanced resistance with age to antitumor agents Increased expression of the multidrug resistance gene has been reported in some older patients Other proteins that result in drug efflux have been shown to have prognostic importance, but age-associated changes have not been described Increased tumor hypoxia with age has been observed in a murine model
Toxicity	Mucositis, cardiotoxicity, and peripheral and central neurotoxicity become more common and more severe with aging Cardiotoxicity is a complication of anthracyclines and anthraquinone, mitomycin C, and high-dose cyclophosphamide; the incidence of cardiotoxicity also increases with age Peripheral neurotoxicity with vincristine is more common and more severe in older patients The incidence of cerebellar toxicity from high-dose cytosine arabinoside increases with age
Myelotoxicity	Chemotherapy-related myelotoxicity may become more severe and more prolonged with aging, but moderately toxic treatment regimens, such as CMF (cyclophosphamide, methotrexate, fluorouracil), cisplatin and fluorouracil, and cisplatin and etoposide are tolerated by many patients aged 70 and older without life-threatening neutropenia or thrombocytopenia However, infections are markedly increased among older acute leukemia patients undergoing intensive induction treatment; in these cases it is possible that the disease itself, rather than an age-associated change in "marrow reserve," is responsible for the depletion of hemopoietic stem cells
Recent advances	Granulocyte colony-stimulating factor and granulocyte-macrophage colony-stimulating factor have reduced the incidence of neutropenic infections in patients receiving intensive treatment, and their effectiveness does not appear to be diminished with advancing patient age Certain new drugs or new formulations may be particularly suitable to the aged patient, eg, oral etoposide and fludarabine, gemcitabine, vinorelbine, capecitabine, paclitaxel protein-bound particles, and liposomal doxorubicin

gistic with chemotherapy in the management of malignant melanoma. Currently used hormonal agents are listed in Table 59.4. Most of these are well tolerated by older persons and commonly are the treatment of choice in this age group. Diethylstilbestrol is an estrogenic compound with serious cardiovascular risks (stroke, heart attack, thromboembolism) when used to treat prostate cancer in older men.

Biologic Therapy

Modulation of immune response is a particularly attractive option in treating the older person, whose natural defenses against cancer may be impaired by immune senescence. Only a limited number of options are clinically available, and these are clearly inadequate to restore a normal immune response in the aged person.

Recombinant α-interferon at moderate doses (eg, 3 million units, three times weekly) is reasonably well tolerated by patients of all ages. At higher doses α-interferon causes myelodepression, severe fatigue, flu-like illness, malaise, fever, neuropathy, and abnormalities of liver enzymes. There are reports of delirium, depression, and dementia following α-interferon use in persons aged 65 and older. More information on the safety of this compound in the elderly patient would be desirable. This is particularly important because interferon has been shown to be effective therapy for chronic myeloid leukemia, hairy cell leukemia, and multiple myeloma, hematologic malignancies that occur more commonly among elderly people. It may also prolong survival after chemotherapy for follicular lymphoma. It is being tested at higher, more toxic doses in patients with stage II melanoma after surgical resection of the primary lesion. About 15% of patients with metastatic melanoma may experience a partial response from α-interferon.

Interleukin-2 is used to treat metastatic melanoma and renal cancer. When administered daily at 3 million units per square meter, it may produce partial responses in about 15% of patients and complete remissions in about 5% of patients, many of which responses are long lasting. Interleukin-2 can produce severe dose-related toxicity, including capillary leak syndrome, hypotension, adult respiratory distress syndrome, cardiac arrhythmias, peripheral edema, renal failure (prerenal), cholestatic liver dysfunction, skin rashes, and thrombocytopenia. These complications tend to appear gradually in less severe form; generally, patients do not suddenly deteriorate. The toxicities reverse completely within a few days of stopping the drug. It is a strong clinical impression that interleukin-2 toxicities are less severe and develop later in older patients.

Monoclonal antibodies directed against CD20 (rituximab) expressed on B-cell lymphomas and against HER-2/*neu* (trastuzumab) expressed on breast cancer and other epithelial malignancies are effective treatments. In most patients the antibodies are given just before combination chemotherapy; the antibodies appear to augment the response to the drugs. These humanized antibodies generally have mild toxicities. Patients may develop hypotension or shortness of breath with the first infusion because of complement fixation. Symptoms clear when the infusion rate is slowed down, and such symptoms rarely recur. Other antibodies against cancers are in development.

Radiation Therapy

Radiation therapy provides palliation for virtually all cancers, and it may be part of a treatment plan for lymphomas and cancers of the prostate, bladder, cervix, esophagus, breast, and head and neck area. In combination with cytotoxic chemotherapy, radiation therapy has allowed organ preservation in cancers of the anus, bladder, and larynx, and in extremity sarcomas. A central issue for radiation therapy in the older patient is safety. There has been a trend for almost five decades to use radiation therapy as an alternative to surgery in poor surgical candidates, mainly patients aged 65 and older, with the implied expectation that such an approach is less toxic. In fact, published reports have indicated that radiation therapy is both safe and effective in older patients. However, there remains concern when treatment involves irradiation of the whole brain (fear of neurologic sequelae, including dementia) or pelvis (fear of marrow aplasia or myelodysplasia or radiation enteritis), but no systematic investigation has categorically substantiated these concerns.

Advances in radiation therapy include techniques that allow a more restricted radiation field, especially partial brain irradiation, new applications of brachytherapy (insertion of radiation sources into the tumor bed), the development of radiosurgery (gamma

Table 59.4—Hormonal Agents Commonly Used in Treating Cancer

Site	Hormonal Agents
Breast	Antiestrogens: tamoxifen, toremifene
	Progestational agents: medroxyprogesterone acetate
	Aromatase inhibitors: aminoglutethimide, letrozole, anastrozole, exemestane
Prostate	LH-RH analogs: goserelin, leuprolide
	Estrogens: diethylstilbestrol
	Antiandrogens: flutamide, bicalutamide
Endometrium	Progestational agents
	Antiestrogens

ray knife, a precisely focused external beam of radiation) that allows destruction of small lesions (diameter ≤ 4 cm) of the central nervous system without craniotomy, and the development of new radiosensitizers.

Surgery

Concerns related to cancer surgery in the older person are safety and rehabilitative potential. Several reports indicate that age itself is not a risk factor for elective cancer surgery, but the length of hospital stay and the time to full recovery become more prolonged with advancing age of the patient. Similar results have been reported both from referral centers and community hospitals.

Advances in anesthesia and surgery have benefited the older patient. Included among these are new endoscopic procedures that provide valuable palliation for the many tumors of the gastrointestinal tract, and the more widespread use of spinal anesthesia for major abdominal interventions, with a substantial decline in perioperative complications and mortality. More widespread use of laparoscopic surgical techniques and application of laser and photodynamic therapy is also broadening the surgical armamentarium and providing more older patients with potential palliation and cure.

The trend to manage cancer without deforming surgery may preclude the need for complex rehabilitation and may be of special value for older people. Organ preservation without compromise of treatment outcome is obtainable for cancer of the anus and of the larynx, and is being studied for cancers of the oropharynx, the esophagus, the bladder, and the vulva. Also, the use of initial (neoadjuvant) chemotherapy before primary surgery has been shown to be effective in patients with large primary breast and lung cancers. Such an approach results in less extensive and potentially more curative surgical procedures.

See also "Perioperative Care" (p 99).

Quality-of-Life Issues

Several studies have determined that the perception of quality of life is highly subjective and is poorly reproduced by external observers, even when these are close relationships or health care providers are very familiar with a person's physical condition. Furthermore, there is considerable discrepancy between the physician's determination of the patient's quality of life and the patient's own assessment; physicians tend to underestimate the patient's quality of life.

Early assessments of quality of life focused on functional status and freedom from pain, but these factors, though important, are inadequate to evaluate far-reaching consequences of serious diseases on all domains of life. In the past decade several instruments for the measurement of quality of life have been validated and have been successfully used to study specific problems, such as the effects on quality of life of intensive care, the consequences of limb amputation, of partial and total mastectomy, and of iatrogenic impotence. These instruments are questionnaires requesting a person to rate his or her own well-being in several dimensions with a categorical or a visual analogue scale. Unfortunately, these instruments have not been adjusted to the special needs of the older person. It is reasonable to assume that the importance of some factors, such as professional or job satisfaction, may decline with age, while the importance of others, including social support and the perception of family burden, may become more prominent.

Other problems related to assessing quality of life include the complexity of some questionnaires, which may overburden some older persons. In addition, little progress has been made in the assessment of quality of life in cognitively impaired persons. Studies of pain in demented persons have demonstrated the reliability of repetitive behavioral testing in the assessment of discomfort, even in patients with cognitive impairment. Perhaps the same principles may be applied to the assessment of quality of life in demented patients.

At present, the main application of quality-of-life assessment in clinical decision making concerns the choice between interventions yielding comparable survival. An area of potential use is in medical decisions involving limited survival benefits at the price of a decline in quality of life. At present, the value of this trade-off is evaluated with measures known as "quality of life adjusted survival" or "quality-adjusted time without symptoms or toxicity," both of which include complex interviews of limited application to persons aged 70 and older.

SPECIFIC CANCERS

Breast Cancer

Controversy surrounds several critical issues in the management of this most common malignancy in older women. These issues include the following.

Postoperative Irradiation Following Lumpectomy

Although irradiation following lumpectomy is safe in women aged 65 and older, it may be a source of significant inconvenience and cost to them. The value of postoperative irradiation has been questioned because the local recurrence rate of breast cancer may decrease with age, and the inconvenience of daily radiation treatment protocols may outweigh the limited benefits for some.

Need for Axillary Lymphadenectomy

Given the benefits regardless of nodal status of adjuvant tamoxifen in all postmenopausal women with estrogen-receptor positive breast cancer, axillary dissection when the axilla is clinically negative may add unnecessary morbidity. This is particularly true if the procedure requires general anesthesia. However, proponents of lymphadenectomy claim that the procedure not only has a staging function but may also improve the curability of breast cancer or reduce the duration of adjuvant tamoxifen treatment. In some centers, axillary dissection is being replaced by biopsy of the *sentinel node*, the first lymph node draining the area of the breast that harbors the cancer. This is determined at operation by injecting a dye into the site of the resected lump and removing the first node that turns blue. Early data suggest that sentinel node sampling is just as accurate as axillary dissection but considerably less toxic.

Adjuvant Hormonal Treatment

A meta-analysis of randomized trials established that adjuvant treatment with tamoxifen for at least 2 years prolongs both the disease-free survival and the overall survival of postmenopausal women. The benefits and risks of more prolonged treatment, especially for women over 70, are still controversial. Aromatase inhibitors are currently licensed as second-line hormonal treatment for patients who have progressed on tamoxifen. Recent trials of aromatase inhibitors have established them as first-line treatment in women with estrogen-receptor positive tumors. They are both more effective and less toxic than tamoxifen.

Initial Management of Metastatic Breast Cancer

Women aged 65 and older with metastatic, hormone receptor-positive breast cancer are likely to have effective palliation with hormonal therapy, such as tamoxifen. Hormonal treatment has also been shown to benefit older patients with hormone receptor–poor tumors, but chemotherapy has been shown to be safe and effective in this group of patients, as well.

Lung Cancer

Lung cancer is becoming increasingly common in older women for reasons that are not completely understood. The increase may be due to the more widespread smoking among women. In addition, some data suggest that women are at greater risk of developing lung cancer per unit of tobacco exposure. Lung cancer currently is the leading cause of cancer death in men and women. Early recognition and surgical resection remain the best chance for cure. For patients with lesions in a location that precludes surgery, occasionally localized radiation produces long-term survival. Over the past decade chemotherapy has been shown to produce clinical responses and provide effective palliation for a portion of the patients with metastatic disease. Prolongation of survival has been demonstrated, but the added increment is measured in weeks to months. New chemotherapeutic agents, such as vinorelbine and gemcitabine, and more established agents such as paclitaxel or docetaxel used in lower-dose weekly schedules, have proven to be effective treatments for older patients with lung cancer.

Colon Cancer

Two thirds of colon cancer cases occur in persons aged 65 years and over. With advancing age, there is a greater likelihood of right-sided lesions and presentations with anemia rather than pain. Colonoscopy has become the mainstay of diagnosis, primarily because it enables the gastroenterologist to directly visualize and biopsy the entire colon. Surgical excision may be adequate for lesions confined to the colon, but if extension to regional nodes is observed, postoperative adjuvant chemotherapy (usually 5-fluorouracil plus leucovorin) has been found to reduce recurrence by 40% to 50%. Survival of patients with disease metastatic to liver or other organs remains disappointing, despite the appearance of new drugs, such as irinotecan, capable of inducing partial remissions in a subset of patients. New drugs that target a tyrosine kinase (an integral enzyme for cellular proliferation) within tumor cells and neutralize vascular endothelial growth factor (thought to promote angiogenesis) are currently in development, and these offer great promise for future patients. Surgical excision of solitary hepatic lesions has been shown to offer survival advantage for selected patients, primarily those with smaller lesions, five or fewer lesions confined to a single hepatic lobe, and a longer interval from original tumor resection until the diagnosis of hepatic metastasis.

Prostate Cancer

See "Prostate Disease" (p 423).

Hematologic Malignancies

Leukemias

Acute myeloid leukemia (AML) following myelodysplastic syndromes, as occurs more commonly among elderly patients, is more likely to be refractory to treatment and to have a smoldering course, requiring only supportive care. What is not clear is whether the prevalence of unfavorable cytogenetic abnormalities and of multilineage neoplastic involvement increases with age in de novo AML. The subset of myelodysplasia patients who do not have excess blasts or overt leukemia but are neutropenic and have recurrent infections may benefit from intermittent granulocyte colony-stimulating factor.

In a trial with older patients with AML, the effectiveness of delayed treatment was found to be much inferior to that of immediate treatment. Although this study established the value of timely chemotherapy, the choice of treatment (whether full-dose induction or low-dose cytarabine) remains controversial. In one study the survival of older patients with leukemia treated with low-dose cytarabine was found to be superior to the survival of those receiving standard induction, because of lower treatment-related mortality. Others have obtained different results and claimed the superiority of standard treatment.

Chronic Lymphocytic Leukemia

Chronic lymphocytic leukemia (CLL) is the most common form of leukemia in the Western world; about 12,500 cases are diagnosed each year in the United States. The incidence is declining for unknown reasons. The median age at diagnosis is 61 years. The diagnosis is most often made incidentally when a peripheral white blood cell count reveals leukocytosis with a small lymphocyte count above 4,000/μL. Treatment is generally withheld until it is required to control a life-threatening or symptomatic complication. The major complications of the disease are infection and marrow failure. Because about 25% of patients develop autoimmune anemia or thrombocytopenia some time in the course of the disease, it is important to investigate the mechanism of any decline in peripheral blood cell counts. Autoimmune mechanisms can be treated with glucocorticoids or splenectomy, whereas marrow infiltration by tumor cells requires antitumor therapy. Chlorambucil and fludarabine are the two most active agents. Median survival varies with the stage of disease. Once anemia or thrombocytopenia develop as a consequence of marrow failure, median survival is about 18 months.

Non-Hodgkin's Lymphoma

The prognosis of low- and intermediate-grade non-Hodgkin's lymphoma worsens with age, but the explanation remains unclear. It is possible that older patients have more aggressive variants or, equally likely, that older patients are increasingly susceptible to the complications of intensive treatment.

The treatment of older persons with intermediate-grade large cell lymphoma is controversial. As many as 30% of such patients obtain a durable complete remission with standard treatment (CHOP, ie, cyclophosphamide, doxorubicin, vincristine, prednisone). Administration of lower-than-normal doses results in a poorer outcome. Whether hematopoietic growth factors can lessen the hematopoietic toxicity of treatment has not been specifically addressed in the aged population. The outcome of CHOP treatment in the most common form of lymphoma (diffuse large B-cell lymphoma) appears to be significantly improved by the addition of rituximab, a monoclonal antibody directed at CD20 expressed on B cells.

Hodgkin's Disease

Hodgkin's disease exhibits a curious bimodal age-incidence curve, with a second peak late in life. There have been earlier reports that older patients with advanced disease respond less well to therapy and that their survival is shorter. Several factors may contribute: more extensive disease at presentation, biologic differences from authentic Hodgkin's disease, greater toxicity with standard treatment regimens, or the provision of less aggressive treatment. Each of these factors may be involved. Most older patients tolerate full doses of ABVD (ie, doxorubicin, bleomycin, vinblastine, dacarbazine) without life-threatening bone-marrow toxicity.

Multiple Myeloma

Multiple myeloma is diagnosed in about 14,400 people each year in the United States. The median age at diagnosis is 68 years; it is rare in people younger than 40 years. Black Americans have twice the incidence of white Americans. The classic triad of myeloma is marrow plasmacytosis (> 10%), lytic bone lesions, and a serum or urine, or both, monoclonal gammopathy. Monoclonal gammopathy is common in older people, estimated at 6% of persons aged 70 or older. Distinguishing myeloma from monoclonal gammopathy of uncertain significance is important. When an abnormal paraprotein is discovered on serum immunoelectrophoresis, the best diagnostic test to identify myeloma is a skeletal survey. However, if the skeletal survey is normal, a bone marrow biopsy is still indicated to determine the presence of marrow plasmacytosis. Patients with monoclonal gammopathy of uncertain significance do not have lytic bone lesions and usually do not have the other features of myeloma, including hypercalcemia, renal failure, anemia, or susceptibility to infection, and marrow plasma cells are less than 10% of the total cell number. Patients with myeloma require treatment when the lytic bone lesions become symptomatic or progressive, recurrent infections occur, or the serum paraprotein increases. Standard treatment consists of intermittent pulses of an oral alkylating agent and prednisone given for 4 to 7 days every 4 to 6 weeks. Supportive care includes bisphosphonates to decrease bone turnover, erythropoietin and other hematinics for the anemia, intravenous immunoglobulin for recurrent infections, radiation to specific symptomatic bone lesions, maintenance of hydration to preserve renal function, and adequate analgesia.

PRINCIPLES OF MANAGEMENT

Both the incidence and prevalence of cancer increase with age, and older persons more often present with advanced-stage disease. Efforts to screen the older population for common cancers (such as colon, breast, and prostate) before they experience symptoms are likely to discover earlier and more curable lesions. Older patients may have less physiologic reserve than younger patients, but unless a specific comorbid illness is influencing baseline organ function, cancer treatments with curative or palliative potential should be offered to most patients in most settings, regardless of age. Curative surgical procedures may require more prolonged convalescence, but recovery from most procedures is expected. Radiation therapy is safe and effective in the same settings it is used in younger patients. Chemotherapy may need to be adjusted to the individual patient's level of tolerance of the adverse effects, but usually the changes should be made in the face of toxicities actually encountered rather than toxicities anticipated. Biologic therapies are usually safe; some produce less toxicity in older than in younger patients.

See also "Dermatologic Diseases and Disorders" (p 309) for the diagnosis and treatment of skin cancers, and "Persistent Pain" (p 140) and "Palliative Care" (p 133) for the management of pain and end-of-life care.

ANNOTATED REFERENCES

■ Bach PB, Schrag D, Brawley OW, et al. Survival of blacks and whites after a cancer diagnosis. *JAMA.* 2002; 287(16):2106–2113.

> This meta-analysis involving over 220,000 patients suggests that the cancer-specific hazard ratio for deaths in blacks relative to whites was only 1.07 when both received similar treatment. Of the 14 cancers examined, death rates for cancer of the breast, uterus, and bladder were higher among blacks than whites.

■ Balducci L, Lyman GH, Ershler WB et al., eds. *Comprehensive Geriatric Oncology.* 2nd ed. Philadelphia: Lippincott Williams and Wilkins; 2004.

> This authoritative text by more than 75 contributing authors provides a thorough discussion of the issues of aging and cancer. Exhaustive in certain areas, the volume is a reference resource for the accumulated wisdom in this developing clinical subspecialty. Several chapters are focused on general management of cancer in the older patient; others cover rehabilitation and supportive care; and many cover specific cancers. This is the most comprehensive resource available on the topic of geriatric oncology.

■ Muss HB, Longo DL, eds. Cancer in the elderly. *Semin Oncol.* 2004;31:125–296.

> This indexed, multiauthor volume provides a useful resource on issues of geriatric oncology. Chapters on medical-legal issues and end-of-life care are included with reviews of specific tumor types and general treatment considerations. Aging-related effects on chemotherapy, radiation therapy, and surgery efficacy and toxicity are also discussed.

■ Sundararajan V, Grann VR, Jacobson JS, et al. Variations in the use of adjuvant chemotherapy for node-positive colon cancer in the elderly: a population-based study. *Cancer J.* 2001;7:213–219.

> This novel analysis depended upon the merging of the National Cancer Institute's Surveillance, Epidemiology, and End Results (SEER) database with Medicare records and found the very disturbing information that only about one half of patients with node-positive colon cancer who are aged 65 or over actually receive life-extending adjuvant therapy with a 5-fluorouracil-based regimen. Elderly black Americans were even less likely to receive such therapy than were elderly white Americans (41% versus 51%). The basis for this failure of the health care delivery system must be discerned and corrected.

William B. Ershler, MD
Dan L. Longo, MD

APPENDIX CONTENTS

ANTICOAGULATION

Warfarin Therapy

Prescribing Warfarin

- For anticoagulation in nonacute conditions, initiate therapy by giving warfarin (Coumadin, Carfin, Sofarin) 2–5 mg/day as fixed dose [T: 1, 2, 2.5, 3, 4, 5, 6, 7.5, 10]; reduce dose if INR > 2.5 on day 3.
- Half-life is 31–51 hours; steady state is achieved on day 5–7 of fixed dose.
- Warfarin therapy is implicated in **many** adverse drug-drug interactions.
- Some drugs that **increase** INR in conjunction with warfarin:

alcohol (with concurrent liver disease)	cimetidine	metolazone
amiodarone	clofibrate	miconazole
androgens	clotrimazole	piroxicam
antibiotics (many)	fluconazole	propafenone
acetaminophen (> 1.3 g/day > 1 week)	flu vaccine	propranolol
acetylsalicylic acid or aspirin (> 3 g/day)	isoniazid	sulindac
chloral hydrate	ketoprofen	tolmetin
		trimethoprim

- Some drugs that **decrease** INR in conjunction with warfarin

barbiturates	dicloxacillin	rifampin
carbamazepine	etretinate	sucralfate
cholestyramine	griseofulvin	trazodone
cyclosporine	nafcillin	vitamin K

Indications for Anticoagulation in the Absence of Active Bleeding or Severe Bleeding Risk

Condition	Target INR	Duration of Therapy
Hip or major knee surgery	2.0–3.0	At least 7–10 days
Idiopathic venous thromboembolism (includes pulmonary embolism)	2.0–3.0	At least 6–12 months*
Atrial fibrillation	2.0–3.0	Indefinitely
Mitral valvular heart disease with history of systemic embolization or left atrial diameter > 5.5 cm	2.0–3.0	Indefinitely
Cardiomyopathy with ejection fraction < 25%	2.0–3.0	Indefinitely
Mechanical aortic valve with normal left atrial size and sinus rhythm	2.0–3.0**	Indefinitely
Mechanical aortic valve with enlarged left atrium or atrial fibrillation or both	2.5–3.5**†	Indefinitely
Mechanical mitral valve	2.5–3.5**†	Indefinitely
Caged ball or caged disk valve	2.5–3.5‡	Indefinitely
Bioprosthetic heart valve	2.0–3.0	3 months
Acute myocardial infarction complicated by severe left ventricular dysfunction, heart failure, previous emboli, mural thrombus on echocardiography	2.0–3.0	1–3 months

* For first event of idiopathic deep-vein thrombosis or pulmonary embolism, consider indefinite anticoagulation, particularly after cases of life-threatening embolism or in patients with thrombophilia such as Factor V Leiden mutations.

** If additional risk factors are present or if there is systemic embolism despite anticoagulation treatment, target INR is 2.5–3.5 and aspirin 80–100 mg/day should be added.

† Alternative target INR 2.0–3.0 with addition of aspirin 80–100 mg/day.

‡ With addition of aspirin 80–100 mg/day.

Treatment of Warfarin Overdose

INR	Clinical Situation	Action
≥ 3.5 and < 5.0	No significant bleeding	Omit next warfarin dose or lower dose or both
≥ 5.0 and < 9.0	No significant bleeding	Omit next 1–2 doses of warfarin and restart therapy at lower dose; alternatively, omit 1 dose and give VK 1.0–2.5 mg po
≥ 9.0	No significant bleeding	Discontinue warfarin and give VK 3.0–10.0 mg po; give additional VK po if INR is not substantially reduced in 24–48 hours. Restart warfarin at lower dose when INR is therapeutic.
Any elevation	Serious bleeding	Discontinue warfarin; give VK 10.0 mg by slow IV infusion, supplemented with fresh frozen plasma or prothrombin complex concentrate depending on urgency of situation; check INR every 6 hours; repeat VK every 12 hours as needed
Any elevation	Life-threatening bleeding	Discontinue warfarin; give VK 10.0 mg by slow IV infusion, supplemented with prothrombin complex concentrate; repeat this treatment as needed

NOTE: IV = intravenous; po = by mouth; VK = vitamin K.

SOURCE: Data from American College of Chest Physicians Consensus Panel on Antithrombotic Therapy: Ansell J, Hirsch J, Pollar L, et al. The pharmacology and management of the vitamin K antagonists.. In: Seventh ACCP Conference on Antithrombotic and Thrombolytic Therapy. *Chest.* 2004; 126:204S–233S.

Acute Anticoagulation

Anticoagulants for Deep-Vein Thrombosis or Pulmonary Embolism Prophylaxis and Treatment

Class, Agent	Prophylaxis Dosage By Condition Type	Treatment Dosage	Comments
Heparin			
Unfractionated heparin (Hep-Lock)	General surgery: 5000 U SC 2 h before and q 12 h after surgery	5000 U/kg IV bolus followed by 15 mg/kg/h IV*	Bleeding, anemia, thrombocytopenia, hypertransaminasemia, urticaria (L, K)
Low-Molecular-Weight Heparin			
Enoxaparin (Lovenox)	THA, HFX: 30 mg SC q 12 h or 40 mg SC qd KR: 30 mg SC q 12 h AS: 40 mg SC qd	Outpatient treatment of DVT: 1 mg/kg SC q 12 h; inpatient treatment of DVT ± PE: 1 mg/kg SC q 12 h or 1.5 mg/kg SC qd*	Bleeding, anemia, hyperkalemia, hypertransaminasemia, thrombocytopenia, thrombocytosis, urticaria, angioedema (K)
Dalteparin (Fragmin)	Low-risk THA: 2500–5000 U SC before surgery, 5000 U SC qd after surgery Abdominal surgery: 2500–5000 U SC before and after surgery	DVT: 100 U/kg SC q 12 h; also indicated for anticoagulation in acute coronary syndrome	Same (K)
Tinzaparin (Innohep)	NA	175 anti-Xa IU/kg SC qd*	Same (K)
Heparinoid			
Danaparoid (Orgaran)	THA, HFX, HIT: 750 anti-Xa U SC bid	NA	Same as LMWH (K)
Factor Xa Inhibitor			
Fondaparinux (Arixtra)	THA, HFX, KR: 2.5 mg SC qd beginning 6–8 h after surgery	Weight < 50 kg: 5 mg SC qd; weight 50–100 kg: 7.5 mg SC qd; weight > 100 kg: 10 mg SC qd	Contraindicated if CrCl <30 mL/min (K)

(table continued on next page)

Anticoagulants for Deep-Vein Thrombosis or Pulmonary Embolism Prophylaxis and Treatment (continued)

Class, Agent	Prophylaxis Dosage By Condition Type	Treatment Dosage	Comments
Direct Thrombin Inhibitors			
Argatroban	HIT: 2 µg/kg/min IV infusion	HIT: 2 µg/kg/min IV infusion	Decrease dosage if hepatic impairment (L)
Lepirudin (Refludan)	HIT: 4 mg/kg bolus, then 0.15 mg/kg/h	HIT: 4 mg/kg bolus, then 0.15 mg/kg/h	Decrease bolus to 0.2 mg/kg if CrCl < 60
Thrombolytics			
Streptokinase (Kabikinase, Streptase)	NA	250,000 U IV over 30 min, then 100,000 U/h for 24 h†	Risk of hemorrhage increased with age and higher BMI; HTN, hallucination, agitation, confusion, serum sickness (L)

NOTE: AS = aortic stenosis; bid = twice a day; BMI = body mass index; CrCl = creatinine clearance; d = day(s); DVT = deep-vein thrombosis; H = hepatic elimination; h = hour(s); HFX = hip fracture surgery; HIT = heparin-induced thrombocytopenia; HTN = hypertension; IV = intravenous(ly); K = renal elimination; KR = knee replacement; LMWH = low-molecular-weight heparin; NA = not applicable; q = each, every; SC = subcutaneous(ly); THA = total hip arthroplasty (hip replacement).

* Also indicated for anticoagulation in acute coronary syndrome.

† Dose in acute myocardial infarction is 1.5 million U IV over 60 minutes.

Source

Reuben DB, Herr KA, Pacala JT, et al. *Geriatrics At Your Fingertips 2006*. 8th ed. New York: The American Geriatrics Society; 2006:18–20. Reprinted with permission.

ASSISTED LIVING FACILITIES POSITION STATEMENT

Health Care Systems Committee, American Geriatrics Society

Background

The American Geriatrics Society (AGS) believes that Assisted Living Facilities (ALF) can offer seniors an environment that could enhance their health status over other possible living arrangements. This Position Statement is to provide policymakers, administrators, health care professionals, and consumers with guidance for achieving optimum outcomes with regards to ALFs.

Positions

The following principles are essential to realizing the potential benefits of ALFs.

1. ALFs have a responsibility to provide complete information to prospective residents to assure that an appropriate match is made between resident and facility.

Rationale: Consumers of ALFs need to have detailed information regarding the services provided and any associated costs. In contrast to nursing facilities whose primary payor are the states through Medicaid, ALF payors tend to be the residents themselves. As a result, ALFs are subject to less state and federal regulation and are more affected by market pressures. In order for consumers to make optimal decisions, ALFs need to disclose fully the services provided, the limitations of their facility, how much functional decline they can handle effectively, and especially the criteria residents must continue to meet to remain in the ALF. In addition, the staffing levels and expertise should be discussed with all potential ALF residents.

Reference: Hawes C, Phillips C, Rose M. (2000) High Service or High Privacy Assisted Living Facilities, their Residents and Staff: Results from a National Survey. Miriam Rose, Myers Research Institute. U.S Department of Health and Human Services, Office of the Assistant Secretary for Planning and Evaluation, Office of Disability, Aging, and Long-Term Care Policy (ASPE) and Research Triangle Institute, November.

2. Residents entering an ALF should have a baseline evaluation, completed within 30 days of their admission, of their physical, medical and psychosocial needs, and a detailed review of all medications, prescription, nonprescription, herbal and other remedies, completed by a qualified, licensed practitioner experienced in the care of older adults. This culturally sensitive evaluation should be the basis for the development of a care plan that indicates resident physical and psychosocial needs along with resident preferences for treatment and strategies for meeting identified needs. This care plan should be available to the resident and to the ALF staff. The ALF should clearly indicate, preferably prior to admission, the specific elements of the care plan that the ALF will meet and is willing to accommodate as well as the responsibility of the resident/family.

Rationale: A resident's move to assisted living is a critical life-change event. This event offers a special opportunity for a comprehensive review of the resident's health and social needs. This move to an ALF often signals some medical, cognitive or functional need for the senior, which makes a comprehensive assessment all the more crucial at this transition of care. It also offers the opportunity to provide optimum interventions designed to maintain independence and prevent pre-existing conditions from deteriorating.

3. ALF staff should be knowledgeable and skilled in carrying out important components of geriatric care, including, but not limited to, safe medication administration, falls prevention, incontinence care, communication techniques, dementia care, skin care, and able to recognize the changes that can signal acute illness, delirium, and depression.

Rationale: Staffing levels and expertise do vary between ALFs. In a national study of ALFs, 40% reported having full-time registered nurse staff, 55% had a registered nurse either full or part time, and 71% had a registered nurse or licensed practical nurse on staff full or part time. About half (52%) used outside agencies to supply registered or licensed practical nurses. Staff working on-site should be sufficient in numbers and experience to meet the ongoing needs of the residents at all times. Staff should be knowledgeable regarding safe medication administration, falls prevention, incontinence care, communication techniques, dementia care, skin care, and recognition of the changes that can signal acute illness/delirium.

Reference: Phillips, Munoz, Sherman et al. (2003) Effects of Facility Characteristics on Departures from Assisted Living: Results from a National Study. *Gerontologist* 42 (5): 690–696.

Reference: Ambulatory Geriatric Clinical Care and Services Position Statement. Developed by the AGS Health Care Systems Committee and approved May 2000 by the AGS Board of Directors. *Journal of the American Geriatrics Society*, 48:845-846.

4. A primary care provider (includes geriatric nurse practitioners as well as physicians) experienced in geriatrics care should be available within each ALF to help direct staff in optimizing outcomes for each resident.

Rationale: The benefit of clinical leadership within long-term-care facilities was noted in 1978 in the *Journal of the American Geriatrics Society* and later supported by a 1993 AGS position statement on the Physician's Role in the Long-Term Care Facility, which illustrated the importance of this involvement. This benefit is true in all long-term-care facilities, including ALFs, extended-care units, skilled nursing facilities, intermediate care facilities, and residential units caring for frail residents. More recently the work of the Assisted Living Workgroup highlighted the link between these clinical services and outcome for ALF residents.

Reference: Ingman SR, Lawson IR, Carbon D. (1978) Medical Direction in Long-term Care. *Journal of the American Geriatrics Society* 26(4);157–166.

Reference: Assisted Living Workgroup Report to US Senate Special Committee on Aging 2003. Available at: www.aahsa.org/alw.htm (accessed November 2005).

5. ALFs need to become aligned with other facilities, providers, and systems of care to produce optimum outcomes for seniors.

Rationale: A comprehensive system of care is able to accommodate seniors with varied needs as they traverse through different levels of health and function in their aging lifetime. Key to coordination of care is communication at each transition of care.

Reference: Improving the Quality of Transitional Care for Persons with Complex Care Needs Position Statement. Developed by the AGS Health Care Systems Committee and approved May 2002 by the AGS Board of Directors. The American Geriatrics Society, New York, NY.

6. ALF resources need to be within the reach of those living in rural and low-income communities.

Rationale: The lack of noninstitutional, long-term-care services in many rural areas may explain why residents of nursing homes in rural areas tend to be younger and less disabled than their urban counterparts. Part of this can be accomplished with continued funding of the 1915[c] Home and Community Based Services waiver program to provide needed services. The 1915[c] Home and Community Based Services waiver is the primary Medicaid funding vehicle for low-income persons requiring assisted-living services.

Reference: Spector W, et al. (1996) Appropriate placement of nursing home residents in lower levels of care. *Millbank Quarterly*. 74:139–160.

Credits

American Geriatrics Society and approved by the AGS Board of Directors in May 2004. Written by the AGS Health Care Systems Committee, with special thanks to Drs. Richard Stefanacci, Leslie Wooldridge, and Kenneth Brummel-Smith. AGS, The Empire State Building, 350 Fifth Avenue, Suite 801, New York, NY 10118.

SOURCE: American Geriatrics Society. Assisted Living Facilities: American Geriatrics Society Position Paper, AGS Health Care Systems Committee. *J Am Geriatr Soc.* 2005;53(3):536–537. Reprinted by permission of Blackwell Science, Inc.

DEPRESSION: THE GERIATRIC DEPRESSION SCALE (SHORT FORM)

Choose the best answer for how you felt over the past week.

1. Are you basically satisfied with your life?	yes/**no**
2. Have you dropped many of your activities and interests?	**yes**/no
3. Do you feel that your life is empty?	**yes**/no
4. Do you often get bored?	**yes**/no
5. Are you in good spirits most of the time?	yes/**no**
6. Are you afraid that something bad is going to happen to you?	**yes**/no
7. Do you feel happy most of the time?	yes/**no**
8. Do you often feel helpless?	**yes**/no
9. Do you prefer to stay at home, rather than going out and doing new things?	**yes**/no
10. Do you feel you have more problems with memory than most?	**yes**/no
11. Do you think it is wonderful to be alive now?	yes/**no**
12. Do you feel pretty worthless the way you are now?	**yes**/no
13. Do you feel full of energy?	yes/**no**
14. Do you feel that your situation is hopeless?	**yes**/no
15. Do you think that most people are better off than you are?	**yes**/no

NOTE: Score bolded answers. One point for each of these answers. Cut-off: normal = 0–5; above 5 suggests depression. For additional information on administration and scoring, refer to the following references:
1. Sheikh JI, Yesavage JA. Geriatric Depression Scale: recent evidence and development of a shorter version. *Clin Gerontol.* 1986;5:165–172.
2. Yesavage JA, Brink TL, Rose TL, et al. Development and validation of a geriatric depression rating scale: a preliminary report. *J Psych Res.* 1983;17:27.

SOURCE: Courtesy of Jerome A. Yesavage, MD.

FALLS: GUIDELINES FOR PREVENTION

Recommendations from the American Geriatrics Society

The aim of this guideline is to assist health care professionals in their assessment of fall risk and in their management of older patients who are at risk of falling and those who have fallen. The Panel on Falls Prevention assumes that health care professionals will use their general clinical knowledge and judgment in applying the general principles and specific recommendations of this document to the assessment and management of individual patients. Decisions to adopt any particular recommendation must be made by the practitioner in light of available evidence and resources. (The key to strength of recommendations, indicated by letters A–D, is located in the note on next page.)

Assessment

Approach to older persons as part of routine care (not presenting after a fall):

- All older persons who are under the care of a health professional or their caregivers should be asked at least once a year about falls.

- All older persons who report a single fall should be observed as they stand up from a chair without using their arms, walk several paces, and return (ie, the "Get Up and Go Test"). Those demonstrating no difficulty or unsteadiness need no further assessment.

- Persons who have difficulty or demonstrate unsteadiness performing this test require further assessment.

Approach to older persons presenting with one or more falls or who have abnormalities of gait or balance or both, or who report recurrent falls:

- Older persons who present for medical attention because of a fall, report recurrent falls in the past year, or demonstrate abnormalities of gait or balance, or both, should have a fall evaluation performed. This evaluation should be performed by a clinician with appropriate skills and experience, which may necessitate referral to a specialist (eg, geriatrician).

- A fall evaluation is defined as an assessment that includes the following: a history of fall circumstances, medications, acute or chronic medical problems, and mobility levels; an examination of vision, gait and balance, and lower extremity joint function; an examination of basic neurologic function, including mental status, muscle strength, lower extremity peripheral nerves, proprioception, reflexes, tests of cortical, extrapyramidal, and cerebellar function; and assessment of basic cardiovascular status, including heart rate and rhythm, postural pulse and blood pressure, and, if appropriate, heart rate and blood-pressure responses to carotid sinus stimulation.

Multifactorial Interventions

- Among *community-dwelling* older persons (ie, those living in their own homes), multifactorial interventions should include: gait training and advice on the appropriate use of assistive devices (B); review and modification of medication, especially psychotropic medication (B); exercise programs, with balance training as one of the components (B); treatment of postural hypotension (B); modification of environmental hazards (C); and treatment of cardiovascular disorders, including cardiac arrhythmias (D).

- In *long-term care and assisted-living settings*, multifactorial interventions should include: staff education programs (B); gait training and advice on the appropriate use of assistive devices (B); and review and modification of medications, especially psychotropic medications (B).

- The evidence is insufficient to make recommendations for or against multifactorial interventions in *acute hospital* settings.

Single Intervention: Exercise

- Although exercise has many proven benefits, the optimal type, duration, and intensity of exercise for falls prevention remain unclear (B).

- Older people who have had recurrent falls should be offered long-term exercise and balance training (B).

- Tai Chi C'uan is a promising type of balance exercise, although it requires further evaluation before it can be recommended as the preferred balance training (C).

Single Intervention: Environmental Modification

- When older patients at increased risk of falls are discharged from the hospital, a facilitated environmental home assessment should be considered (B).

Single Intervention: Medications

- Patients who have fallen should have their medications reviewed and altered or stopped, as appropriate, in light of their risk of future falls. Particular attention to medication reduction should be given to older persons taking four or more medications and to those taking psychotropic medications (C).

Single Intervention: Assistive Devices

- Studies of multifactorial interventions that have included assistive devices have demonstrated benefit. However, there is no direct evidence that the use of assistive devices alone will prevent falls. Therefore, while assistive devices may be effective elements of a multifactorial intervention program, their isolated use without attention to other risk factors cannot be recommended (C).

Single Intervention: Behavioral and Educational Programs

- Although studies of multifactorial interventions that have included behavioral and educational programs have demonstrated benefit, when used as an isolated intervention, health or behavioral education does not reduce falls and should not be done in isolation (B).

NOTE:

Key to Strength of Recommendation: A: Directly based on Class I evidence; B: Directly based on Class II evidence or extrapolated recommendation from Class I evidence; C: Directly based on Class III evidence or extrapolated recommendation from Class I or II evidence; D: Directly based on Class IV evidence or extrapolated recommendation from Class I, II, or III evidence.

Key to Categories of Evidence: Class I: Evidence from at least one randomized controlled trial or a meta-analysis of randomized controlled trials; Class II: Evidence from at least one controlled study without randomization or evidence from at least one other type of quasi-experimental study; Class III: Evidence from nonexperimental studies, such as comparative studies, correlation studies, and case-control studies; Class IV: Evidence from expert committee reports or opinions and/or clinical experience of respected authorities.

SOURCE: Adapted from American Geriatrics Society, British Geriatrics Society, and American Academy of Orthopaedic Surgeons Panel on Falls Prevention. Guidelines for the prevention of falls in older persons. *J Am Geriatr Soc* 2001;49(5):664–672. Reprinted by permission of Blackwell Science, Inc.

INCONTINENCE: BEHAVIORAL PREVENTION AND MANAGEMENT

Behavioral treatment for urinary incontinence depends on careful instruction of the patient. The following tools are examples of patient education materials for bladder training, bladder urge control, and pelvic muscle (Kegel's) exercises that have been found to be clinically useful. See "Urinary Incontinence" (p 184) for discussion of the use of behavioral approaches.

Bladder Training

Bladder training involves following a strict schedule for bathroom visits during the day. The schedule starts with bathroom visits every 2 hours or so, but the time between visits is gradually increased. The longer stretch of time between bathroom visits gives you increased bladder control and independence.

If you have a habit of using the bathroom more than once every 2 hours due to urgency—with or without urge incontinence—you may benefit from bladder training. Bladder training has been shown to be effective for both stress and urge incontinence.

Goals

Bladder training has several goals. It helps you

- Lengthen the amount of time between bathroom visits.

- Increase the amount of urine that the bladder can comfortably hold.

- Improve self-control over bladder urges by voiding on a schedule, not when the urge strikes.

- Reduce or eliminate incontinence.

- Increase independence in bladder management.

How To Do Bladder Training

Bladder training requires motivation for starting and maintaining a schedule for voids. Each week, as incontinence decreases, the schedule is changed slightly so that your bathroom visits occur less often. Bladder training will take between 6 and 8 weeks for success, but noticeable improvements will occur early in the program.

- Start with a Bladder Diary. Record your bathroom visits and urine leaks on the Bladder Diary for 48 hours. Measure the urine you produce during bathroom visits with a calibrated cup. This will help determine the amount of urine your bladder is able to hold.

- Review the Bladder Diary with your clinician, who will set a bladder training schedule according to the amount of time between your usual bathroom visits. For many people, the bathroom visits are scheduled for every 1 to 2 hours.

- For the first week, use the bathroom strictly according to the schedule. If a strong bladder urge strikes, use the Bladder Urge Control Procedure (below) to regain control and wait until the next scheduled time to void. If the urge is too strong and it cannot be entirely suppressed, use the bathroom, but then resume the bladder schedule.

- Each week, increase the time between bathroom visits by 30 minutes, as tolerated. As incontinence decreases week by week, the schedule can be further increased. For many individuals, bathroom visits every 3 to 6 hours is desirable. For most older persons, every 3 to 4 hours is optimal.

- Monitor the number of urine leaks each day and for the entire week. Also monitor the amount of each leak. For example, a person may have two leaks a day, but instead of large leaks that saturate a pad, they are small dribbles that slightly dampen the pad. This is considered good improvement.

- If the number of urine leaks does not lessen in 1 week, then maintain the same bladder training schedule for another week. Adjust the schedule in the next week when urine leaks decrease.

Bladder Urge Control Procedures

When a bladder urge strikes, you may be tempted to rush to the bathroom to prevent incontinence. This response can cause more harm than good, since the already overactive bladder becomes more stimulated and irritated with the rushed movement to the toilet. To get control over the bladder, practice the Bladder Control Procedure when the urge strikes. In this procedure, you

- Stand quietly or sit still. This prevents overstimulation of the bladder.

- Take slow, relaxed breaths.

- Contract the pelvic floor muscles repeatedly (see pelvic muscle exercises below). This helps keep the urethra closed to prevent urine from leaking. This also calms the bladder through special signals that are carried to the brain.

- Concentrate on making the urge go away. Use mental imagery and self-talk to help suppress the urge. Think to yourself, "I am in control of my bladder and this bladder has one job only and that is to hold urine until I am ready to go to the toilet." Imagine the urge as a wave that has peaked and now is fading away.

- Use mental distraction to reduce the awareness of the discomfort of the urge. Hum a tune or do mathematical calculations (subtract 7 from 100, then continue subtracting 7).

- When the urge subsides, do not use the toilet until the next scheduled void.

- If the urge does not completely subside, you may use the toilet.

When used with every urge, this procedure becomes more effective and gives you greater control over your bladder. Be encouraged by even small improvements in your symptoms. Although progress may seem slow, you are developing entirely new habits for bladder control. These healthy bladder habits will remain an important part of your life style. This takes both time and patience, but the rewards are worth the effort.

Pelvic Muscle (Kegel's) Exercises

Pelvic muscles, like other muscles, can become weak or damaged. Pelvic muscle exercises strengthen weak muscles around the bladder.

- Start by doing your pelvic muscle exercises 3 to 4 times each week. Usually it takes about 10 minutes to do the exercises. Your clinician will give you exact instructions about how many times you should perform the exercises and the number of times a day.

- Practice anywhere and any time. It is usually best to begin practicing them when lying on your bed. Once you have mastered the exercises lying down, practice them sitting in a chair. Then advance to practicing them standing. Soon you will be able to do them anywhere.

- Never use your stomach, thigh, or buttock muscles. To find out whether you are also contracting your stomach muscles, place your hand on your abdomen while you squeeze your pelvic muscle. If you feel your abdomen move, then you are also using these muscles.

- Avoid holding your breath. Inhale and exhale slowly while counting. In time, you will learn to practice effortlessly.

- If you forget to do your exercises for several days, do not be discouraged. When you have realized you have forgotten, begin your program again as instructed. Do not try to make up for lost days by doing more exercises or you will have sore muscles.

After 4 to 6 weeks of following your prescribed exercise routine, you will begin to notice that you are having fewer urinary accidents. After 3 months, you will see an even bigger difference. It may help to keep a diary of the times you practice your exercises and the times that you leak urine. This will give you a picture of the progress you are making. If you are having problems, your clinician may suggest biofeedback, weighted vaginal cones, or electrostimulation to help you with pelvic muscle exercises.

SOURCE: Adapted from Busby-Whitehead J, Kinkade J, Granville L. *Urinary Incontinence: Management in Primary Practice*. Tool Kit 2, Practicing Physician Education Project, Robinson BE, ed. New York: The John A. Hartford Foundation and The American Geriatrics Society; 2000. Reprinted with permission.

NUTRITION SCREENING: DETERMINE YOUR NUTRITIONAL HEALTH CHECKLIST

The nutrition screen is based on these warning signs of poor nutrition:

Disease

Eating poorly

Tooth loss, mouth pain

Economic hardship

Reduced social contact

Multiple medicines

Involuntary weight loss or gain

Need for assistance in self-care

Elderly (age > 80)

The mnemonic DETERMINE represents the warning signs and the questions in the screen.

Read the statements below. Circle the number in the "YES" column for those that apply to you or someone under your care. For each "YES" answer, score the number listed. Total your nutrition score.

	YES
1. I have an illness or condition that made me change the kind and/or amount of food I eat.	2
2. I eat fewer than 2 meals per day.	3
3. I eat few fruits or vegetables, or milk products.	2
4. I have 3 or more drinks of beer, liquor, or wine almost every day.	2
5. I have tooth or mouth problems that make it hard for me to eat.	2
6. I don't always have enough money to buy the food I need.	4
7. I eat alone most of the time.	1
8. I take 3 or more different prescribed or over-the-counter drugs a day.	1
9. Without wanting to, I have lost or gained 10 pounds in the last 6 months.	2
10. I am not always physically able to shop, cook, and/or feed myself.	2
TOTAL _____	

NOTE: Scoring: 0–2 = good; 3–5 = moderate nutritional risk; 6 or more = high nutritional risk.

SOURCE: DETERMINE Your Nutritional Health Checklist. Reprinted with permission of the Nutrition Screening Initiative, a project of the American Academy of Family Physicians, the American Dietetic Association, and the National Council on Aging, Inc., and funded in part by a grant from Ross Products Division, Abbott Laboratories Inc.

Terms Used to Interpret Screening and Diagnostic Tests

Term	Definition, Description
Positive test	Condition present = true positive (a)
	Condition absent = false positive (b)
Negative test	Condition present = false negative (c)
	Condition absent = true negative (d)
Sensitivity	Proportion of persons with the condition who test positive: $a / (a + c)$
Specificity	Proportion of persons without the condition who test negative: $d / (b + d)$
Positive predictive value	Proportion of persons with a positive test who have the condition: $a / (a + b)$
Negative predictive value	Proportion of persons with a negative test who do not have the condition: $d / (c + d)$
Positive predictive value (PPV)	Depends on sensitivity and specificity of the test and the prevalence of the disease: $\text{PPV} = prevalence \times sensitivity / (prevalence \times sensitivity) + (1 - prevalence)(1 - specificity)$

NOTE: For conditions, like cancer, that are relatively uncommon in asymptomatic people, a test for a low prevalence condition that is only modestly specific will result in many more positive tests than there are individuals who actually have cancer. This is the main difficulty with screening, as a positive test must be followed by more specific tests that are usually more invasive and associated with morbidity.

RESOURCES

What Can You Find on the AGS Website?
http://www.americangeriatrics.org
e-mail: info.amger@americangeriatrics.org

- **What is the American Geriatrics Society**? AGS mission and goals, current activities, history, AGS staff/contact information, list of Board of Directors and Committee Chairs and their affiliations.

- **All New MyAGS: An AGS Members Only Resource**
  Created by the American Geriatrics Society, My AGS offers members access to exclusive members only tools and resources while enabling them to navigate the regular AGS website at the same time. Resources include one click access to the Journal of the American Geriatrics Society, Access to the Online Members Directory, free support materials for the American Board of Internal Medicine (ABIM) geriatrics modules under the ABIM Self-Evaluation Process, AGS Legislative Toolkit, AGS Practice Management Toolkit and more.

- Information on all AGS publications, including the *Geriatrics Review Syllabus: A Core Curriculum in Geriatric Medicine (GRS), Geriatric Nursing Review Syllabus, GRS Teaching Slides, Case Based Geriatrics Review, Doorway Thoughts,* and *Geriatrics At Your Fingertips.*

- **Geriatrics-For-Specialists Website**—To respond to the need for better geriatric training, the American Geriatrics Society (AGS), with funding from the John A. Hartford Foundation, established the Geriatrics for Specialists Project. Launched in 1994, the project is expanding geriatrics expertise in 10 surgical and related medical specialties.

- **Professional Education** opportunities, including free online CME opportunities, information on the **Geriatrics Recognition Award (GRA)**, and listings of continuing education courses and AGS co-sponsored events.

- **Patient Education**—Link to the AGS Foundation for Health in Aging (FHA) which strives to make trustworthy and practical health care information available to the public. Its many pamphlets, fact sheets, consumer tools, books and website are designed to inform your patients about multiple chronic illnesses and promote disease prevention and healthy living.

- **Public Policy**—an overview of AGS public policy and legislative activities.

- **Council of State Affiliates Representatives (COSAR)**—information on AGS state affiliates promoting geriatrics at the local level.

- **Links** to dozens of aging/health/education-related Web sites.

- **AGS Annual Meeting Information**

- **Junior Faculty Development Opportunities**—An updated listing of junior faculty award opportunities, including the **Hartford Geriatrics Health Outcomes Research Scholars Award Program** and the **T. Franklin Williams Research Scholars Award**.

- Access to other AGS publications including the *Journal of the American Geriatrics Society*, the *Annals of Long-Term Care: Clinical Care and Aging*, the *AGS Newsletter*, and full-text versions of AGS Position Papers, Statements, and Guidelines.

Directory of Agencies and Organizations for Geriatric Clinicians

While this list represents a comprehensive guide to organizations that address the clinical care needs of older people, it is not a resource of all social service agencies and organizations assisting older citizens. If you have questions that do not specifically relate to one of the following organizations, please contact your state and/or area agency on aging as listed by the Administration on Aging (AOA). These agencies provide information on, and refer callers to, local services for senior citizens. To locate state and area agencies on aging, visit the AOA Web site at http://www.aoa.dhhs.gov/agingsites/state.html or call the Eldercare Locator service (1-800-677-1116) operated by the National Association of Area Agencies on Aging.

Note: The organizations on this list are arranged in categories in the following order:
- *GENERAL AGING*
- *END-OF-LIFE ISSUES*
- *EDUCATION*
- *LEGAL ISSUES AND ELDER ABUSE*
- *RESOURCES ON SPECIFIC HEALTH PROBLEMS:*
  - Cancer
  - Complementary and Alternative Medicine
  - Diabetes Mellitus
  - Digestive Problems
  - Head and Neck Problems
  - Hearing Problems
  - Heart and Circulation Problems
  - Joint, Muscle, and Bone Problems
  - Lung and Breathing Problems
  - Memory and Thinking Problems
  - Neurologic Problems
  - Nutritional Concerns
  - Pain
  - Psychological Problems
  - Sexuality and Sexual Concers
  - Sight Problems
  - Skin Problems
  - Urinary Problems

GENERAL AGING

Administration on Aging
330 Independence Avenue, SW
Washington, DC 20201
Tel: (202) 619-0724
Fax: (202) 401-7620 or (202) 537-3555
Web site: http://www.aoa.gov
E-Mail: aoainfo@aoa.gov or aoainfo@aoa.hhs.gov

National Aging Information Center (NAIC)
(A Service of the Administration on Aging)
330 Independence Avenue, SW, Room 4656
Washington, DC 20201
Telephone: (202) 619-7501
TTY: (202) 401-7575
Fax: (202) 401-7620
Web site: http://www.aoa.gov/naic
E-Mail: naic@aoa.gov

Agency for Health Care Research and Quality (AHRQ), formerly the Agency for Health Care Policy and Research
540 Gaither Road
Rockville, MD 20850
Tel: (301) 427-1364
On-line retrieval: http://www.ahrq.gov

Aging Network Services
Topaz House
4400 East-West Hwy., Suite 907
Bethesda, MD 20814
Tel: (301) 657-4329
Fax: (301) 657-3250
Web site: http://www.agingnets.com
E-Mail: ans@agingnets.com

Alliance for Aging Research
2021 K Street, NW, Suite 305
Washington, DC 20006
Tel: (202) 293-2856
Fax: (202) 785-8574
Web site: www.agingresearch.org
Email: info@agingresearch.org

American Academy of Home Care Physicians
PO Box 1037
Edgewood, MD 21040
Tel: (410) 676-7966
Fax: (410) 676-7980
Web site: www.aahcp.org
E-Mail: aahcp@comcast.net

American Association of Homes & Services for the Aging
2519 Connecticut Avenue, NW
Washington, DC 20008-1520
Tel: (202) 783-2242
Fax: (202) 783-2255
Web site: www.aahsa.org
E-Mail: info@aahsa.org

American Association of Retired Persons
601 E Street, NW
Washington, DC 20049
Tel: (800)424-3410 or (888) OUR-AARP (687-2277)
Web site: www.aarp.org
E-Mail: member@aarp.org

American College of Health Care
Administrators
300 N. Lee Street, Suite 301
Alexandria, VA 22314
Tel: (703) 739-7900 or (888)
88-ACHCA (882-2422)
Fax: (703) 739-7901
Toll Free: (888) 888-ACHCA
(22422)
Web site: www.achca.org
E-Mail: info@achca.org

American Federation for Aging
Research
70 West 40th St., 11th Floor
New York, NY 10018
Tel: (212) 703-9977
Fax: (212) 832-2298
(212)-997-0030
Web site: www.afar.org
E-Mail: info@afar.org

American Geriatrics Society
The Empire State Building
350 Fifth Avenue, Suite 801
New York, NY 10118
Tel: (212) 308-1414
Fax: (212) 832-8646
Web site:
www.americangeriatrics.org
E-Mail:
info.amger@americangeriatrics.org

American Health Care Association
1201 L Street, NW
Washington, DC 20005
Tel: (202) 842-4444
Fax: (202) 842-3860
Toll Free for Publications Only
(800) 321-0343
Web site: www.ahca.org

American Hospital Association
1 North Franklin
Chicago, IL 60606
Tel: (312) 422-3000
Fax: (312) 422-4796
Web site: www.aha.org

American Medical Directors
Association
10480 Patuxent Parkway, Suite 760
Columbia, MD 21044
Tel: (410) 740-9743
Toll Free: (800) 876-2632
Fax: (410) 740-4572
Web site: www.amda.com
Email: info@amda.com

American Occupational Therapy
Association
4720 Montgomery Lane, PO Box
31220
Bethesda, MD 20824-1220
Tel: (301) 652-2682 or (800)
372-8555
Fax: (301) 652-7711
Web site: www.aota.org

American Red Cross
American Red Cross National
Headquarters
2025 E. Street, NW
Washington, DC 20006
Tel: (202) 303-4498
Web site: www.redcross.org

American Senior Fitness Association
PO Box 2575
New Smyrna Beach, FL 32170
Tel: (800) 243-1478
Web site: www.seniorfitness.net
E-Mail: sfa@ucnsb.net

American Seniors Housing
Association
1850 M Street, NW, Suite 540
Washington, DC 20036
Tel: (202) 974-2300
Fax: (202) 775-0112
Web site: www.nmhc.org
E-Mail: info@nmhc.org

American Social Health Association
Hotlines under the auspices of the
ASHA American Social Health
Association
CDC National AIDS Hotline
(English)—Toll Free (800)
342-AIDS PO Box13827
CDC National AIDS Hotline
(Spanish)—Toll Free: (800)
344-7432
CDC National AIDS Hotline—TTY
Toll Free: (800) 243-7889 Tel:
(919) 361-8400
CDC National STD Hotline—Toll
Free: (800) 227-8922 Fax: (919)
361-8425
CDC National Immunization
Information Hotline—Toll Free:
(800) 232-2522
Web site: www.ashastd.org

American Society on Aging
833 Market Street, Suite 511
San Francisco, CA 94103-1824
Tel: (415) 974-9600 or (800)
537-9728
Fax: (415) 974-0300
Web site: www.asaging.org
E-Mail: info@asaging.org

American Society of Consultant
Pharmacists
1321 Duke Street
Alexandria, VA 22314-3516
Tel: (703) 739-1300
Fax: (703) 739-1321
Toll Free Tel: (800) 355-2727
Toll Free Fax: (800) 707-ASCP
Fast Fax: (800) 220-1321 or (703)
739-1321
Web site: www.ascp.com
E-Mail: info@ascp.com

Assisted Living Federation of
America
11200 Waples Mill Road, Suite 150
Fairfax, VA 22030
Tel: (703) 691-8100
Fax: (703) 691-8106
Web site: www.alfa.org
E-Mail: info@alfa.org

B'nai B'rith
International Headquarters
2020 K Street, NW, 7th Floor
Washington, DC 20006
Tel: (202) 857-6600
Fax: (202) 857-1099
Toll Free: (888) 388-4224
Senior Housing
Tel: (202) 857-6581
Fax: (202) 857-0980
E-Mail: senior@bnaibrith.org

Catholic Charities
1731 King Street, Suite 200
Alexandria, VA 22314
Tel: (703) 549-1390
Fax: (703) 549-1656
Web site:
www.catholiccharitiesusa.org

Children of Aging Parents
PO Box 167
Richboro, PA 18954
Tel: (800) 227-7294
Toll Free Information/Referral:
(800) 227-7294
Web site: www.caps4caregivers.org
Email: info@caps4caregivers.org

CDC National Prevention
Information Network
For information on HIV, AIDS,
STD, TB
PO Box 6003
Rockville, MD 20849-6003
Tel: (301) 562-1098
Toll Free Tel: (800) 458-5231
Toll Free Fax: (888) 282-7681
Toll Free TTY: (800) 243-7012
Web site: www.cdcnpin.org
E-Mail: info@cdcnpin.org

Commission on Accreditation for
Rehabilitation Facilities (CARF)
4891 East Grant Road
Tucson, AZ 85712
Tel: (520) 325-1044 or
(888) 281-6531
Fax: (520) 318-1129
Web site: www.carf.org

Department of Veteran Affairs
Office of Public Affairs
810 Vermont Avenue, NW
Washington, DC 20420
Tel: (202) 273-5700
Fax: (202) 273-6705
Web site: www.va.gov

Disabled American Veterans
807 Maine Avenue, SW
Washington, DC 20024
Tel: (202) 554-3501
Fax: (202) 554-3581
Web site: www.dav.org

Family Caregivers Alliance
180 Montgomery St., Suite 1100
San Francisco, CA 94104
Tel: (415) 434-3388 or
(800) 455-8106
Fax: (415) 434-3508
Toll Free: (800) 445-8106
Web site: www.caregiver.org.
E-Mail: info@caregiver.org

Gerontological Society of America
1030 15th Street NW, Suite 250
Washington, DC 20005
Tel: (202) 842-1275
Fax: (202) 842-1150
Web site: www.geron.org
Email: geron@geron.org

Healthcare Information and
Management Systems Society
230 East Ohio Street, Suite 500
Chicago, IL 60611-3269
Tel: (312) 664-4467
Fax: (312) 664-6143
Web site: www.himss.org
Email: himss@himss.org

Interfaith Caregivers Alliance
One West Armour Blvd.
Suite 202
Kansas City, MO 64111
Tel: (816) 931-5442
Fax: (816) 931-5202
Web site:
www.interfaithcaregivers.org
E-Mail: info@interfaithcaregivers.org

Joint Commission on Accreditation
of Healthcare Organizations
(JCAHO)
One Renaissance Boulevard
Oakbrook Terrace, IL 60181
Tel: (630) 792-5000
Fax: (630) 792-5005
Web site: www.jcaho.org

Medicare Hotline
Toll Free English & Spanish:
(800) MEDICARE (633-4227)
7500 Security Boulevard Baltimore,
MD 21244-1850
Web site: www.medicare.gov

National Adult Day Services
Association
2519 Connecticut Ave., NW
Washington, DC 20008
Tel: (202) 508-1205 or
(800) 558-5301
Fax: (202) 783-3255
Web site: www.nadsa.org
info@nadsa.org

National Asian Pacific Center on
Aging
Melbourne Tower, Suite 914
1511 Third Avenue
Seattle, WA 98101
Tel: (206) 624-1221
Fax: (206) 624-1023
Web site: www.napca.org

National Association of Area
Agencies on Aging
1730 Rhode Island Ave., NW
Suite 1200
Washington, DC 20036
Tel: (202) 872-0888
Fax: (202) 872-0057
Web site: www.n4a.org
E-Mail: rseay@n4a.org
Toll Free Eldercare Locator:
(800) 677-1116, operated as a
cooperative partnership of the
Administration on Aging, the
National Association of Area
Agencies on Aging, and the
National Association of State Units
on Aging.

National Association of Directors of
Nursing Administration
10101 Alliance Road, #140
Cincinnati, OH 45242
Tel: (513) 791-3679
Fax: (513) 791-3699
Toll Free: (800) 222-0539
Web site: www.nadona.org
Email: info@nadona.org

National Association for Home Care
228 7th Street, SE
Washington, DC 20003
Tel: (202) 547-7424
Fax: (202) 547-3540
Web site: www.nahc.org

National Association of Professional
Geriatric Care Managers
1604 North Country Club Road
Tucson, AZ 85716
Tel: (520) 881-8008
Fax: (520) 325-7925
Web site: www.caremanager.org

National Association for the Support
of Long Term Care
1321 Duke Street, Suite 304
Alexandria, VA 22314
Tel: (703) 549-8500
Fax: (703) 549-8342
Web site: www.NASL.org

National Caucus and Center on
Black Aged, Inc.
1220 L Street, NW, Suite 800
Washington, DC 20005
Tel: (202) 637-8400
Fax: (202) 347-0895
Web site: www.ncba-aged.org
E-Mail: info@ncba-aged.org

National Citizens' Coalition for
Nursing Home Reform
801 L Street, NW Suite 801
Washington, DC 20036-2211
Tel: (202) 332-2275
Fax: (202) 332-2949
Web site: www.nccnhr.org
E-Mail: nccnhr1@nccnhr.org

National Council on the Aging
300 D Street, SW, Suite 801
Washington, DC 20024
Tel: (202) 479-1200
Fax: (202) 479-0735
Web site: www.ncoa.org
E-Mail: info@ncoa.org

National Council on Patient
Information and Education
4915 Saint Elmo Avenue
Suite 505
Bethesda, MD 20814-6053
Tel: (301) 656-8565
Fax: (301) 656-4464
Web site: www.talkaboutrx.org
Email: ncpie@ncpie.info

National Family Caregivers
Association
10400 Connecticut Avenue # 500
Kensington, MD 20895-3944
Tel: (301) 942-6430
Fax: (301) 942-2302
Toll Free: (800) 896-3650
Web site: www.nfcacares.org
E-mail: info@nfcacares.org

National Health Information Center
PO Box 1133
Washington, DC 20013-1133
Tel: (301) 565-4167
Toll Free: (800) 336-4797
Fax: (301) 884-4256
Web site:
http://www.health.gov/nhic
E-Mail: info@nhic.org

National Indian Council on Aging
10501 Montgomery Boulevard NE
Suite 210
Albuquerque, NM 87111-3846
Tel: (505) 292-2001
Fax: (505) 292-1922
Web site: www.nicoa.org
E-Mail: dave@nicoa.org

National Institute on Aging
Building 31, Room 5C27
31 Center Drive MSC 2292
Bethesda, MD 20892-2292
Tel: toll free (800) 222-4225 or
(301) 496-1752
Fax: (301) 496-1072
Web site: www.nih.gov/nia

National Institute on Disability and
Rehabilitation Research
ABLEDATA
8630 Fenton Street
Suite 930
Silver Spring, MD 20910
Tel: (301) 608-8998
Fax: (301) 608-8958
Toll Free: (800) 227-0216
Web site: www.abledata.com
Email: adaigle@macroint.com

National Rehabilitation Information
Center
4200 Forbes Boulevard, Suite 202
Lanham, MD 20706
Toll Free: (800) 346-2742
Fax: (301) 459-5900 or
(301) 459-5984
Web site: www.naric.com
Email: naricinfo@heitechservices.com

National Subacute Care Association
7315 Wisconsin Avenue, Suite 424E
Bethesda, MD 20814
Tel: (301) 961-8680
Fax: (301) 961-8681
Web site: www.nsca.net
E-Mail: nsca@tiac.net

Projecto Ayuda
1452 West Temple Street, Suite 100
Los Angeles, CA 90026
Tel: (213) 487-1922
Fax: (213) 202-5905

United Seniors Health Cooperative
409 Third Street SW
Washington, DC 20024
Tel: (202) 479-6973
Fax: (202) 479-6660
Web site: unitedseniorshealth.org

Visiting Nurse Associations of
America
99 Summer St., Suite 1700
Boston, MA 02110
Tel: (617) 737-3200
Fax: (617) 227-4843
(617) 737-1144
Web site: www.vnaa.org
Email: vnaa@vnaa.org

Well Spouse Foundation
63 West Main St., Suite H
Freehold, NJ 07728
Tel: (732) 577-8899 or
(800) 838-0879
Fax: (732) 577-8644
Toll Free: (800) 838-0879
Web site: www.wellspouse.org
E-Mail: info@wellspouse.org

END-OF-LIFE ISSUES

Americans for Better Care of the
Dying
3720 Upton St. NW, Rm. B147
Washington, DC 20016
Tel: (202) 895-2660
Fax: (202) 966-5410
Web site: www.abcd-caring.com
E-Mail: info@abcd-caring.org

Center to Improve Care of the
Dying
Rand Corporation
1200 South Hayes Street
Arlington, VA 22202
Tel: (703) 413-1100
Web site: www.medicaring.org

Choice in Dying, Inc.
1035 30th Street, NW
Washington, DC 20007
Tel: (202) 338-9790
Fax: (202) 338-0242
Toll Free: (800) 989-WILL (9455)
Web site: partnershipforcaring.org

Compassion in Dying
6312 SW Capital Hwy, Suite 415
Portland, OR 97239
Tel: (503) 221-9556
Fax: (503) 228-9160
Web site:
www.compassionindying.org
E-Mail:
info@compassionandchoices.org

GriefNet
Internet Address: www.rivendell.org

Hospice Association of America
228 Seventh Street, SE
Washington, DC 20003
Tel: (202) 546-4759
Fax: (202) 547-9559
Web site: www.hospice-america.org

Hospice Education Institute
3 Unity Square, PO Box 98
Machiasport, ME 04655
Tel: (207) 255-8800
Fax: (207) 255-8000
Toll Free for Publications:
(800) 331-1620
Hospice Link Referral Service—Toll
Free: (800) 331-1620
Web site: www.hospiceworld.org
E-Mail: info@hospiceworld.org

Hospice Foundation of America
2001 S Street NW, Suite 300
Washington, DC 20009
Tel: (202) 638-5419
Toll Free: (800) 854-3402
Fax: (202) 638-5312
Web site:
www.hospicefoundation.org
E-Mail: hfa@hospicefoundation.org

The Last Acts Campaign
Barksdale Ballard & Co.
1951 Kidwell Drive, Suite 205
Vienna, VA 22182
Tel: (703) 827-8771
Fax: (703) 827-0783
Web site: www.lastacts.org

Life With Dignity
1744 Riggs Place NW Suite 300
Washington, DC 20009
Tel: (202) 986-0118
Web site: www.lifewithdignity.org
E-Mail: lwdfdn@aol.com

National Hospice and Palliative Care
Organization
1700 Diagonal Road, Suite 625
Alexandria, VA 22314
Tel: (703) 837-1500
Fax: (703) 837-1233
Web site: www.nhpco.org
E-Mail: nhpco_info@nhpco.org

EDUCATION

Association for Gerontology in
Higher Education
1030 15th Street, NW, Suite 240
Washington, DC 20005-1503
Tel: (202) 289-9806
Fax: (202) 289-9824
Web site: www.aghe.org

Association of American Medical
Colleges
2450 N Street, NW
Washington, DC 20037-1126
Tel: (202) 828-0400
Fax: (202) 828-1125
Web site: www.aamc.org
Email: rsherrod@aamc.org

LEGAL ISSUES AND ELDER
ABUSE

Legal Services for the Elderly
130 West 42nd Street, 17th Floor
New York, NY 10036
Tel: (212) 391-0120
Fax: (212) 719-1939
E-Mail: hn4923@handsnet.org

National Academy of Elder Law
Attorneys
1604 North Country Club Road
Tucson, AZ 85716
Tel: (520) 881-4005
Fax: (520) 325-7925
Web site: www.naela.org
E-Mail: info@naela.com

National Center on Elder Abuse
A consortium of the following six
partners with NASUA the lead
agency:
National Association of State Units
on Aging (NASUA)
Commission on Legal Problems of
the Elderly of the American Bar
Association (ABA)
The Clearinghouse on Abuse and
Neglect of the Elderly of the
University of Delaware CANE)
The San Francisco Consortium for
Elder Abuse Prevention of the
Goldman Institute on Aging
(GIOA)
The National Association of Adult
Protective Services Administrators
(NAAPSA)
The National Committee to Prevent
Elder Abuse (NCPEA)
1201 15th Street, NW, Suite 350
Washington, DC 20005
Tel: (202) 898-2586
Fax: (202) 898-2583
Web site: www.elderabusecenter.org
E-Mail: ncea@nasua.org

National Association of State Units
on Aging
1201 15th Street, Suite 350
Washington, DC 20005
Tel: (202) 898-2578
Fax: (202) 898-2583
Web site: www.nasua.org
E-Mail: info@nasua.org

National Clearinghouse on Elder
Abuse (Literature)
University of Delaware
College of Human Resources,
Education and Public Policy
Department of Consumer Studies
211 Allison Annex
Newark, DE 19716
Tel: (302) 831-3525
Fax: (302) 831-6081

National Committee for Prevention
of Elder Abuse (Research)
Institute on Aging
UMASS Memorial Health Care
119 Belmont Street
Worcester, MA 01605
Tel: (508) 334-6166
Fax: (508) 334-6906
Web site:
www.preventelderabuse.org

National Senior Citizens Law
Center
1101 14th Street, NW, Suite 400
Washington, DC 20005
Tel: (202) 289-6976
Fax: (202) 289-7224
Web site: www.nsclc.org
E-Mail: nsclc@nsclc.org

RESOURCES ON SPECIFIC HEALTH PROBLEMS

Cancer

American Cancer Society, Inc.
National Headquarters
1599 Clifton Road, NE
Atlanta, GA 30329
Tel: (404) 320-3333
Fax: (404) 329-5787
Toll Free National Cancer
Information Center:
(800) 227-2345
Web site: www.cancer.org

National Cancer Institute
Public Inquiries Office
Building 31, Room 10A31
31 Center Drive, MSC 2580
Bethesda, MD 20892-2580
Tel: (301) 435-3848
Toll Free: (800) 4-CANCER
(422-6237)
Web site: www.nci.nih.gov
E-Mail: cancergovstaff@mail.nih.gov

Complementary and Alternative Medicine

Department of Health and Human
Services, Public Health Service
Healthfinder
PO Box 1133
Washington, DC 20013-1133
Web site: www.healthfinder.gov
E-Mail: healthfinder@nhic.org

The Evidence-Based
Complementary and Alternative
Web site for Health Care
Professionals
19 Russell Street
Toronto, ON M5S 2S2
Fax: (416) 978-1833
Web site: www.camline.org
E-Mail: cam.line@utoronto.ca

HerbMed by the Alternative
Medicine Foundation, Inc.
PO Box 60016
Potomac, MD 20859
Tel: (301) 340-1960
Fax: (301) 340-1936
Web site: www.herbmed.org
Email: info@amfoundation.org

National Center for Complementary
and Alternative Medicine
NCCAM Clearinghouse
PO Box 7923
Gaithersburg, MD 20898
Toll Free: (888) 644-6226
Tel: (301) 519-3153
TTY: (866) 464-3615
Fax: (866) 464-3616
Web site: www.nccam.nih.gov
E-Mail: info@nccam.nih.gov

Natural Medicines Comprehensive
Database
3120 W. March Lane
PO Box 8190
Stockton, CA 95208
Tel: (209) 472-2244
Fax: (209) 472-2249

WebMD Inc.
Corporate Headquarters
669 River Drive
Elmwood Park, NJ 07407
Tel: (201) 703-3400
Fax: (201) 703-3401
Web site: www.WebMD.com

Diabetes Mellitus

American Diabetes Association
Attn: Customer Service
1701 North Beauregard Street
Alexandria, VA 22311
Tel: (703) 549-1500
Fax: (703) 549-6995
Toll Free: (800) DIABETES
(232-3472)
Web site: www.diabetes.org
E-Mail:
customerservice@diabetes.org

National Diabetes Information
Clearinghouse
1 Information Way
Bethesda, MD 20892-3560
Tel: (301) 654-3327 or
(800) 860-8747
Fax: (301) 907-8906
Web site: www.niddk.nih.gov
E-Mail: ndic@info.niddk.nih.gov

Digestive Problems

American Liver Foundation
75 Maiden Lane, Suite 603
New York, NY 10038
Toll Free: (800) GO LIVER
(465-4837)
Web site: www.liverfoundation.org
E-Mail: info@liverfoundation.org

National Digestive Disease
Information Clearinghouse
2 Information Way
Bethesda, MD 20892-3570
Tel: (301) 654-3810 or
(800) 891-5389
Fax: 703-738-4929
Web site: www.niddk.nih.gov
E-Mail: nddic@info.niddk.nih.gov

United Ostomy Association
19772 MacArthur Boulevard
Suite 200
Irvine, CA 92612-2405
Tel: (949) 660-8624
Fax: (949) 660-9262
Toll Free: (800) 826-0826
Web site: www.uoa.org
E-Mail: info@uoa.org

Head and Neck Problems

American Academy of
Otolaryngology—Head and Neck
Surgery, Inc.
1 Prince Street
Alexandria, VA 22314-3357
Tel: (703) 836-4444
Fax: (703) 683-5100
TTY: (703) 519-1585
Web site: www.entnet.org

American Council for Headache
Education
19 Mantua Road
Mt. Royal, NJ 08061
Tel: (856) 423-0258
Toll Free: (800) 255-ACHE (2243)
Fax: (856) 423-0082
Web site: www.achenet.org
E-Mail: achehg@talley.com

American Dental Association
211 East Chicago Avenue
Chicago, IL 60611
Tel: (312) 440-2500
Fax: (312) 440-2800
Web site: www.ada.org

American Society for Geriatric
Dentistry
401 North Michigan Avenue
Chicago, IL 60611
Tel: (312) 527-6764
Fax: (312) 673-6663
Web site: www.foscod.org
E-Mail: SCD@SCDonline.org

National Headache Foundation
428 West St. James Place, 2nd
Floor
Chicago, IL 60614-2750
Tel: (773) 388-6399
Toll Free: (888) NHF-5552
Fax: (773) 525-7357
Web site: www.headaches.org
E-Mail: info@headaches.org

National Institute of Dental &
Craniofacial Research
National Institute of Health
Bethesda, MD 20892-2190
Tel: (301) 496-4261
Fax: (301) 496-9988
Web site: www.nidcr.nih.gov
E-Mail: nidcrinfo@mail.nih.gov

Hearing Problems

American Tinnitus Association
65 SW Yamhill Street
Portland, OR 97204
Tel: (503) 248-9985
Fax: (503) 248-0024
Toll Free: (800) 634-8978
Web site: www.ata.org
E-Mail: tinnitus@ata.org

Better Hearing Institute
515 King Street, Suite 420
Alexandria, VA 22314
Toll Free: (800) EARWELL
(327-9355) or (703) 684-3391
Fax: (703) 750-9302
Web site: www.betterhearing.org
E-Mail: mail@betterhearing.org

International Hearing Society
16880 Middlebelt Road, Suite 4
Livonia, MI 48154
Tel: (734) 522-7200
Fax: (734) 522-0200
Toll Free Hearing Aid
Helpline: (800) 521-5247
Web site: www.ihsinfo.org

National Institute on Deafness and Other Communication Disorders
National Institute of Health
31 Center Drive, MSC 2320
Bethesda, MD 20892-2320
Tel: (301) 496-7243
Fax: (301) 402-0018
Toll Free NIDCD Information Clearinghouse: (800) 241-1044
Web site: www.nidcd.nih.gov
E-Mail: nidcdinfo@nidcd.nih.gov

Self Help for Hard of Hearing People
7910 Woodmont Avenue, Suite 1200
Bethesda, MD 20814
Tel: (301) 657-2248
Fax: (301) 913-9413
TTY: (301) 657-2249
Web site: www.shhh.org
E-Mail: national@shhh.org

Heart and Circulation Problems

American Association of Cardiovascular and Pulmonary Rehabilitation
National Office
401 North Michigan Avenue, Suite 2200
Chicago, IL 60611
Tel: (312) 321-5146
Web site: www.aacvpr.org
E-Mail: aacvpr@smithbucklin.com

American Heart Association
7272 Greenville Avenue
Dallas, TX 75231
Tel: (214) 373-6300
Toll Free Tel: (800) 242-8721
Web site: www.americanheart.org
AHA's Stroke Connection: (800) 553-6321

Courage Stroke Network
3915 Golden Valley Road
Golden Valley, MN 55422
Tel: (763) 520-0520 or (800) 553-6321
Fax: (763) 520-0577

National Heart, Lung and Blood Institute
Office of Prevention, Education and Control
31 Center Drive, MSC 2480
Bethesda, MD 20892-2480
Tel: (301) 496-5437
Fax: (301) 402-2405
Web site: www.nhlbi.nih.gov
E-Mail: nhlbiinfo@nhlbi.nih.gov

National Institute of Neurological Disorders and Stroke
NIH Neurological Institute
PO Box 5801
Bethesda, MD 20824
Toll Free: (800) 352-9424 or (301) 496-5751
Web site: www.ninds.nih.gov

National Stroke Association
9707 E. Easter Lane
Englewood, CO 80112
Tel: (303) 649-9299
Fax: (303) 649-1328
Toll Free: (800) STROKES (787-6537)
Web site: www.stroke.org

Joint, Muscle, and Bone Problems

American Academy of Orthopedic Surgeons
6300 North River Road
Rosemont, IL 60018-4262
Tel: (847) 823-7186
Toll Free: (800) 346-AAOS (2267)
Fax: (847) 823-8125
Web site: www.aaos.org
E-Mail: custserv@aaos.org

American Podiatric Medical Association
9312 Old Georgetown Road
Bethesda, MD 20814
Tel: (301) 571-9200
Fax: (301) 530-2752
Toll Free for Patient Education Literature only: (800) FOOT-CARE
Web site: www.apma.org
E-Mail: askapma@apma.org

Arthritis Foundation
PO Box 7669
Atlanta, GA 30357
Tel: (404) 872-7100
Toll Free Information: (800) 283-7800
Fax: (404) 872-0457
Web site: www.arthritis.org
E-Mail: help@arthritis.org

Lupus Foundation of America
2000 L Street, NW, Suite 710
Washington, DC 20036
Tel: (202) 349-1155
Toll Free Line for Information Packet: English (800) 558-0121, Spanish (800) 558-0231
Fax: (202) 349-1156
Web site: www.lupus.org

National Arthritis and Musculoskeletal and Skin Diseases Information Clearinghouse
National Institutes of Health
1 AMS Circle
Bethesda, MD 20892-3675
Tel: (301) 495-4484
Toll Free: (877) 22-NIAMS (226-4267)
Fax: (301) 718-6366
Web site: www.nih.gov/niams
E-Mail: niamsinfo@mail.nih.gov

National Osteoporosis Foundation
1232 22nd Street NW
Washington, DC 20037-1292
Tel: (202) 223-2226
Fax: (202) 223-2237
Toll Free Info: (800) 223-9994
Web site: www.nof.org
E-Mail: customerservice@nof.org

Lung and Breathing Problems

American Association of Cardiovascular and Pulmonary Rehabilitation
401 North Michigan Avenue, Suite 2200
Chicago, IL 60611
Tel: (312) 321-5196
Web site: www.aacvpr.org
E-Mail: aacvpr@smithbucklin.com

American Lung Association
61 Broadway, 6th Floor
New York, NY 10019
Tel: (212) 315-8700
Fax: (212) 265-5642
Toll Free: (800) LUNG-USA
(800-586-4872)
Web site: www.lungusa.org
E-Mail: info@lungusa.org

National Heart, Lung and Blood
Institute
Office of Prevention, Education and
Control
31 Center Drive, MSC 2480
Bethesda, MD 20892-2480
Tel: (301) 496-5437
Fax: (301) 402-2405
Web site: www.nhlbi.nih.gov
E-Mail: nhlbiinfo@nhlbi.nih.gov

Memory and Thinking Problems

Alzheimer's Association
225 North Michigan Avenue
Floor 17
Chicago, IL 60601
Toll Free Information:
(800) 272-3900
Tel: (312) 335-8700
TTY: (312) 335-8882
Fax: (312) 335-1110
Web site: www.alz.org
E-Mail: info@alz.org
Safe Return Program
(identification tags, medical alert
bracelets): (888) 572-8566

Alzheimer's Disease Education and
Referral Center
PO Box 8250
Silver Spring, MD 20907-8250
Tel: (301) 495-3311
Fax: (301) 495-3334
Toll Free Information Service:
(800) 438-4380
Web site: www.alzheimers.org
E-Mail: adear@alzheimers.org

Neurologic Problems

American Academy of Neurology
1080 Montreal Avenue
St. Paul, MN 55116
Tel: (651) 695-2717 or
(800) 879-1960
Fax: (651) 695-2791
Web site: www.aan.com
E-Mail: memberservices@aan.com

American Parkinson's Disease
Association
1250 Hylan Boulevard
Suite 4B
Staten Island, NY 10305-1946
Tel: (718) 981-8001
Toll Free Information Hotline:
(800) 223-2732
Fax: (718) 981-4399
Web site: www.apdaparkinson.org
E-Mail: apda@apdaparkinson.org

Epilepsy Foundation of America
4351 Garden City Drive
Landover, MD 20785
Tel: (301) 459-3700
Toll Free Information & Referral:
(800) 332-1000
Fax: (301) 577-2684
Web site: www.efa.org

Huntington's Disease Society of
America
505 Eighth Avenue, Suite 902
New York, NY 10018
Tel: (212) 242-1968
Fax: (212) 239-3430
Toll Free Hotline: (800) 345-4372
Web site: www.hdsa.org
E-Mail: hdsainfo@hdsa.org

National Institute of Neurological
Disorders and Stroke
NIH Neurological Institute
PO Box 5801
Bethesda, MD 20824
Toll Free: (800) 352-9424 or
(301) 496-5751
Web site: www.ninds.nih.gov
(for other stroke information, see
Heart & Circulation)

Parkinson's Disease Foundation
1359 Broadway, Suite 1509
New York, NY 10018
Tel: (212) 923-4700
Toll Free: (800) 457-6676
Fax: (212) 923-4778
Web site: www.pdf.org
E-Mail: info@pdf.org

Nutritional Concerns

Food and Nutrition Information
Center
US Department of Agriculture
National Agriculture Library
Building
10301 Baltimore Avenue
Room 304
Beltsville, MD 20705-2351
Tel: (301) 504-5719
Fax: (301) 504-6409
Web site:
http://www.nal.usda.gov/fnic
E-Mail: fnic@nal.usda.gov

Meals On Wheels Association of
America
203 S. Union Street
Alexandria, VA 2231
Tel: (703) 548-5558
Fax: (703) 548-8024
Web site: www.mowaa.org
E-Mail: mowaa@tbq.dqsys.com

Pain

American Chronic Pain Association
PO Box 850
Rocklin, CA 95677
Tel: (916) 632-0922
Fax: (916) 632-3208
Web site: www.theacpa.org
E-Mail: acpa@pacbell.net

American Geriatrics Society
The Empire State Building
350 Fifth Avenue, Suite 801
New York, NY 10118
Tel: (212) 308-1414
Fax: (212) 832-8646
Web site:
www.americangeriatrics.org
E-Mail:
info.amger@americangeriatrics.org

American Pain Society
4700 West Lake Avenue
Glenview, IL 60025
Tel: (847) 375-4715
Fax: (847) 375-7777
Web site: www.ampainsoc.org
E-Mail: info@ampainsoc.org

City of Hope Pain Resource Center
City of Hope National Medical
Center
Dept. of Nursing Research &
Education
1500 East Duarte Road
Duarte, CA 91010
Tel: (626) 359-8111 ext. 3829
Web site: www.cityofhope.org
E-Mail: media@coh.org

National Chronic Pain Outreach
Association
PO Box 274
Millboro, VA 24460-9606
Tel: (540) 862-9437
Fax: (540) 862-9485
Email: ncpoa@cfw.com
Web site: www.chronicpain.org

Psychological Problems

American Association for Geriatric
Psychiatry
7910 Woodmont Avenue, Suite
1050
Bethesda, MD 20814-3004
Tel: (301) 654-7850
Fax: (301) 654-4137
Web site: www.aagpgpa.org
E-Mail: main@aagpgpa.org

National Alliance for the
Mentally Ill
Colonial Place Three
2107 Wilson Blvd.
Suite 300
Arlington, VA 22201-3042
Tel: (703) 524-7600
Fax: (703) 524-9094
Toll Free: (800) 950-6264
Web site: www.nami.org

National Institute of Mental Health
Information Resources & Inquiries
6001 Executive Blvd., Room 8184,
MSC 9663
Bethesda, MD 20892-9663
Tel: (301) 443-4513
Fax: (301) 443-5158
Web site: www.nimh.nih.gov
E-Mail: nimhinfo@nih.gov

National Mental Health Association
2001 N. Beauregard Street, 12th
Floor
Alexandria, VA 22311
Tel: (703) 684-7722
Fax: (703) 684-5968
Toll Free Information:
(800) 969-NMHA (6642)
Web site: www.nmha.org

Sexuality and Sexual Concerns

American College of Obstetricians
and Gynecologists
409 12th Street, SW PO Box
96920
Washington, DC 20090-6920
Tel: (202) 638-5577
Fax: (202) 484-1595
Web site: www.acog.com
E-Mail: resources@acog.org

American Urological Association
1000 Corporate Boulevard
Linthicum, MD 21090
Tel: (410) 689-3700 or (866)
RING AUA (746-4282)
Fax: (410) 689-3800
Web site: www.auanet.org
E-Mail: aua@auanet.org or
executiveadministration@auanet.org

Hysterectomy Educational
Resources and Services Foundation
422 Bryn Mawr Avenue
Bala Cynwyd, PA 19004
Tel: (610) 667-7757
Fax: (610) 667-8096
Web site: www.hersfoundation.com
E-Mail: HERSFdn@earthlink.net

Sexuality Information and
Education Council of the
United States
130 West 42nd Street, Suite 350
New York, NY 10036
Tel: (212) 819-9770
Fax: (212) 819-9776
Web site: www.siecus.org
E-Mail: siecus@siecus.org

Sight Problems

American Academy of
Ophthalmology
PO Box 7424
San Francisco, CA 94120
Tel: (415) 561-8500
Fax: (415) 561-8533
Toll Free: (800) 222-3937
Web site: www.eyenet.org
E-Mail: comm@aao.org

American Foundation for the Blind
11 Penn Plaza, Suite 300
New York, NY 10001
Tel: (212) 502-7600
Toll Free: (800) AFB LINE
(232-5463)
Fax: (212) 502-7777
Web site: www.afb.org
E-Mail: afbinfo@afb.net

American Optometric Association
243 North Lindbergh Blvd.
St. Louis, MO 63141
Tel: (314) 991-4100
Fax: (314) 991-4101
Toll Free: (800) 365-2219
Web site: www.aoanet.org

Better Vision Institute
1700 Diagonal Road, Suite 500
Arlington, VA 22314
Tel: (703) 548-4560
Toll Free: (800) 642-3253
Fax: (703) 548-4580
Web site: www.visionsite.org
E-Mail: vca@visionsite.org

Foundation for Glaucoma Research
490 Post Street, Suite 1472
San Francisco, CA 94104
Tel: (415) 986-3162 or
(800) 826-6693
Fax: (415) 986-3763
Web site: www.glaucoma.org or
info@glaucoma.org

National Eye Institute
Information Office
2020 Vision Place
Bethesda, MD 20892-3655
Tel: (301) 496-5248
Fax: (301) 402-1065
Web site: www.nei.nih.gov
E-Mail: 2020@nei.nih.gov

Prevent Blindness America
211 West Wacker Drive, Suite 1700
Chicago, IL 60606
Toll Free: (800) 331-2020
Web site: www.preventblindness.org
E-Mail: info@preventblindness.org

Skin Problems

American Academy of Dermatology
1350 First St., NW, Suite 870
Washington, DC 20005-2355
Tel: (202) 842-3555
Toll Free: (888) 462-DERM (3376)
Fax: (202) 842-4355
Web site: www.aad.org
E-Mail: yurbikas@aad.org

American Academy of Facial Plastic
and Reconstructive Surgery
310 South Henry Street
Alexandria, VA 22314
Tel: (703) 299-9291
Fax: (703) 299-8898
Toll Free: (800) 332-FACE
Web site: www.aafprs.org
E-Mail: info@aafprs.org

American Social Health Association
Herpes Resource Center
PO Box 13827
Research Triangle Park, NC 27709
Tel: (919) 361-8400
Fax: (919) 361-8425
Web site: http://www.ashastd.org
E-Mail: phidra@ashastd.org

National Arthritis and
Musculoskeletal and Skin Diseases
Information Clearinghouse
National Institutes of Health
1 AMS Circle
Bethesda, MD 20892-3675
Tel: (301) 495-4484
Toll Free: (877) 22-NIAMS
(226-4267)
Fax: (301) 718-6366
Web site: www.nih.gov/niams
E-Mail: niamsinfo@mail.nih.gov

The Skin Cancer Foundation
245 5th Avenue, Suite 1403
New York, NY 10016
Tel: (212) 725-5176
Toll Free: (800) SKIN-490
(754-6490)
Fax: (212) 725-5751
Web site: www.skincancer.org
E-Mail: info@skincancer.org

Urinary Problems

National Association for Continence
(NAFC)
PO Box 1019
Charleston, SC 29402
Tel: (843) 377-0900
Toll Free: (800) BLADDER
(252-3337)
Fax: (843) 377-0905
Web site: www.nafc.org
E-Mail: memberservices@nafc.org

National Kidney and Urologic
Diseases Information Clearinghouse
3 Information Way
Bethesda, MD 20892-3560
Tel: (800) 891-5390
Fax: (703) 738-4929
Web site: www.niddk.nih.gov
E-Mail: nkudic@info.niddk.nih.gov

National Kidney Foundation
30 East 33rd Street
Suite 1100
New York, NY 10016
Tel: (212) 889-2210
Toll Free: (800) 622-9010
Fax: (212) 689-9261
Web site: www.kidney.org
E-Mail: info@kidney.org

The Simon Foundation for
Continence
PO Box 815
Wilmette, IL 60091
Tel: (847) 864-3913
Toll Free: (800) 23-SIMON
(237-4666)
Fax: (847) 864-9758
Web site: www.simonfoundation.org
E-Mail:
simoninfo@simonfoundation.org

INDEX

Page references followed by *t* and *f* indicate tables and figures, respectively.

Allergic conjunctivitis, 153
α-Adrenergic agonists
    adverse effects of, 152, 152t
    and incontinence, 185t
α-Adrenergic antagonists or a-blockers
    for benign prostatic hyperplasia, 424, 424t,
        425
    for hypertension, 365
    and incontinence, 185t
Alprazolam, 245t
Alprostadil, 420, 421–422, 421t
Alteplase, 461
Altered mental status. See Delirium
Alternative medicine, 80–86
Alzheimer's disease
    behavioral problems in, 233
    deaths due to, 5, 6t
    dementia associated with, 83, 224, 224t,
        233
    diagnostic features of, 224t
    differential diagnosis of, 224
    general progression of, 226t
    genetic testing and, 29
    pharmacologic treatment of, 228–229
    protective factors for, 222t
    risk factors for, 222t
AMA. See American Medical Association
Amantadine, 245t, 464
Ambulance services, 34t
Ambulatory electrocardiographic monitoring,
    171
American Academy of Family Physicians
    joint guidelines, 95–96
    Nutrition Screening Initiative, 177
    recommendations for management of AF,
        356–357
American Academy of Neurology
    recommendations for physical activity,
        58t
American Academy of Ophthalmology
    recommendations for comprehensive eye
        examinations, 149
American Academy of Orthopaedic Surgeons
    (AAOS)
    recommendations for antibiotic
        prophylaxis, 340
    recommendations for physical activity, 58t
American Cancer Society recommendations
    for prostate cancer screening, 426
American College of Cardiology (ACC)
    guidelines for coronary revascularization in
        treatment of unstable angina or
        non-Q-wave myocardial infarction,
        347, 348t
    guidelines for diagnosing CAD, 346
    guidelines for perioperative cardiovascular
        evaluation for noncardiac surgery, 100
    indications for automatic implantable
        cardioverter-defibrillator, 356t
    indications for early invasive treatment of
        unstable angina or non-Q-wave
        myocardial infarction, 348t
    indications for permanent pacemaker
        implantation in bradyarrhythmias, 358t
American College of Obstetrics and
    Gynecology (ACOG) classification of
    pelvic organ prolapse, 413, 413t

American College of Physicians
    joint guidelines, 95–96
    recommendations for management of AF,
        356–357
    recommendations for prostate cancer
        screening, 426
American College of Rheumatology
    diagnostic criteria for fibromyalgia,
        432–433
    diagnostic criteria for giant cell arteritis,
        439
    diagnostic criteria for osteoarthritis, 436t
    diagnostic criteria for systemic lupus
        erythematosus, 442
    recommendations for treating
        osteoarthritis, 437
American College of Sports Medicine
    recommendations for physical activity,
        58t, 62
American Dental Association
    recommendations for antibiotic
        prophylaxis, 340
American Diabetes Association
    diagnostic criteria for diabetes mellitus,
        383
    recommendations for physical activity, 58t
American Dietetic Association, 177
American Geriatrics Society (AGS)
    assisted living facilities position statement,
        494–495
    guidelines for prevention of falls
        recommendations, 497–498
    guidelines for research using cognitively
        impaired persons as subjects, 26, 26t
    recommendations for physical activity, 58t
    recommendations for treating
        osteoarthritis, 437
    Web site resources, 503
American Heart Association (AHA)
    guidelines for coronary revascularization in
        treatment of unstable angina or
        non-Q-wave myocardial infarction,
        347, 348t
    guidelines for diagnosing CAD, 346
    guidelines for perioperative cardiovascular
        evaluation for noncardiac surgery, 100
    guidelines for prophylactic antibiotics to
        prevent bacterial endocarditis, 354,
        355
    indications for automatic implantable
        cardioverter-defibrillator, 356t
    indications for early invasive treatment of
        unstable angina or non-Q-wave
        myocardial infarction, 348t
    indications for permanent pacemaker
        implantation in bradyarrhythmias, 358t
    recommendations for driving after syncope,
        173
    recommendations for endocarditis
        prophylaxis, 340
    recommendations for physical activity, 58t
    Web site, 102
American Medical Association (AMA)
    recommendations for fair process, 331
    Web site, 90
American Medical Directors Association, 123
American Society of Anesthesiologists (ASA)
    classification of physical status, 100, 100t

American Urogynecologic Association
    classification of pelvic organ prolapse,
        413
American Urological Association
    recommendations for prostate cancer
        screening, 426
Amiodarone, 357
Amitriptyline, 245t
Amputation
    for circulatory system disorders, 38t
    rehabilitation for, 117
Amyotrophic lateral sclerosis, 468
Anakinra, 442
Analgesia. See also Pain management;
        Palliative care
    and incontinence, 185t
    narcotic, 185t
Androgen ablation, complete, 429
Androgens
    adrenal, 377–378
    in men, 212
Anemia, 471–476
    causes of, 472t
    of chronic disease, 473
    diagnosis of, 474f
    hemolytic, 472t, 473, 476
    hypoproliferative, 472t, 473–475
    macrocytic, 475
    physiologic classification of, 472t
    presentation of, 472
    work-up of, 472–473
Aneurysm, aortic abdominal, 66t, 67
Aneurysms and dissections, 358–359
Angina pectoris
    screening for, 69t
    stable, 347
    unstable, 347, 348t
Angiodysplasia, 397
    colonic, 397–398
Angioplasty, percutaneous transluminal
        coronary, 349
Angiotensin-converting enzyme inhibitors
    drug interactions, 77t
    for heart failure, 352
    for hypertension, 364
    and incontinence, 185t
Angiotensin II type 1 receptor antagonists,
        352–353
Angiotensin-receptor blockers, 364
Anhedonia, 269
Ankle-brachial index (ABI), 359
Anorexia, 137
Anserine bursitis, 435
Antacids, 177t
Anthropometrics, 175
Antiarrhythmics
    drug interactions, 77t
    and incontinence, 185t
Antibiotic therapy
    guidelines for prophylactic antibiotics to
        prevent bacterial endocarditis, 354,
        355
    for infections, 334, 335t
    minimum criteria for initiation in
        long-term care settings, 334, 335t
    nutrient interactions, 177t
    for prostatitis, 429

management of, 449
 physical examination of, 447–448, 448*t*
Baclofen (Lioresal), 143*t*
Bacteremia, 335
Bacterial endocarditis, 354, 355
Bacterial meningitis, 341
Bacteriuria, asymptomatic, 337–338
Baker cyst, 435–436
Balance assessment, 47
Balance training, 59, 61–62
Balanced Budget Act of 1997 (BBA 97),
 40–41, 121, 125
Balanced Budget Revision Act of 1999, 42
Barbiturates, 245*t*
Barthel ADL Index, 113
Basal cell carcinoma, 317–318, 318*f*
Beclomethasone, 328*t*
Bedsores. *See* Pressure ulcers
Behavioral interventions. *See also* Cognitive
 behavioral therapy
 for dementia care, 233–234, 233*t*
 for insomnia, 237, 237*t*
 programs for prevention of falls, 498 for
  urinary incontinence, 188*t*, 190–191,
  190*t*, 191*t*, 499–500
Behavioral problems
 adaptive difficulties, 305
 assessment of, 232–233
 basic approach to treatment of, 233–234
 clinical features of, 231–232
 in dementia, 231–238, 235*t*
 differential diagnosis of, 232–233
 disorders in aging adults with mental
  retardation, 305–306
 drugs to treat depressive features of,
  234–235, 235*t*
 with manic features, 234–235, 235*t*
 manic-like syndromes, 234–235, 235*t*
Bell's palsy, 342
Benign cutaneous growths, 316–317
Benign positional vertigo, 163
 Epley's maneuver for, 163, 164*f*
 management of, 166
Benign prostatic hyperplasia, 423–425
 CAM treatments for, 84
 diagnosis of, 423–424
 epidemiology of, 423
 lower urinary tract symptoms of, 423
 management options for, 424, 424*t*
 medical treatment of, 424–425
Benzodiazepines, 276
 for anxiety disorders, 284
 chronic use of, 257
 and delirium, 245*t*
 drug interactions, 77*t*
 for insomnia, 257*t*
 for mania and manic-like symptoms, 278*t*
Benztropine, 245*t*
Bereavement, 18
 assessment of, 48
 differential diagnosis of, 271
 and sleep problems, 251
 therapy for, 272, 272*t*
β-Blockers
 for acute MI, 348
 adverse effects of, 152, 152*t*
 for anxiety disorders, 284*t*
 for heart failure, 353

for hypertension, 365
 after myocardial infarction, 348–349
 perioperative, 100
 for stable angina pectoris, 347
 for unstable angina pectoris and
  non-Q-wave myocardial infarction,
  348
 for ventricular arrhythmias, 356
Betamethasone, 439
Biceps tendinitis, 433
Biguanides, 386, 387*t*
Biliary disease, 393–394
Bioavailability, 72
Biofeedback for urinary incontinence, 191*t*
Biologic therapy
 for cancer, 484
 safety of agents, 85
Biology
 of aging, 8–16
 of cancer, 480–481
Biopsy, kidney, 403–404
Biotin, 175*t*
Biphosphate emollient enema (Fleet), 105*t*
Bipolar disorder
 clinical presentation and diagnosis of, 270
 management of, 277–279
Bisacodyl (Dulcolax), 105*t*
Bisphosphonates
 instructions for administration of, 216*t*
 for osteoporosis prevention and treatment,
  215–216, 216*t*
Black Americans
 CAM use by, 81
 cancer diagnosis and survival, 481, 481*t*
 cancer incidence in, 481, 481*t*
 hypertension in, 361
 intracerebral hemorrhage in, 460
 leading causes of death for, 5, 6*t*
 life expectancy of, 1, 2*t*
 multiple myeloma in, 487
 nursing-home population, 120
 oral cancer in, 323
 perceived health of Medicare beneficiaries,
  4, 5*t*
 poverty rates in, 2
 prostate cancer in, 425
 self-reported functional limitations of
  Medicare beneficiaries, 4–5, 6*f*
 social status and health of, 18–19
Bladder cancer
 racial differences in diagnosis and survival,
  481, 481*t*
 screening for, 71*t*
Bladder diary, 189, 191
Bladder outlet obstruction, 187, 193
Bladder training, 190, 190*t*, 191*t*, 499
Bladder urge control procedures, 500
Bleeding
 And anticoagulation, 491*t*
 gastrointestinal, 397
 postmenopausal vaginal, 414–415, 414*t*
 upper gastrointestinal, 112*t*
Bleeding diatheses, 477
Blood chemistry panels, annual, 71*t*
Blood pressure. *See also* Hypertension;
 Hypotension
 CAM use for, 82–83

classification of, 361–362, 362*t*
 screening, 66*t*
Body composition changes, 174
Body mass index, 47, 65, 175, 175*t*
Body size classification, 175, 175*t*
Bone, Paget's disease of, 375–376
Bone formation changes, 212
Bone infections, 341
Bone loss, 210–211. *See also* Osteomalacia;
 Osteoporosis
Bone mineral density testing, 66*t*, 67,
 213–214
 indications for, 213*t*
Bone remodeling, 210–211, 214
Bone resources, 511
Borderline personality disorder
 features of, 291, 292*t*
 therapeutic strategies for, 293–295, 294*t*
Brachytherapy, 428, 428*t*
Braden Scale, 260
Bradyarrhythmias, 357–358
Bradykinesia, 463
Brain disease, structural, 271
Brain imaging, 223
Breast cancer, 485–486
 adjuvant hormonal treatment of, 486
 biologic therapy for, 484
 CAM treatment for, 84
 characteristics of, 480–481
 ethnic and racial differences in incidence,
  481, 481*t*
 hormonal therapy for, 484*t*
 metastatic, 486
 racial differences in diagnosis and survival,
  481, 481*t*
 recommended preventive services for, 66*t*
 screening for, 67
Breathing, sleep-disordered, 251–252, 329
Breathing disorders resources, 511–512
Breathlessness, 138
British Geriatrics Society recommendations
 for physical activity, 58*t*
Bromocriptine, 464
Budesonide, 328*t*
Bullous pemphigoid, 312–313, 313*f*
Bunions, 452*t*
Bupropion (Wellbutrin SR), 235*t*, 275, 276*t*
Burning mouth syndrome, 324
Burns, 66*t*
Bursitis, anserine, 435
Buspirone, 284
Bypass surgery
 coronary artery, 100, 349
 lower extremity, 360

C

Cachexia, 137
CAGE Questionnaire, 301, 301*t*
Calcaneal spur, 452*t*
Calcitonin, 216*t*, 217
Calcium, 179
 counseling for intake of, 66*t*
 deficiency of, 211
 disorders of metabolism of, 373–376
 drug interactions, 177*t*
 foods containing, 215*t*
 homeostasis alterations, 373, 375*t*

Fluvastatin, 351*t*

Fluvoxamine, 274

Folate

  deficiency, 475, 476–477

  drug interactions, 177*t*

  RDAs for persons aged 71 and older, 175*t*

Folic acid, 179

Folstein Mini-Mental State Examination (MMSE), 24, 47, 223, 240, 241*t*

Fondaparinux (Arixtra), 492*t*

Food and Nutrition Board of the Institute of Medicine macronutrient guidelines, 174–175

Food guide pyramid, 174

Foods, calcium-containing, 215*t*

Foot care, 457

Foot disorders, 451–458, 452*t*

  disorders of the skin and nails, 453–456

  orthopedic, 451–453

  systemic diseases and, 456–457

Foot drop, 196*t*

Foot slap, 196*t*

Forefoot disorders, orthopedic, 451–453

Foreign-born population, older, 3

Forgoing and discontinuing interventions, 27

Formoterol, 328*t*

Foster care, adult, 132

Fractures, 61–62

  of hip, 38*t*, 115–116

  osteoporotic sacral fractures, 447

  osteoporotic vertebral, 446–447

  pathologic, 38*t*

  of pelvis, 38*t*

  prediction of, 212–214

  rehabilitation for, 115–116

  risk factors for, 212

  surgical care of, 115

  vertebral compression, 446–447

Fragile X syndrome, 306, 306*t*

Fragmin (dalteparin), 492*t*

Frail, older residents of long-term care facilities, 334, 334*t*

Frontal lobe damage, 306, 306*t*

Frontotemporal dementia

  behavioral problems in, 233

  diagnostic features of, 224*t*

  differential diagnosis of, 224–225

Frozen shoulder syndrome, 434

Functional adrenocortical adenoma, 377, 377*t*

Functional Independence Measure (FIM), 109, 113

Functional reach test, 204–206

Functional status

  assessment of, 46–47

  epidemiologic trends in, 4–5

  impairments in hospitalized patients, 92*t*, 93

  limitations of Medicare beneficiaries, 4–5, 6*f*

  performance-based assessment of, 199

  rapid screening followed by assessment and management of, 45–46, 45*t*

FUO. *See* Fever, of unknown origin

Futility, 331

G

Gabapentin (Neurontin)

  for epilepsy, 468*t*

  for persistent pain, 143*t*, 147

Gait apraxia, 197

Gait impairment, 195–201

  abnormalities, 196*t*, 198*t*

  assessment of, 197–199

  conditions that contribute to, 196–197

  epidemiology of, 195–196

  history and physical examination, 197–199

  interventions to reduce, 199–201

Gait speed, 47

Galantamine, 228

Gallstones, 393–394

Gastroesophageal reflux disease, 391–392

Gastrointestinal bleeding, occult, 397

Gastrointestinal diseases and disorders, 390–400

  angiodysplasia, colonic, 397–398

  biliary disease, 393–394

  bleeding, 112*t*, 393, 393*t*, 397

  Clostridium difficile infection, 398

  colon cancer, 398–399, 481, 481*t*, 486

  colonic, 394–399

  constipation, 104, 105*t*, 135, 394–395, 396

  diverticular disease, 395–396

  dyspepsia, 392–393

  dysphagia, 390–391

  esophageal, 390–392

  fecal incontinence, 395

  gastroesophageal reflux disease, 391–392

  irritable bowel syndrome, 396–397

  infections, 342

  NSAID-induced, 393, 393*t*

  peptic ulcer disease, 393

  postoperative management of, 104

  pseudo-obstruction, acute colonic, 398

  polyps, colonic, 398–399

  and urinary incontinence, 185, 186*t*

Gastrostomy, percutaneous endoscopic, 183

Gaze-evoked nystagmus, 165

GEM units. *See* Geriatric evaluation and management units

Gemfibrozil, 351*t*

Gender issues, cross-cultural, 54

Gene expression, 12–13, 13*t*

Generalized anxiety disorder, 283, 284*t*

Genetic testing, 29

Genitourinary imaging, 403–404

Genu recurvatum, 196*t*

GERD. *See* Gastroesophageal reflux disease

Geriatric Depression Scale (short form), 496

Geriatric evaluation and management (GEM) units, 97

Geriatric syndrome of late-life depression, 269–270. *See also* Depression

  psychotherapy for, 272, 272*t*

Get Up and Go test, 45*t*, 46–47, 199, 206

Giant cell (temporal) arteritis, 439–440

  diagnostic criteria for, 439

  headache due to, 461

Ginkgo biloba, 82*t*, 83, 228–229

Glaucoma, 152, 152*t*

Gleason grading system, 426

Glipizide (Glucotrol, Glucotrol XL), 387*t*

Glipizide and metformin (METAGLIP), 388*t*

Glomerular filtration rate, 103

Glomerulonephritis, 406

Glucocorticoid hypersecretion, subclinical, 377

Glucophage (metformin), 387*t*

Glucophage XR (metformin), 387*t*

Glucosamine

  for osteoarthritis, 437

  safety issues, 82*t*

Glucose screening, 66*t*

α-Glucosidase inhibitors, 386, 387*t*

Glucotrol (glipizide), 387*t*

Glucotrol XL (glipizide), 387*t*

Glucovance (glyburide and metformin), 388*t*

Glutathione, 83

Glyburide (Diaβeta, Micronase)

  for diabetes mellitus, 387*t*

  micronized (Glynase), 386, 387*t*

Glyburide and metformin (Glucovance), 388*t*

Glyset (miglitol), 387*t*

Gout

  pseudogout, 438–439

  rheumatoid, 437–438

Grand mal seizures, 467

Graves' disease, 371, 372*f*

Grief. *See* Bereavement

Group homes, 132

Group therapy, 225

Growth factors, 12–13, 13*t*

Growth hormone, 380

Growth regulatory genes, 12–13, 13*t*

Gustatory dysfunction

  drugs that cause, 324, 324*t*

  nonpharmacologic causes of, 324, 325*t*

Gynecologic diseases and disorders, 410–415

H

H$_2$-blocking agents, 244, 245*t*

HAART (highly active antiretroviral therapy), 341

Habit training for urge incontinence, 190*t*, 191*t*

Haglund's deformity, 452*t*

Hallucinations, 285–286

  antipsychotic agents for, 236–237, 236*t*

  in delirium, 288

  in dementia, 236–237, 236*t*

  evaluation of person with, 286, 286*f*

  isolated, 289–290

Hallucinosis, organic, 289–290

Hallux abducto valgus, 452*t*, 453*f*

Hallux limitus and rigidus, 452*t*

Hallux valgus, 452*t*

Haloperidol

  for agitated delirium, 246, 246*t*

  dosing and side effects, 288*t*

Hammertoe, 451–453, 453*f*

Harris-Benedict equations, 174, 174*t*

Harris Hip Questionnaire, 113, 115

Head and neck problems. *See also* Back pain; Headaches

  head and neck cancer, 481, 481*t*

  resources, 510

Head-shaking, 165

Headaches, 38*t*, 461–462

Mixed urge and stress incontinence, 191t

MMSE. *See* Mini-Mental State Examination

Mobility aids, 117–118, 201

Mobility status
   and prevention of pressure ulcers, 262
   rapid screening followed by assessment and management of, 45–46, 45t
   and rehabilitation, 111

Modafinil (Provigil), 276t

Moderators of stress, 20–21

Mono-Gesic (salsalate), 143t

Monoamine oxidase inhibitors, 275

Mood disorders, 269–307
   in dementia, 234
   psychotic symptoms in, 288
   treatment of, 234

Mood stabilizers, 234–235, 235t

Morbidity, 6–7

Morphine, immediate release (MSIR, Roxanol), 144t

Morphine, sustained release (MSContin, Kadian), 144t

Morton's syndrome, 452t

Motor neuron disease, 468

Motor vehicle accidents. *See also* Driving
   death rates, 5
   recommended preventive services for, 66t

Movement disorders, 461–467
   drug-induced, 466

MSAs. *See* Medical savings accounts

MSContin (morphine, sustained release), 144t

MSIR (morphine, immediate release), 144t

MTB. *See* Mycobacterium tuberculosis

Mucosal problems, oral, 323–324

Multidensity inserts for shoes, 457

Multiple myeloma, 212t, 487–488

Multiple sclerosis, 185, 186t

Multiple system atrophy, 464–465

Musculoskeletal diseases and disorders, 430–444
   CAM treatment for, 81–82
   diagnosis of, 430–431
   exercise treatment of, 431
   and incontinence, 185, 186t
   malignancy, 38t
   resources, 511

MUSE (medicated urethral system for erection), 421t, 422

Mycobacterium tuberculosis (MTB), 338–339

Myelodysplastic syndromes, 475–476, 487

Myelopathy, 469

Myeloproliferative disorders, chronic, 478–479

Myelotoxicity, 483t

Myocardial infarction
   ACC/AHA guidelines for coronary revascularization in treatment of, 347, 348t
   ACC/AHA indications for early invasive treatment of unstable angina, 348t
   acute, 38t, 347–348, 491t
   coronary revascularization after, 349
   non-Q-wave, 347, 348t
   preventive activities for, 69t
   recommended preventive services for, 66t

risk factors for coronary events after, 349, 349t

risk stratification after, 349, 349t

screening for, 69t

treatment after, 348–349

Myofascial pain, 141

Myofascial trigger points, 432

Myopathy, 470

N

Nail problems, 454–456

Narcissistic personality disorder
   features of, 292t
   therapeutic strategies for, 293–295, 294t

Narcotic analgesics, 185t

Narcotics Anonymous, 302

Nateglinide (Starlix), 387t

National Center on Elder Abuse Web site, 90

National Cholesterol Education Program Expert Panel (3rd Report)
   recommendations for physical activity, 58t

National Council on Aging, Inc. Nutrition Screening Initiative, 177

National Institutes of Health (NIH)
   guidelines regarding body size classification, 175, 175t

National Osteoporosis Foundation
   recommendations for BMD testing, 213

Native Americans
   burning mouth syndrome in, 324
   CAM use by, 81
   nursing-home population, 120

Nausea and vomiting
   postoperative, 104
   in terminal illness, 136–137, 136t

Neck pain, 445, 449–450
   assessment of, 450
   causes of, 449–450
   diagnostic imaging of, 450
   management of, 450

Nedocromil, 328t

Neglect. *See also* Elder mistreatment
   key indicators of, 88t
   self-neglect, 89

Neoplasia, vulvar, 413

Nephritis
   acute interstitial, 406
   deaths due to, 5, 6t

Nephropathy, 404, 406

Nephrosis, 5, 6t

Nephrotic syndrome, 404
   deaths due to, 5, 6t

Nepro, 183t

Neuralgia, post-herpetic, 315

Neurodermatitis, 311

Neuroendocrinologic theory of aging, 9t, 10

Neuroimaging, 166. *See also* Imaging

Neurologic diseases and disorders, 458–470
   associated with incontinence, 185, 186t
   CAM treatment for, 83–84
   cerebrovascular disease, 5, 6t, 38t, 185, 186t, 459–461
   epilepsy, 467
   headaches, 461–462
   motor neuron disease, 468

movement disorders, 462–467

myelopathy, 469

myopathy, 470

peripheral neuropathy, 469–470

degenerative disorders of, 38t

radiculopathy, 469

resources, 512

subdural hematoma, 461

Neurologic testing, 172

Neurontin (gabapentin), 143t

Neuropathic pain, 141

Neuropathy, peripheral, 469–470

Neuropsychiatry
   diseases associated with incontinence, 185, 186t
   disorders in aging adults with mental retardation, 305–306
   preoperative concerns, 103
   and sleep problems, 250–251

Neurosyphilis, 341–342

Niacin
   drug interactions, 177t
   for dyslipidemia, 351t
   RDAs for persons aged 71 and older, 175t

Nifedipine, 354

NIH Stroke Scale, 114, 459, 461

Nitrates, 77t

Nitroglycerin, 347

Nociceptive pain, 141

Nodular melanoma, 318

Nodular thyroid disease, 373, 374f

Non-Hodgkin's lymphoma, 487

Nonadherence to medications, 79

Nonsteroidal anti-inflammatory drugs
   for chondrocalcinosis, 439
   drug interactions, 77t
   gastric complications with, 393
   for gout, 438
   and incontinence, 185t
   kidney diseases associated with use of, 407
   medications to avoid in older adults, 147
   for osteoarthritis, 437
   for persistent pain, 145
   for rheumatoid arthritis, 440–441
   risk factors for upper gastrointestinal adverse events with, 393, 393t

Nonverbal communication, cross-cultural, 52

Normal-pressure hydrocephalus
   effect on incontinence, 185, 186t
   interventions for, 200

Norpramin (desipramine), 143t, 275t

Norton Scale, 260

Nortriptyline (Aventyl, Pamelor), 274, 275t
   for depressive features of behavioral disturbances in dementia, 235t
   for persistent pain management, 143t

Novolin (insulin), 389t

Novolin 70/30 (isophane insulin & regular insulin), 389t

NovoLog (insulin aspart), 389t

Numeric Rating Scale for pain, 141

Nurse practitioners, health insurance coverage for, 34t

Nursing care trends, 7

Nursing-home acquired pneumonia, 336–337. *See also* Pneumonia

nursing-home care responsibilities, 123, 124*t*

nursing-home practice, 123–124

Pick's disease, 233

Pioglitazone (Actos), 387*t*

Pirbuterol, 328*t*

Plantar fasciitis, 452*t*, 453

Plaque, dental, 321

Platelets, 477–478

Pleurisy, 38*t*

Pneumococcal vaccination
in hospitalized patients, 92*t*, 96–97
recommendations for, 66*t*, 69

Pneumonia, 38*t*, 335–337
aspiration, 182
causes of, 335–336, 336*f*
community-acquired, 336
deaths due to, 5, 6*t*
hospital-acquired, 336–337
in hospitalized patients, 92*t*
nursing-home acquired, 336–337
and rehabilitation, 111–112, 112*t*

Polycarbophil (FiberCon, others), 105*t*

Polycythemia vera, 478

Polyethylene glycol (MiraLax), 105*t*

Polymyalgia rheumatica, 439

Polymyositis, 431, 443–444

Polyps, colonic, 398–399

Polysomnography, 250

Popliteal cyst, 435–436

Post-herpetic neuralgia, 315

Postacute care
health insurance coverage for, 34*t*
nursing-home care, 120–121
primary diagnoses for which "early" discharges from hospitals are regarded as "transfers" to, 37, 38*t*

Postacute rehabilitation, 37–38
fee for service, 38–39
managed care, 38

Posttraumatic stress disorder, 282–283, 284*t*

Postvoiding residual volume measurement, 189

Potassium, 77*t*, 177*t*

Potassium supplements, 77*t*

PPD skin tests, 339

PPOs. *See* Preferred provider organizations

Prader-Willie syndrome, 306, 306*t*

Pramipexole, 464

Pramlintide (Symlin), 388*t*

Prandin (repaglinide), 387*t*

Pravastatin, 351*t*

Pre-renal acute renal insufficiency, 405

Prealbumin, 176

Precose (acarbose), 387*t*

Prednisone (Deltasone, Liquid Pred, Orasone)
for headache due to giant cell (temporal) arteritis, 461
for persistent pain management, 143*t*
for polymyalgia rheumatica, 439
for polymyositis and dermatomyositis, 443–444

Preferred provider organizations (PPOs), 40

Pregabalin (Lyrica), 143*t*

Prehypertension, 361–362, 362*t*

Preoperative assessment and management, 100–103

Preoperative cardiac care, 100, 101*f*

Presbycusis, 156

Presbyesophagus, 181

Prescribing
Cascade, 76
factors associated with inappropriate prescribing or overprescribing, 75, 75*t*
optimizing, 75
principles of, 78–79, 78*t*

Prescription drugs. *See* Drugs; Pharmacotherapy

Pressure Sore Status Tool, 266

Pressure Ulcer Scale for Healing, 266

Pressure ulcers, 259–268
assessment of, 262–264
Braden Scale, 260
complications from, 267
control of infections in, 266–267
dressings for, 264, 265*t*
epidemiology of, 259–260
incidence of, 260
management of, 262–267, 263*t*
monitoring healing, 266
Norton Scale, 260
prevalence of, 260
prevention of, 261–262, 261*t*
risk-assessment scales, 260
risk factors for, 260
staging system for, 262–264, 263*t*
support surfaces for persons at risk for, 262, 262*t*
surgical repair of, 264
treatment of, 264–267

Presyncope, 164

Prevention, 64–71
aspirin therapy, 347
of atherosclerotic complications of diabetes mellitus, 385–386
atherosclerotic stroke prevention, 459–460
of delirium, 247
delivery of services, 71
of elder mistreatment, 86–87
of falls, 66*t*, 206–207
health insurance coverage for services, 34*t*
of hip fracture recurrence, 116
of microvascular complications of diabetes mellitus, 386
physical activity effects, 56–57
potentially beneficial services lacking evidence, 69, 69*t*
recommended services, 64–71, 66*t*, 69*t*
services not indicated in older adults, 70–71, 71*t*

Primidone, 245*t*

Private FFS plans, 41

Problem solving therapy for depression, 272, 272*t*

Problem substance use, 298

Progesterone, 237

Program of All-inclusive Care of the Elderly (PACE), 39–40, 130

Progressive supranuclear palsy, 465

Prompted voiding, 190*t*, 191*t*

Propoxyphene (Darvon), 147

Propulsion, 196*t*

Prospective payment system (PPS), 39, 125

Prostaglandins, 152, 152*t*

Prostate cancer, 425–429
CAM treatment for, 84–85
diagnostic tests, 426
ethnic and racial differences in incidence, 481, 481*t*
grading, 426
hormonal therapy for, 484*t*
incidence and epidemiology, 425
locally advanced, 428
management of advanced disease, 429
management of localized disease, 427–428, 428*t*
screening for, 69*t*, 70, 426
staging systems for, 426–427, 427*t*
symptoms, 425

Prostate disease, 423–430

Prostate-specific antigen testing, 426

Prostatectomy, radical, 427–428, 428*t*

Prostatic hyperplasia, benign, 423–425
CAM treatment for, 84
management options for, 424, 424*t*

Prostatism, 423

Prostatitis, 429

Prosthesis, penile, 421*t*, 422

Prosthetic device infections, 340

Protein-energy undernutrition, 178

Protein needs, 174–175, 174*t*

Proteinuria, 402–403

Provider-sponsored organizations (PSOs), 41

Provigil (modafinil), 276*t*

Proxy, health care, 25

Prozac (fluoxetine), 274*t*

Pruritus, 313

Pseudo-addiction, 146

Pseudoclaudication, 446

Pseudogout, 438–439

Pseudomembranous colitis, 398

Psoriasis, 313–314, 314*f*

PSOs. *See* Provider-sponsored organizations

Psychiatric diseases and disorders. *See also* specific disorders
associated with incontinence, 185, 186*t*
in aging adults with mental retardation, 305–306
preoperative concerns, 103
and sleep problems, 250–251

Psychoactive medications, 229

Psychogenic dizziness, 163

Psychologic mistreatment, 88–89

Psychologic assessment, 48

Psychologic problems, 513

Psychosis
antipsychotic agents for, 236–237, 236*t*
in dementia, 236–237, 236*t*, 288–289
and incontinence, 185, 186*t*

Psychosocial issues, 16–22
and sleep disorders, 250–251

Psychotherapy
for anxiety disorders, 284–285
for dementia, 225
for geriatric syndrome of late-life depression, 272, 272*t*

Psychotic depression, 277

Psychotic disorders, 285–290

Strontium ranelate, 218
Subacute befuddlement. *See* Delirium
Subclinical glucocorticoid hypersecretion, 377
Subclinical hyperthyroidism, 371
Subclinical hypothyroidism, 369, 370*f*
Subdural hematoma, 461
Substance abuse
  alcohol abuse, 298–304
  at-risk use, 298, 303
  brief interventions for, 303
  definitions of, 298–299
  drug abuse, 298–304
  excess physical disability with, 300–301
  identifying disorders of, 301–302
  mental health problems with, 301
  outpatient management of, 302–303
  risks and benefits of, 300–301
  treatment of, 302–303
Substance Abuse and Mental Health Services
    Administration, 303
Substance dependence, 298
Subungual heloma, 456
Suicide, 5
  physician-assisted, 27–28
Sulfa drugs, 77*t*
Sulfasalazine, 441
Sulfonylureas, 2nd-generation, 386, 387*t*
Supplemental Security Income (SSI),
    131–132
Support surfaces and pressure ulcers, 262,
    262*t*
Support systems, social, 48
Supranuclear palsy, progressive, 465
Surgery
  ACC/AHA guideline for perioperative
      cardiovascular evaluation for
      noncardiac surgery, 100
  for benign prostatic hyperplasia, 424*t*, 425
  for cancer, 485
  coronary artery bypass, 100, 349
  hip fracture, 115
  indications for anticoagulation in absence
      of active bleeding or severe bleeding
      risk, 491*t*
  lower extremity bypass, 360
  overview of operative therapy, 99
  perioperative care, 99–107
  postoperative delirium, 242–243
  postoperative management, 103–107
  preoperative assessment and management,
      100–103
  preoperative cardiac care, 100, 101*f*
  for pressure ulcers, 264
  for prolapse, genital, 414
  for stress incontinence, 192*t*, 193
  total hip and knee arthroplasty, 116–117
Surveillance for prostate cancer, 427–428
Suspiciousness, isolated, 289
Swallowing, 181–182
Symlin (pramlintide), 388*t*
Syncope, 168–173
  causes of, 169, 169*t*
  classes of, 170, 171*t*
  evaluation of, 170–172
  history, 170
  natural history of, 169–170
  physical examination of, 170–171
  treatment of, 172–173

Syndrome of inappropriate antidiuretic
    hormone, 376
Syphilis, 341–342
Systemic lupus erythematosus, 442
  diagnostic criteria for, 442
  exercise treatment of, 431
  laboratory testing for, 431

T

T₃ thyrotoxicosis, 371
Tacrine, 228
Tadalafil, 420–421, 421*t*
Tai Chi Chuan, 62, 206
Tailor's bunion, 452*t*
Taste dysfunction
  drugs that cause, 324, 324*t*
  nonpharmacologic causes of, 324, 325*t*
Teeth, 319–320, 320*f*, 320*t*
Tegretol (carbamazepine), 143*t*, 278*t*
Telemedicine, 130–131
Telomerase, 12
Telomeres, 12
Temazepam, 257*t*
Temporal arteritis, 439–440, 461
Temporal lobe lesions, 306, 306*t*
Tenosynovitis, 452*t*
Terbinafine, 455
Teriparatide, 216*t*, 218
Terminal illness
  anorexia in, 137
  cachexia in, 137
  communicating news about, 135
  constipation in, 135
  cough in, 139
  delirium in, 137
  depression in, 137–138
  diarrhea in, 137
  dyspnea in, 138–139
  nausea and vomiting in, 136–137, 136*t*
  palliative care, 133–140
Terminology
  foot disorders, 452*t*
  gait abnormalities, 196*t*
  to interpret screening and diagnostic tests,
      502
  preferred terms for cultural identity, 51
Testamentary competence, 24
Testosterone, 378
Testosterone supplementation, 378, 379*t*
  for erectile dysfunction, 422
  for female sexual dysfunction, 416–417,
      417
Tetanus booster, 66*t*
Tetanus vaccination, 69
Theophylline
  for asthma, 327
  drug interactions, 77*t*
  nutrient interactions, 177*t*
Thiamin, 175*t*
Thiazolidinediones
  for diabetes mellitus, 386, 387*t*
  and incontinence, 185*t*
Thrombin inhibitors, 493*t*
Thrombocythemia, essential, 478–479
Thrombolytics, 493*t*
Thrombopathy, 477

Thrombotic thrombocytopenic purpura, 476
Thyroid disorders, 369–373
  cancer, 373
  nodular, 373, 374*f*
  screening for, 69*t*, 70
Thyroid-stimulating hormone, 371, 372*f*
Thyroiditis, 371, 372*f*
Thyrotoxicosis, 371
Thyroxine (T₄), 369
  exogenous, 371, 372*f*
  high T₄ syndrome, 371
Tiagabine, 468*t*
Tilt-table testing, 172
Timed Get Up and Go (TUG) test, 45*t*,
    46–47, 199
Tinea pedis, 455*f*
Tinzaparin (Innohep), 492*t*
Tiotropium, 328*t*
TMP-SMX. *See*
    Trimethoprim-sulfamethoxazole
α-Tocopherol, 175*t*
Toenails
  disorders of the, 454–456
  ingrown, 455–456
Tolterodine, 190*t*, 191, 192
Toothlessness, 66*t*, 321–322
Topiramate, 468*t*
Total hip and knee arthroplasty, 116–117
  assessment of, 116
  management of, 116–117
  natural history of, 116
Toxic encephalopathy, 239
Toxic nodular goiter, 371, 372*f*
Toxicity
  chemotherapy issues, 483*t*
  warfarin overdose, 492*t*
Tracheostomy, 38*t*
Tramadol (Ultram), 144*t*, 147
Transcription factors, 12–13, 13*t*
Transdermal fentanyl (Duragesic), 144*t*
Transesophageal echocardiography, 339–340,
    357
"Transfers" to postacute care, 37, 38*t*
Transient ischemic attacks, 66*t*
Transitions in care, 38*t*, 66*t*, 106–107
Transplantation, renal, 408–409
Transthoracic echocardiography, 339
Trauma, psychologic
  history of traumatic experiences, 52
  posttraumatic stress disorder, 282–283,
      284*t*
Trazodone (Desyrel), 276*t*
  for anxiety disorders, 284*t*
  for depressive features of behavioral
      disturbances in dementia, 235*t*
  for insomnia, 257*t*
  for sleep disturbances, 237, 256–257
Treatment decisions, 29–30
Tremor, essential, 466–467
Trendelenburg gait, 196*t*, 197, 198*t*
Triamcinolone, 328*t*, 439
Triazolam, 245*t*, 256
Tricosal (choline magnesium trisalicylate),
    143*t*